ELECTRICAL THERAPY FOR CARDIAC ARRHYTHMIAS

Pacing, Antitachycardia Devices,
Catheter Ablation

Edited by

SANJEEV SAKSENA, M.D.

Director, Cardiac Electrophysiology,
Newark Beth Israel Medical Center;
Director, Arrhythmia and Pacemaker Service,
General Hospital Center at Passaic;
Clinical Associate Professor of Medicine,
University of Medicine and Dentistry of New Jersey—
New Jersey Medical School, Newark, New Jersey

NORA GOLDSCHLAGER, M.D.

Director, Coronary Care Unit,
San Francisco General Hospital;
Professor of Clinical Medicine,
University of California, San Francisco,
San Francisco, California

1990

W. B. SAUNDERS COMPANY

HARCOURT BRACE JOVANOVICH, INC.

Philadelphia, London, Toronto, Montreal, Sydney, Tokyo

W. B. SAUNDERS COMPANY

Harcourt Brace Jovanovich, Inc.

The Curtis Center
Independence Square West
Philadelphia, PA 19106

Library of Congress Cataloging-in-Publication Data

Electrical therapy for cardiac arrhythmias / edited by Sanjeev
Saksena, Nora F. Goldschlager.

p. cm.

1. Arrhythmia—Treatment. 2. Cardiac pacing.
   I. Saksena, Sanjeev. II. Goldschlager, Nora. [DNLM:
   1. Arrhythmia—therapy. 2. Cardiac Pacing, Artificial.
   3. Electrotherapy. 4. Pacemaker, Artificial. WG 330
   E375]

RC685.A65E43 1990   616.1′280645—dc19

ISBN 0–7216–2451–0   88–39757

Acquisition Editor: William Lamsback

Manuscript Editor: Bonnie Boehme

Production Manager: Frank Polizzano

Illustration Coordinator: Kenneth Green

Indexer: Nancy Weaver

Electrical Therapy for Cardiac Arrhythmias   ISBN 0–7216–2451–0

Copyright © 1990 by W. B. Saunders Company.

Printed in the United States of America.

Last digit is the print number: 9   8   7   6   5   4   3   2   1

"I am a part of all that I have met . . .
Tho' much is taken, much abides . . .
That which we are we are—
One equal temper of heroic heart . . .
    strong in will
To strive, to seek, to find and not to yield."

Alfred, Lord Tennyson

"For all those whose cares have been our
concern, the work goes on, the cause endures,
the hope still lives and the dream shall never die."

Edward Kennedy, August 13, 1980

Dedication

To Diane, Arnie, our parents and children with respect, love, and gratitude.

Acknowledgment

We wish to thank the many project participants at W.B. Saunders Company and Mrs. Ina Ellen Wendler for their indefatigable efforts and support in this enterprise.

CONTRIBUTORS

HUANLIN AN, M.D.
Research Associate, University of Medicine and Dentistry of New Jersey, New Jersey Medical School, Newark Beth Israel Medical Center, Newark and Eastern Heart Institute, Passaic, New Jersey.
Electrophysiologic Mechanisms in Electrical Therapy of Ventricular Tachycardia; Ablation Using Radiofrequency Current and Low-Energy Direct-Current Shocks

STANLEY M. BACH, Jr., B.S.E.E., M.D.
Senior Medical Engineer, Cardiac Pacemakers, Inc., St. Paul, Minnesota.
Engineering Aspects of Implantable Defibrillators

S. SERGE BAROLD, M.B., B.S., F.R.A.C.P., F.A.C.P., F.A.C.C.
Professor of Medicine, University of Rochester School of Medicine and Dentistry; Chief of Cardiology, The Genesee Hospital, Rochester, New York.
Electrocardiography of Contemporary DDD Pacemakers

ALAN D. BERNSTEIN, Eng.Sc.D., F.A.C.C.
Director of Technical Research, Department of Surgery, and Technical Director, Pacemaker Center, Newark Beth Israel Medical Center, Newark, New Jersey.
Engineering Aspects of Pulse Generators for Cardiac Pacing

SAROJA BHARATI, M.D.
Professor of Pathology, Rush Medical School, Rush-Presbyterian-St. Lukes Medical Center, Chicago; Director, Congenital Heart and Conduction System Center, Heart Institute for Children of the Christ Hospital, Oak Lawn, Illinois.
Pathologic Aspects of Electrical Ablation

MARTIN BORGGREFE
Med. Universitätsklinik und Poliklinik, Abt. Innere Medizin C, Münster, German Democratic Republic
Catheter Ablation for Ventricular Tachycardia

E.G.C.A. BOYD, Ph.D.
Principal Physicist, Guy's Hospital, London, England.
Physical and Experimental Aspects of Ablation with Direct-Current Shocks

GÜNTER BREITHARDT, M.D.
Professor of Medicine and Director of the Cardiology Department, Med. Universitätsklinik und Poliklinik, Abt. Innere Medizin C, Münster, German Democratic Republic.
Catheter Ablation for Ventricular Tachycardia

THOMAS BUDDE, M.D.
Med. Universitätsklinik und Poliklinik, Abt. Innere Medizin C, German Democratic Republic.
Catheter Ablation for Ventricular Tachycardia

A. JOHN CAMM, M.D., F.R.C.P., F.A.C.C.
Professor of Clinical Cardiology, St George's Hospital Medical School, London, England.
Recognition of Tachyarrhythmias by Implantable Devices

PENG-SHENG CHEN, M.D.
Assistant Professor of Medicine, Department of Medicine, University of California, San Diego; Staff Cardiologist, San Diego Veterans Administration Hospital, San Diego, California.
Physiologic Effects of Electrical Stimulation in Cardiac Muscle

JOHN W. DANFORTH, M.D.
Assistant Clinical Professor, Division of Cardiology, University of California, San Francisco, and San Francisco General Hospital, San Francisco, California.
Indications for Permanent Cardiac Pacing in the Adult Patient

DEBRA S. ECHT, M.D.
Assistant Professor of Medicine, Vanderbilt University School of Medicine; Director, Cardiac Electrophysiology Laboratory, Vanderbilt University Hospital, Nashville, Tennessee.
Implantation and Intraoperative Assessment of Antitachycardia Devices

NABIL EL-SHERIF, M.D.
Professor of Medicine and Physiology, State University of New York Health Science Center at Brooklyn; Chief, Cardiology Division, Brooklyn Veterans Administration Medical Center; Director, Electrophysiology Program, SUNY/Health Science Center at Brooklyn.
Electrocardiography of Single-Chamber Pacemakers; Electrophysiologic Mechanisms of Electrical Therapy of Ventricular Tachycardia

G. THOMAS EVANS, M.D.
Assistant Clinical Professor of Medicine, University of California, San Francisco; Attending Physician, Moffitt-Long Hospitals, Courtesy Staff Physician, San Francisco General Hospital, San Francisco, California.
Catheter Ablation for Patients with Supraventricular Tachycardia

MICHAEL D. FALKOFF, M.D.
Associate Professor of Medicine, University of Rochester School of Medicine and Dentistry; Chief, Electrophysiology Laboratory, The Genesee Hospital, Rochester, New York.
Electrocardiography of Contemporary DDD Pacemakers

GÉRARD FARENQ, M.D.
Staff Member, Service de Rythmologie et de Stimulation Cardiaque, Hôpital Jean Rostand, Ivry Sur Seine, France.
Catheter Ablation for Ventricular Tachycardia

JOHN D. FISHER, M.D.
Professor of Medicine, Albert Einstein College of Medicine; Acting Director, Cardiology Division, and Director, Cardiac Arrhythmia Service, Montefiore Medical Center, Henry and Lucy Moses Hospital Division, Bronx, New York.
Antitachycardia Pacing in the Acute Care Setting; Clinical Results with Implanted Antitachycardia Pacemakers

GUY FONTAINE, M.D., F.A.C.C.
Director of the Department, Service de Rythmologie et de Stimulation Cardiaque, Hôpital Jean Rostand, Ivry Sur Seine, France.
Catheter Ablation for Ventricular Tachycardia

ROBERT FRANK, M.D.
Assistant Professor, Service de Rythmologie et de Stimulation Cardiaque, Hôpital Jean Rostand, Ivry Sur Seine, France.
Catheter Ablation for Ventricular Tachycardia

DAVID W. FRAZIER, M.D.
Internal Medicine Resident, Duke University Medical Center, Durham, North Carolina.
Physiologic Effects of Electrical Stimulation in Cardiac Muscle

SEYMOUR FURMAN, M.D.
Professor of Surgery, Albert Einstein College of Medicine; Attending Surgeon, Montefiore Medical Center, Bronx, New York.
Principles of Outpatient Follow-up of the Cardiac Pacemaker Patient

YVES GALLAIS, M.D.
Staff Member, Service de Rythmologie et de Stimulation Cardiaque, Hôpital Jean Rostand, Ivry Sur Seine, France
Catheter Ablation for Ventricular Tachycardia

CLIFFORD GARRATT, M.A., M.R.C.P.
Clinical Research Fellow, Department of Cardiological Sciences, St. George's Hospital Medical School; Honorary Clinical Registrar, St. George's Hospital, London, England.
Rate-Responsive Pacing and Sensors

EDWARD W. GERTZ
Professor of Medicine, Radiology and Medical Information Sciences, University of California, San Francisco, California.
Principles of Outpatient Follow-up of the Cardiac Pacemaker Patient

PAUL C. GILLETTE, M.D.
Professor of Pediatrics and Surgery, Medical University of South Carolina; Director, Pediatric Cardiology, Director, South Carolina Childrens Heart Center, Charleston, South Carolina.
Pediatric Cardiac Pacing

NORA GOLDSCHLAGER, M.D.
Professor of Clinical Medicine, University of California, San Francisco; Director, Coronary Care Unit and Electrocardiographic Laboratory, San Francisco General Hospital, San Francisco, California.
Indications for Permanent Cardiac Pacing in the Adult Patient; Temporary Cardiac Pacing; Considerations in the Selection of Cardiac Pacing Systems; Hemodynamic Effects of Cardiac Pacing; Principles of Outpatient Follow-up of the Cardiac Pacemaker Patient

JERRY C. GRIFFIN, M.D.
Associate Professor of Medicine, University of California, San Francisco; Associate Director, Electrocardiography and Clinical Cardiac Electrophysiology, Moffitt-Long Hospital, San Francisco, California.
Follow-up Techniques for Patients with Implanted Antitachycardia Devices

YVES GROSGOGEAT, M.D., F.A.C.C.

Professor of Cardiology, Chairman of the Board, Service de Rythmologie et de Stimulation Cardiaque, Hôpital Jean Rostand, Ivry Sur Seine, France.
Catheter Ablation for Ventricular Tachycardia

PETER M. GUZY, M.D., Ph.D

Associate Professor of Medicine, University of California, Los Angeles; Director, Pacemaker Clinic, University of California, Los Angeles, California.
Considerations in the Selection of Cardiac Pacing Systems

JOHN W. HAMMON, M.D.

Associate Professor of Surgery, Vanderbilt University School of Medicine; Director of VA Cardiac and Thoracic Surgery, Vanderbilt University Hospital, Nashville, Tennessee.
Implantation and Intraoperative Assessment of Antitachycardia Devices

ROBERT G. HAUSER, M.D., F.A.C.C.

Director, Pacemaker Surveillance Clinic, Minneapolis Heart Institute, Minneapolis, Minnesota.
Complications of Permanent Pacing Systems: Diagnosis and Management

DAVID L. HAYES, M.D.

Assistant Professor of Medicine, Mayo Medical School, Mayo Clinic – Mayo Foundation, Rochester, Minnesota.
Pacemaker Implantation Techniques

JAMES J. HEGER, M.D.

Fort Wayne Cardiology, Fort Wayne, Indiana.
Clinical Results with Transvenous Cardioversion

ROBERT A. HEINLE, M.D., F.A.C.C.

Clinical Associate Professor of Medicine, University of Rochester School of Medicine and Dentistry; Director, Cardiac Catheterization Laboratory, The Genesee Hospital, Rochester, New York.
Electrocardiography of Contemporary DDD Pacemakers

RICHARD W. HENTHORN, M.D.

Assistant Professor of Medicine, Case Western Reserve University School of Medicine; Staff Physician, University Hospitals of Cleveland, Cleveland, Ohio.
Supraventricular Tachycardias

DAVID R. HOLMES, Jr., MD.

Professor of Medicine, Mayo Medical School, Mayo Clinic – Mayo Foundation, Rochester, Minnesota.
Pacemaker Implantation Techniques

P. M. HOLT, M.D., M.R.C.P.

Consultant Cardiologist, Guy's Hospital, London, and Maidstone Hospital, Kent, England.
Physical and Experimental Aspects of Ablation with Direct-Current Shocks

RAYMOND E. IDEKER, M.D., Ph.D.
Professor of Pathology, Assistant Professor of Medicine, Duke University Medical Center, Durham, North Carolina.
Physiologic Effects of Electrical Stimulation in Cardiac Muscle

MARK E. JOSEPHSON, M.D.
Robinette Professor of Medicine (Cardiovascular Disease), University of Pennsylvania School of Medicine; Chief, Section of Cardiology, Hospital of the University of Pennsylvania, Philadelphia, Pennsylvania.
Complications of Implantable Antitachycardia Devices: Diagnosis and Management

LINDA M. KALLINEN, R.D.C.S.
Technical Director, Pacemaker Surveillance Clinic, Minneapolis Heart Institute, Minneapolis, Minnesota.
Complications of Permanent Pacing Systems: Diagnosis and Management

HELMUT KLEIN, M.D.
Associate Professor of Cardiology, Department of Cardiology, Hannover Medical School and University Hospital, Hannover, German Democratic Republic.
Diagnostic Evaluation of the Prospective Antitachycardia Device Patient

LAWRENCE S. KLEIN, M.D.
Assistant Professor of Medicine, Indiana University School of Medicine and Krannert Institute of Cardiology; Staff Physician, Indiana University Hospital and Roudebush Veterans Administration Medical Center, Indianapolis, Indiana.
Clinical Results with Transvenous Cardioversion

WANDA KRASSOWSKA, Ph.D.
Research Assistant Professor, Department of Biomedical Engineering, Duke University, Durham, North Carolina.
Physiologic Effects of Electrical Stimulation in Cardiac Muscle

RYSZARD B. KROL, M.D.
Attending Cardiac Electrophysiologist, Newark Beth Israel Medical Center, Newark, New Jersey.
Ventricular Tachycardia

RALPH LAZZARA, M.D.
George Lynn Cross Research Professor of Medicine, University of Oklahoma Health Sciences Center; University of Oklahoma College of Medicine, Oklahoma City, Oklahoma; Chief, Cardiovascular Section, Oklahoma Memorial Hospital, Veterans Administration Medical Center.
Mechanisms of Arrhythmogenesis in Cardiac Muscle

JOHN T. LEE, M.D.
Assistant Professor of Medicine, Vanderbilt University School of Medicine; Director, Heart Station, Vanderbilt University Hospital, Nashville, Tennessee.
Implantation and Intraoperative Assessment of Antitachycardia Devices

MAURICE LEV, M.D.

Professor of Pathology, Rush Medical School, Rush-Presbyterian-St. Lukes Medical Center, Chicago; Associate Director, Congenital Heart and Conduction System Center, Heart Institute for Children of the Christ Hospital, Oak Lawn, Illinois.
Pathologic Aspects of Electrical Ablation.

MARTIN LILAMAND

Computer Engineer, Service de Rythmologie et de Stimulation Cardiaque, Hôpital Jean Rostand, Ivry Sur Seine, France.
Catheter Ablation for Ventricular Tachycardia

BRUCE D. LINDSAY, M.D.

Assistant Professor of Medicine, Cardiology Division, Washington University School of Medicine; Attending Physician, Barnes Hospital, St. Louis, Missouri.
Programmed Stimulation and Transvenous Cardioversion-Defibrillation

FRANCIS E. MARCHLINSKI, M.D.

Associate Professor of Medicine, Department of Medicine, University of Pennsylvania School of Medicine; Co-Director of the Electrophysiology Laboratory, Director of the Arrhythmia Evaluation Center, Hospital of the University of Pennsylvania, Philadelphia, Pennsylvania.
Complications of Implantable Antitachycardia Devices: Diagnosis and Management

RAHUL MEHRA, Ph.D.

Senior Staff Scientist, Medtronic Inc., Minneapolis, Minnesota.
Electrical Stimulation Techniques for Prevention of Ventricular Tachyarrhythmias

WILLIAM M. MILES, M.D.

Research Associate Krannert Institute of Cardiology, Indiana University School of Medicine; Roudebush Veterans Administration Medical Center, Indianapolis, Indiana.
Clinical Results with Transvenous Cardioversion

MICHEL M. MIROWSKI, M.D.

Professor of Medicine, The Johns Hopkins University School of Medicine; Director, Coronary Care Unit, Sinai Hospital of Baltimore, Baltimore, Maryland.
Clinical Results with Implantable Defibrillators

FRED MORADY, M.D.

Professor of Internal Medicine and Director of the Electrophysiology Laboratory, University of Michigan Medical Center, Ann Arbor, Michigan.
Catheter Ablation for Patients with Supraventricular Tachycardia

MORTON M. MOWER, M.D.

Associate Professor of Medicine, The Johns Hopkins University School of Medicine; Chief of Cardiology, Sinai Hospital of Baltimore, Baltimore, Maryland.
Clinical Results with Implantable Defibrillators

NAVIN C. NANDA, M.D.

Professor of Medicine, University of Alabama in Birmingham; Director, Heart Station and Echocardiography-Graphics Laboratory, University Hospital, University of Alabama in Birmingham, Alabama.
Use of Noninvasive Cardiac Diagnostic Techniques in Patients with Cardiac Pacemakers

LING S. ONG, M.D., F.A.C.C.
Assistant Professor of Medicine, University of Rochester School of Medicine and Dentistry;
Director, Interventional Cardiology, The Genesee Hospital, Rochester, New York.
Electrocardiography of Contemporary DDD Pacemakers

VICTOR PARSONNET, M.D., F.A.C.C.
Clinical Professor of Surgery, University of Medicine and Dentistry of New Jersey – New
Jersey Medical School; Director of Surgery, Department of Surgery, and Director, Pacemaker
Center, Newark Beth Israel Medical Center, Newark, New Jersey.
Engineering Aspects of Pulse Generators for Cardiac Pacing

VINCE PAUL, B.S., M.R.C.P.
Research Registrar, Department of Cardiological Sciences, St. George's Hospital Medical
School, London, England.
Recognition of Tachyarrhythmias by Implantable Devices

GILBERT J. PERRY, M.D.
Assistant Professor of Medicine, University of Alabama in Birmingham; Director, Heart
Station and Acting Chief of Cardiology, Birmingham Veterans Administration Medical Center,
Birmingham, Alabama.
Use of Noninvasive Cardiac Diagnostic Techniques in Patients with Cardiac Pacemakers

ERIC N. PRYSTOWSKY, M.D.
Consulting Professor of Medicine, Duke University Medical Center, Durham, North Carolina;
Director of Electrophysiology, St. Vincent's Hospital, Indianapolis, Indiana.
Clinical Results with Transvenous Cardioversion

JAMES A. REIFFEL, M.D.
Professor of Clinical Medicine, Columbia University, College of Physicians and Surgeons;
Attending Physician and Associate Director, Arrhythmia Control Unit, and The Clinical
Electrophysiology and Pacemaker Laboratory, The Presbyterian Hospital, Columbia Presby-
terian Medical Center, New York, New York.
Clinical Evaluation of the Prospective Pacemaker Patient

MICHAEL R. ROSEN, M.D.
Professor of Pharmacology and Pediatrics, Columbia University College of Physicians and
Surgeons; Attending Physician, Presbyterian Hospital, New York, New York.
Mechanisms of Cardiac Impulse Initiation and Propagation

MARK E. ROSENTHAL, M.D.
Clinical Assistant Professor of Medicine, University of Pennsylvania School of Medicine;
Attending Physician, Abington Memorial Hospital; Director, Pacemaker Evaluation Center,
Hospital of the University of Pennsylvania, Philadelphia, Pennsylvania.
Complications of Implantable Antitachycardia Devices: Diagnosis and Management

BERTRAND A. ROSS, M.D.
Assistant Professor of Pediatrics, Medical University of South Carolina, Charleston, South
Carolina.
Pediatric Cardiac Pacing

ISABELLE ROUGIER, M.D.
Staff Member, Service de Rythmologie et de Stimulation Cardiaque, Hôpital Jean Rostand, Ivry Sur Seine, France.
Catheter Ablation for Ventricular Tachycardia

SANJEEV SAKSENA, M.D., F.A.C.C.
Clinical Associate Professor of Medicine, University of Medicine and Dentistry of New Jersey – New Jersey Medical School; Director, Cardiac Electrophysiology, Beth Israel Medical Center, Newark, and Director, Arrhythmia and Pacemaker Service, Eastern Heart Institute, Passaic, New Jersey.
Hemodynamic Effects of Cardiac Pacing; Electrophysiologic Mechanisms Underlying Termination and Prevention of Supraventricular Tachyarrhythmias; Programmed Stimulation and Transvenous Cardioversion-Defibrillation; Diagnostic Evaluation of the Prospective Antitachycardia Device Patient; Ventricular Tachycardia; Implantable Antitachycardia Devices—the Next Generation; Ablation Using Radiofrequency Current and Low-Energy Direct-Current Shocks

MELVIN M. SCHEINMAN, M.D.
Professor of Medicine, University of California, San Francisco; Chief, Electrocardiography and Cardiac Electrophysiology Section, Moffitt-Long Hospital, San Francisco, California.
Catheter Ablation for Patients with Supraventricular Tachycardia

J. EDWARD SHAPLAND, Ph.D.
Director, Applied Research, Cardiac Pacemakers, Inc., St. Paul, Minnesota.
Engineering Aspects of Implantable Defibrillators

IGOR SINGER, M.B.B.S., F.R.A.C.P., F.A.C.P.
Assistant Professor of Medicine and Director of Electrophysiology, Humana Hospital and University of Louisville, Louisville, Kentucky.
Clinical Results with Implantable Defibrillators

DONALD F. SWITZER, M.D.
Clinical Assistant Professor of Medicine, University of Buffalo; Director of Electrophysiology, Millard Fillmore Hospital, Buffalo, New York.
Supraventricular Tachycardias

GERALD C. TIMMIS, M.D.
Clinical Professor of Health Sciences (Internal Medicine), Oakland University, Rochester, Michigan; Staff Cardiologist, Medical Director, Clinical Research Division of Cardiology, William Beaumont Hospital, Royal Oak, Michigan.
The Electrobiology and Engineering of Pacemaker Leads

JOELCI TONET, M.D.
Staff Member of the Department, Service de Rythmologie et de Stimulation Cardiaque, Hôpital Jean Rostand, Ivry Sur Seine, France.
Catheter Ablation for Ventricular Tachycardia

NICHOLAS G. TULLO, M.D.
Attending Cardiac Electrophysiologist, Newark Beth Israel Medical Center; University Hospital, University of Medicine and Dentistry of New Jersey, Newark, New Jersey.
Ablation Using Radiofrequency Current and Low-Energy Direct-Current Shocks

SHANTHA URSELL, M.D., F.A.C.C.
Associate Professor of Medicine, State University of New York, Health Science Center at Brooklyn; Director, Coronary Care Unit, SUNY Health Science Center, Brooklyn, New York.
Electrocardiography of Single-Chamber Pacemakers

ENRICO P. VELTRI, M.D.
Assistant Professor of Medicine, The Johns Hopkins University School of Medicine; Director, Sudden Death Prevention Program and Director, Cardiac Electrophysiology Laboratory, Co-Director, Coronary Care Unit, Sinai Hospital of Baltimore, Maryland.
Clinical Results with Implantable Defibrillators

ALBERT L. WALDO, M.D.
The Walter H. Pritchard Professor of Cardiology, Professor of Medicine, and Professor of Biomedical Engineering, Case Western Reserve University School of Medicine; Attending Physician, University Hospitals of Cleveland, Cleveland, Ohio.
Supraventricular Tachycardias

DAVID WARD, M.D., M.R.C.P., F.A.C.C.
Consultant Cardiologist, St. George's Hospital, London, England.
Rate-Responsive Pacing and Sensors; Recognition of Tachyarrhythmias by Implantable Devices

JAY WARREN, M.S.E.E.
Science Advisor, Camino, California.
Complications of Permanent Pacing Systems: Diagnosis and Management

J. MARCUS WHARTON, M.D.
Assistant Professor of Medicine, Division of Cardiology, Duke University Medical Center; Director, Clinical Cardiac Electrophysiology, Duke University Medical Center, Durham, North Carolina.
Temporary Cardiac Pacing; Physiologic Effects of Electrical Stimulation in Cardiac Muscle

VICKI L. ZEIGLER, R.N., B.S.N.
Pediatric Pacemaker, Clinical Coordinator, South Carolina Childrens Heart Center, Medical University of South Carolina, Charleston, South Carolina.
Pediatric Cardiac Pacing

DOUGLAS P. ZIPES, M.D.
Professor of Medicine, Indiana University School of Medicine, Senior Research Associate, Krannert Institute of Cardiology, Indiana University School of Medicine; Roudebush Veterans Administration Medical Center, Indianapolis, Indiana.
Clinical Results with Transvenous Cardioversion

PREFACE

This work resulted from a perceived need for a comprehensive and contemporary text addressing all major aspects of electrical therapy as applied to cardiac arrhythmias. Antiarrhythmic therapy in the last decade of the twentieth century encompasses pharmacologic and nonpharmacologic options for many different arrhythmias. Electrical therapies form the major component of presently available nonpharmacologic techniques and are being applied to a rapidly expanding patient population. Implantable antiarrhythmic device therapy, once synonymous with cardiac pacing systems for patients with bradycardias requiring rate support, is now being widely used for patients with tachyarrhythmias. It has been estimated that device therapy for tachyarrhythmias will exceed that for bradycardias before the turn of the century. Cardiac pacemakers for bradycardias have become increasingly complex. Initially, they were relatively simple standby devices for patients with a failing intrinsic cardiac rhythm; they now attempt to provide physiologic electrical stimulation, a goal increasingly achieved by monitoring a variety of biosensors that reflect metabolic and circulatory demands and automatically adjusting cardiac rate and output. Electrode catheter ablation techniques are being increasingly applied for tachycardia control, often in conjunction with implantable antitachycardia and antifibrillatory device therapy. The knowledge base in all these fields has been expanding at an astonishing rate. A few reference books and monographs on individual therapies suitable for advanced students in this field have become available. This textbook evolved from our view that these therapies are not only closely interrelated, sharing as they do common physical and physiologic principles, but they also form a single discipline. It is our expectation that present-day and future students will be trained in this manner. Equally important is the need for this discipline to find a relevant and well-defined role in modern medical practice. Thus, this book is designed for reference use by the student and practitioner of clinical medicine and cardiology as well as the specialist in cardiac pacing and electrophysiology.

The individual contributions reflect the international interest in this science. Distinguished experts from 30 centers with records of major scientific achievement in this area have provided the core of this text. A sectional approach dealing with basic concepts and individual therapies has been used to preserve continuity. Physical and physiologic elements relevant to each therapy introduce each section. Individual chapters provide current concepts and state-of the-art information. Numerous illustrations and detailed bibliographies have been encouraged. It is our hope that this textbook will help to coalesce and consolidate an important cardiologic discipline.

SANJEEV SAKSENA, M.D.
NORA GOLDSCHLAGER, M.D.

CONTENTS

I

PATHOPHYSIOLOGY OF CARDIAC ARRHYTHMIAS

1

MECHANISMS OF CARDIAC IMPULSE INITIATION AND PROPAGATION

MICHAEL R. ROSEN

The initiation and propagation of the cardiac impulse are readily understood at the level of the single cardiac cell. By considering the determinants of the cardiac impulse at this level, as well as the interactions of groups of cardiac cells functionally connected to one another, one can begin to comprehend not only the basis for the control of electrical activity in the normal heart but also the derangements that occur as a result of cardiac disease. With this in mind, Chapter 1 will concentrate on the normal control of cardiac rhythm and will provide a basis for the discussion in Chapter 2 of arrhythmogenic mechanisms.

THE TRANSMEMBRANE POTENTIAL

Cardiac fibers have an electronegative transmembrane potential: The inside of the cell has a negative charge ranging from approximately -90 mV in cells of the ventricular specialized conducting system to -50 mV in cells of the sinus node. The basis for the transmembrane potential is provided by a disparate distribution of ions across the cell membrane (Fig. 1–1). The membrane itself is a lipid bilayer that functions both as an insulator and as a barrier to the ready flow of ions.[4] However, the membrane contains channels, aqueous pores through which the flow of ions is regulated, as well as biochemical pumps that can distribute

ions across the membrane using a process that requires energy.[4] One such pump is Na^+,K^+-ATPase, an enzyme that exchanges sodium and potassium across the membrane, using adenosine triphosphate (ATP) as its source of energy. This pump is electrogenic in nature: When operating at its highest efficiency, three Na^+ are pumped out of the cell for every two K^+ pumped in.[7, 11] There is a high concentration of K^+ and a low concentration of Na^+ inside the cell, the result of Na^+,K^+ pumping. Moreover, a number of the positively charged ions inside the cell are bound to proteins. The result of these processes is an excess of negative charge inside the cell and a negative transmembrane potential.

The cell behaves much like a potassium electrode[1, 6]; its membrane potential *(E)* is a function of the intracellular and extracellular K ions, as described in the *Nernst equation*:

$$E = RT/f \ln ([K^+]_i/[K^+]_o)$$

where R = the gas constant, T = absolute temperature, and f = the Faraday constant

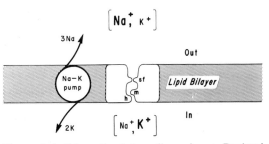

Figure 1–1. Schematic of the cell membrane. Depicted are the lipid bilayer, the sodium-potassium pump, and a fast sodium channel. Sf = the selectivity filter; m and h = channel gates. See text for description.

Certain of the studies referred to were supported by USPHS-NHLBI Grants HL-28223, HL-28958, and HL-33727.

At $[K^+]_o$ greater than 5 mM, the relationship between $[K^+]_o$ and membrane potential is linear. Only in the range of $[K^+]_o$ less than 5 mM does the relationship between membrane potential and $[K^+]_o$ deviate from linearity, implicating the activity of ions other than potassium (e.g., calcium, sodium) in modulating membrane potential here.

THE ACTION POTENTIAL

As already described, the cell membrane is a lipid bilayer that is interposed between two aqueous solutions, the intracellular and extracellular spaces. Each of these spaces has a different concentration of ions, in large part a reflection of ionic pumping and exchange mechanisms. Intracellularly, the major cation is potassium, with lesser concentrations of sodium and calcium.

If sodium and potassium were permitted to equilibrate across the membrane ad libitum, their concentration gradients are such that we would expect sodium to enter the cell and potassium to leave it. There is an electrical gradient across the cell membrane as well—given the negative charge inside the cell—which would favor the retention of potassium intracellularly as well as the entry of sodium. The lipid bilayer of the cell membrane acts to prevent the concentration and electrical gradients from being expressed. The ionic gradients in a very real sense constitute the driving force behind the generation of the transmembrane potential; indeed, were the membrane solely a lipid bilayer with only the ability to insulate and separate, no electrical activity would be generated.

As already stated, the energy-requiring pumps that exist in the cell membrane permit one means of ionic exchange. The other structures housed in the membrane that facilitate the passage of ions are the channels (Fig. 1–1). These are proteins that traverse the membrane, providing an aqueous pathway through which ions may travel.[4] The most completely studied channels to date are those specific for sodium and potassium. There are a number of distinguishing features about these channels that determine their function and their ionic specificity. Each type of channel has, near its external surface, a selectivity filter. This may be thought of as a narrowing of the channel. The narrowing is such that it favors the passage of one type of ion with its water of hydration more specifically than other ions. However, it

will not admit one ion exclusively. For example, sodium channels will also admit hydrogen ions, calcium channels, sodium ions, and so forth. But the specificity of the filter is such that of the ions usually found in the body, the particular ionic species for which the channel is named finds passage most readily.

If all the channel encompassed was an aqueous pore and a selectivity filter, the ions and charges would soon equilibrate across the membrane, leaving an inactive and inexcitable system. Clearly, something is needed to limit the flow of ions. This limiting activity is provided by channel "gates" (Fig. 1–1).[4, 5, 8, 9] These are substructures of the channel protein that may be in open or closed positions. When open, they will permit the flow of ions across the cell membrane. This flow will be a passive event, the ions simply following their concentration and charge gradients. In contrast, when the channels are closed, no ions of that species can traverse the membrane.

Let us now synthesize this information in a manner that permits us to understand the transmembrane action potential (Fig. 1–2). We will refer only to sodium, potassium, and calcium channels in this discussion and will use the Purkinje fiber as an example. In the resting state, with a fiber at -90 mV of membrane potential, sodium and calcium channels tend to be closed. Some potassium channels are open, however, permitting this ion to leave via a concentration gradient (carrying with it a positive charge) that favors the persistence of a high level of negativity within the cell. Channels have characteristics of voltage sensitivity, and if a depolarizing stimulus is delivered to the cell, its sodium channels will open and its potassium channels close. With opening of the sodium channel, this positively charged ion

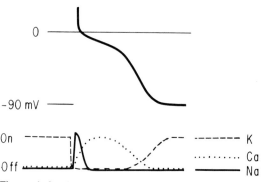

Figure 1–2. The Purkinje fiber transmembrane potential and its relationship to rapid inward sodium, slow inward calcium, and repolarizing potassium currents. This figure is not meant to be temporally accurate. See text for description.

can enter the cell along its electrical and concentration gradients, thereby depolarizing it, and in fact carrying the cell to relatively positive potentials ($+20$ to $+40$ mV). The depolarization of the membrane has several secondary effects. The calcium channels begin to open and so do the potassium channels. A transient outward current carried by potassium along voltage and concentration gradients is responsible for phase 1 repolarization of the membrane. A diminishing inward sodium current also contributes here. This repolarizing trend is interrupted by an inward current carried by calcium, as well as a persisting inward current carried by sodium, resulting in the plateau phase of the action potential. The subsequent phase 3 repolarization is caused by an increasing ionic flow out of the potassium channel and lesser inward flow through the calcium and sodium channels. Finally, as a result of potassium leaving the cell, repolarization is complete.

It is apparent that if this ongoing pattern of sodium entry and potassium loss during the action potential continued unabated, the result would be the accumulation of sodium inside the cell and potassium outside the cell, the loss of membrane potential, and electrical quiescence and inexcitability. What renders the process self-regenerating is the action of the ionic pumps, moving the ions across the membrane to restore and maintain their initial gradients.

The extent to which a channel can move from one state to another is controlled by so-called "gates," the function of which is complex. We shall use the sodium channel as an example (Fig. 1–3). This channel has two gates[9]: One, an activation gate, is responsible for opening the channel and is referred to as "m"; the other, an inactivation gate, is referred to as "h." When the cell is in the resting state, "m" is closed and "h" is open. When the membrane is initially stimulated, the "m" gate opens, permitting positive charge to enter. Almost immediately thereafter, "h" begins to close, resulting in an inactivated state of the channel. As the cell returns to its resting state, "h" again opens and "m" closes.

Another complicating factor is that channels of the same type do not open, inactivate, and close with complete uniformity. Rather, there are random openings and closings of channels, and while they are open, ions can pass through them.[4] However, the likelihood that channels of a given type will be open at a given time and voltage is consistent and predictable. Hence, during the resting state of the membrane, most sodium channels are closed; only occasional random openings occur. When the membrane is brought to its threshold potential, most of the sodium channels are in the open state, and during repolarization most are in the inactivated state, returning to the resting state as excitability returns.

Thus far, I have described a membrane in which the interposition of pumps and channels permits the maintenance of a high resting potential, as well as the occurrence of an action potential. Not all cells generate the same type of action potential, however. The sodium-dependent action potential already discussed (in Fig. 1–2), also called the fast response because of the rapid phase 0 depolarization and rapid propagation that characterize it, is representative of normal cells in the atrial and ventricular myocardium and specialized conducting system. Cells in the sinus and atrioventricular nodes, as well as cells on the atrial surfaces of the atrioventricular valves, have a very different action potential. At the normal level of membrane potential of these cells, positive to -70 mV, most fast sodium channel activity is inactivated. The major channel capable of carrying inward current here is the calcium channel. This channel generates an action potential having a slow rate of rise and one that propagates slowly (Fig. 1–4). Hence, it has been called the *slow response*. This same type of action potential can be seen in fibers of the myocardium and specialized conducting systems as a result of depolarization induced by

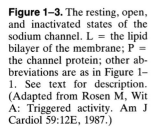

Figure 1–3. The resting, open, and inactivated states of the sodium channel. L = the lipid bilayer of the membrane; P = the channel protein; other abbreviations are as in Figure 1–1. See text for description. (Adapted from Rosen M, Wit A: Triggered activity. Am J Cardiol 59:12E, 1987.)

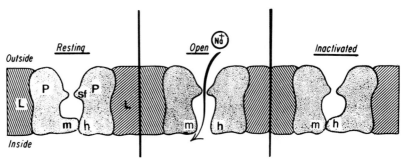

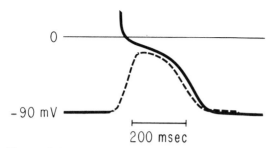

Figure 1–4. The fast-response action potential *(solid trace)*, having a rapid rate of rise and high amplitude, contrasted with the slow response *(interrupted trace)*, having a lower rate of rise and amplitude.

cardiac disease. In this event, the slow response (or action potentials having characteristics intermediate between the slow and fast responses) can play a role in arrhythmogenesis. This role will be detailed in Chapter 2.

The Initiation of the Action Potential

In discussing the action potential thus far, I have described an electrical potential that is generated as the result of electrical stimulation of a cell. However, certain cardiac fibers have the property of "automaticity," the ability to generate an action potential de novo.[11] This property determines the pacemaker function of the sinus node (which has the fastest intrinsic pacemaker rate), as well as the pacemaker potential of cells in the atrial, atrioventricular junctional, and ventricular specialized conducting systems. Again, I shall use the Purkinje system as an initial example. On the completion of full repolarization in the Purkinje system, there is the onset of an inward current, carried by sodium, thorough a channel designated i_f.[2] This channel carries positive charge into the cell, and if it accumulates faster than pump activity can remove it, the cell will reach threshold potential, at which time the fast sodium channels open and an action potential is initiated (Fig. 1–5). A similar current exists in the sinus node, but of probably greater importance is a decay in outward current carried by potassium that has the same end result,[10] that is, depolarization of the membrane and attainment of threshold. Hence, by two somewhat dissimilar means (an increasing inward current and a decreasing outward current) two different tissues of the heart generate their pacemaker potentials.

A question that is often asked is why specialized conducting fibers in the ventricle do not generate their pacemaker function more readily, thereby inducing ectopic activity. The

answer in part lies in the different kinetics of the pacemaker currents and in part is attributable to a specialized function of pacemaker tissues, referred to as overdrive suppression.[12, 13] This term refers to the stimulation of a pacemaker fiber at a rate faster than its intrinsic automatic rate, resulting in suppression of its pacemaker activity (Fig. 1–5). When one paces a cardiac fiber rapidly, there is an initial phase of depolarization of the membrane. This depolarization is the result of extracellular potassium accumulation, secondary to potassium egress during phase 3 repolarization. The depolarization is followed by a period of hyperpolarization, resulting from stimulation of the sodium-potassium pump. The stimulus for this is sodium entry via phase 0 of the action potential. In fibers having a high level of membrane potential, there is considerable sodium entry during phase 0; the resulting heightened pump function creates an outward current that persists for some time after overdrive pacing has ceased and serves to counteract the depolarizing effect of phase 4 depolarization. In cells having low membrane potential and less sodium entry during phase 0 (such as the sinus node), there is less of a stimulus for Na^+,K^+ pumping and a lower degree of overdrive suppression than occurs in the ventricle. Hence, via its intrinsic relatively rapid rate of impulse initiation and its ability to overdrive suppress other cardiac pacemaker tissues, the sinus node is the primary pacemaker of the heart.

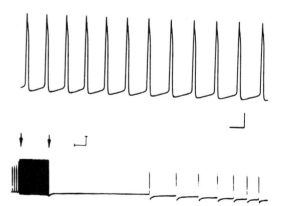

Figure 1–5. *Upper panel:* An automatic Purkinje fiber is seen, showing depolarization during phase 4. *Lower panel* (different gain and sweep speed): The first four beats are spontaneous and are followed by a period of overdrive pacing. On cessation of pacing, automatic activity has terminated. It subsequently recommences and gradually increases in rate. (Reproduced, with permission, from: Rosen M, Reder R: Does triggered activity have a role in the genesis of cardiac arrhythmias? Ann Intern Med 94:794–801, 1981.)

THE CONDUCTION OF THE CARDIAC IMPULSE

Thus far, all I have described is related to the function of individual cells. The question that now arises is how the signal generated in one cell or one group of cells can propagate to the rest of the heart. In describing the characteristics of the individual cell, I mentioned that it is encased in a lipid bilayer. Since the bilayer is an excellent insulator, current cannot flow readily between the highly conductive aqueous solutions in the cell interior and in the extracellular space.

Let us consider a chain of cells and the properties that would be ideal for the conduction of an impulse. The simplest model would be a copper electrical wire, ensheathed in an insulator. Given an electrical power source or battery interposed in the cable, we would have a means for electrons to flow. If we interposed a variable resistor, we could now control the relationship between current and voltage and generate a signal.

A chain of cells has the potential to act much as the cable above. It has that potential not only because of the highly conductive internal ionic milieu but also because of the intrinsic power source that is present (i.e., the transmembrane potential) and the ability of some cells—via automaticity—to "turn on" the power source. The final essential ingredient, after one cell has initiated an impulse, is a pathway of low resistance through which current can flow from cell to cell. Such a pathway is provided by the nexal junctions, at which cardiac cells are tightly apposed and through which minute low-resistance pathways communicate between cells.[9] As a result, when the first cell in a chain depolarizes and generates an action potential, the current flow generated between this cell and the next in sequence may be sufficient to depolarize that cell to threshold potential, at which time its sodium channels open, it generates an action potential, and it depolarizes the next cell in the sequence (Fig. 1–6).

The velocity of propagation of this signal depends on a number of factors. First is the structure of the fiber itself,[11] that is, the velocity of propagation increases with the square of the radius of a fiber. Hence, fibers of large diameter, such as those in the Purkinje system, conduct more rapidly than those of small diameter, such as those in the atrioventricular node. A second factor is the signal that is generated. The sodium-dependent fast response produces a larger and more rapidly

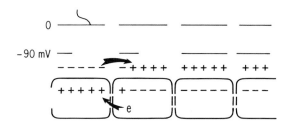

Figure 1–6. A series of four cells, joined via low-resistance junctions (spaces). The cell on the left has generated an action potential, resulting in a reversal of the polarity across the cell membrane. Electrons (e) flow from areas of negative charge to those of positive charge, and this results in a beginning change in the charge across the second cell membrane. This change will be sufficient to bring the cell to threshold potential, resulting in opening of the sodium channels, and the initiation of the action potential. The combination of excitation of the membrane, secondary to the flow of electrons, and the upstroke of the action potential (resulting from fast Na⁺ entry) determines the propagation of the action potential.

depolarizing signal than the calcium-dependent slow response and hence is a more efficient stimulus. Considering the efficiency of the stimulus brings us to several related factors. First is the relationship of the membrane potential of a fiber to its threshold potential.[3] The greater the disparity between these two variables, the greater the displacement of membrane potential that will be needed to depolarize the membrane to threshold. Also of importance is the ratio of the source of electrical activity to the unexcited area into which it is propagating. If a cell that is generating a large signal is tightly connected to just one or two cells, it may readily depolarize them. However, if it is connected to a larger number of cells, its current flow may be dispersed among them in a way that is sufficient to displace membrane potential slightly, but not enough to bring any fiber to threshold. The result will be the failure of propagation. The final factor to be considered is the coupling of fibers to one another. A signal that is normally adequate to permit propagation from one fiber to the next may become inadequate if fibers are uncoupled, as a result of either separation or interposition of a poor conducting medium (such as connective tissue) in some portion of the circuit.

All these factors will determine whether or not an impulse can propagate, as well as the velocity with which it propagates. The other important determinant to consider is the direction the impulse takes. For example, the bundle branches lie within the mass of the ventricular septum, in close proximity to ventricular myocardial fibers. What prevents the activation of the septum concurrently with the bundle branches is the insulation existing between the two tissue types, as well as the low resistance to antegrade conduction. It is the similar organization of high- and low-resistance pathways throughout the heart that determines the direction of electrical activation and the organization of cardiac conduction along approximately the same pathway from one cycle to the next. A variety of factors can serve to disorganize the pathways and to disrupt conduction. These are to be discussed in Chapter 2.

REFERENCES

1. Burgen ASV, Terroux KG: The membrane resting and action potentials of cat auricle. J Physiol 119:139–152, 1953.
2. DiFrancesco D: A new interpretation of the pacemaker current in calf Purkinje fibers. J Physiol 314:359–376, 1981.
3. Dominguez G, Fozzard HA: Influence of extracellular K^+ concentration on cable properties and excitability of sheep cardiac Purkinje fibers. Circ Res 26:565, 1970.
4. Hille B: Ionic Channels of Excitable Membranes. Sunderland, MA, Sinauer Associates, 1984.
5. Hodgkin AL, Huxley AF: A quantitative description of membrane current and its application to conduction and excitation in nerve. J Physiol 117:500–544, 1952.
6. Hoffman BF: Electrophysiology of single cardiac cells. Bull NY Acad Med 35:689–706, 1959.
7. Hoffman BF, Cranefield PF: Electrophysiology of the Heart. New York, McGraw-Hill, 1960.
8. Hondeghem L, Katzung B: Time and voltage dependent interactions of antiarrhythmic drugs with cardiac sodium channels. Biochem Biophys Acta 472:373–398, 1977.
9. Jack JJB, Noble D, Tsien RW: Electric Current Flow in Excitable Cells. Oxford, England, Clarendon Press, 1975.
10. Noma A, Irasawa H: A time- and voltage-dependent potassium current in the rabbit sinoatrial node cell. Pflugers Arch 366:251–258, 1976.
11. Rosen MR, Hoffman BF: Electrophysiologic determinants of normal cardiac rhythms and arrhythmias. In Rosen MR, Hoffman BF (eds): Cardiac Therapy. Boston, Martinus Nijhoff, 1983, pp 1–19.
12. Vassalle M: Electrogenic suppression of automaticity in sheep and dog Purkinje fibers. Circ Res 27:361–377, 1970.
13. Vassalle M: The relationship among cardiac pacemakers: Overdrive suppression. Circ Res 41:269–277, 1977.

2

MECHANISMS OF ARRHYTHMOGENESIS IN CARDIAC MUSCLE

RALPH LAZZARA

Disorders of the rate and rhythm of the heartbeat can be classified as tachyarrhythmias or bradyarrhythmias. Linguistic purists advocate the term "dysrhythmias," but the term "arrhythmias" remains the common usage for disorders of the cardiac rhythm. In the context of clinical practice, a classification of arrhythmias into tachyarrhythmias and bradyarrhythmias is incomplete, since certain disturbances of the cardiac rhythm—for example, accelerated ventricular rhythms or bigeminy—may have net rates that are within the normal range, neither tachycardia or bradycardia. From the standpoint of mechanisms, tachyarrhythmias can be considered to reflect those processes that act to usurp the control of the heartbeat for one or more cycles from the normal pacemaker locus in the sinus node. The bradyarrhythmias reflect processes that interfere with the control of the heart by the sinus node at normal heart rates, resulting in slow heart rates.

TACHYARRHYTHMIAS

The processes that generate tachyarrhythmias can be classified as follows:

A. Regenerative propagation

    1. Reentry
    2. Reflection
    3. Reexcitation during repolarization

B. Autoactivation

    1. Accelerated automaticity
    2. Abnormal automaticity
       a. Depolarized Purkinje fibers
       b. Automatic myocardial cells
    3. Afterpotentials and triggered firing

Reentry

The archetypical model of a reentry circuit consists of a conducting ring around an inexcitable center or "hole," illustrated in Figure 2–1. This model originated as a literal translation of the first operating reentry circuits formed in rings cut from the medusa of the jellyfish.[35, 36] The model incorporates certain essential elements. To initiate reiterative propagation, it is necessary to have a locus of unidirectional block. Upon arrival at this locus during the first transit, the earliest of two excitation fronts is terminated while the later one approaching from the opposite direction is transmitted. In this manner, a single excitation front remains and it can circle repetitively.

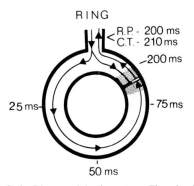

Figure 2–1. Ring model of reentry. The circuit forms around an impenetrable barrier for propagation, a "hole." The stippled area represents a site of slow conduction and of unidirectional block represented by a bar partly filled and partly empty. At this locus of unidirectional block, the initial impulse is blocked but the later impulse approaching from the other direction is transmitted. The refractory period (R.P.) and conduction times (C.T.) at the entry site are shown, as well as the conduction times at different loci in the circuit. For reentry to occur at the entry site, the total conduction time in the circuit must be longer than the refractory period.

Given the normal conduction velocities and normal durations of refractory periods of myocardial cells and specialized conducting cells, for the transit time in the circuit to exceed the refractory periods of all the elements of the circuit, the circuit would be expected to be at least 10 cm long. For smaller circuits to form, the conduction velocity must be abnormally slow in all or part of the circuit, or the refractory periods must be abnormally brief throughout the circuit and throughout the myocardium activated by the circuit. It is far easier to satisfy the requirement of abnormally slow conduction in a small part of the circuit than that of abnormally brief refractoriness in the whole circuit and its connecting myocardium. Therefore, the ring model commonly includes a segment of slow conduction. However, the model can be conceived as a ring with uniformly slow conduction velocity and a locus of unidirectional block.

In the ring model the relationship between the transit time, determined by the conduction velocity of the circulating wave front, and the duration of the refractory period can be represented by a "head" of the traveling excitation followed by a "tail" of refractoriness, the length of which is equal to the duration of the refractory period or periods divided by the conduction velocity. The length of the tail of refractoriness is important in relation to the length of the entire circuit, as illustrated by the examples in Figure 2–2. If the tail is short, occupying a relatively small portion of the circuit, there would be a large "excitable gap." Another excitation front could enter the circuit during the gap and possibly reset the circuit. Repetitive entering impulses could "entrain" the circuit by driving it at a rate somewhat higher than its intrinsic rate, since each new entering excitation front would begin a new circuit before the prior one would complete the circuit.[55] Since the natural rate of the reentry circuit is the reciprocal of the natural total transit time, the repetitive initiation of new circuits at intervals less than the natural transit time would drive the circuit at a higher rate.

An operating circuit could be disturbed and terminated by the entrance of a properly timed excitation front into the circuit at a point in time when the excitation front encounters a part of the tail that represents the relative refractory period. The new entering excitation front might fail to conduct in one direction during the relatively refractory tail and collide with the head of the circulating excitation front

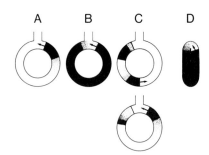

Figure 2–2. Relationships between activation front, refractory wake, and circuit length in reentry circuits. The activation front is represented by the arrow. Absolute refractory tissue is black, and relative refractory tissue stippled. The excitatory gap is the part of the circuit that is excitable. In *A* the excitatory gap is large because the refractory wake or tail is relatively short in relation to the length of the circuit. In *B* the excitatory gap is short and only relative because the activation front is continually activating relatively refractory tissue. In *C*, as in the ring model of Figure 2–1, a segment of the circuit has distinctive properties. In this case, the segment not only slows conduction but also has longer refractory periods because the tissue is depressed. At the top, the wave front has proceeded away from the segment, leaving most of it absolutely refractory and some relatively refractory. At the bottom, the wave front has proceeded further along the circuit, and more of this segment has recovered into the relatively refractory state. In *D* the circuit lacks an impenetrable barrier or "hole" and the limbs of the circuit abut one another, but absolute refractoriness prevents the impulse from crossing the line of block. The activation front turns the corner when absolute refractoriness recedes. It is thought that this type of circuit, representing the leading circle concept, tends to have a brief excitatory gap.

in the other direction, terminating the circuit. The circuit could also be terminated if the entering excitation front, meeting the relatively refractory tail, became blocked in both directions and left a segment of absolute refractoriness, which could block the circulating excitation front. These relationships are shown in Figure 2–3.

The application of the ring model, which is composed of linear elements, to the cardiac syncytium, which permits conduction in three

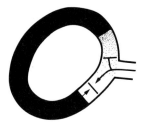

Figure 2–3. Interruption of reentry. A new activation front entering the circuit during the relative refractory tail of the circulating activation front may block in one direction and collide in the other direction, terminating the reentry. See text for details.

Leading Circle

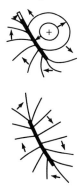

Figure 2–4. The leading circle model of reentry. The formation of the circuit is shown at the top. An impulse initiated at the site represented by a plus sign spreads in concentric wave fronts until an interface of refractory tissue is encountered, represented by a bar. The wave fronts proceed around the edge of the bar to activate the tissue on the other side and begin the circuit. The sustained circuit is shown below. The areas of tissue on one side and the other are alternatively activated or refractory. See text for details.

dimensions, requires contrived conditions to isolate the linear pathways. Recently, the pattern of activation has been mapped in reentry circuits formed in the cardiac syncytium. Multidimensional models of reentry applicable to the cardiac syncytium have emerged.

In the "leading circle" model[3] shown in Figure 2–4, an interface between excitable and refractory tissue forms the barrier for encirclement. The circuit is begun when an approaching wave front encounters refractory tissue and blocks at an interface, which is depicted by a "line" of block in a two-dimensional, that is, planar, representation of the activation sequence. This interface of block also could be represented by a surface in a three-dimensional model. The wave fronts turn around one extremity of the interface when refractoriness recedes and proceed to activate the initially refractory tissue on the other side of the interface, progressing in a direction generally parallel to the line of block. During this progress of the wave fronts of activation, the interface of block remains intact because tissue on the side activated on the initial approach of the wave front is now in the refractory state. The wave fronts turn back again at the other extremity of the line of block when refractoriness recedes, to "reenter" the tissue on the side initially activated. The second activation proceeds in a direction generally parallel to the line of block. The process is repetitive, and the line of block separates two sides that are alternatively undergoing activation or resting

in the refractory state. This model was demonstrated in atrial myocardium, which is thin enough that the activation sequence can be considered in the context of a surface.

The "figure-of-eight" model shown in Figure 2–5 incorporates basic elements of the leading circle model with certain variations in the spatial configuration. Studies in dogs of reentry in the thin epicardial layer of ischemically injured myocardium overlying infarction have elucidated the features of the figure-of-eight model.[13, 58] Reentry is initiated when the wave fronts of activation encounter refractory tissue at a convex interface in the shape of an arc in a two-dimensional representation. The arc forms in an area of sharp gradient of increasing refractoriness within the ischemically injured zone.[19] The wave fronts proceed around both ends of the arc of block when refractoriness recedes and pursue the receding refractoriness to activate the myocardium adjoining the concave face of the arc. The two sets of wave fronts approach each other near the center of the arc, coalesce, and turn back to penetrate the arc near its center, where there is earliest recovery from refractoriness of the myocardium activated on the initial approach, that on the convex side of the arc. After reentering the originally activated tissue, the wave front diverges, forming two sets of wave fronts that travel toward the ends of the two segments of

Figure of Eight

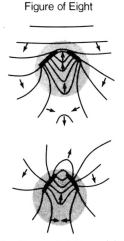

Figure 2–5. The figure-of-eight model of reentry. The initiation of the circuit is shown at the top, and its maintenance at the bottom. Wave fronts of activation approaching an abnormal region (stippled circle) encounter a curved interface of refractory tissue, the "arc of block." Wave fronts circle both edges of the arc and merge to penetrate the center of the arc in the other direction when the tissue recovers from refractoriness. The circuit is maintained by wave fronts circling two segments of the arc, as shown at the bottom. See text for details.

the arc. At the ends they turn back toward the concave surface, and the process is repeated. In this model the circuit forms around two segments of interface rather than one.

The slow conduction essential to the formation of these circuits is largely the result of activation of myocardium during the relatively refractory period. In abnormal myocardium—for example, ischemically injured myocardium—the relatively refractory period can be prolonged by postrepolarization refractoriness, which is absolute or relative refractoriness outlasting the action potential.[31] Postrepolarization refractoriness can be the result of slow removal of inactivation from depressed sodium channels. Postrepolarization refractoriness is prolonged during cardiac cycles when early stimulation produces poor responses and exaggerated slowing of conduction. Comparison between a normal action potential with normal refractory properties and abnormal responses with postrepolarization refractoriness is shown in Figure 2–6.

In ischemically injured myocardium, the most common source of ventricular arrhythmias in the clinical setting, the fast sodium channel is depressed because cells are partially depolarized, resulting in more inactivation of the channels, and because of the operation of some depressant factor that reduces the fast current at any level of membrane potential, that is, shifts the membrane responsiveness curve downward.[31] The result of this intrinsic depression is that there is diminished excitatory current, reflected in the maximal upstroke velocity of the action potential. $\dot{V}_{max}$, and slowed conduction velocity at any level of resting potential. In addition, excitatory current of low intensity can be generated at membrane potentials where normal cells are inexcitable because inactivation is complete. The shifts in membrane responsiveness are illustrated in Figure 2–7. The result is a propensity to slow conduction, especially at shorter cycle lengths. The observation of action potentials

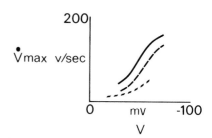

Figure 2–7. Membrane responsiveness curves, representing relationships between maximal upstroke velocity ($\dot{V}_{max}$) and membrane potential (V). A shift of the normal membrane responsiveness (continuous curve) downward indicates reduction of the fast sodium current. A downward and leftward shift indicates that fast channels can be activated at more positive levels of membrane potential. Examples of these shifts are shown by interrupted curves.

with very slow upstrokes generated at levels of membrane potential between -60 and -40 mV suggested that excitatory current might be generated via the slow calcium channels,[51] which can be activated in this range of membrane potentials and transmit less intense current than the fast channels. To date, most of the evidence favors the operation of depressed fast channels rather than slow channels in the generation of excitatory current in ischemically injured myocardium.[30]

In addition to abnormalities of excitatory current and refractory properties, recent investigators have detected evidence of increased intracellular impedance, that is, cell uncoupling, especially in ischemia and hypoxia.[52, 59] It appears that increased resting intracellular concentrations of free Ca^{2+} in the cytosol raise the resistance of tight junctions.[10] Increase of intracellular Na^+ and H^+ can produce the same effects.[11, 12] Since the maintenance of low concentrations of Ca^{2+}, Na^+, and H^+, requires energy, concentrations of these ions tend to rise in ischemia and hypoxia. In addition, interspersed fibrosis tends to separate cardiac cells in more chronic ischemia.[17] Cell uncoupling reduces conduction velocity and enhances anisotropy of propagation. The role of anisotropic conduction related to fiber orientation recently has been investigated.[50] It has been shown that conduction is more rapid but there is less reserve (safety factor) in a direction parallel to the long axes of fiber bundles in comparison to a direction perpendicular to the long axes. When excitatory current is depressed, block tends to occur during propagation in the direction of the alignment of the fibers, forming a line of block perpendicular

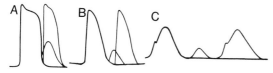

Figure 2–6. Representations of normal *(A)*, mildly abnormal *(B)*, and markedly abnormal *(C)*, action potentials of myocardial cells. Prematurely stimulated action potentials shown in the lighter line mark the end of the absolute and relative refractory periods in each panel. Note the pronounced postrepolarization refractoriness in *C*.

to the long axes. Very slow conduction is more likely in the direction normal to a long axis. At this time, the importance of fiber bundle orientation and anisotropy of propagation in the formation of reentry circuits is uncertain.

Reflection

Reflection is a disorder of propagation in which a viable but inexcitable segment of cardiac tissue narrowly separates two excitable regions but allows excitatory current to flow between them.[4] The model proposed, illustrated in Figure 2–8, is essentially linear based on experiments with Purkinje strands. Multidimensional counterparts can be conceived, but the realization of concrete examples appears more difficult. An approaching activation front generates an action potential on one side of the inexcitable segment, but no action potentials are generated within the segment. Excitatory current transmitted across the segment causes an electrotonic response on the other (distal) side that depends, among other things, on the resistance of the extracellular space that completes the local circuit of the electrotonic current flow. In experimental studies of this mechanism, this extracellular resistance is artificially inserted and varied. If

the delay necessary for the electrotonic response to reach threshold is sufficient, the second action potential will return current to the initial (proximal) side when the cells have repolarized enough to be reexcitable. A secondary response can be generated on the initial side, an "extrasystole." The process can "see-saw" back and forth, causing a tachyarrhythmia.

It has been suggested that reflection may operate in the first few minutes following coronary occlusion.[23] The suggestion is based primarily on experiments that fail to demonstrate continuous propagation and reentry preceding ectopic beats and on calculations that local extracellular injury currents measured in the myocardium during early ischemia are sufficiently intense to excite. At this time, there has not been a direct conclusive demonstration of reflection in vivo.

Reexcitation During Repolarization

Hypothetically, current could flow between nearby cells at different levels of intracellular potential during repolarization because of different rates of repolarization. This current could excite the more rapidly repolarizing cell when it became excitable, that is, when the absolute refractory period was terminated. There have been no definite demonstrations of this type of reexcitation.

Accelerated and Abnormal Automaticity

The normal pacemaker current in Purkinje fibers, which flows through a cation channel activated at relatively negative levels of membrane potential,[9] can be stimulated by various factors, including catecholamines. If global or local stimulation of the current were sufficiently intense, Purkinje pacemakers could fire fast enough to control the heart, causing an accelerated idioventricular rhythm. When Purkinje fibers are abnormally depolarized, the normal pacemaker current might not flow, but other currents, such as calcium currents, might serve a pacemaker function at levels of membrane potential between −60 and −40 mV. Ischemically injured Purkinje fibers show enhanced pacemaker activity at various levels of diastolic potential. It has been proposed that excess automatic activity of ischemically injured Purkinje fibers accounts for most of the spontaneous ventricular tachyarrhythmias 24 hours after coronary occlusion in experimental animals.[44] It is possible that a variety of cur-

Reflection

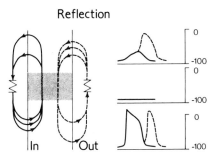

Figure 2–8. Model of reflection. On the left is shown a conduction pathway *(vertical lines)* containing an inexcitable segment *(stippled)*. On the right are shown transmembrane potentials recorded from the various segments of the pathway. The excitable segment below is activated, generating an action potential *(continuous curve below right)*. The current is transmitted across the segment *(continuous local circuits on the left)* to cause an electrotonic deflection in the membrane potential of the excitable region above the segment *(continuous curve above right)*. The electronic deflection reaches threshold, and an action potential occurs with some delay in the upper segment *(interrupted curve above right)*. This action potential generates local current spread back toward the bottom segment *(interrupted local circuits on the left)*. This current can reexcite the segment below *(interrupted curve below right)* if the action potential has repolarized sufficiently. Variable extracellular resistances incorporated in this model are represented by herringbone symbols.

rents may produce cyclic diastolic depolarization in cardiac cells at different levels of membrane potentials under different pathologic conditions. Pacemakers at different levels of diastolic potential may have different pharmacologic sensitivities. Purkinje pacemakers at more negative levels of diastolic potential (-90 to -60 mV) are suppressed by lidocaine, while those at more depolarized levels are unaffected.[2] Conversely, pacemakers operating at more depolarized levels can be sensitive to ethmozine, whereas more negative ones are insensitive.[8] Therefore, the identification of the precise pacemaker processes operating in vivo could be of practical importance. There have been indications that normally nonautomatic myocardial cells may manifest pacemaker currents under some abnormal conditions.[26, 48]

Afterpotentials and Triggered Firing

Afterpotentials in cardiac muscle were discovered almost 50 years ago.[46] However, these phenomena did not receive attention until the early 1970s, when it was discovered that cardiac glycosides, commonly used clinically, could induce afterpotentials in vitro, and it was suggested that these might be the mechanism for glycoside-induced arrhythmogenesis in vivo.[16, 42] The descriptive classification of Cranefield is in common usage.[7] Afterdepolarizations are transient depolarizing (positive) shifts of the membrane potential. Early afterdepolarizations (EADs) are transient retardations in the course of repolarization, like secondary plateaus, or transient reversals of repolarization in the positive direction. Delayed afterdepolarizations (DADs) are transient positive shifts after repolarization is complete, usually in early diastole. Examples are shown in Figure 2–9.

DADs induced by cardiac glycosides have been studied most intensively. Glycosides block sodium-potassium pumping, leading to increase in the concentration of Na^+ in the cytosol.[45] This increase in the cytosol reduces the transsarcolemmal gradient of concentration of Na^+, which is a prime driving force for Ca^{2+} extrusion via the Na^+-Ca^{2+} exchanger.[41, 47] As the result of the reduced driving force for Ca^{2+} extrusion, Ca^{2+} concentration increases in the cell and loads the sarcoplasmic reticulum (SR). The loaded SR tends to oscillate, releasing Ca^{2+} secondarily after the primary release that triggers contraction in systole.[24, 53] The secondary releases and increases of free Ca^{2+} in the cytosol generate inward

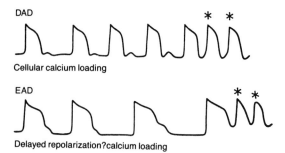

Figure 2–9. Representations of delayed (DAD) and early (EAD) afterdepolarizations. DADs are thought to be manifestations of calcium loading and are more prominent at higher heart rates. Triggered action potentials are shown by asterisks. EADs can occur if repolarization is delayed and may also be influenced by calcium loading. They are more prominent at slower heart rates. Relationships between cycle lengths and the size of the afterdepolarizations can be seen for both DADs and EADs.

transsarcolemmal current by the Na^+-Ca^{2+} exchanger, which operates to extrude the excess Ca^{2+} by exchange with Na^+ moving into the cell. The exchange is not electroneutral. Na^+ is in excess, and net inward current is generated.[38] The secondary Ca^{2+} release also may activate nonspecific cation channels that transmit inward current.[24] Other interventions besides cardiac glycosides can augment cellular Ca^{2+} and induce DADs. For example, beta-adrenergic stimulation increases slow inward current of Ca^{2+},[40] as well as SR uptake and release,[25] and can induce DADs in ordinary myocardium.[43] DADs have been observed after coronary occlusion in ischemically injured Purkinje fibers.[15] It has been proposed that DADs, rather than automatic mechanisms, are the predominant bases for ventricular tachyarrhythmias in dogs 1 to 3 days after coronary occlusion. However, the relative importance of DADs versus automatic mechanisms in this phase of myocardial infarction has not been resolved.[34]

When the amplitudes of DADs reach the level of the threshold potential, triggered excitation occurs. DADs and triggering become more prominent at higher heart rates[16, 42] because diastole, when calcium is extruded, is shortened relative to systole, when calcium is gained. Thus, the cells gain more calcium. In addition, the coupling interval of the DAD to the preceding action potential is shortened at higher heart rates. With glycoside-induced DADs, the amplitude of the primary DAD reaches a peak at rates of 100 to 120 and then declines. The pattern of response of glycoside-induced DADs has been suggested as a paradigm for identifying arrhythmias in vivo that are generated by DADs. However, it is not clear at this time that Ca^{2+} loading induced by other means, such as adrenergic stimulation, would produce DADs with the same pattern of response to heart rate.

EADs have excited growing interest following the recent demonstration that an arrhythmia identical with polymorphic ventricular tachycardia, called *torsades de pointes,* in the long Q-T syndromes can develop from EADs caused by suppression of repolarizing potassium currents by cesium.[5] EADs have been shown to develop under various conditions that upset the normal dominance of outward potassium currents during repolarization. When potassium channels are blocked, as by cesium, reducing outward repolarizing potassium currents, repolarization is prolonged and EADs develop. In addition, if weak inward currents, normally dominated by potassium currents during repolarization, are augmented, repolarization is prolonged and EADs can emerge. For example, aconitine can enhance the late flow of sodium ions through the fast channel by interfering with inactivation and other properties of the channel, retarding repolarization and generating EADs.[39]

In contrast to DADs, EADs are more prominent at slower heart rates because repolarizing potassium currents are reduced at slower rates.[5] The conditions that commonly have been implicated in the induction of *torsades de pointes* and long QTU intervals, such as administration of type 1a antiarrhythmic agents and hypokalemia, reduce outward potassium currents. Arrhythmias under these conditions are known to be aggravated at slower heart rates. Distinctive alteration of the TU wave observed after long cycles may reflect accentuation of afterpotentials after long cycles.

BRADYARRHYTHMIAS

Pacemaker Failure

Pacemaker cells in the interior of the sinus node control the heartbeat because their intrinsic firing rate is higher and because overdrive suppression tends to inhibit further the escape rate of subsidiary pacemakers.[54] Subsidiary pacemakers exist in the atria, atrioventricular (AV) junction, and His-Purkinje system.[20, 22] When sinus node pacemakers fail, subsidiary pacemakers in the atria or AV node usually assume control, accelerating during a brief period of recovery from overdrive suppression. Sinus node pacemakers can fail because of intrinsic depression of pacemaker activity, conduction block from the central pacemaker region to the atrial myocardium, or extrinsic factors depressing sinus node function. It has been shown that cells in the center of the sinus node lack fast channels and generate weak excitatory current by the slow channel.[18] Consequently, conduction block may occur within the node: sinoatrial (SA) block. When block occurs, only a fraction of the pacemaker impulses successfully reach the atrial myocardium, and bradycardia ensues.

Extrinsic depressors of sinus node pacemakers are numerous, including excess vagal (cholinergic) stimulation from various causes, hypoxia, ischemia, and toxic effects of various pharmacologic agents. There can be various causes of excess vagal stimulation, including lesions in the central nervous system; carotid sinus hypersensitivity; abnormal stimulation of intracardiac receptors activating vagal efferents, as in inferior posterior infarction; and certain emotional responses, as in vasovagal reactions.

The intrinsic rate of pacemakers in the His bundle and proximal bundle branches is 35 to 45 beats per minute, but pacemakers in the peripheral Purkinje network fire very slowly and erratically.[22] In general, pacemakers in the His-Purkinje system are less sensitive to vagal influences in vivo than are supraventricular pacemakers.[29] Subsidiary pacemakers can be depressed along with the sinus node pacemaker when extrinsic factors have a global effect on the heart or when there is diffuse pathologic involvement of the conduction system, as in sick sinus syndrome. In these circumstances dangerous cardiac slowing can occur.

HEART BLOCK

Once the wave front of activation enters the AV node, it is confined to a relatively small mass of conducting tissue, made up of the AV node, His bundle, and proximal bundle branches, which is not freely connected with the mass of ordinary myocardium.[1, 33] Midway down the septum the bundle branches begin to connect with the myocardium and to ramify in the freely communicating Purkinje network. Heart block can result from interruption of conduction in the AV node, His bundle, or proximal bundle branches.

The activation front normally propagates slowly in the AV node. Although the evidence is not yet definitive, there are strong indications that AV nodal cells, especially near the center of the node, generate excitatory current through slow channels rather than fast channels.[60, 67] As a result, upstrokes of action potentials are slow and conduction is very slow. In keeping with the slow recovery from activation of slow channels, the AV node has a relatively long period of postrepolarization refractoriness, during which conduction is further slowed.[21] The characteristic type of intermittent conduction block in the AV node is classified as Mobitz I or Wenckebach,[37, 56, 57] in which there is progressive slowing of conduction with each cycle until one cycle shows AV nodal block. AV nodal conduction is very sensitive to autonomic influences.[21] It is depressed by vagal stimulation and facilitated by sympathetic (beta) stimulation. The AV node is also highly sensitive to certain pharmacologic agents, notably those that affect slow inward current: beta agonists and blockers, cholinergic agonists and antagonists, calcium entry blockers, and cardiac glycosides. Blockers of the fast channel—that is, antiarrhythmic agents of type 1, such as lidocaine and quinidine—have little effect. The AV node, with its low level of excitatory current and marked sensitivity to autonomic and pharmacologic influences, commonly is the site of intermittent or complete AV block that is transitory. However, permanent block in the AV node is relatively uncommon.

The His-Purkinje system is specialized for rapid conduction and wide dissemination of the impulse.[29] Among the various types of cardiac cells, Purkinje fibers show the most intense sodium current, the most rapid upstrokes, and the fastest conduction. Propagation in Purkinje fibers is virtually insensitive to autonomic influences or blockers of calcium channels. It is sensitive to blockers of the fast channels, that is, antiarrhythmic agents of type 1. However, the depression of conduction by these agents is modest unless the cells are abnormal or the agents are in high concentration. Intermittent block in the His-Purkinje system is characterized by apparent constancy of conduction punctuated by intermittent single cycles with complete block: Mobitz II block.[28] Close analysis of conduction in abnormal His-Purkinje cells, mostly ischemically damaged fibers, indicated that partially depolarized cells acquire certain characteristics of AV nodal cells: slow upstrokes with slow conduction and delayed recovery from inactivation, with relatively long relative refractory periods outlasting repolarization.[14, 32] When

these characteristics are pronounced, the type of intermittent block seen is manifestly of the Wenckebach type, readily apparent on observation of the P-R intervals on the electrocardiogram. When the abnormalities are less pronounced, intermittent block still is generally of the Wenckebach type, but the progressive conduction delays may be slight and inapparent except at high recording resolution. This finding has led to the assertion that intermittent conduction block is always of the Wenckebach type, but in the His-Purkinje system it may be inapparent at the usual recording resolution of the electrocardiogram.[19] This failure to appreciate the progressive delays gave rise to the classification of Mobitz II, which has turned out to be a useful indication of block in the His-Purkinje system. Transitory block caused by extrinsic factors is less common in the His-Purkinje system than in the AV node. On the other hand, chronic heart block is more commonly due to disease in the His-Purkinje system, usually sclerodegenerative disease of the conduction system.

Abnormal pacemaker fibers can demonstrate depressed propagation linked to abnormal pacemaker activity. When depressed cells are operating at partially depolarized levels of membrane potential, they may demonstrate conduction block late in diastole, when diastolic depolarization has progressed substantially, but not early in diastole, when the cells are relatively more polarized.[49] The diastolic depolarization and a positive shift of the threshold potential result in action potentials with upstrokes too diminutive and slow to propagate. Such a phenomenon has been termed "phase four block" and has been offered as the mechanism for certain instances of bradycardia-dependent block, that is, a block of conduction occurring at slow heart rates observed clinically.[6, 27]

REFERENCES

1. Abramson DL, Margolin S: Purkinje conduction network in the myocardium of the mammalian ventricle. J Anat 70:250–259, 1936.
2. Allen JD, Brennan JF, Wit AL: Actions of lidocaine on transmembrane potentials of subendocardial Purkinje fibers surviving in infarcted canine hearts. Circ Res 43:470–480, 1978.
3. Allessie MA, Bonke FIM, Schopman FJG: Circus movement in rabbit atrial muscle as a mechanism of tachycardia. III. The "leading circle" concept: A new model of circus movement in cardiac tissue without the involvement of an anatomical obstacle. Circ Res 41:9–18, 1977.

4. Antzelevitch C, Jalife J, Moe GK: Characteristics of reflection as a mechanism of reentrant arrhythmias and its relationship to parasystole. Circulation 61:182–191, 1980.
5. Brachmann J, Scherlag BJ, Rosenshtraukh LV, Lazzara R: Bradycardia-dependent triggered activity: Relevance to drug-induced multiform ventricular tachycardia. Circulation 68:846–856, 1983.
6. Castellanos A, Khuddus SA, Sommer LS: His bundle recordings in bradycardia-dependent AV block induced by premature beats. Br Heart J 37:570, 1975.
7. Cranefield PF: Action potentials, afterpotentials and arrhythmias. Circ Res 41:415–423, 1977.
8. Dangman KH, Hoffman BF: Antiarrhythmic effects of ethmozin in cardiac Purkinje fibers: Suppression of automaticity and abolition of triggering. J Pharmacol Exp Ther 227:578, 1983.
9. DeFrancesco D, Ojeda C: Properties of the current i_f in the sinoatrial node of the rabbit compared with those of the current i_{k2} in Purkinje fibers. J Physiol (Lond) 308:353–367, 1980.
10. DeMello WC: Effect of intracellular injection of calcium and strontium on cell communication in heart. J Physiol 250:231–245, 1975.
11. DeMello WC: Influence of the sodium pump on intracellular communication in heart fibers: Effect of intracellular injection of sodium ion on electrical coupling. J Physiol 263:171–197, 1976.
12. DeMello WC: Intracellular injection of H^+ on the electrical coupling in cardiac Purkinje fibers. Cell Biol Int Rep 4:51–58, 1980.
13. El-Sherif N, Mehra R, Gough WB: Ventricular activation pattern of spontaneous and induced ventricular rhythms in canine one-day-old myocardial infarction. Evidence for focal and reentrant mechanisms. Circ Res 51:152–166, 1982.
14. El-Sherif N, Scherlag BJ, Lazzara R: Pathophysiology of second degree atrioventricular block: A unified hypothesis. Am J Cardiol 35:421–434, 1975.
15. El-Sherif N, Gough WB, Zeiler RH, Mehra R: Triggered ventricular rhythms in 1-day-old myocardial infarction in the dog. Circ Res 52:566–579, 1983.
16. Ferrier GR, Saunders JH, Mendez CA: Cellular mechanism for the generation of ventricular arrhythmias by acetylstrophanthidin. Circ Res 32:206–214, 1973.
17. Gardner MD, Ursell PC, Fenoglio JJ Jr, Wit AL: Electrophysiologic and anatomic basis for fractionated electrograms recorded from healed myocardial infarcts. Circulation 72:596–611, 1985.
18. Giles W, van Ginneken A, Shibata EF: Ionic currents underlying cardiac pacemaker activity: A summary of voltage-clamp data from single cells. In Nathan RD (ed): Cardiac Muscle: The Regulation of Excitation and Contraction. Orlando, FL, Academic Press, 1986, pp 1–27.
19. Gough WB, Mehra R, Restivo M, et al: Reentrant ventricular arrhythmias in the late myocardial infarction period in the dog. Circ Res 57:432–442, 1985.
20. Hoffman BF, Cranefield PF: Electrophysiology of the Heart. New York, McGraw-Hill, 1960, pp 104–130.
21. Hoffman BF, Cranefield PF: Electrophysiology of the Heart. New York, McGraw-Hill, 1960, pp 132–174.
22. Hope RR, Scherlag BJ, El-Sherif N, Lazzara R: Hierarchy of ventricular pacemakers. Circ Res 39:883–888, 1976.
23. Janse MJ, van Capelle FJL, Morsink H, et al: Flow of "injury" current and pattern of excitation during early ventricular arrhythmias in acute regional myocardial ischemia in isolated porcine and canine hearts: Evidence for two different arrhythmogenic mechanisms. Circ Res 47:151–165, 1980.
24. Kass RS, Lederer WM, Tsien RW: Role of calcium ions in transient inward currents and aftercontractions induced by strophanthidin in cardiac Purkinje fibers. J Physiol (Lond) 281:187–208, 1978.
25. Katz AM, Tada M, Kirchberger MA; Control of calcium transport in the myocardium by the cyclic AMP–protein kinase system. Adv Cyclic Nucleotide Res 5:453–472, 1975.
26. Katzung BO, Morgenstern JA: Effects of extracellular potassium on ventricular automaticity and evidence for a pacemaker current in mammalian ventricular myocardium. Circ Res 40:105–111, 1977.
27. Langendorf R: The role of spontaneous diastolic depolarization in second degree A-V block: The mechanism of "paroxysmal" A-V block and a new form of pseudosupernormal A-V conduction [editorial]. Chest 63:652, 1973.
28. Langendorf R, Pick A: Atrioventricular block, type II (Mobitz)—its nature and clinical significance. Circulation 38:819–821, 1968.
29. Lazzara R: Electrophysiology of the specialized conduction system: Selected aspects relevant to clinical bradyarrhythmias. In Samet P, El-Sherif N (eds): Cardiac Pacing. 2nd ed. New York, Grune and Stratton, 1980, pp 37–66.
30. Lazzara R, Scherlag BJ: The role of the slow current in the generation of arrhythmias in ischemic myocardium. In Zipes DP, Bailey JC, Elharrar V (eds): The Slow Inward Current and Cardiac Arrhythmias. The Hague, Martinus Nijhoff, 1980, pp 399–416.
31. Lazzara R, Scherlag BJ: Cellular electrophysiology and ischemia. In Sperelakis N (ed): Physiology and Pathophysiology of the Heart. The Hague, Martinus Nijhoff, 1984, pp 443–458.
32. Lazzara R, El-Sherif N, Scherlag BJ: Disorders of cellular electrophysiology produced by ischemia of the canine His bundle. Circ Res 36:444–453, 1975.
33. Lazzara R, Yeh BK, Samet P: Functional anatomy of the canine left bundle branch. Am J Cardiol 33:623–631, 1974.
34. LeMarec H, Dangman KH, Danilo P Jr, Rosen MR: An evaluation of automaticity and triggered activity in the canine heart one to four days after myocardial infarction. Circulation 71:1224–1236, 1985.
35. Mayer AG: Rhythmical pulsation in scyphomedusae. Washington, DC, Carnegie Institution of Washington, Publication No. 47, 1906.
36. Mayer AG: Rhythmical pulsation in scyphomedusae. In Papers from the Tortugas Laboratory of the Carnegie Institution of Washington 1:113–131 (Carnegie Institution of Washington, Publication No. 102, Part VII), 1908.
37. Mobitz W: Uber die unfallständige Störung der Erregungsüberleitung zwischen Vorhof und Kammer des Menschlichen Herzens. Z Ges Exp Med 41:180–237, 1924.
38. Mullins LJ: The generation of electric currents in cardiac fibers by Na/Ca exchange. Am J Physiol (Cell Physiol) 236:C103–C110, 1979.
39. Peper K, Trautwein W: The effect of aconitine on the membrane current in cardiac muscle. Pflugers Arch 296:328, 1967.
40. Reuter H: Localization of beta adrenergic receptors and effects of noradrenalin and cyclic nucleotides on action potentials, ionic currents, and tension in mammalian cardiac muscle. J Physiol (Lond) 242:429–451, 1974.
41. Reuter H, Seitz N: The dependence of calcium efflux from cardiac muscle on temperature and external

ion composition. J Physiol (Lond) 195;451–470, 1968.

42. Rosen MR, Gelband H, Hoffman BF: Correlation between effects of ouabain in the canine electrocardiogram and transmembrane potentials of isolated Purkinje fibers. Circulation 47:65–72, 1973.

43. Schechter E, Freeman C, Lazzara R: Afterdepolarizations as a mechanism for the long QT syndrome: Electrophysiological studies of a case. J Am Coll Cardiol 3:1556–1561, 1984.

44. Scherlag BJ, El-Sherif N, Hope RR, Lazzara R: Characterization and localization of ventricular arrhythmias resulting from myocardial ischemia and infarction. Circ Res 35:372–383, 1974.

45. Schwartz A, Lindenmayer GE, Allen JC: The sodium-potassium adenosine triphosphatase: Pharmacological, physiological and biochemical aspects. Pharmacol Rev 27:1–134, 1975.

46. Segers M: Le rôle des potentiels tardifs du coeur. Mem Acad R Med Belg (Series II) 1:1–30, 1941.

47. Sheu SS, Fozzard HA: Transmembrane Na^+ and Ca^{2+} electrochemical gradients in cardiac muscle and their relationship to force development. J Gen Physiol 80:325–351, 1982.

48. Singer DH, Baumgarten CM, Ten Eick RE: Cellular electrophysiology of ventricular and other dysrhythmias: Studies on diseased and ischemic heart. Prog Cardiovasc Dis 24:97–156, 1981.

49. Singer DH, Lazzara R, Hoffman BF: Interrelationships between automaticity and conduction in Purkinje fibers. Circ Res 21:537, 1967.

50. Spach MS, Miller WT III, Geselowitz DB, et al: The discontinuous nature of propagation in normal canine cardiac muscle. Circ Res 48:39–54, 1981.

51. Spear JF, Horowitz LN, Hodess AB: Cellular electrophysiology of human myocardial infarction. I. Abnormalities of cellular activation. Circulation 59:247–256, 1979.

52. Spear JF, Michelson EL, Moore EN: Reduced space constant in slowly conducting regions of chronically infarcted canine myocardium. Circ Res 53:176, 1983.

53. Tsien RW, Kass RS, Weingart R: Cellular and subcellular mechanisms of cardiac pacemaker oscillations. J Exp Biol 81:205–215, 1979.

54. Vassalle M: The relationship among cardiac pacemakers. Overdrive suppression. Circ Res 41:269–277, 1977.

55. Waldo AL, Plumb VJ, Arciniegas JG, et al: Transient entrainment and interruption of A-V bypass pathway type paroxysmal atrial tachycardia. A model for understanding and identifying reentrant arrhythmias in man. Circulation 67:73, 1982.

56. Wenckebach KF: Zur Analyse des unregelmassigen Pulses. Z Klin Med 37:475–488, 1899.

57. Wenckebach KF: Beiträge zur Kenntis der menschlichen Herztätigkeit. Arch Anat Physiol (Physiol Abtheilung) 297–354, 1906.

58. Wit AL, Allessie MA, Bonke FIM: Electrophysiologic mapping to determine the mechanism of experimental ventricular tachycardia initiated by premature impulses: Experimental approach initial results demonstrating reentrant excitation. Am J Cardiol 49:166–185, 1982.

59. Wojtczak J: Contractures and increase in internal longitudinal resistance of cow ventricular muscle induced by hypoxia. Circ Res 44:88–95, 1979.

60. Zipes DP, Fischer JC: Effects of agents which inhibit the slow channel on sinus node automaticity and atrioventricular conduction in the dog. Circ Res 34:184–192, 1974.

61. Zipes DP, Mendez C: Action of manganese ions and tetrodotoxin on AV nodal potentials in isolated rabbit hearts. Circ Res 32:447–454, 1973.

II

ELECTRICAL THERAPY FOR BRADY-ARRHYTHMIAS

3

ENGINEERING ASPECTS OF PULSE GENERATORS FOR CARDIAC PACING

ALAN D. BERNSTEIN *and* VICTOR PARSONNET

Cardiac pacing is an interdisciplinary field. In addition to surgery, cardiology, and cardiac electrophysiology, it involves the practical application of a variety of concepts drawn from physics, mathematics, electrical engineering, chemistry, materials sciences, and computer science. Clearly, a solid background in all of these disciplines is not required in the practice of day-to-day clinical pacing, just as a thorough understanding of the thermodynamics of the internal combustion engine is not required in operating an automobile. On the other hand, when a technical problem arises, an understanding of one or more of these scientific disciplines may be crucial.

The primary objective of this chapter is to assist the reader in visualizing pulse-generator operation and in understanding some important related technical concepts. The discussion presented herein will therefore concentrate on describing what pulse generators do in various circumstances, without pretending to explain adequately how they do it, which would require mathematics and circuit theory beyond the scope of this book. The message inherent in this restriction is that part of the skill required in dealing with pacing problems of a technical nature is recognizing when it is time to seek technical advice.

The basic "building blocks" of an antibrady-arrhythmia-pacemaker will be described, and the function and, in most cases, limitations of each will be discussed. A brief description of each of the standard modes of antibradyarrhythmia pacing will then be presented from the standpoint of pulse generator operation.

NOTATION CONVENTIONS AND CODES

Several techniques exist that can simplify the task of visualizing the pacemaker's interaction with the heart in each of the various modes described below and in Chapter 7. In this chapter it will be assumed that the reader is familiar with the NASPE/BPEG Generic (NBG) Code.[1] There will also be occasion to use electrocardiograms with diagnostic overlays to illustrate important aspects of pulse generator design and behavior in various situations.[1]

THE BASIC FUNCTIONAL ELEMENTS OF A PULSE GENERATOR

In the block diagram shown in Figure 3–1, a conventional single-chamber pacemaker pulse generator is broken down into several important functional elements whose nature and purpose should be understood. Each will be considered in turn.

The Power Source

In the simplest possible terms, a pulse generator may be regarded as an electric battery equipped with an automatic switch that connects the battery to the heart for about a millisecond once every second or so. The power source does two things: It provides electric current to run the electric circuitry of the pulse generator, and it causes an electric

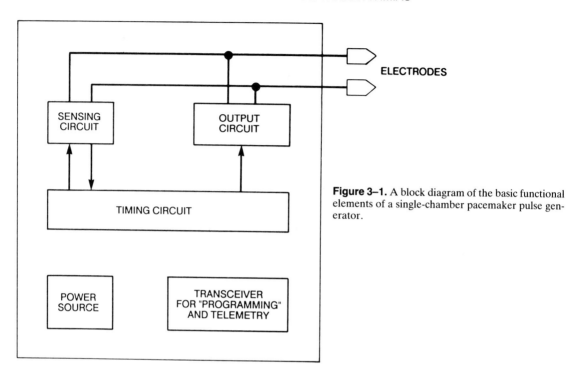

Figure 3–1. A block diagram of the basic functional elements of a single-chamber pacemaker pulse generator.

current to flow periodically through a portion of myocardial tissue to stimulate cardiac depolarization.

Whatever its chemical composition or the nature of its operation, the power source can be regarded as a reservoir of electric charge. Its capacity is usually measured in units of charge (ampere-hours), and it passes charge through an electric circuit in the form of current (charge per unit time) by converting chemical potential energy into electrical potential energy. All of the charge drawn from a power source as current returns to the source, but the source's ability to pump charge through an external load decreases as it becomes "depleted," at which time the voltage (electrical potential energy per unit charge) at its terminals becomes too low to be useful.

Tabulated values of battery capacity can be misleading, since they usually refer to the *theoretical* quantity of charge that can be drawn from the battery as current. Before that amount of charge has been drawn, the terminal voltage may become too low to operate an electric circuit. In clinical pacing, the only battery capacity of practical interest is the capacity up to the point where the terminal voltage is too low to provide a stimulus capable of producing a cardiac depolarization. Unfortunately, battery capacity defined in this way is usually not tabulated in pulse generator manuals or other sources of information. It is important, therefore, to have a way of detecting imminent battery depletion so that the pulse generator can be replaced in a timely fashion.

The power sources used in implantable pulse generators differ somewhat in several important ways. First, there is considerable variation in battery capacity. The actuarial survival of pulse generators using mercury-zinc batteries (now obsolete) and various lithium-chemistry cells is summarized in Figure 3–2.[3–6] Radioactive plutonium-238 power sources are not shown in the figure, but recent data indicate that 88 per cent of implanted "nuclear-powered" pulse generators survive after 12 years.[6]

A second important difference in power sources is the behavior of the terminal voltage as a function of time as the battery becomes depleted. Mercury-zinc batteries provide relatively invariant terminal voltage throughout the useful life of the battery, but this voltage drops somewhat abruptly at the end of the battery's life, so that battery depletion is relatively difficult to anticipate and actual pacemaker failure is more likely to occur than with lithium-chemistry batteries, whose terminal voltage decreases more gradually, permitting routine tracking as part of pacemaker follow-up and, in turn, timely replacement of the pulse generator when battery failure is imminent. In some pulse generators, the battery voltage is monitored internally, and the user

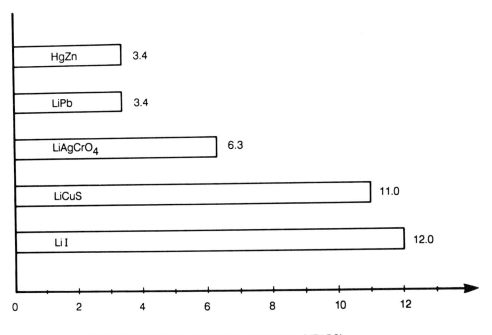

APPROXIMATE 50% ACTUARIAL SURVIVAL (YEARS)

Figure 3–2. Fifty per cent actuarial survival of pulse generators powered by mercury-zinc batteries and by cells of various lithium-chemistry formulations.[3-6] Plutonium-238 sources are not represented in the figure because the 50 per cent survival point has not yet been reached even after 16 years of "nuclear" pacing. HgZn = mercury-zinc; LiPb = lithium-lead; $LiAgCrO_4$ = lithium–silver chromate; LiCuS = lithium–cupric sulfide; LiI = lithium-iodine.

is warned (via a change in the magnet-mode rate, for example) that the battery is approaching the end of its life.

A third difference is related to battery chemistry. The reactions by which mercury-zinc and lithium–cupric sulfide batteries function produce gas, which must escape, or the cell will crack or explode. The gas can permeate epoxy resin, but its production precludes the enclosure of the battery or the entire pulse generator in a hermetically sealed can. Plutonium sources are hermetically sealed in multiple encapsulations but must be protected from extreme heat (as in cremation, for example), which might disrupt the shielding encapsulation.

Cardiac Stimulation and Output Circuits

Several important variables are involved in stimulating the heart by passing an electric current through excitable cardiac tissue. The stimulus current density (current per unit of cross-sectional area) must be sufficiently high, and the stimulus must be of sufficient duration, to depolarize a large enough group of cells to initiate myocardial impulse propagation of the kind that occurs during spontaneous organized cardiac depolarization. This is accomplished by applying a voltage across two electrodes connected to the body. In bipolar pacing, the two electrodes are in close proximity and in direct contact with myocardial tissue; in unipolar pacing, one electrode is in contact with the heart and the other (usually all or part of the metal housing of the pulse generator) is elsewhere in the body. The two electrode configurations behave somewhat differently in terms of both stimulation and the detection of spontaneous cardiac events, as will be discussed below.

The threshold of stimulation—the current, voltage, energy, or charge required for reliable cardiac capture during electrical diastole with a stimulus of given duration—determines the stimulus parameters required for pacing. Figures 3–3 to 3–5 depict the behavior of the stimulation threshold as a function of the stimulus duration in terms of each of these stimulus-amplitude parameters. Because the concept of stimulation threshold is sometimes misunderstood, it should be emphasized that the behavior of *each* parameter—voltage, current, energy, or charge—depends upon the duration of the stimulus, as may be readily

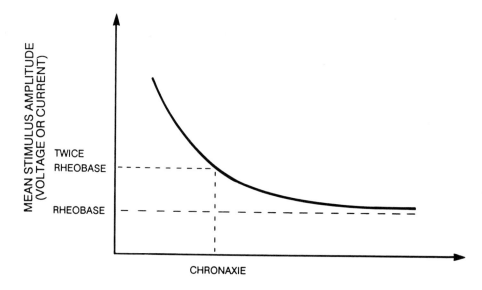

Figure 3–3. A "strength-duration" curve representing the threshold of cardiac stimulation. Capture may be achieved by any combination of mean amplitude and stimulus duration whose corresponding point on the strength-duration plane lies above the threshold curve. The *rheobase* is the threshold amplitude as the stimulus duration becomes infinite; the *chronaxie* is the duration of a stimulus at the threshold of stimulation whose mean amplitude is twice the rheobase.

seen in the figures. Thus, the value of whatever amplitude parameter is chosen at the threshold of stimulation depends upon the duration of the stimulus.

The two types of pulse-generator output circuits in common use behave somewhat differently and may have important clinical implications in the event of lead-insulation leakage.

Most pulse generators perform *voltage-source pacing,* as illustrated in Figure 3–6. The commonly used term "constant-voltage pacing" is erroneous and misleading, as may be seen in the figure: The stimulus voltage and stimulus current both decay during the stimulus as the charged capacitor C discharges through the cardiac impedance Z_H. It should be emphasized that the peak values V and I of the stimulus voltage and current, respectively, are greater than the corresponding mean values $\overline{V}$ and $\overline{I}$ used in establishing a safety margin relative to the "strength-dura-

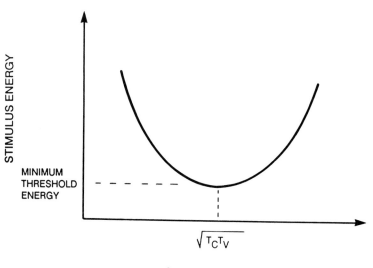

Figure 3–4. A curve representing the stimulus energy at the threshold of cardiac stimulation, as a function of the stimulus duration. The minimal energy required for capture is achieved with a duration equal to the geometric mean of the current chronaxie (T_I) and the voltage chronaxie (T_V).

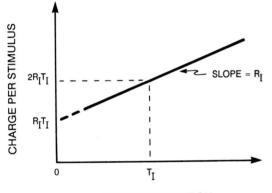

Figure 3–5. A curve representing the charge per stimulus at the threshold of cardiac stimulation, as a function of the stimulus duration. The relation is linear and is completely determined by the current rheobase (R_I) and the current chronaxie (T_I). Less charge is required for capture with briefer stimuli, but higher current or voltage may be needed. (See Fig. 3–3.)

tion" curve of Figure 3–3. The more rapid the decay, the lower the mean values, even though the peak values remain the same.

In voltage-source pacing, if a current leak develops in the outer insulation of a unipolar lead or the septal insulation of a bipolar lead, the peak voltage remains the same, but the peak current *through the heart* is decreased, the voltage and current both decay more rapidly, and the mean voltage and current are lower. Therefore, if the only stimulus-amplitude parameter observed during follow-up is the peak amplitude of the stimulus artifact seen across the surface-lead electrocardiography electrodes, the existence of an insulation failure may not be noticed before capture is lost.

Current-source pacing is illustrated in Figure 3–7. In this instance, the commonly used term "constant-current pacing" is appropriate because the current through the series combination of the coupling capacitor C and the heart impedance Z_H is indeed constant for the duration of the stimulus, as is the stimulus voltage. Because there is no decay, the mean values of voltage and current are the same as

the corresponding peak values, which simplifies relating measured amplitudes to the voltage or current threshold, as reflected in Figure 3–3.

In current-source pacing, if a current leak develops in the outer insulation of a unipolar lead or the septal insulation of a bipolar lead, the stimulus voltage and current are both reduced. The current source is attempting to pump charge through a lower composite resistance and may be unable to do so at a constant rate throughout the duration of the stimulus, producing a distortion in the rectangular shape of the stimulus (or stimulus-artifact) waveform. Even if the waveform remains rectangular, an insulation leak whose electrical resistance is approximately the same as that of the heart will cause the stimulus voltage and current to be halved. This halving will reduce the capture safety margin and may result in loss of capture, but the drop in stimulus amplitude will be more readily detected in pacemaker-clinic follow-up before clinical consequences become manifest.

Sensing Circuits

The intended role of the pulse generator's sensing circuit is the detection of spontaneous cardiac depolarizations. Depending on the electrode configuration (unipolar or bipolar), other electrical signals may be detected and wrongly interpreted as cardiac depolarizations.

To understand the normal and abnormal operation of pacemaker sensing, it is important to consider both how sensing is achieved and what may be there to be sensed. Sensing was defined above, in a restricted fashion, as the detection of real or apparent spontaneous cardiac depolarizations. It must be distinguished clearly from the measurement of a physiologic variable, such as blood temperature, stimulus–to–T-wave interval, or mechanical vibration, that is used to control rate modulation in the manner described in Chapter 16.

A conventional sensing circuit has three basic functional elements, as shown in Figure 3–8. The *sensing amplifier* magnifies the volt-

Figure 3–6. Voltage-source pacing. A charged capacitor (C) discharges through the heart. i = instantaneous current; v = instantaneous voltage; I_0 = initial current; V_0 = initial voltage; $\bar{I}$ = mean current; $\bar{V}$ = mean voltage; Z_H = heart impedance; T = stimulus duration.

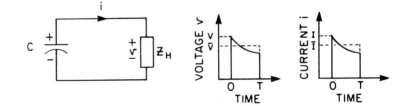

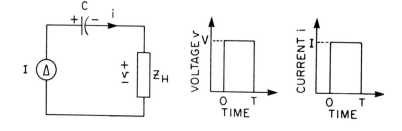

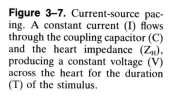

Figure 3–7. Current-source pacing. A constant current (I) flows through the coupling capacitor (C) and the heart impedance (Z_H), producing a constant voltage (V) across the heart for the duration (T) of the stimulus.

age difference that appears across the electrodes. This difference, which may range from less than a millivolt to approximately 40 mV, is converted to a larger voltage difference that can be handled by the subsequent circuitry without undue corruption by the low-voltage electrical noise normally generated in the circuits themselves. To avoid having the amplifier affected by an anticipated high-amplitude input signal, such as an atrial stimulus "seen" by the ventricular-channel sensing circuit connected with the ventricular electrodes of a dual-chamber pacemaker, the amplifier can be disabled (in effect, turned off) deliberately for a short period, called a *blanking period.*

A *bandpass filter* is included to isolate the components of the amplified input signal that most clearly signify cardiac depolarization: the rapid deflection (sometimes referred to as the "intrinsic deflection"), illustrated in Figure 3–9. This deflection lasts on the order of 10 msec and is followed by a slow deflection, which is useful during pervenous lead implantation in verifying good mechanical contact between an electrode and the endocardial surface. The slow deflection may be of considerable amplitude immediately after electrode placement,

reflecting a so-called "current of injury," but the amplitude may decrease markedly as the electrode-tissue interface matures. The bandpass filter rejects relatively slow-moving signal components (to avoid responding to the slow deflection) as well as very rapidly moving signal components (to reduce the likelihood of responding to myopotentials and ambient electrical noise). It functions somewhat like the tone controls on a high-fidelity phonograph, attenuating tones that are higher or lower in pitch than those that fall within the range selected.

When a spontaneous depolarization occurs, the filter output is of reasonable amplitude, because of the amplifier, and consists mainly of the rapid-deflection components that remain after filtering. A *threshold comparator* then performs the actual detection by comparing the instantaneous voltage at the filter output with a fixed reference voltage, producing a logic signal (a voltage pulse) whenever the filter output exceeds the reference voltage in amplitude. This logic signal can be used by the control circuitry of the pulse generator for resetting the pacemaker's escape timing or for other purposes. An interval during which the

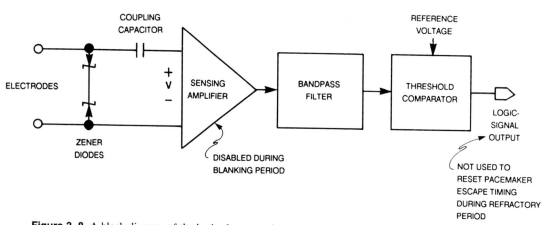

Figure 3–8. A block diagram of the basic elements of a conventional analog sensing circuit, showing Zener diodes (for protection against high applied voltages, such as those occurring during defibrillation), the sensing amplifier, the bandpass filter, and the threshold comparator. The sensing amplifier is disabled during a *blanking period,* and the logic output is not used to reset pacemaker escape timing during a *refractory period.*

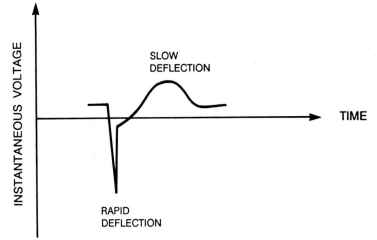

Figure 3–9. Two major components of the intracardiac-electrogram signal, as seen by the sensing circuit of the pulse generator upon cardiac depolarization: a rapid deflection (sometimes called the "intrinsic deflection") followed by a slow deflection.

logic signal produced by sensing is ignored by the timing circuitry is called a *refractory period.*

When a pulse generator is adjusted ("programmed") to increase or decrease its sensitivity to spontaneous waveforms, what is usually changed is the gain of the sensing amplifier, with the threshold-detection reference voltage held constant. On the other hand, the pulse generator manual often specifies the available values of the *sensing threshold.* This number represents an approximation of the minimal rapid-deflection amplitude that will be detected at a given sensitivity setting. The amplifier gain is *increased* to raise the sensitivity, or lower the sensing threshold, and *decreased* to lower the sensitivity, or raise the sensing threshold.

The Function of Blanking and Refractory Periods

It should be emphasized that there are *two* ways of disabling the sensing function of the pulse generator. First, the sensing amplifier itself may be disabled (turned off) during a *blanking period* to avoid its being driven into saturation (a condition of maximal output) by an anticipated high input voltage resulting from a stimulus delivered elsewhere in the heart. This means that the amplifier can be reenabled (turned on again) a moment later and used immediately for sensing without having to wait for it to recover from its saturated state. Second, *refractory periods* may be incorporated in the pulse generator's timing-control logic so that the device will not respond to a sensing-system output by resetting the pacemaker's escape timing during those portions of

the cardiac cycle when one may safely anticipate that what is actually triggering the sensing circuit is an appropriate signal. In this way, T waves following ventricular pacing can be prevented from being sensed as R waves by the ventricular channel, and intracardiac QRS complexes following atrial pacing and retrograde P waves after ventricular events can be prevented from affecting the atrial channel.

Figure 3–10 shows blanking and refractory periods in DDD pacing. The blanking period in the ventricular channel is intended to prevent interchannel *crosstalk,* as a result of which the ventricular channel would sense the atrial stimulus or its electrical aftermath (the electrical polarization of the atrial electrode-tissue interface as a result of the stimulus) and respond as though a spontaneous ventricular

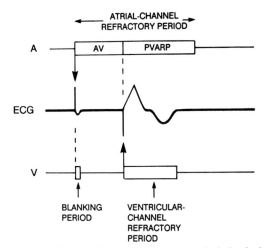

Figure 3–10. Blanking and refractory periods in dual-chamber pacing. The pacing mode illustrated here is DDD. AV = atrioventricular interval; PVARP = postventricular atrial refractory period.

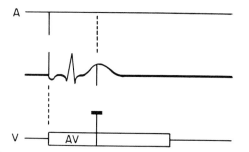

Figure 3–11. "Committed" DVI pacing. Because the ventricular channel is refractory throughout the AV interval, the spontaneous ventricular response to the evoked atrial depolarization does not reset the pacemaker escape timing, and the pending ventricular stimulus is therefore not inhibited.

depolarization had been detected. Some pulse generators produce biphasic (negative, then positive) stimulation pulses to alleviate this problem further. The shorter the blanking period can safely be made, the sooner the sensing amplifier can be reactivated so that sensing (and waveform telemetry if the pulse generator has this capability) can be resumed.

An awareness of the refractory-period structure of the ventricular channel can be helpful in understanding the operation of DVI and DDD pacemakers. As Figure 3–11 shows, if the ventricular channel is refractory throughout the atrioventricular (AV) interval, a spontaneous ventricular response to a paced atrial depolarization is not "seen" by the pulse generator and cannot be used to inhibit a ventricular stimulus. Such a system, in which a ventricular stimulus is inevitable once the atrium has been stimulated, performs what is known as "committed" ventricular stimulation.

Pacemaker Circuit Protection

The back-to-back Zener diodes shown across the electrode terminals of the pulse generator in Figure 3–8 deserve comment. A diode is an electronic circuit component that conducts current readily in one direction but blocks its passage in the opposite direction. A Zener diode can conduct in the reverse direction as well, but not until the voltage across its terminals exceeds a design parameter known as the Zener voltage. The Zener diodes in Figure 3–8 are normally electrically "invisible," behaving like an open circuit and thus playing no role in the operation of the pacemaker. No current flows through them unless the voltage across the electrode terminals reaches an abnormally high value (exceeds the Zener voltage), which may occur during cardioversion, defibrillation, or electrocautery. When this happens, as shown in Figure 3–12 for a unipolar pacing system, the Zener diodes conduct, and the voltage across the sensing-amplifier input is *limited* to a safe value (the Zener voltage), ensuring that the circuitry will not be damaged as long as the Zener diodes themselves remain undamaged. But this protection is achieved by shunting current through the Zener diodes *and through the heart* via the cardiac electrode, with possible thermal damage to the electrode-tissue interface.

For example, supposing that the applied voltage is 2000 V (reasonable in defibrillation), the tissue resistance is 200 ohms for each applied electrode, the cardiac impedance is 500 ohms, and the Zener voltage is 10 V, the voltage across the sensing amplifier is safely

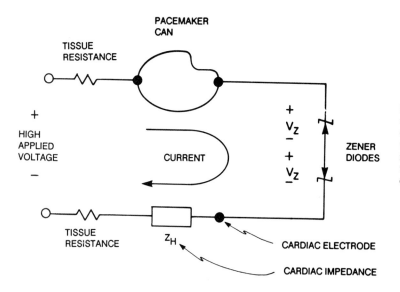

Figure 3–12. A schematic circuit diagram of a mechanism whereby extremely large currents may pass through the cardiac electrode-tissue interface when the Zener diodes that protect the pulse generator circuitry conduct during defibrillation.

limited to 10 V, but the voltage across the heart exceeds 1100 V and the current passing through it is greater than 2.2 A. Because the surface area of the cardiac electrode is small, on the order of 10 mm², the current density in this situation is extremely high and thermal damage may occur. Thus, protecting the pacemaker is not enough; the electrode-tissue interface may be affected sufficiently to raise the threshold of stimulation, perhaps to the point where capture is lost.

Undersensing and Oversensing

Although the standard pacing modes are usually thought of in terms of the pacemaker's response to the sensing of spontaneous atrial and ventricular depolarizations, what the sensing system actually "sees" may include an impressive array of other signals as well. The simplicity of the sensing system described above is achieved at the cost of a kind of electronic stupidity, because the system may interpret as a cardiac depolarization any of the signals listed in Tables 3–1 and 3–2, provided those signals can get through the filter with sufficient amplitude. The sensing of anything other than spontaneous depolarizations causes problems that may be dealt with by special mechanisms designed into the pulse generator (such as "noise" modes or "ventricular safety pacing"), but only if the device recognizes or assumes *a priori* that what is being detected is not a spontaneous cardiac depolarization of the type expected.

Undersensing is a useful term that means what it says: The signal applied to the sensing-circuit input during a spontaneous depolarization is of inadequate amplitude or inappropriate waveshape to pass through the sensing filter with adequate amplitude to trigger the

TABLE 3–1. SIGNALS THAT MAY BE SENSED VIA AN ATRIAL LEAD

Signals Arising in the Atrium
  P waves
  Retrograde P waves
  Ectopic atrial depolarizations
  Atrial flutter
  Atrial fibrillation
Signals Arising Elsewhere
  Skeletal-muscle potentials
  Far-field cardiac signals (e.g., R waves)
  Stimuli from the ventricular channel of the same pulse
    generator
  Stimuli from another implanted device
  Stimuli from an external device
  Electromagnetic interference

TABLE 3–2. SIGNALS THAT MAY BE SENSED VIA A VENTRICULAR LEAD

Signals Arising in the Ventricle
  R waves
  Ectopic ventricular depolarizations
  T waves
  Ventricular flutter
  Ventricular fibrillation
  Ventricular-tissue repolarization signals following
    ventricular stimuli
Signals Arising Elsewhere
  Skeletal-muscle potentials
  Stimuli from the atrial channel of the same pulse
    generator
  Stimuli from another implanted device
  Stimuli from an external device
  Electromagnetic interference

threshold detector, and the pacemaker fails to sense the spontaneous depolarization. This situation can sometimes be corrected by increasing the sensitivity of the sensing system (lowering the sensing threshold), provided this can be done without undue sensing of spurious signals, such as those listed in Tables 3–1 and 3–2. If not, physical relocation of the cardiac electrode can often solve the problem. Of course, this phenomenon is different from *normal* failure to sense a spontaneous event that occurs during a blanking period (when the sensing amplifier is deliberately disabled) or to respond to a spontaneous event that takes place during a refractory period. Such "failures" may not always provide the best therapy, but they are neither pacemaker malfunctions nor instances of inappropriate adjustment of the sensing threshold.

Oversensing, which sounds like the opposite of undersensing, is actually an unfortunate misnomer with an entirely different meaning. (We might suspect this; after all, how can the sensing circuit get too much of an R wave or a P wave?) This misleading term refers to an important and sometimes difficult problem in pacing: the sensing of unwanted signals (see Tables 3–1 and 3–2). The problem is considerably less prone to occur with bipolar pacing systems because the closely spaced electrodes make the sensing system relatively insensitive to far-field (distant) signals. This observation makes sense when it is recalled that the sensing amplifier looks at the voltage *difference* across the electrodes. The closer the electrodes, the closer an electrical disturbance must be for this difference to be significant; a far-field signal looks much the same to each of the closely spaced electrodes of a bipolar system, so the voltage difference is small.

The process of identifying and correcting

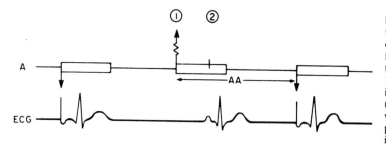

Figure 3–13. Failure to sense a spontaneous atrial depolarization as a result of previous sensing of electrical interference in the AAI mode. Sensed electrical interference ("noise," event 1) resets the AA interval. The ensuing spontaneous atrial depolarization (event 2) is not sensed because it falls within the pulse generator's refractory period (*short vertical line*), and the AA interval is therefore not reset.

sensing problems is usually much easier when the pacemaker's sensing mechanism is understood. For example, when an atrial pacemaker resets its escape timing upon sensing an extraneous signal, such as pectoral muscle potential, a spontaneous atrial depolarization may be missed because it falls in the pacemaker's refractory period, as shown in Figure 3–13. This phenomenon is easily understood as normal pulse generator behavior in the AAI mode (described later).

Timing Circuits

The basic intervals intrinsic to the design of the various pacing modes are discussed in Chapter 12. They include the AA and VV intervals between successive atrial and ventricular stimuli in single-chamber atrial and ventricular pacing, respectively, and the AV and VA interstimulus intervals in dual-chamber pacing. The electronic timing circuit that counts out these intervals produces a logic pulse at the end of each such interval that can be used to trigger an output circuit to produce a stimulus, as illustrated in Figure 3–1. As the block diagram shows, the timing circuit also produces signals that control the blanking and refractory periods that characterize the operation of the sensing circuit.

When sensing takes place, the sensing circuit produces a logic-pulse output, as described above, which serves as an input to the timing circuit. Depending upon the pacing mode, the timing circuit responds by reinitiating a timing interval or in some other way.

Programming and Telemetry Circuits

A transceiver (transmitter and receiver) circuit (see Fig. 3–1) in the pulse generator permits bidirectional communication with an associated pacemaker-"programming" device. The medium of communication is usually pulsed radio-frequency (RF) signals or a pulsed mag-

netic field. In programming a pacemaker, coded signals produced by the programming device are transmitted to the pulse generator, where they are decoded and used to change the programmable-parameter choices that are stored in the pulse generator's electronic memory and "looked up" by the timing and logic circuitry as needed.

Strictly speaking, telemetry means "measurement at a distance." In pacing, this term is used somewhat more broadly. A pulse generator may have the ability to acknowledge the receipt of instructions from an external programming device; to report the values to which its adjustable parameters are currently set; to provide the results of measurements performed internally, such as the terminal voltage of the battery or the electrical resistance of the lead system as seen by the pulse generator (this is true telemetry); or even to provide telemetered intracardiac-electrogram signals acquired by the sensing circuits.

PULSE GENERATOR OPERATION IN REPRESENTATIVE PACING MODES

AOO (Asynchronous Atrial Pacing)

In asynchronous pacing (Fig. 3–14) there is no sensing function, and therefore no refractory or blanking periods are required. The AOO mode is characterized completely by a single basic interval (AA). When this interval elapses, an atrial stimulus is released and the AA interval is reinitiated. The atrial stimuli are represented by arrows in the overlay diagram of Figure 3–14.

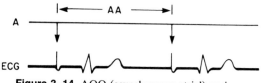

Figure 3–14. AOO (asynchronous atrial) pacing.

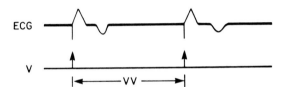

Figure 3–15. VOO (asynchronous ventricular) pacing.

VOO (Asynchronous Ventricular Pacing)

The VOO mode (Fig. 3–15) is identical with AOO except that the stimuli are delivered to the ventricle instead of the atrium. A pulse generator suitable for AOO pacing can thus be used equally well in the ventricle. Arrows are used in the overlay diagram of Figure 3–15 to denote the ventricular stimuli.

AAI (Inhibited Atrial Pacing)

The AAI mode (Fig. 3–16) is characterized by a single basic interval (AA). A refractory period following the delivery of a stimulus or the detection of a spontaneous atrial depolarization is included in the design to prevent the anticipated spontaneous ventricular response to an evoked (paced) or spontaneous atrial depolarization from being sensed by the pulse generator and interpreted erroneously as a spontaneous atrial depolarization.

The numbered events in the example of Figure 3–16 are as follows:

1. Upon timeout of the AA interval (i.e., when the AA interval elapses), an atrial stimulus is released (which captures the atrium, although the pulse generator does not "know" this). The AA interval is reinitiated.

2. A spontaneous atrial depolarization is sensed. The AA interval is reinitiated without the release of a stimulus.

3. The pending atrial stimulus (short vertical line) is inhibited because in reinitiating the AA interval the pulse generator has "forgotten" it.

4. The AA interval times out (elapses), the atrium is paced, and the AA interval is reinitiated.

VVI (Inhibited Ventricular Pacing)

The VVI mode (Fig. 3–17) is functionally identical with AAI except that the ventricle is sensed and stimulated instead of the atrium. In addition, the sensitivity setting may be different, and the characteristics of the sensing filter used to isolate the intracardiac R wave are usually slightly different from those of the filter used to isolate the intracardiac P wave. The example of Figure 3–17 is the ventricular-pacing analog of the AAI example just discussed.

1. Upon timeout of the VV interval, a ventricular stimulus is released (which captures the ventricle, although the pulse generator does not "know" this). The VV interval is reinitiated.

2. A spontaneous ventricular depolarization is sensed. The VV interval is reinitiated without the release of a stimulus.

3. The pending ventricular stimulus (short vertical line) is inhibited because in reinitiating the VV interval the pulse generator has "forgotten" it.

4. The VV interval times out, the ventricle is paced, and the VV interval is reinitiated.

DOO (Asynchronous AV-Sequential Pacing)

Two basic intervals (AV and VA) characterize this mode (Fig. 3–18); their sum (AA or VV) is the overall duration of the pacing cycle (sometimes referred to inappropriately as the cycle "length"). There is no sensing function and therefore no need for refractory or blanking periods. In Figure 3–18, the atrial channel of the pulse generator is represented above the electrocardiogram, the ventricular channel below it.

Figure 3–16. AAI (inhibited atrial) pacing.

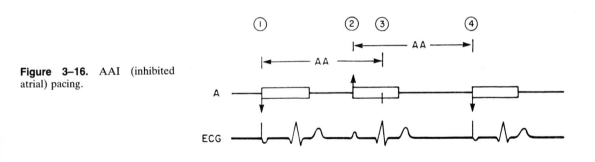

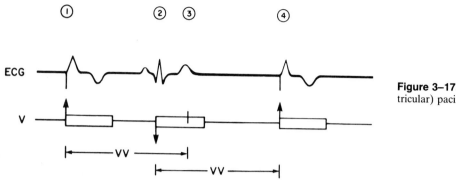

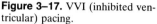

Figure 3–17. VVI (inhibited ventricular) pacing.

VAT (Atrial-Synchronous Ventricular Pacing)

As in the previous example, this mode (Fig. 3–19) is characterized by two basic intervals, AV and VA. Only the atrial channel has sensing capability; hence refractory periods are not shown in the ventricular channel.

1. The AV interval times out, the ventricle is paced, and the VA interval begins.

2. A spontaneous P wave is sensed, the VA timing is abandoned, and the AV internal is reinitiated.

3. The AV interval times out, the ventricle is paced, and the VA interval begins.

4. The pending ventricular stimulus shown by the short vertical line in the ventricular channel is inhibited because the spontaneous P wave sensed earlier (event 2) has reset the pulse generator's escape timing, as described.

5. The ventricle depolarizes spontaneously, but the pulse generator is unaware of this because there is no sensing function in the ventricular channel.

6. The AV interval times out, a ventricular stimulus is released (which fails to capture the ventricle), and the VA interval begins.

DVI ("Committed" AV-Sequential Ventricular-Inhibited Pacing)

In this mode (Fig. 3–20) both atrium and ventricle are paced, but sensing takes place only in the ventricular channel. As is the case with all of the dual-chamber modes, DVI pacing is characterized by two fundamental intervals, AV and VA. In the example of Figure 3–20, the structure of the refractory period shows that the pulse generator has a "committed" ventricular output (see Fig. 3–11 and the discussion of blanking and refractory periods, above).

1. The VA interval times out, the atrium is paced, and the AV interval begins.

2. The ventricle responds spontaneously to the evoked atrial depolarization, but the conducted intracardiac R wave falls in the ventricular-channel refractory period (short vertical line, ventricular channel) and is not sensed. The AV interval continues undisturbed.

3. The AV interval times out, a ventricular stimulus is released, and the VA interval begins. The stimulus fails to capture the ventricle, which is refractory after having depolarized spontaneously.

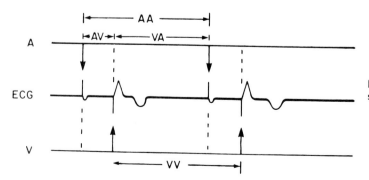

Figure 3–18. DOO (asynchronous AV-sequential) pacing.

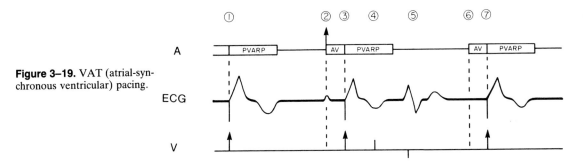

Figure 3–19. VAT (atrial-synchronous ventricular) pacing.

4. An ectopic ventricular depolarization is sensed, and the VA interval is reinitiated without the release of a stimulus in either channel. Note the refractory period following ventricular sensing.

5. The pending atrial stimulus is inhibited as a result of resetting the escape timing (event 4).

6. The pending ventricular stimulus is inhibited as a result of resetting the escape timing (event 4).

7. The VA interval times out, the atrium is paced, and the AV interval begins.

8. The AV interval times out, the ventricle is paced, and the VA interval begins, as in event 1.

DDD ("Uncommitted" Atrial-Synchronous AV-Sequential Dual-Chamber–Inhibited Pacing)

In this "universal" or "physiologic" mode (Fig. 3–21) pacing and sensing occur in both the atrium and the ventricle. As before, however, the basic pacemaker timing is completely characterized by two fundamental intervals, AV and VA. In the example of Figure 3–21, the ventricular channel has a brief blanking period following an atrial stimulus but is not refractory throughout the AV interval. Thus, the ventricular stimulus is not "committed," as in the previous example.

1. The VA interval times out, the atrium is paced, and the AV interval begins.

2. The AV interval times out, the ventricle is paced, and the VA interval begins.

3. A retrograde atrial depolarization occurs, but the intracardiac retrograde P wave (short vertical line, atrial channel) falls within the postventricular atrial refractory period (PVARP) and is ignored by the pulse generator. The timing is not affected.

4. A spontaneous atrial depolarization is sensed, and the AV interval begins immediately. Note that there is no need for a ventricular-channel blanking period after a *spontaneous* atrial depolarization.

5. A spontaneous ventricular depolarization is sensed during the AV interval (this could not happen with a "committed" system), and the VA interval begins immediately.

It should be reiterated that the preceding is not a comprehensive presentation of all existing antibradyarrhythmia pacing modes. DDI pacing, used in the presence of unstable atrial rhythms, has not been discussed, nor have the (primarily diagnostic) triggered modes, such as VVT and DDT.

CONCLUSIONS

In this chapter some of the basic "building blocks" of a pacemaker pulse generator have

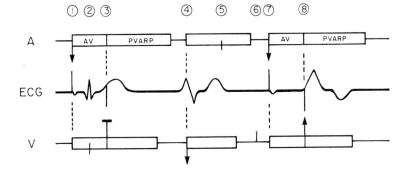

Figure 3–20. DVI ("committed" AV-sequential ventricular-inhibited) pacing.

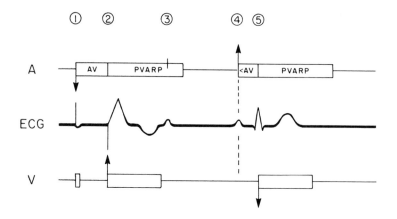

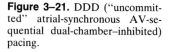

Figure 3–21. DDD ("uncommitted" atrial-synchronous AV-sequential dual-chamber–inhibited) pacing.

been discussed, and examples of pulse generator operation in each of several standard antibradyarrhythmia pacing modes have been presented.

The interpretation of paced electrocardiograms, particularly in dual-chamber pacing, is often facilitated by considering the interaction of the pacemaker with the cardiac conduction system *from the standpoint of the pulse generator*. In the absence of rate hysteresis, rate modulation, or other special features, the simplicity of pacemaker timing can be used to advantage in electrocardiogram interpretation, particularly by identifying an atrial or ventricular stimulus and working *backward* to determine the event that initiated the AV or VA interval immediately preceding that stimulus. Those pulse generators that can provide intracardiac-waveform telemetry can make it far easier to visualize events as the pacemaker "sees" them, as can timing diagrams constructed by a pacemaker-programming device from timing information or marker signals transmitted by the implant. It should be emphasized, however, that the discussion presented here has been limited to fairly common pulse generator attributes. The technical details (such as the pulse generator's response to ventricular ectopics) that vary from device to device should be taken into account to avoid being misled by a pacemaker "pseudomalfunction" that is actually an example of entirely normal, but unfamiliar, behavior.

REFERENCES

1. Bernstein AD, Camm AJ, Fletcher RD, et al: The NASPE/BPEG Generic Pacemaker Code for antibradyarrhythmia and adaptive-rate pacing and antitachyarrhythmia devices. PACE 10:794–799, 1987.
2. Bernstein AD, Parsonnet V: Notation conventions and overlay diagrams for analysis of paced electrocardiograms. PACE 6:73–80, 1983.
3. Bilitch M, Hauser RG, Goldman BS, et al: Performance of cardiac pacemaker pulse generators. PACE 5:139–144, 1982.
4. Bilitch M, Hauser RG, Goldman BS, et al: Performance of cardiac pacemaker pulse generators. PACE 8:276–282, 1985.
5. Bilitch M, Hauser RG, Goldman BS, et al: Performance of implantable cardiac rhythm management devices. PACE 9:256–267, 1986.
6. Bilitch M, Hauser RG, Goldman BS, et al: Performance of implantable cardiac rhythm management devices. PACE 10:389–398, 1987.

4

THE ELECTROBIOLOGY AND ENGINEERING OF PACEMAKER LEADS

GERALD C. TIMMIS

The evolution of pacemaker leads largely reflects the pacemaker industry's growing sophistication in its understanding of the electrobiology of the heart as the medical community has concurrently become more conversant with design, engineering, and manufacturing concepts. This chapter will attempt to chronicle this exchange of information and the results that have issued from it. Knowledge about the electrobiology of the heart is essential for comprehending the electrophysiology of pacing. An understanding of this relationship and of the interface between the electrode and endomyocardium has led to improvements in the design and manufacture of pacemaker systems. These concepts will be discussed in a clinically manageable fashion in the course of focusing on the bioengineering of pacemaker leads. Although epimyocardial leads and electrodes will briefly be reviewed, the major emphasis will be on endocardial leads because since 1981, 95 per cent of all pacemaker leads have been implanted transvenously.[161]

The pacemaker lead is the connecting link between the heart and the power source required to stimulate it when abnormalities of impulse formation or conduction exist (Fig. 4-1).[86] It consists of an electrode, which actually contacts the heart; the intervening conductor coil; and a proximal terminal pin for connection with the pacemaker generator. The entire assembly is encased in insulating material, from the terminal pin to the point of electrode contact, to ensure the efficient transfer of energy from the generator to the heart.

As early as 1952, John A. Hopps was studying transvenous endomyocardial stimulation using a bipolar electrode located on the distal tip of a small catheter.[99] At that time, no commercially made catheter electrodes were

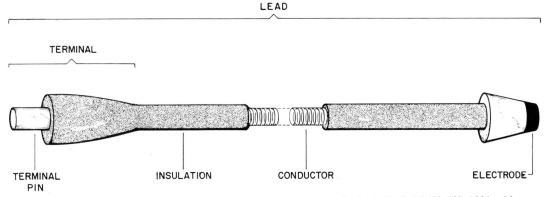

Figure 4–1. Pacemaker lead. (From Harthorne JW: Pacemaker leads. Int J Cardiol 6:423–429, 1984; with permission.)

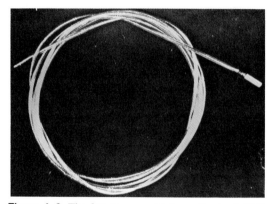

Figure 4–2. The first permanent intracardiac lead, 1962. (From Lagergren H: How it happened: My recollection of early pacing. PACE 1:140–143, 1978; with permission.)

available. However, shortly thereafter in 1958, Furman and Robinson reported the clinical use of an intracardiac endocardial lead system for the correction of total heart block.[69] The first totally implantable system employing endocardial electrodes was reported in 1962 by Lagergren.[123] This electrode, depicted in Figure 4–2, was tunneled subcutaneously from the entry jugular vein to the left groin. It was connected externally with a generator, along with an anodal stainless steel plate implanted below the left costal arch, the lead to which was also exteriorized. Several days later, the intracardiac portion of the lead was cut to the left of the umbilicus, where it remained sterile in subcutaneous tissue and was ultimately connected with a permanently implanted subcutaneous pulse generator (Fig. 4–3). Other historical landmarks in lead development are listed in Table 4–1.[208] Since then, lead technology has become increasingly complex, resulting in numerous conflicting claims of the superiority of one system over another. These issues will be analyzed in an attempt to define in clinically meaningful terms the state of the art as it concerns pacemaker leads and electrodes.

THE BIOLOGY OF PACING AND SENSING

The Biology of Pacing

CELLULAR POLARIZATION, DEPOLARIZATION, AND THE ACTION POTENTIAL. Understanding the process of cellular polarization as distinct from polarization incident to artificial stimulation is basic to the comprehension of myocardial excitability. Electrochemical polar-

ization results from the separation of one species of charge from another species of opposite charge.[191] This phenomenon contributes to both pacing and sensing impedance and, as will be discussed later in this chapter, is a direct function of pulse duration and an inverse function of electrode size. It develops when electrodes are charged and is due to the difference in the charge of the carriers at the electrode surface (electrons) and in the tissue-fluid conducting medium (ions).

The polarization process referred to in this section is that resulting in a resting membrane potential from which the action potential is generated in the course of depolarization. A variety of influences affect cellular polarization and will be dealt with below in discussing the metabolism and pharmacology of myocardial excitation. There are large differences in the concentration of ions both within and outside living cell membranes. In the myocardium, the potassium concentration is 35 times greater than that in the extracellular compartment, while sodium concentration is almost 5 times greater in the extracellular compartment than it is within the cell. Concentration gradients tend to force potassium out and sodium into the cell in proportion to their respective concentration gradients.[191] However, other forces exist that oppose this. Electrical forces exist because of a difference in electrical potential

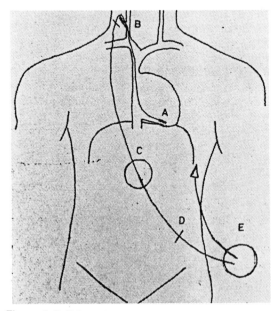

Figure 4–3. Schematic illustration of the operative technique employed by Lagergren. (From Lagergren H: How it happened: My recollection of early pacing. PACE 1:140–143, 1978; with permission.)

TABLE 4–1. MAJOR ADVANCES IN TRANSVENOUS LEAD DESIGN FOR IMPROVED PACING THRESHOLDS

YEAR REPORTED	ADVANCE	PRIMARY INVESTIGATOR(S)
1958	First endocardial leads	Furman
1961	Coil conductors	Chardack
1963	Transvenous endocardial leads adapted to implantable systems	Lagergren, Parsonnet
1965	Widespread use of pacing systems with transvenous leads	Greatbach, Chardack
1966	Differential current density (DCD) electrode	Lewin, Parsonnet
1968	Electrode size impact on thresholds characterized	Furman, Parker
1968	Nonexcitable tissue effect on thresholds ("virtual" electrode)	Thalen/Parker, Furman
1971	Dielectric pacemaker electrode (DPE) for reduced polarization	Schaldach
1971	Lead flexibility impact on thresholds	Driller
1975	Smooth pyrolytic carbon electrodes	Helland, Stokes
1976	High current density over a large surface area (birdcage electrode)	Lagergren
1976	Ring-tip electrode (high current density over a large surface area)	Thalen
1978	Totally porous electrode	Amundson
1979	Lead stability as an influence on thresholds	Gordon, Timmis
1979	Low-resistance, multifilar conductor coils	Upton
1979	Vitreous (activated, porous) carbon electrode	Beck-Jansen
1979	Porous-surfaced electrode	MacGregor
1983	Platinized microporous target-tip electrode	Bornzin, Stokes
1983	Carbon vapor–coated porous titanium electrode	Sleutz
1983	Steroid-eluting electrode	Stokes/Timmis, Gordon/Parsonnet

across the cell membrane. In resting myocardial cells, there is a negative potential of about -90 mV compared with the extracellular compartment. This difference is due largely to the difference in potassium concentration on either side of the membrane (the equilibrium potential of potassium). This electrical force tends to displace cations, such as sodium and potassium, to the inside of the cell while displacing anions, such as chloride, to the outside in proportion to the voltage gradient. In addition, there is an active sodium-potassium exchange pump, which facilitates accumulation of intracellular potassium by the extracellular displacement of sodium; this results in membrane polarization. When the resting transmembrane potential increases to -60 mV in automatic cells, or to -70 mV in certain cells of the ventricular specialized conduction system such as Purkinje fibers, the process of depolarization ensues, as shown in Figure 4–4,[177] with sodium rapidly entering the cell through fast sodium channels; this produces the steeply rising phase 0 of the action potential, peaking at a positive potential that terminates phase 1. At this point, other cations, such as calcium, enter the cell through slower channels. This entry initiates a flat, nearly isoelectric portion of the action potential in phase 2, during which the slow inward movement of sodium and

extracellular displacement of potassium occur simultaneously. The point at which the action potential becomes rapidly negative heralds the intracellular return of potassium; during this third phase the membrane repolarizes. In phase 4, the sodium-potassium exchange pump, catalyzed by sodium-potassium adenosine triphosphatase (ATPase), moves sodium out of the cell, facilitating intracellular entry of potassium.

THE CONDUCTION SYSTEM. Assuming that a critical mass of cells has been depolarized by raising the resting membrane potential from an approximate -90 mV to -60 mV, and assuming further that whatever conduction system disease that may exist is upstream from the point of myocardial stimulation, conduction will progress as the wave front of depolarization is propagated. Both the ventricular specialized conduction system and the specialized conduction pathways within the atrium are relatively resistant to noxious influences such as ischemia. Even if these major conduction pathways are impaired, propagation of a wave front may occur in the ventricular Purkinje network, albeit through a circuitous pathway, resulting in a prolonged ventricular activation time. In addition, the Purkinje network may be affected by metabolic acidosis and especially severe hyperkalemia. Resting mem-

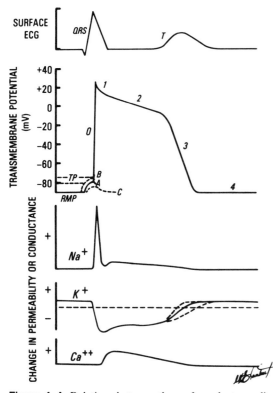

Figure 4–4. Relations between the surface electrocardiogram (ECG) and the transmembrane potential, and diagrams of the relative changes in ion permeability (or conductance), that are responsible for the action potential. The (0 to 4) phases of a typical fast action potential are indicated, the resting membrane potential (RMP) being phase 4. The threshold potential (TP) is also shown: C represents a subthreshold stimulus (nonpropagated), A is a threshold stimulus, and B is a threshold stimulus at a lower (less negative) threshold potential (*dashed line*). The large, rapid increase in Na$^+$ conductance during phase 0 is shown, together with the sustained, small increase in Na$^+$ conductance (slow Na$^+$ current) during phase 2 of the action potential. The large, less rapid drop in K$^+$ conductance during phase 0 of the action potential is indicated, and the dashed lines of altered K$^+$ conductance during phase 3 indicate induced changes in K$^+$ permeability (P_K). The dashed horizontal line indicates that K$^+$ conductance is above zero at rest. The increased Ca^{++} conductance during phase 2 of the action potential is shown. (From Ross J Jr, Covell JW: Electrical impulse formation and conduction in the heart. *In* Vardoulakis MK [ed]: Best and Taylor's Physiological Basis of Medical Practice. 11th ed. pp 148–162, © 1985, The Williams & Wilkins Co, Baltimore; with permission.)

brane potentials may be shifted toward zero by high potassium levels. Although the stimulation threshold may initially be reduced, ultimately the rate of depolarization falls with shortening of the action potential duration, resulting not only in impaired conduction but also in a measurably and potentially threatening increase in threshold.[58] Nevertheless, our major concern in electrically exciting the heart

with energy that is not native to this organ involves the initial depolarization of myocardial cells that are juxtaposed to a well-arborized conduction pathway in which, even though it may be abnormal, the development of a wave front of myocardial excitation will generally take care of itself. It is this stimulation-conduction paradigm that will be employed in subsequent discussions of the biology, physics, and pharmacology of pacing.

MYOCARDIAL STIMULATION. Purkinje fibers will depolarize at a potential of about − 70 mV, which may be achieved either spontaneously by the transmembrane cation movement or by the alteration of the electrical potential across the membrane resulting from an artificial stimulus. In the latter instance, the ensuing depolarization represents the process of electrostimulation.[109] Thus, the artificially created change in an external electrical field, until it reaches a critical level to incite cellular activity, requires an electromotive force about equal to that which spontaneously occurs. The minimal amount of electrical stimulation required to elicit consistently a response in the cell, in its fully polarized state, is called the *threshold.*

The endomyocardial stimulation threshold changes spontaneously in a variety of physiologic states, such as sleeping and eating, both of which may increase the stimulation threshold. In contrast, exercise and postural changes decrease threshold. These events mediate their effect through changes in sympathetic tone.[58] These phenomena are usually not clinically important unless an electrode-endomyocardial interface has been established. In the first several weeks after implantation of an endocardial pacing system, thresholds progressively rise, peaking between the second and fourth weeks, after which thresholds tend to fall. When thresholds are at their highest, the aforementioned influences affecting excitation may become clinically germane.

METABOLISM, EXCITABILITY, AND STIMULATION THRESHOLDS. Metabolic abnormalities, such as electrolyte shifts involving potassium, acid-base imbalance, and hyperglycemia, affect myocardial excitability. The last, if severe, can produce more than a 50 per cent increase in stimulation threshold, whereas hypoglycemia has little, if any, effect.[221] Hyperkalemia in excess of 7.0 mEq/L may increase thresholds substantially.[77, 128, 196] On the other hand, intravenous administration of potassium has been employed to increase myocardial excitability.[218] This increase is explained by the fact that if the serum potassium level is normal or only mildly elevated, the acute decrease in the potassium gradient across the cell membrane incident to the infusion of this cation may have a salutary influence on the stimulation threshold.[168] The increase in excitability depends additionally on the rate at which the potassium is administered.[197] Although both sodium and calcium ions may be useful in correcting some of the effects of hyperkalemia, impaired conduction occurs independently of serum sodium and calicum levels, pH, PO_2, and PCO_2,[197] at least in animals. Accordingly, the elevation in serum potassium level must be specifically treated using, for example, intravenous infusions of glucose and insulin or cation-exchange resins. A significant rise or fall in pH can increase the threshold by 70 per cent or more.[100] Inadequate respiratory gas exchange, resulting in a fall in PO_2 or retention of carbon dioxide, may increase the stimulation threshold. Both factors should be considered independently in conjunction with general anesthesia for patients who have pacemakers or in the course of cardiopulmonary resuscitation.

Just as hypothyroidism may produce conduction defects, it may increase the threshold of myocardial excitation.[17, 182] Thyroxine repletion may correct this condition. Adrenocortical hormones of the glucocorticoid type may lower the threshold to block.[168] Endogenous catecholamines decrease the stimulation threshold.[97] Their congeners, such as isoproterenol, have also been shown to decrease the excitation threshold and have been used both intravenously and sublingually in the treatment of pacing unresponsiveness (exit block).[129]

The effects of these metabolic shifts and humoral influences were much more important before noninvasive multiple-parameter programming was available. Nevertheless, this feature alone is often incapable of correcting exit block (failure of electrical stimulation to initiate a contraction) resulting from serious metabolic abnormalities.

THE PHARMACOLOGY OF MYOCARDIAL STIMULATION. As indicated earlier, endogenous catecholamines and corticosteroids have a variable effect on endomyocardial thresholds. Extrapolations of these basic observations have led to the use of synthetic analogs for the therapeutic manipulation of myocardial excitation. As previously suggested, intravenous or sublingual isoproterenol has been used to restore capture in exit block.[129] Glucocorticoids, such as prednisolone, have also been used for this purpose, with considerable success in many patients.[147, 150, 169] Steroids have been used successfully, but only when thresholds are abnormally high, as may occur with unusual inflammatory reaction at the electrode-endomyocardial interface. Steroids probably have little effect on stimulation thresholds within the normal range. However, steroid analogs have been used not only to correct exit block but also to reduce early threshold peaking after pacemaker implantation and have even been incorporated into an eluting core of lead-electrode assemblies to lower the excitation threshold chronically, as will be discussed later in this chapter.[206] The effects of glucocorticoids on myocardial excitation are complex. It has long been suspected that corticosteroids alter cellular membrane permeability, producing significant and sustained threshold changes that abet pacing.[168] They may increase cellular efflux of potassium, decreasing the transmembrane gradient of this cation, which has been shown to increase excitability. However, since the effects of glucocorticoids and mineralocorticoids are antagonistic, with respect to excitability, potassium shifts are unlikely to mediate this effect of steroids on thresholds.[168] Moreover, the electrophysiologic response to glucocorticoids is not particularly striking. Thus, Kreitt and his colleagues found that dexamethasone sodium phosphate had minimal effects on the electrophysiologic properties of rabbit atrium (J. M. Kreitt and colleagues, unpublished observations). The electrophysiologic effect of steroid hormones may be mediated by the initial binding of the hormones to stereospecific intracellular receptor proteins in the cytoplasm of target cells. Glucocorticoid-binding sites have been demonstrated in both dog and rat hearts.[60] As of this writing, however, the mechanism by which corticosteroids decrease pacing thresholds is not completely understood.

Antiarrhythmic drugs have a variable effect on excitation threshold and conduction. All type 1A agents (Vaughn-Williams) alter transmembrane potential, particularly the maximal rate of rise of the action potential upstroke (phase 0; V_{max}), and decrease excitability. Certain type 1C agents may also increase the stimulation threshold. Flecainide, which, unlike other 1C agents, may display class III properties by prolonging the action potential duration, increases the ventricular effective refractory period and may block sodium fast channels.[29] It has been shown to alter threshold measurably.[90, 91] Lidocaine, a type 1B agent, probably has little effect on thresholds in the absence of underlying disease. However, in some pathologic states, lidocaine has been shown to induce, in a manner similar to that of procainamide, sufficient increases in threshold to produce pacemaker latency.[148] Amiodarone, a class III agent, affects automaticity, especially with chronic oral administration, and lengthens the action potential. It also increases conduction time and refractoriness of the His-Purkinje interval.[103, 146] As yet, however, its effect on stimulation thresholds has not been established.

The Biology of Sensing

THE GENERATION OF ELECTROGRAPHIC SIGNALS. Detection of intracardiac electrograms is achieved by one or more electrodes that are separated from the endocardium by a layer of blood; thus, electrographic signals can best be understood if we think of the electrode as a point in a conductive medium, at a point near the endomyocardium generating this signal, with a second neutral electrode remote to the point of electrographic generation. A schematic of the relationship of such an electrode to the endomyocardium is depicted in Figure 4–5.[108] Assuming that the wave front of excitation proceeds from one end of this layer of myocardium to the other polarized segment of myocardium, there is a transverse dipole representing the intracellular positive charge and the transient extracellular negative charge resulting from the depolarization process. Downstream from the electrode the opposite is true; the intracellular charge in the still-polarized myocardium remains negative in reference to the positive extracellular charge. This results in a dipole of opposite polarity. There is an additional longitudinal dipole parallel to the surface of the endomyocardium that is produced by the juxtaposition of the negative extracellular charge upstream from the electrode with the positive extracellular charge downstream from the electrode. A fourth dipole representing the upstream-downstream juxtaposition of an intracellular positive charge in the depolarized segment and an intracellular negative charge in the still-polarized downstream segment contributes to an overall quadripole.[108] Because of the high transmembrane impedance of the still-repolarized myocardium, the transmembrane dipole of the still-polarized myocardial layer and the intracellular longitudinal dipole contribute little, if anything, to current fields without the body. Therefore, the transmembrane dipole in the depolarized segment and the longitudinal extracellular dipole remain the major forces contributing to the intracardiac electrogram. Figure 4–6 is a schematic of potentials due to an uniformly moving dipole, resulting in the biphasic signal as shown. Figure 4–7 displays the monophasic signal reflecting the transverse dipole, which is generated by the wave front of depolarization, spreading not only across the endocardium but also from the endocardium outward to the epicardial surface through myocardium, as "viewed" by the electrode in axial alignment with this dipole. The superposition of the effects of these two dipoles yields the resultant endocardial electrogram.[108] Given the difference in wall thickness between the atrium and the ventricles, the contribution of the transverse dipole to the overall electrographic morphology will be considerably greater in the ventricle.

In addition to morphology and relative amplitude of the electrogram, another important

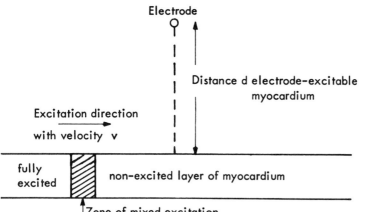

Figure 4–5. Abstraction of the electrode-myocardium system: point electrode with distance, *d,* to a one-dimensional, homogenous layer of excitable tissue. (From Irnich W: Intracardiac electrograms and sensing test signals: Electrophysiological, physical, and technical considerations. PACE 8:870–888, 1985; with permission.)

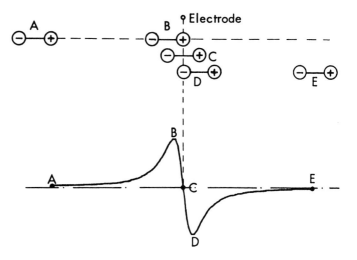

Figure 4–6. The field of the longitudinal dipole. This diagram illustrates how an electrical potential at the electrode is generated by the moving dipole. The charge closest to the electrode will determine polarity; its magnitude will progressively increase as it approaches the electrode axis, which is perpendicular to the endocardium. As it crosses this axis, the potential falls to zero and becomes reciprocally negative in mirror image to the antecedent positive component. (From Irnich W: Intracardiac electrograms and sensing test signals: Electrophysiological, physical, and technical considerations. PACE 8:870–888, 1985; with permission.)

characteristic of cardiac signals is excitation velocity, that is, the velocity of accession of the wave front of depolarization. This velocity will affect the slew rate of the electrogram and its frequency content. *Slew rate* is defined as the first derivative of a waveform, that is, the rate of change of potentials generated over the time-base of the electrical signal. Waveform morphology, amplitude, slew rate, and spectral content may all be employed in the development of electric circuitry for the detection of intracardiac signals. These variables will be discussed under "Electrophysiology of Sensing," further on.

The neurohumoral control of the sinoatrial node is such that when its function is normal, its rate of automaticity provides the ultimately

physiologic modulation of heart rate, whether spontaneous or stimulated. In the latter circumstance, atrial signals issuing from spontaneous atrial depolarization can be tracked by existing sensing circuitry; through linkage with rate-adjustable ventricular pacing systems, truly physiologic pacing can be achieved with maintenance of atrioventricular synchrony. Such systems are useful in about half of all potential pacemaker candidates who, in spite of abnormalities of impulse formation and conduction, retain normal sinus node function.[173]

Although most physiologic pacing systems that maintain atrioventricular synchrony vary heart rate in direct response to sensed spontaneous changes of the sinoatrial discharge rate, some pacemakers employ detectors that

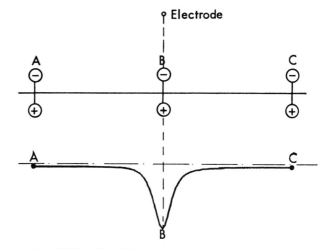

Figure 4–7. The field of the transverse dipole. In this illustration, a transverse dipole is assumed to reflect the negative extracellular charge on the endocardial surface juxtaposed to a positive charge within the intracellular space and, indeed, within the myocardial wall. The transverse wave front, which progresses from endocardium to epicardium, creates a transverse dipole, which will be added to the longitudinal dipole content of the electrogram. This transverse component is always negative. Algebraic summation of the transverse component with the longitudinal component of the electrogram will tend to increase the negative amplitude of the recorded electrogram at the expense of the antecedent positive deflection. One would expect this effect to be more striking at the ventricular level than in the atrium. An offsetting influence that tends to maintain the biphasic morphology of acute ventricular electrograms is the acute current of injury arising from the electrode-endocardial interface. This current of injury tends to amplify the positive deflection at the expense of the negative deflection. However, as the interface matures, the injury vector dissipates, with the result that over half of chronically recorded ventricular electrograms are monophasic and negative. (From Irnich W: Intracardiac electrograms and sensing test signals: Electrophysiological, physical, and technical considerations. PACE 8:870–888, 1985; with permission.)

sense *average atrial rate;* this value is then utilized to adjust ventricular stimulation rate. Experience with this system has apparently not been very satisfactory.[180]

In the presence of sinus rhythm, the *Q-T interval* has long been known to vary inversely with heart rate, but is this true of the pacemaker-dependent patient whose Q-T interval is evoked by myocardial stimulation? Other factors have been shown to affect Q-T interval, whether it results from a spontaneous or an evoked depolarization process. Catecholamine blood levels also affect the Q-T interval to a degree that is considerable and independent of the intrinsic heart rate.[61] Thus, exercise induces a humorally mediated decrease in both the intrinsic and the evoked Q-T interval, with opposite changes when the patient is in repose. Accordingly, with the anticipation that the Q-T interval will reflect alterations in metabolic rate and effort- or stress-related increases in physiologic demand, systems have been developed to detect changes in the Q-T interval as the physiologic trigger to alter pacemaker discharge rate.[174]

NONELECTROGRAPHIC BIOLOGIC SIGNALS TO MODULATE STIMULATION RATE. A variety of new single-chamber, rate-responsive pacing systems that have been developed depend on the detection of physiologic signals reflecting changing levels of physical effort or metabolic demand. Nonelectrical signals that herald changes in activity or metabolism include the temperature, pH or oxygen saturation of mixed venous blood, ventricular volumes, and even the physical consequences of exercise, such as the ballistics of body movement and the low-frequency noise of skeletal muscle.

First conceptualized in the late 1970s,[220] *temperature sensing* for adjustment of the pacemaker discharge rate has been studied by a number of investigators,[2, 82, 113, 122, 195] and microcomputer-based temperature-sensitive cardiac pacemaker systems have subsequently been developed.[63, 112, 195] These systems detect the increase in mixed venous blood temperature upon exertion of effort by the patient and its resolution at lower levels of activity. The capacity to increase pacemaker discharge rate in response to a sensed temperature increase in central venous blood, and conversely to decrease discharge rate as blood cools, provides a physiologic matching of heart rate with metabolic requirements that is not possible with conventional fixed-rate pacing, even with multiprogrammable systems.

Carbon dioxide production is closely related

to skeletal muscle activity and, by generating a *pH shift* that is detectable by electronic circuitry, provides another physiologic stimulus for altering pacemaker discharge rate. During exercise, a fall in the pH of mixed venous blood reflects the effort-related peripheral production of carbon dioxide. An electrode has been developed to detect this fall in mixed venous pH and has been successfully employed to accelerate the generator stimulation rate.[45]

Although mixed venous oxygen saturation is not directly affected by heart rate, oxygen transport is clearly facilitated by an increase in heart rate. Sensors are currently under study for detecting changes in *oxygen saturation* that have been reciprocally linked to variations in the discharge rate of permanent pacing systems, for the purpose of optimizing cardiac output and tissue oxygenation.[223]

The ballistics of *whole-body* activity as a physiologic trigger has attracted a good deal of interest in the past several years.[5] Systems that incorporate sensors sensitive to low-frequency sonic impulses have been developed. As these impulses increase with physical activity, the pacemaker discharge rate increases. Given a reasonably stable stroke volume, cardiac output would therein be more physiologically matched to metabolic needs.

Other physically driven rate-responsive sensing systems have been investigated. Parallel unidirectional changes in heart rate and *respiratory rate* have been employed to optimize circulatory performance. The increase in carbon dioxide production that renders venous blood more acidic is sensed by endogenous chemoreceptors as a stimulus for an increased respiratory rate. This relationship between carbon dioxide production and ventilation is markedly more dependable than that between minute ventilation and oxygen uptake. The relationship of respiration to heart rate, which was previously conceptualized by Ionescu, among others,[47, 104] has led to the clinical development of a fully automatic pacing system.[178, 179, 181]

All of the above physiologic signals have direct or indirect relationships to metabolic and circulatory requirements. They reflect, with variable fidelity and timeliness, instantaneous circulatory changes that would normally occur under physiologic circumstances. Physiologic pacing is defined as the artificial stimulation of the heart that maintains not only the normal atrioventricular activation sequence but also a physiologic rate response.[179] In those circumstances when maintenance of atrioven-

TABLE 4–2. PHYSIOLOGIC RESPONSIVE PACING SYSTEMS COMPARED

PHYSIOLOGIC PARAMETER	SPEED OF RESPONSE			SENSOR RELIABILITY	SYSTEM SPECIFICITY
	Physiology	Sensor	System		
Temperature	Slow	Fast	Slow	High	Medium
QT interval	Fast	Fast	Slow	High	Medium
Respiratory rate	Fast	Fast	Slow	High	Medium
Oxygen saturation	Fast	Fast	Slow	Low	High
pH	Fast	Fast	Slow	Low	High
Activity	Fast	Fast	Fast	High	Medium

tricular synchrony employing conventional sensing of atrial signals is impossible, as, for example, in atrial fibrillation, detection of the aforementioned nonelectrographic signals reviewed in this section may also be employed for physiologic pacing, although in a manner less fastidious than just defined. The sensors of these signals have various response times, reliability, and specificity, as seen in Table 4–2.[78]

The Endomyocardial Basis of Threshold Maturation

THE HISTOLOGY AND PATHOPHYSIOLOGY OF THE ELECTRODE-ENDOMYOCARDIAL INTERFACE. Electrode-endocardial contact results in sufficient abrasion and trauma to injure endocardial cells, causing acute inflammation and subsequent fibrin deposition. Guarda and colleagues concluded that this fibrin layer is not sufficient to fix the electrode tip, which continues to rub the endocardial surface; thus, the inflammation already in progress may worsen, and further deposition of fibrin may occur.[83] This process takes up to 3 months, with the ultimate formation of a fibrous capsule of up to 2 mm in thickness.[105]

The initial injury of the cell alters membrane permeability to sodium and potassium transfer. This alteration in permeability may decrease the difference between the resting membrane potential and threshold potential to the point where less energy may be required for electrostimulation of the myocardium; that is, the stimulation threshold may actually fall within the first few minutes of intracardiac electrode placement.[134] The subsequent inflammation, fibrin deposition, and capsule formation may all contribute to an early increase in threshold in the first several weeks after implantation, as shown for the 6971 lead in Figure 4–8. As inflammation resolves, a secondary, more stable fall in threshold ensues. The intensity of this interface reaction and the amplitude of the threshold variations are a function of the

degree of tissue response. The more rapidly electrode fixation occurs at the interface, the less the degree of inflammation and the less luxuriant the early tissue response and subsequent scar formation. Both fixation and certain electrode modifications, such as the steroid-eluting lead, to be discussed later in this chapter, may have a salutary effect on the fibrous capsule.

The fibrous capsule was studied at length by Thalen and coworkers[200] and Parker and associates.[157] They showed that the effect of electrode size, which is inversely related to electrical field strength and directly to stimulation thresholds, is influenced by the thickness of the electrode capsule, which is nonexcitable but conductive. Thus, the "virtual electrode" concept has arisen[70] wherein the net size of a hemispheric electrode is defined not by the radius of the electrode itself but by the extension of that radius to the nearest excitable tissue, as shown in Figure 4–9. This figure depicts why the stimulation threshold increases for the first several months after implantation. Excluding the early threshold peaking in the first several weeks after implantation, which, as indicated above, involves more complex tissue reactions, the difference between acute and chronic thresholds is otherwise largely a measure of capsule thickness.[106]

BIOENGINEERING CONCEPTS

Electrophysiology of Pacing

ELECTRODE-ENDOMYOCARDIAL INTERFACE. The design and manufacture of an efficient pacemaker lead require a thorough understanding of the electrophysiology extant at the interface in the course of phasic stimulation. Both chemical and physical phenomena are involved and must be understood to resolve the apparently disparate effects of electrode porosity increasing its functional area to improve sensing performance, while the outer geometric area for pacing (inversely propor-

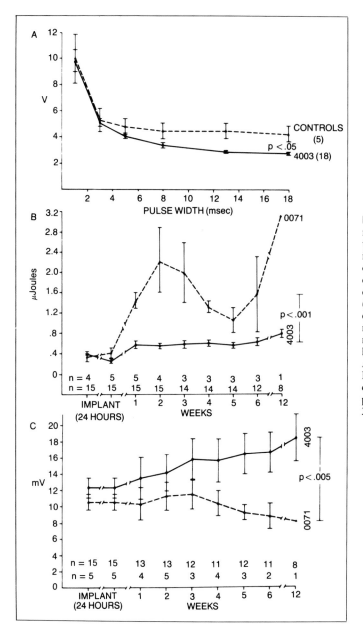

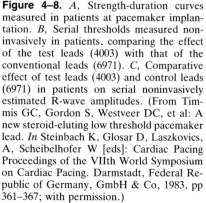

Figure 4–8. *A,* Strength-duration curves measured in patients at pacemaker implantation. *B,* Serial thresholds measured noninvasively in patients, comparing the effect of the test leads (4003) with that of the conventional leads (6971). *C,* Comparative effect of test leads (4003) and control leads (6971) in patients on serial noninvasively estimated R-wave amplitudes. (From Timmis GC, Gordon S, Westveer DC, et al: A new steroid-eluting low threshold pacemaker lead. *In* Steinbach K, Glosar D, Laszkovics, A, Scheibelhofer W [eds]: Cardiac Pacing Proceedings of the VIIth World Symposium on Cardiac Pacing. Darmstadt, Federal Republic of Germany, GmbH & Co, 1983, pp 361–367; with permission.)

tionate to the density of the field of current) remains small. Understanding the basic electrophysiologic and electrochemical issues involved in pacing is essential to determine what aspects of an electrode modification is truly responsible for the electrode's new and different performance. Since many electrode modifications are multiple, and tested multiply, there is confusion regarding how electrode material, geometry, size, polarization characteristics, or pharmacologic effluents are operative in effecting changes in pacing or sensing. Unfortunately, we have seen too frequently a lead tested in both animals and humans with-

out specific focus on the individual effects of its multiple new revisions.

The electrophysiology of pacing depends on the *electrochemistry* at the interface. As previously indicated, the charge carrier of a solid electrode is different from that of the tissue fluid that immediately surrounds it. Conduction within the electrode depends on electrons, while ions are responsible for conduction within the electrolytic tissue fluid. When these elements are in contact with each other, charge flows from one phase to the other until the potentials in each phase are equal. This flow of charge results in the development of a very

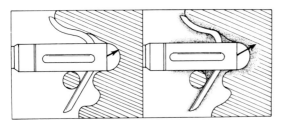

Figure 4–9. The "virtual electrode" concept. Acutely (*left*), the radius of a hemispheric electrode extends only to its surface. Chronically (*right*), the radius of the effective electrode extends to the nearest excitable tissue. Thus, fibrotic maturation of the electrode-tissue interface increases pacing thresholds. Chronic thresholds are lower from small electrodes, despite the fact that the increment in chronic thresholds is largest for small electrodes. (From Timmis GC, Helland J, Westveer DC, et al: The evolution of low threshold leads. Clin Prog Pacing Electrophysiol 1:313–334, 1983; with permission.)

thin charge layer around the electrode, known as the "Helmholtz layer," which performs electrically as a capacitor; it is in parallel with an ohmic resistance pathway (Warburg resistor), conduction through which depends on the frequency of stimulation and the density of current.[107] These concepts are schematically characterized in Figure 4–10. As shown in the diagram, there is another element, polarization voltage, which involves many different processes; it consists of that voltage arising from the potential difference of charge carriers at the electrode-tissue interface that occurs during stimulation.

POLARIZATION. Polarization is an electrochemical reaction resulting from the phasic accumulation of oppositely charged particles at the electrode-heart interface. It increases throughout the duration of the stimulation pulse, becoming a progressively higher fraction of the residual voltage at the end of the stimulation waveform. This factor may be a nuisance by contributing in a major way to sensing impedance, but it has an arguably variable effect on myocardial stimulation. Irnich has shown that stainless steel electrodes, which contribute significantly to polarization, display lower voltage and current threshold than does the somewhat toxic but relatively nonpolarizing silver–silver chloride electrode.[107] Thus, in some situations, polarization may actually facilitate pacing.

Polarization is affected by a variety of influences, including the unipolar versus bipolar mode of stimulation, electrolytic variations at the interface, electrode material, current, amplitude and pulse duration of the stimulus, and the maturity of the tissue reaction at the interface.[15] It is also significantly affected by electrode size, increasing as the outer area of the electrode decreases. With higher currents, polarization impedance accounts for relatively less of the total resistance than is the case with lower currents, when it may constitute up to 70 per cent of the total resistance for a small electrode.[15, 73] Because polarization is relatively small in the first milliseconds of the stimulation pulse and rises progressively throughout the duration of the pulse, impedance progressively increases throughout the duration of the stimulus, as shown in Figure 4–11. During constant-current stimulation, voltage rises exponentially throughout the duration of the pulse; however, because of polarization impedance, it is primarily the initial voltage amplitude of the stimulus that is available to excite the heart. Thus, there are those who take a different position from that expressed by Irnich above[107]; that is, polarization results in wasted energy. In contrast to the much more powerful effect of polarization on sensing, the effect of resistive polarization elements on myocardial stimulation is relatively smaller, so that sufficient current at the leading edge of the pacing pulse is available for stimulation. Nevertheless,

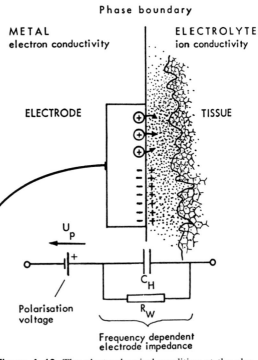

Phase boundary

METAL
electron conductivity

ELECTROLYTE
ion conductivity

ELECTRODE

TISSUE

U_P

Polarisation voltage

C_H

R_W

Frequency dependent electrode impedance

Figure 4–10. The electrochemical condition at the electrode-tissue interface. U_p = polarization voltage; C_H = capacitor; R_W = Warburg-resistor. (From Irnich W: The electrode myocardial interface. Clin Prog Electrophysiol Pacing 3:338–348, 1985; with permission.)

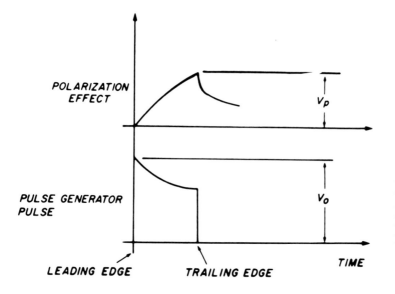

Figure 4–11. Polarization effect. The polarization effect is essentially zero at the leading edge of the pulse (capacitor-coupled constant-voltage waveform) and increases to the trailing edge, after which it dissipates by diffusion. The vertical scale represents relative voltage, and the horizontal scale represents time. V_p = polarization voltage; V_o = voltage output of pulse generator. (From Barold SS, Ong LS, Heinle RA: Stimulation and sensing thresholds for cardiac pacing: Electrophysiologic and technical aspects. Prog Cardiovasc Dis 24:1, 1981; with permission.)

the direct-current (DC) polarization components of electrodes of small area exert a profound effect on the energy delivered to the heart, tending to make small electrodes inefficient in this regard. These effects are generally offset by the lower pacing threshold due to a higher current density at the interface, as will be discussed below.[213] Accordingly, early in the development of pacemaker leads, efforts were made to devise low-polarizing electrodes, such as that of Lewin and colleagues, shown in Figure 4–12.[130]

Sensing or source impedance may be as high as 2500 ohms. Its components include tissue resistance, wire resistance, and, importantly, the effects of polarization. Accordingly, as is the case for pacing, sensing impedance is also related inversely to electrode surface area and directly to the duration of the stimulus. Fischler studied the polarization characteristics of platinum-iridium and Elgiloy pacemaker (El-

giloy Limited Partnership, Elgin, Illinois) electrodes of small surface area and their implications for sensing.[64] In testing electrodes in the size range of 10.0 to 12.5 mm^2, he found that the absolute electrode polarization impedance of platinum-iridium electrodes at 10 Hz (the lower end of the frequency range for the ventricular electrogram) ranged from 2.5 to 5.0 kilo-ohms, whereas for the Elgiloy electrodes it was considerably higher. These high sensing impedances at the electrode-tissue interface require a much higher input impedance in the sensing circuitry than was being manufactured in the 1970s because of loss of electrographic amplitude, distortion, and sensing failures, which will otherwise occur.

IMPEDANCE AFTERPOTENTIALS. Impedance at the electrode-tissue interface is complex, consisting of resistive (including polarization) and reactive (capacitive) components, which represent energy that is both dissipated and

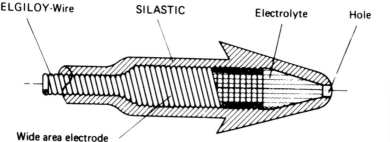

Figure 4–12. The differential current density (DCD) electrode. It is constructed of a helical coil of platinum-iridium or Elgiloy, which is widened at its tip to form a cylinder with a surface area exceeding 1 cm^2. It is encased in a silicone rubber capsule, which extends beyond the coil and is open at the very tip. The large surface area of the wire coil results in a minimization of polarization while the current applied to the coil passes through the encapsulated electrolytic body fluids, which in turn contact excitable tissue through the small hole at the tip. This contact produces high current densities and low excitation thresholds. (From Timmis GC, Helland J, Westveer DC, et al: The evolution of low threshold leads. Clin Prog Pacing Electrophysiol 1: 313–334, 1983; and Lewin G, Myers GH, Parsonnet V, et al: Differential current density [DCD] electrodes for pacemakers. *In* Engineering in Medicine and Biology. Proceedings of the 19th Annual Conference, 1966, p 165; with permission.)

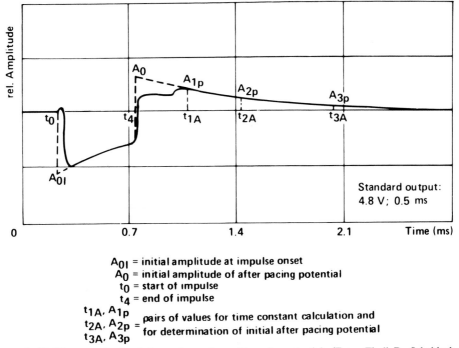

A_{0I} = initial amplitude at impulse onset
A_0 = initial amplitude of after pacing potential
t_0 = start of impulse
t_4 = end of impulse

t_{1A}, A_{1p}
t_{2A}, A_{2p} = pairs of values for time constant calculation and for determination of initial after pacing potential
t_{3A}, A_{3p}

Figure 4–13. Diagram of stimulating pulse and resulting afterpotential. (From Thull R, Schaldach M: Electrochemistry of after-pacing potentials on electrodes. PACE 9:1191–1196, 1986; with permission.)

stored at the electrode-tissue interface, respectively. Resistance and capacitance vary with frequencies of stimulation (or alternation of current), both being larger at lower frequencies and smaller at higher frequencies.[219] The stored capacitor charge may result in a post-stimulus voltage artifact of about 1 V at its highest amplitude; this may mask recording the evoked electrogram. This "afterpotential" is at its maximum just beyond the trailing edge of the stimulation pulse and is of opposite sign. It slowly dissipates over a time-base that is considerably longer than that of the stimulation pulse, as shown in Figure 4–13.[202] Afterpotentials superimposed on portions of the intracardiac signal may provide the basis for oversensing.

CATHODAL AND ANODAL STIMULATION. Cathodal stimulation is usually employed for myocardial excitation; that is, the stimulus usually arises from the negative pole of the battery. Cathodal stimulation is more likely to depolarize cell membranes than is anodal current; the latter may actually hyperpolarize the membrane and hence inhibit depolarization. Alternately, when anodal extracellular current is used for myocardial stimulation, it may depolarize certain parts of the cell membrane or certain cells and hyperpolarize other parts; if hyperpolarization is too great, the action potential generated at the site of depolarization may not be propagated through the hyperpolarized region.[40] Another undesirable feature of anodal stimulation is that myocardial responsiveness to it occurs earlier than is the case with cathodal stimulation after the absolute refractory period has expired. Moreover, sensitivity to anodal stimulation is greater during the vulnerable period than is sensitivity to cathodal stimulation. This factor may result in repetitive responses or ventricular fibrillation. Simply stated, an anodal stimulus can initiate an arrhythmia over a greater portion of the cardiac cycle and at a lower threshold than can a cathodal stimulus.[68] Of course, cathodal stimulation is possible only with a bipolar lead in which the cathode and anode are both contained within the heart.

CURRENT DENSITY AND FIELD STRENGTH. The electrical force affecting depolarization and myocardial excitation is the function of an exogenic electrical field. Electrical fields can be visualized with the aid of small filaments of acetate, which Irnich suspended in carbon tetrachloride. By applying an electrical stimulus to the electrode, he was able to demonstrate the relatively homogeneous radial field of a hemispheric electrode, as shown in Figure 4–14.[107] He also showed that with columnar electrodes the density of the electrical field was

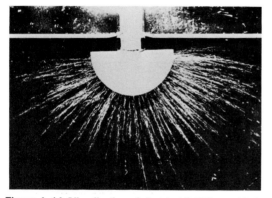

Figure 4–14. Visualization of electrical field lines with the aid of small filaments of acetates suspended in carbon tetrachloride. The regular radial field of a hemispheric electrode is shown. (From Irnich W: The electrode myocardial interface. Clin Prog Electrophysiol Pacing 3:338–348, 1985; with permission.)

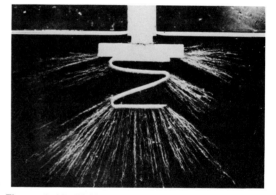

Figure 4–16. Field lines concentrated at the points of sharp angulation and tip of a helical electrode. (From Irnich W: The electrode myocardial interface. Clin Prog Electrophysiol Pacing 3:338–348, 1985; with permission.)

greatest at the edges (Fig. 4–15) and at the tip and bend points of spiral electrodes (Fig. 4–16). When a voltage is applied to electrodes, maximal field strength is produced at the surface of the electrode and diminishes throughout the myocardium as a function of the square of the distance; it is independent of conductivity. Field strength increases with decreasing electrode size and, as indicated above, is greatest at the point of highest electrode curvature and especially at sharp edges thereof. It dissipates faster than with larger electrodes. The minimal field strength capable of myocardial stimulation is partly dependent on the pulse duration; it also depends on the thickness of nonexcitable tissue around the electrode, as shown in Figure 4–9. Irnich found that the voltage threshold is at its minimum when the radius of the electrode is equal to the thickness

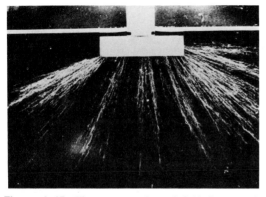

Figure 4–15. The concentration of field lines at the corners of a columnar electrode is shown. (From Irnich W: The electrode myocardial interface. Clin Prog Electrophysiol Pacing 3:338–348, 1985; with permission.)

of the nonexcitable tissue.[107] The effect of the nonexcitable layer can be expressed as follows:

$$E = V/r_o \ (r_o/r)^2$$

where E is the electrical field strength, r is the radius from the center of the electrode to the nearest excitable tissue, r_o is the radius of the electrode itself, and V is the voltage applied to the electrode.

Current density is the quotient of current and electrode area. Incorporating the virtual electrode concept displayed in Figure 4–9, it equals I/A_c, where I equals current and A_c equals the surface area of virtual electrode, including the interposed fibrotic, nonexcitable tissue. This expains why threshold increases occurring in the first several months after pacemaker implantation are largely determined by the thickness of the nonexcitable layer. Ripart and Mugica found that in contrast to the dominant effect of polarization on sensing, stimulation thresholds were primarily affected by the thickness of fibrosis, loss of electrode efficiency to polarization losses, and electrode surface area, in that order.[175] Fischler defined electrode efficiency as the relationship between the useful energy expended in the process of myocardial stimulation and that wasted on the "electrode-tissue" load.[64] As the size of an electrode decreases, polarization impedance increases nearly in inverse proportion to the reduction in area; tissue resistance increases in inverse proportion to the square root of the electrode area. Nevertheless, this effect of the electrode size on polarization impedance and on tissue resistance is largely offset by the effect of small electrode size on thresholds. In spite of the larger polarization losses, the higher current density and field strength are actually achieved with relatively little increase in tissue resistance.[61]

Both electrode materials and electrode stabilization, which are discussed on pages 59 and 68, respectively, will have an effect on myocardial fibrosis and the thickness of the nonexcitable layer. As previously shown by Guarda, the more rapidly the physical stability of the electrode-endomyocardial interface is established, the less inflammation edema and fibrin layering that occur at the interface.[83] A variety of active- and passive-fixation devices have been employed to effect this, as shown in Figures 4–17 to 4–20.[192] Physical stresses at the electrode-endomyocardial interface may be greater with small electrodes, in which axial force is transmitted through the conductor portion of the lead to the electrode tip. This increased stress may exacerbate the foreign-body reaction at the interface.

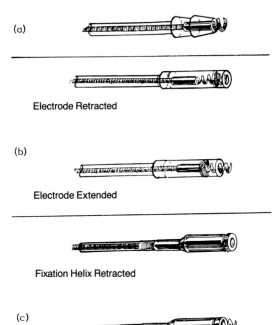

(a)

Electrode Retracted

(b)

Electrode Extended

Fixation Helix Retracted

(c)

Fixation Helix Extended

Figure 4–18. Examples of currently used transvenous ventricular pacing leads with active-fixation designs: (a) Osypka Screw-in (Osypka); (b) Medtronic 6957 (Bisping); and (c) Medtronic 6959 (Dutcher). (From Stokes K, Stephenson NL: The implantable cardiac pacing lead—just a simple wire? *In* Barold SS, Mugica J [eds]: The Third Decade of Cardiac Pacing: Advances in Technology and Clinical Applications. Mount Kisco, NY, Futura Publishing Co, 1982; pp 365–416; with permission.)

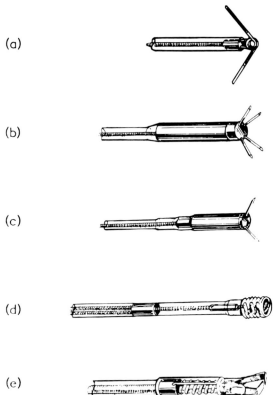

(a)

(b)

(c)

(d)

(e)

Figure 4–17. Early transvenous ventricular leads with active-fixation devices: (a) Biotronic IVE-85 (Schaldach); (b) Vitatron MIP 2000 (Schmitt); (c) Biotronic IE-651 (Irnich); (d) Medtronic 6954 (Helland); and (e) Coratomic Endo-Loc L-40. (From Stokes K, Stephenson NL: The implantable cardiac pacing lead—just a simple wire? *In* Barold SS, Mugica J [eds]: The Third Decade of Cardiac Pacing: Advances in Technology and Clinical Applications. Mount Kisco, NY, Futura Publishing Co, 1983, pp 365–416; with permission.)

STIMULATION THRESHOLDS. Threshold has been defined as the minimal amount of electricity required to stimulate a response in a cell.[109] As previously discussed, stimulation thresholds are affected by factors such as the duration of the stimulus, the size and material of the electrode, maturation of the electrode-endomyocardial interface, and the characteristics of the generator producing the electrical stimulus. Thresholds are usually measured in terms of current (ampere or coulombs per second) or voltage. Thresholds may also be measured in units derived from current, voltage, and resistance, such as *energy* or *charge*. Energy is the product of voltage, current, and the time over which it is delivered; charge is the total quantity of current consumed during the time the stimulus is applied. The unit of energy is joules, and the unit of charge is the coulomb. The time over which the stimulus is applied defines the *pulse duration*. The electrical pulse is applied to a segment of myocardium through two electrodes. The cathodal or negative electrode is usually in physical contact with the heart, whereas the positive or anodal electrode, while always remote to the cathode, may be in, on, or removed from the heart, in which case it is referred to as an "indifferent" or "inactive" electrode that is not involved in the direct electrical stimulation of the heart. The average measured current over the duration of the pulse, which consistently depolarizes the myocardium, defines current (usually expressed milliamperes [mA]) threshold, and the average measured voltage across the duration of the pulse defines voltage thresholds. In a study of the precision of pacemaker thresholds, Timmis and colleagues found that

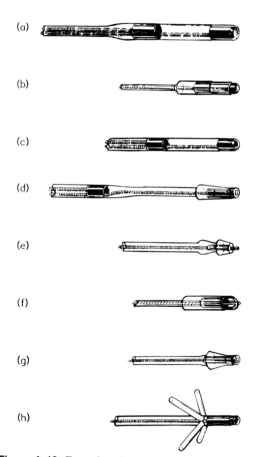

Figure 4–19. Examples of some early transvenous ventricular pacing leads: (a) Medtronic 5816 (Chardack); (b) Elema 588D (Lagergren); (c) Medtronic 5818 (Chardack); (d) Medtronic 6901R; (e) Medcor Microtip P56 MTF; (f) Elema 588K (Lagergren); (g) Vitatron 2147 LOE (Thalen); and (h) Medtronic 6951 (Citron). (From Stokes K, Stephenson NL: The implantable cardiac pacing lead—just a simple wire? *In* Barold SS, Mugica J [eds]: The Third Decade of Cardiac Pacing: Advances in Technology and Clinical Applications. Mount Kisco, NY, Futura Publishing Co, 1982, pp 365–416; with permission.)

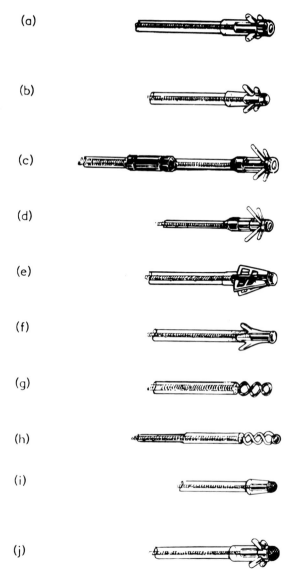

Figure 4–20. Currently used transvenous ventricular pacing leads with passive-fixation modifications: (a) Medtronic 6961/6962 (Helland); (b) Intermedics 476-02/477-02; (c) Medtronic 6972 (Stokes); (d) Medtronic 6971 (Stokes); (e) Cordis Fin-tip; (f) Telectronic Trailing Tine; (g) Vitatron Helifix; (h) Vitatron Helifix Ball Tip (Babotai); (i) CPI 411/4226 Porous (Amundson); and (j) CPI 4130/4230 Porous Tined (Amundson). (From Stokes K, Stephenson NL: The implantable cardiac pacing lead—just a simple wire? *In* Barold SS, Mugica J [eds]: The Third Decade of Cardiac Pacing: Advances in Technology and Clinical Applications. Mount Kisco, NY, Futura Publishing Co, 1982, pp 365–416; with permission.)

varying voltage at a constant pulse duration and varying pulse duration at a constant voltage routinely yielded lower thresholds with decremental suprathreshold stimuli than with incremental subthreshold stimuli.[211] That gain-of-capture thresholds were higher than main-

GENERALIZED THRESHOLD STRENGTH-DURATION CURVE

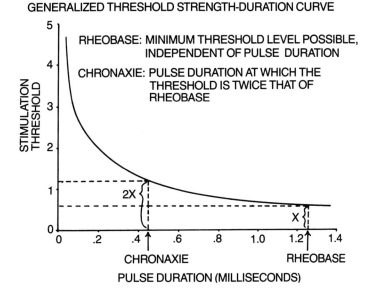

Figure 4–21. Diagram of a strength-duration curve of the type characterizing voltage and current thresholds. (From Timmis GC, Helland J, Westveer DC, et al: The evolution of low threshold leads: Clin Prog Pacing Electrophysiol 1:313–334, 1983; with permission.)

tenance-of-capture thresholds is probably a manifestation of the Wedensky effect, reflecting the influence of electrotonic conditioning.[48] At implant this difference is approximately 0.15 mA in humans.

STRENGTH-DURATION CURVES. The effect of varying pulse duration on threshold defines the strength-duration curve, which more accurately characterizes the response to electrostimulation at the electrode-tissue interface. As shown in Figure 4–21,[191] shortening the duration of the stimulus increases threshold and vice versa. In the steep initial portion of both the voltage and current strength-duration curves, minor changes in pulse duration can have a major impact on thresholds. The term *rheobase* is defined as the lowest intensity of the stimulus at any pulse duration sufficient to cause myocardial excitation (or the excitation of any electrically responsive tissue). *Chronaxie* is defined as the pulse duration at which threshold is twice that of the rheobase. When comparing the threshold of different electrodes, it is not sufficient to measure them at only one pulse duration. One electrode with a flatter strength-duration curve may look efficient at shorter pulse durations but perform less well than another electrode with a steeper strength-duration curve at pulse durations near the rheobase, as shown in Figure 4–22.[106] Solid electrodes with small surface areas of about 8 mm² exhibit lower chronaxie points than do larger (approximately 12 mm²) similar electrodes[8]; so do steroid-eluting leads compared with conventional ring-tipped electrodes.[206]

In contrast to the descending hyperbolic configuration of both voltage and current

Figure 4–22. Comparison of two curves with different chronaxie times and rheobase values: Electrode A is more favorable in region I; in region II the situation is reversed. (From Irnich W: Comparison of pacing electrodes of different shape and material—recommendations. PACE 6:422–426, 1983; with permission.)

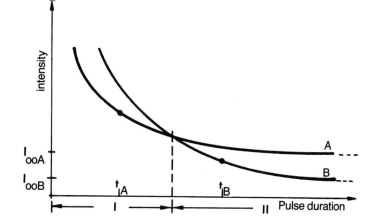

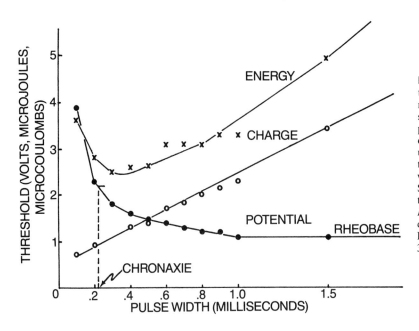

Figure 4–23. Relationships between chronic ventricular (canine) constant-voltage threshold strength-duration curves expressed in terms of potential, charge, and energy for a tined unipolar lead with a 8-mm^2 ring tip. Thresholds were obtained with increasing stimuli. (From Stokes K, Bornzin G: The electrode-biointerface: Stimulation. *In* Barold SS [ed]: Modern Cardiac Pacing. Mount Kisco, NY, Futura Publishing Co, 1985, p 33; with permission.)

strength-duration curves, the charge strength-duration curve is upsloping and linear, and the energy strength-duration curve has a parabolic shape with its convexity downward (Fig. 4–23).[191]

THRESHOLD AS INFLUENCED BY THE NATURE OF THE STIMULUS. Some clinically relevant variables affecting the electrostimulation pulse itself include its amplitude, duration, cathodal or anodal charge, and the threshold-lowering influence of the Wedensky effect on the stimulus; these have already been discussed. Still to be reviewed are the output characteristics of pulse generators. Most units in clinical use at this time employ a stimulus, the voltage of which is maintained at a relatively constant level, at least in the earlier portion of the stimulus, as shown in Figure 4–24.[15] With this type of stimulus, current is largely dependent on impedance. The latter increases over the duration of the stimulus because of polarization, so that current flow falls from its initial level throughout the duration of the pulse (Fig. 4–25). The implantable generators of some manufacturers have employed constant-current circuitry, in which cur-

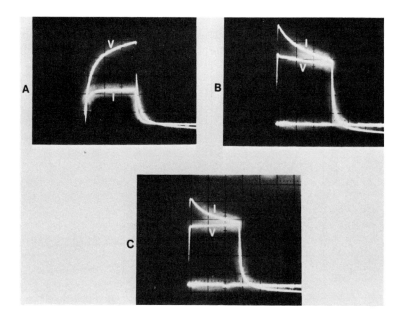

Figure 4–24. *A,* Voltage and current waveform with the application of a constant-current impulse. *B,* Voltage and current waveforms with a constant-voltage (capacitor-coupled) impulse. *C,* Voltage and current waveforms with a true constant-voltage impulse applied. I = current; V = voltage; pulse width was 0.6 msec for all recordings. (From Barold SS, Ong LS, Heinle RA: Stimulation and sensing thresholds for cardiac pacing: Electrophysiologic and technical aspects. Prog Cardiovasc Dis 24:1, 1981; with permission.)

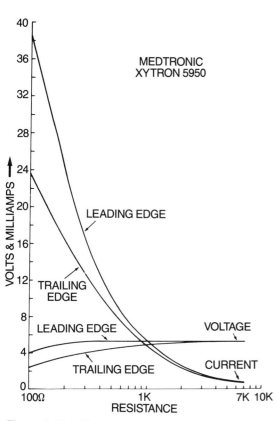

Figure 4–25. Voltage and current waveforms of a constant-voltage (capacitor-coupled) implantable pulse generator (Medtronic 5950) for different resistive loads. Note that only the leading edge of the voltage remains constant with all resistances over 200 ohms but that current falls as the resistance increases. The graph illustrates that any constant-voltage source may cease to remain constant when the load is very low because the battery then becomes unable to supply all the current required to maintain a steady voltage. However, such a low range of resistance is unlikely to be encountered clinically. K = 1000 ohms. (From Barold SS, Winner JA: Techniques and significance of threshold measurement for cardiac pacing. Chest 70:760, 1976; with permission.)

rent flow remains relatively constant throughout much of the stimulus. To achieve this in the face of the rising impedance, which inevitably occurs because of increasing polarization throughout the pulse delivery, voltage rises sharply, as shown in Figures 4–24 and 4–26. Certain external pulse generators employ constant-current circuitry as well. The delivery of current by constant-voltage pulse generators is much more impedance dependent than is that by constant-current units. A constant-voltage generator cannot compensate for higher lead impedance as well as a constant-current device can because voltage requirements are directly proportionate to the product of current and resistance.

Barold has described several scenarios detailing the strengths and weaknesses of each type of unit.[15] In the presence of high resistance of several thousand ohms, the nominal voltage output (5 V) of many units currently in use may not be able to achieve a current threshold of 1 to 2 mA. On the other hand, constant-current units may be a problem in the more clinically realistic scenario of high current thresholds in the range of 10 mA in the presence of low impedances of 200 to 300 ohms, as may occur with an insulation break or with intramyocardial leads. We repeatedly encountered the latter situation in our initial experience with screw-in leads.[204] In these instances, a constant-voltage generator would be preferable.

UNIPOLAR VERSUS BIPOLAR THRESHOLDS. The preference of unipolar to bipolar electrode configurations has been based on the putative superiority of sensing by unipolar systems, since electrographic amplitudes were allegedly larger and sensing failure occurred less frequently. Because of extraneous signals that have proved to be a problem with unipolar systems, interest in the bipolar systems has been rekindled.[87] This is particularly true in the context of physiologic bifocal pacing systems, since the detection of noise and crosstalk has been a problem that occurs less frequently with bipolar leads. There is little evidence that stimulation thresholds in one system are superior to those of the other. In one of the few studies systematically comparing unipolar and bipolar thresholds in patients, Breivik and associates found that although unipolar thresholds were lower in the constant-current pacing mode, there were no significant differences during constant-voltage pacing.[35] On the other hand, bipolar leads in the past were considered to be relatively undesirable because of their size. Revisions in engineering techniques have resulted in the manufacture of smaller-caliber bipolar leads, which are now as facile as their unipolar equivalents.

THRESHOLDS AND ELECTRODE CONFIGURATION. As previously indicated, the shape of an electrode will affect the current density and therefore thresholds. Current density is greatest at the points of greatest curvature or angulation or at the edge of an electrode. This characteristic has been employed in the pursuit of the dual goals of lowering thresholds by modulating current density and field strength and of securing electrode stability at the interface. The larger the electrode, the less likely a perforation will occur. However, large electrodes yield lower field strength, manifested by higher pacing thresholds. An early modifi-

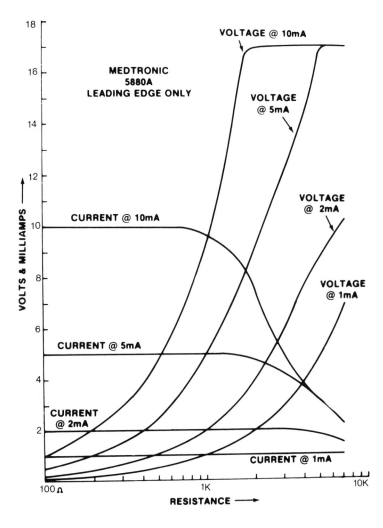

Figure 4–26. Current and voltage output curves (leading edge only) of a constant-current pulse generator (Medtronic 5880A) at various resistive loads. Corresponding current and voltage curves are shown for current settings of 1,2,5, and 10 mA. K = 1000 ohms. Resistance is shown in the log scale. (From Barold SS, Winner JA: Techniques and significance of threshold measurement for cardiac pacing. Chest 70:760, 1976; with permission.)

cation was to abandon columnar electrodes for a ring-tip design, as shown in Figure 4–19, examples d and g. This design achieved retention of the nonpenetrating electrode bulk while allowing for a decrease in its size, imparting an edge and lowering thresholds. The effect of current density on thresholds was particularly evident in our early studies with the screw-in helical electrode, in which both acute and chronic thresholds were extremely low, with electrical exposure of only 3.8 mm^2 of the tip.[204]

THRESHOLD SAFETY MARGINS. Because of changes in myocardial excitability throughout the day, variable responses to pharmacologic influences and metabolic changes, and threshold changes associated with electrode-tissue interface maturation, there must be sufficient slack between stimulus strength, excitability requirements, and generator output. Ideally, the acute voltage threshold should, at most, be 15 per cent of the voltage output rating for the implanted pulse pacemaker generator.[15] The safety factor depends on how thresholds are being determined. If energy thresholds reported in microjoules (μJ) are being employed, the pacing generator's capacity to deliver this energy should be three-fold that required at the time of threshold measurement, since energy requirements may vary by as much as 50 per cent above or below nominal threshold levels.[169] Under physiologic circumstances, energy thresholds may vary by as much as 50 per cent, from roughly 2.5 to 7.5 μJ.[168, 169, 187] Generally, a voltage threshold safety margin need be only 2 to 1. The reason why the energy safety factor must be higher is that a 4-fold increase in current measured in milliamperes would be equivalent to a 16-fold increase expressed in microjoules. Thus, in accordance with Ohm's law, energy is not only the product of voltage, current, and pulse duration, but also the product of resistance, time, and square of current (I^2RT). Pulse duration may also be employed as a noninvasive variable for threshold measurement. Accordingly, a threshold safety factor using pulse duration may be a particularly useful measurement with chronically implanted leads. However, voltage and pulse-width thresholds are not interchangeable. Although strength-duration curves show that voltage and pulse duration are inversely related, this is a nonlinear relationship; thus, doubling the pulse duration does not decrease the voltage threshold by one half. This is particularly apparent when studying the steepest and flattest portions of the voltage strength-duration curve, as shown in Figure 4–21. It has been recommended that a reasonable safety factor can be achieved by tripling the pulse duration over threshold at half-amplitude.[191]

Electrophysiology of Sensing

SIGNAL AMPLITUDE POLARIZATION AND THE EFFECT OF IMPEDANCE ON SENSING. As stated earlier in this chapter, source or sensing impedance at the electrode is largely influenced by polarization and electrode size, to which it is inversely proportionate, and is considerably higher than pacing impedance. Pacemaker sensing circuitry incorporates as a major component a resistive impedance component that produces a drop in the voltage of the sensed signal as it enters the generator. This drop is what the generator "sees." If electrode impedance at the signal source is very high, a considerable voltage drop will occur at that point, resulting in a relatively small signal ultimately presenting itself at the generator. A low input impedance at this point will result in a relatively small drop in voltage; thus, a small voltage drop of a small signal that has lost most of its voltage at the electrode-tissue interface will be poorly detected, if at all, by sensing circuitry. To maximize the voltage drop at the generator, therefore, a high input impedance is required. Clinically dependable "impedance matching" requires that input impedance be 20 kilo-ohms or more. High input impedances also have an effect on the electrographic spectral content (frequency components of the signal) and shift the band width of the sensing system downward. On the other hand, low-frequency content of the signal is selectively attenuated at the electrode-tissue interface, shifting the band width upward.[210] Although the band width of atrial and ventricular signals is different,[108, 152] most sensing circuitry in clinical use is suitable for either

signal. Kleinert and associates confirmed this by measuring the spectral densities of unipolar P waves in the atrium and R waves in the ventricle.[118] They found that the band width of maximal spectral density was between 10 and 30 Hz for both R waves and P waves and concluded that the same filter characteristics of the sensing circuitry may be employed for either purpose. Sensing circuitry filters out the low-frequency T waves, which have a spectral content below 10 Hz, usually 3 Hz. However, myopotentials arising from skeletal muscle activity have a spectral content in the 50-Hz range (30 to 70 Hz), which can be detected by existing sensing circuitry.[118]

SLEW RATE. For an electrographic signal to be detected by the sensing circuitry of the pacemaker, it must have both sufficient amplitude and slew rate. The latter term is defined for clinical purposes as the rate of change of voltage from the positive to negative peak of the electrogram, as shown in Figure 4–27, or in that part of the electrogram moving most rapidly away from the isoelectric line if the signal is monophasic. Even if the amplitude of a deflection is sufficiently high, it will not be sensed if the slew rate is excessively low. Slew rates should preferably exceed 1.0 V/sec at implant, since they may fall by as much as 50 per cent as the fibrous capsule at the electrode-tissue interface matures.[52] Slew rates of 0.5 V/sec or less should be rejected and the lead repositioned, especially when sensing amplitudes approach the highest gain setting of the pulse generator.

BIPOLAR VERSUS UNIPOLAR SENSING. Sensing is achieved by the two different electrodes detecting a difference in the voltage registered by myocardial signal. With unipolar systems, most of the changes in potential occur in the neighborhood of the intracardiac electrode, while very little change occurs near the remote electrode, which is actually the metallic "can" of the generator. In contrast, with intracardiac bipolar electrodes, both electrodes may "see" the signal equally well, with relatively little difference in the voltage registered at each electrode by the sensed signal. This is likely to be the case when the origin of the signal is proximate to and similarly approaches both electrodes. The capacity of each of the two electrodes of an intracardiac bipolar system to detect the difference in a potential that is being registered by signals arising from skeletal muscle (myopotentials) is negligible. However, the voltage difference of deltopectoral myopotentials registered between the immediately ad-

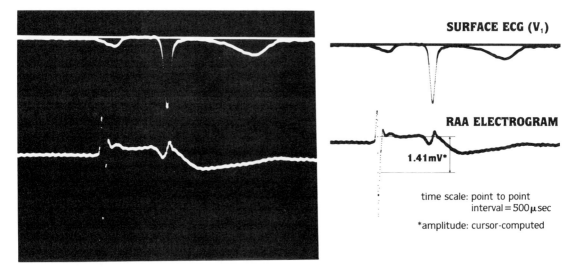

SURFACE ECG (V₁)

RAA ELECTROGRAM

1.41mV*

time scale: point to point
interval = 500 μsec

*amplitude: cursor-computed

Figure 4–27. Typical surface and electrographic complexes recorded in a single patient. The artifacts resulting from time-division multiplexing of the oscilloscopic recording beam produce an electrographic reconstruction consisting of discrete dots recorded at 0.5-msec intervals. Employing two-point cursor identification, these time marks are used, along with the automatically calibrated voltage displacement, for computerized measurements of slew rates. RAA = right atrial appendage. (From Timmis GC, Westveer DC, Gadowski G, et al: The effect of electrode position on atrial sensing for physiologically responsive cardiac pacemakers. Am Heart J 108:909–916, 1984; with permission.)

jacent indifferent electrode (the generator casing itself) and a widely separated unipolar intracardiac electrode is considerable. This difference in potential registered between the two electrodes permits sensing of myopotentials. As indicated above, filtration circuitry fails to screen out the spurious input, which has a frequency spectrum overlapping that of P waves and R waves.[152] Breivik and Ohm found that 85 per cent of unipolar pacemakers from different manufacturers could be suppressed by myopotentials.[34] These same systems are uniquely vulnerable to exogenous interference signals arising from electrocautery, metal detectors, microwaves, and radar waves. Because bipolar leads have been downsized to the dimensions of unipolar leads, owing to polyurethane and thin silicone insulators, some of the dissatisfaction with bipolar leads has largely waned, even though the amplitude of bipolar signals is generally smaller than that of unipolar signals. This smaller amplitude is due in part to the higher signal source impedance of bipolar versus unipolar leads.[81] Nevertheless, DeCaprio and colleagues found that for all practical purposes there was no significant difference between unipolar and bipolar electrograms and that bipolar electrodes have a superior signal-to-noise ratio.[52] More recently, Breivik and his colleagues found that bipolar electrograms displayed higher amplitudes than did unipolar signals in the majority of their

patients.[35] Accordingly, the major difference in unipolar and bipolar signals is confined to the surface electrocardiogram and is clinically less important in the circuitry of sensing systems.

Some pacemaker leads employing bipolar orthogonal floating electrodes, as shown in Figure 4–28, do not actually contact the endocardium. This type of bipolar electrode has been found to discriminate far better between the amplitude of intraatrial P waves and far-field QRS complexes (voltage difference of 15 to 1).[10] It was also better able to discriminate between whatever differences there were in the spectral frequency content of P waves and QRS complexes than was possible with unipolar leads.[9] We also have found that bipolar leads do a better job for the electrographic discrimination between the atrial electrograms and far-field R-waves.[210]

AFTERPOTENTIALS. The residual wasted energy of the stimulus that is stored at the electrode-tissue interface has a charge opposite to that of the stimulus and may have considerable voltage, which decays slowly.[202] Accordingly, it may be sensed inappropriately, suppressing and recycling the pulse generator. Afterpotentials are greater with higher-strength stimuli and pulses of longer duration. Both of these variables are noninvasively programmable in many currently used systems and should be readjusted when inappropriate slow-

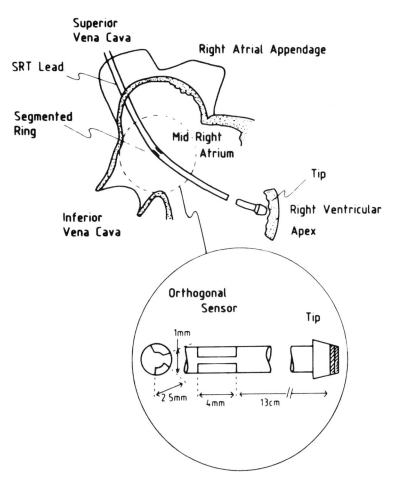

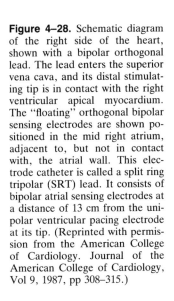

Figure 4–28. Schematic diagram of the right side of the heart, shown with a bipolar orthogonal lead. The lead enters the superior vena cava, and its distal stimulating tip is in contact with the right ventricular apical myocardium. The "floating" orthogonal bipolar sensing electrodes are shown positioned in the mid right atrium, adjacent to, but not in contact with, the atrial wall. This electrode catheter is called a split ring tripolar (SRT) lead. It consists of bipolar atrial sensing electrodes at a distance of 13 cm from the unipolar ventricular pacing electrode at its tip. (Reprinted with permission from the American College of Cardiology. Journal of the American College of Cardiology, Vol 9, 1987, pp 308–315.)

ing or recycling occurs, especially in recently implanted pacemakers.

ELECTRODE SIZE AND POSITION. Large electrodes facilitate sensing because of lower source impedance. Nevertheless, there has been a tendency to employ smaller electrodes ranging from 8 mm^2 to 12 mm^2. With the use of circuitry to detect high impedance, as described above, and programmable pacemaker sensitivity, these smaller electrodes have not been a problem. As previously indicated, sensing occurs when each electrode "sees" the voltage generated by the approaching "wall" of the depolarization wave front differently. The major difference detected by intracardiac bipolar leads is due to the difference in time at which the wave front approaches each electrode; thus, this difference is most likely to occur when the axis of the bipolar leads is perpendicular to the approaching "wall" and unlikely to occur when the axis of two electrodes is parallel to the wave front. In contrast, because of the remote location of the indifferent electrode in unipolar systems, the differ-

ence in voltage seen by the two electrodes is primarily a result of the distance of the indifferent electrode from the signal source rather than attributable to the electrode axis–wave front relationship. Proximity to the endocardium or myocardium also facilitates sensing because of larger amplitudes. Thus, as the electrode moves away from the endocardium, especially at the right ventricular apex, R-wave amplitudes tend to decrease.[101] The same phenomenon is operative at the atrial level. Nevertheless, as previously indicated, floating bipolar orthogonal electrodes have been proved to be clinically effective.[9, 10]

Pacing and Sensing Threshold Changes over Time

Chronic thresholds may be serially measured directly at the time of generator replacement or indirectly employing the noninvasive adjustment of pacemaker output (Vario; Fig. 4–29)[198] or stimulus duration. Most studies have shown an increase in both voltage and current

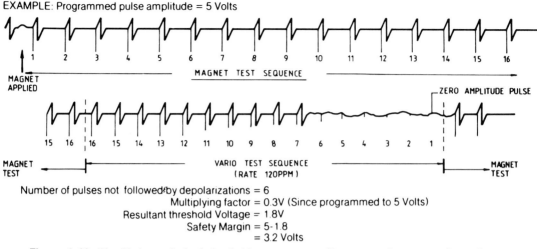

EXAMPLE: Programmed pulse amplitude = 5 Volts

Number of pulses not followed by depolarizations = 6
Multiplying factor = 0.3V (Since programmed to 5 Volts)
Resultant threshold Voltage = 1.8V
Safety Margin = 5-1.8
= 3.2 Volts

Figure 4–29. The Vario method of threshold measurement. Sixteen asynchronous pacing pulses are decrementally applied, beginning with 5 V in this example, with sequential drops of 0.3 V until capture is lost. (From Telectronics Physician's Manual 100-537. Englewood, CO, Telectronics, January 1985; with permission.)

thresholds over time. Angello and coworkers found that the mean acute current threshold in 61 patients of 0.81 ± 0.33 mA increased two to five times over a period of up to 10 years, while chronic voltage threshold increased considerably less; impedance derived from current and voltage data remained relatively stable.[7] Using direct threshold measurements over a period of up to 11 years, Luceri and colleagues found that 20 per cent of patients with permanent pacemakers exhibited a progressive increase in pacing threshold, whereas the thresholds in the remainder, after the anticipated early rise in the first several months, displayed stable thresholds; 107 of their 120 patients had endocardial leads.[133] Using programmable pulse duration, Scoblionko and Rolett detected an early 2 to 10 fold threshold increase in 22 patients over 8 to 12 weeks, which tended to level off thereafter.[183] Platia and Brinker, employing invasively validated telemetric data in patients with fully automatic, multiprogrammable bifocal pacing systems, found that both atrial and ventricular pacing impedance fell from about 540 ohms to about 480 ohms.[167] Stimulation thresholds averaging slightly over 1 V at implant rose approximately 0.2 V in both the atrium and the ventricle at 13 months. The amplitude of telemetered electrograms did not change significantly over this period. All patients had unspecified endocardial unipolar pacing leads. Using similar telemetered data for serial R-wave sensing and noninvasively adjustable output and pulse duration for seri-

alizing stimulation thresholds, we found that with conventional ring-tip (8 mm²) electrodes (6971), voltage, especially energy thresholds, progressively rose over a 12-week period in 23 patients, while steroid-eluting leads (4003) displayed a much less striking rise in threshold (Fig. 4–8B). The amplitude of telemetered electrograms gradually fell with the conventional lead while actually increasing with steroid leads.[206] In a chronic pulse-duration threshold study comparing smooth 8-mm² ring-tip electrodes, 8-mm² ball-tip electrodes, 17.5-mm² conventional columnar electrodes, and 7.5-mm² electrodes employing a textured porous surface rather than a polished surface (see "Microstructure [Electrode Surface]," further on), Breivik and associates found no significant difference between the various electrodes at 18 months; the ball-tip electrode tended to give the best long-term results, and the porous electrode the poorest.[36]

Chronic pulse-duration thresholds have been used to compare transvenous and myoepicardial leads. Henglein and colleagues found that although at the atrial level transvenous thresholds were lower than those of epimyocardial leads, the difference became significant only at the ventricular level.[93] They concluded that transvenous leads had a "slight advantage," as estimated by this threshold-serializing technique. In a long-term study of 74 patients with permanent pacemakers noninvasively programmable to either a unipolar or a bipolar electrode configuration, both pacing and sensing thresholds were found to mature in similar fashion. There were no clinically significant differences in pacing or sensing between bipolar and unipolar thresholds over a period of 9.3 months. High threshold and loss of capture were corrected in two patients by reprogramming to the unipolar configuration.[155]

Electrode Design and Manufacture

ELECTRODE SIZE. Recognition of the inefficiencies of large electrodes—ranging as they did, 15 to 20 years ago, up to 80 to 90 mm^2 in surface area[73]—has led to a progressive reduction in electrode size, as demonstrated in Figure 4–30. This size reduction holds true for both unipolar and bipolar electrodes, particularly those at the cathodal position on the lead tip. As previously indicated, the trade-off for the higher pacing impedance of small electrodes is their delivery of higher current densities and field strength, which result in a net reduction in stimulation thresholds. We found that both voltage and current thresholds were lower when the distal electrode of a bipolar pair was 3.8 mm^2 than it was with larger 6.3 mm^2 electrodes (0.80 V versus 0.83 V and 0.70 mA versus 0.94 mA). Not unexpectedly, lead impedances were high for the smaller electrode (1230 ohms versus 950 ohms).[73] However, high impedances may have a favorable effect on current drain. Source or sensing impedance is, of course, considerably higher than pacing impedance because of its reciprocal relationship to the frequency (spectral content) of the sensed signal, which is even more affected by downsizing electrodes.

Between 20 and 70 mm^2, the relationship between electrode size and threshold may be somewhat less clear than with the two extremes of size.[36] On the other hand, some studies have shown a measurably lower chronaxie point for 8-mm^2 solid-tip electrodes than with similar 12-mm^2 electrodes.[211] Irnich[105] and Parker and colleagues[157] suggested that there was little improvement in thresholds on further reducing the radius of a hemispheric electrode to less than 0.6 to 1.0 mm. This dimension roughly corresponds to the thickness of the fibrous capsule that ultimately forms at the electrode-tissue interface.

ELECTRODE MATERIALS. In selecting electrode material, issues such as corrosion, electrolysis, tissue toxicity, and electrochemical reactions at the interface must all be considered. A variety of metallic ions, such as cobalt, silver, lead, copper, and mercury, are toxic to tissue.[40, 191] A silver–silver chloride electrode exhibits extremely low polarization properties, but because of its potential toxicity and failure to yield chronic stimulation thresholds less than those in clinical use, it has not been used to a great extent clinically. Zinc also evokes a severe tissue reaction and high thresholds.[94] Even platinum in its pure form may be toxic.[40]

Traditionally, electrode material has consisted of either corrosion-resistant noble metals and alloys or different types of carbon. Steel alloys, such as Elgiloy, can be used clinically only as a cathode because of rapid electrolysis at the anode.[216] Titanium and tantalum are excellent electrode materials, but they tend to accumulate insulating surface oxides, which produce a dielectric capacitor effect at the interface. This impedes the capacitor-coupling

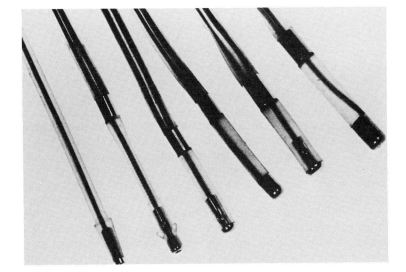

Figure 4–30. Modifications of electrode size and configuration over 19 years by a single manufacturer (Medtronic). Leads from left to right are identified by model number and electrode size: 6907, 11-mm^2 cylindrical (1969); 6962, 8-mm^2 ring tip (1977); 6904, 23-mm^2 cylindrical (1973); 5818, 48-mm^2 cylindrical (1966); 6902, 28-mm^2 cylindrical (1973); and 5816, 85-mm^2 cylindrical (1964). (From Timmis GC, Helland J, Westveer DC, et al: The evolution of low threshold leads. Clin Prog Pacing Electrophysiol 1:313–334, 1983; with permission.)

function of the electrode-tissue interface and diminishes the transfer of electrical energy.[192] The alloy of platinum and iridium (90 per cent and 10 per cent, respectively) has been used frequently as an electrode material because of its corrosion resistance, biocompatibility, and relatively low polarizing effect.[40, 165] Most clinically implanted electrodes were made of this alloy in the late 1970s. Platinum has also been applied to titanium; this process of platinizing the surface lowers polarization at the interface.

Carbon electrodes are also very biologically inert and durable. They, too, are corrosion resistant and tend to reduce polarization losses. They also tend to be more porous than polished metal surfaces, as will be discussed under "Microstructure (Electrode Surface)," further on. However, Stokes found that carbon electrodes suffer from degradative mechanisms that cause electrode pitting during stimulation. He found that in contrast to the experience of other manufacturers they are difficult to produce in volume.[192] By roughening the surface of vitreous carbon ("activation") electrodes, a double layer with a capacitance of approximtely 20 to 40 mF results. As a result, current is conducted across this barrier, capacitively eliminating the electrochemical charge-transfer reaction at the surface, which would otherwise contribute to polarization[171] (see "Polarization" above). In animal studies comparing activated carbon electrodes with platinum-iridium and Elgiloy electrodes, the platinum-iridium and Elgiloy ones displayed early current-threshold increases of 90 per cent and 190 per cent, respectively, versus only 40 per cent for carbon. A multicenter clinical study of 287 carbon-tipped leads showed that current-voltage thresholds at 18 months averaged 1.2 V. This threshold was lower than the thresholds measured at 1 month and was significantly better than comparable chronic data for metal electrodes ($P < .001$).[176] Another carbon electrode process consists of layering pyrolytic carbon (pyrocarbon) over a graphite core, to a thickness of 100 to 150 μm. This surface layer may be further modified by an "activation" process similar to that employed with vitreous carbon to reduce further the already low polarization characterizing electrodes of this material. This activation process has been shown to produce the same tissue ingrowth and reduction of capsule thickness as does porous platinum-iridium and less than that of polished metal electrodes.[75] In animal studies, consistently lower stimulation thresholds were seen at 6 weeks in pyrocarbon compared with

platinum-iridium electrodes (0.7 V versus 0.9 V and 0.75 μJ versus 0.91 μJ). Chronic Vario thresholds were shown to be consistently low and less than 1.5 V in almost half of all 121 patients studied. These results were anticipated by low rheobase values for both current and voltage thresholds at implant.[76]

MACROSTRUCTURE (ELECTRODE GEOMETRY). As previously indicated in discussing the electrophysiology of lead geometry (p. 47), current densities may be homogeneously distributed in an electrical field or have a more focused distribution, depending on their origin from electrode edges, points of greater curvature, or pointed electrode tips (Figs. 4–15 and 4–16). Accordingly, in 1976 Lagergren introduced a birdcage electrode design (Fig. 4–19, example f)[125] to utilize these concepts. Thalen introduced an annular or ring electrode configuration (Fig. 4–19, example g).[199] Babotai introduced a closed-loop helical electrode (Fig. 4–20, example g).[11] Although most of these designs continue to be clinically utilized, the ring-tip electrode has had the most extensive use in the United States. It displays lower thesholds and better R-wave sensing than do ball-tip and hemispheric electrodes of similar size[49] and lower impedances than do electrodes with both smooth and porous surfaces.[215]

Although recently electrode materials have been employed as much as geometric revisions and electrode shape to reduce polarization, this controversial determinant (among others) of pacing thresholds was perceived in the 1960s as an energy-wasting nuisance by some investigators. Lewin, Parsonnet, and their colleagues devised an electrode yielding differential current densities in an effort to reduce polarization (Fig. 4–12).[130] This electrode is constructed of a helical coil of platinum-iridium or Elgiloy, which is widened at its tip to form a cyclinder with a surface area of more than 1 cm^2. It is encapsulated in silicone rubber, with an opening at the very tip of the electrode. The large area of the wire coil results in a major reduction in polarization, and the small hole at the tip of the capsule focuses current passing through the coil, increasing its density at the electrode-tissue interface to lower excitation thresholds. Tyers and his colleagues studied this electrode extensively and confirmed lower polarization losses in association with notably higher impedances than that achieved with a variety of solid metal electrodes of various shapes.[212, 213]

Other innovations employed the focusing of current density at electrode edges and curva-

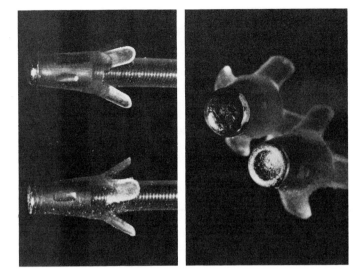

Figure 4–31. The high-impedance dish electrode (Telectronics Pty.). The dish electrode (030-227) is at the bottom in each illustration. It has a diameter of 2.3 mm, with a central concavity and a surface area of 6 mm². Apart from its shape, it is identical with the standard electrode (030-220) at the top of each illustration. (From Mond H, Holley L, Hirshorn M: The high impedance dish electrode—clinical experience with a new tined lead. PACE 5:529–534, 1982; with permission.)

tures. A dish-shaped electrode developed by Mond and associates was designed with this concept in mind (Fig. 4–31).[144] This proved to be a current-sparing high-impedance electrode. Bornzin and colleagues introduced, with Stokes, a new electrode shape that maximized the edge–current density relationship (Fig. 4–32).[30] This lead will be discussed later in this chapter.

MICROSTRUCTURE (ELECTRODE SURFACE). The term "microstructure" is employed to characterize changes in electrode surface as opposed to revisions of electrode shape. It does not necessarily refer to microscopic surface alterations, although it will be shown that microscopy illustrates these changes in bold relief. Throughout the 1960s and 1970s, most electrodes consisted of a polished metal surface. In the late 1970s, techniques were devel-

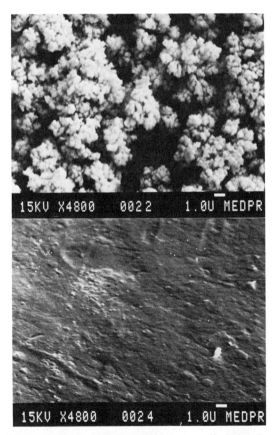

Figure 4–33. Surface electron microscopy displaying the texture imparted to a platinum electrode by the deposition of platinum black granular particles (*Top*). This is the surface used with the target-tip electrode shown in Figure 4–32. The lower micrograph displays a similarly magnified polished platinum-iridium surface. A comparison of the two surfaces graphically demonstrates how the actual surface of the platinized electrode is significantly greater; this has a favorable effect on pacemaker sensing.

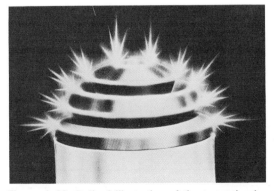

Figure 4–32. Stylized illustration of the target-tip electrode, showing the effect of the electrode edge on current density, as seen also in Figure 4–15.

oped to impart a textured quality to the electrode's surface. This texturing was developed to enhance electrode stability and to create a large surface for electrolytic contact (to reduce polarization losses) and improve both impulse and source signal transmission (Fig. 4–33). In 1978, Amundson and colleagues employed an electrode consisting of a porous body of platinum-iridium fibers compacted into a configuration similar to that of conventional solid electrodes and documented that human tissue ingrowth did indeed occur in the porous interstices of the electrode.[3] These observations were confirmed by MacGregor and his colleagues, who concluded that tissue fixation and a thinner fibrous capsule were the basis for superior long-term stimulation thresholds, which averaged less than one third of those displayed by Elgiloy electrode tips in canine atria.[137] In contrast to the Amundson electrode, theirs was produced by powder metallurgy technique. The histologic studies of

Guarda and associates and others confirmed that these new electrodes were stable and rapidly fixed and evoked a thinner fibrous capsule than did smooth platinum-iridium electrodes.[81, 83] A variety of porous electrodes have subsequently been developed; these range from porous wire baskets housing wire mesh (totally porous) to electrodes whose surface only is of a porous texture (surface porous), as shown in Figures 4–34 and 4–35.[26, 135] Surface modification has been achieved by depositing Elgiloy or platinum granules ranging from 20 to 100 μm on a solid metal surface (Fig. 4–35),[26, 65] by compacting platinum spheres ranging in size from 177 to 250 μm to impart a network of cavities and crevices (Fig. 4–36, left), or by employing a laser technique to drill holes of about 130 μm in diameter through the shell of a platinum electrode (Fig. 4–36, right).[95]

Chronic stimulation thresholds of various porous electrodes have been shown by a num-

POROUS ELECTRODE DESIGNS

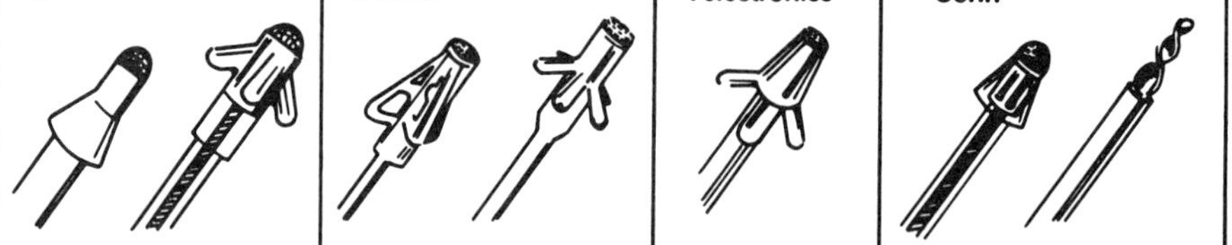

	Totally porous	Porous surface		
	CPI	Cordis	Telectronics	Sorin
Model	4116 4129-31	"Encor"	"Laserpor"	S80 S90
Material	Platinum - Platinum - Iridium Iridium	Elgiloy	Platinum	Platinum - Iridium
Distal electrode Surface area	7.5 mm² 8-9 mm²	8.8 mm²	8 mm²	8 mm² 7 mm²
Porous Technology	Coiled wire mesh with basket screen	Sintered micro spheres	"laser" pores	Sintered surface

Figure 4–34. A selection of porous electrodes is available, including those with surface porosity only as well as electrodes whose entire substance is porous (totally porous). (From MacCarter DJ, Lundborg KM, Corstjens JPM: Porous electrodes: Concept, technology and results. PACE 6:427–435, 1983; with permission.)

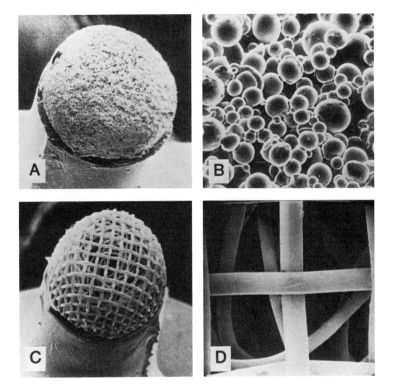

Figure 4–35. Scanning electron micrographs of the surfaces of the porous-surfaced electrode (*A*, original magnification × 20; *B*, original magnification × 500) and the totally porous electrode (*C*, original magnification × 20; *D*, original magnification × 200) showing the size of the porosity inherent in both designs. (From Bobyn JD, Wilson GJ, Mycyk TR, et al: Comparison of a porous-surfaced with a totally porous ventricular endocardial pacing electrode. PACE 4:405–416, 1981; with permission.)

ber of investigators to be as good as or better than those of polished electrodes at both the atrial and the ventricular levels.[26, 65, 81, 137] Although the impedance of these electrodes was

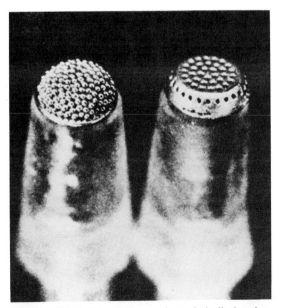

Figure 4–36. A sintered porous electrode is displayed on the left. A laser electrode is shown on the right (Telectronics Pty.). (From Hirshorn MS, Holley LK, Skalsky M, et al: Characteristics of advanced porous and textured surface pacemaker electrodes. PACE 6:525–536, 1983; with permission.)

demonstrated to be no higher than that of conventional electrodes, the polarization loss was found to be less than half (16 per cent) of that exhibited by solid electrodes (37 per cent).[12, 96] However, not all studies confirm the superior performance of porous electrode designs. Burman and associates compared 7.5-mm^2 totally porous electrodes with 8-mm^2 polished ring-tip electrodes; both consisted of platinum-iridium.[21] Strength-duration curves at implant and chronic pulse-duration thresholds were not significantly different. Breivik and colleagues compared the same porous electrodes having a stimulation area of 7.5 mm^2 and an effective sensing area of 50 mm^2 with solid electrodes 8 mm^2 and 17 mm^2 in size and found that while porous electrodes exhibited lower acute stimulation thresholds, chronic pulse-duration thresholds at 18 months were no better and sometimes worse.[36] These findings were subsequently confirmed by Antunez and colleagues.[8]

THE EFFECT OF ELECTRODE MATERIAL ON MICROSTRUCTURE. Vitreous carbon electrodes have been used in the past for muscle stimulation. Other forms of carbon that have been employed for stimulation include carbon deposited by vapor on titanium; pyrolytic carbon, as has been used in prosthetic heart valves; and carbon fiber.[175]

The primacy of materials over microstruc-

TABLE 4–3. MAIN CHARACTERISTICS OF THE LEADS STUDIED

LEAD	ELECTRICAL MATERIAL	ELECTRODE SHAPE	ELECTRODE SURFACE (mm^2)	COIL RESISTANCE (Ω)
PMCF 860, ELA Medical	Vitreous carbon	Annular	8	50
PMAF 860, ELA Medical	Platinum	Annular	8	50
S 100, Sorin	Pyrolytic carbon	Annular	7	35
BCT 112, Daig	Platinum	Annular	8	110
411S/412S, Siemens	Vitreous carbon	Hemispheric	12	125

ture is unsettled. In a double-blind study of 150 patients comparing two porous-tipped leads, one made of vitreous carbon and the other of Elgiloy (12 mm^2 and 8 mm^2, respectively), it was shown that although the current strength-duration curve was higher for carbon (1.3 mA versus 0.9 mA at a pulse-duration of 0.5 msec; $P < .0005$), impedance was considerably less (473 ohms versus 716 ohms; $P < .0005$) and that R-wave amplitudes were greater (10.2 V versus 6.8 V; $P < .0005$). Chronic stimulation thresholds were similar (1.9 versus 1.5 [Vario]) for carbon and Elgiloy electrodes, respectively.[141]

State-of-the-art Electrodes Reflecting the Interaction of Material, Macrostructure, and Microstructure

CARBON RING-TIP ELECTRODE. Several manufacturers have combined ring-tip technology with either vitreous or pyrolytic carbon, as shown in Table 4–3. The PMCF 860 ELA Medical electrode (ELA Medical, Minnetonka, MN) is displayed in Figure 4–37. The carbon surface has been further processed by "activation" to improve surface porosity. Mugica and his colleagues, comparing different carbon electrodes with polished platinum electrodes, found significantly lower chronic thresholds with only the macrostructure-microstructure-material combination. In contrast, 12-mm^2 vitreous carbon hemispheric leads failed to show significantly better thresholds.[151] Although this observation conflicts with previous studies,[176] it is supported by others.[141]

CARBON-COATED POROUS TITANIUM ELECTRODE. Vapor deposits of carbon bond strongly to titanium. This concept has been employed in the development of a new carbon-coated porous titanium electrode (Fig. 4–38).[185] Animal studies of a similar electrode employing unmodified, polished titanium showed little difference in rheobase voltage

thresholds compared with a variety of smooth and porous electrodes.[208] More recently, the new carbon-titanium porous complex was shown to be significantly better than the polished platinum ring-tip electrode in terms of voltage and current thresholds; chronic source impedance was less, and R-wave amplitude was greater. This finding achieved statistical significance, however, only for chronic stimulation thresholds, as shown in Table 4–4. As has been demonstrated with the pyrolytic carbon ring-tip electrode,[76] afterpotentials were much smaller and the histologic reaction less luxuriant than with the platinum ring-tip electrode.[185]

LASER POROUS DISH ELECTRODE. Laser-drilled surface porosity has been combined with a modified annulus-like electrode employing a dish configuration to achieve the dual

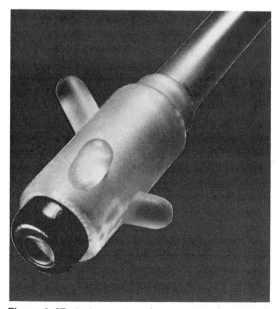

Figure 4–37. A vitreous 8-mm^2 carbon electrode employing the additional advantage of an annular configuration (PMCF 860). (Courtesy of ELA Medical, Minnetonka, MN.)

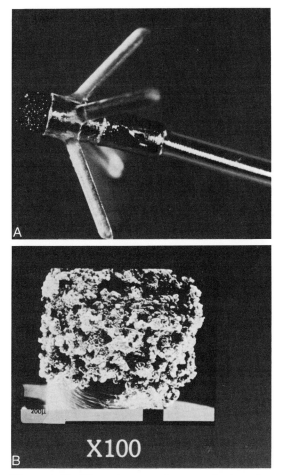

Figure 4–38. The carbon-coated porous titanium electrode (*A*). The electron micrograph (*B*) displays the spongelike structure resulting from proprietary powder metallurgy and a carbon-coating process (Intermedics). The tip consists of pure titanium particles ranging in size from 38 to 75 μm. The effective surface area is approximately 11 mm². (From Timmis GC, Helland J, Westveer DC, et al: The evolution of low threshold leads. Clin Prog Pacing Electrophysiol 1:313–334, 1983; with permission.)

advantages of edge focusing of current and an increase in effective sensing area, along with reduced polarization incident to porosity (Fig. 4–39). Mond and colleagues compared the

clinical performance of a 7.5-mm² laser porous dish electrode (Telectronics, Englewood, CO) with that of an 8-mm² solid-tip and a 12-mm² vitreous carbon electrode over an 1-year period. They found that average impedance was higher with the test electrode (701 ohms) than with the solid-tip (630 ohms) and carbon (610 ohms) electrodes ($P < .05$ for both). This electrode was specifically designed to be a high-impedance current-sparing device. Serial thresholds are given in Table 4–5. They were significantly lower with the laser porous dish electrode than with the other two varieties.[145]

TARGET-TIP ELECTRODE. Still another multifaceted design innovation incorporates the low polarizing characteristics of platinized titanium with the geometric edge-induced concentration of current density and field strength. Bornzin and colleagues investigated such an electrode, which consists of a grooved platinum surface coated with platinum black particles of less than 1 μm (Figs. 4–32 and 4–33).[30] Animal studies showed greatly reduced peaking of thresholds with fewer threshold increases in 12 weeks than was the case with a control platinum-iridium ring-tip electrode, as shown in Table 4–6.[33] Djordjevic and associates compared the performance of the target-tip 8.4-mm² electrode in 292 patients with that of a 8.0-mm² conventional ring-tip electrode in 150 patients and a 12-mm² hemispheric vitreous carbon electrode in 52 patients.[57] They found that in contrast to acute pacing and sensing thresholds, which were similar with all three electrodes, chronic Vario thresholds were about 0.7 V for the target-tip electrode compared with 1.44 V and 1.20 V for the ring-tip ($P < .01$) and carbon electrodes ($P < .05$), respectively.

STEROID-ELUTING ELECTRODE. A truly unique technologic advance in pacing electrodes was clinically introduced in 1983 by Timmis and coworkers and Parsonnet's group.[160, 206] This electrode employed a revo-

TABLE 4–4. THE CARBON VAPOR–COATED POROUS TITANIUM ELECTRODE COMPARED WITH THE PLATINUM RING-TIP ELECTRODE IN DOGS (*N* = 6)*

	VOLTAGE THRESHOLD (V)		CURRENT THRESHOLD (mA)		IMPEDANCE (Ω)		R WAVE (mV)	
ELECTRODE	**Acute**	**Chronic**	**Acute**	**Chronic**	**Acute**	**Chronic**	**Acute**	**Chronic**
Carbon-coated porous titanium	0.53 ± 0.16	0.62 ± 0.08	0.09 ± 0.26	1.23 ± 0.27	587 ± 95	521 ± 101	21.9 ± 4.9	17.9 ± 5.8
Platinum ring-tip	0.58 ± 0.12 NS	1.25 ± 0.16 $P < .01$	0.97 ± 0.21 NS	2.10 ± 0.42 $P < .05$	610 ± 92 NS	602 ± 90 NS	19.9 ± 5.6 NS	16.2 ± 5.9 NS

*Analysis for unpaired data; "chronic" refers to 6-month data; NS = not significant.

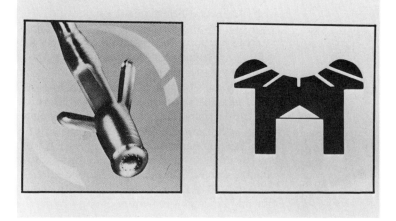

Figure 4–39. A high-impedance electrode modified with laser-bored porosity (Laserdish 030-436). (Courtesy of Telectronics, Englewood, CO.)

lutionary concept of impregnating with steroids an eluting core communicating directly with a porous channel in contact with the electrode's surface, as shown in Figure 4–40. The core consists of silicone rubber, which in a physiologic environment has been shown to release drugs at a uniform rate in a controlled and predictable fashion. Substances such as dexamethasone sodium phosphate have long been known to diffuse into and out of silicone rubber. Considering the amount of steroid adsorbed to the surface of the electrode and the porous channel as well as that in the silicone core, there is approximately 1 mg of dexamethasone sodium phosphate in the entire complex. The elution process governed by the kinetics of a concentration gradient was initially thought to occur in exponential fashion

over a period of 2 weeks. More recently, it has been suggested that this process may take up to 6 years or more.[19] The remainder of the electrode complex consists of an 8-mm[2] hemispheric titanium electrode, the surface of which has been rendered porous by sintering titanium particles both on the surface and in the channel and overlaying this with a thin layer of platinum. The remaining assembly consists of a polyurethane-tined lead.

Animal studies showed that the threshold peaking that occurs with conventional leads in the first several weeks after implantation was not seen with the steroid-eluting lead. Moreover, direct serial measurements of source impedance were significantly less than with both conventional platinum-iridium ring-tipped electrodes and identically configured

TABLE 4–5. MEAN VARIO THRESHOLDS (V)

LEAD	NO.	IMPLANT	DAY 1	2 WK	6 MO	1 YR
Solid-tip	20	0.12 ± 0.15 $P < .05$	0.23 ± 0.17 NS	1.01 ± 0.42 NS	0.93 ± 0.37 $P = .01$	0.88 ± 0.30 $P < .01$
Vitreous carbon	10	0.27 ± 0.17	0.30 ± 0	1.38 ± 0.94	1.28 ± 0.38	
Laser porous dish	20	0.21 ± 0.14 NS	0.21 ± 0.14 NS	0.90 ± 0.46 $P < .05$	0.67 ± 0.26 $P < .005$	0.62 ± 0.28

NS = not significant

TABLE 4–6. SERIAL VOLTAGE THRESHOLDS FOR THE MICROPOROUS TARGET-TIP LOW-THRESHOLD, LOW-POLARIZING PLATINIZED ENDOCARDIAL ELECTRODE*

CHAMBER	LEAD	VOLTAGE THRESHOLD (0.5 MSEC)			
		Implant	Peak	12 Wk	6 Mo
Ventricle	6971†	0.32 ± 0.05	1.50 ± 0.33	1.50 ± 0.75	—
Ventricle	1X461A‡	0.40 ± 0.13	0.61 ± 0.24	0.53 ± 0.14	0.47 ± 0.15
Atrium	6991U†	0.40 ± 0.09	2.40 ± 0.75	1.00 ± 0.18	—
Atrium	1X071A†	0.29 ± 0.08	1.00 ± 0.43	0.41 ± 0.13	0.38 ± 0.13

*$n = 9$ for ventricular leads; $n = 8$ for atrial leads.
†Standard leads, polished platinum electrodes.
‡Platinized grooved electrode leads.

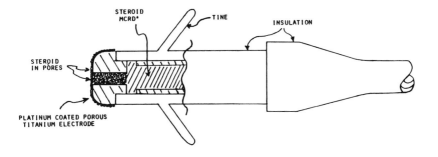

*MCRD = MONOLITHIC CONTROLLED RELEASE DEVICE.

A

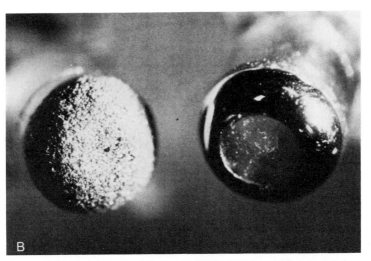

B

Figure 4–40. A steroid-eluting electrode (Medtronic 4003). This is a platinum-coated porous titanium electrode with an effective surface area of 8 mm². Its core consists of a silicone rubber, monolithic, controlled-release device that is impregnated with dexamethasone sodium phosphate (*A*). It is displayed with a conventional ring-tip electrode (6971) with a similar surface area (*B*). (From Timmis GC, Helland J, Westveer DC, et al: The evolution of low threshold leads. Clin Prog Pacing Electrophysiol 1:313–334, 1983; with permission.)

steroid-free control electrodes. Initial clinical studies on the absence of threshold peaking confirmed the observations in animals (Fig. 4–8).[206] A follow-up study was performed in two institutions in 28 patients with the steroid-eluting lead and on 14 patients with an identically configured steroid-free control lead. Serial pulse-duration thresholds at one-quarter generator output (1.35 V) showed that over a period of 18 months thresholds were consistently lower with the steroid-eluting lead than with the control lead (0.15 ± 0.05 msec versus 0.27 ± 0.004 msec; $P = .023$, ANOVA).[209] Mond and colleagues conducted a double-blind study of the steroid lead and the same control lead that we used. They employed the identical threshold tracking method and found that although there were no significant differences at implant, thresholds became significantly lower with the steroid lead shortly thereafter and were maintained throughout the study. Their pulse-duration thesholds at 26 weeks were almost identical with ours at 18 months.[142] This electrode has been shown to exhibit Vario stimulation thresholds over a period of 12 months that never exceeded 1 V at either the atrial or the ventricular level.[120] The steroid electrode has been used successfully by a number of investigators for the management of exit block.[18, 88, 116, 142]

The mechanism by which corticosteroids consistently reduce stimulation thresholds and source impedance both acutely and chronically is conjectural. It is generally assumed that glucocorticoids will suppress inflammation at the electrode-endomyocardial interface and ultimately reduce the thickness of the fibrous capsule. However, acute pharmacologic effects may also be operative via corticosteroid receptors on the endocardium or in the myocardium, which mediate an effect on the cell membrane and on myocardial excitation. These concepts are further discussed under "The Pharmacology of Myocardial Stimulation," above.

Electrode Stabilization

The stability of permanent transvenous pacing leads with no active- or passive-fixation devices was initially a grievous clinical problem; repositioning the lead in the first several weeks after implant was required in up to 30 per cent of cases in the early 1970s.[208] The necessity for lead revisions to prevent this was obvious. Accordingly, numerous stabilization devices were developed. In addition to resolving the lead dislodgment problem to varying degrees, depending on the individual modification, an additional advantage largely recognized only after the introduction of these modified leads was the reduction in the luxuriant inflammatory and fibrotic responses at the electrode-tissue interface that were seen with earlier, less stable leads. These responses are discussed under "The Histology and Pathophysiology of the Electrode-Endomyocardial Interface," above.

ACTIVE-FIXATION DEVICES. These devices include springs, deployable radiating pins or needles, and endocardial claws and screws (Fig. 4–17). The endocardial screw-in electrode evoked considerable interest, and a variety of such devices have been studied. The screw has been variously employed as a combined anchor and electrode[24, 162] or as an anchor only. The earliest screw-in electrode permanently extended from the lead and for the purpose of venous passage was shrouded by a pleated silicone skirt, which collapsed against the shank of the lead as the pointed helix was screwed into the myocardium (Fig. 4–41).[204] Other screws were retractable into the insulating sheath of the lead (Fig. 4–18).[24] These devices were first introduced in 1976—in the atrium, by Bisping and Rupe, and in the ventricle, by our own group.[204] Subsequently, they have been used with considerable success in both the atrium and the ventricle.[25, 33, 203] This device has proved to be particularly useful for patients with dilated ventricles, for those requiring difficult atrial placements, and for those who have had atrial appendectomies. Active-fixation leads have been used successfully for atrial stabilization, even without the popular preformed distal curvature to facilitate placement in the right atrial appendage.[203] Helical screw-in leads have been employed for securing ventricular leads, the insertion of which has been rendered circuitous or difficult, as with a persistent left superior vena cava.[92] Stenzl and colleagues, reporting an experience with more than 700 Bisping electrodes, had a 1 per cent dislodgment rate in the ventricle and 2.5 per cent rate in the atrium.[189] This has

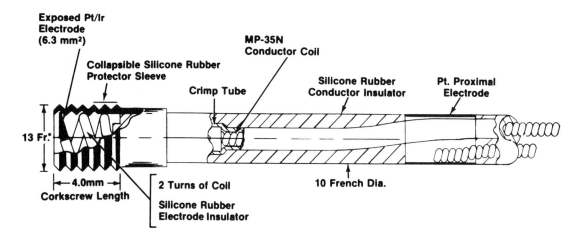

* **Fits through a 12 French tube**

Figure 4–41. A bipolar transvenous endocardial screw-in electrode (Medtronic 6954). (From Timmis GC, Gordon S, Helland J: Enhanced electrode stability: The endocardial screw. *In* Watanabe Y [ed]: Cardiac Pacing: Proceedings of the Vth International Symposium. Amsterdam, Excerpta Medica, 1977, pp 516–526; with permission.)

generally been the experience of all who have used these types of leads. If infection or other complications develop, necessitating removal of such leads, they can usually be "unscrewed," although in some cases prolonged traction may be required to extricate the lead-electrode assembly from its fibrous sheath.

PASSIVE-FIXATION DEVICES. In 1976, Lagergren introduced a basket-shaped electrode of large surface area (47 mm²) (Fig. 4–19, example f) for passive stabilization.[125] It was designed to accommodate tissue ingrowth for improved anchoring. In his follow-up report of 1985, Lagergren concluded that it was a useful revision that contributed to a reduction in lead complications, including dislodgments, to 1.2 per cent.[124] Another successful passive-stabilization lead employed a silicone fin assembly (Fig. 4–20, example e) and has been used with some success since 1976.[137] This lead was also designed for acute trabecular trapping. All four fins were connected with the column of the distal lead immediately behind the electrode. Dislocation rates were further reduced using a subsequent modification that disconnected the proximal end of two of the fins from the shank of the lead.[84] The most recently reported lead dislodgment rate was less than 0.5 per cent for 407 transvenous ventricular leads.[62]

In 1977, Babotai introduced a closed-loop helical coil electrode (Fig. 4–20, example g).[11] Acute intratrabecular fixation was achieved by a clockwise rotation and reversed by counterclockwise rotation. Such rotation avoided the snagging of endocardial structures and achieved a stabilization rate of 97 per cent. In 1979, Sloman and colleagues introduced an electrode assembly with a gas-filled balloon of small circumference located 10 mm proximal to the electrode tip.[184] It was theorized that stabilization would be achieved by insinuating the distal assembly with its balloon into the trabecular network. Unfortunately, the lead failed to fulfill its stabilization objectives and was abandoned. At about the same time, tined leads (Figs. 4–19 example h, and 4–20, examples b, c, d, and j) were introduced. One of the earliest clinical evaluations was reported by Gordon and associates in 1979.[80] Since then, tine leads have become the most commonly used stabilization device. Four radially located tines are usually employed and have gradually decreased in length and caliber as the change-over from silicone to polyurethane insulation has been made. Tined leads initially reduced reoperation rates for dislodgment to 1.5 per

cent or less.[98] More recently, others have claimed that it has virtually eliminated dislodgment.[143, 186]

There have been a number of reports detailing the difficulty of extracting both atrial and ventricular tined leads.[74, 138] A variety of reasons exist for removal of such leads, including unacceptable pacing or sensing thresholds, insulation breaks, wire fractures, and infection. If the lead system itself is infected, its removal is imperative; on the other hand, a nonfunctioning lead that remains clean and unfragmented may be left in place.[67] The experienced implanter of pacemakers has endured many problems in attempting to remove impacted leads, including insulation tears and dangerous uncoiling of the conductors, not to mention the traction placed on the heart itself, the risk of arrhythmias, myocardial trauma, valvular tears, chordal rupture, and vessel rips. Thus, the discretion advised by Furman is often the wisest course.[67]

In a comparison of a variety of active- and passive-stabilization leads, including projecting pins, flanges (the first passive-stabilization modification; Fig. 4–19, examples d, e, and g), and tines, Furman and colleagues, in two different reports involving a total of over 500 implants, failed to establish the clear superiority of one fixation device over another.[71, 72]

Lead Insulation

The lead insulator should have a high dielectric strength and high volume resistivity that persist after exposure to moisture; there should be no leakage of current in the physiologic environment. A variety of other factors, such as its biocompatibility, lubricity, tensile strength, resistance to clot formation, capacity for sterilization, and absence of toxicity, are all essential characteristics. Teflon, polyethylene, and polyester urethanes were all initially used but, in one way or another, lacked one or more of the aforementioned essential qualities of a lead insulator. Ultimately, silicone became the insulation of choice, since it fulfilled the necessary criteria for clinical use. It was the insulator employed by virtually all lead manufacturers in the 1960s and early 1970s, displaying few disadvantages and relatively few insulation failures. One disadvantage was its relatively low tear and tensile strength, which necessitated a thicker layer of insulating silicone to ensure its clinical durability. With bipolar leads and their two separate conductors, the outer dimensions of the silicone-insulated lead assembly were large and difficult to manage clinically in some cases. This factor led to their loss of popularity in favor of unipolar leads. Recently, a new high-performance platinum-cured silicone has been utilized. Compared with the older peroxide-cured silicone, it has greater strength, permitting a thinner insulating layer and smaller diameter leads.

In the mid 1970s, a search for an insulator with higher tear strength and elastic modulus was concluded with the discovery that in contrast to polyester urethane, the polyether variety of this polymer was extremely tough and elastic and displayed all the other desirable characteristics of an insulator. This finding led to a revolutionary changeover to this polymer as the insulator of choice. However, insulation failures began to appear months to a year or two after implant, sometimes at alarming rates, which ranged from 6.6 per cent to 15.0 per cent at the ventricular level.[85, 170] Most of these failures occurred at the extracardiac vascular tie-down point and involved a single bipolar lead (Medtronic 6972, Medtronic, Minneapolis, MN). In the meantime, Byrd and his colleagues, who were exclusively using a unipolar polyurethane ventricular lead (6971), found that the insulation failure rate of 454 such leads was only 0.2 per cent.[42] In contrast, they found that a unipolar polyurethane atrial lead (Medtronic 6991U) displayed the same high insulation failure rate that was being seen with the 6972 lead; insulation failures occurred in 7 per cent of their 74 atrial implants.[42] The insulation failure occurred at the point of maximal J curvature in the distal atrial lead or at the ligation site or both. Only one other manufacturer reported insulation failures (Cordis atrial lead, Miami, FL).[43] With all of these leads, the polyurethane was of the 80A variety (the number defines the polyurethane type; the letter defines its hardness). The 80A polyurethane leads of other manufacturers have been used extensively without insulation failures, but all explanted polyurethane has displayed surface changes regardless of its integrity as an insulator. These changes have been described macroscopically as "frosting" and microscopically as surface cracking. Scanning electron microscopy has shown that the surface cracks and fissures extend approximately 10 to 20 μm into the outer layers of the polyurethane.[205, 207]

Even though there had been only 104 failures in a worldwide experience with 225,000 polyurethane leads (0.044 per cent), at the time of these findings many investigators were concerned.[207] In addition, we found that there was a 10 per cent reduction in the tensile strength of polyurethane in explanted No. 4 French leads and a 33 per cent reduction in No. 6 French leads.[205] Neither electron spectroscopy nor infrared spectroscopy identified a chemical cause for the surface changes. Physiologic substances such as protein, sugars, and lipids were also exonerated. Stokes proposed environmental stress cracking as a cause.[194] When a thermoplastic material such as polyurethane is melted and extruded in a cold mold for its insulator function, surface molecules become "frozen" in conformations different from those of the core molecules.[50, 51, 66] This "freezing" results in residual intrinsic differential stresses between the skin and the core of polyurethane tubing. These stresses are compounded by the absorption of physiologic fluids, which cause the polymer to swell to the extent allowed by the tensile strength of its molecular entanglements.[190] When this limit is exceeded, the swelling force may produce breaks, especially at the interface of the soft-segment (polyether) and hard-segment hydrogen-bonding thiocyanate derivatives (polyurethane linkages). This two-phase material differs in composition between the skin (more soft segments) and the core (more hard segments) because of the manufacturing process.[53]

Surface fissures may be made worse by the application of extrinsic forces that propagate inward to the core of the polyurethane tubing. Such extrinsic forces include those from snugly stretching the polymer over the conduction coil ("interference fitting"), to which may be added the stresses of the vascular ligature and bend flexion and torsion in the distal J of an atrial lead.[163] In addition, heavy metal catalysts, such as silver ions, that are found in drawn-brazed-stranded conductor coils may induce a process of metal-catalyzed oxidation.[201] This oxidation can lead to insulation failure even at sites of lesser stress than that resulting from vascular ligation or flexion of the atrial J. It is at this latter point that polyurethane is placed over the conduction coil in a solvent-expanded state. The solvent is then removed, allowing the tubing to shrink to its original size. This process results in unusual stresses at the outer curvature of the atrial J.[43] Phillips and Thoma have recently incriminated a polyurethane–metal ion interaction that may result in a loss of key mechanical properties, such as tensile strength and flex-fatigue resistance, and may add further to environmental stress cracking. They specifically noted calcium, which is apparently selectively extracted by the polyurethane polymer, especially its soft segment.[164]

With the growing recognition that the lead must be treated gently, especially at the ligature point and especially after revisions in the manufacturing process to remove built-in stresses, the overall performance of polyurethane leads has remained clinically acceptable.[193] Hayes and colleagues reported that the prerevision failure rate of the 6972 lead was 8.8 per cent, compared with 3.9 per cent for more recently manufactured leads.[89] Beyersdorf and coworkers, reporting on their 8-year experience with 2578 polyurethane leads (Medtronic 6959 ventricular and 6957 ventricular-atrial; Bisping screw-in leads), had no insulation failures.[22] However, the polyurethane was exposed to smaller stresses, since it less snugly encased the conduction coil and screw-deploying channel assembly in these models. In describing their 5-year experience with 82 unipolar 6971 leads, Pirzada and colleagues reported two patients with insulation failure.[166] Since 1978, Byrd and associates have implanted more than 3000 polyurethane leads, over half of which use the harder (and stiffer) 55D polymer. They found that the 55D polyurethane was more durable than the 80A polymer.[43]

At the present time, polyurethane leads have a wide clinical use, and their performance compares favorably even with that of the new high-performance silicone leads.

Conductors and Connectors

CONDUCTORS. A fractured wire conductor in the body of the lead was a common reason for lead replacement in the early years of pacing. The need for replacement has been drastically reduced by using a conducting coil rather than a straight wire; this practice decreases the stresses to which the straight conducting wire was exposed. Modification of the single-wire coil (unifilar) to three (trifilar) or four (quadrifilar) wires, as shown in Figure 4–42, increased conductor flex life and decreased the high resistance inherent in unifilar coil designs. Stainless steel, because of corrosion, and alloys of platinum, because of cost, were largely abandoned. A fatigue-resistant alloy of nickel, cobalt, chromium, and molybdenum (MP35N; Dupont) and a similar alloy containing the same constituents plus iron (Elgiloy) have been used to reduce the very high early fracture rates to 1.5 per cent to 2.0 per cent

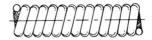

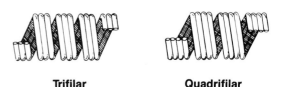

Unifilar

Trifilar   **Quadrifilar**

Figure 4–42. Schematic drawing of single, triple, and quadruple conductor coils.

per year.[192] Subsequently, General Electric introduced the drawn-brazed-stranded (DBS) stainless steel filamentous wire, which could be woven into multistrand units (Fig. 4–43). It was extremely resistant to flex stresses, and fracture rates fell to less than 0.1 per cent.[192] Upton described it as the 'tinsel wire conductor'' and found that its resistance was very low, in the range of 10 ohms, in contrast to resistances ranging from 75 to 150 ohms with MP35N and Elgiloy.[214] This low resistance rendered the conductor more energy efficient, with smaller energy losses in the conductor itself. The resultant increase in the generator current drain was shown to remain relatively small (11 per cent or less).

The silver matrix of the DBS wire tinsel proved to be a problem because of its proclivity to complex (as does calcium) with the soft polyether segments of polyurethane. This complexing was found to reduce the polymer's tensile strength and flex-fatigue resistance.[164] As previously explained, this exacerbates the process of superficial environmental stress

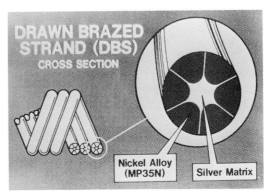

Figure 4–43. A schematic of the drawn-brazed-stranded (DBS) conductor coil. (Courtesy of Medtronic, Minneapolis, MN.)

cracking to the point where insulation failures ultimately ensue. For this reason, the use of the DBS conductor in polyurethane leads has been abandoned; however, it can apparently be used safely with silicone rubber.

CONNECTORS. A variety of proximal connector pins joining the lead to the generator have been in clinical use. These may be single or double, depending on the unipolar or bipolar configuration of the lead. More recent bipolar leads have been rendered coaxial, with a single connector pin equipped with two insulator-separated points of contact with the generator. A great deal of clinical difficulty has arisen over the nonstandard nature, caliber, length, and points of contact of connector pins, not to mention how they are secured within the generator. This nonuniformity prohibits the interchange of one manufacturer's generator with another; at times, such interchangeability is highly desirable and indeed essential when clinically important revisions have been newly engineered into a particular manufacturer's pacemaker. The industry has been variably aware of, and sympathetic with, the need for standardization. A plea was recently made for an industry-wide, voluntary standardization of the size of the connector. At the behest of Dr. Eckard Alt of the German Pacing Group, the major pacemaker manufacturers met in Torremolinos, Spain, in 1985. At this meeting, agreement was reached on the need for a voluntary standard.[44] Subsequent meetings were held by a coalition of manufacturers and physicians, who ultimately reconvened in Chicago at a meeting of the Ad Hoc Committee of Pacemaker Manufacturers in September of 1985 and finally adopted a voluntary standard. A major difference of opinion arose over the location of the sealing mechanism for the connection of the lead with the pacemaker. One group felt that the sealing rings should be on the lead (Fig. 4–44), and the other group believed as fervently that they should be in the connector cavity of the generator (Fig. 4–45). The former design was ultimately sanctioned, and virtually every manufacturer has subscribed to this voluntary standard.[44] This agreement represents a landmark in pacing, with the promise of a new spirit of cooperation throughout the pacemaker industry.

Special-Purpose Leads

ATRIAL LEADS. Many unipolar and bipolar pacing leads have been developed for atrial pacing. They basically consist of several fundamental design elements. Most leads employ a preformed distal J curvature variably maintained by the conduction coil, insulator, or both for securing the position and stability of the distal electrode either in the right atrial appendage or at its base if an appendectomy has been performed.[28, 115] The J curvature may be straightened by insertion of a guide wire for transvenous passage of the lead. The J curvature is reestablished on removal of the guide wire by the "memory" of the insulator-conductor complex.[121] Stabilization of the distal lead electrode assembly may also be secured by radially positioned tines or by an endomyocardial screw-in device, such as the Bisping lead. These stabilizing assemblies are discussed under "Electrode Stabilization," above.

The early and late efficacy of three types of transvenous atrial leads was studied by Pehrs-

SEALS ON THE LEAD

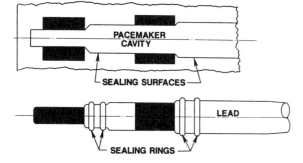

- ELECTRICAL CONTACT

Figure 4–44. Connector-pin assembly with the sealing rings on the pin. This is the configuration of the international standard (IS-1 connector assembly) that has recently been endorsed by virtually the entire pacemaker industry. (From Calfee RV, Saulson SH: A voluntary standard for 3.2 mm unipolar and bipolar pacemaker leads and connectors. PACE 9:1181–1185, 1986; with permission.)

SEALS IN THE PACEMAKER CAVITY

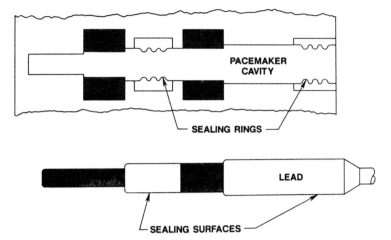

Figure 4–45. Connector-pin assembly with sealing rings within the pacemaker cavity. (From Calfee RV, Saulson SH: A voluntary standard for 3.2 mm unipolar and bipolar pacemaker leads and connectors. PACE 9:1181–1185, 1986; with permission.)

son and his colleagues.[162] Analyzing the performance of 30 screw-in leads (Vitatron Helifix-12; Dieren, the Netherlands), 40 J leads (Intermedics Lifeline 483-01), and a straight tined lead (Medtronic 6961), they were unable to identify clearly superior pacing or sensing function in any of the leads. Stimulation thresholds ranged from 0.25 to 2.50 V and were not significantly different between electrodes. Early dislodgments were confined to five Lifeline and two Helifix leads; there were no late dislodgments over a mean follow-up period of 14 months. It may be reasonably concluded that a variety of leads, some of which can be used interchangeably in the ventricle, reliably stimulate the atrium.

Atrial sensing is generally satisfactory with conventional unipolar or bipolar electrodes. Goldreyer and associates introduced an orthogonal arrangement of electrodes that were sufficiently proximal to the distal right ventricular electrode to be located in the atrium in the vicinity of its lateral wall but not in contact with it (floating), as shown in Figure 4–46.[79] "Orthogonal" refers to the circumferential location of the sensing electrodes on the pacemaker lead; this electrode arrangement is oriented on a plane perpendicular to the wave front of depolarization. The configuration of the intraatrial sensing electrode component is shown in Figure 4–47 (Cardiac Pacemakers Inc.; Minneapolis, MN). This electrode provided excellent discrimination of the atrial electrogram from the far-field QRS complex; the P/QRS amplitude ratio was approximately 32:1.[79] It has been employed for P wave–responsive ventricular pacing. A similar elec-

trode configuration has also been developed for leads designed both to pace and to sense in the atrium (Fig. 4–48).[10] The sensing electrodes with this device are also floating. Aubert and coworkers felt that these orthogonal electrodes offered superior sensing characteristics because of the large amplitude of sensed P waves and the discriminating power between P and QRS deflections (P/QRS voltage ratio of 15:1).[10] However, the atrial electrographic amplitude with either type of orthogonal lead is less than that which can often be achieved with a conventional bipolar electrode that has been stably located in the right atrial appendage.[210] Accordingly, orthogonal leads are probably most useful in certain clinically difficult circumstances of the type previously referred to.

The current selection of transvenous atrial electrodes can be implanted rapidly and reliably. The rate of dislocation of passive-anchoring atrial electrodes is similar to that of ventricular electrodes (very low); active-fixation screw-in electrodes may reduce this rate even further. The screw-in electrode offers the option of selecting other regions of the right atrium if the atrial appendage, for one reason or another, proves unsatisfactory.[117] Other options for atrial pacing are discussed in the next section.

MYOCARDIAL LEADS. Sutureless and suture-type leads have been developed for epimyocardial implantation at both the atrial and the ventricular levels. Interest in these leads was primarily the result of the early lead malposition problem, which has since been virtually solved by modifications that stabilize the en-

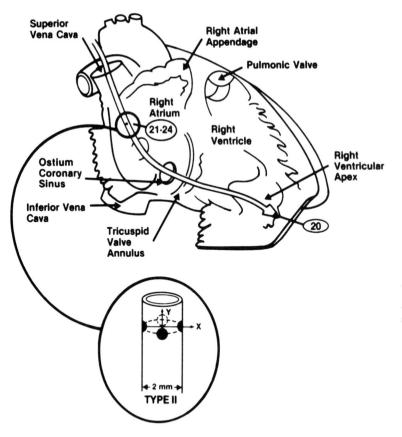

Figure 4–46. A schematic diagram of the right side of the heart is shown and labeled. An electrode catheter enters the superior vena cava, where the distal stimulating tip (20) is in contact with the right ventricular apical myocardium. Orthogonal sensing electrodes 21 to 24 are shown positioned in the high lateral right atrium adjacent to, but not in contact with, the atrial wall. (From Goldreyer BN, Olive AL, Leslie J, et al: A new orthogonal lead for P synchronous pacing. PACE 4:638–644, 1981; with permission.)

docardial lead. Nevertheless, the odd endocardial threshold problem or the opportunity to implant permanent (prophylactic) pacemaker leads at the time of surgery is such that there has been a continued interest in epimyocardial leads. In addition, it has become clinically routine to place both atrial and ventricular temporary leads at the time of surgery for postoperative atrioventricular synchronous pacing or for antiarrhythmic purposes.

Myocardial leads with suture-electrodes are inserted using a needle, which is subsequently removed, as shown in Figures 4–49 and 4–50 (Telectronics 030-168).[110] This type of electrode has been used for both temporary and permanent pacing. In contrast to the screw-in electrode, suture-electrodes are implanted by many surgeons in the right ventricle. Similar leads, used primarily for temporary pacing, are available from other manufacturers (Fig.

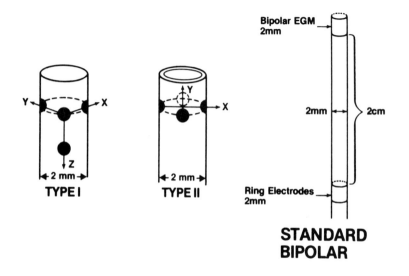

Figure 4–47. Types I and II atrial sensing orthogonal electrode configurations are demonstrated. Catheter diameter is 2 mm. In the type I catheter, poles oriented at 90 degrees represent X and Y axes; the Z axis is reflected by the electrode 2 mm more distal on the catheter. In the type II catheter, X and Y vectors are oriented 180 degrees to one another. A standard bipolar catheter with a 2-mm catheter diameter and ring electrodes placed 2 cm apart from one another is shown for comparison. (From Goldreyer BN, Olive AL, Leslie J, et al: A new orthogonal lead for P synchronous pacing. PACE 4:638–644, 1981; with permission.)

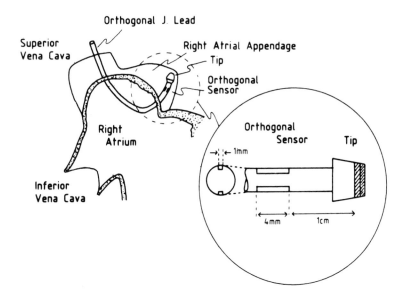

Figure 4–48. Schematic diagram of the right atrium, shown with an orthogonal J lead. The lead enters the superior vena cava, and its distal stimulating tip is in contact with the myocardium of the right atrial appendage. The orthogonal bipolar sensing electrodes are shown positioned in the right atrial appendage adjacent to, but not in contact with, the wall. (Reprinted with permission from the American College of Cardiology. Journal of the American College of Cardiology, Vol 9, 1987, pp 308–315.)

4–51).[39] The electrodes of single-pass myocardial suture-type leads range in area from 7.5 mm^2 (Medtronic 6400) to 25.0 mm^2 (Telectronics 030-168). Two myocardial suture-electrodes may be placed in parallel on either the atrium or the ventricle for bipolar pacing, although one electrode usually suffices, with the second electrode in an extracardiac location serving as a reference lead.[37] Breivik's group found that at the atrial level constant-current bipolar temporary pacing thresholds after cardiac surgery ranged from 0.65 mA to 2.30 mA.[38] Parsonnet and Bhatti have employed a single myocardial wire with two separate electrodes for tempo-

rary postoperative dual-chamber bipolar pacing.[159] With the availability of external physiologic atrioventricular sequential pacing generators (e.g., Medtronic model 5330), only two wires, rather than four—one at the atrial level and the other at the ventricle—need to be employed. This arranagement was found to be facile and reliable. Comparisons of the Medtronic 6400 7.5-mm^2 electrode with the Davis and Geck electrode, which is 4 cm long (Fig. 4–51), have shown that right ventricular current thresholds were significantly lower with the smaller 6400 electrode (3.4 mA versus 10.0 mA; $P < .001$).[39, 222] Suture-type leads may be

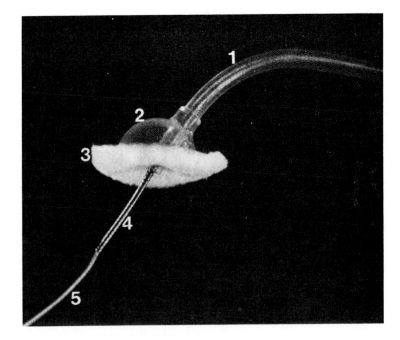

Figure 4–49. The lead (1), silicone-half bubble (2), Dacron felt patch (3), stimulating electrode (4), and suture (5). (From Jausseran J, Timpone G, Formichi M, et al: Clinical use of a new myocardial electrode. PACE 5:495–500, 1982; with permission.)

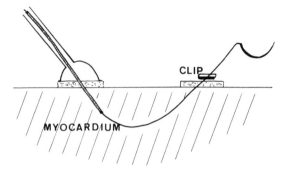

Figure 4–50. Method of implantation of the leads shown in Figure 4–49 (Telectronics 030-168). (From Jausseran J, Timpone G, Formichi M, et al: Clinical use of a new myocardial electrode. PACE 5:495–500, 1982; with permission.)

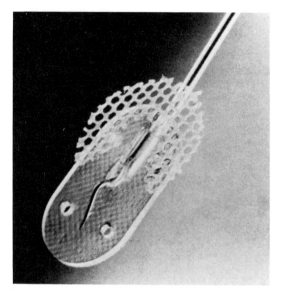

Figure 4–52. The Medtronic Model 4951 "stab-in" or "fish hook" epicardial pacing lead, viewed obliquely from the myocardial aspect. (From Michalik RE, Williams WH, Zorn-Chelton S, et al: Experience with a new epimyocardial pacing lead in children. PACE 7:831–838, 1984; with permission.)

removed by gentle traction or left in situ after the maximal length of external segment has been surgically severed at the skin using gentle traction.

Sutureless leads have employed a "stab-in" electrode with a fish hook configuration at the atrial level (Fig. 4–52)[140] and a corkscrew electrode shape at the ventricular level (Fig. 4–53)[55]; the former electrode (Medtronic 4951) may also be used at the ventricular level. Acute voltage thresholds using a stimulation duration of 1 msec remained 1.5 V or less within the first 9 days in 26 consecutive human adult atrial implants.[27] Similar results were reported for 10 atrial and 18 ventricular stab-in leads implanted in 16 infants and children.[140] Implant voltage thresholds were 1 V or less at a pulse

duration of 0.5 msec in all but two cases. In a study of more than 100 patients, the sutureless screw-in electrode displayed mean implant thresholds of less than 1 V in over 80 per cent of patients, with R-wave amplitudes of 4 mV or more.[54] The screw-in lead may be implanted using either a transmediastinal approach or the riskier subxyphoid approach. The latter approach has a total hospital mortality of 4 per cent, although hospital morbidity is less than that with the transmediastinal procedure.[16] Recent results have shown that late critical elevation of the pacing threshold is surprisingly frequent, especially when a two-turn screw-in variety of electrode (versus the three-turn type) has been employed (Fig. 4–54).[119] In a comparison of the screw-in (Medtronic 6917-35A) and suture-type (Telectronics 030-170) epimyocardial electrodes (Fig. 4–53), DeLeon and associates found that exit block was more likely to occur with the screw-in lead.[55] Other ventricular and atrial sutureless leads are shown in Figures 4–55 and 4–56, respectively.[192]

Although many surgeons prefer to use the right ventricle even for epidmyocardial pacing, others feel that because of its greater thickness the left ventricle is a distinctly superior site for pacing.[119] The electrode should be implanted in a healthy-appearing segment of myocardium devoid of vessels or epicardial fat.[153]

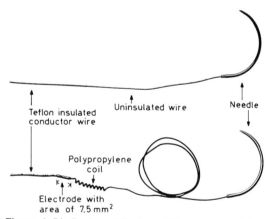

Figure 4–51. Davis and Geck multifilamentous stainless steel heart wire (*top*) and Medtronic Model 6400 temporary pacing lead (*bottom*). (From Breivik K, Engedal H, Segadal L, et al: New temporary pacing lead for use after cardiac operations. J Thorac Cardiovasc Surg 84:787–794, 1982; with permission.)

Figure 4–53. Sutureless (SLE) and suture-type (STE) electrodes. The SLE had a larger head (H), measuring 7 × 14 mm (height × length). The Dacron patch was trimmed to show the head clearly. The surface area (*arrow*) is smaller (11 mm²). The STE has a smaller head or collar (C), measuring 3 × 6 mm (height × length). The surface area (*arrow*) is larger (55 mm²). The Mersilene suture attached to the tip was cut. (From DeLeon SY, Ilbawi MN, Koster N, et al: Comparison of the sutureless and suture-type epicardial electrodes in pediatric cardiac pacing. Ann Thorac Surg 33:273–276, 1982; with permission.)

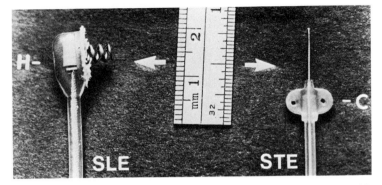

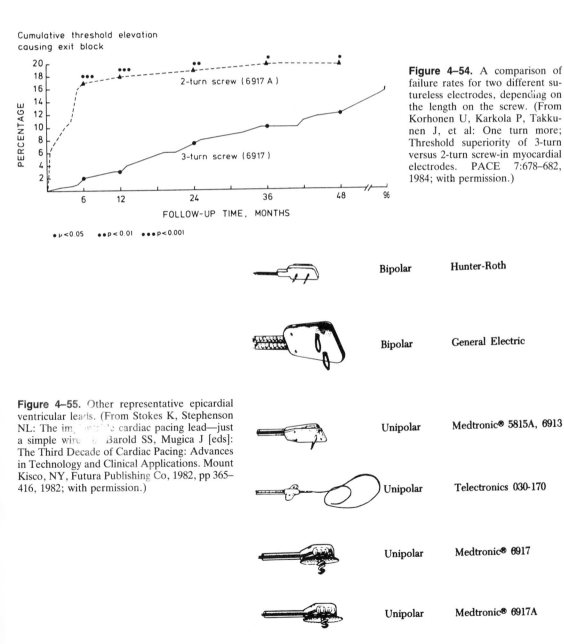

Figure 4–54. A comparison of failure rates for two different sutureless electrodes, depending on the length on the screw. (From Korhonen U, Karkola P, Takkunen J, et al: One turn more; Threshold superiority of 3-turn versus 2-turn screw-in myocardial electrodes. PACE 7:678–682, 1984; with permission.)

Figure 4–55. Other representative epicardial ventricular leads. (From Stokes K, Stephenson NL: The implantable cardiac pacing lead—just a simple wire? *In* Barold SS, Mugica J [eds]: The Third Decade of Cardiac Pacing: Advances in Technology and Clinical Applications. Mount Kisco, NY, Futura Publishing Co, 1982, pp 365–416, 1982; with permission.)

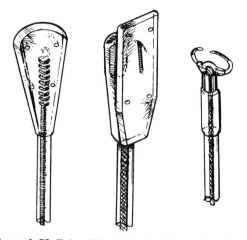

Figure 4–56. Epicardial atrial leads. Left to right, Cordis "9-turn," Medtronic 5815A (Modified), and Medtronic 6995 ("Pinch-on"). (From Stokes K, Stephenson NL: The implantable cardiac pacing lead—just a simple wire? *In* Barold SS, Mugica J [eds]: The Third Decade of Cardiac Pacing: Advances in Technology and Clinical Applications. Mount Kisco, NY, Futura Publishing Co, 1982, pp 365–416, 1982; with permission.)

TEMPORARY LEADS. Temporary myocardial leads may be implanted at the time of cardiac surgery for conventional asynchronous demand pacing, for sequential atrioventricular pacing, or for antiarrhythmic purposes. In the nonsurgical setting, most temporary leads are of the endocardial type and are usually inserted at the bedside with the guidance of intracardiac electrography on portable fluoroscopy. Filamentous small-caliber catheter-electrode assemblies and balloon-mounted flow-directed

catheters have been employed for this purpose. Pacing wires may be passed through a flow-directed catheter, such as the Swan-Ganz Paceport catheter (model 98-100H, American Edwards Laboratories, Santa Ana, CA; Chandler Transluminal V-Pacing Probe). The same manufacturer (American Edwards Laboratories) designed a balloon-mounted flow-directed single-pass bifocal pacing catheter for physiologic pacing, as shown in Figure 4–57 (balloon not shown at tip). Semirigid standard bipolar electrode catheters may be inserted in the catheter laboratory. In a study comparing the latter type of pacing catheter with balloon-tipped flow-guided leads for ventricular pacing, Lang and colleagues found that the flow-guided devices were superior to the semirigid catheter electrodes in four respects: shorter insertion time (6 minutes and 45 seconds versus 13 minutes and 30 seconds), fewer displacements (13 per cent versus 32 per cent), longer stability interval (4.4 days versus 1.4 days), and fewer arrhythmias (1.5 per cent versus 20.4 per cent). These differences were all statistically significant.[127] Temporary transvenous pacing leads may be inserted peripherally into veins in the arm or groin or more centrally via percutaneous entry into the subclavian vein.[132]

A variety of transesophageal leads are available for either atrial or ventricular pacing as well as physiologic P wave–synchronous ventricular pacing. If atrial pacing is intended, the stimulation electrode should be placed 7 to 11 cm above the gastroesophageal junction; for ventricular pacing, it is placed 2 to 4 cm above

Final Catheter Position

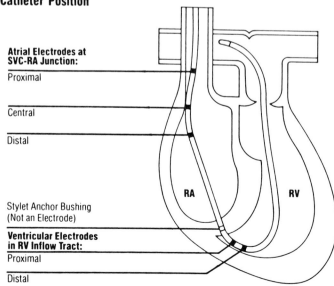

Atrial Electrodes at SVC-RA Junction:

Proximal

Central

Distal

Stylet Anchor Bushing (Not an Electrode)

Ventricular Electrodes in RV Inflow Tract:

Proximal

Distal

RA   RV

Figure 4–57. Flow-directed multipolar temporary pacing lead. The balloon located at the distal tip of this multipurpose Swan-Ganz thermodilution catheter is not shown. SVC = superior vena cava; RA = right atrium; RV = right ventricle. (American Edwards Laboratories, reprinted with permission. Swan-Ganz® is a registered trademark of American Edwards Laboratories.)

the junction.[4] Although the mean distance from the nostrils to the atrioventricular groove is about 40 ± 4 cm, this distance is highly variable from individual to individual. The esophageal electrogram may also be employed to locate the stimulating electrode.[149] However, there are those who have found that neither the amplitude nor the configuration of the atrial electrogram is useful in determining the position of esophageal electrodes.[23] Virtually any pacemaker lead may be employed for esophageal pacing. Quadripolar catheters have been found to be useful for bipolar pacing while at the same time recording bipolar esophageal electrograms.[114] The esophageal "pill," which has been used for transesophageal atrial electrography, has recently been found to be useful for pacing as well.[111] The pill electrode is contained within a gelatin capsule, which is tethered to a filamentous pacing wire that can be swallowed. Its location can be determined by the esophageal electrogram. Current levels of 25 mA were found to be effective in sustaining capture with long-term pacing (4 hours). Currents of greater than 60 mA were shown to produce esophageal injury in animals; however, this level considerably exceeds clinical thresholds.[111]

PHYSIOLOGIC SINGLE-CHAMBER PACING. The cardiovascular system has been finely tuned to accommodate changes in metabolic needs. One component of this fundamental property is the change in heart rate that occurs in response to a variety of neurohumoral and metabolic stimuli. Heart rate inversely "conditions" the QT interval, shortening it at higher heart rates. Catecholamines, which increase during exercise and stress, may independently shorten the QT interval even in pacemaker-dependent patients. This relationship of an evoked QT interval to changing humoral and metabolic conditions was studied by Rickards and Norman in 1981.[174] In 1982, an evoked T-wave–sensing generator was introduced into clinical trials (Quintech, Vitatron/Medial, Dieren, the Netherlands). The system employs a conventional unipolar pacing electrode with a pacemaker that is capable of measuring the timing interval from the pacing pulse to the evoked T-wave following a stimulated ventricular depolarization.[59] This lead, paired with sensing circuitry equipped with a multiply adjustable sensing gain (0.5 to 5.0 mV), has been found by a number of investigators to achieve rate-responsive pacing, which more physiologically reflects changing metabolic burdens.[56, 61, 173] Boute and colleagues found that the evoked T-wave amplitude was

higher than 0.75 mV in more than 94 per cent of 1500 patients with pacemakers.[31] They showed that certain electrode characteristics, such as a surface area of less than 12 mm[2], a porous surface structure (especially carbon), and atraumatic passive fixation, facilitated T-wave sensing.

A variety of nonelectrographic biologic signals may be detected to adjust pacemaker discharge rate. Variation in ventricular volume may be measured by an impedance technique using a conventional quadripolar catheter electrode assembly in the right ventricle. By emitting a very high-frequency, low-amplitude electric field using the most distal and proximal electrodes, while employing two intervening electrodes to sense impedance changes, a continuous measurement may be derived that is related to the volume of blood between the sensing electrodes and therein to right ventricular volume.[41, 172] Humorally mediated decreases in end-systolic volume during exercise may be similarly detected for an appropriate adjustment in stimulation rate.[172] This system has not as yet been in clinical trials.

Electrodes that are sensitive to changes in the temperature of mixed venous blood (for example, during exercise) have been under development for several years. Leads with a thermistor located 30 to 50 mm proximal to a distal stimulating electrode have been able to detect changes ranging from 0.60 to 0.75°C at intermediate levels of physical effort and as much as 1.35°C at high levels of physical activity (Fig. 4–58).[122] These temperature changes were shown to begin 20 to 40 seconds following the onset of exercise. The almost parallel relationship between central venous temperature and heart rate has been repeatedly reconfirmed both in animals[1, 112] and, more recently, in humans (Fig. 4–59).[2] Temperature-sensitive leads have been linked to a microcomputer-based cardiac pacemaker control system.[63, 197] Fully implantable systems are now in clinical trials in Europe. A schematic of the temperature-sensitive lead component of this system is shown in Figure 4–60.[13]

One of the earliest metabolically sensitive systems to have been implanted in humans was the pH-triggered pacemaker, first described by Cammilli and associates in 1978.[45] This system employed a standard right ventricular unipolar pacing lead and an iridium oxide electrode in the right atrium for sensing changes in blood pH.[156] The pH-sensing loop is closed by a silver–silver chloride reference electrode on the generator can. The relationship of blood

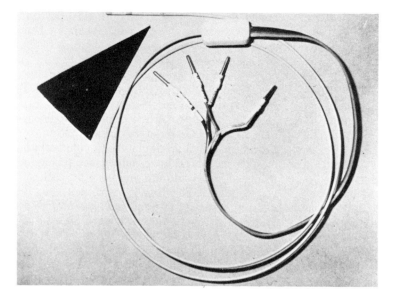

Figure 4–58. Bipolar pacing lead with integrated thermistor (*arrowhead*). (From Laczkovics A: The central venous blood temperature as a guide for rate control in pacemaker therapy. PACE 7:822–830, 1984; with permission.)

acidity over time to exercise is shown in Figure 4–61. A fall in pH triggers an increase in heart rate and presumably cardiac output. In seven human implants, acute rate control was found to be satisfactory, as was the case in at least one chronic (14 months) implant.[45, 46] There has been some concern expressed that the elements of acidity may prove destructive to the sensing electrode over time.[6]

In 1983, Rossi and colleagues described a fully implantable automatic heart rate adjustable pacemaker system triggered by changes in respiratory rate.[179] Since under physiologic circumstances the respiratory rate, reflecting carbon dioxide production, tends to change in parallel with heart rate, it has been employed to trigger adjustments in pacemaker stimula-

tion rate in patients with abnormalities of impulse formation or conduction. A fully implantable system (Biorate, Bologna, Italy) has been under study since 1983; its general configuration is shown in Figure 4–62.[179] The respiratory rate is detected by changes in electrical impedance between the pacemaker can and the auxillary electrode. Myocardial stimulation is achieved with any new or previously implanted conventional pacemaker lead. This system has been used clinically at both the atrial and especially the ventricular level, resulting in the achievement of consistently higher levels of physical activity than was possible with fixed-rated ventricular pacing.[178] More recently, efforts to confine the system to a totally intracardiac location have been under

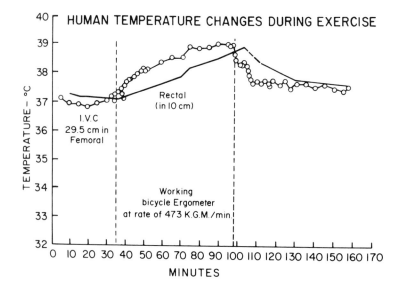

Figure 4–59. Human inferior vena cava (IVC) and rectal temperatures recorded during rest and during exercise on a bicycle ergometer. (Redrawn from data of Bazett. From Jolgren D, Fearnot N, Geddes L: A rate-responsive pacemaker controlled by right ventricular blood temperature. PACE 7:794–801, 1984; with permission.)

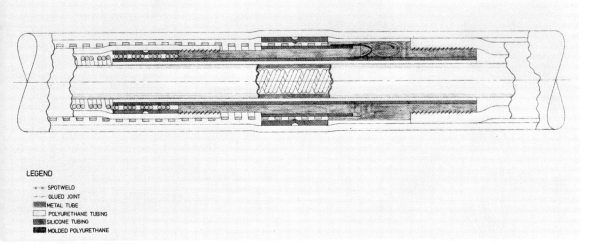

LEGEND

- ✶✶ SPOTWELD
- ⌒⌒ GLUED JOINT
- ▓ METAL TUBE
- ▢ POLYURETHANE TUBING
- ▨ SILICONE TUBING
- ▦ MOLDED POLYURETHANE

Figure 4–60. Diagram of the portion of the temperature-sensing lead where the thermistor is connected. A metal tube provides a rigid anchor and strain relief for the small thermistor wires. (From Baker RG Jr, Phillips RE, Frey ML, et al: A central venous temperature sensing lead. PACE 9:965, 1986; with permission.)

study. Using a quadripolar arrangement, Nappholtz and coworkers have shown that a current field can be established between a right ventricular floating electrode and the pacemaker can and that voltage and impedance measurements can be achieved with sensing electrodes in the superior vena cava and the pacemaker can.[154] Recent studies showed that

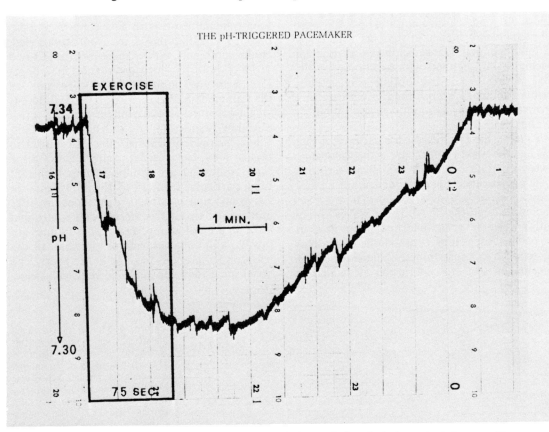

Figure 4–61. Variations of venous blood pH before, during, and after physical exercise in humans. (From Cammilli L, Alcidi L, Papeschi G, et al: Preliminary experience with the pH-triggered pacemaker. PACE 1:448–457, 1978; with permission.)

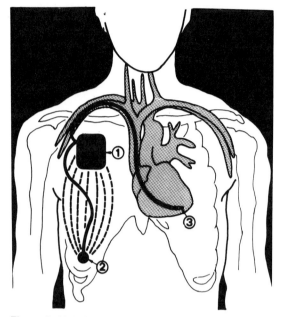

Figure 4–62. Diagram of the respiration-dependent pacemaker system. (1) Pacemaker, (2) auxiliary lead, and (3) pacing lead. (From Rossi P, Plicchi G, Canducci G, et al: Respiratory rate as a determinant of optimal pacing rate. PACE 6:502–507, 1983; with permission.)

aerobic threshold ($P < .001$), oxygen uptake ($P < .001$), and cardiac output ($P < .05$) were all significantly higher in patients with respiration-dependent rate-responsive ventricular pacing than in patients with fixed-rate ventricular pacing.[181] Cardiac output was actually higher (about 12 L/min) than in patients with atrioventricular synchronous pacing (about 11 L/min).

To date, the rate-responsive pacemaker that has had the widest clinical use is the Medtronic Activitrax unit.[5] This is a ballistic-sensitive system that detects low-frequency mechanical resonances or pressure waves that are conducted through the body. These waves, along with movement of the pacemaker can itself in its pocket, as well as contractions of muscles adjacent to it, cause minute deflections of the pacemaker can, to the inside of which is

bonded a piezoelectric sensor. The sensor transforms mechanical energy into electrical energy, which triggers increments in the basic stimulation rate.[102] Thus, the sensing system is the can itself with the modifications described. Pacing can be achieved with either a conventional unipolar or a bipolar electrode.[131] Initial studies suggested that while exercise duration and maximal oxygen consumption were similar in the activity-sensing and fixed-rate modes, anaerobic threshold and cardiac output were higher in the former.[102] More recently, a multiinstitutional study of 120 patients whose pacemakers could be programmed from a fixed rate to an activity mode showed that exercise time was longer in the latter ($P < .001$).[131]

Recent comparative studies have shown that the physiologic performance of the QT-sensitive (Quintech), respiratory-dependent (Biorate), and activity-sensitive (Activitrax) pacing systems is comparable, although each system has its special attributes and weak points.[139, 223]

A more complete discussion of the biologic aspects of nonelectrographic physiologic signal sensing may be found on page 42.

SINGLE-PASS DUAL-CHAMBER PACING LEADS. These leads are available from the major manufacturers in this country and include a conventional tined ventricular electrode combined with a more proximal tined atrial J, both of which are carried in a single sheath to the point of the J curvature, as diagrammed in Figure 4–63.[20, 126] A different single-pass bifocal lead configuration was introduced by Wainwright and colleagues in 1983.[217] Their "Crown of Thorns" lead, displayed in Figure 4–64, has a radial arrangement of three atrial spines that are variably located (constant for a particular lead) 10 to 16 cm proximal to the ventricular electrode. Electrodes are situated at the tip of the three radial spines and have an area of about 5 mm². These spines are flexible and collapse back on the shaft of the lead for transvenous passage to the heart. The atrial spines and conventional ventricular elec-

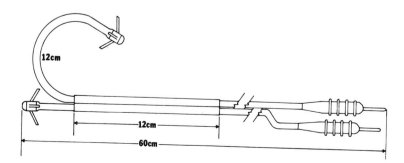

Figure 4–63. A polyurethane sheath (12 cm in length) is attached to the atrial J electrode (French No. 6). It is big enough to admit the smaller ventricular electrode (French No. 4), preserving its sliding characteristics. (From Lajos TZ: Transvenous physiological pacing—a new atrioventricular electrode. PACE 5:264–267, 1982; with permission.)

12cm

12cm
60cm

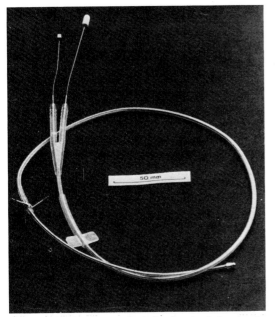

Figure 4–64. Single-pass dual-chamber lead showing the radial arrangement of the three atrial spines ("Crown of Thorns"). (From Wainwright R, Cricle J, Sowton E: Clinical evaluation of a single-pass implantable electrode for all modes of pacing. The "Crown of Thorns" lead. PACE 6:210–220, 1983; with permission.)

trodes are employed for both pacing and sensing. Clinical experience has shown that these leads can be passed with ease from either the cephalic or the jugular vein.[188] Three separate signals arise from the atrial spines. The final sensed signal passes through a mixed circuit for signal averaging; atrial signals average about 2.2 mV. There have been no complications related to lead passage in more than 270 patients. The Crown of Thorns can be used for long-term physiologic pacing with currently available atrioventricular synchronous generators.[188]

Since survival of atrial electrodes now approximates that of electrodes in the ventricle, it has been suggested that the time has come to implant leads routinely in both chambers. This recommendation is based on the fact that it is not always possible to determine in an individual case who will require physiologic pacing and who can survive having no morbidity with single-chamber fixed-rate pacing. There are times when patients display all the physiologic qualifications for asynchronous single-chamber pacing, only to display subsequently the need for a physiologic pacemaker. Accordingly, given the availability of a single-pass bifocal pacing lead, but even if two separate leads are required, this practice has been recommended.[158]

CONCLUSIONS

The pacemaker electrode has become progressively smaller as we have come to understand the importance of current density and especially field strength in the process of myocardial stimulation. We have additionally learned that electrode shape, especially when characterized by edges, sharp curvatures, and pointed tips, accentuates (focuses) current density. This observation has led to the design of a variety of electrodes, the configuration of which represents a major departure from their initial columnar or hemispheric shapes. Thus, cages, ball points, helical screws, ring tips, and other designs capitalizing on the interplay between electrode edge and current density have emerged. The very material from which the electrode is constructed has led to a reduction in polarization losses, which contribute to impedance. Reduction of polarization by the use of certain materials, including carbon and platinum black, has improved pacemaker sensing, and possibly stimulation as well, although the latter issue is still unresolved. Changing from polished metal to textured electrode surfaces has improved pacemaker sensing, since the latter yields a larger effective electrode area for signal detection. It also promotes tissue growth into the microinterstices of the electrode to facilitate stabilization while reducing the thickness of the fibrous capsule at the electrode-tissue interface. Thus, the introduction of electrodes that incorporate revisions in size, shape, and material and even steroid-eluting assemblies has provided us with a variety of state-of-the-art systems.

Other major advances have been made as well. The problem of electrode stabilization has been largely resolved by both active- and passive-stabilization devices, such as screw-in electrodes and especially by radially placed tines located immediately proximal to the electrodes; the latter are designed for intratrabecular insinuation and maintenance of intracardiac lead position. Fracture of the conductor that joins the distal electrode to the proximal connecting pin has been remedied by changing from single wires to multiple coils made from flex-resistant alloys of nickel, cobalt, chromium, and molybdenum, as well as iron in some instances. The multiplicity of connecting pin sizes, shapes, and contact points has heretofore prevented the interchangeability of generators, some possibly equipped with desirable new features with another manufacturer's lead. This problem has now been largely solved by

TABLE 4–7. SUGGESTED NOMENCLATURE CODE FOR CARDIAC PACING LEADS

POSITION I MODE	POSITION II LOCALIZATION	POSITION III FIXATION ELEMENTS	POSITION IV MATERIAL	POSITION V TIP FORM	POSITION VI SHAPES	POSITION VII POLARITY

E = endocardial
M = myocardial
p = epicardial
m = epimyocardial
	A = atrial
	V = ventricular
	D = double
	Cs = coronary
	  sinus
		S = screw-in
		Sr = screw-in
		  (retractable)
		Sd = double
		  screw-in
		A = anchored
		H = helicoid
		T = tined
		F = flanged
		O = none,
		  without
		  fixation
			C = carbon
			V = vitreous
			  carbon
			P = platinum
			Pi = platinum-
			  iridium
			E = Elgiloy
			A = alloy
				C = cylindrical
				R = ring
				S = spherical
				P = porous
				M = multiedge
				V = various
					J = J-shaped
					O = without
					  shape
					  memory
						U = unipolar
						B = bipolar
						M = multipolar

a collaborative effort between the medical community and virtually all packmaker manufacturers that has resulted in a commitment to a single standardized connector pin and generator sheath. This practice will enable patients to profit from essential advances in pacemaker design sooner than would be possible if they were rigidly restricted to using a given manufacturer's lead. Finally, advances in lead insulation have refocused interest on the bipolar electrode, which in many ways is more desirable, especially for physiologic dual-chambered pacing. Polyurethane is an insulator that continues to enjoy wide use in spite of initial insulation failures. The latter were found to be due to avoidable stresses resulting from the combined effects of certain manufacturing processes, practices, surgical excesses (especially at the venous ligature site), and undesirable metal complexing with the polymer, all of which have been largely corrected. Use of the newer forms of silicone rubber, such as platinum-cured silicone, has also permitted reduction in lead caliber.

CODE FOR PERMANENT PACEMAKER LEADS. A code for permanent pacing leads was recently devised by Bredikis and Stirbys.[32] Though cumbersome (Table 4–7), it provides a reasonably precise and succinct characterization of pacemaker leads as they currently exist.

REFERENCES

1. Alt E, Hirgstetter C, Heinz M: Measurement of right ventricular blood temperature during exercise as a means of rate control in physiological pacemakers. PACE 9:970, 1986.
2. Alt E, Hirgstetter C, Heinz M, et al: Rate control of physiologic pacemakers by central venous blood temperature. Circulation 73:1206–1212, 1986.
3. Amundson DC, McArthur W, Mosharrafa M: The porous endocardial electrode. PACE 2:40–50, 1979.
4. Andersen HR, Pless P: Trans-esophageal pacing. PACE 6:674–679, 1983.
5. Anderson K, Humen D, Klein GJ, et al: A rate variable pacemaker which automatically adjusts for physical activity. PACE 6:A–12, 1983.
6. Anderson KM, Moore AA: Sensors in pacing. PACE 9:954, 1986.
7. Angello DA, McAnulty JH, Dobbs J: Characterization of chronically implanted ventricular endocardial pacing leads. Am Heart J 107:1142, 1984.
8. Antunez F, Goicolea A, Belaza J: A comparison study of chronaxie, rheobase and threshold values for solid, porous and carbon tip electrodes. PACE 6:A–60, 1983.
9. Aubert AE, Ector H, Denys BG, et al: Sensing characteristics of unipolar and bipolar orthogonal floating atrial electrodes: Morphology and spectral analysis. PACE 9:343–359, 1986.
10. Aubert AE, Goldreyer BN, Wyman MG, et al: Sensing and pacing with floating electrodes in the right atrium and right atrial appendage. J Am Coll Cardiol 9:308–315, 1987.
11. Babotai I, Meier W: Erste klinische Ehrfahrungern mit der neuen intrakardialen Electrode "Helifix." Schweiz Med Wochenschr 107:1592, 1977.
12. Babotai I, Barberis L, Braun M, et al: Solid versus porous tip electrodes—experimental study in the dog. PACE 6:A–63, 1983.
13. Baker RG Jr, Phillips RE, Frey ML, et al: A central venous temperature sensing lead. PACE 9:965, 1986.
14. Barold SS, Winner JA: Techniques and significance of threshold measurement for cardiac pacing. Chest 70:760, 1976.
15. Barold SS, Ong LS, Heinle RA: Stimulation and sensing thresholds for cardiac pacing: Electrophysiologic and technical aspects. Prog Cardiovasc Dis 24:1, 1981.
16. Bashore TM, Burks JM, Wagner GS: The epicardial screw-on electrode. PACE 5:59–66, 1982.
17. Basu D, Chatterjee K: Unusually high pacemaker threshold in severe myxedema: Decrease with thyroid hormone therapy. Chest 70:677–679, 1976.

18. Beanlands DS, Akyurekli Y, Keon WJ: Prednisone in the management of exit block. *In* Meere C (ed): Proceedings of the VIth World Symposium on Cardiac Pacing. Montreal, PACESYMP, 1979.

19. Benditt DG, Stokes KB, Marrone JM: Long-term canine performance of a porous steroid electrode. *In* Aubert AE, Ector H (eds): Pacemaker Leads. Amsterdam, Elsevier Science Publishers, 1985, pp 323–330.

20. Benditt DG, Benson DW Jr, Stokes KB, et al: A combined atrial/ventricular lead for permanent dual-chamber cardiac pacing applications. Chest 83:929–931, 1983.

21. Berman ND, Dickson SE, Lipton IH: Acute and chronic clinical performance comparison of a porous and a solid electrode design. PACE 5:67, 1982.

22. Beyersdorf E, Kreuzer J, Zegelman M: Polyurethane insulated cardiac pacing leads: An overview after eight years. Clin Prog Pacing Electrophysiol 4:199–204, 1986.

23. Binkley PF, Bush CA, Kolibash AJ, et al: The anatomic relationship of the esophageal lead to the left atrium. PACE 5:853–859, 1982.

24. Bisping HJ, Rupp M: A new permanent transvenous electrode for fixation in the atrium. *In* Proceedings of the Vth International Symposium on Cardiac Pacing, Tokyo 1976. Amsterdam, Excerpta Medica, 1976, pp 543–547.

25. Bisping HJ, Kreuzer J, Birkenheier H: Three-year clinical experience with a new endocardial screw-in lead with introduction protection for use in the atrium and ventricle. PACE 3:424–435, 1980.

26. Bobyn JD, Wilson GJ, Mycyk TR, et al: Comparison of a porous-surfaced with a totally porous ventricular endocardial pacing electrode. PACE 4:405–416, 1981.

27. Bognolo D, Stokes K, Wiebush W, et al: Experimental and clinical study of a new permanent myocardial atrial sutureless pacing lead. PACE 6:113–118, 1983.

28. Bognolo DA, Vijayanagar RR, Eckstein PF, et al: Permanent transvenous atrial pacing after heart surgery. PACE 5:870–872, 1982.

29. Borchard U, Boisten M: Effect of flecainide on action potentials and alternating current–induced arrhythmias in mammalian myocardium. J Cardiovasc Pharmacol 4:205–212, 1982.

30. Bornzin GA, Stokes KB, Wiebush WA: A low threshold, low polarization platinized endocardial electrode. PACE 6:A–70, 1983.

31. Boute W, Derrien Y, Wittkampf FHM: Reliability of evoked endocardial T-wave sensing in 1,500 pacemaker patients. PACE 9:948–953, 1986.

32. Bredikis JJ, Stirbys PP: A suggested code for permanent cardiac pacing leads. PACE 8:320–328, 1985.

33. Bredikis J, Dumcius A, Stirbys P, et al: Permanent cardiac pacing with electrodes of a new type of fixation in the endocardium. PACE 1:25–30, 1978.

34. Breivik K, Ohm O: Myopotential inhibition of unipolar QRS-inhibited (VVI) pacemakers, assessed by ambulatory Holter monitoring of the electrocardiogram. PACE 3:470–478, 1980.

35. Breivik K, Engedal H, Ohm O: Electrophysiological properties of a new permanent endocardial lead for uni- and bipolar pacing. PACE 5:268–274, 1982.

36. Breivik K, Ohm O, Engedal H: Acute and chronic pulse-width thresholds in solid versus porous tip electrodes. PACE 5:650–657, 1982.

37. Breivik K, Engedal H, Resch F, et al: Clinical and electrophysiological properties of a new temporary pacemaker lead after open-heart surgery. PACE 5:600–606, 1982.

38. Breivik K, Engedal H, Resch F, et al: Bipolar atrial application of a new temporary pacing lead after cardiac operations. J Thorac Cardiovasc Surg 85:625–631, 1983.

39. Breivik K, Engedal H, Segadal L, et al: New temporary pacing lead for use after cardiac operations. J Thorac Cardiovasc Surg 84:787–794, 1982.

40. Brummer SB, Robblee LS, Hambrecht FT: Criteria for selecting electrodes for electrical stimulation: Theoretical and practical considerations. Ann NY Acad Sci 405:159–171, 1983.

41. Burkhoff D, Van Der Velde E, Kass D: Accuracy of volume measurement by conductance catheter in isolated, ejecting canine hearts. Circulation 72:440–447, 1985.

42. Byrd CL, McArthur W, Stokes K, et al: Implant experience with unipolar polyurethane pacing leads. PACE 6:868–882, 1983.

43. Byrd CL, Schwartz SJ, Sivina M, et al: Degradation of polyurethane endocardial pacing leads: An 8 year retrospective analysis. *In* Planck H, Syre I, Dauner M, Egbers G (eds): Progress in Biomedical Engineering: 3 Polyurethanes in Biomedical Engineering II. Amsterdam, Elsevier Science Publishers, 1987, pp 65–74.

44. Calfee RV, Saulson SH: A voluntary standard for 3.2 mm unipolar and bipolar pacemaker leads and connectors. PACE 9:1181–1185, 1986.

45. Cammilli L, Alcidi L, Papeschi G, et al: Preliminary experience with the pH-triggered pacemaker. PACE 1:448–457, 1978.

46. Cammilli L, Ricci D, Risani R, et al: pH-Triggered pacemaker: Design and clinical results. *In* Meere C (ed): Proceedings of the VIth World Symposium on Cardiac Pacing. Montreal, PACESYMP, 1979.

47. Casaburi R, Whipp BJ, Wasserman K, et al: Ventilatory and gas exchange dynamics in response to sinusoidal work. J Appl Physiol: Respir Environ Exerc Physiol 42:300–311, 1977.

48. Castellanos A Jr, Lemberg L, Johnson D, et al: The Wedensky effect in the human heart. Br Heart J 28:276–283, 1966.

49. Chen P, Myers GH, Parsonnet V: Electrode geometry and pacemaker function. *In* Engineering in Medicine and Biology: Proceedings of the 29th Annual Conference, Boston, 1976, p 24.

50. Crouthamel DL, Isayev AI, Wang KK: Effect of processing conditions on the residual stress in the injection molding of amorphous polymers. Soc Plast Eng 28:295–297, 1982.

51. Deanin RD, Hauser DI: Recent developments in environmental stresscrack resistance of plastics. Polym Plast Technol Eng 17:123–137, 1981.

52. DeCaprio V, Hurzeler P, Furman S: A comparison of unipolar and bipolar electrograms for cardiac pacemaker sensing. Circulation 56:750–755, 1977.

53. DeCosta VS, Brier-Russel D, Salzman EW, et al: ESCA studies of polyurethanes: Blood platelet activation in relation to surface composition. J Colloid Interface Sci 80:445–452, 1981.

54. DeFeyter PJ, Majid PA, Hoitsma HFW: Permanent

cardiac pacing with sutureless myocardial electrodes: Experience in first one hundred patients. PACE 3:144–149, 1980.

55. DeLeon SY, Ilbawi MN, Koster N, et al: Comparison of the sutureless and suture-type epicardial electrodes in pediatric cardiac pacing. Ann Thorac Surg 33:273–276, 1982.

56. De Oro AG, Ayza MW, DeLaLlana R, et al: Rate-responsive pacing: Clinical experience. PACE 8:322–328, 1985.

57. Djordjevic M, Stojanov P, Velimirovic D, et al: Target lead—low threshold electrode. PACE 9:1206–1210, 1986.

58. Dohrmann ML, Goldschlager NF: Myocardial stimulation threshold in patients with cardiac pacemakers: Effect of physiologic variables, pharmacologic agents, and lead electrodes. Cardiol Clin 3:527–537, 1985.

59. Donaldson RM, Rickards AF: Rate responsive pacing using the evoked QT principle: A physiological alternative to atrial synchronous pacemakers. PACE 6:1344–1349, 1983.

60. Duval D, Funder JW, Devynck M, et al: Arterial glucocorticoid receptors: The binding of tritiated dexamethasone in rabbit aorta. Cardiovasc Res 11:529–535, 1977.

61. Fananapazir L, Rademaker M, Bennett DH: Reliability of the evoked response in determining the paced ventricular rate and performance of the QT or rate responsive (TX) pacemaker. PACE 8:701–714, 1985.

62. Fananapazir L, Martin TS, Martin V, et al: Experience with 407 transvenous, finned pacing leads with a sintered porous-surfaced electrode. PACE 7:132–135, 1984.

63. Fearnot NE, Jolgren DL, Tacker WA, et al: Increasing cardiac rate by measurement of right ventricular temperature. PACE 7:1240–1245, 1984.

64. Fischler H: Polarization properties of small-surface-area pacemaker electrodes—implications on reliability of sensing and pacing. PACE 2:403–416, 1979.

65. Freud GE, Chinaglia B: Sintered platinum for cardiac pacing. Int J Artif Organs 4:238–242, 1981.

66. Fujiyama M, Azuma K: Skin/core morphology and tensile impact strength of injection-molded polypropylene. J Appl Pol Sci 23:2807–2811, 1979.

67. Furman S: Pacemaker lead extraction. PACE 7:937, 1984.

68. Furman S: Basic concepts. In Furman S, Hayes DL, Holmes DR Jr (eds): A Practice of Cardiac Pacing. Mount Kisco, NY, Futura Publishing Co, 1986, p 27.

69. Furman S, Robinson G: The use of an intracardiac pacemaker in the correction of total heart block. Surg Forum 9:245, 1958.

70. Furman S, Hurzeler P, Parker B: Clinical thresholds of endocardial cardiac stimulation: A long-term study. J Surg Res 19:149–155, 1975.

71. Furman S, Pannizzo F, Campo I: Comparison of active and passive adhering leads for endocardial pacing. PACE 2:417–427, 1979.

72. Furman S, Pannizzo F, Campo I: Evaluation of new equipment. PACE 4:78–83, 1981.

73. Furman S, Parker B, Escher D, et al: Decreasing electrode size and increasing efficiency of cardiac stimulation. J Surg Res 11:105–110, 1971.

74. Furstenberg S, Bluhm G, Olin C: Entrapment of an atrial tined pacemaker electrode in the tricuspid valve—a case report. PACE 7:760–762, 1984.

75. Gadaleta G, Lunati M, Guarda F, et al: A comparison of histological reactions caused by leads of different design: Polished platinum, sintered platinum and pyrolytic carbon. PACE 6:A–69, 1983.

76. Garberoglio B, Inguaggiato B, Chinaglia B, et al: Initial results with an activated pyrolytic carbon tip electrode. PACE 6:440–447, 1983.

77. Gettes LS, Shabetai R, Downs TA, et al: Effect of changes in potassium and calcium concentrations on diastolic threshold and strength-interval relationships of the human heart. Ann NY Acad of Sci 167:693–705, 1969.

78. Gillette P: Critical analysis of sensors for physiological responsive pacing. PACE 7:1263–1266, 1984.

79. Goldreyer BN, Olive AL, Leslie J, et al: A new orthogonal lead for P synchronous pacing. PACE 4:638–644, 1981.

80. Gordon S, Timmis GC, Ramos RG, et al: Improved transvenous pacemaker electrode stability. In Meere C (ed): Proceedings of the VIth World Symposium on Cardiac Pacing. Montreal, PACE-SYMP, 1979.

81. Gould L, Patel C, Becker W: Long-term threshold stability with porous tip electrodes. PACE 9:1202–1205, 1986.

82. Griffin JC, Jutzy KR, Claude JP, et al: Central body temperature as a guide to optimal heart rate. PACE 6:498–501, 1983.

83. Guarda F, Galloni M, Assone F, et al: Histological reactions of porous tip endocardial electrodes implanted in sheep. Int J Artif Organs 5:267–273, 1982.

84. Hakki A, Horowitz LN, Reiser J, et al: Improved pacemaker fixation and performance using a modified finned porous surface tip lead. Int Surg 69:291–294, 1984.

85. Hanson JS: Sixteen failures in a single model of bipolar polyurethane-insulated ventricular pacing lead: A 44-month experience. PACE 7:389–394, 1984.

86. Harthorne JW: Pacemaker leads. Int J Cardiol 6:423–429, 1984.

87. Hauser RG: Bipolar leads for cardiac pacing in the 1980s: A reappraisal provoked by skeletal muscle interference. PACE 5:34–37, 1982.

88. Hayes DL, Broadbent JC, Holmes DR, et al: Steroid-tipped leads: 1-year follow-up. In Aubert AE, Ector H (eds): Pacemaker Leads. Amsterdam, Elsevier Science Publishers, 1985, pp 317–322.

89. Hayes DL, Holmes DR Jr, Merideth J, et al: Bipolar tined polyurethane ventricular lead: A four-year experience. PACE 8:192–196, 1985.

90. Hellestrand KJ, Burnett PJ, Milne JR, et al: Effect of the antiarrhythmic agent flecainide acetate on acute and chronic pacing thresholds. PACE 6:892–899, 1983.

91. Hellestrand KJ, Nathan AW, Bexton RS, et al: Electrophysiologic effects of flecainide acetate on sinus node function, anomalous atrioventricular connections, and pacemaker thresholds. Am J Cardiol 53:30B–38B, 1984.

92. Hellestrand KJ, Ward DE, Bexton RS, et al: The use of active fixation electrodes for permanent endocardial pacing via a persistent left superior vena cava. PACE 5:180–184, 1982.

93. Henglein D, Gillette PC, Shannon C, et al: Long-term follow-up of pulse width threshold of transvenous and myo-epicardial leads. PACE 7:203–214, 1984.

94. Hirshorn MS, Holley LK, Hales JR, et al: Screening

of solid and porous materials for pacemaker electrodes. PACE 4:380–390, 1981.

95. Hirshorn MS, Holley LK, Skalsky M, et al: Characteristics of advanced porous and textured surface pacemaker electrodes. PACE 6:525–536, 1983.

96. Hirshorn MS, Holley LK, Skalsky M, et al: Effect of pore size on threshold and impedance of pacemaker electrodes. PACE 6:A–63, 1983.

97. Hoffman BF, Siebens AA, Cranefield PF, et al: The effect of epinephrine and norepinephrine on ventricular vulnerability. Circ Res 3:140–146, 1955.

98. Holmes DR Jr, Nissen RG, Maloney JD, et al: Transvenous tined electrode systems: An approach to acute dislodgement. Mayo Clin Proc 54:219–222, 1979.

99. Hopps JA: The development of the pacemaker. PACE 4:106–108, 1981.

100. Hughes HC, Tyers GFO, Torman HA: Effects of acid-base imbalance on myocardial pacing thresholds. J Thorac Cardiovasc Surg 69:743, 1975.

101. Hughes HC, Brownlee RR, Bertolet RD, et al: The effects of electrode position on the detection of the transvenous cardiac electrogram. PACE 3:651–655, 1980.

102. Humen DP, Kostuk WJ, Klein GJ: Activity-sensing, rate-responsive pacing: Improvement in myocardial performance with exercise. PACE 8:52–59, 1985.

103. Ikeda N, Nademanee K, Kannan R, et al: Electrophysiologic effects of amiodarone: Experimental and clinical observation relative to serum and tissue drug concentrations. Am Heart J 108:890–898, 1984.

104. Ionescu VL: An "on demand pacemaker" responsive to respiration rate. PACE 3:375, 1980.

105. Irnich W: Engineering concepts of pacemaker electrodes. In Schaldach M, Furman S, Hein F, Thull R (eds): Advances in Pacemaker Technology. New York, Springer-Verlag, 1975, p 241.

106. Irnich W: Comparison of pacing electrodes of different shape and material—recommendations. PACE 6:422–426, 1983.

107. Irnich W: The electrode myocardial interface. Clin Prog Electrophysiol and Pacing 3:338–348, 1985.

108. Irnich W: Intracardiac electrograms and sensing test signals: Electrophysiological, physical, and technical considerations. PACE 8:870–888, 1985.

109. Irnich W, Parsonnet V, Meyers GH: Compendium of pacemaker technology: II, Definitions and Glossary (part I). PACE 2:88–93, 1979.

110. Jausseran J, Timpone G, Formichi M, et al: Clinical use of a new myocardial electrode. PACE 5:495–500, 1982.

111. Jenkins JM, Dick M, Collins S, et al: Use of the pill electrode for transesophageal atrial pacing. PACE 8:512–527, 1985.

112. Jolgren D, Fearnot N, Geddes L: A rate-responsive pacemaker controlled by right ventricular blood temperature. PACE 7:794–801, 1984.

113. Jolgren D, Fearnot N, Geddes L, et al: A rate responsive pacemaker controlled by right ventricular blood temperature. J Am Coll Cardiol 1:720, 1983.

114. Kerr CR, Chung DC, Cooper J: Improved transesophageal recording and stimulation utilizing a new quadripolar lead configuration. PACE 9:644–651, 1986.

115. Kerr CR, Mason MA, Tyers GFO, et al: Transvenous atrial pacing following amputation of the

atrial appendage at open heart surgery. PACE 8:497–501, 1985.

116. King DH, Gillette PC, Shannon C, et al: Steroid-eluting endocardial pacing lead for treatment of exit block. Am Heart J 106:1438–1440, 1983.

117. Kleinert M: Permanent atrial leads. PACE 3:487–491, 1980.

118. Kleinert M: Elmqvist H, Strandberg H: Spectral properties of atrial and ventricular endocardial signals. PACE 2:11–19, 1979.

119. Korhonen U, Karkola P, Takkunen J, et al: One turn more: Threshold superiority of 3-turn versus 2-turn screw-in myocardial electrodes. PACE 7:678–682, 1984.

120. Kruse I, Terpstra B: Acute and long-term atrial and ventricular stimulation thresholds with a steroid-eluting electrode. PACE 8:45–49, 1985.

121. Kruse IB, Ryden L, Ydse B: A new lead for transvenous atrial pacing and sensing. PACE 3:395–405, 1980.

122. Laczkovics A: The central venous blood temperature as a guide for rate control in pacemaker therapy. PACE 7:822–830, 1984.

123. Lagergren H: How it happened: My recollection of early pacing. PACE 1:140–143, 1978.

124. Lagergren H: A comparison between conventional and basket transvenous electrodes. PACE 8:181–185, 1985.

125. Lagergren H, Edhag O, Wahlberg I: A low threshold non-dislocating endocardial electrode. J Thorac Cardiovasc Surg 72:259, 1976.

126. Lajos TZ: Transvenous physiological pacing—a new atrioventricular electrode. PACE 5:264–267, 1982.

127. Lang R, David D, Klein HO, et al: The use of the balloon-tipped floating catheter in temporary transvenous cardiac pacing. PACE 4:491–496, 1981.

128. Lee D, Greenspan K, Edmands RE, et al: The effect of electrolyte alteration on stimulus requirement of cardiac pacemakers. Circulation 38:1–124, 1968.

129. Levick CE, Mizgala HF, Kerr CR: Failure to pace following high dose antiarrhythmic therapy—reversal with isoproterenol. PACE 7:252–256, 1984.

130. Lewin G, Myers GH, Parsonnet V, et al: Differential current density (DCD) electrodes for pacemakers. In Engineering in Medicine and Biology: Proceedings of the 19th Annual Conference, 1966, p 165.

131. Lindemans FW, Rankin IR, Murtaugh R, et al: Clinical experience with an activity sensing pacemaker. PACE 9:978–986, 1986.

132. Littleford PO, Pepine CJ: A new temporary atrial pacing catheter inserted percutaneously into the subclavian vein without fluoroscopy: A preliminary report. PACE 4:458–464, 1981.

133. Luceri RM, Furman S, Hurzeler P, et al: Threshold behavior of electrodes in long-term ventricular pacing. Am J Cardiol 40:184–188, 1977.

134. MacCarter DJ, Jenewein CG, Schyma DH: Spontaneous subacute reduction in myocardial stimulation thresholds. In Meere C (ed): Proceedings of the VIth World Symposium on Cardiac Pacing. Montreal, PACESYMP, 1979.

135. MacCarter DJ, Lundberg KM, Corstjens JPM: Porous electrodes: Concept, technology and results. PACE 6:427–435, 1983.

136. MacGregor DC, Wilson GJ, Dutcher RG, et al: A new positive fixation endocardial pacemaker lead using an extendable/retractable helix. In Meere C

(ed): Proceedings of the VIth World Symposium on Cardiac Pacing. Montreal, PACESYMP, 1979.

137. MacGregor DC, Wilson GJ, Lixfeld W, et al: The porous-surfaced electrode. J Thorac Cardiovasc Surg 78:281–291, 1979.

138. Madigan NP, Curtis JJ, Sanfelippo JF: Difficulty of extraction of chronically implanted tined ventricular endocardial leads. J Am Coll Cardiol 3:724–731, 1984.

139. Maisch B, Langenfeld H: Rate adaptive pacing—clinical experience with three different pacing systems. PACE 9:997–1004, 1986.

140. Michalik RE, Williams WH, Zorn-Chelton S, et al: Experience with a new epimyocardial pacing lead in children. PACE 7:831–838, 1984.

141. Molajo AO, Bowes RJ, Fananapazir L, et al: Comparison of vitreous carbon and Elgiloy transvenous ventricular pacing leads. PACE 8:261–265, 1985.

142. Mond H: Experiences with Medtronic CapSure™ steroid-eluting leads. Medtronic News, Winter 1986, p 3.

143. Mond H, Sloman G: The small-tined pacemaker lead—absence of dislodgement. PACE 3:171–177, 1980.

144. Mond H, Holley L, Hirshorn M: The high impedance dish electrode—clinical experience with a new tined lead. PACE 5:529–534, 1982.

145. Mond H, Stewart S, Chan W, et al: Laser drilled porous electrode: Comparative study with conventional electrodes to assess chronic pacing thresholds. J Cardiac Soc Aust N Z, May 1985.

146. Morady F, DiCarlo LA Jr, Krol RB, et al: Acute and chronic effects of amiodarone on ventricular refractoriness, intraventricular conduction and ventricular tachycardia induction. J Am Coll Cardiol 7:148–157, 1986.

147. Morris JD, Judge RD, Leininger BJ, et al: Clinical experience and problems encountered with an implantable pacemaker. J Thorac Cardiovasc Surg 50:849–856, 1965.

148. Moss AJ, Goldstein S: Clinical and pharmacological factors associated with pacemaker latency and incomplete pacemaker capture. Br Heart J 31:112–117, 1969.

149. Moura P, Demorizi NM, MacMillan RM, et al: Esophageal P-synchronous pacing. PACE 8:374–377, 1985.

150. Mowry FM, Judge RD, Preston TA, et al: Identification and management of exit block in patients with implanted pacemakers. Circulation [Suppl] 31–32:II–157, 1965.

151. Mugica J, Henry L, Attuel P, et al: Clinical experience with 910 carbon tip leads: Comparison with polished platinum leads. PACE 9:1230–1238, 1986.

152. Myers GH, Kresh YM, Parsonnet V: Characteristics of intracardiac electrograms. PACE 1:90–103, 1978.

153. Naclerio EA, Varriale P: The sutureless electrode for cardiac pacing: Problems, advantages and surgical technique. PACE 3:232–235, 1980.

154. Nappholtz T, Valenta H, Maloney J, et al: Electrode configurations for a respiratory impedance measurement suitable for rate responsive pacing. PACE 9:960–964, 1986.

155. Nielsen AP, Cashion R, Spencer WH, et al: Long-term assessment of unipolar and bipolar stimulation and sensing thresholds using a lead configuration programmable pacemaker. J Am Coll Cardiol 5:198–204, 1985.

156. Papeschi G, Bordi S, Carla M, et al: An iridium–

157. Parker B, Furman S, Hurzeler P, et al: Electrode geometry and the evolution of long-term endocardial threshold. In Engineering in Medicine and Biology: Proceedings of the 27th Annual Conference, 1974, p 98.

158. Parsonnet V: Routine implantation of permanent transvenous pacemaker electrodes in both chambers. A technique whose time has come. PACE 4:109–112, 1981.

159. Parsonnet V, Bhatti M: A technique for postoperative application of a newly designed temporary bipolar dual-chamber pacemaker electrode. J Thorac Cardiovasc Surg 89:456–458, 1985.

160. Parsonnet V, Werres R: Clinical experience with a porous-tip steroid-loaded ventricular pacing electrode. PACE 6:319, 1983.

161. Parsonnet V, Crawford CC, Bernstein AD, et al: The 1981 United States Survey of Cardiac Pacing Practices. J Am Coll Cardiol 3:1321–1332, 1984.

162. Pehrsson SK, Bergdahl L, Svane B: Early and late efficacy of three types of transvenous atrial leads. PACE 7:195–202, 1984.

163. Phillips R, Frey M, Martin RO: Long-term performance of polyurethane pacing leads: Mechanisms of design-related failures. PACE 9:1166–1172, 1986.

164. Phillips RE, Thoma RJ: Metal ion complexation of polyurethane: A proposed mechanism for calcification. In Planck H et al (eds): Polyurethanes in Biomedical Engineering II: Proceedings of the 2nd International Conference on Polyurethanes in Biomedical Engineering. Amsterdam, Elsevier Science Publishers, 1987, pp 91–108.

165. Pioger G, Garberoglio B: Pacemaker electrodes and problems related to cardiac pacing and sensing: Current solutions and future trends. Life Support Syst 2:169–182, 1984.

166. Pirzada FA, Seltzer JP, Blair-Saletin D, et al: Five-year performance of the Medtronic 6971 polyurethane endocardial electrode. PACE 9:1173–1180, 1986.

167. Platia EV, Brinker JA: Time course of transvenous pacemaker stimulation impedance, capture threshold, and electrogram amplitude. PACE 9:620–625, 1986.

168. Preston TA, Judge RD: Alteration of pacemaker threshold by drug and physiological factors. Ann NY Acad Sci 167:686–692, 1969.

169. Preston TA, Fletcher RD, Lucchesi BR, et al: Changes in myocardial threshold: Physiologic and pharmacologic factors in patients with implanted pacemakers. Am Heart J 74:235–242, 1967.

170. Raymond RD, Nanian KB: Insulation failure with bipolar polyurethane pacing leads. PACE 7:378–380, 1984.

171. Richter GJ, Weidlich E, Rao JR, et al: Chronic threshold of stimulating electrodes: Comparison of activated vitreous carbon with conventional platinum-iridium electrodes in animal tests. Med Prog Technol 8:67–76, 1981.

172. Rickards AF: Rate-responsive pacing. In Barold SS (ed): Modern Cardiac Pacing. Mount Kisco, NY, Futura Publishing Co, 1985, pp 799–809.

173. Rickards AF, Donaldson RM: Rate responsive pacing. Clin Prog Pacing Electrophysiol 1:12–19, 1983.

174. Rickards AF, Norman J: Relation between QT interval and heart rate: New design of a physiologically adaptive cardiac pacemaker. Br Heart J 45:56, 1981.

175. Ripart A, Mugica J: Electrode-heart interface: Def-

inition of the ideal electrode. PACE 6:410–421, 1983.

176. Ross AM, Hohler H, Gundersen T: Siemens Elema tined carbon tip lead: A multicenter study of acute and long term thresholds as measured by the vario function of the Siemens Elema Model 668 pacemaker. PACE 6:A–68, 1983.

177. Ross J Jr, Covell JW: Electrical impulse formation and conduction in the heart. *In* Vardoulakis K (ed): Best and Taylor's Physiological Basis of Medical Practice. 11th ed. Baltimore, The Williams & Wilkins Co, 1985, pp 148–162.

178. Rossi P, Aina F, Rognoni G, et al: Increasing cardiac rate by tracking the respiratory rate. PACE 7:1246–1256, 1984.

179. Rossi P, Plicchi G, Canducci G, et al: Respiratory rate as a determinant of optimal pacing rate. PACE 6:502–507, 1983.

180. Rossi P, Rognoni G, Aina F, et al: Permanent physiological pacing. G Ital Cardiol 14/11:784–787, 1984.

181. Rossi P, Rognoni G, Occhetta E, et al: Respiration-dependent ventricular pacing compared with fixed ventricular and atrial-ventricular synchronous pacing: Aerobic and hemodynamic variables. J Am Coll Cardiol 6:646–652, 1985.

182. Schlesinger Z, Rosenberg T, Stryjer D, et al: Exit block in myxedema, treated effectively by thyroid hormone therapy. PACE 3:737–739, 1980.

183. Scoblionko DP, Rolett EL: Short-term threshold behavior of human ventricular pacing electrodes: Noninvasive monitoring with a multiprogrammable pacing system. PACE 4:631–637, 1981.

184. Sloman JG, Mond HG, Bailey B, et al: The use of balloon-tipped electrodes for permanent cardiac pacing. PACE 2:579–585, 1979.

185. Sluetz J, Spehr P, Haubold A, et al: New carbon coated porous tip electrode for low energy pacing. PACE 6:A–56, 1983.

186. Snow N: Elimination of lead dislodgement by the use of tined transvenous electrodes. PACE 5:571–574, 1982.

187. Sowton E, Barr I: Physiological changes in threshold. Ann NY Acad Sci 167:679, 1979.

188. Sowton E, Wainwright RJ, Crick JCP: "Crown of Thorns" single pass lead—clinical results. PACE 6:470–474, 1983.

189. Stenzl W, Tscheliessnigg KH, Dacar D, et al: Four years experience with the Bisping transvenous pacemaker electrode. PACE 6:A–58, 1983.

190. Stokes K: The long-term biostability of polyurethane leads. Stimucoeur 10:205–212, 1982.

191. Stokes K, Bornzin G: The electrode-biointerface: Stimulation. *In* Barold SS (ed): Modern Cardiac Pacing. Mount Kisco, NY, Futura Publishing Co, 1985, p 33.

192. Stokes K, Stephenson NL: The implantable cardiac pacing lead—just a simple wire? *In* Barold SS, Mugica J (eds): The Third Decade of Cardiac Pacing: Advances in Technology and Clinical Applications. Mount Kisco, NY, Futura Publishing Co, 1982, pp 365–416.

193. Stokes KB, Church T: Ten-year experience with implanted polyurethane lead isulation. PACE 9:1160–1165, 1986.

194. Stokes KB, Frazer WA, Christofferson RA: Environmental stress cracking in implanted polyurethanes. Proceedings of the Second World Congress on Biomaterials, 10th Annual Meeting of the Society for Biomaterials, Washington, DC, 1984, p 254.

195. Sugiura T, Itoh Y, Mizushina S, et al: Microcomputer-based cardiac pacemaker–control system through blood temperature. J Med Eng Technol 8:267–269, 1984.

196. Surawicz B: Role of electrolytes in etiology and management of cardiac arrhythmias. Prog Cardiovasc Dis 8:364–386, 1966.

197. Surawicz B, Chlebus H, Reeves JT, et al: Increase of ventricular excitability threshold by hyperpotassemia. JAMA 191:71–76, 1965.

198. Telectronics Physician's Manual (100-537, Issue 1). Englewood, CO, Telectronics, January 1985.

199. Thalen HJT: Stimulation electrodes, past, present, future. *In* Norman J, Richards A (eds). Proceedings of the Pacemaker Colloquium. Arnhem, The Netherlands, Vitatron Medical, 1976.

200. Thalen HJT, Van den Berg JW, Homan Van der Heide JN, et al: The Artificial Cardiac Pacemaker: Its History, Development and Clinical Application. Springfield, IL, CC Thomas, 1969, p 177.

201. Thoma RJ, Phillips RE: Note: Studies of poly(ether)urethane pacemaker lead insulation oxidation. J Biomed Mater Res 21:525–530, 1987.

202. Thull R, Schaldach M: Electrochemistry of after-pacing potentials on electrodes. PACE 9:1191–1196, 1986.

203. Timmermans AJM, van Hemel NM, Defauw J, et al: Results of non-preshaped screw-in leads for atrial pacing and sensing in 89 patients (pts.). PACE 6:A–58, 1983.

204. Timmis GC, Gordon S, Helland J: Enhanced electrode stability: The endocardial screw. *In* Watanabe Y (ed): Cardiac Pacing: Proceedings of the Vth International Symposium. Amsterdam, Excerpta Medica, 1976, pp 516–526.

205. Timmis GC, Westveer DC, Martin R: The significance of surface changes on explanted polyurethane pacemaker leads. PACE 6:845–857, 1983.

206. Timmis GC, Gordon S, Westveer DC, et al: A new steroid-eluting low threshold pacemaker lead. *In* Steinbach K, Glogar D, Laszkovics A, Scheibelhofer W (eds): Cardiac Pacing: Proceedings of the VIIth International Symposium. Darmstadt, Federal Republic of Germany, GmbH & Co, KG, 1983, pp 361–367.

207. Timmis GC, Gordon S, Westveer DC, et al: Polyurethane as a pacemaker lead insulator. *In* Steinbach K, Glogar D, Laszkovics A, Scheibelhofer W (eds): Cardiac Pacing: Proceedings of the VIIth International Symposium. Darmstadt, Federal Republic of Germany, GmbH and Co, KG, 1983, pp 303–310.

208. Timmis GC, Helland J, Westveer DC, et al: The evolution of low threshold leads. Clin Prog Pacing Electrophysiol 1:313–334, 1983.

209. Timmis GC, Parsonnet V, Gordon S, et al: The late effects of steroid-eluting leads. J Am Coll Cardiol 7:3A, 1986.

210. Timmis GC, Westveer DC, Gadowski G, et al: The effect of electrode position on atrial sensing for physiologically responsive cardiac pacemakers. Am Heart J 108:909–916, 1984.

211. Timmis GC, Westveer DC, Helland J, et al: Precision of pacemaker thresholds: The Wedensky effect. PACE 6:A–60, 1983.

212. Tyers GFO, Brownlee RR, Hughes HC, et al: Myocardial stimulation impedance: The effects of electrode, physiological, and stimulus variables. Ann Thorac Surg 27:63–69, 1979.

213. Tyers GFO, Torman HA, Hughes HC Jr: Comparative studies of "state of the art" and presently

used clinical cardiac pacemaker electrodes. J Thorac Cardiovasc Surg 67:849–856, 1974.

214. Upton JE: New pacing lead conductors: *In* Meere C (ed): Proceedings of the VIth World Symposium on Cardiac Pacing. Montreal, PACESYMP, 1979.

215. Vachon B, Forbath P, Hart J: Acute and long term electrophysiological performance of smooth, porous, ring tip electrodes. PACE 6:A–70, 1983.

216. Van Heeckeren DW, Hogan JF, Glenn WWL: Engineering analysis of pacemaker electrodes. Ann NY Acad Sci 167:774, 1969.

217. Wainwright R, Crick J, Sowton E: Clinical evaluation of a single-pass implantable electrode for all modes of pacing. The "Crown of Thorns" lead. PACE 6:210–220, 1983.

218. Walker WJ, Elkins JT, Wood LW, et al: Effect of potassium in restoring myocardial response to a subthreshold cardiac pacemaker. N Engl J Med 271:597, 1964.

219. Walton C, Gergely S, Economides AP: Platinum pacemaker electrodes: Origins and effects of the electrode-tissue interface impedance. PACE 10:87–99, 1987.

220. Weisswang A, Csapo G, Perach W, et al: Frequenzsteuerung von Schrittmachern durch Bluttemperatur. Verh Dtsch Ges Kreislaufforsch 44:152, 1978.

221. Westerholm CJ: Threshold studies in transvenous cardiac pacemaker treatment. Scand J Thorac Cardiovasc Surg [Suppl] 8:1, 1971.

222. Wigneswaran WT, Jamieson MPG: Temporary pacing leads in cardiac surgery. J Cardiovasc Surg 27:609–612, 1986.

223. Wirtzfeld A, Heinze R, Liess HD, et al: An active optical sensor for monitoring mixed venous oxygen-saturation for an implantable rate-regulating pacing system. PACE 6:494–497, 1983.

224. Zegelman M, Beyersdorf F, Kreuzer J, et al: Rate responsive pacemakers: Assessment after two years. PACE 9:1005–1009, 1986.

5

INDICATIONS FOR CARDIAC PACING

A. Indications for Permanent Cardiac Pacing in the Adult Patient

JOHN DANFORTH *and* NORA GOLDSCHLAGER

Over the past 30 years, the indications for permanent cardiac pacing have changed substantially, and hence the frequency of permanent cardiac pacemaker implantation procedures has increased exponentially[20, 135, 159] (Biomedical Business International, Tustin, CA, personal communication; Scientific and Technical Information Branch, National Center for Health Statistics, Bethesda, MD, personal communication). At present, the implantation of a permanent pacing system represents one of the most commonly performed operations involving the heart and certainly the most successful cardiac procedure involving the implantation of a prosthetic device.[159] The increase in the frequency of cardiac pacemaker implantation procedures stems in large part from technologic developments and improved surgical techniques that have contributed to the safety, efficacy, reliability, and longevity of permanent pacing systems (Table 5–1). As a result of technologic improvements in pacing leads, power sources, and generator design (see Chapters 3 and 4), the incidence of once relatively common pacing system–related complications, such as lead wire fracture, electronic component failure, "open-circuit" failure (due to leaks in battery casing, or fluid absorption in the epoxy potting material), and premature power source depletion, have decreased dramatically.[53, 112, 159] Surgical techniques have evolved to the extent that the

morbidity associated with this procedure approaches zero.[159] The most important developments in this regard include the virtually universal adoption of the transvenous approach and the discontinuation of general anesthesia for induction during pacemaker implantation.[13, 22, 69, 159, 184] As a result, the therapeutic potential and hence the clinical utility of permanent pacemaker therapy have increased dramatically. With continuing technologic developments, it is likely that this trend will continue. This first part of Chapter 5 summarizes the recognized indications for permanent cardiac pacing in the 1980s.

POTENTIAL FOR OVERUTILIZATION OF CARDIAC PACING SYSTEMS

In 1970, syncope in association with complete heart block constituted the predominant indication for the implantation of a permanent cardiac pacing system[186] (Scientific and Technical Information Branch, National Center for Health Statistics, Bethesda, MD, personal communication). Currently, however, symptomatic high-degree and complete atrioventricular (AV) block represents the principal indication in fewer than 25 per cent of pacemaker recipients.[4, 88] Coincident with the recognition of the broadened therapeutic potential of per-

TABLE 5–1. PERMANENT PACEMAKER THERAPY: HISTORICAL PERSPECTIVE

Gerbezius	1719	Noted slow pulse among patients with apoplexy
Galvani	1791	Determined fundamentals of electrical cardiac stimulation
Bichat	1798	Electrically stimulated human hearts following decapitation
Aldini	1819	Attempted cardiac electrical stimulation to arouse the dead
Walshe	1862	Proposed cardiac galvanic current
Gaskell	1883	Postulated the existence of a cardiac conduction system
Kent and His	1893	First described the cardiac conduction system
Tawara	1906	First described the atrioventricular (AV) node
Keith and Flack	1907	First described the sinoatrial (SA) node
Gould	1929	Resuscitated a baby by direct electrical stimulation of the heart
Butterworth and Poindexter	1942	Described an experimental synchronous pacemaker
Bigelow and Callaghan	1951	Developed a functional pacemaker
Zoll	1952	Restarted a human heart with electrical pacing
Hopps and Bigelow	1954	Described transvenous endocardial pacing in animals
Furman and Robinson	1958	Reported transvenous endocardial pacing
Elmquest and Senning	1959	Described the first completely implantable permanent cardiac pacemaker
Lagergren	1964	First described the transvenous approach for permanent pacemakers
Keleor	1964	Developed a synchronous atrial-ventricular pacemaker
Goetz	1966	Developed a "demand" pacemaker
Tarjan	1972	Developed external programmability

manent pacemaker therapy, several authors have expressed concern regarding the increasing number of patients in whom permanent pacemakers are implanted without *apparent* clinical benefit and have suggested that this phenomenon might relate to the overutilization of this therapeutic approach.[87, 88, 134] Clearly, the insertion of a pacing system will not influence the frequency of symptoms that are noncardiac in origin. The distinction of symptoms as being cardiac or noncardiac in origin is not always clear from the medical history or the diagnostic workup. Hence, prior to pacing system implantation, every effort should be made to determine the pathophysiology and natural history of the condition for which pacemaker therapy is being considered and to confirm that the condition will benefit from such therapy. For example, it is now recognized that syncope, a symptom previously considered sufficient in and of itself to warrant the implantation of a permanent pacing system,[14] is multifactorial in origin. In some reports,[84] cardiac conditions account for fewer than 40 per cent of all episodes of syncope in elderly subjects. Autonomic insufficiency, cerebrovascular disease, diabetes, and the use of various pharmacologic agents (such as sedatives, diuretics, vasodilators, and beta blockers) probably account for the majority of syncopal events in these individuals.[16, 98] In contrast, vasodepressor (and/or "psychogenic") phenomena, with or without associated bradycardia, account for up to 50 per cent of syncopal episodes in younger subjects.[41] Moreover, in many patients in all age groups, the etiology of the syncope is not established either at the time of initial presentation or by the time of hospital discharge.[14, 84]

In patients with cardiac syncope due to dysrhythmia, it is acknowledged that many of the responsible rhythm disturbances are not amenable to permanent antibradycardia pacemaker therapy. Ventricular tachycardia undoubtedly represents the most common cause of arrhythmogenically mediated cardiac syncope in certain groups of patients, particularly those with significant left ventricular dysfunction, with or without acute or chronic myocardial ischemia.[54, 131] Supraventricular tachycardias also account for syncopal spells, according to the results of some,[18, 38, 65, 108] but not all,[3, 74, 116] clinical studies. In response to legitimate concerns regarding pacemaker overutilization, a subcommittee of the Task Force on Assessment of Cardiovascular Procedures that is evaluating pacemaker implantation practices has recommended that "the decision to implant a pacemaker must be reached by scrupulous adherence to a fundamental principle of clinical medicine which demands a careful, thoughtful analysis of each individual patient by the responsible physician."[50]

In patients with recurrent syncope of unclear origin, who are, by virtue of a high recurrence rate, considered potential candidates for permanent pacemaker therapy, electrophysiologic

TABLE 5–2. INCIDENCE OF PERSISTENCE OF SYMPTOMS FOLLOWING IMPLANTATION OF A PERMANENT CARDIAC PACING SYSTEM

INVESTIGATORS	INCIDENCE (%)
Hartel et al.[70]	1.3
Chokshi et al.[24]	8.3
Conde et al.[27]	9.7
Rokseth and Hatle[143]	19.0
Gross-Fengels et al.[64]	30.0

testing should be performed if noninvasive evaluation procedures (ambulatory electrocardiography, exercise testing, patient-activated event recordings) prove nondiagnostic[38, 65, 74, 131] (see Chapter 6). The rationale for this recommendation is based on studies that indicate that noninvasive diagnostic approaches are frequently unrewarding in patients with ventricular tachycardia.[25, 56] Provoking sustained ventricular tachycardia by means of electrical stimulation in the electrophysiology laboratory has been shown to correspond to the spontaneous occurrence of this arrhythmia.[39, 99, 105, 171] Furthermore, the suppression of induced ventricular tachycardia in the laboratory following the administration of antiarrhythmic therapy has been shown to have prognostic significance with regard to recurrence of syncopal episodes[80, 106, 131] (see Chapters 6 and 22).

Despite assiduous preoperative evaluation, symptoms of dizziness, palpitations, near-syncope, and frank syncope can persist with relative frequency following pacemaker implantation, with a reported incidence of up to 10 per cent[24, 27, 64, 70, 79, 143] (Table 5–2). Persistence of symptoms in patients extensively evaluated underscores the nonspecificity of reported symptoms (Table 5–3) and the difficulty in achieving a definite correlation between symptoms and electrocardiographic data and does not invalidate this therapeutic approach.

TABLE 5–3. NONSPECIFIC SYMPTOMS THAT SUGGEST (BUT DO NOT PROVE) AN ARRHYTHMIC ORIGIN

Syncope
Dizziness
Weakness
  May be episodic
  May be profound
Palpitations
Breathlessness
  Episodic, at rest
  With effort
Fatigue on effort

EFFECT OF AGE

The majority of the recipients of permanent cardiac pacing devices tend to be older than 70 years of age.[3, 14] A number of factors might contribute to this circumstance. For example, progressive cellular dropout and fibrous tissue replacement occur within the sinoatrial (SA) node as a result of aging. Davies has reported that only 10 per cent of SA nodal pacemaker cells remain viable in individuals 75 years of age.[30] Similar degenerative processes occur within the left bundle branch system; only about 50 per cent of the fibers remain in individuals over 60 years of age. Presumably as a result of these and other age-related phenomena, bradycardia and AV block tend to occur more commonly among the elderly.[84] Hence, the causes of syncope will relate in part to the age of the individual. In patients older than 65 years, syncope is more commonly cardiac in origin, whereas in individuals younger than 65 years of age, a vasovagal etiology is more common.[146, 147, 179] Given the low surgical morbidity and the substantial therapeutic potential for permanent pacemaker therapy in the elderly, the current consensus is that advanced age should not be considered a factor in the decision to proceed with this therapeutic approach.[14, 163, 170]

SICK SINUS SYNDROME

The phrase "sick sinus syndrome" refers to a symptom complex of dizziness and/or syncope in association with any of the following dysrhythmias: (1) episodic sinus arrest resulting in either an escape rhythm or asystole; (2) persistent unexplained marked sinus bradycardia; (3) inability of sinus rhythm to resume following cessation of a supraventricular tachycardia; or (4) marked sinus bradycardia alternating with a supraventricular, junctional, or ventricular tachycardia (the bradycardia-tachycardia syndrome). Symptoms in these individuals generally develop in response to abrupt changes in the heart rate.[42, 100] In the majority of cases, syncope develops coincident with the conversion from a tachycardia to a bradycardia.[27] Sinus node dysfunction was first described by MacKenzie in 1902.[102] Soon after, Laslett reported the development of Stokes-Adams syncope as a result of sinus bradycardia,[92] a phenomenon subsequently observed by others.[42, 120]

At present, the precise pathophysiology of

the rhythm disturbances associated with the sick sinus syndrome remains unclear.[27, 70] The process of aging might contribute to the development of these arrhythmias,[31] although the condition has been observed in children and young adults. In this regard, Evans and colleagues[46] have determined that atrophy or enhanced fibrous tissue proliferation is frequently evident within the sinus node of individuals having the clinical diagnosis of sick sinus syndrome. Although it is intriguing to speculate that the development of vascular changes within the SA artery (the only source of perfusion to the sinus node) might further contribute to the development of rhythm disturbances in these individuals,[27] Evans and coworkers were unable to identify SA vascular pathology.[46] Some investigators have proposed that the sick sinus syndrome develops as a result of a diffuse sclerodegenerative process involving not only the conduction system but also the cardiac skeleton.[51, 123] There is clinical evidence in support of this hypothesis: Up to one third of patients with sinus node dysfunction have conduction abnormalities involving the AV node and/or bundle branches.[27, 46] Other investigators have suggested that the rhythm disturbances associated with the sick sinus syndrome might represent an intermediate phase in the evolution of chronic atrial fibrillation.[89, 167] The symptoms of palpitations, weakness, dizziness, and syncope associated with the sick sinus syndrome commonly resolve following the development of established atrial fibrillation,[26, 89, 172, 183] in which a more stable QRS rhythm exists.

The use of permanent cardiac pacing in the management of the sick sinus syndrome has increased exponentially over the course of the past 20 years,[11, 15, 70] to the extent that this syndrome currently represents the most common indication for permanent pacemaker therapy in many centers.[4, 159] Although there exists little doubt that this therapeutic approach offers some symptomatic relief in most patients,[166] the effectiveness of pacemaker therapy depends upon the nature and frequency of the underlying rhythm disturbances. Thus, as expected, permanent cardiac pacing has been particularly effective in patients with symptoms due predominantly to bradyarrhythmias.[24, 27, 70, 89, 185] In the series of Conde and associates,[27] 87 per cent of patients with symptomatic bradyarrhythmias had symptomatic relief following the insertion of a permanent pacemaker. However, permanent pacing in the management of patients with the bradycardia-tachycardia syndrome has been less gratifying,[148] particularly in patients with symptomatic tachyarrhythmias that are relatively refractory to suppression with vigorous antiarrhythmic therapy.[24, 47, 143] In some circumstances, the insertion of a permanent pacemaker programmed to a reasonable rate can compensate for the anticipated negative chronotropic influence of some required antiarrhythmic agents.[27, 148] Permanent pacing from the atrium, rather than from the ventricle, might also serve to mitigate the frequency of the supraventricular tachyarrhythmias, if their occurrence is bradycardia dependent.

Permanent cardiac pacing has not been found to influence either the overall cardiac mortality or the incidence of sudden death in patients with sick sinus syndrome.[6, 9, 70, 75, 153, 156, 157] The prognosis for this population of patients is relatively poor, with an anticipated 2-year mortality ranging between 32 per cent and 42 per cent.[9, 89, 141, 185] In contrast to patients with more severe manifestations of sinus node dysfunction, such as sinus pauses and/or the bradycardia-tachycardia syndrome, the presence of sinus bradycardia alone has been found to have little impact on mortality; the 15-year survival for elderly patients with sinus bradycardia alone has been found to compare favorably with that of a population without evidence of bradyarrhythmias.[55] It is not clear why more advanced degrees of sinus node dysfunction are associated with a poorer prognosis. These rhythm disturbances are not accurate predictors of either presence or severity of structural heart disease. It is possible, although unproved, that the proclivity to atrial fibrillation, and the systemic and pulmonary emboli that result from alternating atrial bradycardia and tachycardia, have an impact on morbidity and mortality. The mortality in patients with sick sinus syndrome more clearly does depend upon the presence and severity of concomitant underlying cardiovascular disease.[6, 9, 141, 153, 157] The majority of patients with sick sinus syndrome have evidence of either peripheral or coronary artery disease.[27, 70, 119, 155] According to one report,[6] most patients with sick sinus syndrome die of complications sustained as a result of coronary artery disease.

Permanent pacemaker therapy should be reserved for individuals with the sick sinus syndrome who are symptomatic (Fig. 5–1). In this regard, a variety of atrial bradyarrhythmias, including SA exit block, sinus bradycardia, and sinus pauses, have all been observed in asymptomatic, presumably healthy individ-

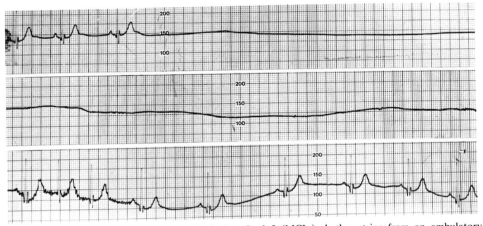

Figure 5–1. Continuously recorded modified chest lead 5 (MCL$_5$) rhythm strips from an ambulatory electrocardiographic (ECG) recording in a 63-year-old woman with episodic weakness and dizziness. Sinus bradycardia with an irregular rate begins and ends the rhythm strip. A markedly prolonged pause in sinus rhythm is present. Note the probable myopotentials recorded at the termination of the pause (bottom strip). The patient did not activate at the event marker on the recording apparatus and, indeed, throughout the recording period noted only generalized weakness in her diary. It is tempting to speculate that the myopotentials recorded at the termination of the pause in cardiac rhythm were due to body motion caused by falling. Although this patient did not have a history of frank syncope or even near-syncope, a permanent cardiac pacemaker was implanted. Her symptoms were only minimally improved.

uals; hence, these arrhythmias alone do not constitute an indication for permanent pacemaker therapy.[2, 5, 19, 44, 78, 107, 148, 160] Mazur and Friedman[107] and others[19, 160] have reported that pauses in sinus rhythm of less than 2 seconds have no clinical significance, and Hilgard and colleagues[75] have shown that pauses of 3 seconds have no prognostic significance. In symptomatic individuals, it is necessary to determine (within feasible limits) that the symptoms are related to an irreversible bradyarrhythmia before proceeding with the insertion of a permanent pacemaker (Table 5–4). On occasion, an argument can be made[43] for empiric insertion of a permanent pacing system in individuals with pauses in sinus rhythm exceeding 3

TABLE 5–4. REVERSIBLE ETIOLOGIES OF SINUS NODE DYSFUNCTION

Enhanced vagal tone
Myocardial ischemia (especially involving the
  area supplied by the right coronary artery)
Surgical injury
Myocarditis
Hypothyroidism
Electrolyte abnormality
Pharmacologic therapy
  Digoxin (with concomitant increased vagal
    tone)
  Quinidine
  Procainamide
  Beta-blocking agents
  Calcium channel blocking agents (verapamil,
    diltiazem)

seconds, even though precise correlative documentation is not established, since at times many of these patients will have symptoms suggestive of cerebral hypoperfusion (Fig. 5–2).

Electrophysiologic evaluation of patients with evidence of sinus node dysfunction should be reserved for those patients who are asymptomatic throughout the noninvasive monitoring period.[5, 82] However, it must be emphasized that the sensitivity of electrophysiologic testing for detecting the presence of sinus node dysfunction is relatively low (26 per cent to 69 per cent for sinus node recovery time and 29 per cent to 75 per cent for SA conduction time).[12, 55, 86, 139] The specificity of electrophysiologic testing is somewhat better, although wide variations have been reported (88 per cent to 100 per cent for sinus node recovery time; 57 per cent to 100 per cent for SA conduction time).[12]

The insertion of an AAI pacing system (or an AAI rate-responsive system when these become available) is currently considered most appropriate in the management of patients with sick sinus syndrome. Peripheral embolization,[166] atrial fibrillation,[195] and congestive heart failure[145] have all been reported to occur less frequently in patients with AAI pacemakers compared with those having VVI pacing systems. Several possibilities have been proposed to account for these observations. Rosenqvist and coworkers[145] have suggested

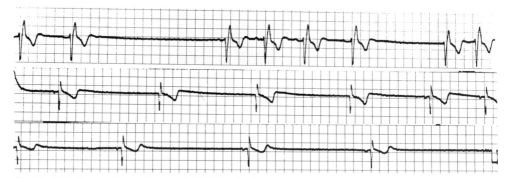

Figure 5–2. Noncontinuously recorded MCL$_1$ rhythm strips from a 72-year-old man with documented three-vessel coronary artery disease, poor left ventricular function (ejection fraction of 36 per cent), dizzy spells, and a single episode of loss of consciousness. Despite the pauses in sinus rhythm, marked sinus bradycardia, and junctional escape rhythms established by these recordings, the patient's symptoms were not clearly correlated with bradycardias. Permanent pacing was undertaken nevertheless, with significant improvement in clinical status.

that the AV asynchrony that commonly results from VVI pacing in patients with sinus rhythm might provoke atrial dilatation and thus promote the development of atrial fibrillation. Furman and Cooper[52] have proposed that retrograde ventriculoatrial conduction, a relatively common occurrence in individuals with sick sinus syndrome who have VVI pacing systems,[130] might permit the occurrence of atrial depolarizations in addition to those originating from the sinus node; these depolarizations might provoke the development of atrial fibrillation if they fall in the atrial vulnerable period. Finally, it is possible that atrial bradycardia per se can contribute to the development of atrial tachyarrhythmias (bradycardia-dependent tachycardia), a circumstance that is precluded by atrial pacing. Given the reported low risk of progression to advanced AV block (3.4 per cent in a 15-year follow-up study),[73] it appears that DDD pacing systems are not indicated for patients with sick sinus syndrome if AV conduction is demonstrated to be intact at the time of pacing system implantation (see Chapter 7).

CAROTID SINUS HYPERSENSITIVITY

The performance of carotid sinus massage in normal individuals generally results in a moderate reduction in mean blood pressure and heart rate.[1, 104, 169] If the response is excessive, the individual is considered to have carotid sinus hypersensitivity.[103, 149, 168] Although uncommon (33 per million patients),[118] carotid sinus hypersensitivity must be considered in the differential diagnosis of syncope because it

is potentially treatable.[28, 103] Two major types of carotid sinus hypersensitivity are identified: the cardioinhibitory type and the vasodepressor type.[28, 168, 178] The performance of carotid sinus massage in patients with the cardioinhibitory type of carotid sinus hypersensitivity results in the development of either transient asystole, having a duration of at least 3 seconds, or a profound bradycardia.[103] The response is mediated by the vagus nerve, and hence it is relatively sensitive to the intravenous administration of atropine. Performance of carotid sinus massage in patients with the vasodepressor type results in a disproportionate reduction in the blood pressure relative to heart rate.[28, 103] Typically, these individuals sustain a fall in systolic blood pressure exceeding 50 mm Hg, without developing a significant bradycardia.[28, 103] Blood pressure should be determined with the patient in the erect position if blood pressure abnormalities with the patient supine are not demonstrated. The hypotension in this form of carotid sinus hypersensitivity is not responsive to the administration of atropine,[28] nor does the prevention of any associated bradycardia affect the vasodepressor response. The incidence of the cardioinhibitory type of carotid sinus hypersensitivity is substantially higher than that of the vasodepressor type. A mixed form, with features of both types, is also recognized and is relatively common.

Classically, patients with carotid sinus hypersensitivity of the cardioinhibitory type develop syncope, blurred vision, lightheadedness, and/or confusion as a result of turning their head.[8, 28, 81, 168] Symptoms related to orthostatic phenomena are described by patients with the vasodepressor type of carotid sinus hypersensitivity. However, many patients cannot recall any precipitating factors[40, 77] or trigger points.[175] Moreover, the symptoms associated with this condition tend to wax and wane over time.[165, 175]

The precise pathophysiology of carotid sinus hypersensitivity remains unknown. Although hypersensitivity within the carotid sinus reflex arc has been proposed to account for the development of the profound bradycardia seen in individuals with the cardioinhibitory type, the specific site of the hypersensitivity within this reflex arc remains to be determined. In brief, the carotid sinus reflex arc consists of afferent fibers located within the carotid sinus nerve, a branch of the glossopharyngeal nerve that extends into the cardioinhibitory center of the medulla; the vagus nerve constitutes the efferent limb of this reflex arc. In this regard, some patients with disabling carotid sinus hypersensitivity refractory to pacing and fluid therapy have responded to resection of the glossopharyngeal nerve. Excessive vagal tone, as well as local compressive factors, such as tumors, lymph nodes, and scars, that impinge upon the carotid sinus,[37, 178] have been proposed to account for the development of carotid sinus hypersensitivity, although additional contributing mechanisms, such as excessive release of acetylcholine or inadequate cholinesterase activity, may be operative. Reed and Scott[142] have shown that unilateral vagotomy in animals results in an exaggerated cardioinhibitory response to stimulation of the carotid sinus; the clinical significance of this finding, however, remains to be determined. Although it is intriguing to speculate that the pathophysiology of the carotid hypersensitivity syndrome and that of the sick sinus syndrome are interrelated, the current consensus is that the two conditions are clinically distinct.[29, 71, 117, 118, 175]

Understanding of the pathophysiology of the vasodepressor response is relatively limited. Most investigations suggest that the hypotension develops in response to a transient reduction in peripheral vascular resistance,[45, 61, 180] which presumably results from transient inhibition of sympathetic responsiveness.[61] The mechanism or mechanisms by which the responsiveness of the sympathetic nervous system can be influenced, however, remain unknown. Although the symptoms tend to be the same in both types of carotid sinus hypersensitivity, they last longer in individuals with the vasodepressor type, reflecting the usually longer

duration of the hypotensive episodes compared with the periods of bradycardia.[101, 169]

Screening patients for the presence of carotid sinus hypersensitivity often presents a clinical dilemma. Many patients cannot recall a trigger episode.[175] Carotid sinus hypersensitivity unassociated with clinical symptoms can be provoked in approximately 30 per cent of older men with atherosclerotic coronary artery disease or hypertensive heart disease or both.[29, 71, 128, 154, 168, 175] Moreover, carotid sinus massage resulting in abnormal bradycardia or hypotension or both frequently does not provoke the patient's presenting symptom,[137, 175] particularly when performed with the patient in the supine position, in which intravascular volume is maximal.[137, 168, 178] Carotid sinus massage should be performed following a thorough evaluation for the presence of carotid artery bruits. The absolute criteria for the diagnosis of carotid sinus hypersensitivity are the provocation of a 3-second pause in rhythm and a 50 mm Hg fall in systolic blood pressure. The pause in QRS rhythm elicited by carotid sinus massage can be due to sinus bradycardia (or arrest) or to transient advanced AV block. Borderline criteria include the development of a 30 mm Hg reduction in systolic blood pressure, a 30 to 50 per cent reduction in heart rate, and ventricular asystole of 2 seconds' duration.[81, 168] The coexistence of the cardioinhibitory and vasodepressor responses to carotid sinus massage can be determined by administering atropine intravenously prior to the carotid massage. A significant reduction in blood pressure in the presence of a normal heart rate is diagnostic of a vasodepressor component.[101, 169, 175] In patients in whom atropine is contraindicated (such as those with glaucoma), the insertion of a temporary pacemaker may be required.[164]

In patients with *symptomatic* carotid sinus hypersensitivity of the cardioinhibitory type, the implantation of a permanent cardiac pacemaker is the treatment of choice.[29, 73, 118, 137, 175] Alternative approaches have included the use of anticholinergic drugs,[165, 175] the use of sympathomimetic agents,[118, 168] carotid sinus irradiation,[63] and the excision of focal mass lesions impinging on the carotid sinus, such as tumors and lymph nodes.[168] Only about two thirds of patients respond to radiation therapy or surgical intervention.[63, 169] Furthermore, the majority of individuals cannot tolerate the large doses of anticholinergic drugs required in the pharmacologic management of this disorder.[174]

Morley and colleagues[118] have reported that 83 per cent of patients with the cardioinhibitory type of carotid sinus hypersensitivity sustain symptomatic relief following insertion of a permanent pacemaker. Although recurrence of symptoms following cardiac pacemaker implantation has been reported,[136, 158, 175] this recurrence probably reflects the coexistence of a vasodepressor component that is not affected by the insertion of a pacemaker.[103, 118, 136] The type of pacing system recommended will depend upon the frequency of the symptoms. Rare episodes are effectively treated with VVI systems. AAI pacing is generally not advised, even in patients who exhibit only profound sinus bradycardia during carotid massage, owing to the relatively high incidence of AV block. Moreover, maintenance of atrial rate by pacing can unmask AV block that is absent at slow atrial rates but present at faster atrial rates. Dual-chamber pacing is preferred in patients whose symptoms are frequent; this pacing mode has been reported to be associated with smaller and less abrupt falls in blood pressure.[103]

Very little can be offered to patients with symptomatic vasodepressor carotid sinus hypersensitivity.[28] The condition is unresponsive to permanent pacemaker therapy. Patients with mild cases may respond to volume loading achieved by means of mineralocorticoid therapy. Cheng and Norris[23] have reported symptomatic relief in one instance following adventitial stripping of the carotid bifurcation, and Thomas[168] has suggested that ephedrine might be useful. The use of pressure gradient hosiery has been advised, although the benefit appears to be marginal.

DISORDERS OF ATRIOVENTRICULAR CONDUCTION

First-Degree Atrioventricular Block

The term "first-degree AV block" refers to a delay in conduction between the atria and the ventricles, resulting in prolongation of the PR interval. All impulses are conducted to the ventricles. The PR interval comprises intraatrial conduction, intra–AV nodal conduction, intra–His bundle conduction, and His-Purkinje conduction.[17, 58, 59, 94, 95, 125, 140, 152] The usual cause of PR interval prolongation is delay in conduction within the AV node. The clinical significance of PR interval prolongation depends upon the presence or absence of underlying heart disease and additional conduction system abnormalities; by itself, this condition is benign[17, 122] and hence is not an indication for permanent pacemaker therapy. Hiss and Lamb[78] have suggested that enhanced vagal tone probably accounts for the development of isolated first-degree AV block in the majority of cases. Progression to higher grades of AV block is extremely unusual, occurring in fewer than 2 per cent of cases.[122] The presence of first-degree AV block in the setting of either left or right bundle branch block, however, frequently reflects the presence of infra-His block.[96]

Second-Degree Atrioventricular Block

In second-degree AV block, not all supraventricular impulses are conducted to the ventricles. At the turn of the century, Wenckebach determined that there were two different types of second-degree heart block by analyzing the jugular venous patterns of individuals with this conduction abnormality.[181, 182] His original impressions based on physical examination were subsequently confirmed by Mobitz,[114] who used electrocardiographic criteria to distinguish type I from type II second-degree AV block.

Type I (Mobitz I) second-degree AV block is characterized by progressive delay in impulse conduction, with periodic failure of conduction.[17, 58, 59, 94, 125, 152] It is a relatively stable condition and is thus usually benign. Symptomatic type I second-degree AV block can occur in the presence of slow sinus rates and low AV conduction ratios, such as 3:2 or 2:1. Type I second-degree AV block is most often recognized in the setting of acute myocardial ischemia and infarction.[85] Chronic isolated type I AV block occurs infrequently,[17, 62, 78, 132] with an estimated prevalence of approximately 0.003 per cent.[78] The reported prevalence will reflect the population under study; for example, trained athletes having high vagal tone not uncommonly have type I second-degree AV block, in addition to slow and often irregular sinus rates. The prognostic significance of this conduction abnormality is dependent upon the extent of coexisting organic heart disease. In the absence of organic heart disease, type I second-degree AV block is a benign rhythm disturbance that does not warrant the insertion of a permanent pacemaker.[91, 113, 161]

Atypical forms of type I second-degree AV block can occur in response to high vagal tone; in this circumstance, sinus bradycardia with sinus arrhythmia is usually present. AV block due to hypervagotonia does not constitute an indication for permanent cardiac pacing, since the phenomenon is usually transient and related to specific maneuvers, such as swallowing (deglutition bradycardia),[83, 124] yawning, or micturition or defecation. Occasionally, atropine-responsive vagotonic AV block is observed in the absence of specific vagal maneuvers.[162] Despite the transient nature of the condition, bradyarrhythmias mediated by enhanced vagal tone are, on occasion, life threatening. If such bradyarrhythmias are documented, permanent cardiac pacing should be undertaken despite the possible evanescence of the problem.

Type II Second-Degree Atrioventricular Block

Type II (Mobitz II) second-degree AV block generally indicates the presence of a conduction abnormality distal to the AV node. Given the recognized instability of AV conduction in this rhythm disturbance, type II second-degree AV block is generally considered an indication for permanent cardiac pacing, even in asymptomatic individuals.[60]

If 2:1 AV conduction is present, the conduction block could lie either within the AV node or within the His-Purkinje system. Maneuvers that increase the AV conduction ratio, such as the administration of intravenous atropine, are often helpful in establishing the level of conduction block. Occasionally, His bundle electrography and pacing are required for precise localization of the conduction delay (see Chapter 13). Generally, in patients with 2:1 AV conduction, if the PR interval of conducted sinus impulses is prolonged and the QRS complexes are narrow and normal appearing, the area of conduction block is in the AV node. If, however, the PR interval of the conducted sinus impulses is normal and intraventricular conduction delay (or delays) is (or are) present, the conduction block is infra–AV nodal, often within the fascicles.

Block Within the His Bundle

Conduction delay or block within the His bundle accounts for 16 to 29 per cent of all cases of advanced second- and third-degree AV block.[7, 66, 67, 126] Typically, patients with this disorder are elderly and have advanced athero-sclerotic cardiovascular disease.[7, 68, 126] The majority are symptomatic, with either recurrent syncope or congestive heart failure.[7] Intravenously administered atropine can be used to screen patients for this abnormality, since this agent does not substantially influence conduction within the His bundle. However, the response is often variable and unpredictable even in the same patient at different times; thus, caution should be used in the interpretation of a given response. The variability in response to atropine can probably be accounted for by the site of conduction block within the His bundle, as well as by prevailing autonomic tone.[68] Frequently, electrophysiologic testing is required to confirm the diagnosis. A split His potential is considered pathognomonic for His bundle block.[127] Given the instability and unpredictability of AV conduction in this circumstance in some patients, the insertion of a permanent pacing system is generally indicated if symptoms are present.[68]

Advanced and Complete Atrioventricular Block

Advanced or complete AV block represents one of the principal indications for the implantation of a permanent pacemaker. The development of symptoms in patients with this disorder is dependent upon the age and activity level of the patient the intrinsic rate of the QRS rhythm, and the responsiveness of the focus of origin of the rhythm to sympathetic stimulation. Both the rate and the responsiveness of the escape focus tend to decrease with a progressively more distal location of this focus within the conduction system. The majority of individuals who develop paroxysmal or established complete AV block become symptomatic[60]; there exists little argument that permanent cardiac pacing is particularly effective in alleviating these symptoms (Fig. 5–3).

Debate continues concerning the rationale for pacemaker implantation in asymptomatic individuals with chronic, stable complete AV block as well as in those with symptoms that do not suggest bradycardia-related cerebral hypoperfusion[109] (Fig. 5–4). The conduction delay in these patients often involves the AV node, and hence the escape rhythm is frequently junctional in origin. Junctional escape mechanisms are often relatively stable over time and responsive to physiologic demands. Escape rhythms originating in Purkinje or ventricular tissue, however, are less stable over

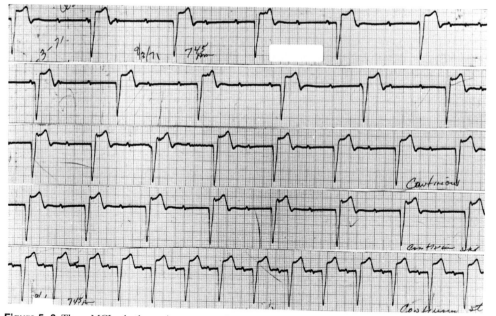

Figure 5–3. These MCL₁ rhythm strips were continuously recorded from a patient admitted after a syncopal episode. They illustrate the rapid devolution from complete atrioventricular (AV) block to 1:1 AV conduction. The atrial rhythm is sinus. In the top two strips, complete AV block is present, with a ventricular rate of 32 per minute. The duration of the QRS complex is 0.12 second, and the configuration is that of left bundle branch block. The QRS complexes suggest an origin in the Purkinje system because of their slow rate and prolonged duration; subsequent rhythm strips prove that these complexes in fact originate from a higher focus, presumably within the bundle of His.

A 2:1 AV conduction is present in the third and fourth rhythm strips; the PR interval of the (presumably) conducted complexes is markedly prolonged at 0.60 second. In the bottom strip, 1:1 AV conduction with first-degree AV block is present. Myocardial infarction was ruled out. Electrophysiologic studies suggested that the site of conduction block was within the His bundle. A permanent cardiac pacemaker was implanted.

time and tend to have a slower rate and an attenuated responsiveness to catecholamine stimulation; hence, permanent pacing is usually recommended (Fig. 5–4). Many patients who are considered to be asymptomatic prior to permanent pacemaker implantation are able to define a much improved quality of life after pacing system insertion, again emphasizing that the decision to institute pacemaker therapy in the absence of symptoms is a difficult clinical dilemma.

On occasion, the presence of bradycardia-dependent ventricular tachycardia, with or without QT interval prolongation, can be of pathogenetic significance (Fig. 5–5). Permanent cardiac pacing has been employed for this condition with good results (J. Griffin, personal communication).

Bundle Branch Block

Considerable controversy still exists concerning the rationale for permanent pacemaker therapy in patients with bifascicular and documented trifascicular block who have symptoms suggestive of cerebral hypoperfusion. The impetus to consider permanent pacemaker therapy stems from observations that these patients have a relatively poor 5-year prognosis[93, 109] as well as an increased risk for sudden death,[32, 111, 151] thus suggesting a potential predisposition to the development of complete AV block. To date, however, no data exist to demonstrate that the increase in mortality in this population derives from the development of progressive AV conduction system disease.[49, 110, 138] The implantation of a permanent pacing system has not influenced the mortality in symptomatic individuals with bundle branch block and electrophysiologic evidence of infranodal conduction delay.[111] Recent studies demonstrate that the enhanced mortality in this population of patients derives primarily from the high prevalence of underlying myocardial disease.[111, 138] In the study of Peters and coworkers,[138] 88 per cent of deaths in patients with bifascicular or trifascicular

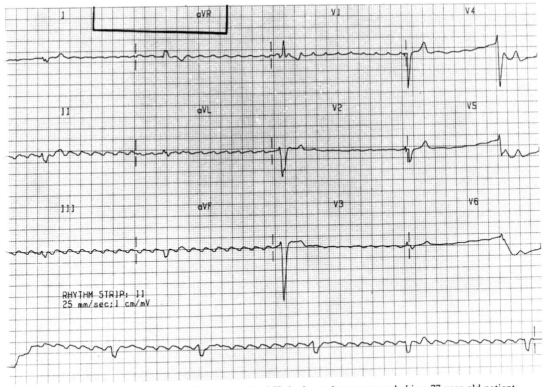

Figure 5–4. This 12-lead electrocardiogram and lead II rhythm strip were recorded in a 77-year-old patient receiving no medications, who had presented to the emergency room with spells of lightheadedness. The atrial rhythm is flutter. The QRS rhythm is markedly slow at 31 per minute; the morphology suggests a focus of origin in the left posterior fascicle of the left bundle branch. Blood pressure was normal on admission, and no orthostatic changes were present. Myocardial infarction was ruled out. Despite the nonspecificity of the clinical symptom of episodic lightheadedness, a permanent VVI pacing system was implanted, and the patient's spells disappeared completely.

Figure 5–5. Sequentially reconstructed rhythm strips obtained from telemetric monitoring equipment in a patient who died during the recording. Bursts of polymorphic ventricular tachycardia finally degenerate into sustained ventricular tachycardia and fibrillation. Each tachycardia burst is preceded by a relative increase in RR cycle length and is thus bradycardia related. The long QT interval observed in these rhythm strips was not present on admission but developed during the occurrence of this arrhythmia. The patient had ischemic heart disease; no antiarrhythmic therapy was being administered, and serum potassium and magnesium levels were normal. Permanent cardiac pacing should be considered in such individuals.

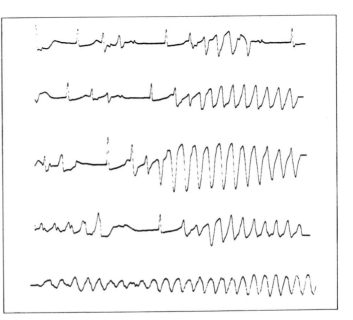

disease could be attributed to the coexistence of congestive heart failure or atherosclerotic coronary artery disease. McAnulty and colleagues[109] similarly reported that the 5-year prognosis for these patients was profoundly influenced by the coexistence of coronary artery disease. In a 3-year prospective study by Denes and colleagues[32] of 277 patients with chronic bifascicular block, sudden death occurred in 30 patients and followed the onset of ventricular fibrillation rather than abrupt advanced AV block. If, in fact, progression to complete heart block accounts for some of the mortality in the population of patients at recognized risk for sudden death, there currently exists no reliable means of identifying them.[110] No element of the clinical history, including the occurrence of syncope, has been found to correlate with an enhanced risk for sudden death in either retrospective[115, 144] or prospective studies.[33, 34] Analysis of the electrocardiogram has similarly been found to be of limited value in this regard. For example, the identification of individuals with combined right bundle branch block and left posterior fascicular block (an allegedly "malignant" form of conduction block[21, 90]) has not been helpful in predicting increased risk for sudden death on prospective analysis.[35] Even electrophysiologic evaluation, with specific attention to the HV interval as a marker for diffuse conduction system disease, has provided little insight with respect to risk stratification for, and prediction of, sudden death. Dhingra and coworkers[36] have reported that prolongation of the HV interval beyond 80 msec has no prognostic significance in this population of patients and no relationship to the occurrence of syncope. However, not all investigators are in agreement on this point.[150] Lichstein and colleagues[97] have reported that the prognosis tends to be worse among individuals with a progressively diminishing HV interval, concluding that this electrophysiologic finding identifies a subgroup of individuals with extensive coronary artery disease and hence a poor prognosis.

Given the inability to stratify patients accurately with respect to risk of progression to advanced and complete AV block, as well as the inability to predict death in patients with bradycardia, permanent pacemakers should not be implanted as a prophylactic measure in this population of patients; rather, this therapeutic approach should be reserved for patients with demonstrated symptomatic bradyarrhythmias in the setting of bifascicular and trifascicular block. It should also be reiterated that this population is particularly prone to the development of ventricular tachycardia as the underlying mechanism for syncope.[115]

PERMANENT CARDIAC PACING IN PATIENTS WITH ATRIOVENTRICULAR CONDUCTION DISORDERS DURING ACUTE MYOCARDIAL INFARCTION

Patients with bundle branch block and acute myocardial infarction have higher short-term and long-term mortality than do those without bundle branch block (see the second part of this chapter, "Temporary Cardiac Pacing"). Most of these deaths appear to be due to ventricular tachyarrhythmias and pump failure.[76, 177] Some studies,[10, 76, 177] but not all,[57, 72, 121, 129] have suggested that permanent cardiac pacing in patients who develop transient high-grade AV block in the setting of acute myocardial infarction has improved survival. In the multicenter study of Hindman and associates, the risk of sudden death or recurrent high-grade AV block was 65 per cent in patients who did not receive a permanent pacemaker, compared with only 10 per cent in those who did.[76] On the basis of these data, these investigators recommended permanent cardiac pacing for all individuals with acute myocardial infarction complicated by bundle branch block and high-grade AV block, despite the fact that the AV block almost always resolved during recovery.[76] However, a number of smaller studies of better design, in which patients were matched for age, infarct location, and type of conduction system disturbance, have not confirmed that permanent pacing has a significant effect on long-term survival[57, 72, 121, 129, 176]; this observation can almost certainly be explained by sudden death that results from ventricular tachycardia-fibrillation rather than from bradycardia. Furthermore, permanent cardiac pacing does not appear to alter long-term prognosis in patients with myocardial infarction and bundle branch block who do not develop transient high-grade AV block but who do have a prolonged HV interval.[133] This issue remains somewhat controversial as well. In patients who do receive a permanent pacing system, interrogation of the pulse generators should allow the clinician to assess whether pacing has been required in these patients, so that the natural history of this complication can be scientifically evaluated.

REFERENCES

1. Abel FL, McCutcheon ET: Cardiovascular Function: Principles and Applications. Boston, Little, Brown, 1979, pp 319–320.
2. Agruss NS, Rosin EY, Adolph RJ, Fowler NO: Significance of chronic sinus bradycardia in elderly people. Circulation 46:924–930, 1972.
3. Akhtar M, Shenasa M, Denker S, et al: Role of cardiac electrophysiologic studies in patients with unexplained recurrent syncope. PACE 6:192–201, 1983.
4. Alpert MA: Indications for permanent cardiac pacing. Am Fam Physician 26:187–197, 1982.
5. Alpert MA, Flaker G: Arrhythmias associated with sinus node dysfunction. JAMA 250:2160–2166, 1983.
6. Alpert MA, Katti SK: Natural history of sinus node dysfunction after permanent pacemaker implantation. South Med J 75:1182–1188, 1982.
7. Amat-y-Leon F, Dhingra R, Denes P, et al: The clinical spectrum of chronic His bundle block. Chest 70:747–754, 1976.
8. Arenberg IK, Cummins GM, Bucy PC, Oberhill HR: Symptomatic hyperirritable carotid sinus mechanism. Laryngoscope 81:253–263, 1971.
9. Aroesty JM, Cohen SI, Morkin E: Bradycardia-tachycardia syndrome: Results in 28 patients treated by combined pharmacologic therapy and pacemaker implantation. Chest 66:257–63, 1974.
10. Atkins J, Leshin S, Blomqvist CG, et al: Ventricular conduction blocks and sudden death in acute myocardial infarction. N Engl J Med 288:281–284, 1973.
11. Bayley PJ: Long-term ventricular pacing in treatment of sinoatrial block. Br Med J 3(5772):456–458, 1971.
12. Benditt DG, Gornick CC, Dunbar D, et al: Indications for electrophysiologic testing in the diagnosis and assessment of sinus node dysfunction. Circulation 75 [Suppl III]:II–93–99, 1987.
13. Benrey J, Gillette DC, Nasrallah AT, Hallman GI: Permanent pacemaker implantation in infants, children and adolescents: Long term follow-up. Circulation 53:245–248, 1976.
14. Berman ND: Antiarrhythmic therapy in the elderly: Pacemakers and drugs. Geriatrics 41:61–72, 1986.
15. Bernstein V, Roten CE, Peretz DI: Permanent pacemakers: 8-year followup study. Ann Intern Med 74:361, 1971.
16. Besdine RW: Geriatric medicine: An overview. Annu Rev Gerontol Geriatrics 1:135–153, 1980.
17. Bexton RS, Camm AJ: First degree atrioventricular block. Eur Heart J 5[Suppl A]:107–109, 1984.
18. Brandenburg RO, Holmes DR, Hartzler GO: The electrophysiologic assessment of patients with syncope [abstract]. Am J Cardiol 47:433, 1981.
19. Brodsky M, Wu D, Denes P, et al: Arrhythmias documented by 24 hour continuous electrocardiographic monitoring in 50 male medical students without apparent heart disease. Am J Cardiol 39:390–395, 1977.
20. Callaghan JC, Bigelow WG: An electrical artificial pacemaker for standstill of the heart. Ann Surg 134:8–17, 1951.
21. Castellanos A, Maytin O, Arcebal AG, Lemberg L: Significance of complete right bundle-branch block with right axis deviation in the absence of right ventricular hypertrophy. Br Heart J 32:85–92, 1970.

22. Chardack WM, Gage A, Frederico AJ, et al: The long-term treatment of heart block. Prog Cardiovasc Dis 9:105–135, 1966.
23. Cheng LH, Norris CW: Surgical management of the carotid sinus syndrome. Arch Otolaryngol 97:395–398, 1973.
24. Chokshi DS, Mascarenhas E, Samet P, Center S: Treatment of sinoatrial rhythm disturbances with permanent cardiac pacing. Am J Cardiol 32:215–220, 1973.
25. Clark PI, Glasser SP, Spoto E: Arrhythmias detected by ambulatory monitoring: Lack of correlation with symptoms of dizziness and syncope. Chest 77:722–725, 1980.
26. Cohen HE, Meltzer LE, Lattimer G, et al: Treatment of refractory supraventricular arrhythmias with induced permanent atrial fibrillation. Am J Cardiol 28:472–474, 1971.
27. Conde CA, Leppo J, Lipski J, et al: Effectiveness of pacemaker treatment in the bradycardia-tachycardia syndrome. Am J Cardiol 32:209–214, 1973.
28. Coplan NL, Schweitzer P: Carotid sinus hypersensitivity: Case report and review of the literature. Am J Med 77:561–565, 1984.
29. Davies AB, Stephens MR, Davies AG: Carotid sinus hypersensitivity in patients presenting with syncope. Br Heart J 42:583–586, 1979.
30. Davies MJ: Pathology of the conducting system. *In* Caird FL, Dall JLC, Kennedy RD (eds): Cardiology in Old Age. New York, Plenum Press, 1976, pp 57–86.
31. Davies MJ, Pomerance A: Quantitative study of aging changes in human sinoatrial node and internodal tracts. Br Heart J 34:150–152, 1972.
32. Denes P, Dhingra R, Wu D, et al: Sudden death in patients with chronic bifascicular block. Arch Intern Med 137:1005–1010, 1977.
33. DePasquale NP, Bruno MS: Natural history of combined right bundle branch block and left anterior hemiblock (bilateral bundle branch block). Am J Med 54:297, 1973.
34. Dhingra RC, Denes P, Wu D, et al: Syncope in patients with chronic bifascicular block: Significance, causative mechanisms, and clinical implications. Ann Intern Med 81:302–306, 1974.
35. Dhingra RC, Denes P, Wu D, et al: Complete right bundle branch block and left posterior hemiblock: Clinical, electrophysiologic and prognostic observations. Am J Cardiol 36:867–872, 1975.
36. Dhingra RC, Denes P, Wu D, et al: Prospective observations in patients with chronic branch block and H-V prolongation. Circulation 53:600–604, 1976.
37. Dickinson AM, Traver CA: Carotid body tumors: Review of the literature with report of two cases. Am J Surg 69:9–16, 1945.
38. DiMarco JP, Garan H, Harthorne JW, Ruskin JN: Intracardiac electrophysiological techniques in recurrent syncope of unknown cause. Ann Intern Med 95:542–548, 1981.
39. Doherty JU, Pembrook-Rogers D, Grogan EW, et al: Electrophysiologic evaluation and followup characteristics of patients with recurrent unexplained syncope and presyncope. Am J Cardiol 55:703–708, 1985.
40. Draper AJ: The cardioinhibitory carotid sinus syndrome. Ann Intern Med 32:700–716, 1950.
41. Eagle KA, Black HR, Cook EF, Goldman I: Evaluation of prognostic classifications for patients with syncope. Am J Med 79:455, 1985.

42. Easley R, Goldstein S: Sino-atrial syncope. Am J Med 50:166–177, 1971.

43. Ector H, Rolies L, De Geest H: Dynamic electrocardiography and ventricular pauses of 3 seconds and more: Etiology and therapeutic implications. PACE 6:548–551, 1983.

44. Ekblom B, Kilbom A, Soltysiak J: Physical training, bradycardia, and autonomic nervous system. Scand J Clin Lab Invest 32:251–256, 1973.

45. Epstein SE, Stampfer M, Beiser GD: Role of the capacitance and resistance vessels in vasovagal syncope. Circulation 37:524–533, 1968.

46. Evans R, Shaw DB: Pathological studies in sinoatrial disorder (sick sinus syndrome). Br Heart J 39:778–786, 1970.

47. Ferrer MI: The sick sinus syndrome. Circulation 47:635–641, 1973.

48. Ferris EB, Capps RB, Weiss S: Carotid sinus syncope and its bearing on the mechanism of the unconscious state and convulsions. Medicine 14:377–456, 1935.

49. Fisch GR, Zipes DP, Fisch C: Bundle branch block and sudden death. Prog Cardiovasc Dis 23:187, 1980.

50. Frye RL, Collins JJ, DeSanctis RW, et al: Guidelines for permanent cardiac pacemaker implantation, May 1984: A report of the Joint American College of Cardiology/American Heart Association Task Force on Assessment of Cardiovascular Procedures (Subcommittee on Pacemaker Implantation). Circulation 70:331A–339A, 1984.

51. Fulkerson PK, Beaver BM, Auseon JC, Graber HL: Calcification of the mitral anulus: Etiology, clinical associations, complications and therapy. Am J Med 66:967–977, 1979.

52. Furman F, Cooper JA: Atrial fibrillation during A-V sequential pacing. PACE 5:133, 1982.

53. Gadboys HL, Lubkan S, Litwak RS: Long-term followup of patients with cardiac pacemakers. Am J Cardiol 21:55–59, 1968.

54. Gang ES, Peter T, Rosenthal ME, et al: Detection of late potentials on the surface electrocardiogram in unexplained syncope. Am J Cardiol 58:1014–1020, 1986.

55. Gann D, Tolentino A, Samet P: Electrophysiologic evaluation of elderly patients with sinus bradycardia: A long-term follow up study. Ann Intern Med 90:24–29, 1979.

56. Gibson TC, Heitzman MR: Diagnostic efficacy of 24-hour electrocardiographic monitoring for syncope. Am J Cardiol 53:1013–1017, 1984.

57. Ginks WR, Sutton R, Oh W, Leatham A: Long-term prognosis after acute anterior infarction with atrioventricular block. Br Heart J 39:186–189, 1977.

58. Gomes JAC, Damato AN: His bundle electrocardiography and intracardiac stimulation. *In* Varriale P, Naclerio EA (eds): Cardiac Pacing. Philadelphia, Lea & Febiger, 1979, pp 97–122.

59. Gomes JAC, El-Sherif N: His bundle recordings: Contributions to clinical electrophysiology. *In* Samet P, El-Sherif N (eds): Cardiac Pacing. New York, Grune and Stratton, 1980, pp 375–407.

60. Gomes JAC, El-Sherif N: Atrioventricular block: Mechanism, clinical presentation, and therapy. Med Clin North Am 68:955–967, 1984.

61. Goldstein DS, Spanarkel M, Pitterman A, et al: Circulatory control mechanisms in vasodepressor syncope. Am Heart J 104:1071–1075, 1982.

62. Graybiel A, McFarland RA, Gates DC, Webster FA: Analysis of the electrocardiograms obtained from 1000 young healthy aviators. Am Heart J 27:524–549, 1944.

63. Greeley HP, Smedal MI, Most W: The treatment of the carotid-sinus syndrome by irradiation. N Engl J Med 252:91–94, 1955.

64. Gross-Fengels W, Schilling G, Neumann G, et al: Ambulantes 24-stunden-EKG bei symptomatischen Schrittmacher Patienten. Herz Kreiflauf 7:405–408, 1987.

65. Gulamhusein S, Naccarelli GV, Ko PT, et al: Value and limitations of clinical electrophysiologic study and assessment of patients with unexplained syncope. Am J Med 73:700–705, 1982.

66. Gupta PK, Lichstein E, Chadda KD: Electrophysiological features of Mobitz type II AV block occurring with the His bundle. Br Heart J 34:1232–1237, 1972.

67. Gupta PK, Lichstein E, Chadda KD: Electrophysiological features of complete AV block within the His bundle. Br Heart J 35:610–615, 1973.

68. Gupta PK, Lichstein E, Chadda KD: Chronic His bundle block: Clinical, electrocardiographic, electrophysiological, and follow-up studies on 16 patients. Br Heart J 38:1343–1349, 1976.

69. Harris A: Permanent pacing for chronic heart block. Geriatrics 30:56–57, 1975.

70. Hartel G, Talvensaari T: Treatment of sinoatrial syndrome with permanent cardiac pacing in 90 patients. Acta Med Scand 198:341–347, 1975.

71. Hartzler GO, Maloney JD: Cardioinhibitory carotid sinus hypersensitivity. Arch Intern Med 137:727–731, 1977.

72. Hauer RNW, Lie KI, Liem KL, Durrer D: Long-term prognosis in patients with bundle branch block complicating acute anteroseptal infarction. Am J Cardiol 49:1581–1585, 1982.

73. Hayes DL, Furman S: Stability of AV conduction in sick sinus node syndrome patients with implanted atrial pacemakers. Am Heart J 107:644–647, 1984.

74. Hess DS, Morady F, Scheinman MM: Electrophysiologic testing in the evaluation of patients with syncope of undetermined origin. Am J Cardiol 50:1309–1315, 1982.

75. Hilgard J, Ezri MD, Denes T: Significance of the ventricular pauses of three seconds or more detected on 24-hour Holter recordings. Am J Cardiol 55:1005–1008, 1985.

76. Hindman MC, Wagner GS, JaRo M, et al: The clinical significance of bundle branch block complicating acute myocardial infarction. 2. Indications for temporary and permanent pacemaker insertion. Circulation 58:689–699, 1978.

77. Hinkle LE, Carver ST, Plakun NA: Slow heart rates and increased risk of cardiac death in middle-aged men. Arch Intern Med 129:732–748, 1972.

78. Hiss RG, Lamb LE: Electrocardiographic findings in 122,043 individuals. Circulation 25:947–961, 1962.

79. Hoffmann A, Jost M, Pfifterer M, et al: Persisting symptoms despite permanent pacing: Incidence, causes and followup. Chest 85:207–210, 1984.

80. Horowitz LN, Josephson ME, Farshidi A, et al: Recurrent sustained ventricular tachycardia: Role of the electrophysiologic study in selection of antiarrhythmic regimens. Circulation 58:986–987, 1978.

81. Hutchison EC, Stock JP: Carotid sinus syndrome. Lancet 2:445–449, 1960.

82. Jordan JL, Mandel WJ: Disorders of sinus function. *In* Mandel WJ (ed): Cardiac Arrhythmias. Philadelphia, JB Lippincott Co, 1980, pp 108–145.

83. Kadish AH, Wechsler L, Marchlinski FE: Swallowing syncope: Observations in the absence of conduction system or esophageal disease. Am J Med 81:1098, 1986.

84. Kapoor W, Snustad D, Peterson J, et al: Syncope in the elderly. Am J Med 80:419–428, 1986.

85. Kastor JA: Atrioventricular block. N Engl J Med 292:462–465, 572–574, 1975.

86. Kay R, Estioko M, Wiener I: Primary sick sinus syndrome as an indication for chronic pacemaker therapy in young adults: Incidence, clinical features, and long-term evaluation. Am Heart J 103:338–342, 1982.

87. Kowey PR: Unnecessary pacemakers [letter]. PACE 6:982–983, 1983.

88. Kowey PR, Mulland DF, Wetstein L: Pacemaker therapy. Surg Clin North Am 65:595–611, 1985.

89. Krishnaswami V, Geraci A: Permanent pacing in disorders of sinus node function. Am Heart J 89:579–585, 1975.

90. Kulbertus H, Collignon P: Association of right bundle-branch block with left superior or inferior intraventricular block: Its relation to complete heart block and Adams-Stokes syndrome. Br Heart J 31:435–440, 1969.

91. Langendorf R, Pick A: Atrioventricular block, type II (Mobitz)—its nature and clinical significance. Circulation 38:819–821, 1968.

92. Laslett EE: Syncopal attacks associated with prolonged arrest of the whole heart. Q J Med 2:347–355, 1909.

93. Lasser RP, Haft JI, Friedberg CK: Relationship of right bundle-branch block and marked left axis deviation (with left parietal or peri-infarction block) to complete heart block and syncope. Circulation 37:429, 1968.

94. Lau SH, Damato AN: Mechanism of A-V block. Cardiovasc Clin 2:49–68, 1970.

95. Lev M, Cuadros H, Paul MH: Interruption of the atrioventricular bundle with congenital atrioventricular block. Circulation 43:703–710, 1971.

96. Levites R, Haft JI: Significance of first degree heart block (prolonged P-R interval) in bifascicular block. Am J Cardiol 34:259–264, 1974.

97. Lichstein E, Ribas-Meneclier C, Naik D, et al: The natural history of trifascicular disease following permanent pacemaker implantation. Circulation 54:780–783, 1976.

98. Lipsitz LA, Pouchino FC, Wei JY, et al: Cardiovascular and norepinephrine responses after meal consumption in elderly (older than 75 years) persons with postprandial hypotension and syncope. Am J Cardiol 58:810–815, 1986.

99. Livelli FD, Bigger JT, Reiffel JA, et al: Response to programmed ventricular stimulation: Sensitivity, specificity and relation to heart disease. Am J Cardiol 50:452–458, 1982.

100. Lown B: Electrical reversion of cardiac arrhythmias. Br Heart J 29:469–489, 1967.

101. Lown B, Levine SA: The carotid sinus: Clinical value of its stimulation. Circulation 23:766–789, 1961.

102. Mackenzie J: The cause of heart irregularity in influenza with a demonstration of the clinical polygraph. Br Med J 4(2183):1411–1413, 1902.

103. Madigan NP, Flaker GC, Curtis JJ, et al: Carotid sinus hypersensitivity: Beneficial effects of dual-chamber pacing. Am J Cardiol 53:1034–1040, 1984.

104. Mancia G, Ferrari A, Gregorini L, et al: Control of blood pressure by carotid sinus baroceptors in human beings. Am J Cardiol 44:895–902, 1979.

105. Mason JW, Winkle RA: Electrode-catheter arrhythmia induction in the selection and assessment of antiarrhythmic drug therapy for recurrent ventricular tachycardia. Circulation 58:971–985, 1978.

106. Mason JW, Winkle RA: Accuracy of the ventricular tachycardia–induction study for predicting long-term efficacy and inefficacy of antiarrhythmic drugs. N Engl J Med 303:1073–1077, 1980.

107. Mazur M, Friedman HS: Significance of prolonged electrocardiographic pauses in sinoatrial disease: Sick sinus syndrome. Am J Cardiol 52:485–489, 1983.

108. McAnulty JH, Li CK, Morton M: Evaluation of syncope in patients with heart disease [abstract]. Clin Res 31:13A, 1983.

109. McAnulty J, Kauffman S, Murphy E, et al: Survival of patients with conduction system disease [abstract]. Circulation 51–52 [Suppl III]:113, 1975.

110. McAnulty JH, Rahimtoola SH, Murphy ES, et al: A prospective study of sudden death in "high-risk" bundle-branch block. N Engl J Med 299:209–215, 1978.

111. McAnulty JH, Rahimtoola SH, Murphy E, et al: Natural history of "high-risk" bundle-branch block: Final report of a prospective study. N Engl J Med 307:137–143, 1982.

112. McGuire LB, O'Brien, Nolan SP: Patient survival and instrument performance with permanent cardiac pacing. JAMA 237:558–561, 1977.

113. McNally EN, Benchimol A: Medical and physiological considerations in the use of artificial pacing. Am Heart J 75:380–398, 1968.

114. Mobitz W: Uber die unvollständige Storung der Erregunggsüberleitung zwischen Vorhol und Kammer des menschlichen Herzens. Z Gesamte Exp Med 41:180, 1924.

115. Morady F, Higgins J, Peters RW, et al: Electrophysiological testing in bundle branch block and unexplained syncope. Am J Cardiol 54:587–591, 1984.

116. Morady F, Shen E, Schwartz A, et al: Long term follow-up of patients with recurrent unexplained syncope evaluated by electrophysiologic testing. J Am Coll Cardiol 2:1053–1059, 1983.

117. Morley CA, Sutton R: Carotid sinus syncope. Int J Cardiol 6:287–293, 1984.

118. Morley CA, Perrins EJ, Grant P, et al: Carotid sinus syncope treated by pacing: Analysis of persistent symptoms and role of atrioventricular sequential pacing. Br Heart J 47:411–418, 1982.

119. Moss AJ, Davis RJ: Brady-tachy syndrome. Prog Cardiovasc Dis 16:439–454, 1974.

120. Muller O, Finkelstein D: Adams-Stokes syndrome due to sinoatrial block. Am J Cardiol 17:433–436, 1966.

121. Murphy E, DeMots H, McAnulty J, Rahimtoola SH: Prophylactic permanent pacemakers for transient heart block during myocardial infarction? Results of a prospective study [abstract]. Am J Cardiol 49:952, 1982.

122. Mymin D, Mathewson FAL, Tate RB, Manfreda J: The natural history of primary first-degree atrioventricular heart block. N Engl J Med 315:1183–1187, 1986.

123. Nair CK, Sketch MH, Desai R, et al: High preva-

lence of symptomatic bradyarrhythmias due to atrioventricular node–fascicular and sinus node–atrial disease in patients with mitral annular calcification. Am Heart J 103:226–229, 1982.

124. Nakagawa S, Hisanaga S, Kondoh H, et al: A case of swallow syncope induced by vagotonic visceral reflex resulting in atrioventricular node suppression. J Electrocardiol 20:65, 1987.

125. Narula OS: Conduction disorders in the AV transmission system. In Dreifus LS, Likoff W (eds): Cardiac Arrhythmias. New York, Grune and Stratton, 1973, pp 259–291.

126. Narula OS: Concepts of atrioventricular block. In Narula OS (ed): His Bundle Electrocardiography and Clinical Electrophysiology. Philadelphia, FA Davis, 1975, pp 139–175.

127. Narula OS, Samet P: Wenckebach and Mobitz type II AV block due to block within the His bundle and bundle branches. Circulation 41:947–965, 1970.

128. Nathanson MH: Hyperactive cardioinhibitory carotid sinus reflex. Arch Intern Med 77:491–503, 1946.

129. Nimetz AA, Shubrooks SJ, Hutter AM Jr, DeSanctis RW: The significance of bundle branch block during acute myocardial infarction. Am Heart J 90:439–444, 1975.

130. Nishimura RA, Gersh BJ, Vlietstra RE, et al: Hemodynamic and symptomatic consequences of ventricular pacing. PACE 5:903, 1982.

131. Olshansky B, Mazuz M, Martins JB: Significance of inducible tachycardia in patients with syncope of unknown origin: A long-term follow-up. J Am Coll Cardiol 5:216–223, 1985.

132. Packard JM, Graettinger JS, Graybiel A: Analysis of the electrocardiograms obtained from 1000 young healthy aviators: Ten year follow-up. Circulation 10:384–400, 1954.

133. Pagnoni F, Finzi A, Valentini R, et al: Long-term prognostic significance and electrophysiological evolution of intraventricular conduction disturbances complicating acute myocardial infarction. PACE 9:91–100, 1986.

134. Parsonnet V: The proliferation of cardiac pacing: Medical, technical and socioeconomic dilemmas. Circulation 65:841–845, 1982.

135. Parsonnet V, Manhardt M: Permanent pacing of the heart: 1952 to 1976. Am J Cardiol 39:250–256, 1977.

136. Patel AK, Yap VU, Fields J, Thomsen JH: Carotid sinus syncope induced by malignant tumors in the neck: Emergence of vasodepressor manifestations following pacemaker therapy. Arch Intern Med 139:1281–1284, 1979.

137. Peretz DI, Gerein AN, Miyagishima RT: Permanent demand pacing for hypersensitive carotid sinus syndrome. Can Med Assoc J 108:1131–1134, 1973.

138. Peters RW, Scheinman MM, Modin G, et al: Prophylactic permanent pacemakers for patients with chronic bundle branch block. Am J Med 66:978–985, 1979.

139. Phibbs B, Friedman HS, Graboys TB, et al: Indications for pacing in the treatment of bradyarrhythmias: Report of an independent study group. JAMA 252:1307–1311, 1984.

140. Puech P, Grolleau R, Guilond C: Incidence of different types of A-V blocks and their localisation by His bundle recordings. In Wellens HJJ, Lei K, Janse MJ (eds): The Conduction System of the Heart: Structure, Function and Clinical Implications. Philadelphia, Lea & Febiger, 1976.

141. Rasmussen K: Chronic sinus node disease: Natural course and indications for pacing. Eur Heart J 2:455–459, 1981.

142. Reed EA, Scott JC: Factors influencing the carotid sinus cardioinhibitory reflex. Am J Physiol 181:21–26, 1955.

143. Rokseth R, Hatle L: Prospective study on the occurrence and management of chronic sinoatrial disease, with follow-up. Br Heart J 36:582–587, 1974.

144. Rosenbaum MB, Elizari MV, Lazzari JO, et al: Intraventricular trifascicular blocks: Review of the literature and classification. Am Heart J 78:450–459, 1969.

145. Rosenqvist M, Brandt J, Schuller H: Atrial versus ventricular pacing in sinus node disease: A treatment comparison study. Am Heart J 111:292–297, 1986.

146. Rowe JW: Aging and renal function. Annu Rev Gerontol Geriatrics 1:161–179, 1980.

147. Rowe JW, Troen BR: Sympathetic nervous system and aging in man. Endocr Rev 1:167–179, 1980.

148. Rubenstein JJ, Schulman CL, Yurchak PM, DeSanctis RW: Clinical spectrum of the sick sinus syndrome. Circulation 46:5–13, 1972.

149. Salomon S: The carotid sinus syndrome. Am J Cardiol 2:342–350, 1958.

150. Scheinman M, Weiss A, Kunkel F: His bundle recordings in patients with bundle branch block and transient neurologic symptoms. Circulation 48:322–330, 1973.

151. Scheinman MM, Peters RW, Sauve MJ, et al: Value of the H-Q interval in patients with bundle branch block and the role of prophylactic permanent pacing. Am J Cardiol 50:1316–1322, 1982.

152. Schuilenburg RM, Durrer D: Conduction disturbances located within the His bundle. Circulation 45:612–628, 1972.

153. Shaw DB, Holman RR, Gowers JI: Survival in sinoatrial disorder (sick sinus syndrome). Br Med J 280:139–141, 1980.

154. Sigler LH: The cardioinhibitory carotid sinus reflex. Am J Cardiol 12:175–183, 1963.

155. Sigurd B, Jensen G, Meibom J, Sandoe E: Adams-Stokes syndrome caused by sinoatrial block. Br Heart J 35:1002–1008, 1973.

156. Simon AB, Zloto AE: Symptomatic sinus node disease: Natural history after permanent ventricular pacing. PACE 2:305–314, 1979.

157. Skagen K, Hansen JF: The long-term prognosis for patients with sinoatrial block treated with permanent pacemaker. Acta Med Scand 199:13–15, 1976.

158. Sklaroff HJ: Carotid sinus hypersensitivity—asystole and hypotension in the same patient [letter]. Am Heart J 97:815, 1979.

159. Smyth NPD: Cardiac pacing. Ann Thorac Surg 27:270–283, 1979.

160. Southall DP, Johnston F, Shinebourne E, et al: Twenty-four hour electrocardiographic study of heart rate and rhythm patterns in population of healthy children. Br Heart J 45:281–291, 1981.

161. Strasberg B, Amat-y-Leon F, Dhingra RC, et al: Natural history of chronic second-degree atrioventricular nodal block. Circulation 63:1043–1049, 1981.

162. Strasberg B, Lam W, Swiryn S, et al: Symptomatic spontaneous paroxysmal AV nodal block due to localized hyperresponsiveness of the AV node to vagotonic reflexes. Am Heart J 103:795, 1982.

163. Strauss HD, Berman ND: Permanent pacing in the elderly. PACE 1:458–464, 1978.
164. Stryger D, Friedensohn A, Schlesinger S: Carotid sinus hypersensitivity: Diagnosis of vasodepressor type in the presence of cardioinhibitory type. PACE 5:793–800, 1982.
165. Sugrue DD, Gersh BJ, Holmes DR, et al: Symptomatic "isolated" carotid sinus hypersensitivity: Natural history and results of treatment with anticholinergic drugs or pacemaker. J Am Coll Cardiol 7:158–162, 1986.
166. Sutton R, Citron P: Electrophysiological and haemodynamic basis for application of new pacemaker technology in sick sinus syndrome and atrioventricular block. Br Heart J 41:600–612, 1979.
167. Sutton R, Kenny R: The natural history of sick sinus syndrome. PACE 9:1110–1114, 1986.
168. Thomas JE: Hyperactive carotid sinus reflex and carotid sinus syncope. Mayo Clin Proc 44:127–139, 1969.
169. Thomas JE: Diseases of the carotid sinus—syncope. In Vinkin PJ, Bruyn GW (eds): Handbook of Clinical Neurology. Vol II. Amsterdam, North-Holland Publishing, 1972, p 532.
170. Timmis GC, Gordon S, Ramos R: Heart block in the aged: Is the patient too old to be permanently paced? Chest 60:113, 1971.
171. Vandepol CJ, Farshidi A, Spielman SR, et al: Incidence and clinical significance of induced ventricular tachycardia. Am J Cardiol 45:725–731, 1980.
172. Vera Z, Mason DT, Awan NA, et al: Improvement of symptoms in patients with sick sinus syndrome by spontaneous development of stable atrial fibrillation. Br Heart J 39:160–167, 1977.
173. Von Maur K, Nelson EW, Holsinger JW, Eliot RS: Hypersensitive carotid sinus syncope treated by implantable demand cardiac pacemaker. Am J Cardiol 29:109–110, 1972.
174. Voss DM, Magnin GE: Demand pacing and carotid sinus syncope. Am Heart J 79:544–547, 1970.
175. Walter PF, Crawley IS, Dorney ER: Carotid sinus hypersensitivity and syncope. Am J Cardiol 42:396–403, 1978.
176. Watson RD, Glover DR, Page AJ, et al: The Birmingham Trial of permanent pacing in patients with intraventricular conduction disorders after acute myocardial infarction. Am Heart J 108:496–501, 1984.
177. Waugh RA, Wagner GS, Haney TL, et al: Immediate and remote prognostic significance of fascicular block during acute myocardial infarction. Circulation 47:765–775, 1973.
178. Weiss S, Baker JP: The carotid sinus reflex in health and disease, its role in the causation of fainting and convulsions. Medicine 12:297–354, 1933.
179. Weissler AM, Warren JV: Vasodepressor syncope. Am Heart J 57:786–794, 1959.
180. Weissler AM, Warren JV, Estes EH, et al: Vasodepressor syncope: Factors influencing cardiac output. Circulation 15:875–882, 1957.
181. Wenckebach KF: Zur Analyse des unregelmaessigen Pulses. Z Kolner Med 37:475, 1899.
182. Wenckebach KF: Beitraege zur Kenntnis der menschlichen Herztaetigkeit. Arch Anat Physiol (Physiol Abtheil) 297, 1906.
183. Wiener L, Dwyer EM: Electrical induction of atrial fibrillation: An approach to intractable atrial tachycardia. Am J Cardiol 21:731–734, 1968.
184. Wise JR, Sensenig DM: Permanent cardiac pacing at a regional medical center. J Thorac Cardiovasc Surg 70:677–686, 1975.
185. Wohl AJ, Laborde NJ, Atkins JM, et al: Prognosis of patients permanently paced for sick sinus syndrome. Arch Intern Med 136:406–408, 1976.
186. Zoll PM, Linenthal AJ, Norman RL, Belgard AH: Treatment of Stokes-Adams disease by external electric stimulation of the heart. Circulation 9:482–493, 1954.

B.   Temporary Cardiac Pacing

J. MARCUS WHARTON *and* NORA GOLDSCHLAGER

Since the introduction of the temporary cardiac pacemaker in 1952 by Zoll,[146] the use of temporary and permanent cardiac pacemakers has markedly expanded. It is estimated from the National Hospital Discharge Survey that the number of new pacemakers implanted has grown from 24,000 in 1970 to 165,000 in 1983.[43] Of the pacemakers inserted in 1983, approximately 60,000 were temporary transvenous or epicardial pacemakers. It has been estimated that 40,000 transthoracic pacemakers are used annually[107]; the frequency of use of external pacemakers has yet to be quantified. Between 10 per cent and 15 per cent of patients admitted to the cardiac intensive care units of a teaching hospital will receive temporary pacemakers.[57] One reason for the increasing utilization of pacemakers is the expanding list of indications for their use. Although initially developed for the treatment of transient or established high-grade atrioventricular (AV) block and symptomatic bradyarrhythmias, current indications

Supported in part by National Institutes of Health research grant HL-07063.

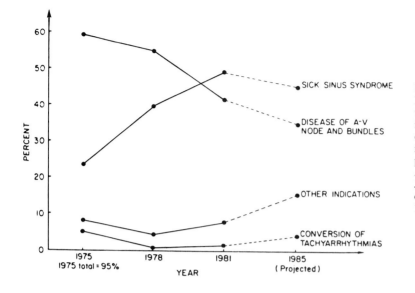

Figure 5–6. Data from the U.S. Pacing Survey of 1981 analyzing the prior 10 years of pacing system insertions. The relative frequency of pacemaker therapy for different indications is illustrated. (Reprinted with permission from the American College of Cardiology. Journal of the American College of Cardiology, Vol 3, 1984, pp 1321–1332.)

include the existence of high risk for the development of significant bradyarrhythmias, in which pacing system insertion is performed as a prophylactic measure against this eventuality; induction, termination, and prevention of several types of atrial and ventricular tachyarrhythmias; and evaluation of coronary reserve and cardiac function.

Increasing knowledge of the effect (or lack of effect) of cardiac pacing in altering the frequency of symptoms or risk of sudden death associated with various conduction disturbances and rhythm disorders has also led to changes in the use of pacemakers. The findings of the U.S. Pacing Survey illustrate this point (Fig. 5–6). Between 1975 and 1985, the percentage of all pacing systems inserted for sinus nodal dysfunction increased from 23 per cent to 48 per cent, whereas the relative frequency of pacemaker insertion for AV nodal dysfunction decreased from 59 per cent to 42 per cent.[99] Over the same time period, the use of pacemakers for control of tachyarrhythmias and "other" undefined indications gradually increased. With increasing concern about cost containment in the delivery of health care, there is greater scrutiny of the indications for insertion of both temporary and permanent pacing systems. Although there are several uncontested indications for pacemaker therapy, controversy still exists in many areas. The purpose of this second part of Chapter 5 is to discuss the various types of temporary cardiac pacemakers and the definite and disputed indications for their use.

TYPES OF TEMPORARY CARDIAC PACING

Temporary cardiac pacing can be achieved by external, transesophageal, or direct myocardial routes. Direct myocardial stimulation can be accomplished by pacing through transvenous, transthoracic (transmyocardial), or epicardial leads. In addition to electrical pacing, temporary external mechanical pacemakers have been developed that stimulate the heart by the transference to the heart of impact energy generated by small pistons on the chest wall[147]; such nonelectrical methods of cardiac pacing have not gained wide acceptance.

External (Transcutaneous) Cardiac Pacing

The oldest form of temporary cardiac pacing is external, or transcutaneous, pacing by passage of current through the heart using electrodes placed on the surface of the chest. This technique was first introduced by Zoll in 1952 as a means of treating asystole and significant bradyarrhythmias.[146] However, the high current densities at the skin electrodes required to pace cardiac tissue in these early devices caused painful stimulation of the cutaneous nerves and underlying skeletal muscle. With the development of transvenous pacing leads later in the 1950s, interest in external pacing waned. Recently, however, there has been a resurgence of enthusiasm for this technique as a result of the recognition of the dire prognosis

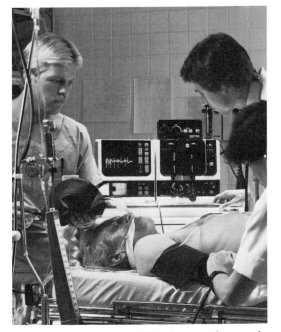

Figure 5–7. Physio-control Lifepak external pacemaker (background), mounted next to a defibrillator, being used in the setting of acute complete heart block. Illustration of Physio-control's Lifepak 8 external pacemaker with external pacing patch electrodes. (Courtesy of Physio-control, Redmond, Washington.)

of patients having cardiac arrest and associated bradycardia and the growing need for readily available temporary pacemakers for use in cardiac catheterization laboratories, intensive care units, emergency rooms, and transport vehicles for patients. Since emergency medical personnel are not trained in the methods of inserting temporary transvenous pacing leads, and since the risk of complications from insertion of temporary leads is greatest in emergency situations, a simple and safe method of pacing the heart that can be rapidly initiated in the cramped compartment of an ambulance or helicopter or that can be quickly applied at the onset of acute rhythm disturbances is needed (Fig. 5–7).

Recent improvements in the design of external pacemakers allow the device to be reasonably well tolerated by the majority of patients.[34, 148] The maximal deliverable current is about 140 mA; generally, only 40 to 70 mA is required to pace cardiac tissue. Whereas the high current densities generated at the surface electrodes in the earlier models were responsible for the majority of intolerable side effects, devices available at present are able to utilize lower current densities by virtue of long

pulse durations of 40 msec, and by the use of two large external electrodes, typically applied to the left subscapular area and to the lower left sternal border or the right upper sternal border and left ventricular apical area. Although cutaneous nerve stimulation is much less of a problem, skeletal muscle stimulation may still occur and may be alleviated by positioning the surface electrodes in areas with less underlying skeletal muscle.

In the studies of Zoll and colleagues,[148] external cardiac pacing was ineffective in 29 of the 134 patients reviewed. The majority of these pacing failures occurred in patients with prolonged cardiopulmonary arrests and terminal circulatory collapse, in whom myocardial stimulation might be anticipated to be more difficult owing to underlying ischemia, hypoxia, and electrolyte abnormalities. The possibility of successful ventricular capture in patients with cardiac arrests exceeding 15 minutes before the institution of external pacing ranges from 33 per cent to 45 per cent.[92, 148] Whether transvenous or transthoracic pacing would be more successful in these individuals is not known. External pacing does not appear to be associated with deleterious hemodynamic effects when compared with transvenous ventricular pacing. Some investigators have found no significant differences between external and transvenous ventricular pacing in measured hemodynamic parameters,[148] whereas others have noted hemodynamic improvement with external pacing.[88, 89] A recent study utilizing esophageal recording electrodes revealed that only the ventricles were directly activated by external pacing stimuli; the atria were activated by retrograde AV conduction.[33] If the hemodynamic performance with external cardiac pacing is superior to that with transvenous pacing, the improvement must be considered to be due to a greater degree of organization of ventricular activation.

Transesophageal Pacing

Shafiroff and Linder first described successful transesophageal atrial pacing in 1957.[120] However, like external cardiac pacing, this technique was eclipsed by the advent of transvenous lead systems. Because placement of esophageal pacing leads is both easy and noninvasive, renewed interest in this modality has occurred, particularly for the treatment of dysrhythmias. Although transesophageal pacing is nearly 100 per cent effective for atrial pacing, it is substantially less effective for ventricular pacing; this constitutes the major limitation to the method. Ventricular pacing using typical esophageal leads is possible in only 3 to 6 per cent of patients.[9, 11, 41, 91] The difference in efficacy between atrial and ventricular pacing is presumably related to the proximity of the left atrium to the esophagus as well as to the greater distance of the base of the left ventricle to the esophagus. Attempts to improve the current distribution generated at the left ventricle either by increasing the current magnitude or by unipolar stimulation have generally resulted in uncomfortable or painful symptoms as well as diaphragmatic stimulation. Some investigators have reported greater success in pacing the ventricles. Sadowski and Szwed[114] were able to pace the ventricles in 75 of 84 patients (89 per cent) using voltage outputs of 10 to 70 V. Using a specially designed balloon electrode to improve contact between the electrode and the esophagus and decrease the distance between the stimulating electrode and the heart, Andersen and Pless were able to pace the ventricle in 54 per cent of their patients.[1]

Until transesophageal pacing techniques can ensure reliable ventricular pacing, they cannot be recommended for the treatment or prophylaxis of high-grade AV block or other situations in which ventricular pacing is required. The method can be used when temporary atrial pacing is indicated. However, given the relative ease of electrode dislodgment with subsequent failure to capture, the limited information on changes in stimulation threshold with prolonged use, and the discomfort, albeit mild, associated with transesophageal pacing, temporary transvenous atrial pacing is not recommended if the requirement for pacing is anticipated to be longer than 10 to 30 minutes or if the patient is dependent upon atrial pacing for hemodynamic support.

Most of the research in transesophageal pacing has been directed toward its use in the diagnosis and treatment of various dysrhythmias. Esophageal pacing has been used to initiate and terminate various supraventricular tachycardias,[9, 12, 41, 66] to test sinoatrial (SA) and AV nodal function,[15, 18] to unmask accessory AV bypass tract conduction,[41] to test serially the efficacy of various antiarrhythmic agents,[10, 13] and to stress the myocardium for detection of ischemia manifested by pacing-induced ventricular wall motion abnormalities assessed echocardiographically.[22] The use of esophageal leads for sensing atrial electrical activity may facilitate the distinction of reentrant paroxys-

mal supraventricular tachycardias that incorporate an accessory AV bypass tract from those that utilize the AV node[12, 40]; of sinus tachycardia from other supraventricular tachycardias, such as atrial flutter[113, 118]; and of ventricular tachycardia from supraventricular tachycardia with aberrant intraventricular conduction.[113, 118]

Bipolar transesophageal pacing (preferably with the cathode proximal to the anode) is more effective than unipolar pacing.[91] Atrial capture is usually best obtained by pacing at or within 2 to 3 cm of the site of the unipolar atrial electrogram having the greatest magnitude.[1, 11, 91] However, the "window," or length of the esophagus over which the atrium can be captured with less than 20 mA, was, in one study, approximately 5 to 8 cm,[11] but this will vary with the type of electrode catheter and interelectrode distance. When ventricular pacing can be achieved, the optimal pacing site is distal to the area at which the largest unipolar atrial electrogram is recorded; this site is usually about 1 to 4 cm above the gastroesophageal junction. Atrial capture can usually be obtained with currents less than 20 mA. Currents greater than 20 to 30 mA usually cause significant discomfort.

A number of esophageal electrode catheters are commercially available (Fig. 5–8). The "pill" electrode consists of a small-gauge flexible wire that causes little pharyngeal irritation; placement is facilitated by covering the tip of the electrode with a gelatin capsule, which allows the patient to swallow the electrode easily.[118]

The pulse generator typically used for transvenous pacing is not suitable for transesophageal pacing. Temporary pacemaker generators designed to be used with transvenous lead

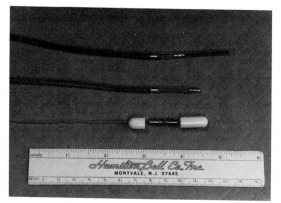

Figure 5–8. Types of esophageal electrodes, including pill electrode.

systems typically have pulse durations of 2 msec or less and a maximal deliverable current of 15 to 20 mA. The strength-duration curve for transesophageal pacing is shifted rightward compared with that for direct myocardial stimulation and does not flatten until pacing stimuli lasting at least 10 msec are delivered (Fig. 5–9).[9] Moreover, current thresholds, even with pacing stimuli of 10 msec duration, not infrequently exceed 20 mA. Thus, the generator for transesophageal pacing must be able to deliver stimuli of up to 30 mA and at least 10 msec duration; several pacemaker manufacturers market generators with these specifications at the present time (Fig. 5–10).

Complications of esophageal pacing are uncommon. Most patients experience substernal or epigastric discomfort similar to indigestion[41, 91]; this discomfort is generally tolerated if the pacing stimulus is less than 20 mA. In a study of 65 patients paced from the esophagus for various reasons, complications other than mild discomfort occurred infrequently: Non-

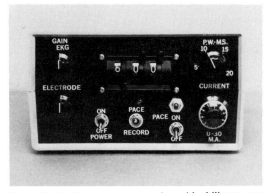

Figure 5–10. Esophageal pacemaker with ability to sense and pace. Note pulse width (P.W.) options of 5, 10, 15, and 20 msec (M.S.) and current options of 0 to 30 mA (M.A.). (Courtesy of Jack Kasall, Durham, NC.)

sustained atrial fibrillation was induced in four patients and ventricular tachycardia in two (both with clinical ventricular tachycardia), and phrenic nerve stimulation occurred in one.[41] Brachial plexus stimulation can occur in infants in whom esophageal electrodes are proximally placed.[9] Esophagogastroscopy has been performed in a small number of patients having esophageal pacing and has not revealed significant erosion or perforation[86, 91]; in two patients paced for 30 and 60 hours respectively, esophagogastroscopy revealed only slight pressure necrosis, similar to that found with prolonged insertion of nasogastric tubes.[19, 86]

Transvenous Pacing

By far, the most commonly used technique of temporary cardiac pacing is by direct myocardial stimulation using either transvenous or transthoracic pacing leads in contact with the endocardium. If transthoracic pacing in truly emergent situations is excluded, 95 per cent of all temporary cardiac pacing is accomplished via the transvenous route.[99] Since the introduction of transvenous pacing in 1959 by Furman and Schwedel for the treatment of Stokes-Adams attacks,[38] indications for transvenous pacing systems have expanded to include all of the situations discussed in this chapter. Transvenous pacing catheters may be positioned in the right atrium, the right ventricle, or both, as well as in other sites such as the coronary sinus. The ability to place catheters in both chambers of the right side of the heart permits dual-chamber sensing and pacing with their attendant hemodynamic benefit in specific clinical situations. Although generally used for pacing, endocardial electrodes, espe-

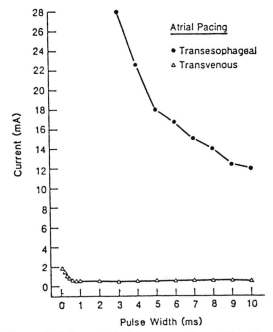

Figure 5–9. Strength-duration curves for atrial pacing using transvenous and transesophageal techniques. With the transvenous approach, increasing the pulse duration beyond 1 msec does not further decrease the low current required for atrial activation. However, with transesophageal atrial pacing, pulse durations exceeding 5 msec do decrease the current required for capture; the strength-duration curve is relatively flat at pulse widths over 10 msec (not shown). (From Benson DW Jr, Dunnigan A, Benditt DG, Schneider SP: Transesophageal cardiac pacing: History, application, technique. Clin Prog Pacing Electrophysiol 2:360–372, 1984; with permission.)

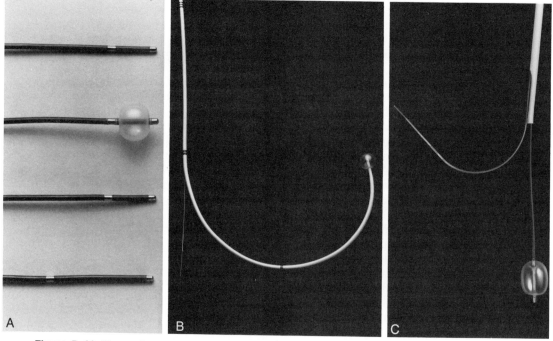

Figure 5–11. Types of temporary transvenous pacing catheters. *A,* From top to bottom: semifloating bipolar pacing electrode; "flow-assisted" bipolar pacing electrode; traditional bipolar pacing electrode; and Goetz bipolar pacing electrode. *B,* Pacing thermodilution catheter system showing the intraluminal ventricular pacing lead extending from the side port. *C,* AV sequential pacing lead showing the atrial J-shaped electrode protruding through the upper port of the insertion sheath and the balloon-tipped bipolar ventricular electrode protruding through the lower port. (All figures courtesy of Bard Critical Care Division, C. R. Bard, Billerica, MA.)

cially atrial, can be used to record atrial and ventricular electrograms in order to diagnose correctly some arrhythmias in a manner identical with that discussed for transesophageal electrodes.

Available lead systems for transvenous right ventricular pacing can be divided into three basic types: balloon flotation, semiflotation, and traditional (Fig. 5–11A). Swan-Ganz catheters containing electrodes built onto the catheter are available, but their use is limited by instability of contact with the endocardium. Recently, Swan-Ganz catheters with side ports through which a pacing wire can be placed have been designed to overcome this problem (Fig. 5–11B). The buoyancy of flotation and semiflotation electrode catheters allows cardiac flow to direct them into the right ventricle. Traditional temporary electrode catheters are stiffer and have greater torque control, which allows manipulation into the ventricle with the aid of fluoroscopy. Temporary atrial leads have been designed whose J shape allows the lead to curl into the right atrial appendage when inserted from an internal jugular or subclavian vein approach.[76] These may be used in con-

junction with ventricular leads for AV sequential pacing (Fig. 5–11C).

Temporary pacing catheters may be inserted easily under direct visualization using fluoroscopy or, if fluoroscopy is not readily available, by recording the unipolar electrogram from the distal electrode during its passage into the heart. To record the intracardiac electrogram, the distal (tip) electrode is connected with the precordial lead of a well-grounded electrocardiographic recorder. The use of a multichannel recorder allows the simultaneous display of both the surface electrocardiogram and the intracavitary electrogram, thereby facilitating recognition of each component of the intracavitary recording. When the catheter tip lies in the right atrium, the magnitude of the recorded atrial electrogram will exceed that of the ventricular electrogram; as the catheter tip passes into the right ventricle, this relationship reverses (Fig. 5–12). Upon contact with right ventricular endocardium, a current of injury manifested as ST-segment elevation will be recorded. The different routes and means of placement of transvenous lead systems are discussed in detail in Chapter 9. Recently,

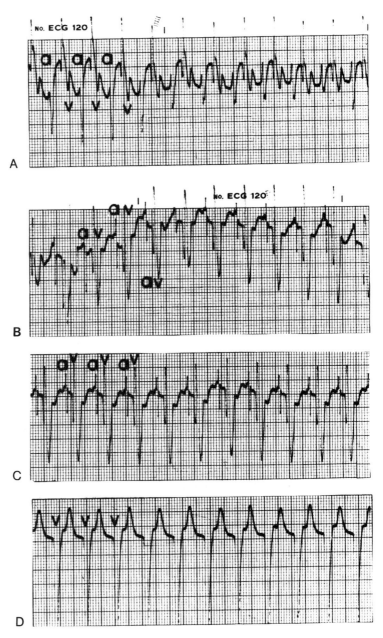

Figure 5–12. Intracavitary electrograms from a 56-year-old woman with acute anterior wall myocardial infarction, intermittent type II second-degree AV block, and new left bundle branch block. *A, B, C,* and *D* illustrate electrograms recorded from the vicinity of the high right atrium, tricuspid valve, right ventricular cavity, and right ventricular endocardium, respectively. Note the decreasing size of the atrial electrogram (a) relative to the ventricular electrogram (v) as the catheter is passed to the low right atrium and tricuspid valve. The atrial electrogram is not expected to be recorded from the body or apex of the right ventricle and is not seen in *D*. Note the ST-segment elevation in *D*, indicating the pattern of injury associated with endocardial contact.

temporary unipolar pacing during percutaneous transluminal angioplasty was achieved using the guide wire within the coronary artery as the electrode.[85] Ventricular capture was achieved in all patients, with a mean stimulation threshold of 5.7 mA; occasionally, some sites within an infarcted area could not be paced. The sensed epicardial electrogram, recorded at various times during the angioplasty procedure, may be more sensitive than the surface electrocardiogram in detecting myocardial injury currents, suggesting a potential use for this technique.

Unlike external and transesophageal pacing,

myocardial stimulation thresholds are generally much lower using transvenous leads, usually less than 2 mA.[9, 29] However, myocardial infarction and ischemia, hyperkalemia, antiarrhythmic drug therapy, and a number of metabolic derangements may increase this threshold.[29] Commercially available temporary pulse generators are all adequate for direct myocardial pacing, since their pulse durations are typically 1 to 2 msec and their maximal output is approximately 20 mA. However, the maximal rate of 120 to 150 per minute is generally not sufficiently high for rapid pacing techniques to convert tachyarrhythmias; specially designed temporary units with higher rates must be used for this purpose.

The reported complication rate of 4 to 20 per cent with insertion of transvenous pacing systems is considerably higher than with either external or transesophageal pacing.[3, 57, 68] Significant complications include pneumothorax, arterial puncture, serious bleeding, pericardial inflammation, myocardial penetration or perforation, arrhythmias, infection, venous thrombosis, pulmonary embolism, and lead dislodgment. The risk of all complications increases when transvenous systems are inserted in emergency situations, such as during cardiopulmonary resuscitation. In a retrospective survey of all patients admitted to the cardiac intensive care unit of the Mayo Clinic over a 5-year period, complications occurred in 13.7 per cent of patients receiving a temporary pacemaker.[57] The incidence of complications varied with the route of insertion, with internal jugular and femoral approaches having fewer clinically evident complications than subclavian or antecubital approaches in this study (Table 5–5). However, other series have noted a 25 to 35 per cent incidence of deep venous thrombosis demonstrated by noninvasive testing (impedance plethysmography and iodine-125–labeled fibrinogen scanning), venography, and autopsy[93, 97] in patients with femoral vein pacing leads. In patients with venographic evidence of thrombosis at the site of the femoral pacing lead, 50 to 60 per cent had evidence of pulmonary emboli as determined by ventilation-perfusion lung scanning.[93] Femoral vein routes may also carry a greater risk of serious infection.[3] For these reasons, the internal jug-

ular vein approach is preferable to the femoral vein route.

In addition to pacemaker-related complications, temporary transvenous pacing is associated with a 14 to 37 per cent incidence of pacemaker malfunction.[3, 57, 68] The malfunction primarily involves failure to capture and is corrected in most cases by increasing the energy output or repositioning the lead. The incidence of lead migration varies with the insertion site used but is probably greatest with the brachial vein approach owing to the motion transmitted to the electrode catheter with arm movements.[3] The percutaneous brachial vein approach is infrequently used; however, it may be the preferred route in anticoagulated patients, since if bleeding occurs at the site, hemostatic pressure can be most easily applied and maintained.

The incidence of pacemaker-related complications and malfunction can be minimized in several ways. Since the risk of complications is inversely related to the experience of the physician inserting the pacemaker, novices should not be allowed to insert them electively without supervision. Portable anteroposterior and transbed lateral roentgenograms and paced 12-lead electrocardiograms should be obtained immediately after insertion and once daily for the duration of use. The chest roentgenograms should be inspected for the presence of pneumothorax (which may be entirely asymptomatic) and lead migration. The 12-lead electrocardiogram should be analyzed for appropriate sensing and pacing function, for stability of the pacing artifact axis, and for morphology of the paced P wave or QRS

TABLE 5–5. ROUTE OF ELECTRODE INSERTION, PACEMAKER-RELATED COMPLICATIONS, AND INCIDENCE OF COMPLICATIONS FOR EACH ROUTE

	ROUTE			
COMPLICATION	Antecubital (N = 606)	Subclavian (N = 177)	Internal Jugular (N = 111)	Femoral (N = 48)
Pericardial friction rub	43	6	5	0
Dysrhythmia*	18	5	0	1
Right ventricular perforation	17	3	0	1
Local infection	6	3	1	2
Inadvertent arterial puncture	5	5	1	0
Diaphragmatic stimulation	8	0	2	0
Phlebitis	6	0	0	0
Pneumothorax	0	1	0	0
Cardiac tamponade	1	0	0	0
TOTAL	104 (17.2%)	23 (13.0%)	9 (8.1%)	4 (8.3%)

*Catheter-induced ventricular flutter or fibrillation that necessitated direct-current cardioversion.

From Hynes JK, Holmes DR Jr, Harrison CE: Five-year experience with temporary pacemaker therapy in the coronary care unit. Mayo Clin Proc 58:125, 1983; with permission.

complex or both. Changes in the latter suggest lead migration or perforation. Stimulation thresholds should be checked several times a day, and marked changes evaluated further to exclude lead migration or disconnection. Pulse generator batteries should be checked frequently and replaced as needed. Recording the unipolar and bipolar endocardial electrograms in patients who are not pacemaker dependent and noting changes in their morphology will also help to detect lead dislodgment or myocardial penetration. Transvenous pacing leads, like other intravascular catheters, should be removed and new leads inserted in a second site every 3 to 4 days, if possible, to decrease the risk of infection and venous thrombosis.[3]

Transthoracic (Transmyocardial) Pacing

Transthoracic pacing is achieved by insertion of a hooked pacing lead through the chest wall or epigastric area and through the adjacent ventricular wall to allow contact of the lead wire with the ventricular endocardium (Fig. 5–13). Since placement of a transthoracic lead requires ventricular puncture, with its associated risks of cardiac tamponade, myocardial and coronary laceration, and pneumothorax,[17] its use has generally been reserved for strictly life-threatening situations in which transvenous pacing cannot be accomplished rapidly and in which external pacing using skin electrodes is not available or not successful. Its most common use is during cardiac arrest, when it is used to treat asystole or agonal bradyarrhythmias. As with external pacing techniques initiated after prolonged and unsuccessful resuscitation efforts, the efficacy of transthoracic pacing will be marginal at best the later it is employed. The reported incidence of successful ventricular capture varies from 5 to 90 per cent, although typically it is 20 to 40 per cent. Electromechanical dissociation occurs in the majority (60 to 100 per cent) of these patients,[31, 107, 127, 141, 142] however, owing to the agonal clinical situations in which the method is used. Furthermore, in almost all published studies, 0 per cent to, at best, 5 per cent of patients survive the resuscitative efforts.[31, 107, 127, 141, 142] The reasons for these poor results are multiple but relate predominantly to the use of transthoracic pacing only as a "last ditch" effort after prolonged, unsuccessful resuscitation maneuvers, at a time when anoxic and metabolic derangements are so severe that recruitable myocardium is not available. This achievement of poor results has led to the recommendation of early use of transthoracic pacing.[142] The risk associated with transthoracic pacing is probably not as high as once thought. In a report by Davison and colleagues,[25] there was a 31 per cent incidence of pericardial effusion assessed by echocardiography or autopsy in 53 patients who had intracardiac injections for the administration of pharmacologic agents or placement of a transthoracic pacing lead during cardiopulmonary resuscitation. No patient had clinical evidence of cardiac tamponade or autopsy evidence of myocardial or coronary artery laceration. In the 40 patients who survived the resuscitation attempt, only 1 had a significant complication, a pneumothorax.[25] Of 21 patients reported by Tintinelli and White, only 1 had a complication (tamponade) from transthoracic pacemaker placement that resulted directly in the patient's death.[127] Despite these encouraging reports, given the potential gravity of the attendant risks, it is difficult to advocate early use of the method in the cardiac arrest situation, unless no other pacing modality is available; cer-

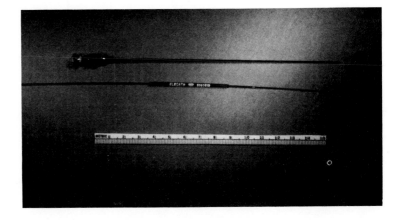

Figure 5–13. Transthoracic pacing lead with insertion set. (Courtesy of Electro-Catheter Corp, Rahway, NJ.)

tainly, the procedure should not be employed in awake or stable patients. Emergency external (transcutaneous) pacing is much safer and probably as effective as transthoracic pacing in the setting of cardiopulmonary arrest and could be used with few, if any, reservations early in the resuscitative effort, even in awake individuals.

Epicardial Pacing

Increasing attention has been focused on the multiple uses of epicardial electrodes temporarily placed on the atria or ventricles or both during and after cardiac surgery. Teflon-coated leads with bared tips can be sutured to the epicardium and exposed externally in a sterile fashion so that pacing and sensing can be accomplished. The leads can be removed from the epicardium with gentle traction when they are no longer required. A pair of closely spaced atrial and ventricular electrode wires are recommended to allow bipolar sensing; in some clinical situations, this facilitates interpretation of the epicardial electrogram relative to surface electrocardiographic events.

The use of epicardial leads in the management of patients after cardiac surgery is increasingly recognized as a helpful adjunct in the diagnosis and treatment of postoperative dysrhythmias.[133, 135] In one large study of 70 consecutive patients who had undergone open heart surgery, temporary atrial epicardial electrodes were used for diagnostic purposes in 8 (11 per cent), for therapeutic reasons in 23 (33 per cent), and for both purposes in 26 (37 per cent); thus, temporary atrial wires were helpful in managing 81 per cent of the patients.[136] Recording the atrial electrogram helps both to identify atrial electrical activity and to establish its association with ventricular electrical activity, thus facilitating the diagnosis of postoperative supraventricular tachycardias and aiding in the differentiation of sinus tachycardia, atrial flutter, atrial fibrillation, and ectopic atrial tachycardia (Fig. 5–14). The method also helps to differentiate supraventricular tachycardias with aberrant intraventricular conduction from ventricular tachycardias with AV dissociation. Temporary ventricular epicardial leads are rarely helpful diagnostically but are useful therapeutically. With the exception of ventricular fibrillation, atrial fibrillation, sinus tachycardia, and type II atrial flutter (flutter rate greater than 340 per minute and positively directed flutter waves in the inferior electrocardiographic leads), virtually all postoperative arrhythmias are potentially treatable or preventable with cardiac pacing.[133, 135] In patients who have undergone surgical ablation of an arrhythmogenic focus, accessory bypass tract, or AV node, atrial and ventricular epicardial wires can be used for postoperative electrophysiologic investigation.

Epicardial electrodes can be used to maintain or improve the hemodynamic status of the patient in the postoperative period. Frequently, patients with limited cardiovascular reserve have a "relative bradycardia," that is, a heart rate that is inappropriately low (although not bradycardiac in a strict definitional

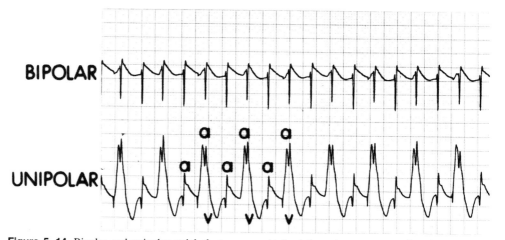

Figure 5–14. Bipolar and unipolar atrial electrograms obtained through temporary epicardial wires in a 73-year-old man 3 days after aortic valve replacement. The atrial rhythm is regular, with a rate of 190 per minute with 2:1 AV conduction. Note the alternans of the atrial electrograms. The atrial rate suggests atrial tachycardia rather than atrial flutter. Rapid atrial pacing failed to correct the bradycardia, but procainamide therapy was successful.

sense) to maintain the cardiac output necessary for the patient's postoperative needs.[133, 135] If both atrial and ventricular epicardial electrodes have been placed, they can be used for AV sequential pacing to optimize cardiac output in hemodynamically compromised patients.[50]

The use of temporary epicardial wires is quite safe. In more than 9000 patients with atrial wires in place, only 3 had a complication—inability to remove the electrode[133]; in all 3, the lead wire was simply clipped at the skin without further problems. Removal of ventricular wires is occasionally associated with mild bleeding, but in only 1 instance in more than 9000 patients was thoracotomy required to control significant bleeding.[133] If the exit site is kept sterile, the risk of infection is very low. Given the utility and safety of temporary epicardial electrodes, they may be recommended routinely after cardiac surgery.

Selection of Route of Temporary Cardiac Pacing

The choice of a specific pacing modality depends upon a number of factors, such as availability of the device, the clinical situation, the indication for pacing, and the expertise of the physician. Table 5–6 summarizes the indications, advantages, and disadvantages of each pacing modality. In many instances, studies comparing pacing modalities are needed to determine which, if any, is the preferred method.

INDICATIONS FOR TEMPORARY CARDIAC PACING

Acute Myocardial Infarction

During acute myocardial infarction, a number of dysrhythmias or conduction disturbances that require temporary pacing may occur. Any bradyarrhythmia that is associated with symptoms or that causes hemodynamic compromise must be treated. Complete AV block, with its associated slow escape rhythms, and type II second-degree AV block, with its associated frequent progression to complete AV block, should be treated. Since placement of a transvenous pacing system may require several minutes during which the patient is hemodynamically jeopardized, and since pacing systems placed during emergency situations have the highest complication rates, it is desirable to be able to determine which patients with acute myocardial infarction are at greatest risk for the development of a significant dysrhythmia, so that pacing leads can be placed prophylactically or, at the very least, the patient can be observed more closely for an impending rhythm change.

TABLE 5–6. COMPARISON OF DIFFERENT MODES OF TEMPORARY CARDIAC PACING

	TRANSVENOUS	TRANSTHORACIC	TRANSESOPHAGEAL	EXTERNAL	EPICARDIAL
Advantages and Disadvantages					
Invasive	+	+	−/+	−	+
Rapidly placed	−/+	+	−/+	+	−
Safe	+	−/+	+	+	+
Prolonged use	+	−	−	−/+	+
Frequent complications	+	+	−	−	−/+
Atrial pacing	+	−	+	−?	+
Ventricular pacing	+	+	−/+	+	+
AV sequential pacing	+	−	−	−	+
Uses					
Sinus bradyarrhythmias	+	+	+	+	+
AV block	+	+	−	+	+
Prophylaxis against AV block	+	−	−	−/+	+
Tachyarrhythmias, diagnosis and treatment	+	−	+	−/+	+
Hemodynamic support	+	−	−	−	+

Correlation of Coronary Artery Anatomy and Rhythm Disturbances

The occurrence of certain types of dysrhythmias or conduction disorders with occlusion of different vascular beds during acute myocardial infarction has long been recognized[37, 58, 112, 116] and can be understood by knowing the blood supply to the impulse-generating tissues and specialized conduction pathways of the heart (Fig. 5–15). The SA node, located on the lateral wall of the right atrium near the junction of the superior vena cava, is supplied by the SA nodal artery, which arises from the proximal right coronary artery in approximately 55 per cent of individuals and from the left circumflex coronary artery in the remainder.[58] The AV node is supplied in approximately 90 per cent of individuals by a small artery (the AV nodal branch) arising from the distal right coronary artery and in the remainder from a small artery arising from the left circumflex coronary artery[58]; normally, collateral flow from adjacent branches of the first septal perforating artery of the left anterior descending artery is not present.[37, 58, 130] The proximal His bundle and the proximal portions of both the left and the right bundle branches usually have a dual blood supply from the AV nodal artery and the first septal perforator of the left anterior descending artery (Fig. 5–

15).[37] Anastomoses between these vessels at the His bundle may allow retrograde collateral flow to the AV node when AV nodal artery flow is decreased.[7, 23] The right bundle branch continues distal to its origin as a discrete bundle for several centimeters and receives its blood supply primarily from branches of the left anterior descending coronary artery. The left bundle, except at its most proximal portion, is anatomically less discrete than the right bundle branch; rather, it fans out shortly after its origin into broad networks of Purkinje fibers.[83] The fibers of the left branch can be divided into two main clusters—the anterior and posterior fascicles; some investigators have described a third centroseptal array of fibers.[27] There is substantial variability, indistinct branching, and frequent interconnections in the left-sided conduction system. Despite this anatomic structure, electrocardiographic definitions describing a bifascicular left-sided conduction system, or, if the right bundle branch is included, a trifascicular conduction system, have become well established (Table 5–7) and have been shown to be useful clinically. The left anterior fascicle, like the left bundle branch, receives its blood supply from branches of the left anterior descending coronary artery and the AV nodal artery.[37, 58] The left posterior fascicle receives its principal

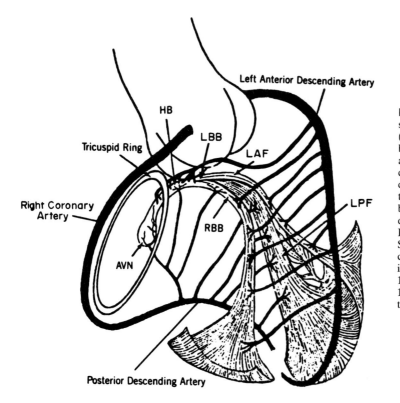

Figure 5–15. Schematic illustration showing the relation of AV node (AVN), His bundle (HB), bundle branches, and fascicles to the aortic and tricuspid valve annuli, and the coronary artery blood supply to the conduction system. LAF = left anterior division of the left bundle branch (LBB); LPF = left posterior division of the left bundle branch; RBB = right bundle branch. (From Scheinman MM, Gonzalez RP: Fascicular block and acute myocardial infarction. JAMA 244:2646–2649, 1980; with permission. Copyright 1980, American Medical Association.)

TABLE 5–7. ELECTROCARDIOGRAPHIC CRITERIA FOR CONDUCTION DISORDERS

TYPE OF BLOCK	PR INTERVAL	QRS DURATION	MEAN FRONTAL PLANE QRS AXIS	QRS MORPHOLOGY
Unifascicular Block				
RBBB	nl	↑	nl	RSR' in V_1; broad S in V_6
LBBB	nl	↑	nl	rS or QS in V_1; monophasic or notched R in V_6
LAFB	nl	nl	LAD	qR in I; rS in III
LPFB	nl	nl	RAD	rS in I; qR in III
Bifascicular Block				
RBBB + LAFB	nl	↑	LAD	RBBB pattern with LAD; qR in I and aVL
RBBB + LPFB	nl	↑	RAD	RBBB pattern with RAD; qR in II and III; rS in I
RBBB + 1° AVB*	↑	↑	nl	RBBB with prolonged PR interval
LBBB + 1° AVB*	↑	↑	nl	LBBB with prolonged PR interval
Trifascicular Block				
Alternating RBBB and LBBB	nl/↑	↑	Varies with conduction delay	RBBB, LBBB
RBBB + alternating LAFB and LPFB	nl/↑	↑	LAD and RAD	RBBB with alternating mean frontal plane axes
RBBB + LAFB + 1° AVB*	↑	↑	LAD	RBBB, LAD, prolonged PR interval
RBBB + LPFB + 1° AVB*	↑	↑	RAD	RBBB, RAD, prolonged PR interval

*The prolonged PR interval may represent AV nodal or intra-His conduction delay, or conduction delay in the contralateral bundle branch.

Abbreviations: RBBB = right bundle branch block; LBBB = left bundle branch block; LAFB = left anterior fascicle block; LPFB = left posterior fascicle block; AVB = AV block; ↑ = increased ≥ 0.12 sec.; nl = normal; LAD = left-axis deviation; RAD = right-axis deviation.

blood supply from the AV nodal artery, the posterior descending coronary artery, and the left circumflex coronary artery.[58]

Since the right coronary artery usually gives off the SA nodal artery and almost always provides the AV nodal artery, an occlusion proximal to their origins may lead to significant dysfunction of the SA or AV node or both. The escape rhythms emerging during significant bradyarrhythmias and heart block in this situation generally arise from a focus at or near the His bundle and thus have narrow QRS-complex morphology (unless prior intraventricular conduction abnormalities exist) and reasonably rapid rates.[56, 110] Although the AV nodal artery frequently provides blood flow to the His bundle, collateral flow from the left anterior descending coronary artery presumably militates against ischemic injury to it.[37] High-grade AV block, right or left bundle branch block, and fascicle blocks may result from injury in the His bundle and proximal bundle branches.[37] Since the His bundle and proximal bundle branches have a dual blood supply, block due to injury of the proximal conducting system more commonly occurs in the setting of combined right and left anterior

descending coronary obstruction.[7, 37] Significant alterations in vagal tone may also cause SA and AV nodal dysfunction (see below), which is usually transient. Occlusion of the left circumflex coronary artery may result in SA and AV nodal dysfunction in patients whose blood supply to these areas derives from this vessel. Occlusion of the left anterior descending coronary artery may result in ischemic damage to the His bundle or, more likely, to the more distal portions of the bundle branches.[58, 112] When high-grade AV block occurs in this situation, the escape rhythms usually arise from distal portions of the Purkinje system or from ventricular myocardium itself; the QRS complex morphology is therefore broad, and the rate is slow and unstable.[56, 110]

Sinus Bradycardia, Sinus Arrest, and Sinoatrial Exit Block

The incidence of sinus bradycardia and sinus node dysfunction occurring during acute myocardial infarction ranges from 5 to 30 per cent in reported series[98, 109, 112] and is more common in the first few hours of infarction. Sinus node dysfunction is at least three times more common in inferoposterior wall myocardial infarction than in anterior wall infarction. This observation is partially explained by coronary artery anatomy, since inferoposterior wall myocardial infarctions are most commonly due to occlusion of the right coronary artery and, to a lesser extent, the left circumflex coronary artery, both of which may give off the SA nodal artery. SA nodal ischemia or infarction, or a localized increase in the metabolites of the ischemic process (such as potassium and adenosine), may contribute to the associated bradycardia.[44, 58, 112] Indirect or direct activation of parasympathetic reflexes and receptors may also contribute; in particular, the Bezold-Jarisch reflex appears to play a major role.[80] In the Bezold-Jarisch reflex, nonmyelinated intracardiac vagal afferent nerves are stimulated by coronary occlusion and cause a marked, but transient, increase in vagal tone with resultant bradycardia or hypotension or both. The preponderance of these vagal receptors in the inferoposterior area of the left ventricle explains the greater frequency of sinus bradycardia with myocardial infarctions at this site. The exact mechanism by which the afferent receptors are stimulated is not known but may be due in part to myocardial fiber stretch generated by systolic bulging (dyskinesia) of the ischemic or infarcted myocardium. The receptors are apparently not activated by either hypoxia or hypercapnia.[81] Activation of the Bezold-Jarisch reflex also occurs with reperfusion of the right (but not the left) coronary artery after a period of occlusion and perhaps explains the higher incidence of bradycardia and hypotension during thrombolytic therapy or mechanical reperfusion in inferior wall myocardial infarction.[32, 140] Other possible etiologies for the occurrence of sinus bradycardia during myocardial infarction include direct stimulation of vagal fibers on or in the right atrium due to atrial infarction; fear and pain; and the use of drugs such as beta blockers, calcium channel blockers, and morphine, which affect SA nodal or autonomic function or both.

Pauses in sinus rhythm and SA exit block occur much less frequently than does sinus bradycardia, with an incidence of approximately 2 to 5 per cent.[109, 112] Direct injury to the SA node and perinodal tissues and increased parasympathetic tone probably contribute to the genesis of these arrhythmias. SA and AV nodal dysfunction may occur together relatively frequently. In the report of Rotman and colleagues, 20 of 539 patients with acute myocardial infarction had sinus pauses or SA exit block; of these 20, 5 had concomitant AV block.[112]

Treatment of sinus bradycardia, sinus pauses, or SA exit block is not necessary unless symptoms, such as worsening ischemia, hypotension, or syncope, result. In some patients, sinus bradyarrhythmias may increase the frequency of ventricular ectopy, including ventricular tachycardia and fibrillation. Since parasympathetic overactivity seems to play a major role in the sinus node dysfunction, most patients respond to intravenous atropine. In unresponsive patients or in those with prolonged periods of bradycardia, intravenous isoproterenol could theoretically be administered but may significantly worsen ischemia because of its positive inotropic action, increase the extent of infarction by causing an increase in myocardial oxygen demand, or exacerbate ventricular ectopy. For this reason, temporary cardiac pacing is the preferred method of treatment when the sinus dysrhythmia is refractory to atropine or unusually severe. In patients having sinus node dysfunction without associated atrial tachyarrhythmias, the risk of significant postinfarction symptomatic bradyarrhythmias appears to be low.[98]

Some reports suggest that patients with sinus bradycardia and acute myocardial infarction have a worse prognosis than those who do not have this dysrhythmia[46]; other studies have shown that the prognosis in such patients is no worse and perhaps even better. In the study of Rotman and colleagues, overall mortality from myocardial infarction was 20 per cent, and the mortality in patients with sinus bradycardia was 10 per cent.[112] The reason for improved survival, if indeed it exists, is not entirely understood but may reflect the increased prevalence of inferior wall myocardial infarction with its associated better prognosis, or lower myocardial oxygen demand with consequent relative myocardial preservation.

Episodes of bradycardia alternating with or following episodes of supraventricular tachycardia (the bradycardia-tachycardia syndrome) may occur during acute myocardial infarction, typically that involving the inferior wall. The bradycardia-tachycardia syndrome has been observed in a small number of patients with acute infarction.[98] Unlike sinus bradycardia and sinus node exit block, this rhythm disturbance has been noted to persist chronically, with most patients requiring permanent cardiac pacing systems for control of symptoms during bradycardiac episodes.[98] Not all investigators have found persistence of the bradycardia-tachycardia syndrome after recovery from acute infarction.[109] Many patients who have a bradycardia-tachycardia syndrome at the time of their myocardial infarction may have had significant, albeit asymptomatic, sinus node dysfunction prior to the infarction, which is exacerbated acutely and chronically by myocardial ischemia and infarction and by medications administered. In some patients, atrial infarction involving the sinus node or sinus node area may result in sinus node dysfunction and atrial tachyarrhythmias.[44, 58, 98] Atrial infarction documented at autopsy occurs in 1 to 42 per cent of patients with infarction[44]; however, its clinical diagnosis can only rarely be made. Treatment of the bradycardia-tachycardia syndrome in the setting of acute myocardial infarction requires pharmacologic treatment of the supraventricular tachycardias (usually atrial fibrillation or flutter or atrial tachycardia). Medicines that are used to treat these tachyarrhythmias, such as digoxin, quinidine, or propranolol, frequently exacerbate the associated bradyarrhythmias. If the latter are symptomatic or become symptomatic, temporary cardiac pacing will be required. If the bradycardias and tachyarrhythmias persist in the postinfarction recovery period and continue to require treatment, permanent cardiac pacing may be required. Rapid atrial pacing and other pacing modes can sometimes be helpful in converting or controlling atrial tachyarrhythmias, especially those refractory to medical therapy (see below and Chapter 21).

Disorders of Atrioventricular Conduction

AV block without associated bundle branch block occurs in 12 to 25 per cent of acute myocardial infarctions,[26, 112, 125] depending on the population of patients studied and the site of infarction. The incidence of first-, second-, and third-degree AV block is 2 to 12 per cent, 3 to 10 per cent, and 3 to 7 per cent, respectively.[26] The majority of AV conduction disorders without associated bundle branch block occur in the setting of acute inferior wall myocardial infarction, in which increased vagal tone and ischemia or infarction of the AV nodal area cause AV nodal dysfunction. In a large series of consecutively studied patients admitted with acute myocardial infarction reported by DeGuzman and Rahimtoola, 76 per cent of instances of AV block without associated bundle branch block occurred during acute inferoposterior infarction; only 18 per

cent occurred during anterior infarction and 6 per cent during infarction showing electrocardiographic changes in both areas (representing either concomitant ischemia or infarction or reciprocal changes).[26] Conversely, of all inferoposterior myocardial infarctions, 12 to 25 per cent are associated with advanced AV block.[119, 125] Recently, it has been observed that patients with inferior wall myocardial infarction and associated right ventricular infarction documented electrocardiographically by recording ST-segment elevation in the right precordial leads and by technetium pyrophosphate imaging have a significantly greater risk of development of high-grade AV block compared with that in patients without right ventricular involvement (48 per cent versus 13 per cent).[16] Since right ventricular infarction is caused by relatively proximal occlusion of the right coronary artery, this greater risk of high-grade AV block is probably due to the increased likelihood of AV nodal ischemia or enhancement of vagal tone or both. Recent pathologic studies of patients with inferoposterior myocardial infarctions have revealed that the occurrence of AV block was not strongly associated with anatomic lesions in either the AV node or the bundle of His but was significantly correlated with infarction of the prenodal atrial myocardium.[14] In another study, 91 per cent of patients who developed some degree of AV block during acute inferior wall myocardial infarction had concomitant obstructive disease in the left anterior descending coronary artery, presumably decreasing potential collateral flow to the prenodal and AV nodal areas.[7]

The development of high-grade AV block in the setting of acute inferoposterior wall myocardial infarction is associated with narrow QRS complex escape rhythms in more than two thirds of patients.[125] These rhythms are considered to originate within the His bundle, which is usually not affected by the infarction process. Since the escape rhythms are usually of adequate rate, hemodynamic stability is often maintained. Moreover, since the escape rates are easily increased with intravenous atropine administration and since the AV block frequently resolves with the use of atropine, temporary cardiac pacing is generally not required.

Several investigators have noted that the occurrence of high-grade AV block in the setting of acute inferior wall myocardial infarction follows a biphasic time course.[35, 119] In the reported studies, high-grade AV block that occurs within 6 hours of symptoms is characterized by abrupt onset, usually without preceding first-degree AV block; short duration (generally less than 24 hours); and responsiveness to intravenous atropine. High-grade AV block that occurs beyond 6 hours after symptoms is characterized by a more gradual onset, often preceded by first-degree AV block; a longer duration of several days; and a lesser likelihood of being atropine responsive. Because of these features, high-grade AV block that develops late in the course of acute inferior infarction is more likely to require temporary pacing,[35] although one group of investigators found less atropine responsiveness and increased pacemaker use in the early-onset group.[119] High-grade AV block occurring with right ventricular infarction is also less often responsive to intravenous atropine.[16] High-degree AV block that fails to resolve with atropine administration is presumably due to severe AV nodal ischemia and injury, whereas AV block that is responsive to atropine is likely to result, in great part, from increases in vagal tone.

The prognosis of patients with inferior wall myocardial infarction and high-grade AV block is worse than that in patients without block. In 144 patients with inferior wall myocardial infarction described by Tans and colleagues, mortality was 22 per cent in those with, and 9 per cent in those without, high-grade AV block.[125] Although most of the increased mortality is due to larger infarct size and associated decreased myocardial function,[112] an increase in mortality is still present if left ventricular failure does not occur.[125] The prognosis of patients with high-grade AV block and inferior myocardial infarction is significantly better than that of patients with anterior wall myocardial infarction and AV block, in large part because left ventricular structural

and functional impairment is less in the former circumstance.[53, 54, 112]

The risk of progression of first-degree AV block to high-grade AV block is approximately 10 to 30 per cent and of second-degree AV block to complete heart block about 36 per cent.[26, 54] Since type I second-degree AV block with normal intraventricular conduction is almost always due to conduction block in the AV node, temporary cardiac pacing is generally not required. However, type I second-degree AV block with a wide QRS complex may in some cases represent conduction block in the His bundle or contralateral "unblocked" bundle branch,[145] especially in the setting of acute anterior wall myocardial infarction. For this reason, it is probably advisable to insert a temporary pacemaker prophylactically in these individuals (see below).

Recently, it has been observed that patients with acute inferior wall myocardial infarction who have alternating Wenckebach periods have a very high incidence of syncope, development of high-grade AV block, hemodynamic deterioration, and death.[74] Alternating Wenckebach periodicity occurs in the setting of 2:1 AV conduction when there is a progressive increase in the PR interval of conducted sinus impulses until two or more consecutive atrial impulses fail to be conducted (Fig. 5–16).[47] Alternating Wenckebach cycles occur in about 2 per cent of patients with inferior wall myocardial infarction. In one study, 83 per cent of these patients required temporary pacemaker placement for hemodynamically significant bradycardias.[74] Unlike the more commonly observed type I second-degree AV block, alternating Wenckebach periods are rarely eliminated or improved and are frequently exacerbated by intravenous atropine administration, presumably owing to enhancement of atrial rate without concomitant en-

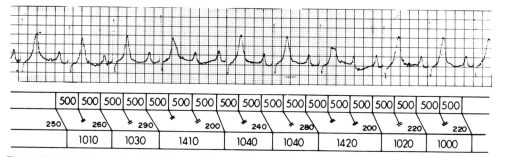

Figure 5–16. MCL_5 monitor lead from a 53-year-old man with acute inferior wall myocardial infarction and alternating Wenckebach periodicity. Ladder diagram illustrates 2:1 AV conduction with progressive prolongation of the PR intervals of conducted P waves and eventual failure of conduction of alternate atrial impulses.

hancement of AV nodal conduction.[20, 74] Since intravenous isoproterenol is also ineffective, temporary cardiac pacing has been recommended in these patients.[74] The severity of the rhythm disturbance has been considered to reflect actual AV nodal injury rather than vagal effect.

Type II second-degree AV block frequently progresses to complete AV block; thus, patients with this conduction disturbance should be prophylactically paced regardless of infarct location. However, a recently published retrospective review of three large population groups with acute myocardial infarction and associated conduction disorders indicated that none of the patients with type II second-degree AV block and *narrow* QRS complexes developed complete AV block while in the hospital.[69] It is possible that some of these cases may actually have represented type I second-degree AV block in which the Wenckebach periodicity was not easily measured[145] or high-grade intra-Hisian block, which possibly has a more benign prognosis than infra-Hisian block. Cases of apparent type II second-degree AV block that occur simultaneously with marked sinus slowing during acute inferior wall myocardial infarction have been shown by His bundle electrography to be due to a block in the AV node (presumably secondary to increased vagal tone) and have a benign prognosis.[82]

Disorders of Intraventricular Conduction

The development of new bundle branch block occurs in 6 to 15 per cent of patients with acute myocardial infarction and is approximately three times more common during anterior infarction than during inferior infarction.[26, 42, 53, 54, 84, 90, 112] Since the left anterior descending coronary artery provides the major blood supply to the His bundle, right and left bundle branches, and left anterior fascicle, the increased frequency of new bundle branch block during anterior infarction is easily explained. In the large multicenter study of Hindman and associates of patients with acute myocardial infarction and bundle branch block, the incidence of left bundle branch block was 38 per cent; of right bundle branch block with left anterior fascicular block, 34 per cent; of right bundle branch block, 11 per cent; of right bundle branch block and left posterior fascicular block, 10 per cent; and of alternating bundle branch block, 6 per cent.[53] The finding of bundle branch block during acute myocar-

dial infarction, especially if it is new, is prognostically important. New-onset bundle branch block is associated with decreased in-hospital and long-term survival, increased risk of congestive heart failure and tachyarrhythmias, increased risk of progression to high-grade AV block in the hospital,[26, 53, 54, 59, 84, 90] and possibly a greater risk of infarct extension.[69] The mortality of patients with acute myocardial infarction and bundle branch block is 30 to 50 per cent compared with the usual overall mortality of 10 to 15 per cent[26, 42, 53, 54, 59, 84, 90, 112, 139]; most of this high mortality is due to the increased prevalence of significant left ventricular dysfunction in these patients, reflecting both the site (anterior wall) and the extent of ischemic damage. In the multicenter study cited above, survival of patients with bundle branch block was directly related to the degree of heart failure: in-hospital mortality for patients in Killip Classes I, II, III, and IV was 8 per cent, 7 per cent, 27 per cent, and 83 per cent, respectively.[53] However, when patients with and without bundle branch block were compared within the same Killip Class, mortality was slightly but significantly greater in those with bundle branch block in Killip Classes I and II, regardless of site of infarction,[53] but was equal in all patients in Killip Classes III and IV. These observations suggest that bundle branch block has prognostic significance in patients without significant left ventricular dysfunction; however, these results have not been confirmed by all investigators.[42, 51, 75, 139]

Several studies have shown that patients with acute myocardial infarction and bundle branch block have a risk of progression to high-grade AV block during their hospital stay that approaches 18 per cent, compared with a 4 per cent incidence in patients without bundle branch block.[26, 42, 53, 54, 59, 90] Since short-term and long-term mortality is higher in the former group of patients, the precise prognostic variables require definition. The increase in mortality may be due to the high-grade AV block itself, in which case permanent cardiac pacing would be expected to lower the mortality. The increase in mortality may be due to hemodynamic deterioration with pump failure. Finally, the increase in mortality may be the result of tachyarrhythmias. The available studies indicate that most of the increase in mortality is caused by the greater degree of myocardial damage resulting from the infarction, which has itself contributed to, if not caused, the conduction disorder by ischemic necrosis of the conduction system.[42, 53, 54, 59, 90] In the study of Hindman and colleagues,[53] 66 per cent of the in-hospital deaths in patients with bundle branch block were due to left ventricular power failure, and only 9 per cent were due to the complete AV block itself.

Notwithstanding these observations, avoidance of bradycardia due to AV block in these patients is an important part of overall management and can be lifesaving. Since progression to high-grade AV block is *relatively* infrequent overall for patients with bundle branch block and acute myocardial infarction, attempts have been made to define various conduction patterns according to risk for development of high-grade AV block. Many studies have addressed this issue but have been limited by a relatively small number of patients, sampling bias, and retrospective rather than prospective analysis. However, three studies are available that include large numbers of patients, albeit retrospectively studied. The first, a multicenter study, involved 432 patients admitted to the hospital with acute infarction between 1967 and 1974.[53, 54] The risk of progression to high-grade AV block did not appear to be related to infarct location except for a slightly lower incidence with infarcts of "indeterminate" location. However, the risk of high-grade AV block was approximately twice as high in patients with bilateral bundle branch block (29 per cent) as in those with unilateral bundle branch block (13 per cent); similarly, a risk for advanced AV block of 24 per cent was present if new bundle branch block developed, compared with 13 per cent if prior bundle branch block existed.[54] The risk of progression to complete heart block was greatest (44 per cent) when alternating bundle branch block was present. AV block risk stratification was best obtained by analysis of three factors: presence or absence of first-degree AV block, bilateral bundle branch block, and new bundle branch block (Fig. 5–17). If none of these were present, the risk of progression to high-grade AV block was low (9 per cent).[54] Patients with first-degree AV block, prior bifascicular block, or new unifascicular block also had a low risk of progression to high-grade AV block (10 to 13 per cent). Patients with either first-degree AV block and new bundle branch block or with first-degree AV block and bifascicular block had intermediate risk of progression to high-grade AV block (19 to 20 per cent). At highest risk (31 per cent) were patients who had new bifascicular block and those who had first-degree AV block and new bifascicular block (38 per cent).[54] In view of the demonstrated risk in these patients, it

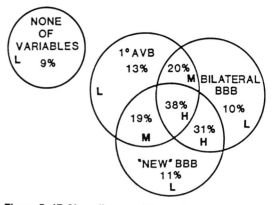

Figure 5–17. Venn diagram of the results of a multicenter study illustrating the risk of progression to high-grade AV block during acute myocardial infarction using three variables to stratify risk: first-degree AV block (AVB), new bundle branch block (BBB), and bifascicular (bilateral) block. See text for discussion. L = low; M = moderate; H = high risk. (From Hindman MC, Wagner GS, JaRo M, et al: The clinical significance of bundle branch block complicating acute myocardial infarction. 2. Indications for temporary and permanent pacemaker insertion. Circulation 58:689–699, 1978; by permission of the American Heart Association, Inc.)

was recommended that patients with new bilateral bundle branch block (with or without first-degree AV block) occurring in the setting of acute myocardial infarction should receive a temporary pacemaker prophylactically.

The second large study involved 257 patients with bundle branch block and acute myocardial infarction culled from 2779 patients with acute infarction who were admitted to the Los Angeles County Hospital from 1966 to 1977, a time period similar to that encompassed in the previously cited report.[26, 53] Similar to the results of the multicenter study, it was found that in the absence of first-degree AV block or new or bilateral bundle branch block the risk of progression to high-grade AV block was low (10 per cent) (Table 5–8). A similar low risk of development of advanced AV block was observed if either isolated new bundle branch block or old prior bilateral bundle branch block was present (16 per cent and 18 per cent risk, respectively)[26] (Fig. 5–18). The risk of occurrence of advanced AV block was high (43 per cent) if all three variables were present and moderate (29 per cent) if first-degree AV block and new bundle branch block were present. However, in contrast to the findings of the multicenter study (Table 5–8), the risk of progression to high-grade AV block in this investigation was moderately high (30 per cent) in patients with isolated first-degree AV block; and if first-degree AV block was

TABLE 5–8. PERCENTAGE OF PATIENTS WITH ACUTE MYOCARDIAL INFARCTION AND BUNDLE BRANCH BLOCK PROGRESSING TO HIGH-GRADE AV BLOCK*

BLOCK	MULTICENTER STUDY (%)	LOS ANGELES COUNTY HOSPITAL STUDY (%)
Overall	22	18
Old BBB only	9	10
1°AVB	13	30
New BBB	11	16
Bifascicular block	10	18
1° AVB + new BBB	19	29
1° AVB + bifascicular block	20	50
New bifascicular block	31	15
1° AVB + new bifascicular block	38	43
Alternating BBB	44	—

*In Hindman et al's multicenter study[54] and the Los Angeles County Hospital Study.[26]

associated with old bilateral bundle branch block, the risk of progression was very high (50 per cent).[26] In addition, a low risk of progression to advanced AV block of 15 per cent was found for patients with new bilateral bundle branch block, substantially less than the 31 per cent incidence found in the multicenter study.[26, 54] The reasons for the discrepancies between these two large studies are not clear but probably reflect differences in populations of patients, electrocardiographic criteria for AV and intraventricular blocks, ascertainment bias, and methods of treatment.

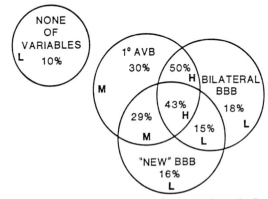

Figure 5–18. Venn diagram of the results from the Los Angeles County Hospital study illustrating the risk of progression to high-grade AV block using same "risk" factors as the multicenter study in Figure 5–17. (From DeGuzman M, Rahimtoola SH: What is the role of pacemakers in patients with coronary artery disease and conduction abnormalities? *In* Rahimtoola SH [ed]: Current Controversies in Coronary Heart Disease. Philadelphia, FA Davis, 1983, pp 191–207; with permission.)

In view of the somewhat conflicting results of these two large studies and the problems in determining how great the risk of progression to high-grade AV block must be to justify the potential risks, complications, and costs of temporary cardiac pacing, it is difficult to provide strict guidelines for prophylactic temporary pacing in acute myocardial infarction. Both studies documented the high risk (38 to 43 per cent) of progression to complete AV block if first-degree AV block is present together with new bilateral bundle branch block; thus, temporary cardiac pacing should be carried out in these patients.

Given the conflicting data in patients with new bilateral bundle branch block and in those with first-degree AV block and old bilateral bundle branch block, we suggest prophylactic pacing in both of these groups of patients until further studies dissipate the confusion. In patients with known prior bilateral bundle branch block and first-degree AV block, His bundle electrography can be helpful in ascertaining the site of conduction delay and thus the indication for temporary pacing, provided that it can be accomplished expeditiously. Patients with documented AV nodal conduction delay generally do not require temporary pacing, whereas those with intra-Hisian or infra-Hisian block probably do. Since the greatest risk of progression to high-grade AV block occurs within the first 4 to 5 days of infarction, temporary cardiac pacing should be instituted for this time period or until the patient's clinical course stabilizes.

Patients with new bundle branch block and first-degree AV block constitute a group at moderate risk (19 to 29 per cent) for advanced AV block. Placement of temporary cardiac pacemakers in these patients is generally not recommended, although some consider the risk that one in five patients will progress to high-grade AV block sufficient to justify temporary pacemaker placement. Temporary pacing is not justified in patients with preexisting bilateral bundle branch block, new isolated bundle branch block, and isolated first-degree AV block. The inclusion of isolated first-degree AV block in this low-risk category, despite the findings of the Los Angeles County Study, reflects the general experience of the authors as well as that of other investigators.[54, 75]

Because of the complexity of assessing the risk of progression to advanced AV block using each of the several possible combinations of conduction disorders, the investigators involved in the Multicenter Investigation of the

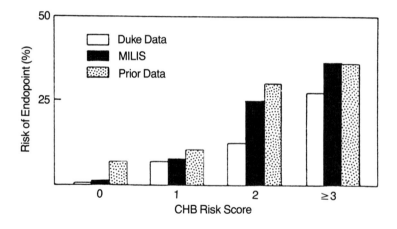

Figure 5–19. Bar graphs showing the incidence of complete AV block predicted by a "risk score" compared with its observed incidence in six published series and the Duke database. The endpoint is AV block. (From Lamas GA, Muller JE, Turi ZG, et al: A simplified method to predict occurrence of complete heart block during acute myocardial infarction. Am J Cardiol 57:1217; 1986; with permission.)

Limitation of Infarct Size (MILIS) have attempted to devise a simpler method of risk stratification based on a retrospective analysis of 698 patients.[69] A "risk score" for complete heart block was obtained by giving one point for each of the following categories of conduction disorder: first-degree AV block, type I (Wenckebach) second-degree AV block, type II second-degree AV block, fascicular block, right bundle branch block, and left bundle branch block. The risk of progression to complete heart block was directly proportional to the "risk score": With scores of 0, 1, 2, and 3 or more, the risk of third-degree AV block was 1.2 per cent, 7.8 per cent, 25.0 per cent, and 36.4 per cent, respectively (Fig. 5–19).[69] These findings have been validated in 3007 patients from other retrospective studies (Fig. 5–19).[69] Thus, this "risk score" seems to be an adequate and much simpler alternative to risk stratification using specific combinations of conduction disorders. Temporary cardiac pacing is not required in individuals with scores of 0 to 1, since the risk of progression to complete heart block is low (less than 10 per cent) relative to the potential complications of temporary transvenous pacing. For patients with a score of 2, recommendations for prophylactic pacing can be based upon infarction location. If the infarction involves the anterior wall, temporary transvenous pacing can be recommended, since if high-grade AV block develops, subsidiary cardiac pacemakers are often inadequate for hemodynamic support. If the infarction involves the inferior wall, subsidiary pacemakers are usually adequate; prophylactic external (transcutaneous) pacing is probably sufficient, if available. All individuals with a score of 3 or more are at high risk (greater than 35 per cent) of developing high-

grade AV block, and temporary pacing is recommended.[69] Whether the risk score could be improved upon by inclusion of other variables, such as time of onset of the conduction disorder, infarction location, or other clinical and hemodynamic variables, has not been studied; however, inclusion of such variables would confound the simplicity of the proposed system.

Little is known about the effect on the risk of progression to high-grade AV block in patients with acute myocardial infarction and first-degree AV block and/or bundle branch block after reperfusion using either thrombolytic agents or angioplasty. Several patients at high risk for conduction disturbances who had successful, acute reperfusion nevertheless developed high-grade AV block (personal observations). The reason for this is not known but may be due to the effects of prolonged ischemia or infarction (such as edema, inflammation, and/or metabolic alterations), which persist up to several days after reperfusion. Until further information is obtained on the natural history of conduction disturbances after successful reperfusion of an infarct area, it is probably prudent to treat patients who are at high risk for AV block by traditional criteria with insertion of a prophylactic pacing system.

Hemodynamic Indications

Temporary cardiac pacing can be used to improve hemodynamic status, particularly in the setting of acute myocardial infarction or after cardiac surgery. Cardiac output is dependent upon not only the rate of ventricular activation but also the stroke volume of each contraction. While temporary pacing from the ventricle will correct the rate deficit generated by bradyarrhythmias consequent to SA and AV nodal dysfunction, it may not be sufficient to increase cardiac output adequately, particularly in the setting of ventricular dysfunction.[21, 50, 128] Synchronized atrial contraction increases ventricular end-diastolic volume, thus increasing contractility by the Frank-Starling mechanism. Since this atrial "kick" is not present during ventricular pacing, cardiac output generally decreases when compared with the same rates during sinus rhythm or during atrial or AV sequential pacing.[72, 115] In addition, when ventriculoatrial conduction is present during ventricular pacing, significant retrograde blood flow into the venae cavae and pulmonary veins may occur when the atria contract against closed AV valves; this may impair ventricular filling and thus further decrease cardiac output. These combined effects may result in a 15 to 20 per cent decrease in cardiac output relative to that in sinus rhythm or that with atrial pacing.[72, 115, 144] Although this decline in resting cardiac output may not be of significance in individuals with normal cardiac reserve, in patients with acute myocardial infarction (or those undergoing major surgery) who have significant diastolic or systolic ventricular dysfunction or both, a fall in cardiac output of this magnitude may make a significant clinical difference. Atrial or AV sequential pacing circumvents this problem.

Chamberlain and colleagues first showed in 1970 that compared with ventricular pacing, AV sequential pacing in patients with heart block and acute anterior or inferior wall myocardial infarction resulted in significant increases in cardiac output and arterial blood pressure, as well as decreases in central venous pressure.[21] More recently, Topol and associates have shown that atrial, but not ventricular, pacing dramatically improves cardiac output in patients with right ventricular infarction accompanied by bradycardia or hypotension or both.[128] The mechanism of hemodynamic improvement in these patients was considered to be due to improved ventricular filling as a result not only of synchronized atrial contraction but also of a decline in intrapericardial pressure. The fall in intrapericardial pressure during atrial (or AV sequential) pacing results from the appropriately timed decline in atrial volume during ventricular end-diastole, thereby providing space within the pericardium for additional filling of the atria from the venae cavae and pulmonary veins. Thus, atrial or AV sequential pacing is the preferred pacing mode in patients with evidence of left or right ventricular dysfunction during acute myocardial infarction. Hartzler and coworkers showed similar hemodynamic benefits from AV sequential pacing in patients following cardiac surgery[50]; these investigators also demonstrated that cardiac output could be further maximized in the majority of patients having AV sequential pacing by the selection of an optimal AV interval.[50]

The hemodynamic benefits of the more physiologic modes of pacing may be attenuated if the pulmonary capillary wedge pressure (an index of left ventricular filling pressure) exceeds 20 mm Hg. In one study of patients with chronic left ventricular dysfunction, atrial pacing had no benefit over ventricular pacing if the pulmonary capillary wedge pressure exceeded 20 mm Hg, but resulted in a 20 to 50 per cent increase in stroke volume if it was less than 20 mm Hg.[45] There are several possible explanations for this observation. First, since the Starling curve tends to be relatively flat in patients with left ventricular dysfunction, the atrial kick contributes little to improvement in contractility. Second, the left ventricle is already maximally or near-maximally volume loaded when end-diastolic pressures are high, again resulting in little additional contribution to the atrial kick. Last, there may be concomitant atrial dysfunction. Notwithstanding these observations, atrial or AV sequential pacing in patients with congestive heart failure and elevated pulmonary capillary wedge pressures is sometimes of substantial benefit. This benefit could reflect differing pressure-volume relationships in a given patient or attenuation or elimination of the effects of an atrial natriuretic factor response to the atrial stretch resulting from AV dyssynchrony during ventricular pacing; however, studies addressing this issue are lacking. More important, the effects of atrial or AV sequential pacing in these patients during conditions other than bed rest are undefined.

Treatment and Prophylaxis of Tachyarrhythmias

Perhaps the most important emerging use of temporary cardiac pacing is in the therapeutic and prophylactic management of cardiac tachyarrhythmias (Fig. 5–20). Cardiac pacing can be applied acutely and chronically for almost all tachyarrhythmias except ventricular fibrillation, atrial fibrillation, sinus tachycardia, and type II atrial flutter.[133, 135] Rhythms that can be

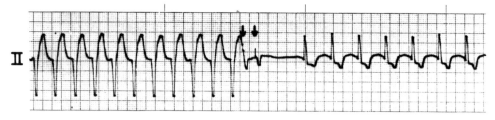

Figure 5–20. Lead II rhythm strip from an elderly woman in the coronary care unit with hemodynamically stable ventricular tachycardia. Two critically timed extrastimuli (*arrows*) terminated the ventricular tachycardia with resumption of sinus rhythm. Single extrastimulus could not terminate her ventricular tachycardia regardless of when it was delivered in the tachycardia cycle.

terminated by or palliated using temporary pacing and the required pacing techniques are listed in Table 5–9 (see also Chapter 21).

The mechanisms by which tachycardia control is achieved are multiple and vary with the underlying rhythm disturbance. Bradycardia-dependent tachyarrhythmias can be effectively terminated and their recurrence prevented by atrial (or ventricular) overdrive pacing. Bradycardia-dependent tachyarrhythmias may be ventricular or atrial; the former are observed more frequently in the acute care setting, in which they may be life threatening. Lown and colleagues noted in 1969 that in the setting of acute myocardial infarction pacing patients at a rate somewhat more rapid than their spontaneous rates could suppress ventricular ectopy.[77] Overdrive pacing may also be helpful in the suppression of transient tachyarrhythmias arising during the initiation of new antiarrhythmic medications and after cardiac surgery. The mechanism by which overdrive pacing is of therapeutic benefit may be a decrease in the dispersion of refractoriness, which is felt to be important in the genesis of reentrant arrhythmias,[49] or may be a suppressive effect on automatic foci.[131] In some situations, the rate of overdrive pacing needed to manage the tachyarrhythmia might have deleterious hemodynamic effects. If such is the case with an atrial tachyarrhythmia, it can sometimes be circumvented by pacing the atria sufficiently rapidly that 2:1 AV block develops, resulting in a reasonable ventricular rate that is unaccompanied by hemodynamic deterioration.[133, 135] A similar effect on ventricular rate can be obtained with ventricular overdrive pacing utilizing paired pacing, in which the second of a pair of pacing stimuli is sufficiently late relative to the prior stimulus to depolarize the heart but sufficiently early relative to the prior mechanical systole such that an effective ventricular contraction does not occur.[133, 135]

TABLE 5–9. PACING TECHNIQUES FOR TREATMENT OF DIFFERENT ARRHYTHMIAS

ARRHYTHMIA	RAS	RVS	ES	OTHER
Sinus tachycardia	–	–	–	–
Atrial flutter, type I	+	–	–	Slow (underdrive) pacing*; conversion to atrial fibrillation
Atrial flutter, type II	–	–	–	Conversion to atrial fibrillation
Atrial fibrillation	–	–	–	–
PSVT	+	+	+	Slow (underdrive) pacing*
Ectopic atrial tachycardia	+	–	–	Very rapid atrial pacing†
Nonparoxysmal atrial tachycardia	+	–	–	Ventricular paired pacing‡
PAD	+	–	–	–
PVC	+	+	–	–
Ventricular tachycardia	+	+	+	Slow pacing, burst pacing, ventricular paired pacing‡
Torsades de pointes	+	+	–	–
Ventricular fibrillation	–	–	–	–

*Pacing below tachyarrhythmia rate effectively interposes extrastimuli at varying coupling intervals.

†Very rapid pacing until 2:1 AV block is obtained, to suppress supraventricular arrhythmia while maintaining relatively normal ventricular rates.

‡Ventricular paired pacing causes rapid ventricular electrical stimulation, but the paired paced depolarization is too early to affect a mechanical event.

Abbreviations: RAS = rapid atrial stimulation; RVS = rapid ventricular stimulation; ES = single or multiple extrastimuli; PSVT = paroxysmal supraventricular tachycardia due either to AV (accessory bypass tract) or to AV nodal reentry; PAD = premature atrial depolarization; PVC = premature ventricular depolarization.

Overdrive pacing may result in entrainment and disruption of reentrant circuits.[94, 134] Paced activation at a rate slightly greater than the tachycardia rate can capture and entrain the reentrant circuit at the pacing rate for the duration of pacing. Upon discontinuing pacing, the spontaneous tachyarrhythmia will resume at its original rate. If the pacing rate is then increased beyond a certain critical rate, block occurs in the reentrant circuit and the spontaneous tachyarrhythmia is terminated. Tachycardia entrainment and disruption have been shown to occur in atrial flutter, paroxysmal supraventricular tachycardia, and ventricular tachycardia.[94, 134] Critically timed single extrastimuli presumably also terminate arrhythmias by depolarizing portions of the reentrant circuit, disallowing maintenance of the rhythm. Another potential mechanism of action of pacing in tachycardia control is by "subthreshold inhibition," in which pacing stimuli below the pacing threshold delivered in the area of the reentrant circuit disallow reentry, presumably by altering refractoriness of a portion of the reentrant loop.[143] Finally, rapid atrial pacing can convert a hemodynamically unfavorable atrial tachyarrhythmia to a more advantageous one; the best example of this is the conversion of atrial flutter to atrial fibrillation, in which the ventricular response is easier to control.[133]

Treatment of Drug-Induced Arrhythmias

A number of pharmacologic agents may produce transient bradyarrhythmias or tachyarrhythmias that require temporary cardiac pacing for the duration of the drug's effect. These arrhythmias may occur at "toxic" serum levels of these agents or as idiosyncratic reactions at normal or even low serum levels. Drugs that cause bradyarrhythmias may decrease automaticity of pacemaker cells in the SA node or subsidiary pacemaker tissue or may create exit block of impulses arising from these pacemaker sites. These effects may be due to a blockade of or reduction in sympathetic tone, an enhancement of parasympathetic tone, a direct action on pacemaker or peripacemaker cells, or a combination of these. AV nodal conduction may be altered by similar means. Drugs such as digoxin, beta-adrenergic blocking agents, calcium channel blocking agents, antiarrhythmic agents, alpha-methyldopa, clonidine, reserpine, and parasympathomimetic agents may all result in significant sinus bradycardia, sinus arrest or exit block, and AV nodal block at toxic levels. In some patients, especially those with the "sick sinus syndrome," SA and AV nodal function may be especially sensitive to the effect of these drugs, so that even "pharmacologic" serum levels result in significant bradyarrhythmias and conduction disorders[105]; however, undue sensitivity to these drug effects does not predict the presence of this syndrome. Temporary pacing is the optimal means of treating the hemodynamic sequelae of the bradyarrhythmias until the offending agent can be counteracted or metabolized. If long-term therapy using these agents is required, a permanent pacemaker will be necessary. In addition to correcting the hemodynamic effects of the bradyarrhythmias, temporary cardiac pacing can be useful in preventing bradycardia-related ventricular ectopy.

Recently, a number of drugs and clinical conditions have been found to underlie the occurrence of a particular type of polymorphic ventricular tachycardia, known as *torsades de pointes,* in which the polarity of the QRS complexes reverses in a sinusoidal fashion[63, 65, 121] (Table 5–10). All of the associated conditions cause delayed myocardial repolarization, reflected in the surface electrocardiogram as marked QT-interval prolongation. Presumably, dispersion of refractoriness in the ventricular myocardium creates the appropriate milieu for microreentry at multiple sites.[121] The polymorphic QRS pattern of *torsades de pointes* is thought to represent changing pat-

TABLE 5–10. DRUGS AND CLINICAL CONDITIONS ASSOCIATED WITH *TORSADES DE POINTES*

Antiarrhythmic agents	Neurologic events
Quinidine	Subarachnoid
Procainamide	hemorrhage
Disopyramide	Encephalitis
Lidocaine (toxic levels)	Head trauma
Amiodarone	Psychoactive agents
Mexiletine	Tricyclic antidepressants
Tocainide	Phenothiazines
Encainide	Liquid protein diets
Aprindine	Antibiotics
Flecainide	Chloroquine
Electrolyte abnormalities	entamidine
Hypokalemia	Amantidine
Hypomagnesemia	Erythromycin
Ischemia or infarction	Trimethoprim-
Myocarditis	sulfamethoxazole
Hereditary long QT	Toxins
syndromes	Organophosphates
Jervell-Lang-Nielsen	Arsenic
Romano-Ward	Anesthetic agents
Bradyarrhythmias	Suxamethonium with
	digoxin

terns of ventricular activation from its initiation from two or more sites.[5] The type IA antiarrhythmic agents (quinidine, procainamide, and disopyramide) will further increase the degree of dispersion of refractoriness, prolong the QT interval, and often exacerbate the rhythm disturbance[121]; thus, these agents are contraindicated in the treatment of *torsades de pointes*. Type IB antiarrhythmic agents, such as lidocaine and phenytoin, shorten the refractory period of ventricular tissue and are occasionally effective in the treatment of *torsades de pointes*.[63, 121] However, overdrive pacing from either atrial or ventricular sites has been shown to be the treatment of choice regardless of etiology.[63, 65, 121] Increasing the rate of ventricular activation is known to shorten refractoriness and decrease the degree of electrical dispersion.[49] Theoretically, atrial pacing, which maintains the normal sequence of ventricular activation, should be associated with less dispersion of refractoriness than ventricular pacing, with its altered ventricular activation sequence; whether this difference is clinically significant is not known. Acceleration of heart rate using intravenous isoproterenol has also been shown to be useful but is less effective than temporary pacing and is frequently associated with significant side effects.

Hypervagotonic States

"Hypervagotonia" exists when there is extreme sensitivity to increases in vagal tone, when abnormal increases in vagal tone occur in response to normal levels of stimulation of vagal reflexes, or when there is marked stimulation of vagal tone in response to pathologic or abnormal mechanical stimuli. Clinical conditions in which hypervagotonia plays a role include the sick sinus syndrome[60, 62]; carotid sinus hypersensitivity[87, 137]; swallowing and cough syncope[6, 73]; and syncope with pharyngeal, esophageal, or gastric manipulation[95] or with glossopharyngeal neuralgia.[123] Rarely, highly trained athletes will develop such excessive vagal tone that syncopal attacks may result.[104] Most of these clinical conditions are due to, or contributed to, by marked increases in vagal tone, which result in a cardioinhibitory, or cardiodecelerator, response manifested by slowing of sinus rate, sinus arrest or exit block, and/or AV nodal block. Cardiac pacing is useful when a cardioinhibitory response dominates the clinical picture. In some vagotonic syndromes, however, there is a sec-ond, less common, vasodepressor response that dominates the clinical picture and that may be unassociated with significant bradycardia. In this vasodepressor response, there is marked vasodilatation and hypotension, presumably caused by inhibition of sympathetic vasomotor tone.[87, 137] The vasodepressor response does not respond to temporary pacing.[87, 137] Both cardioinhibitory and vasodepressor responses may coexist. These may respond to temporary pacing to ensure an adequate heart rate; however, the vasodepressor component must be treated independently. Although the hypervagotonic syndromes tend to be chronic and episodic and often require implantation of a permanent cardiac pacemaker, transient overstimulation of vagal tone occasionally exists in situations such as acute gastric distention; pharyngeal or gastroesophageal manipulation, as occurs during intubation or endoscopy; or increased intracranial pressure; or it may be present when drugs temporarily enhance parasympathetic tone or block sympathetic tone. Generally, the bradycardia and accompanying hypotension are readily reversed with intravenous atropine, and temporary cardiac pacing is rarely required.

Cardiac Catheterization

When intravascular catheters are placed in the right ventricular cavity, the impact of the catheter on the right bundle branch can induce transient right bundle branch block. This block is estimated to occur in approximately 10 per cent of catheterizations of the right side of the heart.[78, 126] The right bundle branch block usually lasts for seconds or minutes until the catheter is removed or repositioned; however, it may last hours to days. Similarly, trauma induced by biopsy of the right side of the interventricular septum may induce temporary and, less commonly, permanent right bundle branch block. If the remainder of the intraventricular conduction system is intact, generally this block is not a problem. However, if there is preexisting left bundle branch block, the occurrence of right bundle branch block will result in complete heart block for the duration of the right bundle branch block.[124] For this reason, a transvenous pacing catheter should be placed prophylactically (preferably with fluoroscopic guidance) before performing catheterizations of the right side of the heart or right ventricular biopsies. Alternatively, an external pacemaker could be used if available. Catheterization of the left side of the heart can induce complete heart block in patients with preexisting right bundle branch block, but its occurrence is rare owing to the short length of the left bundle branch and the broad expanse of the left-sided fascicles[124]; thus, prophylactic pacing is not necessary in this circumstance. There are isolated case reports of catheter-induced complete heart block occurring when catheters in the low right atrium or coronary sinus ostium have impact on the AV nodal area.[102] Since the block in these situations is above the His bundle, the escape rhythm is usually characterized by narrow, normal-appearing QRS complexes occurring at a normal rate. The use of intravascular contrast agents appears to be quite safe in patients with preexisting bundle branch blocks.[70]

Significant bradycardia and asystole may occur during cardiac catheterization, particularly when injecting radiopaque dye in the right coronary artery. Because of this, placement of a temporary pacing system in all individuals undergoing cardiac catheterization has been advocated. However, recent studies have shown that this practice does not alter either morbidity or mortality associated with cardiac catheterization and may even increase the risk of pacing catheter–related ventricular tachyarrhythmias.[71, 96] Similarly, it has been recommended that prophylactic temporary pacemakers be inserted in all individuals undergoing coronary angioplasty. However, since the risk of significant bradyarrhythmias during angioplasty is only 1 to 2 per cent,[30, 85] it is unclear whether prophylactic pacing in this situation will alter morbidity and mortality. Unipolar pacing from the angioplasty guide wire has been described during angioplasty and has been shown to provide an effective option, should the need arise.[85] Given the low incidence of significant bradycardia in these situations as well as its transient nature, temporary pacing using an external pacemaker may be as effective as transvenously inserted pacing catheters, with less associated morbidity and cost.

Perioperative Temporary Pacing

Because of the stress of anesthesia and surgery, with the frequent accompaniment of hypoxemia, hypotension, and electrolyte disturbances, it is conceivable that patients with chronic bifascicular block could develop complete heart block intraoperatively or perioperatively. Thus, the question of the need for prophylactic preoperative temporary pacemaker insertion arises. Several investigations have clearly shown that the incidence of perioperative complete heart block is low and that there is no demonstrable benefit from prophylactic preoperative pacemaker insertion.[8, 100, 132] This finding appears to be true even if first-degree AV block is also present[132] and if the HV interval is documented to be prolonged at preoperative His bundle electrography.[8] Of 98 patients with chronic bifascicular block studied by Bellocci and colleagues,[8] 51 had prolongation of the HV interval; no individual developed complete heart block. This observation is important, since prolongation of the HV interval suggests underlying trifascicular disease and thus a potentially high risk of complete heart block. The reported higher mortality in patients with chronic bifascicular block and a prolonged HV interval is accounted for not by AV block, but by the greater prevalence of heart disease in these patients,[8] with all deaths in this study resulting from ventricular fibrillation, myocardial infarction, and congestive heart failure. Also of importance was the finding that pharmacologic agents that could suppress automaticity or conduction or both, such as digoxin, propranolol, and quinidine, had no clinically significant effect in these patients.

In patients with symptomatic bradyarrhythmias ultimately necessitating permanent pacemaker implantation or with malfunction of an existing permanent pacing system that requires surgical revision, temporary pacing is required perioperatively only if the patient is pacemaker-dependent.

Bacterial Endocarditis

The occurrence of new AV or bundle branch block in the setting of acute bacterial endocarditis suggests that there is a perivalvular, or ring, abscess that has extended to involve the conduction system near the AV node or proximal portion of the His bundle.[2, 36, 108, 138] Septic emboli may also cause these conduction disorders.[138] Wang and associates retrospectively analyzed 142 cases ·of infective endocarditis at the University of Minnesota over a 10-year period and found complete heart block to have occurred in 4 per cent of patients and first- or second-degree AV block in 10 per cent of patients.[138] All but one of the patients who developed complete heart block were found to have mycotic aneurysms and aortocardiac fistulas. In patients with aortic valve endocarditis and valve ring abscess, 19 per cent developed high-grade AV block.[2]

New conduction disorders due to endocarditis occur most commonly with infection involving the aortic valve, especially the noncoronary cusp.[2, 108, 138] This occurrence is understandable, given the proximity of the aortic valve to the AV node and proximal portion of the His bundle (Fig. 5–15). However, extension of infection from the mitral or tricuspid valve may also result in conduction disturbances. Because the onset of new AV or bundle branch block implies perivalvular extension of the infection, these patients should be considered for early operative intervention. There is evidence suggesting that these individuals may be at increased risk for developing complete heart block and for sudden death. In a study by Roberts and Somerville, 18 patients with aortic valve endocarditis had new first-degree AV block[108]; of these, 22 per cent developed complete heart block. Four of six patients with first-degree AV block and left bundle branch block died suddenly, although the cause of death was not stated. All of the studies are flawed because they are retrospective analyses, which typically depend upon identification of patients at surgery or necropsy; this selection process may bias the data toward unfavorable outcomes. Nonetheless, the occurrence of new and unexplained AV block or bundle branch block in the setting of bacterial endocarditis, especially of the aortic valve, should prompt consideration of prophylactic pacing until surgical treatment can be undertaken. Rarely, acute myocarditis of any etiology will result in temporary high-grade AV block requiring temporary pacing.

Neoplasm-Induced Bradyarrhythmias

Not infrequently, involvement of the conduction system by tumor occurs without associated symptoms; progression to high-grade AV block is uncommon. If high-grade AV block develops owing to invasion with tumor tissue that responds poorly to available therapies, a permanent pacing system should be inserted if the clinical situation warrants. However, in treatable tumors, such as some leukemias and lymphomas, high-grade AV block may resolve rapidly with therapy directed against the tumor[79]; thus, temporary pacing

may be all that is necessary. The long-term risk for subsequent return of high-grade AV block in this situation is not known. The SA node is frequently involved with tumor because of its epicardial location; however, the typical rhythm that results is atrial fibrillation rather than significant bradyarrhythmia.

Benign and malignant neck tumors,[101] carotid sinus tumors,[28] and cervical lymphadenopathy[4] may result in a carotid sinus hypersensitivity syndrome when they involve the carotid sinus or Hering's nerve. Temporary cardiac pacing may be required during surgical treatment of these disorders or during radiation or chemotherapy, which result in cellular necrosis and inflammation. Finally, malignant intracranial tumors (or any condition) that produce intracranial hypertension may result in a Cushing reflex with systemic hypertension and bradycardia; temporary pacing may be indicated if the bradycardia is associated with bradycardia-dependent tachycardias.

Temporary Pacing in Diagnostic Testing

Invasive Electrophysiologic Investigation

In 1969, Scherlag and associates described a catheter technique for recording His potentials in humans.[117] Since that time, there has been a marked increase in the use of intravascular electrode catheters for the detection of atrial, His, and ventricular electrograms and for the delivery of programmed electrical stimulation for induction and termination of arrhythmias.[48, 61, 111] These invasive cardiac electrophysiologic investigations have become a useful clinical and research tool (Fig. 5–21). In addition to intravascular catheter electrodes, epicardial[133, 135] or transesophageal[9, 10, 15, 41, 67] electrodes can be utilized. Electrophysiologic investigation may be helpful in a number of clinical conditions in ascertaining the diagnosis of an arrhythmia, in establishing its severity and prognosis, and in directing the appropriate therapeutic intervention (Table 5–11). Electrophysiologic studies can also be used to assess the efficacy of pharmacologic therapy after it is initiated and possibly to detect proarrhythmic effects as well. Furthermore, electrophysiologic studies are essential in directing and testing nonpharmacologic treatment options, such as catheter ablation, permanent anti-tachycardia pacemakers, and implantable defibrillators.

Figure 5–21. Example of data generated by electrophysiologic study. Three narrow complexes of reciprocating tachycardia were induced during electrophysiologic investigation of a patient with Wolff-Parkinson-White syndrome. Fourteen channels of data are collected: five surface ECG leads (I, II, III, V_1, and V_6); bipolar electrograms from the high right atrium (HRA), His bundle area (HBE), right ventricular apex (RVA), proximal coronary sinus (PCS), and distal coronary sinus (DCS); and unipolar electrograms from the four ring electrodes of the coronary sinus catheter (proximal to distal—CS1, CS2, CS3, and CS4). Thus, orthodromic, reciprocating tachycardia involves a reentrant circuit with anterograde AV nodal conduction and retrograde accessory bypass tract conduction. This patient has a left atrioventricular pathway, as indicated by the earliest atrial activation occurring at the CS electrodes, specifically CS3. Numbers before the first set of CS atrial electrograms represent time (in milliseconds) to the onset of atrial activation from the onset at the QRS complex on the surface leads. Atrial electrograms seen on the HBE and HRA are significantly later.

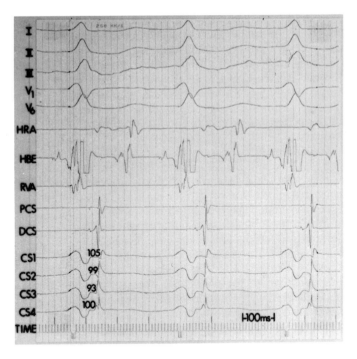

The risk of significant complications with invasive electrophysiologic investigations ranges from 0.6 to 0.7 per cent.[48, 55] The complications are primarily related to the insertion of the intravascular catheters. Despite the fact that there is intentional induction of tachyarrhythmias, occasional precipitation of ventricular fibrillation and frequent cardioversion, the risk of death is very small, and thus the test is safe when conducted by experienced personnel.[48]

TABLE 5–11. CLINICAL SITUATIONS IN WHICH ELECTROPHYSIOLOGIC TESTING MAY BE USEFUL

Sick sinus syndrome
AV conduction disorders and block
Preexcitation syndromes
Paroxysmal supraventricular tachycardias
Nonsustained ventricular tachycardia
Sustained ventricular tachycardia
Wide-complex tachycardia of unknown etiology
Sudden death
Syncope or near-syncope of suspected cardiac origin
Palpitations
Assessing efficacy of pharmacologic therapy
Directing and assessing nonpharmacologic interventions
Assessing asymptomatic individuals in high-risk groups (e.g., idiopathic hypertrophic subaortic stenosis [IHSS], after tetralogy of Fallot repair)

Pacing Stress Test

The treadmill exercise test has been shown to be a very useful tool in diagnosing coronary artery disease and in assessing its severity. However, many patients are unable to perform dynamic exercise because of musculoskeletal deformities, arthritis, peripheral vascular disease, physical deconditioning, and neurologic deficits. In addition, there are a number of relative contraindications to maximal exercise testing, such as unstable angina, recent myocardial infarction, cerebrovascular accidents, and severe hypertension. Last, a number of medications, especially the beta-adrenergic blocking agents, prevent or attenuate an adequate heart rate response to exercise and thus limit the diagnostic utility of the test. For these reasons, other means of stressing coronary reserve have been sought that can be used in the physically disabled and that can be rapidly reversed so that safety is ensured. Sowton and coworkers first used atrial pacing as a means of stressing the coronary reserve of patients with suspected coronary artery disease.[122] Subsequent investigators have shown that atrial pacing stress tests are an effective means of detecting significant coronary obstruction. Early studies suggested that the sensitivity of the pacing stress test was less than or equal to that of the excercise treadmill test and that the pacing test was less specific than the treadmill test[64, 103, 106]; however, more recent investigations suggest an equal sensitivity and specificity for both tests, with patients achieving similar rate-pressure products and experiencing similar frequency of chest pain, electrocardiographic abnormalities, and thallium-201 perfusion defects.[52] Differences in the results of available studies may be due to differences in pacing stress test protocols and in selection of patients.

The treadmill exercise test has been shown to be helpful in identifying patients who are at risk of recurrent infarction and death after acute myocardial infarction. Pacing stress tests have also been used safely after infarction[129] to obtain the same prognostic information. In the study of Tzivoni and colleagues, 85 patients were paced from the atrium approximately 2 weeks post myocardial infarction without complications except for occasional nonsustained atrial fibrillation.[129] The mean paced heart rate was 147 beats per minute, considerably higher than that achieved in treadmill exercise. Perhaps because of this higher heart rate, a 46 per cent incidence of positive pacing stress tests was observed, considerably higher than that usually obtained with limited postinfarction exercise tests. The predictive capability for cardiac events using this technique was similar to that using treadmill exercise. The two advantages of the pacing stress test in the postinfarction period are the ability to include all patients and the immediate reversibility of the stress, should a complication occur. The important disadvantage is that observation of the patient during dynamic exercise is precluded, and thus exercise prescriptions cannot be formulated. At the present time, it appears that thallium scintigraphy using intravenous dipyridamole will replace atrial pacing in patients unable to perform exercise.

REFERENCES

1. Andersen HR, Pless P: Trans-esophageal pacing. PACE 6:674–679, 1983.
2. Arnett EN, Roberts WC: Valve ring abscess in active infective endocarditis: Frequency, location, and clues to clinical diagnosis from the study of 95 necropsy patients. Circulation 54:140–145, 1976.
3. Austin JL, Preis LK, Crampton RS, et al: Analysis of pacemaker malfunction and complications of temporary pacing in the coronary care unit. Am J Cardiol 49:301–306, 1982.
4. Ballantyne F, Vander Ark CR, Hilick M: Carotid sinus syncope and cervical lymphoma. Wis Med J 74:91–92, 1975.
5. Bardy GH, Ungerlieder RM, Smith WM, Ideker RE: A mechanism of torsades de pointes in a canine model. Circulation 67:52–59, 1983.
6. Baron SB, Huang SK: Cough syncope presenting as Mobitz Type II atrioventricular block—an electrophysiologic correlation. PACE 10:65–69, 1987.
7. Bassan R, Maia IG, Bozza A, et al: Atrioventricular block in acute inferior wall myocardial infarction: Harbinger of associated obstruction of the left anterior descending coronary artery. J Am Coll Cardiol 8:773–778, 1986.
8. Bellocci F, Santarelli P, DiGennaro M, et al: The risk of cardiac complications in surgical patients with bifascicular block: A clinical and electrophysiological study in 98 patients. Chest 77:343–348, 1980.
9. Benson DW Jr, Dunnigan A, Benditt DG, Schneider SP: Transesophageal cardiac pacing: History, application, technique. Clin Prog Pacing Electrophysiol 2:360–372, 1984.
10. Benson DW Jr, Dunnigan A, Sterba R, Benditt DG: Atrial pacing from the esophagus in the diagnosis and management of tachycardia and palpitations. J Pediatr 102:40–46, 1983.
11. Benson DW Jr, Sanford M, Dunnigan A, Benditt DG: Transesophageal atrial pacing threshold: Role of interelectrode spacing, pulse width and catheter insertion depth. Am J Cardiol 53:63–67, 1984.
12. Benson DW Jr, Dunnigan A, Benditt DG, et al: Transesophageal study of infant supraventricular tachycardia: Electrophysiologic characteristics. Am J Cardiol 52:1002–1006, 1983.
13. Benson DW Jr, Dunnigan A, Benditt DG, et al: Prediction of digoxin treatment failure in infants with supraventricular tachycardia: Role of transesophageal pacing. Pediatrics 75:288–293, 1985.
14. Bilbao FJ, Zabalza IE, Vilanova JR, Froufe J: Atrioventricular block in posterior acute myocardial infarction: A clinicopathologic correlation. Circulation 75:733–736, 1987.
15. Blomström-Lundqvist C, Edvardsson N: Transesophageal versus intracardiac atrial stimulation in assessing electrophysiologic parameters of the sinus and AV nodes and of atrial myocardium. PACE 10:1081–1095, 1987.
16. Braat SH, de Zwaan C, Brugada P, et al: Right ventricular involvement with acute inferior wall myocardial infarction identifies high risk of developing atrioventricular nodal conduction disturbances. Am Heart J 107:1183–1187, 1984.
17. Brown CG, Gurley HT, Hutchins GM, et al: Injuries associated with percutaneous placement of transthoracic pacemakers. Ann Emerg Med 14:223–228, 1985.
18. Brunetto JF, Sgammini HO, Ledesma RE, et al: Evaluation of sinoatrial node function through the use of transesophageal atrial pacing [abstract]. PACE 2:A–9, 1979.
19. Burack B, Furman S: Transesophageal cardiac pacing. Am J Cardiol 23:469–472, 1969.
20. Castellanos A, Garcia HG, Rozanski JJ, et al: Atropine-induced multilevel block in acute inferior myocardial infarction: A possible indication for prophylactic pacing. PACE 4:528–537, 1981.
21. Chamberlain DA, Leinbach RC, Vassaux CE, et al: Sequential atrioventricular pacing in heart block complicating acute myocardial infarction. N Engl J Med 282:577–582, 1970.
22. Chapman PD, Doyle TP, Troup PJ, et al: Stress echocardiography with transesophageal atrial pacing: Preliminary report of a new method for detection of ischemic wall motion abnormalities. Circulation 70:445–450, 1984.

23. Cohen MV: Coronary Collaterals: Clinical and Experimental Observations. Mount Kisco, NY, Futura Publishing Co, 1985, pp 60–61.
24. Critelli G, Grassi G, Perticone F, et al: Transesophageal pacing for prognostic evaluation of pre-excitation syndrome and assessment of protective therapy. Am J Cardiol 51:513–518, 1983.
25. Davison R, Barresi V, Parker M, et al: Intracardiac injection during cardiopulmonary resuscitation: A low risk procedure. JAMA 244:1111–1112, 1980.
26. DeGuzman M, Rahimtoola SH: What is the role of pacemakers in patients with coronary artery disease and conduction abnormalities? *In* Rahimtoola SH (ed): Current Controversies in Coronary Heart Disease. Philadelphia, FA Davis, 1983, pp 191–207.
27. Demoulin JC, Kulbertus HE: Histopathological examination of concept of left hemiblock. Br Heart J 34:807–814, 1972.
28. Dickinson JM, Traver CA: Carotid body tumors: Review of the literature with report of two cases. Am J Surg 69:9–16, 1945.
29. Dohrmann ML, Goldschlager NF: Myocardial stimulation threshold in patients with cardiac pacemakers: Effect of physiologic variables, pharmacologic agents, and lead electrodes. Cardiol Clin 3:527–537, 1985.
30. Dorros G, Cowley MJ, Simpson J, et al: Percutaneous transluminal coronary angioplasty: Report of complications from the National Heart, Lung, and Blood Institute PTCA Registry. Circulation 67:723–730, 1983.
31. Edhag O, Nyquist O, Orinius E, Paasikivi J: Cardiac pacing through transthoracic electrodes in acute myocardial infarction. Acta Med Scand 192:145–147, 1972.
32. Esente P, Giambartolomei, Gensini GG, Dator C: Coronary reperfusion and Bezold-Jarisch reflex (bradycardia and hypotension). Am J Cardiol 52:221–224, 1983.
33. Falk RH, Ngai STA, Kumaki DJ, Rubinstein JA: Cardiac activation during external cardiac pacing. PACE 10:502–506, 1987.
34. Falk RH, Zoll PM, Zoll RH: Safety and efficacy of noninvasive cardiac pacing: A preliminary report. N Engl J Med 309:1166–1168, 1983.
35. Feigl D, Ashkenazy J, Kishon Y: Early and late atrioventricular block in acute inferior myocardial infarction. J Am Coll Cardiol 4:35–38, 1984.
36. Fenichel NM, Jiminez FA, Polachek AA: 2:1 left bundle branch block in acute bacterial endocarditis with septal abscess. J Electrocardiol 10:287–290, 1977.
37. Frink JR, James TN: Normal blood supply to the human His bundle and proximal bundle branches. Circulation 47:8–18, 1973.
38. Furman S, Schwedel JB: An intracardiac pacemaker for Stokes-Adams seizures. N Engl J Med 261:943–948, 1959.
39. Furman S, Garvey J, Hurzeler P: Pulse duration variation and electrode size as features in pacemaker longevity. J Thorac Cardiovasc Surg 60:382–389, 1975.
40. Gallagher JJ, Smith WM, Kasall J, et al: Use of the esophageal lead in the diagnosis of mechanisms of reciprocating supraventricular tachycardia. PACE 3:440–451, 1980.
41. Gallagher JJ, Smith WM, Kerr CR, et al: Esophageal pacing: A diagnostic and therapeutic tool. Circulation 65:336–341, 1982.
42. Gann D, Balachandran PK, El-Sherif N, Samet P: Prognostic significance of chronic versus acute bundle block in acute myocardial infarction. Chest 67:298–303, 1975.
43. Gillum RF: Trends in cardiac pacing 1970–1983. Am Heart J 112:632–634, 1986.
44. Gordin JM, Singer DH: Atrial infarction: Importance, diagnosis, and localization. Arch Intern Med 141:1345–1348, 1981.
45. Greenberg B, Chatterjee K, Parmley WW, et al: The influence of left ventricular filling pressure on atrial contribution to cardiac output. Am Heart J 98:742–751, 1979.
46. Haden RF, Langsjoen PH, Rapoport MI, McNerney JJ: The significance of sinus bradycardia in acute myocardial infarction. Dis Chest 44:168–173, 1963.
47. Halpern MS, Nau GJ, Levi RJ, et al: Wenckebach periods of alternate beats: Clinical and experimental observations. Circulation 48:41–49, 1973.
48. Hammill SC, Sugrue DD, Gersh BJ, et al: Clinical intracardiac electrophysiologic testing: Technique, diagnostic indications, and therapeutic uses. Mayo Clin Proc 61:478–503, 1986.
49. Han J, Moe GK: Nonuniform recovery of excitability in ventricular muscle. Circ Res 14:44–60, 1964.
50. Hartzler G, Maloney JD, Curtis JJ, Barnhorst DA: Hemodynamic benefits of atrioventricular sequential pacing after cardiac surgery. Am J Cardiol 40:232–236, 1977.
51. Hauer RNW, Lie KI, Liem KL, Durrer D: Long-term prognosis in patients with bundle branch block complicating acute anteroseptal infarction. Am J Cardiol 49:1581–1585, 1982.
52. Heller GV, Aroesty JM, Parker JA, et al: The pacing stress test: Thallium-201 myocardial imaging after atrial pacing. Diagnostic value in detecting coronary artery disease compared with exercise testing. J Am Coll Cardiol 3:1197–1204, 1984.
53. Hindman MC, Wagner GS, JaRo M, et al: The clinical significance of bundle branch block complicating acute myocardial infarction. 1. Clinical characteristics, hospital mortality, and one-year follow-up. Circulation 58:679–688, 1978.
54. Hindman MC, Wagner GS, JaRo M, et al: The clinical significance of bundle branch block complicating acute myocardial infarction. 2. Indications for temporary and permanent pacemaker insertion. Circulation 58:689–699, 1978.
55. Horowitz LN: Safety of electrophysiologic studies. Circulation 73 [Suppl II]:28–31, 1986.
56. Hunt D, Lie JT, Vohra J, Sloman G: Histopathology of heart block complicating acute myocardial infarction: Correlation with the His bundle electrogram. Circulation 48:1252–1261, 1973.
57. Hynes JK, Holmes DR, Harrison CE: Five-year experience with temporary pacemaker therapy in the coronary care unit. Mayo Clin Proc 58:122–126, 1983.
58. James TN: The coronary circulation and conduction system in acute myocardial infarction. Prog Cardiovasc Dis 10:410–449, 1968.
59. Jones ME, Terry G, Kenmure ACF: Frequency and significance of conduction defects in acute myocardial infarction. Am Heart J 94:163–167, 1977.
60. Jordan JL, Yamaguchi I, Mandel WJ: Studies on the mechanism of sinus node dysfunction in the sick sinus syndrome. Circulation 57:217–223, 1978.
61. Josephson ME, Seides SF: Clinical Cardiac Electrophysiology: Techniques and Interpretations. Philadelphia, Lea & Febiger, 1979.

62. Kang PS, Gomes JAC, Kelen G, El-Sherif N: Role of autonomic regulatory mechanisms in sinoatrial conduction and sinus node automaticity in the sick sinus syndrome. Circulation 64:832–838, 1981.
63. Kay GN, Plumb VJ, Arciniegas JG, et al: Torsades de pointes: The short-long initiating sequence and other clinical features: Observations in 32 patients. J Am Coll Cardiol 2:806–817, 1983.
64. Kelemen MH, Gillilan RE, Bouchard RJ, et al: Diagnosis of obstructive coronary disease by maximal exercise and atrial pacing. Circulation 48:1227–1233, 1973.
65. Keren A, Tzivoni D, Gavish D, et al: Etiology, warning signs and therapy of torsades de pointes: A study in 10 patients. Circulation 64:1167–1174, 1981.
66. Kerr CR, Gallagher JJ, Smith WM, et al: The induction of atrial flutter and fibrillation and the termination of atrial flutter by esophageal pacing. PACE 6:60–72, 1983.
67. Krasta T, Sadowski Z, Szwed H: Assessment of sinus node recovery time and sinoatrial conduction time in patients with sick sinus syndrome [abstract]. PACE 2:A-9, 1979.
68. Kreuger SK, Rakes S, Wilkerson J, et al: Temporary pacemaking by general internists. Arch Intern Med 143:1531–1532, 1983.
69. Lamas GA, Muller JE, Turi ZG, et al (MILIS Study Group): A simplified method to predict occurrence of complete heart block during acute myocardial infarction. Am J Cardiol 57:1213–1219, 1986.
70. Langou RA, Sheps DS, Wolfson S, Cohen LS: Intraventricular conduction during coronary arteriography in patients with pre-existing conduction abnormalities. Invest Radiol 12:505–509, 1977.
71. Lehmann MH, Cameron A, Kemp HG Jr: Increased risk of ventricular fibrillation associated with temporary pacemaker during coronary arteriography. PACE 6:923–929, 1983.
72. Leinbach RC, Chamberlain DA, Kastor JA, et al: A comparison of the hemodynamic effects of ventricular and sequential A-V pacing in patients with heart block. Am Heart J 78:502–508, 1969.
73. Levin B, Posner JB: Swallowing syncope: Report of a case and review of the literature. Neurology 22:1086–1093, 1972.
74. Lewin RF, Kusniec J, Sclarovsky S, et al: Alternating Wenckebach periods in acute inferior myocardial infarction: Clinical, electrophysiologic, and therapeutic characterization. PACE 9:468–475, 1986.
75. Lie KI, Wellens HJ, Schuilenberg RM, et al: Factors influencing prognosis of bundle branch block complicating acute antero-septal infarction. Circulation 50:935–941, 1974.
76. Littleford PO, Pepine CJ: A new temporary atrial pacing catheter inserted percutaneously into the subclavian vein without fluoroscopy. PACE 4:458–464, 1981.
77. Lown B, Klein MD, Hershberg PI: Coronary and precoronary care. Am J Med 46:705–724, 1969.
78. Luck JC, Engle TR: Transient right bundle branch block with "Swan-Ganz" catheterization. Am Heart J 92:263–264, 1976.
79. Maguire LC, Burns CP, Brown DD, Tewfik HH: Reversible heart block in acute leukemia. JAMA 240:668–669, 1978.
80. Mark AL: The Bezold-Jarisch reflex revisited: Clinical implications of inhibitory reflexes originating in the heart. J Am Coll Cardiol 1:90–102, 1983.
81. Mark AL, Abboud FM, Heistad DD, et al: Evidence against the presence of ventricular chemoreceptors activated by hypoxia and hypercapnia. Am J Physiol 227:178–182, 1974.
82. Massie B, Scheinman MM, Peters R, et al: Clinical and electrophysiologic findings in patients with paroxysmal slowing of the sinus rate and apparent Mobitz Type II atrioventricular block. Circulation 58:305–314, 1978.
83. Massing GK, James TN: Anatomical configuration of the His bundle and bundle branches in the human heart. Circulation 53:609–621, 1976.
84. McAnulty JH, Rahimtoola SH: Bundle branch block. Prog Cardiovasc Dis 26:333–354, 1983.
85. Meier B, Rutishauser W: Coronary pacing during percutaneous transluminal coronary angioplasty. Circulation 71:557–561, 1985.
86. Montoyo JR, Angel J, Valle V, Gausi C: Cardioversion of tachycardia by transesophageal atrial pacing. Am J Cardiol 32:85–90, 1973.
87. Morley CA, Sutton R: Carotid sinus syncope. Int J Cardiol 6:287–293, 1984.
88. Murdock DK, Moran JF, Speranza D, et al: Augmentation of cardiac output by external cardiac pacing: Pacemaker-induced CPR. PACE 9:127–129, 1986.
89. Niemann JT, Rosborough JP, Garner D, et al: External noninvasive cardiac pacing: A comparative hemodynamic study of two techniques with conventional endocardial pacing. PACE 7:230–236, 1984.
90. Nimetz AA, Shubrooks SJ, Hutter AM Jr, DeSanctis RW: The significance of bundle branch block during acute myocardial infarction. Am Heart J 90:439–444, 1975.
91. Nishimura M, Katoh T, Hanai S, Watanabe Y: Optimal mode of transesophageal atrial pacing. Am J Cardiol 57:791–796, 1986.
92. Noe R, Cockrell W, Moses HW, et al: Transcutaneous pacemaker use in a large hospital. PACE 9:101–104, 1986.
93. Nolewajka AJ, Goddard MD, Brown TC: Temporary transvenous pacing and femoral vein thrombosis. Circulation 62:646–650, 1980.
94. Okamura K, Henthorne RW, Epstein AE, et al: Further observations on transient entrainment: Importance of pacing site and properties of components of the reentry circuit. Circulation 72:1293–1307, 1985.
95. Palmer ED: The abnormal upper gastrointestinal vagovagal reflexes that affect the heart. Am J Gastroenterol 66:513–522, 1976.
96. Palomo AR, Schwartz AM, Trohman RG, et al: Cardiac arrhythmias associated with prophylactic pacing during coronary angiography. Am J Cardiol 58:100–103, 1986.
97. Pandian NG, Kosowsky BD, Gurewich V: Transfemoral temporary pacing and deep vein thrombosis. Am Heart J 100:847–851, 1980.
98. Parameswaran R, Ohe T, Goldberg H: Sinus node dysfunction in acute myocardial infarction. Br Heart J 38:93–96, 1976.
99. Parsonnet V, Crawford CC, Bernstein AD: The 1981 United States Survey of Cardiac Pacing Practices. J Am Coll Cardiol 3:1321–1332, 1984.
100. Pastore JD, Yurchak PM, Janis KM, et al: The risk of advanced heart block in surgical patients with right bundle branch block and left axis deviation. Circulation 57:677–680, 1978.

101. Patel AK, Yap VU, Fields J, Thomsen JH: Carotid sinus syncope by malignant tumors in the neck: Emergence of vasodepressor manifestations following pacemaker therapy. Arch Intern Med 139:1281–1284, 1979.

102. Peters RW, Nussbaum S, Mailhot J, et al: Catheter-induced A-V nodal block occurring during electrophysiologic study. PACE 7:248–251, 1984.

103. Piessens J, van Mieghem W, Kesteloot H, de Geest H: Diagnostic value of clinical history, exercise testing and atrial pacing in patients with chest pain. Am J Cardiol 33:351–356, 1974.

104. Rasmussen V, Hauns S, Skagen K: Cerebral attacks due to excessive vagal tone in heavily trained persons: A clinical and electrophysiologic study. Acta Med Scand 204:401–405, 1978.

105. Reiffel JA: Drugs to avoid in patients with sinus node dysfunction. Drug Ther 12:99–106, 1982.

106. Rios JC, Hurwitz LE: Electrocardiographic responses to atrial pacing and multistage treadmill exercise testing: Correlation with coronary arteriography. Am J Cardiol 34:661–666, 1974.

107. Roberts JR, Greenberg MI: Emergency transthoracic pacemaker. Ann Emerg Med 10:600–612, 1981.

108. Roberts NK, Somerville J: Pathological significance of electrocardiographic changes in aortic valve endocarditis. Br Heart J 31:395–396, 1969.

109. Rokseth R, Hatle L: Sinus arrest in acute myocardial infarction. Br Heart J 33:639–642, 1971.

110. Rosen KM, Loeb HS, Chuquimia R, et al: Site of heart block in acute myocardial infarction. Circulation 42:925–933, 1970.

111. Ross TF, Mandel WJ: Invasive cardiac electrophysiologic testing. In Mandel WJ (ed): Cardiac Arrhythmias: Their Mechanisms, Diagnosis, and Management. Philadelphia, JB Lippincott Co, 1987.

112. Rotman M, Wagner GS, Wallace AG: Bradyarrhythmias in acute myocardial infarction. Circulation 40:703–721, 1972.

113. Rubin IL, Jagendorf B, Goldberg AL: The esophageal lead in the diagnosis of tachycardias with aberrant ventricular conduction. Am Heart J 57:19–28, 1959.

114. Sadowski Z, Szwed H: The effectiveness of transesophageal ventricular pacing in resuscitation procedures of adults [abstract]. PACE 6:A–132, 1983.

115. Samet P, Bernstein WH, Nathan DA, Lopez A: Atrial contribution to cardiac output in complete heart block. Am J Cardiol 16:1–10, 1965.

116. Scheinman MM, Gonzalez RP: Fascicular block and acute myocardial infarction. JAMA 244:2646–2649, 1980.

117. Scherlag BJ, Lau SH, Helfant RH, et al: Catheter technique for recording His bundle activity in man. Circulation 39:13–18, 1969.

118. Schittger I, Rodriguez IM, Winkle RA: Esophageal electrocardiography: A new technology revives an old technique. Am J Cardiol 57:604–607, 1986.

119. Sclarovsky S, Strasberg B, Hirschberg A, et al: Advanced early and late atrioventricular block in acute inferior myocardial infarction. Am Heart J 108:19–24, 1984.

120. Shafiroff BGP, Linder J: Effects of external electrical pacemaker stimuli on the human heart. J Thorac Surg 33:544–550, 1957.

121. Smith WM, Gallapher JJ: "Les torsades de pointes": An unusual ventricular arrhythmia. Ann Intern Med 93:578–584, 1980.

122. Sowton GE, Balcon R, Gross G, Frick MH: Measurement of the angina threshold using atrial pacing. Cardiovasc Res 1:301–307, 1967.

123. St John JN: Glossopharyngeal neuralgia associated with syncope and seizures. Neurosurgery 10:380–383, 1982.

124. Stein PD, Mathur VS, Herman MV, Levine HD: Complete heart block induced during cardiac catheterization of patients with pre-existent bundle-branch block: The hazard of bilateral bundle-branch block. Circulation 34:783–791, 1966.

125. Tans AC, Lie KI, Durrer D: Clinical setting and prognostic significance of high degree atrioventricular block in acute inferior myocardial infarction: A study of 144 patients. Am Heart J 99:4–8, 1980.

126. Thomson IR, Dalton BC, Lappas DG, Lowenstein E: Right bundle branch and complete heart block caused by the Swan-Ganz catheter. Anesthesiology 51:359–362, 1979.

127. Tintinelli JE, White BC: Transthoracic pacing during CPR. Ann Emerg Med 10:113–116, 1981.

128. Topol EJ, Goldschlager N, Ports TA, et al: Hemodynamic benefit of atrial pacing in right ventricular myocardial infarction. Ann Intern Med 96:594–597, 1982.

129. Tzivoni D, Keren A, Gottlieb S, et al: Right atrial pacing soon after myocardial infarction. Circulation 65:330–335, 1982.

130. Van der Hauwaert LG, Stroobandt R, Verhaeghe L: Arterial blood supply of the atrioventricular node and main bundle. Br Heart J 34:1045–1051, 1972.

131. Vassalle M: The relationship among cardiac pacemakers: Overdrive suppression. Circ Res 41:269–277, 1977.

132. Venkataramen K, Madias JE, Hood WB Jr: Indications for prophylactic preoperative insertion of pacemakers in patients with right bundle branch block and left anterior hemiblock. Chest 68:501–506, 1975.

133. Waldo AL, MacLean WAH: Diagnosis and Treatment of Cardiac Arrhythmias Following Open Heart Surgery: Emphasis on the Use of Atrial and Ventricular Epicardial Wire Electrodes. Mount Kisco, NY, Futura Publishing Co, 1980.

134. Waldo AL, Henthorne RW, Plumb VJ, MacLean WAH: Demonstration of the mechanism of transient entrainment and interruption of ventricular tachycardia with rapid atrial pacing. J Am Coll Cardiol 3:422–430, 1984.

135. Waldo AL, Wells JL, Cooper TB, MacLean WAH: Temporary cardiac pacing: Applications and techniques in the treatment of cardiac arrhythmias. Prog Cardiovasc Dis 23:451–474, 1981.

136. Waldo AL, MacLean WAH, Cooper TB, et al: Use of temporarily placed epicardial atrial wire electrodes for the diagnosis and treatment of cardiac arrhythmias following open-heart surgery. J Thorac Cardiovasc Surg 76:500–505, 1978.

137. Walter PF, Crawley IS, Dorney ER: Carotid sinus hypersensitivity and syncope. Am J Cardiol 42:396–403, 1978.

138. Wang K, Gobel F, Gleason DF, Edwards JE: Complete heart block complicating bacterial endocarditis. Circulation 46:939–947, 1972.

139. Waugh RA, Wagner GS, Haney TL, et al: Immediate and remote prognostic significance of fascicular block during acute myocardial infarction. Circulation 47:765–775, 1973.

140. Wei JY, Markis JE, Malagold M, Braunwald E:

Cardiovascular reflexes stimulated by reperfusion of ischemic myocardium in acute myocardial infarction. Circulation 67:796–801, 1983.

141. White JD: Transthoracic pacing in cardiac asystole. Am J Emerg Med 1:201–203, 1983.

142. White JD, Brown CG: Immediate transthoracic pacing for cardiac asystole in an emergency department setting. Am J Emerg Med 3:125–128, 1985.

143. Windle JR, Miles WM, Zipes DP, Prystowsky EN: Subthreshold conditioning stimuli prolong human ventricular refractoriness. Am J Cardiol 57:381–386, 1985.

144. Wirtzfeld A, Schmidt G, Stangl K: Physiologic pacing: Present status and future developments. PACE 10:41–57, 1987.

145. Zipes DP: Second-degree atrioventricular block. Circulation 60:465–472, 1979.

146. Zoll PM: Resuscitation of the heart in ventricular standstill by external electric stimulation. N Engl J Med 247:768–771, 1952.

147. Zoll PM, Belgard AH, Weintraub MJ, Frank HA: External mechanical cardiac stimulation. N Engl J Med 294:1273–1275, 1976.

148. Zoll PM, Zoll RH, Falk RH, et al: External noninvasive cardiac pacing: Clinical trials. Circulation 71:937–944, 1985.

6

CLINICAL EVALUATION OF THE PROSPECTIVE PACEMAKER PATIENT

JAMES A. REIFFEL

The preimplantation evaluation of a prospective pacemaker patient is designed to serve several purposes. The major aim is to establish or verify that a reasonable indication for implanting a permanent pacemaker exists. The common denominator of this aim is the answer "yes" to either or both of the following two questions: (1) In the symptomatic patient, do the symptoms definitely or most probably result from a condition that will be aided by pacemaker implantation? (2) In the patient with an asymptomatic bradycardia or conduction defect, is the dysrhythmia likely to proceed to being symptomatic and is it currently severe enough to justify prophylactic pacing? Once an indication for pacemaker implanta-

tion has been clearly established, however, several additional questions must be answered on the preinsertion evaluation before actual implantation takes place. These are listed in Table 6–1. These questions must be addressed so that we can assure ourselves and the patient that the device can be expected to improve his or her well-being symptomatically and prognostically. The indications for pacing discussed in Chapter 5A are all directly linked to this assurance. In fact, the third-party guidelines for reimbursement[17] have been formulated with this goal in mind. The specific issues raised by the questions noted above will be dealt with in the following three sections of this chapter: clinical assessment, laboratory evaluation, and intraoperative evaluation. These evaluation goals are presented in Table 6–2.

TABLE 6–1. QUESTIONS TO BE ADDRESSED BEFORE PACEMAKER IMPLANTATION

1. Pacing site
   a. Do hemodynamic status or retrograde conduction characteristics mandate a dual-chamber device?
   b. Do atrial arrhythmias preclude a dual-chamber device?
2. Modes, polarity, and timing intervals
   a. What pacing mode should be selected?
   b. Should other modes be available (programmable)?
   c. Are any pacing modes contraindicated?
   d. Should unipolar or bipolar (or programmable) stimulation be used?
   e. What timing intervals and refractory periods should be selected?
3. Additional questions/potential implications
   a. Have potential or actual tachyarrhythmia concerns been addressed?
   b. Will drug-device interactions require consideration?
   c. Have natural history implications been taken into account in answering the above questions?

CLINICAL ASSESSMENT

If the aims of the preimplantation evaluation are focused upon decisions regarding need, site, settings, and functional considerations, by what methods can these aims be achieved? The clinical assessment is the initial and often the most subjective or interpretive phase of the preimplantation evaluation. The physician becomes a detective, looking for clues in the historical and physical evaluation that can help answer any or all of the questions being asked. Although in many patients pacing decisions and justification can most accurately be arrived at with the aid of appropriately selected ancillary studies (see below), these *always* follow a

TABLE 6–2. EVALUATION GOALS

1. Clinical assessment
    a. Document symptoms–bradyarrhythmia interrelationship
    b. Assess etiology and pathophysiology regarding hemodynamics and natural history
    c. Assess rate requirements
    d. Assess lifestyle and environment issues
    e. Assess tachyarrhythmias
2. Laboratory evaluation
    a. Document symptoms–bradyarrhythmia interrelationship
    b. Determine site of block
    c. Detect significant asymptomatic conduction defects
    d. Assess etiology and pathophysiology regarding hemodynamics and natural history
    e. Assess rate requirements
    f. Assess tachyarrhythmias
    g. Assess retrograde conduction
3. Intraoperative evaluation
    a. Assess antegrade conduction
    b. Evaluate retrograde conduction characteristics
    c. Assess sensing and threshold parameters during implantation

pacemaker-oriented history and physical examination.[8, 14, 33] An electrocardiogram and chest radiograph are to be considered part of the initial clinical assessment.

A complete medical history and physical examination for the prospective pacemaker patient can provide important information regarding etiology, nature, and severity of symptoms; hemodynamic issues; lifestyle concerns, and natural history expectations, as well as need. Issues such as these should be viewed from the vantage point of the clinical assessment phase as they relate to the questions regarding indication and the questions posed in Table 6–1.

The first issue to be addressed is one of need. Is the pacer being implanted for symp-tomatic relief or prophylactically or for both reasons? In the symptomatic patient, the history is the initial tool used to assess the link between the symptoms and the bradycardia. Although no symptom complex is pathognomonic for a cardiac dysrhythmia except for sudden cardiac death, certain symptoms are often associated with bradyarrhythmias. Most commonly, these are abrupt, nonvertiginous dizziness or syncope without focal neurologic findings or sequelae. Although the history alone can never document the association of such symptoms with the precipitation of bradycardia, it can be strongly suggestive of a dysrhythmia in general, and a bradycardia in particular, when the symptoms occur in settings of vagal activation (such as swallowing or vomiting) or carotid sinus pressure. The latter can be observed during physical examination by an abnormal response (more than 3-second pause) to carotid sinus massage (5 seconds), with associated symptom development (Fig. 6–1). Blood pressure must also be taken, and if normal while the patient is supine, it must be reassessed with the patient in the upright position, as the hypersensitive carotid sinus syndrome may be manifest as symptomatic bradycardia, symptomatic hypotension (vasodepressor response), or a combination of the two. A permanent pacemaker will relieve symptoms of the bradycardiac type or of the mixed bradycardiac-vasodepressor type—particularly if atrioventricular (AV) sequential pacing is used for the latter. Pacemakers will not relieve symptoms of the pure vasodepressor type. Other symptoms may relate not to an abrupt, transient, severe bradycardia (such as sinus arrest or high-grade AV block) but rather to a lesser, more persistent bradycardia or to an inability to increase heart rate nor-

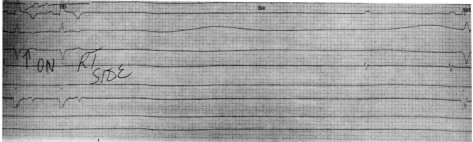

Figure 6–1. Hypersensitive carotid sinus response. Right carotid sinus massage (*arrow* indicates onset of massage) is performed during recording of simultaneous electrocardiographic (ECG) leads I, aV$_F$, and V$_1$, and atrial electrogram (fourth tracing down from the top) and His bundle electrogram (sixth line down from the top). One-second time pips are at the very top edge of the recording paper. Note the marked sinus pause followed by a P wave without atrioventricular (AV) conduction. The patient's symptoms were produced during this procedure.

mally with exercise (chronotropic incompetence). These symptoms are, most commonly, generalized lassitude, exertional fatigue or dyspnea, or subtle personality changes. The history alone in these circumstances will never confirm a bradycardiac cause. In both the symptomatic patient and the asymptomatic patient who is to be prophylactically paced, the history is indispensable in providing important information on the interrelated issues of etiology, hemodynamic considerations, lifestyle concerns, other arrhythmias versus pacing sites, pacing modes, timing intervals, and potential drug-device interactions. In fact, the history and physical examination are more likely to provide essential information regarding these items than they are to document a causal effect between a bradyarrhythmia and a specific symptom.

Etiology and Pathophysiology Considerations

The above-mentioned assessment of underlying etiology and pathophysiology is an extremely important aspect of the preimplantation evaluation because both etiology and pathophysiology have direct implications for pacemaker hemodynamics (see Chapter 8 on the hemodynamic effects of cardiac pacing),[20, 29, 35, 36, 52] necessity for dual-chamber pacing, natural history considerations, timing intervals, and retrograde conduction.

As is discussed in greater detail in Chapter 6, atrial systole is needed to maintain maximal ventricular filling and hence stroke volume. In normal persons, loss of atrial contraction can reduce stroke volume by 10 to 15 per cent. However, in patients with decreased ventricular compliance (Fig. 6–2), loss of atrial contraction can lower stroke volume to a much larger degree (greater than 70 per cent in some patients with idiopathic hypertrophic subaortic stenosis [IHSS]). In patients with a fixed heart rate, this reduction in stroke volume translates directly into a decreased cardiac output. Hence, in patients with left ventricular failure, left ventricular fibrosis, left ventricular hypertrophy, or other causes of decreased compliance, AV sequential pacing is necessary for maximal hemodynamic benefit, whether the pacer is rate responsive or not.

Accordingly, the history and physical examination performed in the preimplantation assessment must focus upon evidence pertaining to these hemodynamic issues. More specifically, one should determine if any signs, symptoms, or past illnesses or conditions indicate ventricular failure, valvular disease, or altered ventricular compliance. For example, does the patient have hypertension; risk factors for, or symptoms of, coronary artery disease; or evidence of an infiltrative or immunologic disorder? Is there an S_4, an S_3, or congestive changes in the pulmonary (rales) or systemic (edema, hepatomegaly, and neck vein distention) venous beds? Is there any evidence of valve disease, which may limit ventricular filling, limit ventricular outflow, or increase ventricular preload—the tolerance of which would decrease if sequential AV systole were lost? More specifically, was there rheumatic fever, is there a murmur of AV valve insufficiency or stenosis, or is there a murmur of aortic valve deformity or of IHSS? Does the electrocardiogram or chest radiograph or both show cardiomegaly, ventricular enlargement, and/or pulmonary vascular congestion? Evidence of

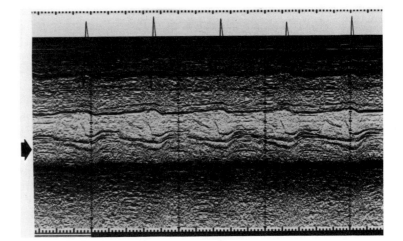

Figure 6–2. Echocardiographic demonstration of left ventricular hypertrophy. An echocardiogram from a patient with decreased left ventricular (LV) compliance due to LV hypertrophy. Note the LV wall thickness (*arrow*) and contrast it with the LV cavity size.

any of these disorders or findings suggests that dual-chamber pacing should be preferable for hemodynamic and hence symptomatic reasons.

Proper timing of atrial systole is also important. If atrial systole follows rather than precedes the QRS, as will occur in patients with VVI pacing and intact ventriculoatrial (VA) conduction, atrial contraction will occur against closed AV valves and result in "cannon A waves" in the systemic and pulmonary venous beds and can result in symptoms of dyspnea, cough, headache, and neck vein pulsations as well as a further drop in cardiac output.[27] The AV valve regurgitation that may accompany the conduction sequence change occurring with ventricular pacing may exacerbate any or all of the above-mentioned hemodynamic alterations. The symptoms from decreased cardiac output (dizziness, fatigue, exercise limitations, and so forth) and from altered venous pulsations are termed "the pacemaker syndrome."[5, 9, 20, 27, 29, 35, 36, 52] They are maximal in patients with elevated atrial pressures (as from decreased ventricular compliance) and intact retrograde conduction (see below for assessment) and can also be prevented with AV sequential pacing.

In assessing ventricular function vis-à-vis dual-versus single-chamber pacing, natural history should also be considered. In the patient with poorly controlled hypertension, ischemic heart disease, or cardiomyopathy, for example, hemodynamic changes might be expected to occur over time, and their implications with regard to pacing modes available in the device to be implanted (e.g., dual-chamber versus single-chamber) should be given forethought if possible. Similarly, natural history considerations can be directly associated with tachyarrhythmias. Ventricular arrhythmias, for example, are commonly encountered over time in patients with primary conduction disease (especially in patients with syncope) or following myocardial infarction. Similarly, atrial tachyarrhythmias commonly develop during the course of sinus node disease and in patients with elevated atrial or ventricular diastolic pressures. These, as noted below, may also affect pacemaker selection. The history and physical examination, therefore, need to focus upon etiology (with regard to the natural history) and evidence of tachyarrhythmias (such as palpitations and nonvagal syncope) as well as upon bradycardiac symptoms.

In addition, considerations of etiology and pathophysiology can affect timing interval and polarity choices. More specifically, one must assess the patient's lifestyle vis-à-vis heart rate requirements[23] and electromagnetic waveform exposure.[54] If a DDD unit is to be implanted, evaluation of exercise habits and physical activity translates directly into a guideline for the upper rate limit selection. Restricted upper rate limits may be needed, for example, in patients with angina, whereas the upper rate limit should be maximized in young, active individuals. Similarly, if the patient has unavoidable exposure to electromagnetic waveforms[54] (such as microwaves), bipolar rather than unipolar stimulation would be preferable. For similar reasons, a lifestyle associated with a high likelihood of unwanted chest wall myopotentials (such as that of a weight lifter) that could cause inappropriate inhibition in a unipolar device would suggest a preference for bipolar pacing.[31] In contrast, if a patient has atrial tachyarrhythmias but requires rate variability because of exercise habits,[23] a non-P-wave-triggered, rate-responsive device that is triggered by such myopotentials would take beneficial advantage of such signals (see Chapters 6 and 14). The same could be true for a patient with persistent sinus bradycardia or chronotropic incompetence who requires an increase in heart rate for exercise.

Many of the above-mentioned hemodynamic considerations have been recognized as important not only by prescribing and implanting physicians, but by third-party carriers as well. Medicare, for example, recognizes the following patients as being suitable candidates for dual-chamber rather than single-chamber pacing[17]: those with evidence of hemodynamic deterioration due to retrograde conduction at the time of initial implantation or generator change; and those in whom even relatively small increases in "cardiac efficiency" will significantly improve the quality of life, for example, patients with congestive heart failure or left ventricular dysfunction.

LABORATORY EVALUATION

When concerns about hemodynamic status or etiology are raised but not definitely addressed by history, physical examination, chest radiograph, or electrocardiogram, further evaluation may be required, and the aid of echocardiography (Fig. 6–2), radionuclide scanning, cardiac catheterization, and/or angiography may be sought. Each of these studies may be used selectively to define further the etiology and pathophysiology relevant to pacemaker selection and natural history. Through demonstration of ventricular hypertrophy, failure, infarction, or diastolic dysfunction, for example, such studies may further solidify the decision to implant a dual-chamber device.

The other major aims of the laboratory evaluation are to define as clearly as possible the link between symptoms and dysrhythmia and to address (further) possible concomitant tachyarrhythmias. These latter aims are generally achieved through noninvasive monitoring methods or electrophysiologic (EP) studies or both. These methodologies are discussed in more detail below.

Ambulatory Electrocardiographic Monitoring and Exercise Testing

Ambulatory electrocardiographic monitoring plays a vital role in the evaluation of the prospective pacemaker patient. The majority of approved pacemaker implantations are for symptomatic bradyarrhythmias or for conduction defects with life-threatening or adverse hemodynamic potential (such as Mobitz II or intermittent complete heart block). Since high-grade AV block or symptomatic episodes are transient in most individuals at the time of evaluation, they are rarely documented by routine electrocardiography. Rather, prolonged (24 hours or longer) electrocardiographic surveillance, often done repeatedly, must be utilized to capture a symptomatic episode. Even so, if clinical symptoms are infrequent, Holter monitoring may not be useful. Alternatively, detection of the transient symptomatic event with ad libitum use of transtelephonic or memory loop electrocardiographic recordings may be tried. Although the technical details of the various modalities of ambulatory electrocardiographic monitoring are beyond the scope of this chapter and can

be found elsewhere,[7] the utility of such an approach must be kept in mind. Thus, in patients with intermittent symptoms in whom documentation of a relationship between symptoms and dysrhythmia is sought or in patients with a bifascicular conduction defect in whom suspicion of transient, advanced AV block exists, ambulatory monitoring is the methodologic intervention of first choice.

The finding of a symptomatic bradyarrhythmia, such as a marked sinus bradycardia, a long sinoatrial pause, or advanced AV block would prompt pacemaker insertion (Fig. 6–3). Similarly, in patients with intermittent symptoms and a conduction defect, asymptomatic Mobitz II (Fig. 6–4 and 6–5), or transient complete heart block during Holter monitoring, pacemaker implantation would be indicated if no reversible cause were evident and if no other cause for symptoms were present. During ambulatory electrocardiographic monitoring, initial and often definitive evidence of concomitant manifest or potential tachyarrhythmias may also be found. In addition, when ventricular premature depolarizations are present, ambulatory monitoring may provide the first evidence of the presence of retrograde VA conduction.

Exercise testing, in contrast, is generally more useful for etiologic assessment (e.g., detection of ischemic heart disease), for unmasking tachycardias,[21] and for evaluation of the range of sinus rates that a patient may experience with activity[23] than it is for assessment of bradycardia or conduction disturbances. There are selected exceptions, however. In my experience, AV block that improves during exercise is most often AV nodal in origin. In contrast, AV conduction defects that increase as sinus rate increases with exercise, such as from 2:1 to 4:1 AV block, are most often His-Purkinje in origin. Similarly, exercise can sometimes be used to evaluate symptoms in

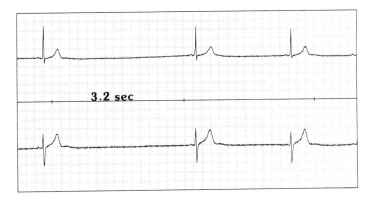

Figure 6–3. Symptomatic pause. A 3.2-second pause is recorded simultaneously on two leads of a Holter monitor recording during an episode of symptomatic sinus bradycardia.

3.2 sec

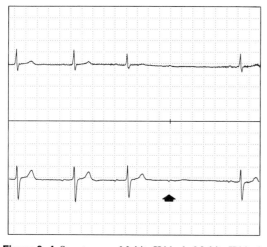

Figure 6–4. Spontaneous Mobitz II block. Mobitz II block (*arrow*) is captured during Holter monitoring in a patient being evaluated for recurrent syncope.

patients with the hypersensitive carotid sinus syndrome. That is, in some such patients we have seen, hypertension that develops during exercise may initiate a vagal reflex, which, immediately at the termination of exercise, produces a profound, symptomatic bradycardiac pause.

When used to assess activity with regard to pacer insertion, exercise testing has a standard protocol (such as the Bruce protocol), which is applied to patients with intact sinus node function who have an AV conduction defect and require a dual-chamber pacer. The sinus rate achieved with a treadmill or bicycle workload equal to the maximal level of activity the patient is likely to achieve spontaneously is noted and is used as a guide to the upper rate limit to be planned for the implanted device. In this way, as the sinus rate increases with physiologic stress, the paced ventricular rate will increase accordingly, to a clinically appropriate degree. One might ask why such testing is necessary for this purpose; that is, why in the patient without angina should any upper

rate limit other than the maximal one available in the pacer be chosen? If the maximal available one were routinely chosen, would not the exercise assessment of heart rate during activity be unnecessary? The answer lies in concerns about potential tachycardias and retrograde conduction. If a patient with a P wave–triggered ventricular pacer develops a supraventricular tachycardia, such as atrial fibrillation, and the pacer's upper rate limit is high, the patient would have constant pacing at this heart rate as long as the arrhythmia persisted (see Chapters 10 and 14). In this sense, for safety and comfort, the patient would be best served by a low upper rate limit. Thus, the exercise test is used to evaluate the maximal rate needed for lifestyle, so that a clinically relevant upper rate may be chosen. The upper rate that is selected is usually less than the maximal one available in the device, particularly in elderly patients. In the patient with ischemic heart disease, the exercise test allows one to assess at what heart rate ischemic changes appear. The upper rate limit of P-wave tracking would then be set at a rate below this level. Concerns about upper rate limits and retrograde conduction issues will be further discussed below.

Exercise tests also can reveal chronotropic incompetence and thus lead to a decision to use a rate responsive pacer.

As with ambulatory electrocardiographic monitoring, exercise testing can also be used to assess tachyarrhythmias in some patients,[21] though exercise-induced tachycardias can usually be predicted by careful interrogation during the history. Last, if ventricular premature depolarizations are present during exercise testing, they should be examined closely. Some patients with ventricular ectopy will be found to have no evidence of retrograde conduction on electrocardiography performance while they are supine but will have VA conduction become manifest with upright posture (Fig. 6–6)[51] or during exercise owing to the effects of

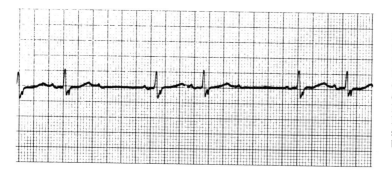

Figure 6–5. Intra-Hisian Wenckebach. Intra-Hisian block of a 3:2 pattern is captured during Holter monitoring in a patient with recurrent dizziness. It was later proved during electrophysiologic studies to be intra-Hisian in origin and is analogous to Mobitz II AV block. Note the very slight increase in PR interval in the beat before the blocked P wave.

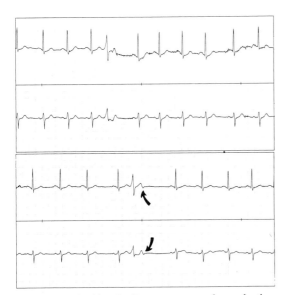

Figure 6–6. Positional effects on retrograde conduction. Two sets of tracings are shown. Each consists of two simultaneously recorded ECG leads during Holter monitoring. The upper two strips were taken with the patient supine. The lower two strips were taken with the patient upright. Note that after the ventricular premature depolarization (VPD) in the lower panel there is a retrograde P wave (*arrows*) at the T-wave terminus that is not evident after the VPD in the upper panel, despite the same VPD configuration and coupling interval.

posture- or activity-altered sympathetic or parasympathetic balance or of circulating catecholamines or of both.

Electrophysiologic (EP) Studies: General Comments

Like ambulatory monitoring, EP studies may play a significant role in the evaluation of the prospective pacemaker patient (Table 6–3).[2, 6, 11–13, 16, 18, 22, 26, 40, 45, 48–50] Utilizing intracardiac electrogram recordings from relevant portions of the specialized conduction system and myocardium in combination with programmable patterns of cardiac stimulation at selected intracardiac or pericardiac sites, EP studies can provide sophisticated diagnostic, therapeutic, and prognostic information in patients with symptomatic and asymptomatic dysrhythmias. More specifically, EP studies may be used to assess the mechanism of symptoms, the prognostic importance of asymptomatic bradyarrhythmias or conduction defects, and the risk of concomitant tachycardias. In addition, EP studies can be used to assess with accuracy retrograde conduction characteristics, the efficacy and risk of antitachycardia stimulation,

and the hemodynamic effects of various rate and AV interval settings prior to implantation. EP studies relating to indication, prognosis, or antitachycardia therapy should be performed as a separate procedure in advance of device implantation. EP studies used to evaluate hemodynamics, retrograde conduction, and timing interval selection can be done either as a preimplantation study or intraoperatively immediately before device implantation or programming or at both times.

Although a detailed review of EP testing is not the subject of this chapter, certain highlights appropriate to the subject at hand will be discussed. It should be kept in mind, however, that EP testing in the evaluation of prospective pacemaker patients is a methodology that should be used in only a selected minority of subjects and is generally used only after noninvasive studies. That is, if noninvasive studies have provided a documented association between symptoms and the conduction disorder, EP studies are not required to reconfirm the diagnosis. Similarly, if noninvasive studies have documented a tachyarrhyth-

TABLE 6–3. INDICATIONS FOR EP STUDY FOR BRADYARRHYTHMIAS

ACTION	SAN	AVN	H-P	PURPOSE
1. Evaluate symptoms (e.g., syncope)	y	y	y	D
2. Confirm suspected dysfunction	y	y	y	D
3. Quantitate dysfunction	y	y	y	D
4. Assess prognosis	y	?	y	D
5. Evaluate VA conduction characteristics	—	y	y	T
6. Assess likelihood and/or types of associated tachyarrhythmias	y	y	y	B
7. Evaluate drug effects	y	y	y	B
8. Verify site of block	—	y	y	D
9. Differentiate Mobitz II from pseudoblock	—	—	y	D
10. Assess relative importance of bradycardia in carotid sinus syndrome	y	y	—	D
11. Assess hemodynamic effects of selected pacing mode and anticipated rate and AV settings	y	y	y	T

SAN = sinoatrial node; AVN = atrioventricular node; H-P = His-Purkinje system; y = yes; ? = uncertain; — = not applicable; D = primarily diagnostic; T = primarily therapeutic, i.e., relates to pacemaker mode or interval settings; B = both D and T.

mia in the chamber or chambers to be paced or sensed, or have documented the presence of retrograde conduction, EP studies are not required merely to reconfirm the observation. EP studies are useful, however, to provide a diagnosis in some patients in whom a dysrhythmia is thought to be the cause of symptoms but the relationship has not been proved by simpler means. As with noninvasive analysis, however, the sensitivity of EP testing for establishing a diagnosis of certainty does not approach 100 per cent.

Electrophysiologic Studies for Diagnosis

Figure 6–7 shows the result of overdrive stimulation (to determine the sinus recovery time[40, 45]) in a patient with sinus bradycardia and intermittent dizziness in whom symptomatic episodes were not captured electrocardiographically. During the long pause following the termination of pacing, the patient's typical symptoms occurred. A permanent pacer was implanted, and in a follow-up now totaling more than 10 years, the symptoms have not recurred. Gann and colleagues,[19] as well as our own group,[40, 43, 45] have shown that when sinus node function testing is abnormal in patients with dizziness or syncope, permanent pacemaker implantation will usually (in more than 85 per cent of cases) prevent symptomatic recurrence. This finding has always been true when symptoms were reproduced during EP testing, as in Figure 6–7, and usually is true when the function test (e.g., sinus recovery time or sinoatrial conduction time) is abnormal but typical symptoms were not present during such testing. Similar observations have been reported for the results of EP testing in patients with recurrent syncope and non–sinus node disorders as well.[1, 15, 16, 26] That is, if abnormalities of rhythm or conduction are

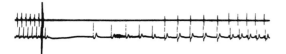

Figure 6–7. A prolonged sinus recovery time. An atrial electrogram (*top*) and simultaneous lead II (*bottom*) are shown during overdrive pacing (to the left of the vertical line, which marks the end of pacing) and during recovery (to the right). Note the junctional escape rhythm and the much longer interval to the onset of atrial activity. The first junctional complex is about 4 seconds after pacing; atrial recovery is about 10 seconds. The patient was symptomatic during the recovery interval.

detected by EP testing in patients with recurrent syncope, and therapy is directed at such abnormalities, symptoms will stop in about 80 per cent of such subjects.[1, 15, 26, 43] Of note, because neither ambulatory monitoring nor EP studies have 100 per cent sensitivity in the evaluation of sinus node function,[46] conduction disease, or syncope,[47] both tests are often required. For patients with AV conduction disturbances, EP testing for diagnostic purposes is performed: (1) to determine the site of block if the body-surface ECG or clinical history does not suggest it with certainty and therapeutic intervention is dependent upon the site of block; (2) to evaluate patients with symptoms compatible with advanced conduction system disease who do not have symptoms present during noninvasive testing (analogous to studies in patients with sinus node disease) and who do not have Mobitz II or complete heart block on ambulatory monitoring[2, 6, 11–13, 18, 22, 32, 48–50]; and (3) to evaluate the status of the AV conduction system in patients who also require pacing for sick sinus syndrome. Some would also suggest EP studies are appropriate for patients who develop persistent bundle branch block with an acute myocardial infarction but who have not had associated Mobitz II or transient complete heart block documented.

When antegrade AV conduction is impaired in patients with sinus node dysfunction, permanent atrial pacing alone (e.g., AAI) is usually not appropriate. When EP studies are used for the first purpose listed above, they are generally employed for an apparent Mobitz block–QRS mismatch (e.g., apparent Mobitz II with a narrow QRS or apparent Mobitz I with a wide QRS) or when a Mobitz II pattern occurs in a patient taking digitalis. Digitalis may produce pseudoblock (concealed His bundle extrasystoles, which impair conduction of the subsequent sinus impulse).[34] The therapy for this is reduction of digitalis, rather than a pacemaker. For apparent Mobitz block–QRS mismatch, the finding of intra-Hisian or sub-Hisian block has the implication of typical Mobitz II with a wide QRS (always sub-Hisian) and should result in permanent pacemaker implantation. In contrast, if AV nodal block is the cause, pacer implantation is guided by current symptoms rather than by the site of block. During studies of AV conduction, induced infra-Hisian block[11] results in permanent pacemaker insertion for relief of symptoms or for prognostic purposes, just as it would if spontaneous sub-Hisian block (e.g., Mobitz II

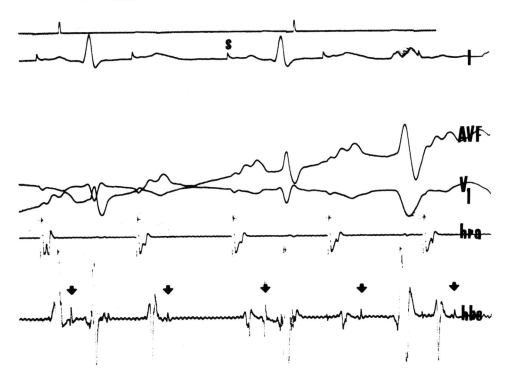

Figure 6–8. Sub-Hisian block. Leads I, aV$_F$, and V$_1$ and a high right atrial (hra) and His bundle (hre) electrogram are shown during atrial pacing. The time pips at the top are 1000 msec apart. S = a stimulus artifact. The arrows are placed over His bundle depolarization. Sub-Hisian Wenckebach with HV intervals greater than 100 msec, as well as sub-Hisian block, is evident.

with a wide QRS) had occurred. Most investigators believe the same should hold true for spontaneous or pacing-induced marked prolongation of HV conduction time in symptomatic patients, even without total infra-Hisian block.[2, 3, 6, 11, 13, 18, 22, 48, 50, 53] What defines a "markedly prolonged" HV interval, however, is controversial. A value greater than 100 msec (Fig. 6–8) is usually agreed to, 80 to 100 msec sometimes is, and less than 80 usually is not.[2, 3, 11, 13, 18, 22, 48, 50, 53] Thus, in this area, therapeutic reactions will not be identical from center to center.

One might assume that the results of EP testing could be anticipated by ambulatory monitoring observations, thus possibly precluding their necessity. That is, one might suspect in the symptomatic patient who is without symptoms during electrocardiographic monitoring, but in whom Holter monitoring reveals asymptomatic sinus bradycardia, sinus pauses, AV Wenckebach, or bundle branch block, that EP studies will merely reveal a more advanced degree of a similar defect and perhaps produce associated symptoms. However, that is often not the case. In fact, in a series of patients with syncope, both our group[47] and Pratt and associates[38] found that it

was infrequent for the results of Holter monitoring to predict the results of the EP study (whether the patient had a bradycardiac, conduction defect, or tachycardiac cause). Equally important, when the results of EP testing are used to guide the therapy of such patients (i.e., those with syncope), as was mentioned above, the reduction in recurrence of symptoms by somewhat less than 80 per cent[1, 15, 16, 26] adds credence to the importance and clinical relevance of the EP findings.

Last, in up to 50 per cent of patients with syncope and bundle branch block, EP studies suggest that the mechanism for syncope is ventricular tachycardia rather than advanced conduction defects. Thus, all patients with conduction disease and symptoms in whom the relationship has not been clearly established by clinical or noninvasive assessment should undergo EP testing rather than have a pacemaker inserted based upon an assumed bradycardiac mechanism.

Comments On Tachyarrhythmias

A tachyarrhythmia assessment should also be an aim of the preimplantation evaluation of the patient with bradyarrhythmia or conduction defect. To understand why this assessment is important, one must ask how a tachyarrhythmia might affect the potential pacemaker and how the pacemaker might affect the tachyarrhythmia. Tachyarrhythmias may affect pacemaker operation or pacemaker choice in several ways. The presence of atrial tachyarrhythmias poses a hazard to or causes discomfort in patients with P wave–triggered ventricular pacing, as they may initiate symptomatically rapid paced ventricular rates. The same may even be true in patients with sinus tachycardia and angina pectoris. Thus, atrial tachycardias may be a contraindication to P wave–triggered ventricular pacing or at least will suggest a restricted upper rate limit. For example, in the patient with paroxysmal atrial fibrillation, one might select an upper rate limit of 100, regardless of exercise concerns. In the patient with angina (as noted earlier), one might similarly choose a restricted upper rate limit (probably with the aid of exercise test guidance) regardless of exercise desires. The presence of paroxysmal atrial tachyarrhythmias is a contraindication to asynchronous atrial pacing, as occurs in the DVI mode, since the nonsynchronized atrial stimulus can initiate the tachyarrhythmia. The presence of persistent atrial tachyarrhythmias, such as fibrillation or flutter, is a contraindication to dual-chamber pacing, regardless of concerns about ventricular functional status (see below), since an atrial stimulus will fail to effect a response and will serve only to drain the batteries prematurely. Thus, in the chamber-paced, individual tachycardias have implications with regard to inadvertent tachycardia stimulation or inability to capture, and in the chamber-sensed, individual tachycardias have implications with regard to upper rate limits. Insofar as tachycardias may alter local electrogram characteristics, they also have implications regarding the potential for malsensing. That is, if local electrogram voltage is reduced during a tachycardia (e.g., due to a change in activation vector) at the site of a sensing electrode, malsensing could occur.

Tachycardia assessment is done in the same sequence as is bradycardia assessment. However, as was indicated earlier, although the history may be suggestive (e.g., if syncope or palpitations are noted), documentation usually requires electrocardiographic monitoring (see "Ambulatory Electrocardiographic Monitoring and Exercise Testing," above) or EP studies. For this purpose, EP studies should be considered if patients have not as yet revealed symptoms compatible with tachyarrhythmias or if tachyarrhythmias have a high likelihood of developing during the natural course of the underlying disease. In this setting, such EP studies can provide data about the type and mechanism of a tachycardia; the ease with which it might be induced by asynchronous stimuli; the efficacy and safety of antitachyarrhythmia pacing in terminating the observed tachyarrhythmia; and, through the use of serial EP studies, the likelihood that drugs can be used to control the tachyarrhythmia effectively. The effects of the tachycardia on local electrograms, which have sensing implications for the implanted device, as discussed above, can also be examined, both before and during serial drug studies. Serial drug studies also allow determination of the effect such drugs may have on stimulation or defibrillation thresholds, tachycardia characteristics, or other potential drug-device interactions.[44]

When serial EP studies to guide drug management of a tachycardia are planned in a patient who is to receive a permanent pacemaker for a bradycardia or conduction defect, they may be done in the manner standard for EP studies in general via the use of temporarily placed electrode catheters and an external programmable stimulator, or they may be done via the implanted permanent pacemaker system itself if a generator with the proper features was chosen prior to implantation. That is, implanted pacemakers that have (programmable) triggered modes and short refractory periods can be used as implanted stimulators for serial EP studies.[41] For this use, the device in the triggered mode can be made to follow external stimuli and thus substitute for repeated catheterizations. However, because of limited availability of such features, the decision to utilize a device with such functions must be made before a pacemaker is implanted. Moreover, at EP study prior to implantation, the stimulating polarity available in the device to be implanted (unipolar or bipolar) must be tested and be shown capable of inducing the tachycardia. An ongoing study in our laboratory has determined that in patients with ventricular tachycardia induced by bipolar stimulation (as is typically used during EP testing) ventricular tachycardia is inducible by unipolar stimulation (Fig. 6–9) in only about 80 per cent of the patients.

In light of the above comments, one could recommend that Holter monitoring and, depending on the history, exercise testing be performed in all patients whose history sug-

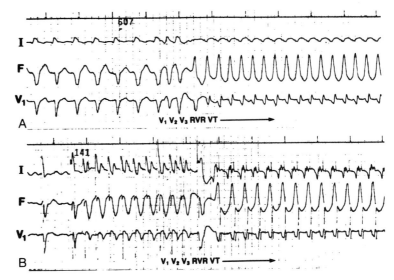

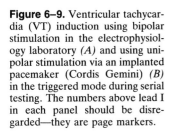

Figure 6–9. Ventricular tachycardia (VT) induction using bipolar stimulation in the electrophysiology laboratory *(A)* and using unipolar stimulation via an implanted pacemaker (Cordis Gemini) *(B)* in the triggered mode during serial testing. The numbers above lead I in each panel should be disregarded—they are page markers.

gests the possibility of a tachycardia (e.g., palpitations), in all patients who are being evaluated for syncope, and in all patients who are being assessed for advanced AV conduction disease, even if the need for a pacemaker is already established. The history or results of noninvasive monitoring, or both, then should be used to decide whether a patient needs EP study specifically for evaluation of a tachyarrhythmia concern. EP studies to determine the risk of a tachycardia should be a part of all EP studies in patients who come to the EP laboratory for evaluation of a bradyarrhythmia, since concomitant tachyarrhythmias are frequently part of the symptom complex and/or natural history. They are also appropriate for patients in whom a chamber is to be paced asynchronously. Finally, EP studies can also be used to assess effects of various AV intervals as they relate to tachycardia induction. For example, in our experience, in some patients with AV nodal or AV reentrant, it may be more difficult for a tachycardia to be initiated in the presence of a short AV interval than in the presence of a longer one. (Similarly, in patients with mitral valve obstruction, the hemodynamic benefit that might be gained by use of a long AV interval rather than a short one can also be assessed.)

INTRAOPERATIVE STUDIES

As was indicated above, EP studies used to assess retrograde conduction, AV conduction

status, hemodynamics, and timing interval selection can be done either during a preoperative study or intraoperatively immediately before device implantation or programming or at both times. However, in most patients, they are done intraoperatively. Hemodynamics and antegrade conduction intervals are interrelated and are discussed fully in Chapter 6. Retrograde and antegrade conduction assessment, however, is appropriate for discussion at this point. Characteristics of retrograde conduction are important to consider because of the role retrograde conduction plays in the following: (1) pacemaker-mediated tachycardia (PMT), a phenomenon that can occur in patients with DDD, VDD, or VAT pacing in the presence of intact VA conduction (see Chapter 12 on pacemaker electrocardiography for dual-chamber devices); (2) the generation of supraventricular arrhythmias in patients prone to them (such as atrial fibrillation or AV reentry in patients with accessory AV connections); (3) the "pacemaker syndrome," a symptomatic consequence that can occur in patients with intact VA conduction who receive VVI pacers (see above); and (4) the choice of an upper rate limit. Since retrograde conduction is much more likely to be present in patients with sinus node dysfunction (about 80 per cent) than in those with AV conduction disturbances (about 10 to 20 per cent) in our experience, as well as in patients with preexcitation, and since these groups of patients frequently have atrial tachyarrhythmias as part of their natural history, this consideration must never be overlooked in these patients.

All patients who, after the clinical assessment and laboratory testing phases of the preimplantation evaluation have been completed, are scheduled to receive a VVI pacemaker, and who have not had retrograde conduction evaluated at a preoperative EP study, must have VA conduction characteristics evaluated intraoperatively prior to implantation of the permanent pulse generator. When VA conduction is absent, symptoms associated with post–QRS atrial contraction, as were discussed earlier, will not be an issue. In the patient without VA conduction in whom ventricular compliance and function are normal, VVI pacing is usually very well tolerated hemodynamically. In the presence of VA conduction or disordered ventricular properties or both, as suggested above, AV sequential pacing will usually result in greater tolerance by the patient, comfort, and function than will VVI stimulation. AV sequential pacing will also minimize the risk of tachyarrhythmia induction secondary to VA conduction. This minimization of risk is most important in patients with AV nodal reentry or accessory AV conduction pathways. The assessment of VA conduction also plays an important role in patients who are to receive P wave–triggered ventricular pacing (e.g., VAT, VDD, and DDD modes). As is discussed in more detail in Chapter 12, when a sensed P wave initiates a ventricular paced event and VA conduction is intact, a ventricular depolarization without a preceding P wave (such as a ventricular premature depolarization) will result in retrograde atrial activation, which, after the programmed AV delay, will result in a ventricular paced QRS, a subsequent retrograde P wave, a subsequent paced QRS, and an endless loop PMT. However, knowledge of VA conduction characteristics may allow this occurrence to be avoided. By setting the postventricular atrial refractory period (PVARP) at an interval that exceeds the VA conduction time, for example, the retrograde P wave will not be sensed and the tachycardia will not be initiated. However, the longer the PVARP (assuming no change in programmed AV interval), the lower will be the maximal upper rate limit available for programming, since P waves that fall during the AV interval or during the PVARP will not trigger a ventricular response. In occasional patients, shortening of the AV interval will result in an atrium still refractory at the time of VA conduction and, therefore, in the absence of a retrograde P wave; alternatively, however, this maneuver will result in retrograde conduction delay through the AV node,

prolongation of the VA conduction time, and a resultant retrograde P wave falling outside the intrinsic or pacemaker atrial refractory period, and thus it is a much less predictable way to deal with PMT. Its effect, however, can be assessed during EP studies.

As the above implies, VA conduction characteristics may be linked to the presence and time sequence of AV conduction. Thus, as we have shown elsewhere,[42] the value determined for the VA conduction interval will be shorter in the presence of AV sequential stimulation than during straight ventricular pacing. Moreover, it will be longer the more rapidly the ventricles are paced in most patients or if ventricular premature stimuli are used to assess it. Since PMT initiation is a phenomenon of P wave–triggered ventricular pacing units, determination of the retrograde refractory period and VA conduction time by programmed stimulation in sinus rhythm or during AV sequential pacing is reasonable. Similarly, for PMT to persist, retrograde conduction must be intact at the rate of the PMT (which cannot exceed and usually equals the programmed upper rate limit of the device). Thus, one might also assess VA conduction during straight ventricular pacing at rates up to the anticipated upper rate limit setting to be used in the pacemaker. This value will usually exceed the one obtained by the former method. The PVARP chosen for the pacer ultimately used should be at least as long as the VA conduction time determined by the initial (AV sequential activation) method and, if it does not unduly limit the choice of an upper rate limit for the patient, would ideally be at least as long as the VA interval demonstrated by the second method. In any case, a setting for the PVARP at least as long as the VA interval determined by the straight ventricular pacing approach should be an available programmed value.

Since VA conduction may be absent during EP studies performed with the patient supine but present with EP studies done during upright activity (see above), one might argue that patients should undergo EP study for retrograde conduction assessment preoperatively rather than intraoperatively, and if there is no evidence of VA conduction when the patient is supine, the assessment should be done again either when the patient is upright or when isoproterenol has been infused. However, because most patients who receive pacemakers do not require preoperative EP studies, because of the availability of programmability of the PVARP, and because PMT is rarely a life-threatening disorder, such additional maneuvers during EP study, which may be theoretically useful but logistically stressful, are typically not performed.

One other advantage of preoperative rather than intraoperative assessment of VA conduction is also linked to the upper rate limit. If the assessment is made preoperatively and retrograde conduction considerations force the upper rate limit to be set at a lower value than would be chosen based upon lifestyle or exercise characteristics, the patient will then be aware preoperatively that his or her maximal activity may be limited to some degree. Fortunately, the development of automatic PVARP extension after ventricular premature depolarizations, which is now available in many units, allows the programmed PVARP to be minimized in many patients, thus reducing the concerns about upper rate limitations.

An additional assessment to be performed intraoperatively, if not done preoperatively, is an evaluation of the status of AV conduction. This evaluation is done in patients with sinus node dysfunction but apparently intact AV conduction. If the AV conduction system is truly normal and chronotropic incompetence is not present, then AAI pacing can be utilized. In contrast, associated abnormal AV conduction would indicate a need for ventricular stimulation (e.g., VVI), whereas the status of hemodynamic values and chronotropic competence would be used to determine the need (or lack thereof) for P wave–triggered or other biosensor-triggered rate-responsive ventricular or dual-chamber pacing (see Chapter 14). AV conduction can be assessed simply by observing the PR interval on the electrocardiogram (or better yet, the AH and HV intervals from a His bundle recording) during incremental atrial pacing (up to rates of 150 beats per minute).[2, 6, 18, 22, 48] The development of AV nodal Wenckebach at an atrial paced rate slower than 120 beats per minute, the presence of a prolonged HV interval, or the development of HV delay or sub-Hisian block should be taken as a sign of impaired AV conduction and should contraindicate AAI pacing.

Assessment of AV conduction is also useful as a guide to the setting of the AV interval in dual-chamber devices. In patients with intact AV conduction, a physiologically reasonable PR interval with spontaneous ventricular depolarization is preferable to a programmed AV interval that results in ventricular pacing. The sequence of ventricular depolarization with ventricular pacing is always abnormal and can result in some degree of decreased cardiac output or AV valve regurgitation or both. Moreover, a paced ventricular complex results in more battery drain than does the sensing of a spontaneous ventricular complex and thus will reduce the longevity of the pacemaker battery. Balanced against these concerns, however, are concerns for upper rate limits. It may be recalled from above that the longer the AV interval for any given PVARP, the slower will be the available upper rate limit. In general, the upper rate limit settings and considerations about retrograde conduction take precedence over the desire to maintain intact AV conduction when the AV interval finally comes to be programmed.

Additional measurements are also performed intraoperatively. These may be done via electrogram recording on a multichannel recorder or via a pacing systems analyzer in conjunction with pacing in the chambers to be assessed. They include the following:[4, 10, 37, 39] (1) measurements to assess sensing thresholds or appropriateness of the signal to be sensed (atrial or ventricular electrogram amplitude and slew rate) or both; (2) documentation of myocardial contact (current of injury); (3) thresholds and resistance calculations (voltage threshold, current threshold, and calculated or measured impedance); and (4) demonstration of capture[30] (by postspike depolarization or fluoroscopic observations or both). However, as these measurements are more a part of the pacemaker implantation process than they are of the clinical assessment of the prospective pacer patient, they will be discussed in Chapter 7, which deals with pacemaker implantation, rather than at this point.

ELECTROPHYSIOLOGIC STUDY AND DRUG-DEVICE INTERACTIONS

Drug-device interactions[41] *in toto* are not within the scope of this chapter. Insofar as they relate to preimplantation (preoperative or intraoperative) EP studies, however, they are appropriate to mention here. Such interactions generally take one of five forms:

1. One needs a pacer to support the use of a drug because of baseline or drug-related bradycardia or AV block. This type has been alluded to earlier.

2. Use of a drug affects the frequency of use or lifespan of the device. For example, a drug may decrease the frequency of a tachyarrhyth-

mia and thus decrease the utilization of an antitachyarrhythmia device, thereby possibly prolonging its battery life. The likelihood of drug efficacy can be assessed with serial preimplantation EP studies. Drugs, however, may raise pacing thresholds and affect capture or battery drain. This factor, too, is assessable with pharmacologic testing during EP studies. If one used a nonprogrammable pacemaker (rare these days), such studies would have to have been completed preoperatively. In general, threshold changes are small and of little clinical relevance. However, in patients with high thresholds at implantation and in patients receiving drugs that have been reported to increase thresholds as much as 300 per cent,[24, 25] such an interaction could be clinically important.

3. Drugs can affect the efficacy or safety of an implanted device. Drug-slowed tachycardias may be easier to terminate or less likely to be accelerated by antitachycardia stimulation.[28] However, drugs may slow a tachycardia or alter local electrograms, so that they no longer meet rate or slew characteristic criteria for recognition by an antitachyarrhythmia device. Similarly, altered electrograms may cause malsensing by pacemakers, improved capture (as noted above), or adverse effects on defibrillation thresholds. Each of these factors can be assessed by preimplantation drug and EP studies.

4. Triggered pacing units may be used for serial drug assessment EP testing. These have been discussed above.

5. Finally, drugs and devices may have additive efficacy, as in some patients with ventricular tachycardia and a congenital long QT syndrome, in whom pacing alone or drugs alone (such as beta blockers or Ib agents) give incomplete relief but AAI overdrive pacing coupled with drugs leads to complete tachycardia suppression. These drug-device interactions may be difficult to assess beforehand, as most patients with the long QT syndrome cannot, with reliability, have their tachycardias induced at EP testing.

CONCLUSIONS

As suggested at the beginning of this chapter, the clinical evaluation of the prospective pacemaker patient is designed (1) to ensure that the patient is an appropriate candidate to receive an implanted device, (2) to ascertain which features of implantable devices should be available in the unit to be received by the patient and which are contraindicated, and (3) to determine what timing intervals are most appropriate. This chapter also suggests that factors that might affect these choices in a given patient over time, such as drug administration or natural history, should be considered, if possible, prior to or at the time of implantation. Finally, this chapter suggests that the preimplantation evaluation is best accomplished by the traditional approaches used throughout medical practice, that is, a thorough history and physical examination and judicious use of well-planned selected laboratory studies.

REFERENCES

1. Akhtar M, Shenasa M, Denker S, et al: Role of cardiac electrophysiologic studies in patients with unexplained syncope. PACE 6:192, 1983.
2. Alpert BL: Role of the electrophysiologic study in pacemaker implantation for bradyarrhythmias. Clin Prog Pacing Electrophysiol 1:109–121, 1983.
3. Altschuler H, Fisher JD, Furman S: Significance of isolated H-V interval prolongation in symptomatic patients without documented heart block. Am Heart J 97:20–25, 1979.
4. Angello DA: Principles of electrical testing for analysis of ventricular endocardial pacing leads. Prog Cardiovasc Dis 27:57–72, 1984.
5. Ausubel K, Boal BH, Furman S: Pacemaker syndrome: Definition and evaluation. Cardiol Clin 3:587–594, 1985.
6. Bauernfeind RR, Welch WJ, Brownstein SL: Distal atrioventricular conduction system function. Cardiol Clin 4:417–428, 1986.
7. Bigger JT Jr, Reiffel JA, Coromilas J: Ambulatory electrocardiography. In Platia E (ed): Non-pharmacologic Management of Cardiac Arrhythmias. New York, JB Lippincott Co, 1986, pp 36–61.
8. Boudoulas H, Weissler AM, Lewis RP, et al: The clinical diagnosis of syncope. Curr Probl Cardiol 7:1–40, 1983.
9. Das G: Pacemaker headaches. PACE 7:802–805, 1984.
10. DeCaprio V, Hurzeler P, Furman S: A comparison of unipolar and bipolar electrograms for cardiac pacemaker sensing. Circulation 56:750–755, 1977.
11. Dhingra RC, Denes P, Wu D, et al: Prospective observations in patients with chronic bundle branch block and marked HV prolongation. Circulation 53:600–604, 1976.
12. Dhingra RC, Palileo E, Strasberg B, et al: Significance of H-V interval in 517 patients with chronic bifascicular block. Circulation 64:1265–1271, 1981.
13. Dhingra RC, Wyndham C, Bauernfeind R, et al: Significance of block distal to the His bundle induced by atrial pacing in patients with chronic bifascicular block. Circulation 60:1455–1464, 1979.
14. DiCarlo LA, Morady F: Evaluation of the patient with syncope. Cardiol Clin 3:499–514, 1985.
15. DiMarco JP, Garan H, Ruskin JN: Approach to the patient with recurrent syncope of unknown cause. Mod Concepts Cardiovasc Dis 52:11, 1983.

16. DiMarco JP, Garan H, Harthorne JW, Ruskin JN: Intracardiac electrophysiologic techniques in recurrent syncope of unknown cause. Ann Intern Med 95:542, 1981.
17. Empire Blue Cross Blue Shield—Medicare coverage changes. Fast Facts for Physicians 29(9):2–3, 1985.
18. Fisher JD: Role of electrophysiologic testing in the diagnosis and treatment of patients with known and suspected bradycardias and tachycardias. Prog Cardiovasc Dis 24:25–90, 1981.
19. Gann D, Tolentino R, Samet P: Electrophysiologic evaluation of elderly patients with sinus bradycardia. Ann Intern Med 90:24–39, 1979.
20. Goldreyer BN: Physiologic pacing: The role of AV synchrony. PACE 5:613–615, 1982.
21. Goldschlager N: Types and prognostic significance of cardiac dysrhythmias occurring during exercise testing. Clin Prog Pacing Electrophysiol 1:205–224, 1983.
22. Greenspan AJ: Electrophysiologic studies for pacemaker selection. Cardiovasc Clin 16:119–137, 1985.
23. Hammond HK, Froelicher VF: Normal and abnormal heart rate responses to exercise. Prog Cardiovasc Dis 27:277–296, 1985.
24. Hellestrand KJ, Burnett PJ, Milne JP, et al: Effect of the antiarrhythmic agent flecainide acetate on acute and chronic pacing thresholds. PACE 6:892, 1983.
25. Hellestrand KJ, Nathan AW, Bexton RS, et al: Electrophysiologic effects of flecainide acetate on sinus node function, anomalous atrioventricular connections, and pacemaker thresholds. Am J Cardiol, 53:30B, 1984.
26. Hess DS, Morady F, Scheinman MM: Electrophysiological testing in the evaluation of patients with syncope of undetermined origin. Am J Cardiol 50:1039, 1982.
27. Holmes DR Jr: Hemodynamics of cardiac pacing. In Furman S, Hayes DL, Holmes DR Jr (eds): A Practice of Cardiac Pacing. Mount Kisco, NY, Futura Publishing Co, 1986, pp 75–95.
28. Keren G, Miura DS, Somberg JC: Pacing termination of ventricular tachycardia: Influence of antiarrhythmic slowed ectopic rate. Am Heart J, 107:638, 1984.
29. Kruse I, Arnman K, Conradson TB, et al: Comparison of the acute and long term hemodynamic effects of ventricular inhibited and atrial synchronous ventricular inhibited pacing. Circulation 65:846–855, 1982.
30. Levine PA: Confirmation of atrial capture and determination of atrial capture thresholds in DDD pacing systems. Clin Prog Pacing Electrophysiol 2:465–473, 1984.
31. Levine PR, Klein M: Myopotential inhibition of unipolar pacemakers: A disease of technologic progress. Ann Intern Med 98:101–102, 1983.
32. McAnulty JH, Rahimtoola SH, Murphy E, et al: Natural history of "high risk" bundle branch block: Final report of a prospective study. N Engl J Med 307:137–143, 1982.
33. Morady F: The evaluation of syncope with electrophysiologic studies. Cardiol Clin 4:515–526, 1986.
34. Narula OS: Current concepts of atrioventricular block. In Narula OS (ed): His Bundle Electrocardiography and Clinical Electrophysiology. Philadelphia, FA Davis, 1975, pp 157–158.
35. Nishimura RA, Gersh BJ, Viletstra RE, et al: Hemodynamic and symptomatic consequences of ventricular pacing. PACE 5:903–910, 1982.
36. Ogawa S, Dreifus LS, Shenoy PN: Hemodynamic consequences of atrioventricular and ventriculoatrial pacing. PACE 1:8–13, 1978.
37. Ohm O, Breivik K, Hammer E, et al: Intraoperative electrical measurement during pacemaker implantation. Clin Prog Pacing Electrophysiol 2:1–23, 1984.
38. Pratt CM, Thornton BC, Magro SA, et al: Spontaneous arrhythmia detected on ambulatory electrocardiographic recordings lacks precision in predicting inducibility of ventricular tachycardia during electrophysiologic study. J Am Coll Cardiol 10:97–104, 1987.
39. Preston JA, Barold SS: Problems in measuring thresholds for cardiac pacing: Recommendations for routine clinical measurement. Am J Cardiol 40:658–660, 1977.
40. Reiffel JA: Electrophysiologic evaluation of sinus node function. Cardiol Clin 4:401–416, 1986.
41. Reiffel JA, Sahar D: The DDT option: Implications of this new pacing feature. Clin Prog Electrophysiol Pacing 4:31–35, 1986.
42. Reiffel JA, Spotnitz HM: Pacemakers, pacemaker mediated tachycardias, and antitachycardia pacemakers. In Vlay S (ed): Practical Management of Cardiac Arrhythmias. Boston, Little, Brown [in press].
43. Reiffel JA, Ferrick K, Bigger JT Jr: Disorders of sinus node function: Diagnostic and therapeutic pacing. Intelligence Rep Cardiac Pacing Electrophysiol 1(3):106–112, 1983.
44. Reiffel JA, Coromilas J, Zimmerman JM, Spotnitz HM: Drug-device interactions: Clinical considerations. PACE 8:369–373, 1985.
45. Reiffel JA, Ferrick K, Zimmerman J, Bigger JT Jr: Electrophysiologic studies of the sinus node and atria. Cardiovasc Clin 16:37–59, 1985.
46. Reiffel JA, Bigger JT Jr, Cramer M et al: Ability of Holter electrocardiographic recording and atrial stimulation to detect sinus nodal dysfunction in symptomatic and asymptomatic patients with sinus bradycardia. Am J Cardiol 40:189–194, 1977.
47. Reiffel JA, Wang P, Bosner R, et al: Electrophysiologic testing in patients with recurrent syncope: Are results predicted by prior ambulatory monitoring. Am Heart J 6:539–544, 1985.
48. Saichin A, Dreifus LS, Michelson EL: Electrophysiologic studies of the AV conduction system and AV nodal arrhythmias. Cardiovasc Clin 16:61–82, 1985.
49. Scheinman MD, Peters RW, Modin G, et al: Prognostic values of infranodal conduction time in patients with chronic bundle branch block. Circulation 56:240–244, 1977.
50. Scheinman MM, Weiss A, Kankel F: His bundle recordings in patients with bundle branch block and transient neurological symptoms. Circulation 48:322–330, 1973.
51. Sensecqua JE, Mann DE, Reiter MJ: Effect of posture on antegrade and retrograde AV nodal conduction. Circulation 74:II–126, 1986.
52. Sutton R, Morley C, Chan SC, et al: Physiologic benefits of atrial synchrony in paced patients. PACE 6:327–328, 1983.
53. Vera A, Mason DT, Fletcher RD, et al: Prolonged His-Q interval in chronic bifascicular block: Relation to impending complete heart block. Circulation 53:46–55, 1976.
54. Warnowicz-Papp MA: The pacemaker patient and the electromagnetic environment. Clin Prog Pacing Electrophysiol 1:166–176, 1983.

7

CONSIDERATIONS IN THE SELECTION OF CARDIAC PACING SYSTEMS

PETER M. GUZY *and* NORA GOLDSCHLAGER

Once the decision has been made to implant a permanent pacing system for the management of symptomatic bradycardias, a specific pacemaker model must be selected from the many available. Each pacemaker manufacturer offers a choice of different models that vary in cost and component features, and new models are constantly being developed. Uncertainty may exist regarding whether a more complicated pacemaker model would be of sufficient benefit to the patient to justify a potentially higher cost. Initially, choosing a pacing system for a specific patient may appear to be very simple, especially if it is assumed that a pacemaker needs only to pace the ventricle and prevent the heart rate from being too slow. On the other hand, the selection process may appear to be unnecessarily complicated to those who are intimidated by the confusing array of complex features that distinguish one pacemaker model from another, even within a single manufacturer's product line. As a result, many physicians recommend only one manufacturer's product line, regardless of track record, or defer the selection to the implanting physician or a manufacturer's representative. To arrive at an ideal decision, a clinical assessment of the patient's physiologic needs must be carried out (see Chapter 6), along with a systematic determination of the pacemaker features that can best meet those needs. The primary clinical objectives should be the restoration and maintenance of optimal cardiac function to enable the patient to continue to be as active as possible. Unless the clinical goals are clearly defined[5] and the physiologic consequences of various pacemaker features

are understood, the pacemaker unit implanted may not fully benefit the patient or may even exacerbate the patient's symptoms.

In the discussion to follow, a clinical approach to selecting a pacemaker will be presented. This approach requires identification of the potential physiologic effects of individual pacemaker features. After acquiring this understanding, any physician, regardless of specialty or degree of experience with patients requiring pacemakers, should be able to participate knowledgeably in the pacemaker selection process.

SINGLE-CHAMBER VERSUS DUAL-CHAMBER PACING SYSTEMS (Fig. 7–1)

The first consideration in the selection of a pacing system is whether a single-chamber pacemaker or a dual-chamber pacemaker will best meet the patient's needs. Although single-chamber atrial pacemaker systems are sometimes implanted, the most common single-chamber pacemaker system utilizes a ventricular lead for backup pacing support. A dual-chamber pacemaker system utilizes both an atrial lead and a ventricular lead and can potentially maintain or restore atrioventricular (AV) synchrony at rest and with varying degrees of exertion if sinus node function is normal (Table 7–1). Since ventricular pacing alone can result in loss of AV synchrony and commonly produces a lower cardiac output than does sinus rhythm or atrial pacing at similar rates, a dual-chamber pacemaker sys-

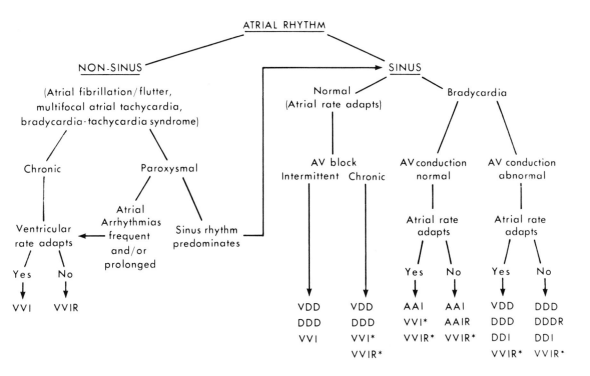

Figure 7–1. Algorithm of pacing system selection. In device selection, the atrial rhythm, rate, and responsiveness to increases in metabolic needs of the body determine the optimal pacing system. Ideal pacing system implantation may require adjustment in elderly, inactive, and/or mentally impaired patients. R = rate adaptive; * = the presence of inadequate atrial signals or atrial unresponsiveness to pacing or both.

tem might be considered a better choice for maintaining AV synchrony. For most patients, superior cardiac performance and an improved subjective sense of well-being result if AV synchrony is maintained or restored. Although patients with reduced ventricular systolic function, impaired ventricular diastolic compliance, mitral or tricuspid valvular insufficiency, or congestive heart failure usually have better cardiac output if AV synchrony is maintained, patients with either normal or above-normal ventricular ejection fractions can also experience symptoms (attributable to a pacemaker syndrome) if only ventricular pacing is provided.

"Pacemaker syndrome" is generally defined as the presence of symptoms of dyspnea, cough, chest discomfort, unpleasant neck or abdominal pulsations, abdominal distention, nausea, poor appetite, peripheral edema, fatigue, poor effort tolerance, palpitations, dizziness, near-syncope, or syncope—all either induced or exacerbated by ventricular pacing.[2] For many patients, one or more of these symp-

toms will lead to initial permanent pacemaker implantation if associated with documented bradycardias. For some of these patients, alleviation of their symptoms will not occur following implantation of a ventricular pacemaker, and for others, including inactive, sedentary individuals, a deterioration of their clinical condition or sense of well-being will occur after ventricular pacemaker implantation. Unless the diagnosis of pacemaker syndrome is considered, most of these patients will continue to be symptomatic despite interventions directed to the treatment of congestive heart failure, postural hypotension, reentrant arrhythmias, or depression. Since the majority of permanent pacemakers are implanted in geriatric patients with multiple medical problems, the symptoms of pacemaker syndrome may be attributed to degenerative aging processes or failure to comply with medical therapy. Some patients with unsuspected pacemaker syndrome are mistakenly told that nothing more can be done to improve their effort tolerance and overall quality of life.

TABLE 7–1. MODES OF PACEMAKER FUNCTION

DESIGNATION	DESCRIPTION OF FUNCTION
1. AOO	Asynchronous (fixed-rate) atrial pacing
2. AAT	Triggered atrial pacing: output pulse delivered into P waves (or any electrical signals sensed by the atrial electrode); paces atrium at preset escape interval
3. AAI	Demand atrial pacing: output inhibited by sensed atrial signals
4. AAIR	AAI pacing with sensor-based increases and decreases in paced atrial rate in response to changes in metabolic demands
5. VOO	Asynchronous (fixed-rate) ventricular pacing
6. VVT	Triggered ventricular pacing: output pulse delivered into R waves (or any electrical signals sensed by the ventricular electrode); paces ventricle at preset escape interval
7. VVI	Noncompetitive (demand) ventricular pacing: output inhibited by sensed ventricular signals
8. VVIR	VVI pacing with sensor-based increases and decreases in paced ventricular rates in response to changes in metabolic demands
9. DVI	Paces in both atrium and ventricle; does not sense P waves; senses R waves
10. DDI	AAI + VVI pacing; tracking of atrial rate by ventricular sensing circuit does not occur
11. VDD	Paces in ventricle; senses in both atrium and ventricle; synchronizes with atrial activity and paces ventricle after a preset AV interval
12. DOO	Asynchronous (fixed-rate) atrial and ventricular pacing at specific AV interval
13. DDD	Paces and senses in both atrium and ventricle; synchronizes with atrial activity and paces ventricle after a preset AV interval
14. DDDR	DDD pacing with sensor-based increases and decreases in paced atrial and/or ventricular rates in responses to changes in metabolic demands

The physiologic consequences constituting the pacemaker syndrome are the result of retrograde ventriculoatrial (VA) conduction induced by ventricular pacing. Virtually all patients with sick sinus syndrome and intact anterograde AV conduction will have evidence of at least intermittent retrograde VA conduction that may be documented by the presence of an inverted P wave in the ST segment or T wave of the surface electrocardiographic leads II, III, and aV_F. Even patients with complete anterograde AV block can have intact retrograde VA conduction. Increased atrial pressures and release of atriopeptin (atrial natriuretic peptide) may result from retrograde atrial depolarization and atrial contraction against closed AV valves. The atriopeptin released may in turn contribute to increased peripheral vasodilation and hypotension.[7] These physiologic mechanisms involving VA conduction induced by ventricular pacing, coupled with the varying degrees of associated mitral and tricuspid valvular insufficiency, can produce the symptoms and the marked deleterious hemodynamic changes observed in the pacemaker syndrome. Finally, retrograde VA conduction may induce or exacerbate reentrant tachyarrhythmias that can be very symptomatic.

The treatment of choice for patients with pacemaker syndrome is a dual-chamber pacemaker. Maintaining AV synchrony is crucial in these patients, since VA conduction and, to a lesser extent, AV dissociation cause the hemodynamic derangements and associated symptoms. Predicting which patients will most likely develop a pacemaker syndrome is difficult. Resting ventricular function does not reliably correlate with susceptibility to the potentially debilitating symptoms of the pacemaker syndrome; and patients with normal ventricular function may develop severe symptoms of pacemaker syndrome with ventricular pacing, while patients with impaired ventricular function may exhibit none. Even children with a single ventricle and complete heart block following a Fontan surgical repair may experience refractory hypotension caused by a pacemaker syndrome during ventricular pacing. Unless dual-chamber pacing support is provided, the refractory hypotension and low cardiac output may persist in these children despite the administration of intravenous vasopressor agents and the use of an external abdominal binder.

Single-chamber ventricular pacing would be the only appropriate pacing approach for patients with chronic atrial fibrillation, atrial standstill, refractory ectopic atrial tachycardias, or refractory atrial flutter (Fig. 7–1). For patients with tachycardia-bradycardia syndrome and intermittent atrial arrhythmias, a dual-chamber pacemaker might be considered, but care must be exercised to ensure that the normal tracking function of these devices does not cause excessively fast ventricular paced rates. Finally, maintaining AV synchrony and preventing VA conduction have been reported to reduce the recurrences of intermittent atrial tachyarrhythmias[8] and may prolong survival in patients having sinus node disease, with and without congestive heart failure.[1, 8]

The patients who would likely benefit from an atrial single-chamber pacemaker system are those with predominant sinus bradycardia and associated normal AV node function (Fig. 7–1). Atrial pacing systems have been used for patients with a prolonged QT interval syndrome and ventricular tachycardias precipitated by slow heart rates, when AV conduction has been satisfactory. Documentation of normal AV node function can be carried out easily by showing that 1:1 AV conduction and a relatively normal PR interval occur with atrial paced rates of 120 per minute or greater. If patients are carefully selected, and repeat testing of AV node function is routinely carried out as part of the outpatient follow-up evaluation, the chances that a patient will develop chronic atrial fibrillation or advanced AV block are relatively small over the long term.[8]

One controversial situation in which the best initial pacemaker system needs to be defined involves the patient with sinus rhythm and infrequent episodes of symptomatic bradycardias due to transient sinus pauses or AV block. In this situation, many physicians advise implantation of a ventricular pacemaker system only and set the backup pacing rate to 50 or 60 beats per minute to minimize the need for pacing support while preventing syncope or near-syncope. On the other hand, other phy-sicians would advise initial dual-chamber pacemaker implantation to preserve AV synchrony and prevent the pacemaker syndrome. Even if infrequent pacing is anticipated initially, the patient's cardiac status may change over time, especially if ischemic heart disease is present. Should an increase in the frequency of ventricular pacing cause untoward symptoms during clinical follow-up, conversion of a ventricular pacing system to a dual-chamber one would involve relatively expensive repeat surgery, atrial lead implantation, and pacemaker generator replacement. However, if a dual-chamber pacemaker had been the initial choice, simply changing the mode of pacemaker function would allow noninvasive optimization of the clinical condition. In these clinical circumstances, preimplantation noninvasive evaluation of the patient assumes great importance (see Chapter 6).

In general, a dual-chamber pacemaker would be most appropriate when preservation of AV synchrony is the top-priority objective in the patient's management. These instances include occurrence of the pacemaker syndrome following implantation of a ventricular pacemaker system, anticipation of a pacemaker syndrome after documentation of retrograde VA conduction during ventricular pacing (Fig. 7–2), and diagnosis of carotid sinus hypersensitivity or marked cardioinhibition associated with paroxysmal but frequent increases in vagal tone. A dual-chamber pacing system is also preferable when even a small increase in car-

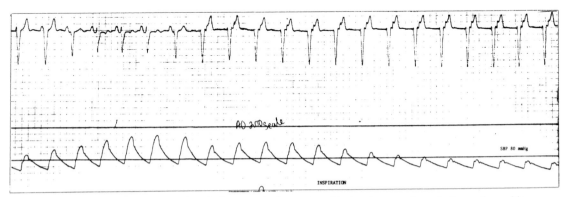

Figure 7–2. Marked hypotension during ventricular pacing. Depicted are surface electrocardiographic (ECG) lead II and the simultaneously recorded intraarterial pressure tracing during ventricular pacing initiated by inspiration. The peak systolic blood pressure during sinus rhythm with normal AV conduction is about 170 mm Hg. During ventricular pacing, there is a gradual fall in systolic pressure to a low of 80 mm Hg, accompanied clinically by dizziness, even though the patient was supine. This 90 mm Hg fall in systolic blood pressure with ventricular pacing suggests that the pacemaker syndrome in this patient could easily have developed if a single-chamber ventricular pacing system had been implanted. Note also the time course of development of the marked hypotension as well as the recovery of the blood pressure after sinus rhythm is restored. Not only is the extent of the hypotension important in the pacemaker syndrome, but also the rate of recovery of normotension.

diac output would benefit a patient with congestive heart failure or when preservation of rate responsiveness with exertion would permit a patient to continue to be fully active. Although a ventricular pacing system may be less expensive, easier to implant, and simpler to understand than a dual-chamber system, these factors do not justify implantation of a ventricular pacemaker when a dual-chamber system is clinically indicated.

PROGRAMMABLE VERSUS NONPROGRAMMABLE PACING SYSTEMS (Tables 7–2 and 7–3)

A programmable pacemaker contains one or more component features that can be adjusted electively and noninvasively after surgical implantation. Although nonprogrammable pacemakers are still manufactured, the majority of pacemaker models have multiple parameters that can be varied with the proper use of a programming device designed for a specific pacemaker manufacturer's product line. Programmable pacemakers are usually more expensive than nonprogrammable models, and dual-chamber programmable pacemakers tend to be much more complicated and more expensive than single-chamber programmable units. However, when comparing different pacemaker models and different manufacturers' products, price alone tends to be an unreliable indicator of technologic sophistication and clinical superiority.

The optimization of the patient's cardiac and clinical status is the justification for and utility of pacemaker programmability. This optimization is accomplished by adjustment of the pacemaker's operating characteristics to accommodate to changes in the patient's condition (Table 7–3). Since the majority of patients with pacemakers have multiple medical problems, including various types of heart disease, changes in the clinical status over time are the rule rather than the exception. Elective adjustment of pacemaker parameters can often produce improved functional capacity, as well as prolong power-source longevity, correct sensing and capture failures, and prevent both spontaneous and pacemaker-mediated arrhythmias (Table 7–3). Programmability can also provide savings in cost by avoiding the need for repeat surgical procedures.[6]

Regardless of the number of programmable features built into a pacemaker model, optimal clinical management and cost savings will not be realized unless a dedicated effort is made during outpatient follow-up to utilize the programmability built into the patient's pacemaker unit (see Chapter 10). Unfortunately, for many patients, the pacemaker's programmable features are never altered from the "nominal settings" established by the manufacturer. Although telephone monitoring of pacemaker function is readily available and some pacemaker models have automatically adjusting features, optimal adjustment of the pacemaker settings requires ongoing clinical follow-up by a physician knowledgeable in cardiac pacing and experienced with various manufacturers' programmers. Without this type of follow-up care, even the most sophisticated programmable pacemaker model functions like a nonprogrammable unit, and potential prolongation of the life of the pacemaker battery and optimization of hemodynamic function are never realized.

UNIPOLAR VERSUS BIPOLAR PACEMAKERS

A unipolar pacemaker utilizes a lead having a single stimulating electrode (cathode); the outer surface of the unipolar pulse generator serves as the anode for the pacing circuit. In contrast, the lead of a bipolar pacemaker system contains both electrodes; the outer surface of the bipolar pulse generator is not part of the pacing circuit. Clinically, both pacemaker types provide similar pacing and sensing functions. However, unipolar pacemakers have some characteristics distinctly different from those of bipolar models.

Since the electric circuit of unipolar pacemakers includes the entire lead and the outer surface of the pacemaker unit, unipolar stimulus output artifacts tend to be large and thus easily seen on the surface electrocardiogram.

TABLE 7–2. SOME PROGRAMMABLE FUNCTIONS OF CARDIAC PACEMAKERS

Rates
  Low rate limit
  AV interval
  Upper rate limit
Energy output*
  Milliamperes, volts, pulse duration
Refractory Period*
Sensitivity*
Hysteresis
Mode of Function (AOO, VOO, DOO, AAI, AAT, VVI, VVT, VAT, VDD, DVI, DDI, DDD)

*In dual-chambered units, these parameters are programmed independently for atrium and ventricle.

**TABLE 7–3. SOME COMMON CLINICAL USES OF PROGRAMMABLE
FEATURES OF PACEMAKERS***

I. Rate (low rate limit)
  A. Decrease
    1. Allow emergence of underlying spontaneous rhythm in order to
      a. Diagnose myocardial ischemia/infarction
      b. Follow natural history of condition for which patient is being paced
      c. Assess sensing function
    2. Allow sinus rhythm to prevail (VVI systems) in order to
      a. Preserve AV synchrony
      b. Alleviate symptoms of pacemaker syndrome
      c. Alleviate pain or discomfort associated with pacing
      d. Minimize angina that occurs at faster paced rates
      e. Preserve battery longevity
  B. Increase
    1. To manage bradycardia-dependent tachycardias
    2. To assess AV conduction (AAI systems)
    3. To assess pacing function (atrium and/or ventricle)
II. AV interval
  A. Increase
    1. To allow normal His-Purkinje conduction to occur in patients with intact AV conduction
    2. To correct for interatrial conduction delay and allow optimal left-sided stroke output
    3. To optimize stroke output in specific patients
  B. Decrease
    1. To optimize stroke output in specific patients
    2. To allow 1:1 tracking of faster atrial rates
    3. To avoid (since total atrial refractory period is composed, in part, of the AV interval) long anterograde conduction time in patients who are capable of associated VA conduction
III. Upper rate limit
  A. Increase
    1. To allow 1:1 tracking of rapid atrial rates
    2. To avoid abrupt, symptomatic slowing of paced ventricular rates at a lower upper rate limit
  B. Decrease
    1. To disallow rapid paced ventricular rates
      a. Palpitations during effort
      b. Angina at rapid paced rates
IV. Sensitivity
  A. Increase
    1. To allow sensing of borderline atrial and/or ventricular intracardiac signals
  B. Decrease
    1. To avoid oversensing (see Table 7–4), thereby eliminating
      a. Pauses in paced rhythm
      b. Pacemaker-mediated tachycardia
V. Energy output
  A. Increase
    1. To overcome elevations in stimulation threshold
      a. Drugs (especially antiarrhythmic agents)
      b. Acute myocardial infarction
      c. Electrolyte abnormalities (specifically hyperkalemia)
      d. Congestive heart failure
  B. Decrease
    1. To increase battery longevity
    2. To ameliorate awareness of pacing
    3. To avoid repetitive ventricular beating associated with pacing
VI. Refractory period
  A. Increase
    1. Ventricular
      a. To avoid T-wave oversensing
    2. Atrial
      a. To avoid 1:1 tracking of rapid native atrial rates
      b. To avoid pacemaker-mediated tachycardia
  B. Decrease
    1. Ventricular
      a. To sense early cycle premature ventricular depolarizations and inhibit
    2. Atrial
      a. To allow 1:1 tracking of rapid sinus rates

*See also Chapters 10 and 12.

Bipolar pacing artifacts, on the other hand, are usually low in voltage amplitude and thus may be difficult to see on any given surface electrocardiographic lead. In unipolar pacing systems, the entire pacemaker lead and the outer surface of the pulse generator serve as the sensing antenna, with a resultant increased sensitivity to electromagnetic or physiologic signals originating from sources other than the heart. As a result, unipolar pacemakers may be influenced by the electrical signals generated by electrical cautery units or by skeletal muscle adjacent to the pulse generator, and inappropriate inhibition or triggering (or both) of pacemaker output pulses may occur, depending on the programmed settings and type of pacemaker unit implanted (Table 7–4). In addition, anodal stimulation of adjacent skeletal muscle may occur with unipolar systems but will not do so with bipolar units unless an inappropriate current leak or a lead insulation break occurs in the connection area of the lead and the pulse generator.

Until recently, unipolar pulse generators were usually smaller than the bipolar units, but the development of coaxial or "in-line" bipolar lead connectors has resulted in little size difference between unipolar and bipolar models. Unfortunately, several different coaxial configurations have been developed by different pacemaker manufacturers; the lack of a uniform standard means that one coaxial bipolar lead connector may not work properly in another manufacturer's pacemaker unit.

TABLE 7–4. CAUSES OF PACEMAKER OVERSENSING

I. Physiologic
   Intracardiac
      QRS complexes (by atrial pacemakers)
      P waves (by ventricular pacemakers)
      T waves (by ventricular pacemakers)
      Concealed extrasystoles (local depolarizations)
   Extracardiac
      Muscle potentials
         Pectoral
         Diaphragmatic
         Abdominal
II. Electromagnetic interference
   Nuclear magnetic resonance
   Electrocautery
   Nerve stimulators
   Electrical defibrillation currents
   Diathermy
   Radio and television transmitters
   Arc-welding equipment
III. Signals generated within the pacing system
   Potential differences originating within the
      generator (autointerference)
   Inactive leads and/or electrode parts
      1. Intermittent contact of metal parts
      2. Electrolysis of dissimilar metals
   Afterpotentials generated by output stimuli

Lead adaptors can be used, but this results in additional connections and extra bulk in the pacemaker site. Although a bipolar lead can be readily converted for unipolar use, a bipolar pacemaker will not function with a unipolar lead unless an anode adaptor plate is implanted and connected with the bipolar pacemaker.

The choice of a unipolar versus a bipolar pacing system is often an arbitrary one, for there are trade-offs of potential advantages and disadvantages for either type. Increasingly, pacemaker generators having built-in polarity programmability options are being produced, and as long as bipolar leads are implanted initially and remain functional, either bipolar or unipolar sensing and pacing modes can be programmed electively during postimplantation follow-up, depending upon the sensing and pacing thresholds in each lead configuration. Except for the fact that most of the pacemaker lead malfunctions in recent years have involved bipolar leads, bipolar leads connected with a polarity programmable pacemaker might provide the best choice and maximal flexibility for the long term. For patients having a separate implanted defibrillating device, a bipolar pacemaker system is the only appropriate choice, because of the potentially conflicting signals generated by unipolar units[3] (see Chapter 27).

TELEMETRY VERSUS NONTELEMETRY

Telemetry is a process of communicating with an implanted pacemaker generator and obtaining direct measurements or recorded data (or both) pertaining to both pacemaker function and the patient's clinical status. These clinical applications have resulted from advances in computer chip technology and microelectronics. Pacemakers with telemetry capability require special microcomputer devices designed specifically for a given pacemaker manufacturer's product line. Some manufacturers have incorporated sophisticated telemetry capabilities into their products, while others have elected to market pacemaker models having little, if any, telemetry capability. Although pacemaker models having telemetry capacity tend to be more expensive than nontelemetry units, the market price alone does not reliably reflect the telemetric sophistication of a specific pacemaker model.

In the simplest telemetry systems, only the programmed pacemaker settings or single pacemaker parameters, such as measured battery voltage, may be provided. More sophisticated telemetry systems supply a variety of directly measured information, such as lead impedance, the current delivered with each pacemaker stimulus, intracardiac electrograms, or central blood temperature changes. The most sophisticated telemetry systems maintain a log of paced events and sensed intrinsic depolarizations, histograms of sensed intrinsic heart rates, intrinsic arrhythmia characteristics, and frequency of utilization of antitachycardia response algorithms. In addition, the more advanced telemetry systems provide the capability for noninvasive electrophysiologic testing via the permanent pacemaker system, telephone transmission of telemetered data directly from the pacemaker unit, and annotated electrocardiograms indicating the specific timing of sensed and paced events.

The added sophistication of telemetry can provide significant benefits to the patient, such as improved troubleshooting capabilities for suspected pacemaker system malfunctions, enhanced capacity for arrhythmia management, prolongation of pacemaker battery life, and optimization of pacemaker function with the patient's changing physiologic needs over time. However, to maximize the utility of telemetry, the patient must receive organized follow-up by knowledgeable physicians having the requisite experience and access to the appropriate programmer device specifically designed for the patient's pacemaker unit.

PULSE GENERATOR SIZE

The smallest pacemaker models available today are single-chamber units weighing 23 to 26 grams and measuring 6 mm in thickness. In contrast, the standard single-chamber units and the smallest dual-chamber models weigh 40 to 50 grams and measure 8 to 10 mm in thickness. Usually, the smaller pacemaker models have smaller-sized batteries, with shorter expected longevity. Reduced battery life may be an acceptable trade-off, however, when the smaller size provides better cosmetic results and less discomfort at the implantation site. Moreover, a smaller unit may be the optimal choice for a young child, for a small adult, or in circumstances in which previous surgery or scars limit the available tissue for subcutaneous implantation of the pacemaker unit.

ACTIVITY-RESPONSIVE PACEMAKERS

A significant number of patients requiring permanent pacemakers have an inability to increase their ventricular rates in response to increases in metabolic demands. These patients have impaired effort tolerance, which can be assessed by exercise testing. Similarly, some patients who have had a heart transplant develop a low-output syndrome postoperatively, despite the presence of two sinus nodes, if their ventricular rate remains inappropriately low at rest or during activity. These patients may derive limited benefit from conventional single- or dual-chamber pacemaker models, as a result of a faster backup pacing rate. However, without an adequate sinus node response to produce an increase in ventricular rate, these patients will still be left with an inability to meet the greater physiologic demands of exertion. In all these cases, the ideal pacemaker is one that responds to a signal other than sinus node–induced atrial depolarizations to provide a faster heart rate response and better cardiac output with activity (Fig. 7–1). An increasing variety of activity-responsive pacemaker models have been developed in recent years, including ones that respond to motion-induced body vibrations, central blood temperature changes, respiratory minute volume, and paced QT-interval changes.[9]

Although only single-chamber units (generally ventricular) with minimal telemetry capability have been available for clinical use, more sophisticated dual-chamber models will be increasingly available in the years ahead.

CONCLUSIONS

In conclusion, selection of the best pacemaker model for a given patient involves consideration of a variety of factors, including determination of the patient's physiologic needs and desired activity level, understanding of the physiologic consequences of the presence and absence of various pacemaker functions, and appreciation of the cost-benefit trade-offs of simple versus sophisticated pacemaker systems. Selection strategies based on the presence or absence of adequate sinus node and AV node function have been recommended.[4] These strategies are useful, but they relate more to how a multiprogrammable pacemaker might be adjusted, rather than how to decide which pacemaker features and which pacemaker model would be most beneficial for the patient in question. Definition of the "best" or "ideal" pacemaker model for a given patient will vary, depending upon a physician's knowledge, experience, and biases regarding pacemaker function and utilization. Since significant differences do exist between different manufacturers' pacemaker products and within each category of single-chamber, dual-chamber, and activity-responsive pacemaker types, and since the track record for one manufacturer's product line may differ markedly from competitors' models, final selection of a pacemaker unit should be made only after carefully consideration of all the options available. The likelihood of a good clinical outcome would appear to depend on the quality and appropriateness of the pacemaker unit selected as well as on the quality of ongoing follow-up monitoring of pacemaker function.[10]

REFERENCES

1. Alpert MA, Curtis JJ, Sanfelippo JF, et al: Comparative survival following permanent ventricular and dual-chamber pacing for patients with chronic symptomatic sinus node dysfunction with and without congestive heart failure. Am Heart J 113:958–965, 1987.

2. Ausubel K, Furman S: The pacemaker syndrome. Ann Intern Med 103:420–429, 1985.
3. Cohen AI, Wish MH, Fletcher RD, et al: The use and interaction of permanent pacemakers and the automatic implantable cardioverter defibrillator. PACE 11:704–711, 1988.
4. Frue RL, Collins JJ, DeSanctis RW, et al: Guidelines for permanent cardiac pacemaker implantation, May 1984. Circulation 70:331A–339A, 1984.
5. Harthorne JW: Cardiac pacemakers. Curr Probl Cardiol 12:649–693, 1987.
6. Ludmer PL, Goldschlager N: Cardiac pacing in the 1980s. N Engl J Med 311:1671–1680, 1984.
7. Needleman P, Greenwald JE: Atriopeptin: A cardiac hormone intimately involved in fluid, electrolyte, and blood-pressure homeostasis. N Engl J Med 314:828–834, 1986.
8. Rosenqvist M, Brandt J, Schuller H: Long-term pacing in sinus node disease: Effects of stimulation mode on cardiovascular morbidity and mortality. Am Heart J 116:16–21, 1988.
9. Rossi P: Rate-responsive pacing: Biosensor reliability and physiological sensitivity. PACE 10:454–466, 1987.
10. Vallario LE, Leman RB, Gillette PC, Kratz JM: Pacemaker follow-up and adequacy of Medicare guidelines. Am Heart J 116:11–15, 1988.

8

HEMODYNAMIC ASPECTS OF CARDIAC PACING

NORA GOLDSCHLAGER *and* SANJEEV SAKSENA

Changes in cardiac rhythm and rate can produce or contribute to significant symptoms or can cause major cardiac events, such as embolism, myocardial infarction, and death. Although symptoms can be related to the electrical disturbance per se, the more common underlying mechanism involves the hemodynamic sequelae of the arrhythmia. These hemodynamic sequelae result in altered cardiocirculatory flow states, which then produce symptoms.

The clinical effects of heart rhythm and rate were mentioned in ancient medical writings. In the seventeenth century,[32] the relationship between the circulation of blood and cardiac rhythm was commented upon by William Harvey. At the beginning of this century, extensive experimental and clinical investigations were undertaken. Thomas Lewis[42] observed in experimental studies that changes in blood pressure and cardiac output occurred with the development of atrial fibrillation. The earliest clinical reports on "Stokes-Adams' disease"[53] noted the association of "epileptiform" attacks, "cardiac asthma," angina pectoris, and "heart shock" with a slow heart rhythm. In the past three decades, the development of artificial cardiac pacemakers designed to correct bradyarrhythmias has resulted in a plethora of iatrogenic alterations in cardiac rhythm and rate. The physiologic basis for the hemodynamic effects of different spontaneous and artificial cardiac rhythms is reviewed in this chapter.

PHYSIOLOGIC EFFECTS OF HEART RATE AND RHYTHM

A major determinant of circulatory stability and tissue perfusion is the systemic arterial pressure. Systemic arterial pressure is determined by cardiac output and peripheral vascular resistance. Cardiac output, in turn, is dependent on heart rate and stroke volume. Alterations in cardiac output are frequent and permit the cardiovascular system to meet the changing metabolic demands of the body. The primary mechanism by which cardiac output responsiveness is achieved is the capability to change heart rate. Secondary mechanisms include alterations in stroke volume and peripheral vascular tone; ventricular systolic and diastolic function and vascular compliance are important determinants of the integrity of these mechanisms. Physiologic increases in circulatory demands, such as those imposed during exercise, are met largely by an increase in heart rate and, to a lesser extent, by an increase in stroke volume and decrease in peripheral vascular resistance. Sinus tachycardia is accompanied by an abbreviation of ventricular diastole and thus of ventricular filling time. Although this decrease in ventricular filling time could result in a reduction in ventricular end-diastolic volume, and secondarily in stroke volume, the effect is offset by the maintenance of the rapid filling phase that occurs during early diastole, by the contribution of atrial systole, and by the enhancement of venous return due to mechanical effects of muscular activity. These effects, concomitant with increased sympathetic stimulation, which enhances cardiac contractility, help maintain and even augment stroke volume.[11, 28, 58, 76] Echocardiographic studies in normal subjects confirm a progressive decrease in end-diastolic and end-systolic left ventricular dimensions with increases in atrial rate from 50 to 150 beats per minute, without change in shortening fraction.[17]

The dependence of stroke volume on left

ventricular filling has been established in experimental and clinical studies.[58, 76] Factors influencing left ventricular filling include filling pressure, diastolic volume, diastolic filling time, left ventricular compliance, and atrioventricular (AV) synchrony. Decreased preload, reduced filling time, and impaired ventricular compliance limit left ventricular filling and thus stroke volume. The atrial contribution to left ventricular filling, which has been referred to as a "booster pump," is an active mechanism by which left ventricular filling and, secondarily, stroke volume is enhanced.[55] Gilmore and coworkers demonstrated the importance of atrial filling to ventricular stroke volume in experimental studies and related it to the sequence of AV contraction.[26] These investigators also noted the role of the specialized conduction system in mediating an optimal sequence of ventricular mechanical contraction, commenting that an altered sequence of ventricular depolarization may also reduce ventricular stroke volume. Earlier observations by Wiggers and Meijler and colleagues, as well as subsequent studies on artificial ventricular pacing, support a role for this factor in maintaining optimal ventricular output.[14, 15, 19, 43, 74, 75, 78] A recent canine study,[79] which specifically assessed the relative effects of left ventricular loading conditions and pacing-induced asynchrony on the rates of left ventricular relaxation and filling, did confirm an independent role of asynchrony in these indices of ventricular function.

The pivotal role of optimal AV sequence of activation is seen in canine studies, in which depression of ventricular function is observed in association with shortening of the interval between atrial and ventricular systole, even prior to loss of AV synchrony. Ventricular pacing without AV synchrony compounds this deterioration in left ventricular function.

It has also been suggested that pacing from left ventricular apical sites has a more favorable effect on peak left ventricular pressure and dP/dt than does pacing from right ventricular apical sites or from basal left ventricular and right ventricular sites.[15] However, not all investigators agree on the issue[59, 61]; Samet and coworkers noted that the development of bundle branch block or ventricular premature depolarizations did not necessarily cause mechanical ventricular asynchrony.[61] Clinical studies in humans have been limited but tend to confirm that hemodynamically significant mechanical ventricular asynchrony may not result from bundle branch block,[10] although it may be observed in individual patients.[9] In contrast to bundle branch block, ventricular premature depolarizations often produce mechanical ventricular asynchrony.[19] The mechanical consequences of asynchronous left ventricular contraction can be of varying importance and will be influenced by preload, rate, compliance, and afterload.

The importance of atrial contribution to cardiac output has been examined in experimental animals, in normal human subjects, and in patients with cardiac disease.[5–7, 18, 29, 45, 48, 52, 63] It is important to understand the significance of this variable as a function of overall cardiac status, including prevailing heart rate, since this may be a key issue in individual patients. In normal subjects, atrial or AV sequential pacing is associated with improved cardiac output, compared with ventricular pacing at identical rates[63]; the rates used in these reports have been generally normal rather than rapid. Atrial contribution to cardiac output is, however, smaller in normal persons than in patients with specific forms of cardiac disease in which left ventricular compliance is reduced. Although initial reports were contradictory,[6, 25, 55] more recent physiologic studies have clarified the issues. Greenberg and coworkers examined the relationship between absolute left ventricular filling pressure and the atrial contribution to cardiac output in chronic disease states.[29] Data derived from their studies and inferences with respect to the role of end-diastolic volume suggest that atrial transport is particularly important in patients with chronic heart disease, normal or minimally elevated left ventricular end-diastolic pressure, normal or mildly increased left ventricular end-diastolic volume, and decreased left ventricular compliance.[16, 29] The relative value of atrial systole declines in patients with very high left ventricular end-diastolic pressures and markedly increased end-diastolic volumes, although exceptions may exist in individual patients. In acute myocardial infarction, the atrial contribution to left ventricular stroke volume is significant in patients with and without a depressed cardiac index and elevated left ventricular end-diastolic volume.[55] However, many patients with primary electrical disturbances, such as chronic complete heart block, have minimal or chronic heart disease with well-preserved left ventricular function, nearly normal end-diastolic volumes, and no congestive heart failure.[65] Atrial synchrony significantly enhances cardiac output in these patients.[36, 60, 65]

Whereas the atrial contribution to left ventricular stroke output is significant at normal or nearly normal heart rates, this contribution declines at more rapid heart rates (in the range of 110 to 120 beats per minute or greater),[52] an observation that has import for the exercising patient. A recent study in which atrial contribution to ventricular systole in patients with various forms of heart disease was assessed by Doppler echocardiographic techniques[39] suggested that the size of the left atrium—and, by inference, its capability to generate an effective "booster pump" action—was a major determinant of the degree of this contribution. In this study, patients with normal left atrial size were more sensitive to the loss of AV synchrony than were those with left atrial enlargement; left ventricular size and overall function were of little importance.

Thus, in analyzing the hemodynamic consequences of dysrhythmias or artificial cardiac pacing in individual patients, the importance of all baseline hemodynamic and disease state variables needs to be carefully assessed, since these variables influence the outcome of the rhythm disturbance to a profound extent and determine its clinical sequelae and response to treatment. Moreover, the various and differing methodologies used to assess these variables (such as intracardiac pressure measurements, radionuclide angiography with ejection fraction and ventricular volume determinations, Doppler echocardiography, and physical work capacity) will have to be taken into consideration when the results of published studies are analyzed.

HEMODYNAMIC EFFECTS OF BRADYARRHYTHMIAS

Sinus Bradycardia

The hemodynamic consequences of sinus bradycardia are primarily related to the slow ventricular rate. Ventricular filling is preserved, and an adequate or enhanced stroke volume will be present in persons who have normal ventricular function. Symptoms are uncommon in patients with resting sinus bradycardia, owing to the low perfusion demands at rest. Samet and colleagues reported an average resting cardiac index in one series of patients of only 1.9 L/min/m².[79] Similar observations are applicable to patients with atrial fibrillation and slow ventricular response due to conduction system disease if left ventricular function is preserved. The adequacy of the response of the sinus rate (or the ventricular rate in the case of atrial fibrillation) to exercise usually determines whether or not symptoms are present. Inadequate heart rate response produces symptoms of inadequate cardiac output relative to metabolic demands. Easy fatigability, limited exercise tolerance, or near-syncope or even syncope during exercise can be observed. In contrast, in asymptomatic individuals an adequate heart rate response to exercise is generally observed (Fig. 8–1). Patients with poor left ventricular function and congestive heart failure tolerate sinus bradycardia poorly. Symptoms of low cardiac output are common at rest and can be profound if the heart rate response during exercise is inadequate.

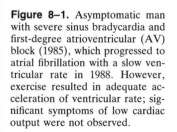

Figure 8–1. Asymptomatic man with severe sinus bradycardia and first-degree atrioventricular (AV) block (1985), which progressed to atrial fibrillation with a slow ventricular rate in 1988. However, exercise resulted in adequate acceleration of ventricular rate; significant symptoms of low cardiac output were not observed.

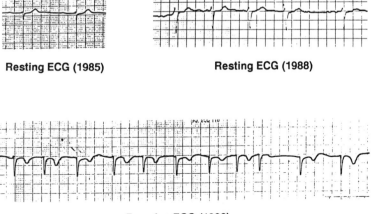

Resting ECG (1985)   **Resting ECG (1988)**

Exercise ECG (1988)

Sinus bradycardia and sinus arrest can be manifestations of vagal stimulation (see Chapter 5) and may thus be episodic and unpredictable in severity and clinical course. Associated hypotension can be due either to the bradycardia or to a loss of peripheral vasomotor tone. Myocardial infarction, particularly of the inferior wall, is often associated with this "vasovagal" disorder. Poor left ventricular compliance and depressed systolic function aggravate the reduction in cardiac output resulting from the bradycardia.

Atrioventricular Block

The hemodynamic consequences of AV block result from two pathophysiologic mechanisms: the effects of the bradycardia (similar to those of sinus bradycardia, discussed above) and the effects of the varying relationships between atrial and ventricular systole. Absence of 1:1 sequential AV contraction impairs ventricular filling; however, in second- and third-degree AV block, stroke volume is usually preserved and may even be increased, owing to prolonged diastole. The heart rate response to exercise or other metabolic stress is usually impaired because of the AV conduction block.[40, 71] In specific clinical syndromes, such as congenital complete heart block, the focus of origin of the ventricular rate can increase its rate in response to exercise and thus minimize symptoms.[34] Cardiac output in these patients is relatively normal, as are intracardiac pressures.[68] In older patients with congenital complete AV block, elevated atrial pressures, with cannon "a" waves, in conjunction with depressed cardiac output and reduced systemic arterial pressures, are often observed, particularly when acquired myocardial disease is present.

The effects of alteration in ventricular rate by artificial cardiac pacing in patients with complete heart block have been extensively studied.[54, 64, 65, 69] In one report,[64] asynchronous ventricular pacing at rates between 40 and 120 beats per minute resulted in an increase in cardiac output in two of every three patients studied. Peak cardiac outputs were generally observed at heart rates of 80 to 105 beats per minute. Stroke volume decreased with increasing paced ventricular rates in all patients, explaining the observation that cardiac outputs did not increase in direct proportion to the increases in paced heart rate. In another report,[65] atrial synchronous pacing increased cardiac output by 10 per cent in patients with complete heart block. However, ventricular

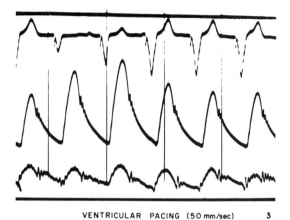

VENTRICULAR PACING (50 mm/sec)   **3**

Figure 8–2. Ventricular pacing in a patient with AV block. The upper trace is electrocardiographic (ECG) lead V_1, the middle trace is systemic arterial pressure, and the lower trace is pulmonary arterial pressure. When the paced QRS complex is clearly preceded by a P wave and an appropriately timed atrial contraction (third pressure waveform), the systemic arterial pressure is significantly higher compared with that accompanying subsequent paced complexes that are not preceded by a P wave and an atrial systole. Minimal change is noted in pulmonary arterial pressures.

rate was also increased by pacing in this study, potentially confounding the results. Benchimol and coworkers demonstrated that AV synchrony improved systemic arterial pressure and left ventricular ejection indices in patients with heart block over a wide range of heart rates (20 to 125 beats per minute)[7] (Fig. 8–2). These early observations have been amply confirmed in more recent hemodynamic and echocardiographic studies performed at rest and during exercise.[23, 36, 37, 54, 69]

Recent investigations of atrial natriuretic peptide in patients with ventricular bradycardia due to advanced AV block have suggested that this factor may play a role in the production of symptoms in these patients.[49] Atrial natriuretic peptide is produced in response to atrial stretch, such as occurs in congestive heart failure and AV dyssynchrony. The diuresis and natriuresis that accompany an increase in serum levels of this peptide can contribute to weakness and impaired effort tolerance. "Normal" levels of atrial natriuretic peptide can be achieved by restoring and maintaining AV synchrony, as well as by treating any underlying cardiac disease that may be present.

The existence of vasodepressor reflex initiated by cannon "a" waves has also recently been described.[21] In the study of Erlebacher and colleagues,[21] AV dyssynchrony resulted in a decline in stroke volume in all 20 patients being investigated, but only in those with cannon "a" waves did systemic hypotension and minimal increase in systemic vascular resistance occur. These investigators suggested that the vasodepressor reflex caused by atrial stretch inhibited the expected increases in systemic vascular resistance and arterial pressure that normally accompany a fall in stroke volume. The relationship of this atrial reflex to atrial natriuretic peptide remains to be clarified.

HEMODYNAMIC EFFECTS OF ARTIFICIAL CARDIAC PACEMAKERS

The hemodynamic consequences of artificial cardiac pacing have been extensively evaluated.[8, 12, 20, 22, 44, 47, 62, 64, 66, 70, 77] Early studies focused on optimal paced heart rates in patients with complete heart block who receive ventricular demand or asynchronous pacemaking.[8, 22, 47, 62, 64, 66, 70] Experimental studies had suggested that cardiac output could be maintained over a wide range of heart rates by altering ventricular rate and stroke volume in inverse proportion.[70, 77] Initial ventricular pacemaker implantations in patients with complete heart block utilized fixed- or variable-rate devices in asynchronous or inhibited modes.[12, 67] Hemodynamic studies indicated that correction of the bradycardia associated with complete heart block usually improved cardiac output and lowered right atrial pressure.[22, 47, 67, 70] The optimal paced rate varies widely among patients, and a variety of rate responses with respect to cardiac output have been observed.[70] A plateau or "flat" rate output curve, in which the cardiac output may remain relatively constant (plus or minus 15 per cent) over a range of ventricular rates, has been reported in 50 per cent of patients.[70] An equal prevalence of "peaked" rate output curves, in which a particular paced rate is associated with a maximal cardiac output, has also been reported.[8, 22, 47, 70] Atrial rates and pressures were observed to be lowest at this rate, and an optimal paced ventricular rate associated with the highest achieved cardiac output and lowest atrial rate or pressure could be defined in a majority of patients.[8, 22, 47, 70] In one study, this optimal rate ranged from 56 to 90 beats per minute, with a mean of 71 beats per minute.[70] During exercise, both flat and peaked types of rate output curves can also be observed. Peaked rate output curves are particularly associated with the presence of myocardial disease.[70] Pacing at a given rate does not preclude

an increase in cardiac output with exercise, since an increase in stroke volume during exercise also occurs. Improved hemodynamic performance with pacing has thus translated into resolution of Stokes-Adams syncopal episodes, refractory congestive heart failure, and angina pectoris, as well as an increase in exercise tolerance and actual work capacity in uncontrolled studies.[22, 47] Subsequent controlled studies in patients with rate-programmable pacemakers have confirmed the results.

Experimental studies have documented the hemodynamic advantages of atrial pacing compared with ventricular pacing. As discussed earlier, an optimal sequence of AV contraction enhances left ventricular filling and thus stroke volume and cardiac output. This atrial "booster pump" effect is of considerable importance in specific acute and chronic clinical conditions. The advantages conferred by atrial pacing seem to be due largely to sequential AV contraction rather than to a normal ventricular contraction pattern.[62] Specific clinical situations in which the benefits of atrial pacing or AV sequential pacing are evident are characterized by impaired left ventricular function and often also by excessive cardiocirculatory demands. Topol and coworkers[73] noted that atrial or AV sequential pacing was essential to establish hemodynamic stability in patients with right ventricular ischemic injury and volume-refractory hypotension; this stability could not be achieved with ventricular pacing alone. Reiter and Hindman observed that AV sequential pacing in patients with left ventricular dysfunction improved the cardiac index by 17 to 29 per cent over ventricular pacing alone at paced rates ranging from 75 to 100 beats per minute.[57] Improved hemodynamic performance with atrial pacing can be predicted by the clinical observation that significant variations in systemic arterial pressure and in pulse pressure occur during ventricular pacing. However, clinical indices of left ventricular function are not generally useful in predicting a given response to atrial pacing, nor are they useful in predicting optimal paced rate. Patients with sinus or junctional rhythm after cardiac surgery can experience deterioration in left ventricular function during ventricular pacing alone, while sequential AV pacing improves cardiac output in most patients.[31] Temporary cardiac pacing in this mode may be particularly important in this clinical circumstance. In 1973, Furman outlined the indications for atrial pacing, which included bradyarrhythmias due to sinus node dysfunc-

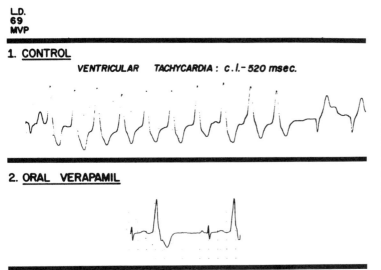

L.D.
69
MVP

1. CONTROL

VENTRICULAR   TACHYCARDIA : c.l.- 520 msec.

2. ORAL VERAPAMIL

3. ATRIAL PACING

Figure 8–3. The use of drug and AAI pacing therapy for suppression of ventricular arrhythmias in a patient with mitral valve prolapse and spontaneous ventricular tachycardia. Oral verapamil converted the ventricular arrhythmia to sinus rhythm with ventricular bigeminy. Atrial pacing at a rate of 90 beats per minute completely suppressed the bigeminy; permanent atrial pacing eliminated the ventricular arrhythmias over the long term.

tion, overdrive suppression of ventricular arrhythmias (Fig. 8–3), improvement of cardiac output, and termination of reentrant supraventricular tachycardias.[24] Currently, the hemodynamic benefits of atrial pacing constitute a major indication for the use of this pacing mode.

The hemodynamic benefits of implanted pacemakers that can function in an AV sequential mode (DDD, VDD, and DVI) compared with a ventricular demand or fixed-rate pacing mode (VVI and VOO) have been documented in a number of randomized, controlled, prospective studies. Cardiac output is improved both at rest and during exercise in AV pacing modes in comparison to fixed-rate ventricular pacing, while stroke volume is comparable at rest but is higher during exercise.[36] Left ventricular filling pressure is reduced by atrial triggered pacing at rest but not during exercise. These hemodynamic advantages are preserved when ventricular paced rates are increased during exercise to match the atrial rates.[8] Thus, although rate-adaptive ventricular pacing (VVIR) has significant advantages over the VVI and VVO pacing modes, atrial synchronous pacing remains the optimal pacing mode, provided that sinus nodal function is normal. The hemodynamic benefits are manifest as improved physical work capacity, which is maintained over time[37]; this improvement occurs in young as well as in elderly patients and in patients both with and without cardiac

disease, although it is more pronounced in the latter. The physiologic variables that are significantly improved include cardiac output, an associated lower AV oxygen content difference and arterial blood lactate level, and cardiac size, which is decreased by physiologic sequential pacing.[56] Patients are subjectively improved to a greater extent, with reduction in symptoms of dyspnea and palpitations.[54, 56]

In addition to the inferior hemodynamic profile of ventricular pacing compared with AV or atrial triggered ventricular pacing, ventricular pacing has an additional specific deleterious hemodynamic consequence related to the presence of retrograde ventriculoatrial (VA) conduction.[4, 27] Retrograde VA conduction may be present in 33 to 50 per cent of individuals with normal antegrade AV conduction[1]; it is usually absent in patients with spontaneous AV block. Retrograde VA conduction can result in a specific clinical condition termed the "pacemaker syndrome." A typical clinical presentation of a patient with this syndrome is continuation of symptoms or development of new ones days to weeks after implantation of the ventricular pacing system. The symptom complex includes manifestations of low cardiac output: fatigue, limited exercise capacity, presyncope or syncope, weakness or lassitude, and breathlessness. The elevated central and pulmonary venous pressures, due in turn both to cannon "a" waves and to mitral and tricuspid regurgitation,[46, 48] can produce symptoms of dyspnea, chest congestion, head and neck pulsations, right upper quadrant tenderness resulting from hepatic congestion, and peripheral edema.[2, 3, 13, 30, 35, 46] An atrial vasodepressor reflex[21, 41, 51] caused by the cannon "a" waves and the AV valve regurgitation may also contribute to the symptoms of hypotension; as discussed earlier, this vasodepressor phenomenon causes a failure of the peripheral vascular resistance to increase appropriately in response to a fall in cardiac output. The relationship of atrial natriuretic factor to the atrial vasodepressor reflex is not entirely clear, but the former may be a mediator of the latter, since natriuretic peptide is known to be increased in patients with ventricular pacing systems and parenteral injection of this factor causes vasodilatation and a fall in systemic vascular resistance.[33]

On physical examination, hypotension, a low pulse amplitude, elevated jugular venous pressure with cannon "a" waves, gallop rhythm, pulmonary rales, accentuation of the pulmonic second heart sound, hepatomegaly, and peripheral edema have been reported. The symptoms can be paroxysmal or chronic, depending on the constancy or intermittency of

VA conduction and on the sinus rate. The resting electrocardiogram during symptoms demonstrates ventricular pacing at an acceptable rate, with inverted P waves in electrocardiographic leads II, III, and aV_F, indicating retrograde atrial depolarization. With demand pacing units, 24-hour ambulatory electrocardiographic recordings may be necessary to demonstrate ventricular pacing and correlate it with symptoms. This syndrome should be suspected whenever a patient with an implanted demand ventricular pacemaker presents with symptoms of low cardiac output or cardiac failure.

The diagnosis of pacemaker syndrome is confirmed by catheterization of the right side of the heart and measurement of hemodynamic performance during sinus rhythm and atrial, AV, and ventricular pacing. Recording of atrial and ventricular electrograms is useful in this regard (Fig. 8–4). Ventricular pacing demonstrates retrograde atrial activation, with the earliest atrial activity recorded in the low right atrium. Retrograde conduction should usually be 1:1 at the programmed pacemaker rate. Uncommonly, decremental VA conduction with varying VA relationships may still be

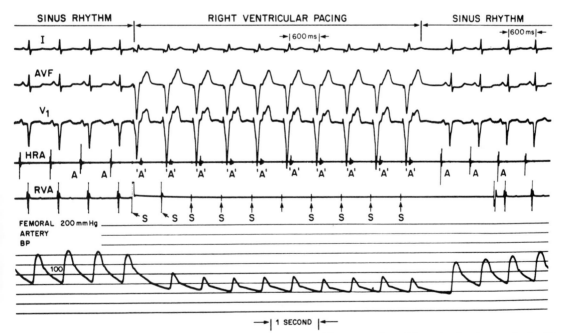

Figure 8–4. Hemodynamic consequences of ventricular pacing with retrograde atrial conduction in a patient with hypertensive heart disease and symptoms of the pacemaker syndrome. The patient is initially in sinus rhythm at 100 beats per minute. Ventricular pacing is begun at the identical rate and is associated with retrograde atrial activation ('A'). Despite a constant identical ventricular rate, an abrupt and marked decline in systolic arterial pressure, from 145 mm Hg to 85 mm Hg, is observed during ventricular pacing. Cessation of ventricular pacing is associated with gradual recovery of normal arterial pressure. HRA = high right atrium; RVA = right ventricular apex; A = antegrade atrial activation; S = pacing stimulus; BP = blood pressure.

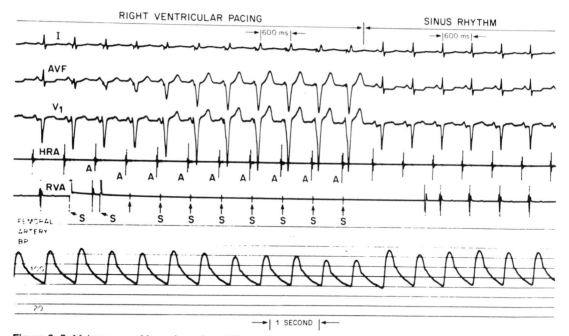

Figure 8–5. Maintenance of hemodynamic stability in the same patient as in Figure 8–4 during ventricular pacing with fortuitous antegrade atrial contraction. Ventricular pacing is begun, and for several complexes, isorhythmically dissociated atrial activity is present prior to the paced depolarization. Note that the systemic arterial pressure remains unchanged but that progressive shortening of the PR interval with a slight decline in arterial pressure is observed toward the end of the pacing sequence. Abbreviations are as in Figure 8–4.

associated with pacemaker syndrome. Ventricular pacing with retrograde atrial depolarization produces an elevation in right and left atrial pressures and in pulmonary capillary wedge pressure, as well as cannon "a" waves due to simultaneous atrial systole during or at completion of ventricular systole. Decreases in left ventricular and aortic systolic pressures and in systemic arterial pulse pressure are observed (Fig. 8–4). A decline in cardiac output during ventricular pacing, compared with that during sinus rhythm or atrial pacing at the same rate, will be present. AV valve regurgitation is not typically present. These findings are pathognomonic and are most often observed in patients with left ventricular dysfunction or reduced left ventricular compliance. Sinus rhythm or atrial or AV sequential pacing alleviates the symptoms and negative hemodynamic effects, and treatment of this disorder is directed at achieving this result. In some patients, the demand ventricular pacemaker may be programmed to a lower rate to allow the emergence of native sinus rhythm. However, AV dyssynchrony will be present and, although this rhythm is hemodynamically superior to 1:1 retrograde VA conduction,[52] may, itself, not restore an asymptomatic state.[50] Infrequent requirement for demand ventricular pacing may eliminate or minimize symptoms. The definitive treatment is revision of the

pacemaker system to an atrial or AV sequential pacing system (Fig. 8–5).

Consideration of the hemodynamic impact of permanent pacemaker implantation should be prospective in nature, using noninvasive methods of evaluation, which include Doppler echocardiography and dynamic exercise testing. This evaluation is particularly important in patients with preexisting cardiac disease and left ventricular dysfunction. In children, younger individuals, and active patients, a combined electrophysiologic and hemodynamic evaluation for optimal pacing mode prior to device implantation is recommended. The development of single- and dual-chamber rate-responsive pacing systems should provide the opportunity for optimal device selection for hemodynamic benefit in virtually all patients.

REFERENCES

1. Akhtar M: Reentry within the His-Purkinje system. *In* Narula OS (ed): Cardiac Arrhythmias. Baltimore, The William & Wilkins Co, 1979, pp 397–418.
2. Alicandri C, Fouad FM, Tarazi RC, et al: Three cases of hypotension and syncope with ventricular pacing: Possible role of atrial reflexes. Am J Cardiol 42:137–142, 1978.
3. Ausubel K, Furman S: The pacemaker syndrome. Ann Intern Med 103:420–429, 1985.

4. Barold S, Linhart J, Samet P: Reciprocal beating induced by ventricular pacing. Circulation 38:330–340, 1968.
5. Benchimol A, Dimond EG: Cardiac function in man during artificial stimulation of the left ventricle, right ventricle and right atrium. Am J Cardiol 17:118–119, 1966.
6. Benchimol A, Ellis JG, Dimond EG: Hemodynamic consequences of atrial and ventricular pacing in patients with normal and abnormal hearts: Effect of exercise at a fixed atrial and ventricular rate. Am J Med 39:911–922, 1965.
7. Benchimol A, Duenas A, Liggett MS, Dimond EG: Contribution of atrial systole to the cardiac function at a fixed and at a variable ventricular rate. Am J Cardiol 16:11–21, 1965.
8. Bevegard S: Observation on the effect of varying ventricular rate on the circulation at rest and during exercise in two patients with artificial pacemakers. Acta Med Scand 172:615–619, 1962.
9. Bourassa MG, Birteau GM, Allenstein BJ: Hemodynamic studies during intermittent left bundle branch block. Am J Cardiol 10:792–799, 1962.
10. Braunwald E, Morrow AG: Sequence of ventricular contraction in human bundle branch block: A study based on simultaneous catheterization of both ventricles. Am J Med 23:205–211, 1957.
11. Braunwald E, Goldblatt A, Harrison DC, Mason DT: Studies on cardiac dimension in intact unanaesthetised man. IV. Effects of muscular exercise. Circ Res 13:460–467, 1963.
12. Chardack WM, Gage AA, Schimert G, et al: Two years clinical experience with the implantable pacemaker for complete heart block. Dis Chest 43:225–239, 1963.
13. Cohen SI, Frank HA: Preservation of active atrial transport: An important clinical consideration in cardiac pacing. Chest 81:51, 1982.
14. Cohn K, Kryda W: The influence of ectopic beats and tachyarrhythmias on stroke volume and cardiac output. J Electrocardiol 14:207–218, 1981.
15. Daggett WM, Bianco JA, Powell WJ, Austen WG: Relative contributions of the atrial systole–ventricular systole interval and of patterns of ventricular activation to ventricular function during electrical pacing of the dog heart. Circ Res 27:69–79, 1970.
16. DeMaria AN, Miller RR, Amsterdam EA, et al: Mitral valve early diastolic closing velocity in the echocardiogram: Relation to sequential diastolic flow and ventricular compliance. Am J Cardiol 37:693–700, 1976.
17. DeMaria AW, Neumann A, Schubart PJ, et al: Systemic correlation of cardiac chamber size and ventricular performance determined with echocardiography and alterations in heart rate in normal persons. Am J Cardiol 43:1–9, 1979.
18. DiCarlo LA, Morady F, Krol RB, et al: The hemodynamic effects of ventricular pacing with and without atrioventricular synchrony in patients with normal and diminished left ventricular function. Am Heart J 114:746, 1987.
19. Eber LM, Berkovits BV, Matloff JM, et al: Dynamic characterization of premature ventricular beats and ventricular tachycardias. Am J Cardiol 33:378–383, 1974.
20. Elmquist R, Landergren J, Patterson SO, et al: Artificial pacemaker for treatment of Adams-Stokes syndrome and slow heart rate. Am Heart J 65:731–748, 1963.
21. Erlebacher JA, Danner RL, Stelzer PE: Hypotension with ventricular pacing: An atrial vasodepressor reflex in human beings. J Am Coll Cardiol 4:550–555, 1984.
22. Escher DJW, Schwedel JB, Eisenberg R, et al: Cardiovascular dynamic responses to artificial pacing of patients in heart block. Circulation 24:928–933, 1961.
23. Fananapazir L, Srinivas V, Bennett DH: Comparison of resting hemodynamic indices and exercise performance during atrial synchronized and asynchronous ventricular pacing. PACE 6:202, 1983.
24. Furman S: Therapeutic uses of atrial pacing. Am Heart J 86:835–840, 1973.
25. Gillespie WJ, Greene DG, Karatzas NB, et al: Effect of atrial systole on right ventricular stroke output in complete heart block. Br Med J 1:75–77, 1967.
26. Gilmore JP, Sarnoff SJ, Mitchell JH, Linden RJ: Synchronicity of ventricular contraction: Observations comparing hemodynamic effects of atrial and ventricular pacing. Br Heart J 25:299–307, 1983.
27. Goldreyer BN, Bigger JT: Ventriculo-atrial conduction in man. Circulation 41:935–946, 1970.
28. Gorlin R, Cohen LS, Elliott WC, et al: Effect of supine exercise on left ventricular volume and oxygen consumption in man. Circulation 32:361–371, 1965.
29. Greenberg B, Chatterjee K, Parmley WW, et al: The influence of left ventricular filling pressure on atrial contribution to cardiac output. Am Heart J 98:742–751, 1979.
30. Haas JM, Strait GB: Pacemaker-induced cardiovascular failure. Am J Cardiol 33:295–299, 1974.
31. Hartzler GO, Maloney JD, Curtis JJ, Barnhorst DA: Hemodynamic benefits of atrioventricular sequential pacing after cardiac surgery. Am J Cardiol 40:232–236, 1977.
32. Harvey W: Exercitatio Anatomica de Motu Cordis et Sanguinis in Animalibus (1628), Willis R (trans). England, Barnes Survey, 1847.
33. Hirata Y, Ishii M, Sugimoto T, et al: The effects of human atrial 28-amino acid peptide on systemic and renal hemodynamics in anesthetized rats. Circ Res 57:634–639, 1985.
34. Ikkos D, Hanson JS: Response to exercise in congenital complete atrioventricular block. Circulation 22:583–590, 1960.
35. Johnson AD, Laiken SL, Engler RL: Hemodynamic compromise associated with ventriculoatrial conduction following transvenous pacemaker placement. Am J Med 65:75–79, 1978.
36. Karlof I: Hemodynamic effect of atrial triggered versus fixed rate pacing at rest and during exercise in complete heart block. Acta Med Scand 197:195–206, 1975.
37. Kruse I, Ryden L: Comparison of physical work capacity and systolic time intervals with ventricular inhibited and atrial synchronous ventricular inhibited pacing. Br Heart J 46:129–136, 1981.
38. Kruse I, Arnman K, Conradson TB, Ryden L: A comparison of the acute and long-term hemodynamic effects of ventricular inhibited and atrial synchronous ventricular inhibited pacing. Circulation 65:846–855, 1982.
39. Labovitz AJ, Williams GA, Redd RM, Kennedy HL: Noninvasive assessment of pacemaker hemodynamics by Doppler echocardiography: Importance of left atrial size. J Am Coll Cardiol 6:196–200, 1985.
40. Levinson DC, Gunther L, Mechan JP, et al: Hemodynamic studies in five patients with heart block and slow ventricular rates. Circulation 12:739–745, 1955.
41. Lewis ME, Sung RJ, Alter BR, Myerburg RJ: Pace-

maker-induced hypotension. Chest 79:354–356, 1981.

42. Lewis T: Fibrillation of the auricles: Its effects upon the circulation. J Exp Med 16:395–398, 1912.

43. Meijler FF, Weiberdink J, Durrer D: L'importance de la position des electrodes stimulatrices au cours du traitement d'un bloc auriculo-ventriculaire postoperativ total. Arch Mal Coeur 55:690–694, 1962.

44. Miller DE, Gleason WK, Whalen RE, et al: Effect of ventricular rate on the cardiac output in the dog with chronic heart block. Circ Res 10:658–661, 1962.

45. Mitchell JH, Gilmore JP, Sarnoff SJ: The transport function of the atrium: Factors influencing the relation between mean left atrial pressure and left ventricular end diastolic pressure. Am J Cardiol 9:237–247, 1962.

46. Morgan DE, Norman R, West RO, Burggraf G: Echocardiographic assessment of tricuspid regurgitation during ventricular demand pacing. Am J Cardiol 58:1025–1029, 1986.

47. Muller OF, Bellet S: Treatment of intractable heart failure in the presence of complete atrioventricular heart block by the use of the internal cardiac pacemaker. N Engl J Med 265:768–772, 1961.

48. Naito M, Dreifus LS, David D, et al: Reevaluation of the role of atrial systole to cardiac hemodynamics: Evidence for pulmonary venous regurgitation during abnormal atrioventricular sequencing. Am Heart J 105:295, 1983.

49. Nakaoka H, Kitahara Y, Imataka K, et al: Atrial natriuretic peptide with artificial pacemakers. Am J Cardiol 60:384–385, 1987.

50. Nishimura RA, Geish BJ, Vlietstra RE, et al: Hemodynamic and symptomatic consequences of ventricular pacing. PACE 5:903–910, 1982.

51. Obata K, Yasue H, Horio Y, et al: Increase of human atrial natriuretic polypeptide in response to cardiac pacing. Am Heart J 113:845, 1987.

52. Ogawa S, Dreifus LS, Shenoy PN, et al: Hemodynamic consequences of atrioventricular and ventriculoatrial pacing. PACE 1:8, 1978.

53. Osler W: On the so-called Stokes-Adams' disease (slow pulse with syncopal attacks, etc.). Lancet 2:516–524, 1903.

54. Perrins EJ, Morley CA, Chan SL, Sutton R: Randomized controlled trial of physiological and ventricular pacing. Br Heart J 50:112–117, 1983.

55. Rahimtoola SH, Ehsani A, Sinno EZ, et al: Left atrial transport function in myocardial infarction: Importance of its booster pump function. Am J Med 59:686–694, 1975.

56. Raza ST, Lajos TZ, Bhayana JN, et al: Improved cardiovascular hemodynamics with atrioventricular sequential pacing compared with ventricular demand pacing. Ann Thorac Surg 38:260–264, 1984.

57. Reiter JM, Hindman MC: Hemodynamic benefits of acute atrioventricular sequential pacing in patients with left ventricular dysfunction. Am J Cardiol 49:687–692, 1982.

58. Ross J Jr, Linhart JW, Braunwald E: Effects of changing heart rate in many by electrical stimulation of the right atrium—studies at rest, during exercise and with isoproterenol. Circulation 32:549–558, 1965.

59. Samet P: Hemodynamic sequelae of cardiac arrhythmias. Circulation 47:399–407, 1973.

60. Samet P, Bernstein W, Levine S: Significance of the atrial contribution to ventricular filling. Am J Cardiol 15:195–202, 1965.

61. Samet P, Bernstein WH, Litwak RS: Electrical activation and mechanical asynchronism in the cardiac cycle of the dog. Circ Res 7:228–232, 1959.

62. Samet P, Castillo C, Bernstein WH: Hemodynamic sequelae of atrial, ventricular and sequential atrioventricular pacing in cardiac patients. Am Heart J 72:725–729, 1966.

63. Samet P, Castillo C, Bernstein WH: Hemodynamic consequences of sequential atrioventricular pacing: Subjects with normal hearts. Am J Cardiol 21:207–212, 1968.

64. Samet P, Bernstein WH, Medow A, Nathan DA: Effect of alterations in ventricular rate on cardiac output in complete heart block. Am J Cardiol 14:477–482, 1964.

65. Samet P, Bernstein WH, Nathan DA, Lopez A: Atrial contribution to cardiac output in complete heart block. Am J Cardiol 16:1–10, 1965.

66. Samet P, Castillo C, Bernstein WH, Fernandez P: Hemodynamic results of right atrial pacing in cardiac subjects. Dis Chest 53:133–137, 1968.

67. Samet P, Jacobs W, Bernstein WH, Shave R: Hemodynamic sequelae of idioventricular pacemaking in complete heart block. Am J Cardiol 11:594–599, 1963.

68. Scarpelli FM, Rudolph AM: The hemodynamics of congenital complete heart block. Prog Cardiovasc Dis 6:327–342, 1964.

69. Segel N, Hudson WA, Harris P, Bishop JM: The circulatory effects of electrically induced changes in ventricular rate at rest and during exercise in complete heart block. J Clin Invest 43:1541, 1964.

70. Sowton E: Hemodynamic studies in patients with artificial cardiac pacemakers. Br Heart J 26:737–746, 1964.

71. Stark MF, Rader B, Sobol BJ, et al: Cardiovascular hemodynamic function in complete heart block and response to isopropylnorepinephrine. Circulation 17:526–531, 1958.

72. Stewart WJ, Dicola VC, Harthorne JW, et al: Doppler ultrasound measurement of cardiac output in patients with physiologic pacemakers: Effects of left ventricular function and retrograde ventriculoatrial conduction. Am J Cardiol 54:308–312, 1984.

73. Topol E, Goldschlager N, Ports TA, et al: Hemodynamic benefit of atrial pacing in right ventricular myocardial infarction. Ann Intern Med 96:594–597, 1982.

74. Torres MAR, Corday E, Meerbaum S, et al: Characterization of left ventricular mechanical function during arrhythmias by two dimensional echocardiography. II. Location of the site of onset of premature ventricular systoles. J Am Coll Cardiol 1:819–829, 1983.

75. Uchiyama T, Corday E, Meerbaum S, et al: Characterization of left ventricular mechanical function during arrhythmias with two dimensional echocardiography. I. Premature ventricular contractions. Am J Cardiol 48:679–689, 1981.

76. Wang Y, Marshall RJ, Shepherd JT: Stroke volume in the dog during graded exercise. Circ Res 8:558–565, 1960.

77. Warner HR, Toronto AF: Regulation of cardiac output through stroke volume. Circ Res 8:549–552, 1960.

78. Wiggers CJ: The muscular reactions of the mammalian ventricles to artificial surface stimuli. Am J Physiol 73:346–350, 1925.

79. Zile MR, Blaustein AS, Shimizu G, Gaasch WH: Right ventricular pacing reduces the rate of left ventricular relaxation and filling. J Am Coll Cardiol 10:702–709, 1987.

9

PACEMAKER IMPLANTATION TECHNIQUES

DAVID R. HOLMES, JR., and DAVID L. HAYES

Implantation of permanent cardiac pacemakers requires personnel skilled in the technical aspects of lead and generator placement, as well as knowledgeable about the clinical condition of the patient and the pacing system to be used. In addition, implantation requires an environment with specialized equipment.

Personnel

The background of the physicians involved in pacemaker implantation has changed substantially over the past decade.[20, 35, 36] Compared with earlier years, when pacemaker implantations were performed almost exclusively by surgeons, a growing number of implantations today are performed by cardiologists trained in these invasive techniques. This change has been the result of many factors, including the widespread use of transvenous systems, which now account for approximately 95 per cent of all pacemaker implantations, the percutaneous approach for lead placement, and the increased complexity of the systems.

In addition to the operator, paramedical personnel are essential. These people act as scrub assistants and help with threshold measurement and evaluation of generator specifications. Ideally, an anesthesia technician or nurse-anesthetist is present during each case. This is of particular importance in older, more debilitated patients and in infants and children.

Implantation Facility

Pacemakers should be implanted in a surgical environment. The requirements for this environment were described in the 1983 Intersociety Commission for Heart Disease Resources.[37] In some institutions, a specially equipped and shielded operating room is suitable; in others, implantation is performed in a catheterization laboratory. In busy pacing practices, a dedicated room is very desirable for ease of scheduling and maintenance (Fig. 9-1). Such a room may also be used for electrophysiologic studies, thus helping to maintain optimal use. High-quality fluoroscopy is essential. The ability to obtain both lateral and anteroposterior projection views is very helpful, particularly in patients in whom atrial positions other than the atrial appendage are needed for atrial pacing.[8] High-quality electrocardiographic monitoring is essential and should be maintained throughout the procedure. Life support equipment is essential, and the capability of intraarterial pressure monitoring is often helpful in special cases. A physiologic recorder is necessary for recording intracardiac electrograms for assessment of ventriculoatrial (VA) conduction and for slew rate measurements.[18] These measurements can alternatively be accomplished with certain commercially available pacing system analyzers.[4, 11]

ANATOMIC APPROACH

A transvenous approach accounts for approximately 95 per cent of all permanent pacemaker implantations. Although epimyocardial placement is still used, it is usually reserved for patients undergoing thoracotomy for an-

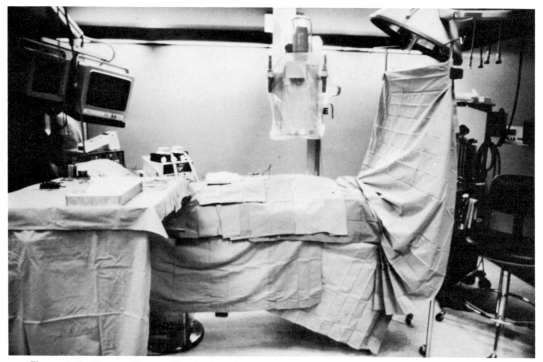

Figure 9–1. Dedicated pacemaker implantation suite. A C-arm fluoroscopy unit is used to enable both anteroposterior (AP) and lateral imaging. The patient's table can be tilted to allow assessment of the effect of upright position on blood pressure and heart rate.

other reason. For transvenous placement, there are several potential approaches, including subclavian and cephalic, most commonly, and the jugular system.

Subclavian Vein Approach

After its introduction in 1979, the subclavian puncture technique became the most commonly utilized method for lead placement.[27, 30] This approach has facilitated the development of the role of the cardiologist as implanting physician. It has also expedited the use of dual-chamber pacing systems.[9, 13, 38]

A modified Seldinger approach is used. After preparation and draping of the sterile field, lidocaine is used for local anesthesia. An incision long enough to accommodate the pulse generator to be used is begun approximately 2 cm below and parallel to the clavicle. This incision is begun at the junction of the middle and inner thirds of the clavicle. Dissection is carried down to the pectoralis fascia, and a pocket is then developed in the prepectoralis fascia, using blunt dissection. The pocket should be placed as medially as possible to prevent axillary migration. The size of the pocket will depend upon the size of the gen-

erator and the leads. Oversizing or undersizing is to be avoided. A sponge soaked in an antibiotic solution, such as neomycin, is then placed in the pacemaker pocket. The sponge serves to tamponade any bleeding in the newly formed pocket; at the end of the procedure the sponge is inspected to assess the pocket for continued bleeding during the procedure.

The approach to the subclavian vein is then undertaken at the junction of the inner and middle thirds of the clavicle (Fig. 9–2). Additional local anesthesia may increase the comfort of the patient. This can be accomplished by injecting lidocaine through the long 18-gauge needle used for subclavian venous entry. Placing the patient in the Trendelenburg position or placing a towel between the scapulae may be helpful for distending and entering the subclavian vein. Prepackaged kits that contain the needle, a guide wire, dilator, and peel-away sheath are available (Fig. 9–3). The needle should be inserted under the clavicle and then advanced toward a position approximately 2 cm cephalad to the clavicular notch (Fig. 9–2). After entry, a guide wire is placed, followed by the dilator sheath set (Fig. 9–4). In elderly patients with calcified costoclavicular ligaments, or in patients with thoracic deform-

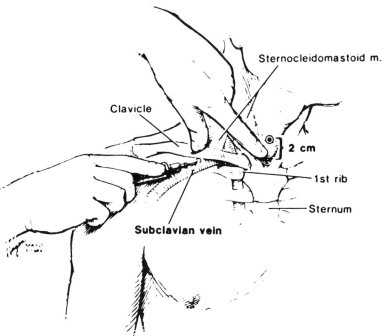

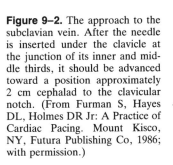

Figure 9–2. The approach to the subclavian vein. After the needle is inserted under the clavicle at the junction of its inner and middle thirds, it should be advanced toward a position approximately 2 cm cephalad to the clavicular notch. (From Furman S, Hayes DL, Holmes DR Jr: A Practice of Cardiac Pacing. Mount Kisco, NY, Futura Publishing Co, 1986; with permission.)

ities, this procedure may be difficult. Injection of contrast through an ipsilateral arm vein during needle placement may be helpful in localizing the vein (Fig. 9–5). After entry into the subclavian vein, the introducer guide wire is advanced into the right side of the heart. During this time, it is important that the patient temporarily suspend breathing to avoid the potential for air embolism.

After placement of the guide wire within the right side of the heart, a number of options are available (Fig. 9–6). These options are based upon whether a single- or dual-chamber pacing system is to be implanted. If a single-chamber pacemaker is to be used, the dilator and sheath are advanced over the guide wire into the subclavian vein and superior vena cava. The size of introducer selected (ranging from No. 8 to 14 French) depends upon the size of the lead or leads to be used. After removal of the guide wire and dilator, the lead can be advanced through the sheath. The

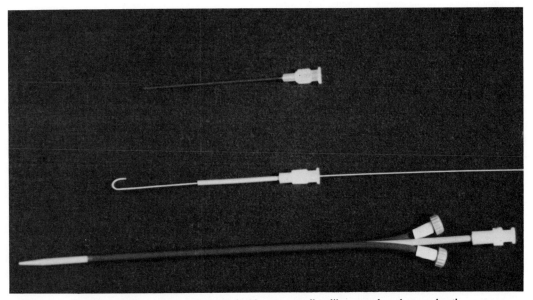

Figure 9–3. Prepackaged kits contain 18-gauge needle, dilator, and peel-away sheath.

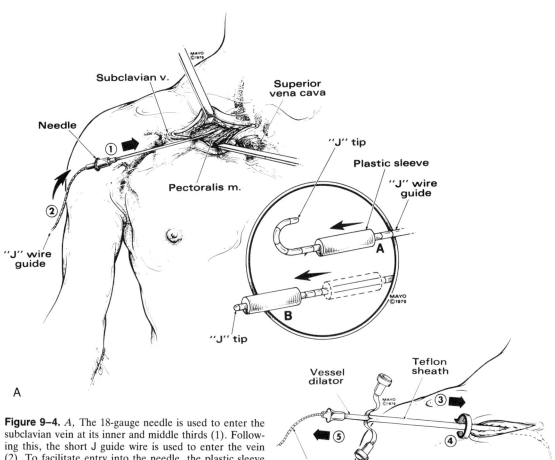

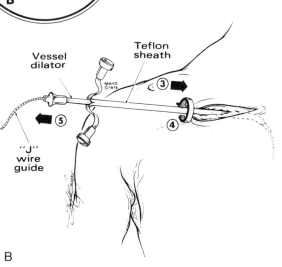

Figure 9–4. *A,* The 18-gauge needle is used to enter the subclavian vein at its inner and middle thirds (1). Following this, the short J guide wire is used to enter the vein (2). To facilitate entry into the needle, the plastic sleeve is used to straighten the J tip (A and B). *B,* After removal of the needle, the prepackaged dilator and sheath are advanced with a rotational motion over the wire into the subclavian vein (3 and 4). The dilator and guide wire are then removed (5). (From Miller FA Jr, Holmes DR Jr, Gersh BJ, Maloney JD: Permanent transvenous pacemaker implantation via the subclavian vein. Mayo Clin Proc 55:309–314, 1980; with permission.)

sheath should be pinched closed during this time to prevent air embolism. In addition, the patient should also suspend respiration. After placement of the lead, the sheath is then peeled away.

If two leads are to be used, one of three approaches may be employed (Fig. 9–6):[5, 9, 13, 38]

1. After the first lead is introduced, a second subclavian puncture is performed in the manner described. A second subclavian puncture increases the potential for complications related to needle entry. In addition, there is some concern that the initial lead could be punctured and damaged during the subsequent venipuncture.

2. Another approach is to use initially an introducer large enough to accommodate both atrial and ventricular leads. Depending on the leads to be used, a No. 12 or 14 French introducer will be necessary to accommodate both leads.

3. A third approach involves replacing the guide wire through the introducer when the first lead is introduced. The first introducer sheath is peeled away, leaving one lead and a guide wire in place. A second introducer is advanced over the guide wire, and the other lead is inserted. This technique avoids both two venipunctures and the use of a larger introducer.[5]

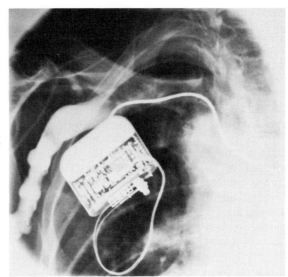

Figure 9–5. If the subclavian vein is difficult to enter, injection of contrast in a vein in the ipsilateral arm may be helpful for vein localization.

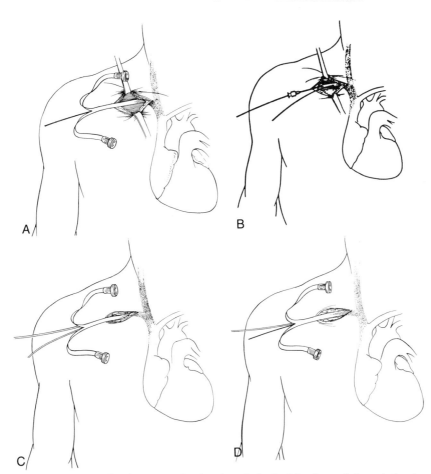

Figure 9–6. *A,* If a single-chamber pacemaker is selected, the lead is advanced through the sheath after removal of the dilator. *B,* For dual-chamber pacing, two subclavian punctures can be performed, the first being placed more medially. *C,* An alternative approach for dual-chamber pacing is the initial use of a sheath large enough to accommodate simultaneous introduction of both leads. *D,* The second alternative involves one vein puncture. When the initial lead is introduced, a second guide wire is also placed. After peeling away the sheath and placing a guide wire and the first lead, a second sheath can be placed. (From Furman S, Hayes DL, Holmes DR Jr: A Practice of Cardiac Pacing. Mount Kisco, NY, Futura Publishing Co, 1986; with permission.)

Cephalic Vein Approach

Prior to the introduction of the subclavian venipuncture technique, the cephalic approach was used in the majority of patients for transvenous implantation. Some centers continue to prefer this approach to avoid the risks associated with subclavian vein puncture.[15] The cephalic vein lies within the deltopectoral groove. It is usually easily identified, particularly in thinner patients, although in a small number of patients it may be too small or friable for use. After careful dissection, it is isolated with two nonabsorbable sutures, and a distal ligature is tied. After venotomy, the pacing lead or leads can be inserted with the aid of a forceps or venous introducer.

Jugular Vein Approach

A jugular approach is rarely necessary unless a subclavian or cephalic approach is not possible because of anatomic deformity or thrombosis due to previous lead placement. For either an internal or an external approach, two incisions are required: supraclavicular and infraclavicular. The infraclavicular incision and pocket are made in the usual fashion. The supraclavicular incision is made over the area between the posterior border of the sternocleidomastoid muscle and the anterior border of the trapezius. Marking the location of the external jugular vein with indelible ink prior to prepping and draping the patient is helpful. The right external jugular vein is often less tortuous than the left and is thus preferred. If a satisfactory external jugular system is not present, the internal jugular vein can be used. Approach to the internal jugular system should be undertaken only with great care. Surgical consultation should be obtained if the operator is not experienced in this approach. The neck incision is extended anterior to the sternal head of the sternocleidomastoid muscle. Beneath the clavicular border of the sternocleidomastoid muscle is the superficial fascia that covers the carotid sheath. After opening the sheath, the internal jugular vein can be isolated, and lead or leads can be introduced.

The jugular approach requires that the leads be tunneled down to the infraclavicular pulse generator pocket. The leads may be tunneled either superficial to or under the clavicle. Neither of these approaches is without risk. Although easier to achieve, tunneling the lead superficial to the clavicle is associated with the potential for erosion or fracture of the lead, particularly in thin patients. Placement deep to the clavicle is more difficult, with the potential for injury to the subclavian artery, but avoids the problem of erosion.

Axillary Vein Approach

This approach is mentioned largely for historical interest. The axillary vein has been used in the past, but now it is rarely, if ever, used in the United States.

CREATING THE PACEMAKER POCKET

Creation of the pacemaker pocket is an integral part of pacemaker implantation. As previously noted, the pocket is usually developed in the prepectoralis fascia. Attempts should be made to place the pocket medially rather than laterally and to make it large enough to allow for easy placement of the pulse generator and leads. A pocket that is not of adequate size, resulting in a tight fit, can cause erosion, and conversely, a pocket that is too large may allow excessive movement and migration. A snug-fitting fabric pouch can be used to encase the pulse generator within the pocket to reduce migration and prevent torsion of the pacing system.[34] In some centers, this is used routinely, while in others it is used only when migration or manipulation of the pacemaker is considered a possible problem.

Pulse generator size has decreased dramatically in recent years. Current units are now small enough that prepectoral positioning can be considered in almost any patient. Size is obviously a major concern in pediatric patients, in adult patients who have a thin, small body frame, and in patients in whom there are specific cosmetic concerns. For these patients, there are several choices.

In the very thin patient with minimal subcutaneous tissue, for whom concern arises regarding potential erosion if the pacemaker is placed in the prepectoral region, the pacemaker can be placed deep to the pectoral muscle. Creating a pacemaker pocket in this position requires special expertise, and the location may also result in a higher incidence of pectoral muscle stimulation or muscle inhibition, especially with a unipolar system. If a position deep to the pectoral muscle is to be used, it is preferable to use a bipolar system.

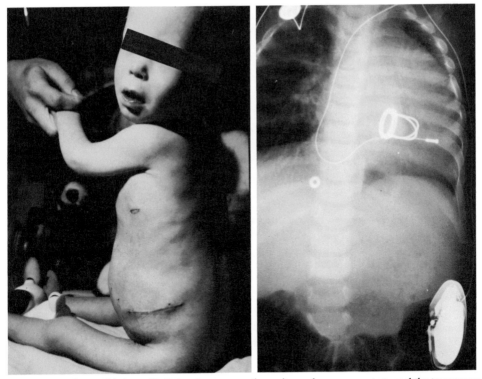

Figure 9–7. In the small infant with little subcutaneous tissue, it may be necessary to tunnel the transvenous lead in the subcutaneous tissue down to the ipsilateral flank for pulse generator placement.

In the infant, endocardial leads can be placed through the transvenous route of choice, and the leads can be tunneled in the subcutaneous tissue to the ipsilateral flank, which would allow more room for pacemaker placement (Fig. 9–7). Again, this is rarely necessary today owing to the availability of very small pulse generators (at this time, VVI devices as small as 24 grams are available).

In female patients in whom there are particular cosmetic concerns about deformity of the pectoral region by the pulse generator itself or deformity from the small incision required for implantation, a retromammary implant can be considered (Fig. 9–8).[6] The small pulse generators available today can be implanted in the retromammary area without causing significant deformity of the breast. If retromammary placement is to be performed, implantation should be done with the patient under light general anesthesia. Unless the operator is experienced with this technique, consultation with a surgical colleague is advisable. If the subclavian vein is used, a very small incision (2 to 3 mm) can be made through which subclavian puncture is performed. After the leads are placed, they should be fastened to the pectoralis fascia with nonabsorbable ligature about the sleeve. An incision is then made in the inframammary fold and carried down to the pectoralis fascia behind the breast. The breast is lifted from the fascia, and a long forceps or other long instrument (e.g., an Adson right angle) is introduced deep to the breast and brought through the small incision made for venous puncture. The leads are then brought to the retromammary incision and connected with the pulse generator. Mammary tissue is resutured anatomically inferior to the pulse generator to provide an additional cushion, and the skin is closed in a routine manner. Subsequently, a pulse generator can be readily replaced through reopening of the inframammary incision.

EPIMYOCARDIAL IMPLANTATION

Epimyocardial systems constitute less than 5 per cent of pacemaker implantation procedures. They are usually used in only two situations: (1) in patients undergoing cardiac surgery for another reason, such as coronary artery bypass graft surgery, valve replacement,

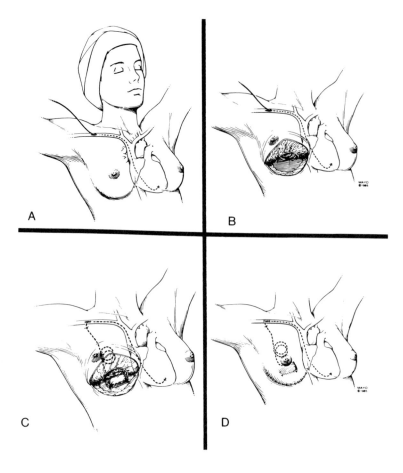

Figure 9–8. For a retromammary approach, subclavian vein puncture and lead placement are performed using a very small incision *(A)*. An inframammary incision is made and carried down to the pectoral fascia *(B)*. The pacing lead is then tunneled down posterior to the breast *(C)*. After testing and connecting the lead, the incision is closed *(D)*. (From Furman S, Hayes DL, Holmes DR Jr: A Practice of Cardiac Pacing. Mount Kisco, NY, Futura Publishing Co, 1986; with permission.)

or correction of congenital heart defects—some of these patients receive epimyocardial systems at the time of their surgery; and (2) in patients with abnormalities of the right side of the heart that preclude stable atrial or ventricular endocardial lead placement.

The specific approach taken varies, depending on the institution and the clinical condition of the particular patient (Fig. 9–9).[25, 33, 40, 41, 43] The most commonly used is a subxyphoid or left costal approach. Both of these provide access to the diaphragmatic surface of the heart, allowing electrode placement on the right ventricle and some portion of the left ventricle. The amount of left ventricle exposed is variable when the subxyphoid approach is selected. A left subcostal incision is sometimes used instead because it results in better exposure of the left ventricle. Left ventricular placement may be required for optimal sensing. Both subcostal and subxyphoid approaches carry with them the potential for cardiac laceration, which may be life threatening.

A left lateral thoracotomy approach is also occasionally used (Fig. 9–9). This approach facilitates implantation of electrodes on the left ventricular epicardium. For implantation, the fifth left intercostal space is used. It is important to avoid placement of the electrode too near the phrenic nerves, which could result in diaphragmatic stimulation.

Selection of epimyocardial pacing may require modification in the personnel and facilities used for pacing. A cardiovascular surgeon is required for epimyocardial lead placement. This practice is in contrast to transvenous pacing which can be performed by a cardiologist skilled in invasive techniques who is trained in pacemaker implantation. In addition, epimyocardial pacing requires a formal operating room suite, whereas transvenous pacing can be performed in a modified catheterization laboratory. For these reasons, as well as the increased incidence of system malfunction in the past with epimyocardial systems, a transvenous approach is preferred in the vast majority of implantations (approximately 95 per cent).

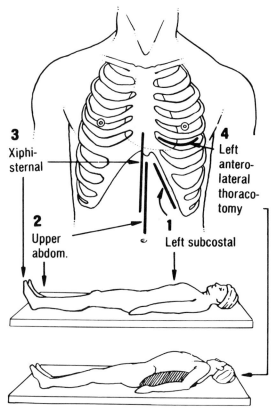

3
Xiphi-
sternal

4
Left
antero-
lateral
thoraco-
tomy

2
Upper
abdom.

1
Left subcostal

Figure 9–9. Several epimyocardial approaches are available. The most commonly used are subxyphoid and left subcostal. (From Furman S, Hayes DL, Holmes DR, Jr: A Practice of Cardiac Pacing. Mount Kisco, NY, Futura Publishing Co, 1986; with permission.)

LEAD PLACEMENT

Ventricular Lead Placement

The goal of right ventricular lead placement is to provide a stable position with adequate pacing and sensing thresholds. A right ventricular apical position is ordinarily used. Placement of the lead requires knowledge of the anatomy of the right side of the heart and catheterization techniques, as well as considerable experience.

There are two general techniques for ventricular lead placement (Fig. 9–10). The first is a relatively straight catheter pass using a gently curved stylet to lift the lead tip up and across the tricuspid valve. Introduction of the lead into the right ventricle can sometimes be accomplished by leaving a straight stylet in the lead but pulling back 5 to 10 cm from the distal end of the lead, leaving it "floppy." With the lead in the right atrium, to-and-fro passage of the lead may allow the floppy end of the

lead to bend over the tricuspid valve and into the right ventricle. Once the tip of the lead is in the right ventricle, the straight stylet can be fully advanced and the lead can be directed toward the right ventricular apex. This procedure may be facilitated by having the patient take a deep inspiration. In a second commonly used approach, a curved stylet is kept in place, and a loop of catheter is made within the right atrium; then the loop is either advanced or rotated across the tricuspid valve.

After entry into the right ventricle, the catheter is usually passed into the right ventricular outflow tract or out into the pulmonary artery (Fig. 9–10C). This ensures right ventricular placement and avoids placement in the coronary sinus. The lead is then withdrawn from the right ventricular outflow tract and positioned in the right ventricular apex. If a curved stylet has been used for entry into the right ventricle, it is usually best to replace it with a straight stylet for positioning in the apex. The straight stylet should be advanced under fluoroscopic guidance as the lead is slowly withdrawn from the right ventricular outflow tract. The stylet should be advanced entirely as the lead is retracted and aimed at the right ventricular apex. With the stylet advanced, the lead can then gently be advanced into the apical portion of the right ventricle. In the proper apical position, there should be a gentle curve within the right atrium and slight systolic cephalad displacement of the catheter segment lying across the tricuspid valve. Stable positioning should be checked during deep inspiration as well as during coughing.

Selection of either technique is dependent upon details of the patient's anatomy, the operator's experience, and the specific lead. For example, passive-fixation leads may become caught in the chordae tendineae during attempts to advance a loop through the tricuspid valve. A straight pass is sometimes easier with these leads.

Atrial Lead Placement

Single-chamber atrial pacing is becoming less common, accounting for less than 5 per cent of implants in the United States. Single-chamber atrial pacing is still used, however, in the setting of symptomatic sinus bradycardia with intact atrioventricular (AV) conduction. More commonly, atrial lead placement is performed as part of dual-chamber pacing.

RIGHT ATRIAL APPENDAGE. The right atrial

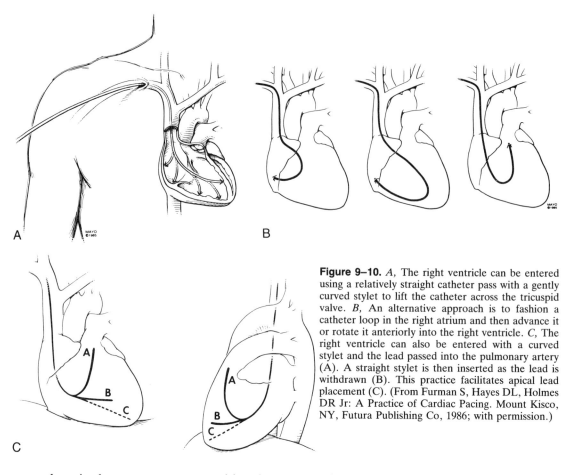

A

B

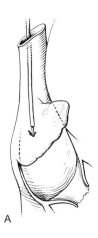

C

Figure 9–10. *A,* The right ventricle can be entered using a relatively straight catheter pass with a gently curved stylet to lift the catheter across the tricuspid valve. *B,* An alternative approach is to fashion a catheter loop in the right atrium and then advance it or rotate it anteriorly into the right ventricle. *C,* The right ventricle can also be entered with a curved stylet and the lead passed into the pulmonary artery (A). A straight stylet is then inserted as the lead is withdrawn (B). This practice facilitates apical lead placement (C). (From Furman S, Hayes DL, Holmes DR Jr: A Practice of Cardiac Pacing. Mount Kisco, NY, Futura Publishing Co, 1986; with permission.)

appendage is the most common position for the atrial lead, although satisfactory pacing can be achieved from a variety of right atrial sites. Placement is the same irrespective of whether a single-chamber atrial or dual-chamber pacemaker is to be used.

Active- or passive-fixation leads, with or without a preformed J configuration, may be used.[7, 28, 29] The lead is advanced, with a gently curved stylet, into the mid right atrium and rotated anteriorly toward the tricuspid valve (Fig. 9–11). If a preformed J lead is used, the stylet is then withdrawn, returning the lead to its J shape. Following this, the lead itself is withdrawn, with medial rotation into the right atrial appendage. Placement of the lead in the right atrial appendage can be recognized by the to-and-fro lateral motion of the catheter

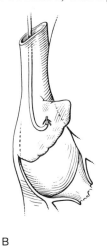

A

B

C

Figure 9–11. For right atrial appendage placement, the lead is advanced over a gently curved stylet into the midatrium and rotated anteriorly (*A* and *B*). After withdrawal of the stylet, the lead returns to its preformed shape to enter the appendage *(C).*

during atrial systole. Lateral fluoroscopy may be helpful in confirming this placement.[8] A stable position is essential and should be checked by noting the effects of torque on the system as well as the effects of deep breathing. During inspiration, the two levels of the J widen toward an L shape but should not exceed approximately 80 degrees. During expiration, the two levels should form an acute angle. If a straight (nonpreformed J) lead is employed, the same procedure is used, with the following exception—a curved stylet is introduced after the lead is passed into the area of the mid right atrium. With the stylet in place, the lead is directed toward the desired position in the atrium. If an active-fixation lead is used, the lead can then be fixed and the stylet removed. Enough slack is left in the atrium to allow the J shape and angulation described above. Many implanters prefer a straight (nonpreformed J) because of increased ease in manipulating the lead to sites other than the atrial appendage. In pediatric patients and certain adults, the atrium may be too small to accommodate certain preformed J leads.

OTHER ATRIAL POSITIONS. Although the atrial appendage is most commonly used, it may not be suitable either because of abnormal anatomy resulting from prior cardiac surgery that involved a ligated atrial appendage or because of poor sensing or pacing thresholds in this location. In these patients, other locations can be used. Lateral fluoroscopy is helpful for exploring the right atrium. With the use of different stylet curvatures, active-fixation leads can be placed in the atrial septum or in the free right atrial wall. Although the coronary sinus has been used for permanent atrial pacing, it is rarely used today. Coronary sinus leads can be difficult to position and, more important, are difficult to maintain in a stable position.

INTRAOPERATIVE THRESHOLD MEASUREMENT

The measurement of pacing and sensing thresholds is an essential part of pacemaker implantation.[2, 3, 14, 17, 42] Although the specific measurements made do vary from laboratory to laboratory, the goal in each case is to ensure satisfactory long-term pacing and sensing. In addition to variability in the specific measurements made, the equipment is also variable. Pacing systems analyzers (PSAs) are available from the pacemaker manufacturers and are

commonly used. Ideally, the PSA utilized should be from the same manufacturer as the pulse generator used because of the markedly different waveform configuration of the various pulse generators and the characteristics of the PSA.[4]

Pacing Threshold

The stimulation threshold (the lowest voltage amplitude or current needed to result consistently in cardiac depolarization) is measured with the same electrode configuration that will be clinically used. For example, if a unipolar system is used, the pacing threshold should be measured in a unipolar mode. A pacing rate that is just faster than the intrinsic rate of the patient is selected. Pacing threshold can be measured in two ways. (1) The output of the PSA is set at 5 V and then gradually decreased to the point at which there is failure to capture. The voltage is then increased to the minimal voltage at which capture is maintained. This is the stimulation, or pacing, threshold. (2) Alternatively, the output of the PSA can be set very low and then increased until capture occurs. It is important to remember that pacing for the measurement of the stimulation threshold may suppress the patient's intrinsic rhythm. This factor is of more concern with ventricular threshold measurements than with atrial threshold measurements. In the patient with a slow ventricular escape rhythm, pacing may further suppress the escape rhythm. In these patients, a temporary pacemaker is commonly placed prior to permanent pacemaker implantation. If a temporary pacemaker is in place, pacing at a faster rate on the permanent lead via the PSA may inhibit the temporary pacemaker. If the output pulse from the PSA is subthreshold, ventricular asystole may occur. It is imperative that the PSA operator be experienced and attentive. At times, it may be advantageous to use the temporary pacemaker in an asynchronous mode.

The stimulation threshold is, in part, a function of the duration of the pacing stimulus. Strength-duration curves are often plotted to allow for analysis of current and voltage thresholds at a specific pulse duration. Strength-duration curves can be developed by varying the pulse duration while keeping the output fixed or by varying the output while keeping the pulse duration fixed (Fig. 9–12). Analysis of the strength-duration curves facilitates selection of the pacing parameters of

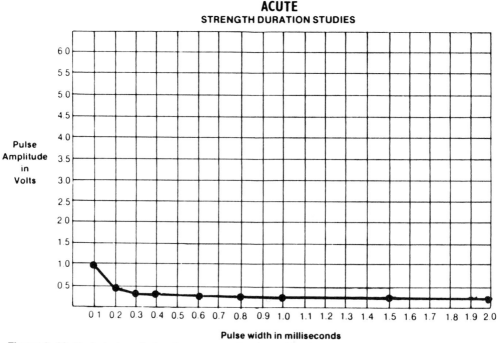

Figure 9–12. Typical strength-duration curve at the time of implantation, which allows selection of the optimal stimulation parameters.

pulse width and output that allow an adequate pacing margin of safety but optimal longevity of the system. The lower the stimulation threshold, the better. Acceptable thresholds for ventricular leads measured at a pulse duration of 0.5 msec are 0.3 to 1.0 V and a current of 0.3 to 2.0 mA. For atrial leads, also measured at 0.5 msec, acceptable thresholds are higher, ranging from 0.6 to 2.0 V and a current of 1.0 to 3.0 mA.

Lead impedance is also measured. This measurement is performed under standardized conditions of 5.0-V output and 0.6-msec pulse duration. Ohm's law (voltage = current × resistance) is used. Measurements of voltage and current are used to solve the equation for lead resistance, which may range from 250 to 1200 ohms. The acute impedance measurement is, in large part, dependent on the geometry of the surface electrode, the lowest values being seen with electrodes of large surface area and the highest with electrodes of small surface area.[42]

Sensing Threshold

Measurement of sensing thresholds is more variable from institution to institution. Either physiologic recorders or a PSA can be used.

If a PSA is used, it is important to match the analyzer with the pulse generator. This practice is necessary because there is no standardization of the sensitivity of pacemaker units. Sensing thresholds, the slew rate of the intrinsic deflection (dV/dt), and intracardiac electrograms are all parameters that may be assessed.

There has been debate about the advantages of unipolar versus bipolar sensing. Unipolar systems were favored for many years because they were felt to be superior for sensing. Not only is there no definite superiority of unipolar sensing, but also the larger distance between electrodes affords a much greater opportunity for sensing of extracardiac signals, especially myopotentials.

The amplitude of the intracardiac signal to be sensed is always measured (Fig. 9–13). The component of the intracardiac electrogram sensed by the pacemaker is the intrinsic deflection. The amplitude of this intracardiac signal is measured in the chamber to be paced and is expressed in millivolts. Adequate sensing thresholds are essential for normal pacemaker function. For atrial lead systems, at least 2 mV is desired to ensure stable sensing. If this signal is not present, the lead should be repositioned. For ventricular leads, a position with a ventricular signal of 6 to 10 mV should

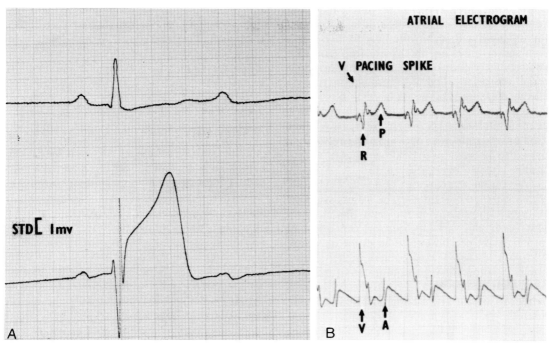

Figure 9–13. *A,* Intracardiac electrograms at the time of implantation. The surface of electrocardiogram is used for timing (*top*). On the bottom, the ventricular electrogram identifies the intrinsic deflection (ID) as well as the current of injury, as demonstrated by ST-segment elevation. *B,* Atrial electrograms are assessed during ventricular pacing. This practice allows measurement of ventriculoatrial (VA) conduction times. In this patient, the VA conduction time is 320 msec. STD = standardization.

be sought. If the ventricular signal is less than 4 mV, the lead should be repositioned.

Other parameters of the intracardiac signal can also be measured, including slew rate, magnitude of the intracardiac signal, and ST-segment deviation. The slew rate is the change in voltage over time (dV/dt). This rate is most important in patients with borderline sensing thresholds. If the largest R wave that can be obtained is only 4 to 5 mV (in the low or borderline range), the finding of a normal slew rate provides some reassurance that accurate sensing is still possible. Slew rates have traditionally been obtained by using a physiologic recorder to record the intracardiac electrogram and then measuring the dv/dt. Newer PSAs make it possible to obtain the slew rate with a printout of the intracardiac waveform via the PSA. Finally, intracardiac electrograms can be measured to document the current of injury that occurs when the electrode is in contact with the endocardial surface. This current of injury is analogous to the ST-segment elevation seen on the surface electrocardiogram early during infarction. It is recognized as the elevation in electrical potential immediately following the intrinsic deflection and indicates adequate endocardial contact.

VENTRICULOATRIAL CONDUCTION

Assessment of VA conduction is an integral part of pacemaker implantation (Fig. 9–13).[24] The pacemaker syndrome has been well described and results from intact VA conduction during ventricular pacing.[1, 12, 32] In the patient in whom ventricular demand pacing is contemplated, evaluation of the hemodynamic effects of this mode is important. If VA conduction is present, ventricular pacing may result in hemodynamic compromise. Assessment of systemic arterial pressure during ventricular pacing and then comparison of this with the hemodynamics during normal sinus rhythm are important in recognizing this problem.[32] Intraarterial pressure recordings are helpful in this regard, but not essential. The effect of upright positioning on hemodynamics using a tilt table in the laboratory should be studied when such equipment is available; in some patients, the adverse effect of VA conduction may be manifest only when the patient is in an upright position. In patients in whom ventricular pacing results in a decrease in arterial pressure by more than 20 to 30 mm Hg, consideration should be given to a dual-chamber system.

VA conduction is assessed while pacing the ventricle at physiologic rates just faster than the intrinsic ventricular rate (Fig. 9–13B). VA conduction times are then measured from the ventricular stimulus to the time of retrograde atrial activation. The VA conduction time is easily measured when dual-chamber pacemakers are to be used and two leads have been implanted. This measurement is then used to determine the optimal atrial refractory period to prevent pacemaker-mediated tachycardia.

AV conduction can also be easily evaluated with atrial lead placement. The atrium is paced at rates just slightly faster than the intrinsic sinus rate, and then up to approximately 120 to 150 beats per minute. The point at which AV block, either Wenckebach or higher grade, occurs is noted. This information is helpful for programming upper rates or in the occasional patient in whom atrial demand units are considered.

COMPLICATIONS

There are two major groups of complications associated with permanent pacemaker implantation. The first group is related to the catheterization techniques used to gain venous access, and the second group is related to placing the lead and fashioning the pocket.[23]

Complications of Venous Entry

The complications of obtaining venous entry are related to the experience of the operator as well as to the route taken. Some centers prefer a cephalic approach for the reason that it avoids the risks of gaining subclavian venous access, which include pneumothorax, hemopneumothorax, and damage to the subclavian artery.[16] With any approach, there is the potential for bleeding, air embolism, and thrombosis. Bleeding is harder to control with the subclavian or internal jugular approach than with the cephalic approach. Despite these concerns, subclavian venipuncture implantations account for the majority of procedures. Fewer than 5 per cent result in clinically recognized complications.

Complications of Lead Placement and Pocket Formation

Lead Dislodgment

Until the widespread use of active- and passive-fixation leads, dislodgment was the most common complication of permanent pacing. This usually occurred within the first month after implantation. With the new leads available, secondary intervention rates for dislodgment should be less than 2 per cent for ventricular leads and less than 5 per cent for atrial leads.

Arrhythmias

Both supraventricular and ventricular arrhythmias are common during lead manipulation. These are usually self-limited, responding to catheter manipulation. In patients with a history of intermittent tachycardia, the arrhythmia may require treatment with either pharmacologic or electrophysiologic techniques. Bradyarrhythmias may also be seen, particularly if a slow intrinsic rhythm is suppressed with overdrive pacing. If this concern exists, a temporary pacemaker should be placed before the procedure.

Perforation

Perforation is fortunately uncommon. It usually manifests as diaphragmatic or chest wall stimulation and increased thresholds. In older patients with thin-walled right ventricles, great care should be taken to avoid excessive force during placement. Should perforation be suspected, echocardiography should be performed. It is uncommon for cardiac tamponade to occur, but a sudden fall in blood pressure, with or without associated chest pain, should raise suspicion of a possible tamponade.

Pacemaker Pocket

There may also be complications related to the pacemaker pocket. The most common is local hematoma formation, which is usually minor. This usually occurs in patients who are taking salicylates or receiving anticoagulants or other antiplatelet agents. Local hemostasis is essential in these patients. It is common to discontinue oral anticoagulants and wait until the prothrombin time has returned to normal before implantation. Anticoagulants can then be restarted 48 to 72 hours after the implantation. For the treatment of hematoma, local conservative therapy is the best (Fig. 9–14). Needle aspiration or placement of a drain should be avoided in most cases because of the increased risk of infection associated with these procedures. If evacuation is required, it should be performed in an operating room setting with strict sterile technique.

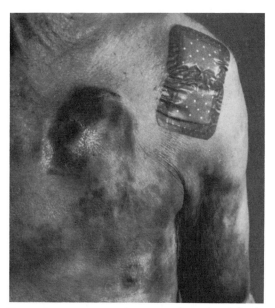

Figure 9–14. Extensive hematoma formation following permanent pacemaker implantation. In such instances, conservative therapy without aspiration is best.

Late Complications

Late complications (more than 1 month post implantation) include erosion, migration, and infection. Erosion and migration usually occur as the result of suboptimal initial implantation technique. A "tight" pacemaker pocket predisposes the patient to erosion. Lateral placement of the pulse generator may allow migration.

Pacemaker Infections

The incidence of infection of permanent pacing systems has been reported to range from 0.5 per cent to 12.6 per cent. Careful attention to surgical details and sterile procedures are of paramount importance in avoiding pacemaker site infection. There has been considerable debate over whether the incidence of infection actually is dependent on whether the procedure is carried out in a surgical suite or in the catheterization laboratory. Although there is no definite consensus regarding where the procedure should be performed, there is certainly evidence that the major factor in avoiding infections of a pacing system is the use of strict sterile technique.

The prophylactic use of antibiotics before implantation and in the immediate postoperative period also remains controversial. Most studies do not show any significant difference in the rate of infection between patients who have had prophylactic administration of antibiotics and those who have not.[21, 39] Irrigation of the pacemaker pocket with an antibiotic solution at the time of pacemaker implantation may decrease the incidence of infection.[19, 22]

Pacemaker infection must be recognized and treated properly. The clinical presentation of a pacemaker infection varies widely; the infection may appear as local inflammation and abscess formation in the area of the pulse generator pocket; erosion of part of the pacing system through the skin with secondary infection; or fever associated with positive blood cultures, with or without a focus of infection elsewhere. Lewis and colleagues have shown that it is actually uncommon for the patient to present with bacteremia.[26] The most common clinical presentation is local inflammation or abscess formation around the pulse generator pocket. Early infections are usually caused by *Staphylococcus aureus*. These infections may be aggressive and are often associated with fever and systemic symptoms. Late infections are commonly caused by *Staphylococcus epidermidis;* these are more indolent and are usually without fever or systemic manifestation. The treatment of either of these requires removal of the entire infected pacing system—pulse generator and leads. There has been some controversy over how to proceed once the infected system has been removed. Some have advocated a one-stage surgical approach that involves implantation of a new pacing system in a distant clean site after explantation of the infected pacing system. Others have promoted removal of the infected system, followed by a period of temporary pacing and antibiotic management, with implantation of a new system at a later date. Previous studies suggest that a one-stage procedure is as successful as the more involved two-stage procedure.[10, 31]

SPECIAL CONSIDERATIONS IN PEDIATRIC PATIENTS

Permanent pacing in pediatric patients raises special issues. These include (1) location of the pulse generator in a very small, thin patient; (2) type of leads that would most likely afford stability in this more active population; (3) how to allow for potential growth of the child; and (4) appropriate transvenous routes in the pediatric patient.

As already mentioned, the prepectoral region is usually sufficient, given the small size of current pulse generators. If, however, it is felt that the infant or child is too small to accommodate the pulse generator in this position, consideration can be given to placing the pacemaker deep to the pectoral muscle or tunneling the leads in a subcutaneous fashion to the flank and placing the pulse generator in this region (Fig. 9–7).

Any standard endocardial lead could potentially be used for pediatric implantation. There may be some advantage to the use of polyurethane leads in such situations only because they are usually of smaller size than their silicone counterparts and it may be easier to introduce two leads into a single vein in a pediatric patient if a dual-chamber implantation is undertaken. Although active- or passive-fixation leads can be used, active-fixation leads may be advantageous for two reasons. First, in the early postimplantation period, an active-fixation mechanism may provide some protection against early dislodgment in the very active child, who cannot be expected to limit his or her activity following pacemaker implantation. Second, it may be easier to re-

move a currently available active-fixation lead than a passive-fixation lead; if the patient is to face a lifetime of permanent pacing and multiple pacing systems, easy lead removal may help prevent the patient from having multiple retained leads in future years.

In the young patient, in whom growth is anticipated, the intracardiac portion of the lead should intentionally be redundant at the time of implantation (Fig. 9–15). This redundancy will allow the system to accommodate somewhat to the patient's growth. The length of the endocardial lead to be used is dependent on the patient's size. In many children, a standard-length (58 cm) pacing lead can be used. However, in a very small child or infant, shorter endocardial leads, which are available form the manufacturer, should be used to avoid excessive lead in the pacemaker pocket.

An additional concern that arises in pacing pediatric patients is the congenital cardiac abnormalities that are frequently present in this population. Currently available active-fixation leads make it possible to pace the heart from

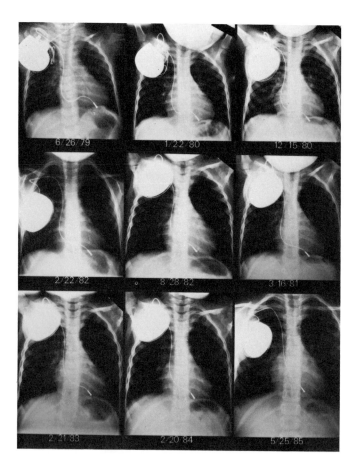

Figure 9–15. In pediatric patients, when growth is expected, the lead system should be redundant. The initial pulse generator was implanted in this 18-month-old child in 1979. Over the subsequent 6 years, as growth occurred, the redundant loop decreased.

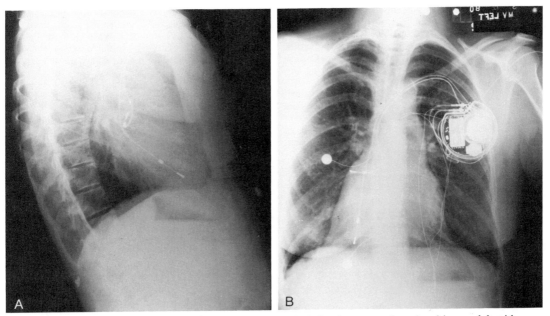

Figure 9–16. Lateral *(A)* and AP *(B)* radiographs of a dual-chamber pacemaker placed in an adult with levotransposition. The passive-fixation atrial lead is positioned in the right atrium, and the ventricular lead is placed in the morphologic left ventricle (venous ventricle).

a variety of positions and make transvenous pacing possible in many patients with congenital defects (Fig. 9–16).

REFERENCES

1. Ausubel K, Furman S: The pacemaker syndrome. Ann Intern Med 103:420–429, 1985.
2. Barold SS, Winner JA: Techniques and significance of threshold measurement for cardiac pacing. Chest 70:760–766, 1976.
3. Barold SS, Ong LS, Heinle RA: Stimulation and sensing thresholds for cardiac pacing: Electrophysiologic and technical aspects. Prog Cardiovasc Dis 24:1–24, 1981.
4. Barold SS, Roehrich DR, Falkoff MD, et al: Sources of error in the determination of output voltage of pulse generators by pacemaker system analyzers. PACE 3:585–596, 1980.
5. Bellot PH: A variation on the introducer technique for unlimited access to the subclavian vein. PACE 4:43–48, 1981.
6. Belott PH, Bucko D: Inframammary pulse generator placement for maximizing cosmetic effect. PACE 6:1241–1244, 1983.
7. Bisping HJ, Kreuger J, Birkenheier H: Three year clinical experience with a new endocardial screw-in lead with introduction protection for use in the atrium and ventricle. PACE 3:424–435, 1980.
8. Bognolo DA, Vijayanagar R, Eckstein PF: Implantation of permanent transvenous atrial "J" lead using lateral view fluoroscopy. Ann Thorac Surg 31:6, 1981.
9. Bognolo DA, Vijayanagar R, Eckstein PF, Janss B: Two leads in one introducer technique for AV sequential implantations. PACE 5:217–218, 1982.
10. Choo MH, Holmes DR Jr, Gersh BJ, et al: Permanent pacemaker infections: Characterization and management. Am J Cardiol 48:559–564, 1981.
11. Duffin E, Rueter J, Anderson K: Dual chamber pacing system analyzer, the Medtronic 5311. Clin Prog Pacing Electrophysiol 4:449–459, 1986.
12. Erlebacher JA, Danner RL, Stelzer PE: Hypotension with ventricular pacing: An atrial vasodepressor reflex in human beings. J Am Coll Cardiol 4:550–555, 1984.
13. Fox S, Toonder FG: Simplified technique for permanent atrioventricular pacing via a single venipuncture. Chest 80:745–747, 1981.
14. Furman S: Basic concepts. *In* Furman S, Hayes DL, Holmes DR (eds) A Practice of Cardiac Pacing. Mount Kisco, NY, Futura Publishing Co, 1986, pp 27–75.
15. Furman S: Subclavian puncture for pacemaker lead placement. [letter from the editor]. PACE 9:467, 1986.
16. Furman S: Venous cutdown for pacemaker implantation. Ann Thorac Surg 41:438–439, 1986.
17. Furman S, Hurzeler P, DeCaprio V: Sensing the endocardial electrogram. Am Heart J 93:794–801, 1977.
18. Furman S, Hurzeler P, DeCaprio V: The ventricular endocardial electrogram and pacemaker sensing. J Thorac Cardiovasc Surg 73:258–266, 1977.
19. Goldman BS, MacGregor DC: Management of infected pacemaker systems. Clin Prog Pacing Electrophysiol 2:220–235, 1984.
20. Hanley PC, Vlietstra RE, Merideth J, et al: Two decades of cardiac pacing at the Mayo Clinic 1961 through 1981. Mayo Clin Proc 59:268–274, 1984.
21. Hartstein AI, Jackson J, Gilbert DN: Prophylactic antibiotics and the insertion of permanent transvenous cardiac pacemakers. J Thorac Cardiovasc Surg 75:219–223, 1978.

22. Hayes DL: Causative organisms and predisposing factors of infection in permanent pacing systems. Clin Prog Pacing Electrophysiol 4:216–222, 1986.

23. Hayes DL: Pacemaker complications. *In* Furman S, Hayes DL, Holmes DR (eds): A Practice of Cardiac Pacing. Mount Kisco, NY, Futura Publishing Co, 1986, pp 253–273.

24. Hayes DL, Furman S: Atrio-ventricular and ventri-culo-atrial conduction times in patients undergoing pacemaker implant. PACE 6:38–46, 1987.

25. Lawrie GM, Seale JP, Morris GC Jr, et al: Results of epicardial pacing by the left subcostal approach. Ann Thorac Surg 28:561–566, 1979.

26. Lewis AB, Hayes DL, Holmes DR Jr, et al: Update on infections involving permanent pacemakers. J Thorac Cardiovasc Surg 89:758–763, 1985.

27. Littleford PO, Spector SD: Device for rapid insertion of a permanent pacing electrode through the sub-clavian vein: Preliminary report. Ann Thorac Surg 27:265–269, 1979.

28. McGoon MD, Maloney JD, McGoon DC: Long-term endocardial atrial pacing in children with postop-erative bradycardia-tachycardia syndrome and lim-ited ventricular access. Am J Cardiol 49:1750–1757, 1982.

29. Messenger JC, Castellanet MJ, Stephenson NL: New permanent endocardial atrial J lead: Implantation techniques and clinical performance. PACE 5:767–772, 1982.

30. Miller FA Jr, Holmes DR Jr, Gersh BJ, et al: Per-manent transvenous pacemaker implantation via the subclavian vein. Mayo Clin Proc 55:309–314, 1980.

31. Muers MF, Arnold AG, Sleight P: Prophylactic anti-biotics for cardiac pacemaker implantation: A pro-spective trial. Br Heart J 46:539–544, 1981.

32. Nishimura RA, Gersh BJ, Vlietstra RE, et al: He-modynamic and symptomatic consequences of ven-tricular pacing. PACE 5:903–910, 1982.

33. Oldershaw PJ, Sutton MG, Ward D, et al: Ten-year experience of 359 epicardial pacemaker systems: Complications and results. Clin Cardiol 5:515–519, 1982.

34. Parsonnet V: A stretch fabric pouch for permanent implanted pacemakers. Arch Surg 105:654–656, 1972.

35. Parsonnet V, Bernstein AD: Cardiac pacing in the 1980's: Treatment and techniques in transition. J Am Coll Cardiol 1:339–354, 1983.

36. Parsonnet V, Crawford CC, Bernstein AD: The 1981 United States Survey of Cardiac Pacing Practices. J Am Coll Cardiol 3:1321–1332, 1984.

37. Parsonnet V, Furman S, Smyth NPD, et al: Optimal resources for implantable cardiac pacemakers. Cir-culation 68:226A–244A, 1983.

38. Parsonnet V, Werres R, Atherley T, et al: Transve-nous insertion of double sets of permanent elec-trodes. JAMA 243:62–64, 1980.

39. Ramsdale DR, Charles RG, Rowlands DB, et al: Antibiotic prophylaxis for pacemaker implantation: A prospective randomized trial. PACE 7:844–849, 1984.

40. Smyth NPD: Techniques of implantation: Atrial and ventricular, thoracotomy and transvenous. Prog Cardiovasc Dis 23:435–450, 1981.

41. Smyth NPD: Pacemaker implantation: Surgical tech-niques. Cardiovasc Clin 14:31–44, 1983.

42. Smyth NPD, Tarjan PP, Chernoff E, et al: The significance of electrode surface area and stimulat-ing thresholds in permanent cardiac pacing. J Thorac Cardiovasc Surg 71:559–565, 1976.

43. Stewart S: Placement of the sutureless epicardial pace-maker lead by the subxiphoid approach. Ann Thorac Surg 18:308–313, 1974.

10

PRINCIPLES OF OUTPATIENT FOLLOW-UP OF THE PACEMAKER PATIENT

EDWARD GERTZ, NORA GOLDSCHLAGER, *and* SEYMOUR FURMAN

In recent years, major advances in technology have resulted in an increasing frequency of implantation of multiprogrammable single-chamber pacing systems, dual-chamber systems, and rate-adaptive devices. The pacemaker clinic, in which most patient follow-up occurs, represents an organized effort to assess normal or abnormal pacemaker function. It has been suggested that pacemaker malfunction can be detected by the clinical history and electrocardiography in more than 95 per cent of patients.[29, 33] It is probably safe to suggest that at the present time the addition of telemetry, transtelephonic monitoring, and ambulatory electrocardiographic monitoring will detect the other few per cent of malfunction cases.

GENERAL PRINCIPLES

Pacemaker follow-up begins at the time the pacing system is implanted and continues until the patient dies or the system is removed. It has been estimated that 1 in every 500 persons in the United States has an implanted pacing system and that approximately 90,000 new implantations are performed each year.[33] Virtually all practicing cardiologists are asked to evaluate patients with pacemakers from time to time, and physicians in all specialties care for these patients. The complexity of pacing systems and their interactions with the patient

has grown rapidly, making it difficult for physicians not specializing in pacing therapy to evaluate system function adequately.

A recent survey of cardiac pacing practices in the United States found that over half of new pacing system implants were for sinus node dysfunction.[33] Because of this indication, failure of a pacemaker system is rarely catastrophic. The major function of a pacemaker follow-up clinic is to detect pacing system malfunction before symptoms develop. Several published reports have demonstrated that careful and intensive follow-up can accomplish this function.[20, 29, 34, 35] Moreover, with the use of thorough troubleshooting techniques, only 11 to 27 per cent of patients who are found to have significant malfunction during follow-up are symptomatic. In a highly organized and experienced follow-up clinic, 64 per cent of patients with serious pacemaker malfunction are able to be treated electively, versus only 10 per cent of patients not participating in an intensive program.[34]

Adequate follow-up is not provided by any single method, but by a combination of techniques. Transtelephonic monitoring can be performed inexpensively, relatively easily, and often. The accuracy of telephone monitoring with electrocardiographic capability is unquestioned for detection of battery depletion, most pacing and sensing problems, and intercurrent arrhythmias.[16] However, direct physician-patient interaction is imperative to produce maximal system longevity and function and to minimize complications. Therefore, the frequency and type of follow-up varies according to the medical condition of the patient and the age and performance characteristics of the pacing systems.[21]

The objectives of a follow-up program are as follows:

1. To maximize pacing system longevity.
2. To predict impending pacing system failure.
3. To determine and correct malfunctions.
4. To maximize system performance to meet the patient's needs.
5. To minimize medical complications from the implanted system.
6. To educate and support the patient.

Even before implantation, the procedure for outpatient follow-up should begin. Education of the patient and family is particularly important,[19] as it serves to allay the anxiety almost all patients feel when they learn they will need a pacing system. Education regarding how the pacemaker works, how it interacts with the environment (for instance, with microwave ovens and airport security alerts) and how the environment may interact with it, and the procedures necessary for adequate follow-up (including pulse checks when indicated, notation of symptoms, and techniques of telephone monitoring) will greatly facilitate the care of the patient.

For patients to be adequately followed, an excellent record-keeping system needs to be in place. Accurate and complete records of the patient's demographic data as well as information regarding the pulse generator, lead (or leads), and sensors, where appropriate, and the implantation sensing and pacing parameters must be obtained. This information should be kept in a file separate from the hospital record. At the time of each follow-up contact, either by telephone or in the office or clinic, this information is updated; the clinic record thus becomes invaluable as a history of the patient and the pacing system. When this information is placed into the general medical chart, either hospital or office, it becomes diluted and difficult to find. The easy access to, and retrieval of, pulse generator and lead serial numbers may prove vital in the management of recalls.[28]

Patients with uncomplicated new pacing system implants are usually discharged from the hospital in 2 to 3 days. Recently, however, data have been collected that suggest that a 24-hour hospitalization might be adequate.[22]

TABLE 10–1. BASIC PROGRAMMABLE FEATURES OF CARDIAC PACEMAKERS*

1. Low rate limit (standby rate)
2. Atrioventricular interval (AVI) (interval between paced or sensed P wave and ensuing ventricular stimulus output)
3. Energy output (current, voltage, pulse duration)
4. Refractory period (atrial, ventricular)
5. Blanking period (ultrashort interval in ventricular circuit during which no electrical signal can be sensed)
6. Mode of function
7. Hysteresis interval (interval between last spontaneous depolarization and first paced depolarization)
8. Upper rate limit
9. Maximal atrial tracking interval (shortest interval at which ventricular pacing will occur following sensed P waves in 1:1 relationship)
10. Ventricular pacing response at upper rate limit
11. Pacemaker-mediated tachycardia-terminating algorithm (if available)
12. Sensor parameters

*The types and ranges of these features will vary with the pulse generator.

At the time of implant, the pulse generator is programmed to appropriate settings, depending upon intraoperative measurements of sensing and pacing thresholds in atria and ventricle and the integrity of sinus and atrioventricular (AV) nodal function (Table 10–1). With dual-chamber units, 24-hour ambulatory ECG monitoring is often performed before discharge, and the unit is reprogrammed as needed.[24] The newer rate-adaptive units require at least one monitored exercise evaluation to program intelligently for maximal benefit to the patient.[4]

At discharge of the patient, a 12-lead electrocardiogram is obtained (preferably using electrocardiographic equipment that displays three channels simultaneously) in the free-running and magnet modes for future reference. The morphology of paced QRS complexes provides clues to lead position. The usual position of a transvenous pacing catheter results in pacing from the right ventricular apical area, producing a paced QRS complex having a superior axis and a left bundle branch block configuration. The bundle branch block pattern may be atypical, especially when active- or passive-fixation leads are used. However, a right bundle branch block pattern with right ventricular pacing is usually abnormal; it can occur when the lead has been positioned in the distal coronary sinus, when the right ventricular free wall or distal interventricular septum has been penetrated, if the lead has entered the left ventricle through a patent foramen ovale, or rarely with normal right ventricular septal pacing. Left ventricular pacing from the epicardium produces a right bundle branch block pattern having a variable mean frontal plane QRS axis, depending on the relationship of cathodal and anodal electrodes. Precise localization of atrial pacing leads is often not possible, since the frontal plane P-wave axis depends both on the electrode location and on the pathway of atrial activation.

In most units, the interstimulus interval, in either the free-running or the magnet mode, is a reliable indicator of battery status; thus, it needs to be accurately measured and recorded soon after implantation. A precision digital counter capable of measuring intervals to the nearest 0.1 beat per minute is mandatory. In some units, a 3 to 5 per cent decline in base pacing rate indicates the need for replacement, whereas in others, a decline in magnet rate is the end-of-life indicator. These small changes in rate over the service life of a pulse generator are impossible to detect by means other than with the digital counter.

Good-quality, highly penetrated chest radiographs in the posteroanterior and lateral views should also be obtained prior to discharge to document lead and pulse generator location as well as to rule out any unrecognized implantation complication, such as pneumothorax. On predischarge radiographs, we have seen large pneumothoraces requiring chest tube insertion that were undetected on the radiographs taken with the portable machine just after implantation.

Immediately before discharge, the implanting physician must check the wound for proper healing and for the presence of hematoma. It has been our practice to close pocket incisions with absorbable subcutaneous suture material and then "butterfly" the skin margins. In the large experience with cephalic vein cutdown for lead introduction, pocket hematoma is rare unless the patient is anticoagulated or is taking aspirin. In most cases, the introducer technique is utilized for lead placement. Although an increased number of pocket hematomas have been reported with this technique, they occur in less than 1 per cent of our patients. When they do occur, unless they are large and interfere with wound healing problems, they are managed by careful observation only.

After discharge, the patients can be followed by telephone monitoring every 2 weeks for 4 to 6 weeks. At that time, the patients should be seen for the first time in the clinic. Unless the patient has a return of symptoms, the visit usually consists of the following:

1. General history since the time of discharge.

2. Examination of the generator pocket with attention to wound healing, hematoma resolution, and evidence of venous thrombosis, infection, or erosion.

3. Twelve-lead electrocardiogram in the free-running and magnet modes (three channels simultaneously recorded is optimal).

4. Electronic rate and pulse width evaluation using the digital counter.

5. Pacing and sensing threshold evaluation.

6. Evaluation for retrograde ventriculo-atrial (VA) conduction.

7. Interrogation of the device to confirm programmed values if the unit is capable.

8. Evaluation of intracardiac electrograms if the unit is capable (Fig. 10–1).

9. Evaluation of other telemetered data, such as lead impedance, if the unit is capable (Fig. 10–1).

10. Evaluation of other stored information, such as rate histograms, in those rate-adaptive units with this capability.

During this first outpatient evaluation, no attempt is made to reprogram generator output for maximal longevity. If any output programming is performed, it is to provide a maximal safety margin for pacing. Although the present generation of electrodes does not appear to have the severe, acute rise in pacing threshold that characterized earlier lead systems, we believe that any battery life saved over the first 6 months does not warrant the potential risk to the patient.

It should always be remembered that during reprogramming most, if not all, pulse generators manufactured today can be programmed to nonphysiologic levels of function. Misprogramming and failure to program can occur. It is therefore imperative that after a programming sequence an electrocardiographic rhythm strip, as well as data regarding pacing rate and pacing impulse duration and any telemetry data that are available, should be obtained.

From this visit until the sixth month after implantation, the patient can be followed by telephone every 4–8 weeks if he or she has a single-chamber non–rate-adaptive unit and every 4 weeks if he or she has a dual-chamber or single-chamber rate-adaptive unit. At 6 months, the patient usually has a second clinic visit. At this visit, all of the procedures of the first visit are repeated, and two are added:

1. The output of the unit is programmed for maximal longevity of the unit and maximal

Pacesetter Systems, Inc.
A Siemens Company © 1986,88
APS: Version 3032 - 0227

[PaRaGON]

Jan 27 1989 2:34 pm
MODEL: 2010   SERIAL: 12891

PATIENT: _____

PHYSICIAN: _____

PROGRAMMED PARAMETERS		
Mode	DDD	
Rate	55	ppm
A-V Delay	175	msec
Max Track	135	ppm
Vent. Pulse Config.	BIPOLAR	
V. Pulse Width	.6	msec
V. Pulse Amplitude	4.0	Volts
V. Sense Config.	BIPOLAR	
V. Sensitivity	2.0	mVolts
V. Refractory	325	msec
Atr. Pulse Config.	BIPOLAR	
A. Pulse Width	.6	msec
A. Pulse Amplitude	4.0	Volts
A. Sense Config.	BIPOLAR	
A. Sensitivity	1.0	mVolts
A. Refractory	350	msec
Blanking	25	msec
V. Safety Option	ENABLE	
PVC Options	+PVARP ON PVC	
PMT Options	127 BEATS >135	
Rate Resp. A-V Delay	ENABLE	
Magnet	TEMPORARY OFF	

MEASURED DATA		
Pacer Rate	55.5	ppm
Ventricular:		
Pulse Amplitude	4.1	Volts
Pulse Current	6.7	mAmperes
Pulse Energy	14	μJoules
Pulse Charge	4	μCoulombs
Lead Impedance	609	Ohms
Atrial:		
Pulse Amplitude	4.0	Volts
Pulse Current	8.8	mAmperes
Pulse Energy	17	μJoules
Pulse Charge	5	μCoulombs
Lead Impedance	460	Ohms
Battery Data: (W.G. 8077 - NOM. 1.8 AHR)		
Voltage	2.86	Volts
Current	20	μAmperes
Impedance	< 1	KOhms

Figure 10–1. Print-out of telemetered data from the Pacesetter Paragon (Pacesetter Systems, Inc., Sylmar, CA). Programmed data describe how the pacemaker was set to perform; measured data indicate how it is, in fact, performing at the time of interrogation. The pulse amplitude, available in both sets of data, should be comparable. Battery data are obtained directly from the power source. Telemetered information varies with the generator manufacturer.

safety of the patient. In voltage output units, a safety margin of 2.0:1 to 2.5:1 is selected. That is, if the pacing threshold in a chamber is measured to be 1.0 V, then the output of the unit is programmed to 2.0 to 2.5 V.

2. In patients with rate-adaptive units, either single-chamber or dual-chamber, an ex-

ercise test should be performed to optimize programming of rate response and to eliminate (in DDD systems) pacing-induced tachyarrhythmias.

All patients are then usually followed by telephone every 8 weeks until the thirty-sixth month after implantation and then every 4 weeks until replacement. Every patient should be seen at least every 6 months in clinic; in many instances, however, only an annual visit may be required, especially if the patient is clinically stable and has adequate medical followup. Unless symptoms develop, the clinic procedure is as outlined for the first visit.

The patient should carry an identification card that specifies the name of the manufacturer; pulse generator model and serial number; lead type, model, and serial number; and the telephone number of the patient's cardiologist. This card, provided to the patient by the manufacturer, specifies certain factory set ("nominal") parameters; since these are likely to be different from the current programmed values, the card must reflect the changes. If the identification card is not up to date, erroneous judgment of pacemaker function or malfunction can be made. For example, a low programmed pacing rate may be misdiagnosed as battery depletion. If the patient has a device that is capable of telemetry, it is wise to provide him or her with a print-out of the most recently programmed information to carry along with the identification card. We also suggest to the patient that he or she carry a copy of the paced electrocardiogram so that any suspicious morphologic features can be compared with a baseline record.

TELEPHONE MONITORING

As the total number of pacemaker patients has grown, it has become harder to follow each patient sufficiently with face-to-face contact. Telephone monitoring, with electrocardiographic capability, has become the most useful and cost-effective technique to follow large numbers of patients over a long period.

The functions of telephone monitoring are as follows:

1. To detect pacing system malfunctions before the patient becomes symptomatic.

2. To detect pulse generator battery depletion before failure of output, possibly with catastrophic results, occurs.

3. To detect intercurrent arrhythmias.

4. To provide technical support for facilities without interest or expertise.

5. To provide follow-up for patients who

cannot travel to a medical facility for regular visits.

Transtelephonic transmission of electrocardiograms is now the standard of care. The pulse generator stimulus either is transmitted directly or, more often, is transmitted as an interruption of the signal. In either case, electronic rate determination can be very accurately determined and displayed. At least 30 seconds of recordings should be made.

High-quality transmission and reception of electrocardiograms is easy to achieve, even with the most inexpensive equipment. However, transtelephonic electrocardiogram transmission can lead to interpretive difficulties and can display artifacts that are similar to those encountered with conventional electrocardiography (Figs. 10–2 and 10–3). A few artifacts are unique to transtelephonic monitoring. The most potentially serious, because interpretive errors can be made, is that created by the use of a single-lead rhythm strip, usually lead I, in which the paced QRS complexes or the pacemaker artifact itself may be isoelectric or otherwise insufficiently diagnostic (Fig. 10–2). Another lead should be selected and the transmission repeated, and this lead system should be used in future transmissions. Telephone noise is frequently picked up from continuous interference and electrical transients; both are generally readily identified as such. Motion artifacts are frequent and are also usually recognizable as such. Troublesome 60-Hz inter-

ference can exist with all systems, although the pacing stimulus and the electrocardiogram can usually be discriminated. Positioning of the magnet over the generator can cause a variety of artifacts, including transient inhibition of the pulse generator due to changing magnetic fields. Respiratory movement is recognized by a rhythmic oscillation of the baseline.

Dual-chamber transtelephonic monitoring is more complex. Some dual-chamber telephonically monitored electrocardiograms are extremely difficult to read (Fig. 10–3), and equipment for interpretation is not as widely available as for single-chamber devices. The increasing use of dual-chamber pacemakers makes monitoring of those devices important despite the associated difficulties. Nevertheless, the transtelephonic electrocardiogram can readily diagnose pacing system malfunctions as well as arrhythmias not associated with the system.[25] Several manufacturers now produce pulse generators with magnet-activated automatic threshold determination that can be evaluated by telephone. Others manufacture units that, upon application of the magnet, increase their rates, shorten their AV intervals, and sense a spontaneous ventricular depolarization if it occurs during the AV interval and then inhibit their ventricular output. The physician overreading or receiving the summary data from the telephone monitoring service must be thoroughly familiar with the response to magnet application of each device implanted in the clinic population. However, no matter how

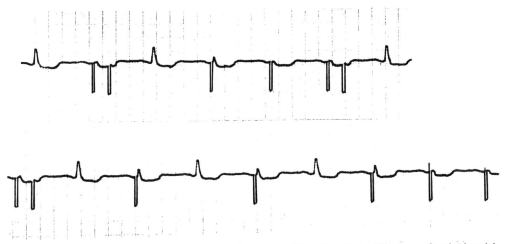

Figure 10–2. Rhythm strips from a transtelephonic monitor, illustrating the inability to confirm both atrial and ventricular capture in a patient with normal sinus rhythm and a DDD pacing system. Where the atrial output stimulus is followed by the ventricular output stimulus, the resulting myocardial depolarizations are each isoelectric to the baseline, and their morphology cannot be discerned. Aside from the atrioventricular (AV) intervals, the AA, VV, and VA times are not clear. A rhythm strip during magnet application would help to confirm the intervals, but verification of capture would still be problematic.

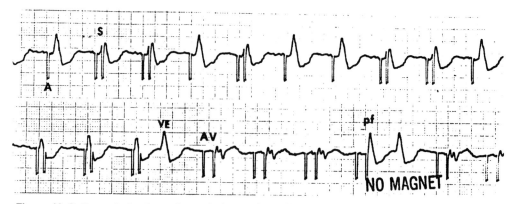

Figure 10–3. Transtelephonic monitor strip in a patient with a DDD pacing system, illustrating some of the difficulties in interpretation. Atrial capture (A) is *never* satisfactorily seen. Ventricular capture is occurring in the bottom strip (AV) at an AV interval of about 200 msec. The paced QRS complexes have an RS morphology. That the very broad, pure R-wave complexes are not paced is confirmed by the occurrence of these complexes in the bottom strip where they are not preceded by pacing artifacts. They are ventricular extrasystoles (VE). Frequent atrial and ventricular pacing artifacts occur at short AV intervals; each of these has the initial portion of a spontaneous QRS complex just within the latter portion of the AV interval. These short AV intervals represent "safety pacing" (S), or the triggering of the ventricular output stimulus at the end of a nonphysiologic AV interval within which a ventricular signal is sensed. The "safety pace" interval is usually in the range of about 110 msec. Finally, some output pulses occur 80 msec prior to the wide, pure R-wave QRS complexes. That these stimuli are not pacing the ventricle is concluded both from their appropriate timing for atrial output delivery and by the morphology of the following broad QRS complex, which has been explained as resulting from its extrasystolic origin. A single pseudo fusion (pf) complex is seen. (Tracing courtesy of Bonnie Sudduth, RN, PA.)

sophisticated this form of follow-up becomes, it does not substitute for patient-physician contact.

The greatest limitation of this technique is the patient. Although most of the transmission devices are simple to use, it must be emphasized that the majority of paced patients are elderly. Hearing, memory impairment, and technical facilities in the home environment may be sufficiently compromised to make follow-up impossible.[11]

Concern is often expressed regarding the potential danger of applying the magnet to pacing systems during telephone transmissions. Pacemaker-induced premature ventricular depolarizations do occur but are almost never sustained (Fig. 10–4); only rarely do multiple extrasystoles require cessation of the use of the magnet. We have never documented an episode of ventricular fibrillation or sustained ventricular tachycardia produced with a magnet in this setting. Pacemaker-mediated tachycardia is occasionally induced in patients with DDD systems; however, termination is usually easily accomplished by reapplication and removal of the magnet. We have seen as many

VOO

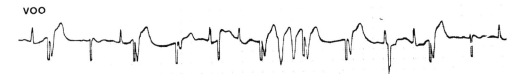

Figure 10–4. VOO pacing during transtelephonic monitoring. A burst of repetitive ventricular beating is caused by a pacing stimulus falling about 430 msec after the previous spontaneous QRS complex, well after the peak of the T wave. The burst is terminated by the delivery of the next pacing stimulus. Sustained, repetitive beating is not expected to occur in the outpatient setting and is more common in acutely ischemic patients and in those with electrolyte disorders or antiarrhythmic drug toxicity. Note also the duration of the inscribed pacing artifact, which is long at about 40 msec. The second, fourth, and eleventh pacing stimuli produce fusion complexes (note their intermediate configuration between the pure sinus-generated QRS complex and the pure paced complex), which are isoelectric to the baseline, making interpretation potentially difficult or erroneous.

cases of magnet-terminated pacemaker-induced tachycardia as we have seen the opposite.

THE PACEMAKER CLINIC VISIT

The function of direct contact with the patient who has a pacing system has changed in the past two decades. Initially, a patient was examined, chest radiographs and electrocardiograms were obtained, and a waveform analysis of pulse generator output was obtained. Today, pulse generators have become more sophisticated, so that clinic visits are more complicated and time consuming.

A general history and physical examination should be performed. The patient should be specifically questioned about symptoms reflecting diminished cerebral perfusion or cardiac output. A return of symptoms similar to those existing prior to pacing system implantation may suggest pacing system malfunction or development of the pacemaker syndrome[34, 35] (see Chapter 6). However, such symptomatology may be nonspecific and attributable to other etiologies, especially in elderly patients. The patient should be directly questioned about symptoms occurring during use of the ipsilateral extremity, which could reflect myopotential oversensing (Table 10–2) (see Chapter 12). Awareness of pacing may not reflect untoward

TABLE 10–2. CLASSIFICATION OF PACEMAKER MALFUNCTION OR APPARENT MALFUNCTION

1. Failure to capture when myocardial tissue is not refractory
   a. Electrode displacement (dislodgment, retraction, myocardial penetration or perforation)
   b. Power source depletion (expected end of life, unanticipated end of life, sudden failure of output)
   c. Increased myocardial stimulation threshold
   d. Lead fracture
   e. Insulation break
   f. Inappropriate (subthreshold) programmed energy output
2. No pacing stimulus observed when generator is not inhibited by native rhythm
   a. Power source depletion (end of life)
   b. Pulse generator component failure
   c. Incomplete circuit (e.g., lead fracture)
   d. Improper (loose) connection of lead to generator
   e. Oversensing
3. Failure to sense (undersensing)
   a. Inadequate intracardiac signal
   b. Power source depletion (end of life)
   c. Pulse generator component failure
   d. Lead fracture
   e. Poor electrode-myocardial interface
   f. Inappropriate programmed sensitivity

problems, or it may be due to pectoral muscle stimulation resulting from lead insulation break or to diaphragmatic muscle stimulation caused by proximity of the ventricular lead tip to the diaphragm. A history of weakness, breathlessness, diminished effort tolerance, orthostatic symptoms, or perception of venous pulsations (cannon waves) in the neck should suggest the presence of the pacemaker syndrome, which is produced by the loss of AV synchrony and atrial contribution to stroke volume and by atrially mediated vasodepressor reflexes (see Chapter 6). Palpitations may be caused by the perception of spontaneous extrasystoles or tachycardias; by inappropriately programmed rate-modulated devices in which the paced rate is not compatible with the patient's activity level; by competitive rhythms caused by sensing malfunction; by hysteresis; and by pacemaker-mediated tachycardias. Pain over the generator pocket may signify improper pocket size, erosion, or infection. Penetration of ventricular myocardium might be suspected if there is a history of chest pain suggestive of pericarditis, hiccups, and diaphragmatic pulsations. However, these symptoms may be unassociated with lead penetration or may result from high stimulus output energy.

During the physical examination, a thorough assessment of the wound, pocket, and area overlying the lead (or leads) should be performed. The unit should be freely moveable, and the overlying skin should be of normal color. Evaluation of the pacemaker pocket for signs of infection, such as pain, swelling, or erythema, which usually occur within the first 6 months of implantation, is required. If infection is suspected, the wound should be irrigated and cultures obtained. To obtain cultures, the skin is cleansed and painted with antiseptic solution (iodine is preferred), and a needle is directed to the pulse generator. The passage of the needle will be stopped by the generator itself, and it will lie in a potential space around the generator. A syringe filled with normal saline (taken from an intravenous infusion packet rather than from solutions used to dilute medications, since these contain bacteriostatic preservatives and will defeat attempts at culture) should be used to irrigate the pacer site. The fluid is then cultured for aerobic and anaerobic organisms. Detection of pocket infection mandates immediate antibiotic therapy to avoid explantation of the pulse generator and leads.[8]

In patients who have VVI pulse generators,

the jugular venous pulsations should be examined for the presence of cannon A waves reflecting atrial contraction against closed AV valves, since loss of AV synchrony is implicated in the genesis of the pacemaker syndrome. Swelling or suffusion of the ipsilateral extremity, neck, or face indicates venous obstruction.[16, 27] Although the subclavian vein is most often involved, the superior vena cava syndrome, with edema of the chest wall and dilatation of superficial collaterals, can occur. Venous thrombosis requires anticoagulation, usually with heparin followed by sodium warfarin (Coumadin); oral anticoagulation is occasionally needed indefinitely. Thrombolysis using streptokinase has also been reported.[28] Rarely, recurrent pulmonary embolism from thrombosis involving the pacing lead will result in the physical findings of pulmonary hypertension.[39] Even more rarely, intracardiac thrombosis around the pacing lead can cause signs of right ventricular failure[32] or constrictive pericarditis.[15]

Cardiac auscultation may reveal a "pacemaker sound" occurring after delivery of the output stimulus that is possibly due to intercostal muscle or diaphragmatic contraction or to myocardial penetration[26]; variable intensity of the first heart sound (due to the variable relationships of atrial systole to ventricular depolarization in patients with VVI pacing systems and to variable AV or PR intervals in patients with dual-chamber pacing systems); a paradoxically split second heart sound (caused by the occurrence of right ventricular depolarization in advance of left ventricular depolarization, mimicking left bundle branch block); a widely split second heart sound during inspiration (due to the occurrence of left ventricular depolarization in advance of right ventricular depolarization in patients with left ventricular epicardial leads, mimicking right bundle branch block); systolic nonejection clicks, possibly caused by slapping of the lead against the tricuspid valve; systolic murmurs (due to hemodynamically insignificant tricuspid valve regurgitation); and a systolic "whoop" or musical murmur, thought to result from movement of the pacing lead within the right ventricular cavity.[7, 18, 30, 37] All of these auscultatory findings are benign, and not unexpected. They must be noted in the medical record, however, and any changes over time specifically looked for. Pacing system revision is virtually never indicated. A pericardial friction rub that develops early after pacing system implantation should suggest myocardial penetration; however, a friction rub of presumed endocardial origin, without evidence of myocardial penetration, has been reported.[18] Clinical evidence of hemodynamically significant pericardial effusion should be sought if a pericardial rub is present. Visible or palpable contractions of the pectoral muscles or diaphragm that occur at the pacing rate should be noted, as they might signify lead insulation defect or too high a generator output for the patient.

The existence of the pacemaker syndrome, suspected from the clinical history, can be confirmed by demonstrating fluctuations in peripheral blood pressure, including orthostatic changes, finding cannon A waves in the jugular venous waves, and hearing the murmurs of AV valve regurgitation. Occasionally, findings of left- and right-sided congestive heart failure may also be present; if they have developed for the first time only after pacing system implantation, they may be assumed to be due to the pacemaker syndrome.

Documentation of myopotential inhibition of pacer output in single-chamber systems, or triggering of pacemaker-mediated tachycardia in dual-chamber ones (see Chapters 10 and 12), requires the provocation of pectoral muscle activity by raising a weight, pulling, or vigorously pressing the hands together (Fig. 10–5). These maneuvers should be performed while the patient is being electrocardiographically monitored; symptoms may or may not occur or be reproduced. Myopotential inhibition and triggering should be specifically sought in patients with unipolar pacing systems, or in those programmed to unipolar configuration, because of the relatively high prevalence of myopotential inhibition and triggering in these circumstances.[36]

A 12-lead electrocardiogram, with and without application of the magnet, should then be performed. The electrocardiograph machine should be an analog writer to avoid errors in interpreting changes in stimulus artifact amplitude and vector, which are often recorded on digitized signal machines and which could lead to an erroneous diagnosis of lead fracture (Figs. 10–6 and 10–7). The electrocardiographic equipment should be checked regularly to avoid "pseudomalfunction" secondary to mechanical problems, such as erratic paper speed. Electrocardiograms should be recorded during performance of the isometric exercises to reveal myopotential inhibition of generator output and during manipulation of the pulse generator within the pocket to elicit a partial lead fracture.

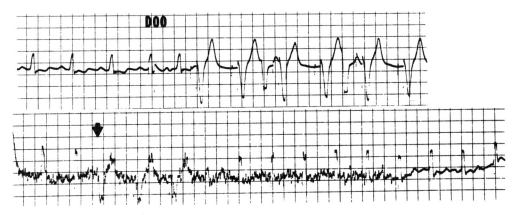

Figure 10–5. *Top*, Onset of DOO pacing shown to illustrate the native P-QRS complexes and the paced ventricular complexes. *Bottom*, A short-lived run of three paced QRS complexes and one fusion complex occurring at the upper rate limit *(arrow)* is triggered by atrial sensing of myopotentials during isometric exercise. Pacemaker-mediated tachycardia did not occur. Reprogramming was not considered necessary.

Testing of the pacing thresholds of the ventricle or atrium, or both, is then performed under electrocardiographic monitoring. Application of the magnet over the pacemaker generator eliminates sensing and results in the asynchronous delivery of pacing stimuli. Magnet application to devices of different manufacturers can produce a variable initial response (e.g., several output pulses at a given rate) prior to pacing at the magnet rate. Variability in response upon removal of the magnet also occurs. Moving a magnet in proximity to some pulse generators can result in changing magnetic fields, with consequent inhibition of pacer output.[38] In VDD and DDD pacing systems, magnet application can cause dissociation between spontaneous sinus depolarizations and paced ventricular rhythm; if ret-

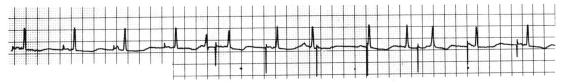

Figure 10–6. AOO pacing using a digital electrocardiograph (ECG) machine. Note the changing amplitude and vector of the atrial output stimuli, caused by the signal processing by the equipment. The pacing output stimulus represents a narrow burst of energy in the time domain that corresponds to a wide frequency in the frequency domain. This signal will be suboptimally sampled by the fixed nyquist sampling rate. The digital reconstruction of the signal in the time doman will contain aliasing artifact, which causes the variation in the amplitude and polarity of the signal, as displayed on the ECG machine.

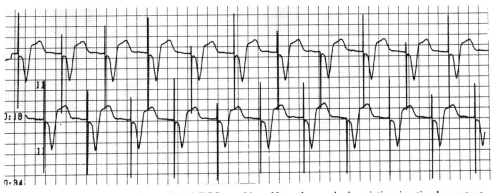

Figure 10–7. VVI pacing using a digital ECG machine. Note the marked variation in stimulus output amplitude and vector.

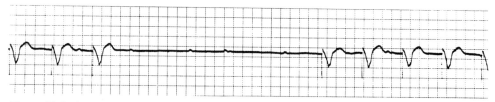

Figure 10–8. Assessment of underlying rhythm and rate by chest wall stimulation in a 48-year-old patient paced for sinus node dysfunction. During chest wall stimulation, stimuli from an external pulse generator are delivered to the body surface through skin monitoring electrodes; these stimuli are sensed by the implanted electrodes and inhibit the implanted unit. In this example, pacemaker dependence is illustrated by the pause in QRS rhythm of nearly 5 seconds despite irregular atrial activity. (The artifacts of the chest wall stimuli are not well seen owing to their very low current [< 0.5 mA].)

rograde VA conduction results, pacemaker-mediated tachycardia can ensue when the magnet is removed. Asynchronous pacing can result in delivery of stimuli in the vulnerable period of the atrium or ventricle, with resulting repetitive rhythms such as atrial fibrillation and ventricular tachycardia.[3, 10, 40] However, arrhythmias due to magnet application are rare, a fact substantiated by the vast experience with transtelephonic monitoring and magnet placement by the patient.

If the patient is not pacer dependent (Fig. 10–8), a 12-lead electrocardiogram of his or her native rhythm should be recorded to document its origin and rate and to follow the natural history of the rhythm for which the pacing system was originally implanted.

In patients with dual-chamber pacing systems who do not have atrial arrhythmias, the presence of retrograde VA conduction should be sought by programming the device to the VVI mode of function and observing inverted P waves in electrocardiographic leads II, III, or aV$_F$ at several ventricular paced rates. The RP interval should be determined to program an appropriate atrial refractory period (see Chapters 10 and 12). Proclivity to pacemaker-mediated tachycardia can be evaluated by causing AV dyssynchrony followed by ventricular pacing (see Chapter 10).

It should be stressed that these evaluations do not always predict actual occurrences; ambulatory electrocardiographic monitoring is a far more sensitive technique for detecting many of these pacemaker-related problems.

Testing of the sensing thresholds of the ventricle or atrium, or both, is then done (Tables 10–2 and 10–3) under electrocardiographic monitoring. Finally, interrogation of the pulse generator's telemetry capabilities is performed.

Telemetry refers to the transmission of data stored within the pulse generator through the programmer to a receiver. At the present time, telemetry of programmed information, data measured directly from the generator itself, and intracardiac electrograms detected by the implanted electrodes can be transmitted. Programmed information refers to those functional parameters, such as mode of operation, that are capable of being altered (Table 10–1) and their present settings (see Fig. 10–1). Measured data, being recorded from the unit itself, indicate pulse generator performance at the time of the interrogation (see Fig. 10–1). The free-running and magnet rates, lead impedance, and actual stimulus output energy, charge, current, and voltage can be measured. Power source information is available, including impedance offered by the battery cell itself, voltage, and current drain. The battery imped-

TABLE 10–3. CAUSES OF PACEMAKER OVERSENSING

1. Physiologic intracardiac signals
   a. T-wave sensing in VVI mode
   b. P-wave sensing in VVI mode
   c. R-wave sensing in AAI mode
2. Extracardiac myopotentials
   a. Pectoral muscles
   b. Diaphragm
3. Electromagnetic interference
   a. Magnetic resonance imaging
   b. Microwave transmission
   c. Electrocautery
   d. Arc welding
   e. Lithotripsy
4. Pacing system itself
   1. Afterpotential sensing (sensing of generator voltage output decay)
   b. "False" signals
      i. Partial lead fracture
      ii. Intermittent contact of metal parts (e.g., two leads)
      iii. Incomplete lead generator circuit (loose connection)
      iv. Magnet application (positioning or removal leading to changing magnetic fields)
      v. Electrolysis of dissimilar metals in lead electrodes
   c. Crosstalk

ance rises over time and may prove useful, along with rate changes, as an end-of-life indicator.[6] Interpretation of changes in these measurements is extremely helpful in the management or anticipation of pacemaker-related problems. For example, a low lead impedance should suggest the possibility of insulation break or a short circuit in a bipolar lead; a high impedance might indicate lead fracture or loose connections between lead and pulse generator.

Some pulse generators can transmit information regarding actual pacemaker use held in memory. The percentage of sensed and paced depolarizations in the atrium and ventricle over a specific period can thus be known, allowing programming (usually of rate or AV interval or both) for optimal function. The number of times the upper rate limit has been reached is also available in some devices, again affording the clinician a means of optimizing patient-device interaction. It is expected that longer-term monitored data, including sensor function in rate-adaptive units, will soon be available.

In patients without symptoms, it is not our policy to reprogram all of the functions of the generator at each clinic visit. Reprogramming of output and sensitivity is performed only if this is the sole means to evaluate pacing and sensing thresholds. With direct telemetry of lead impedance and pulse generator stimulus information, there is no longer need to record the stimulus artifact from surface electrocardiographic information.

Intracardiac electrograms and marker channel information provide extremely useful data.[9] Electrograms provide a direct indication of the quality of the information the pulse generator is receiving from the patient. In cases of possible malfunction, this information is often invaluable. As pulse generators have become more complex, particularly dual-chamber units, the paced electrocardiogram has become extremely difficult to analyze. Unless a physician has continuous exposure to all of the electrocardiograms of each unit, assistance from pacemaker generator markers is always of use.

The endocardial electrogram is the atrial and ventricular electrical signal "seen" by the electrodes, which are usually in contact with the endocardium (Figs. 10–9 to 10–11). Telemetered electrograms provide the magnitude and configuration of these sensed signals; programming of optimal sensitivity can be based upon such information. Since this technique is relatively new, there are few data regarding the

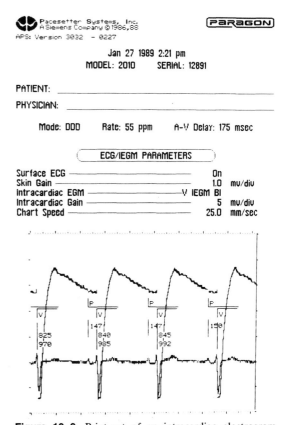

Figure 10–9. Print-out of an intracardiac electrogram recorded from the ventricular electrode, with its corresponding, simultaneously recorded surface electrocardiogram (ECG) in a Pacesetter Paragon pacing system. Whenever feasible, the surface ECG should be recorded with the intracardiac electrogram to relate the events. It is often also advisable to record a surface ECG on a separate ECG machine, on which the surface events may be displayed more clearly. In this example, the intracardiac signal is recorded from a bipolar electrode configuration ("V IEGM BI"); it could also have been recorded from a unipolar configuration, had this been programmed. These capabilities will vary with the manufacturer. Note also that the calibration of the electrogram is provided and can itself be programmed larger or smaller, depending on the amplitude of the electrogram. In this example, marker channel information is available. The designations P and V refer to spontaneous atrial and paced ventricular events, respectively. The numbers refer to the calculated intervals between the sensed or paced atrial and ventricular events and the atrial and ventricular refractory periods.

evolution of the sensed signal over time, or its configurational changes if lead dislodgment or myocardial penetration occurs; however, this information should soon become available as this capability is increasingly used.

Marker channels provide annotated information regarding refractory periods and sensed and paced atrial and ventricular electrical events and the intervals between them (Figs. 10–9 to 10–11). If a surface electrocardiogram is simultaneously telemetered along with

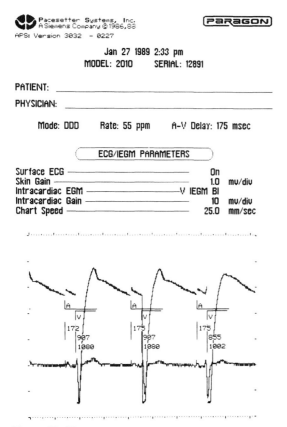

Pacesetter Systems, Inc.
A Siemens Company © 1986,88
APS: Version 3032 — 0227

PARAGON

Jan 27 1989 2:33 pm
MODEL: 2010   SERIAL: 12891

PATIENT: _____
PHYSICIAN: _____

Mode: DDD   Rate: 55 ppm   A-V Delay: 175 msec

ECG/IEGM PARAMETERS

Surface ECG ———————————————— On
Skin Gain ———————————————————— 1.0   mv/div
Intracardiac EGM ———————————— V IEGM BI
Intracardiac Gain ———————————— 10   mv/div
Chart Speed ———————————————— 25.0   mm/sec

Figure 10–10. In this example, AV sequential pacing is occurring at an AV interval of 175 msec.

marker channel information, electrocardiographic interpretation of sensing and pacing function can be facilitated.

Far-field signals that inhibit or trigger pacemaker function can be identified, as can atrial depolarizations that cannot be detected on the surface electrocardiogram (such as retrogradely conducted P waves occurring within the QRST complexes).

DEALING WITH THE PATIENT WHO HAS RETURN OF SYMPTOMS

The most challenging aspect of pacemaker follow-up may be the evaluation of the patient whose symptoms return. In medium- to large-sized practices, roughly 10 per cent of patients with pacing systems will experience what they feel is a return of preimplantation symptoms.[23] Usually, this return of symptoms is unaccompanied by overt evidence of system malfunction. One third of these patients will be found to have a pacing system malfunction, with the remaining two thirds having cardiovascular symptoms unrelated to the pacing system.[14]

Although much has been written about the pacemaker syndrome,[2] we have not encountered this as a major cause of return of symptoms, although it is clear that in a minority of patients it can produce severe symptoms.[1, 12] Because these symptoms (intermittent weakness, dizziness, precordial distress, and/or pounding in the neck and heart) are nonspecific, it is imperative that the symptoms be directly correlated with documented physiologic disturbances.

In general, the return of symptoms can be attributed to either the heart's not being stimulated at a rate adequate to maintain cardiac output or the heart's being stimulated too rapidly to maintain an adequate stroke volume. If the patient can identify an activity that produces the symptoms, this then becomes the easiest malfunction to diagnose. However, in the majority of cases, the patient cannot be specific about what is associated with the symptoms.

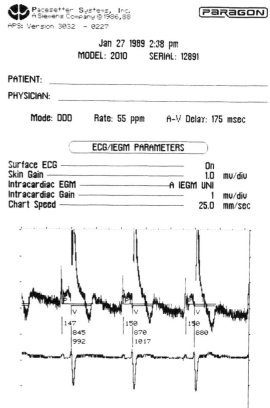

Pacesetter Systems, Inc.
A Siemens Company © 1986,88
APS: Version 3032 — 0227

PARAGON

Jan 27 1989 2:38 pm
MODEL: 2010   SERIAL: 12891

PATIENT: _____
PHYSICIAN: _____

Mode: DDD   Rate: 55 ppm   A-V Delay: 175 msec

ECG/IEGM PARAMETERS

Surface ECG ———————————————— On
Skin Gain ———————————————————— 1.0   mv/div
Intracardiac EGM ———————————— A IEGM UNI
Intracardiac Gain ———————————— 1   mv/div
Chart Speed ———————————————— 25.0   mm/sec

Figure 10–11. This intracardiac electrogram is recorded from the atrial electrode in unipolar configuration, simultaneously with the surface ECG. Although atrial signal magnitude can be accurately determined, the morphology of the signal cannot be seen owing to considerable signal distortion.

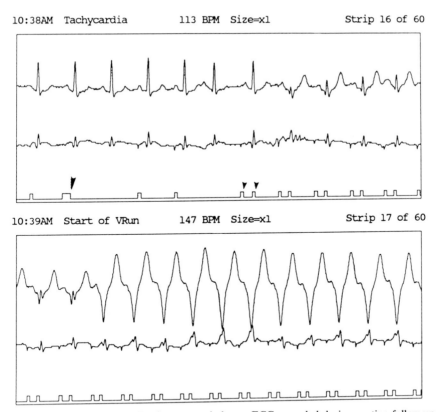

Figure 10–12. Selected rhythm strips from an ambulatory ECG recorded during routine follow-up of an asymptomatic patient who had a Pacesetter Sensolog (Pacesetter Systems, Inc., Sylmar, CA) implanted for malignant vasovagal syndrome. In this ambulatory ECG recording system (Zymed, Camarillo, CA), sensing of the leading and trailing edges of pacing output pulses results in the inscription of small deflections on the rhythm strip *(small arrows)*; a broad deflection *(large arrow)* signifies interference with sensing of the trailing edge of the pulses because of real or potential artifact, alerting the physician to a possible error in pacer spike data. In the top strip, atrial pacing is initially followed by conducted QRS complexes and, at the end of the strip, by ventricular fusion complexes. Since the low rate limit of the pacemaker was set at 65 per minute, this rhythm strip signifies atrial rate-adaptive pacing. In the bottom strip, DDDR pacing is occurring. The first two QRS complexes are fusion complexes (indicated by the annotation of the ventricular pacing pulse below the rhythm); the remainder are purely paced complexes resulting from enablement of the physiologic AV interval, which shortens as rate-adaptive paced atrial rate increases. Pacemaker-mediated tachycardia, with which this can be confused, is excluded by identifying the notated delivery of the atrial output pulse.

In one third of patients with unipolar pacing systems, pectoral muscle stimulation can inhibit the pulse generator.[31] However, of all those who can be inhibited, only one half will be symptomatic. Therefore, just because a patient has symptoms related to a slow heart rate and one can demonstrate inhibition of the generator by muscular activity, one should not automatically assume that the problem is due to myopotential inhibition.

In our experience and that of others, ambulatory electrocardiographic monitoring is the most effective means of correlating symptoms with pacing system function[5, 41] (Fig. 10–12). When one is faced with intermittent symptoms occurring with daily activity, there is no diagnostic technique that is as helpful.[13] Not only

willl this technique capture bradycardia, it also will clearly document the presence of tachycardias producing the symptoms.

In evaluating the patient, chest radiographs, radiographs of the pulse generator, and echocardiography may also be useful (see Chapter 11).

CONCLUSIONS

The complexity of pacing systems is growing at a rapid pace. Equipment that can modify the heart rate under many conditions is either available now or soon will be. The development of this technology will necessitate ever-increasing outpatient surveillance, not only to detect normal and abnormal pacemaker system function but also to optimize the interaction between the device and the patient. Only by doing so will the clinician be assured that the patient is well served.

REFERENCES

1. Alicandri C, Fouad F, Tarazi R: Three cases of hypotension and syncope with ventricular pacing: Possible role of atrial reflexes. Am J Cardiol 42:137–141, 1978.
2. Ausubel K, Furman S: The pacemaker syndrome. Ann Intern Med 103:420–429, 1985.
3. Barold SS, Gaidula JJ, Castillo R: Unusual response of demand pacemakers to magnets. Br Heart J 35:353–358, 1973.
4. Benditt D, Mianulli M, Fetter J: Single chamber cardiac pacing with activity-initiated chronotropic response: Evaluation by cardiopulmonary exercise testing. Circulation 75:185–191, 1987.
5. Breivik K, Ohm O: Myopotential inhibition of unipolar QRS-inhibited (VVI) pacemakers assessed by ambulatory Holter monitoring of the electrocardiogram. PACE 3:470–475, 1980.
6. Castellanet MJ, Garza J, Shaner SP, Messenger JC: Telemetry of programmed and measured data in pacing system evaluation and follow-up. J Electrophysiol 1:360–375, 1987.
7. Cheng TO, Ertem G, Vera Z: Heart sounds in patients with cardiac pacemakers. Chest 62:66–70, 1972.
8. Choo MH, Holmes DR Jr, Gersh BJ, et al: Permanent pacemaker infections: Characterization and management. Am J Cardiol 48:559–563, 1981.
9. Clarke M, Allen A: Use of telemetered electrograms in the assessment of normal pacemaker function. J Electrophysiol 1:388–395, 1987.
10. Cunningham TM: Incessant pacemaker vario operation. Am J Cardiol 61:656–657, 1988.
11. Dreifus L, Pennock R, Feldman M: Experience with 3835 pacemakers utilizing transtelephonic surveillance. Am J Cardiol 35:133–142, 1975.
12. Erlebacher J, Donner R, Stelzer P: Hypotension with ventricular pacing: An atrial vasodepressor reflex in human beings. J Am Coll Cardiol 4:550–558, 1984.
13. Famularo MA, Kennedy HL: Ambulatory electrocardiography in the assessment of pacemaker function. Am Heart J 104:1085–1094, 1982.
14. Fisher J, Escher D, Hurzeler P: Recurrent syncope or dizziness after pacemaker implantation. Clin Res 26:231A, 1978.
15. Foster CJ: Constrictive pericarditis complicating an endocardial pacemaker. Br Heart J 47:497–499, 1982.
16. Furman S: Pacemaker follow-up. In Barold S (ed): Modern Cardiac Pacing. Mount Kisco, NY, Futura Publishing Co, 1985, pp 889–919.
17. Furman S: Pacemaker follow-up. In Furman S, Hayes DL, Holmes DR Jr (ed): A Practice of Cardiac Pacing. Mount Kisco, NY, Futura Publishing Co, 1986, pp 379–412.
18. Glassman RD, Noble RJ, Tavel ME, et al; Pacemaker-induced endocardial friction rub. Am J Cardiol 40:811–814, 1977.
19. Griffin JC, Schuenemeyer TD: Pacemaker follow-up: An introduction and overview. Clin Prog Electrophysiol Pacing 1:481–490, 1983.
20. Griffin JC, Schuenemeyer TD, Hess KR, et al: Pacemaker follow-up: Its role in the detection and correction of pacemaker system malfunction. PACE 9:387–391, 1986.
21. Harthorne JW: Cardiac pacemakers. Current Probl Cardiol 12:679–693, 1987.
22. Hayes D, Vlientstra R, Trusty J, et al: A shorter hospital stay after cardiac pacemaker implantation. Mayo Clin Proc 63:236–240, 1988.
23. Hoffman A, Jost M, Pfisterer M: Persisting symptoms despite permanent pacing: Incidence, causes and follow-up. Chest 85:207–211, 1989.
24. Janosik D, Redd R, Buckingham T, et al: Utility of ambulatory electrocardiography in detecting pacemaker dysfunction in the early postimplantation period. Am J Cardiol 60:1030–1035, 1987.
25. Judson P, Holmes D, Baker W: Evaluation of outpatient arrhythmias utilizing transtelephonic monitoring. Am Heart J 97:759–763, 1979.
26. Korn M, Schoenfeld CD, Ghahramani A, Samet P: The pacemaker sound. Am J Med 49:451–458, 1970.
27. Krug HK, Zerbe F: Major venous thrombosis: A complication of transvenous pacemaker electrodes. Br Heart J 44:158–161, 1980.
28. MacGregor D, Noble E, Morrow J: Management of a pacemaker recall. J Thorac Cardiovasc Surg 74:657–663, 1977.
29. Mantini E, Majors R, Kennedy J: A recommended protocol for pacemaker follow-up analysis of 1,705 implanted pacemakers. Ann Thorac Surg 24:62–68, 1977.
30. Misra KP, Korn M, et al: Auscultatory findings in patients with cardiac pacemakers. Ann Intern Med 74:245–250, 1971.
31. Mymin D, Cuddy T, Sinha S, Winter D: Inhibition of demand pacemakers by skeletal muscle potentials. JAMA 223:527–529, 1973.
32. Nicolosi GL, Charmet PA, Zanuttini D: Large right atrial thrombosis: Rare complication during permanent transvenous endocardial pacing. Br Heart J 43:199–201, 1980.
33. Parsonnet V, Bernstein A, Galasso D: Cardiac pacing practices in the United States in 1985. Am J Cardiol 62:71–77, 1988.
34. Parsonnet V, Myers G, Gilvert L: Prediction of impending pacemaker failure in a pacemaker clinic. Am J Cardiol 25:311–315, 1970.
35. Rubin J, Ellison R, Moore H: Influence of telephone surveillance on pacemaker patient care. J Thorac Cardiovasc Surg 79:218–222, 1980.
36. Secemsky S, Hauser RG, Denes P, Edwards LM: Unipolar sensing abnormalities: Incidence and clinical significance of skeletal muscle interference and undersensing in 228 patients. PACE 5:10–20, 1982.
37. Shirato C, Ishikawa K: Newly developed systolic murmur in patients with a transvenous pacemaker. Am Heart J 99:111–126, 1981.
38. Sinnaeve A, Willems R, Stroobandt R: Inhibition of on demand pacemakers by magnet waving. PACE 5:878–890, 1982.
39. Thompson MF, Arnold RM, Bogart DB, et al: Symptomatic upper extremity venous thrombosis associated with permanent transvenous pacemaker electrodes. Chest 83:274–275, 1983.
40. Van Gelder LM, El Gamal MIH: Magnet application: A cause of persistent arrhythmias in physiological pacemakers. Report of 2 cases. PACE 5:710–714, 1982.
41. Ward D, Camm A, Spurrell A: Ambulatory monitoring of the electrocardiogram: An important aspect of pacemaker surveillance. Biotelemetry 4:109–116, 1977.

11

ELECTROCARDIOGRAPHY OF SINGLE-CHAMBER PACEMAKERS

SHANTHA URSELL *and* NABIL EL-SHERIF

Since the development of implantable pacemakers in 1960, the technology and bioengineering aspects of cardiac pacing have expanded greatly. A basic understanding of pacemaker electrocardiography is crucial for proper follow-up of patients with pacemakers. The purpose of this chapter is to review the various electrocardiographic patterns associated with pacing and to distinguish electrocardiographic manifestations of pacemaker malfunction from variations of normal patterns. It is important to know the design and the programmable functions of the pacemaker to be studied, since the number of manufacturers and types of pacemakers is so large that it is difficult to remember all the specifications of any one type of pacemaker. In addition, since programmability has become a feature of all pacemakers, an accurate recording of these programmable functions should be maintained for follow-up and detection of malfunction.

The Pacemaker Study Group in 1974 recommended a three-letter code to describe pacemaker function.[61] This code has been since modified to a five-letter code to include dual-chamber pacemakers, programmable features, and antitachycardia function.[62] The present chapter will deal only with single-chamber pacing. Electrocardiography of dual-chamber pacemakers will be discussed in Chapter 12. For the following discussion, the first three positions of the recently established five-position NASPE/BPEG generic (NBG) pacemaker code,[10] which are exclusively used for antibradyarrhythmia function, are sufficient. These are as follows:

I. Chamber or chambers paced (0 = none, A = atrium, V = ventricle, D = dual [A + V])

II. Chambers sensed (0 = none, A = atrium, V = ventricle, D = dual [A + V])

III. Response to sensing (0 = none, T = triggered, I = inhibited, D = dual [T + I])

QRS PATTERNS ASSOCIATED WITH VENTRICULAR PACING

The QRS morphology during pacing depends on the site of stimulation. Right ventricular stimulation results in a left bundle branch block (LBBB) pattern, while left ventricular stimulation results in a right bundle branch block (RBBB) pattern. The frontal plane QRS axis is determined by the stimulation site in the ventricle. Right ventricular apical stimulation, commonly seen with transvenous endocardial stimulation, results in an LBBB pattern associated with abnormal left-axis deviation (−30 to −90) because of apex-to-base activation of the ventricles (Fig. 11–1). Left ventricular epicardial implantation is usually done close to the base of the left ventricle. The paced QRS complexes therefore show an RBBB pattern with right-axis deviation (Fig. 11–2). Rarely, the right ventricular outflow tract is used for permanent pacing, and the resulting QRS complex has an LBBB pattern with a normal axis or, uncommonly, a right-axis deviation (Fig. 11–3). Endocardial right ventricular outflow tract pacing is, however, commonly used during electrophysiologic studies.

Although transvenous right ventricular apical stimulation produces an LBBB pattern, RBBB morphology is occasionally seen (Fig. 11–4). If there is a change from an LBBB to

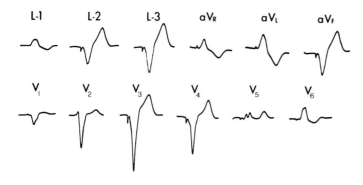

Figure 11–1. Electrocardiographic (ECG) pattern of endocardial pacing of the right ventricular apex, showing a left bundle branch block (LBBB) pattern and abnormal left-axis deviation. The relatively small pacer artifacts are caused by bipolar pacing.

Figure 11–2. ECG pattern of left ventricular epicardial pacing close to the basal portion of the left ventricle, showing a right bundle branch block (RBBB) pattern and right-axis deviation. The relatively large pacer artifacts are caused by unipolar pacing.

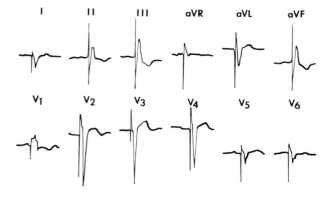

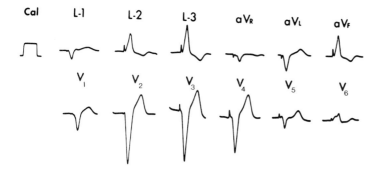

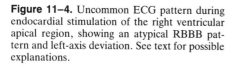

Figure 11–3. Uncommon frontal plane axis during epicardial stimulation of the right ventricular outflow tract. The ECG shows an LBBB pattern and right-axis deviation.

Figure 11–4. Uncommon ECG pattern during endocardial stimulation of the right ventricular apical region, showing an atypical RBBB pattern and left-axis deviation. See text for possible explanations.

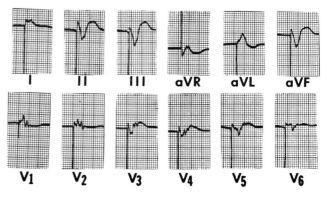

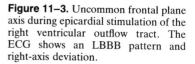

an RBBB pattern, septal perforation by the electrode catheter, causing left ventricular stimulation, should be considered.[17] Loss of capture with no apparent displacement and diaphragmatic or chest wall stimulation may be features of perforation. The electrogram recorded from the tip electrode will show characteristic diminution in the QRS voltage.[2] However, there are two theoretical mechanisms by which RBBB pattern can be produced by ventricular right septal stimulation. Mower and colleagues attributed it to direct selective stimulation of the right bundle branch, with retrograde conduction to the His Bundle and subsequent activation of the left bundle branch.[57] Sodi-Pollares, on the other hand, suggested that the anatomic left septum can extend to the right ventricular endocardium and that stimulation of this area could therefore cause an RBBB pattern.[71] This view is supported by Saksena, who showed an RBBB morphology with right ventricular posteroseptal or inferoposterior pacing and suggested that stimulation of those sites may preferentially excite specialized myocardial fibers in continuity with the left ventricular myocardium.[67] Occasionally, during implantation of a transvenous electrode catheter, it may be inadvertently placed in the coronary sinus or in one of its tributaries. More often, migration or displacement of the catheter into the coronary sinus from its original position in the right ventricular apex can result in stimulation of the left ventricle and result in an RBBB pattern. Radiographs of the chest in both posteroanterior and lateral views will aid in making the diagnosis. When the catheter tip is in the right ventricular apex, the lateral chest radiograph should show the lead to be directed anteriorly, whereas a posterior location of the tip confirms displacement, probably to the coronary sinus.

FUSION BEATS AND PSEUDOFUSION BEATS

True fusion beats occur when the ventricles are simultaneously activated by a spontaneous depolarization and a paced impulse.[18] The spontaneous depolarization can be either a supraventricular beat or an ectopic ventricular impulse. A pseudofusion beat, on the other hand, refers to superimposition of a pacer spike on a QRS complex originating from a single focus.[3] This phenomenon is caused by the discharge of the pacemaker after the onset of the ventricular depolarization in the absolute refractory period of the heart but before the intrinsic ventricular depolarization has reached adequate voltage and slew rate to activate the sensing circuit. A varying portion of the QRS complex may be inscribed in the surface electrocardiogram before the superimposition of the pacemaker spike. When the rate of the spontaneous cardiac rhythm is almost identical with the pacemaker rate, regular alternation of a spontaneous beat and a pseudo fusion beat may occur (Fig. 11–5). This alternation probably occurs because of the slight difference between the pacemaker escape and automatic intervals.

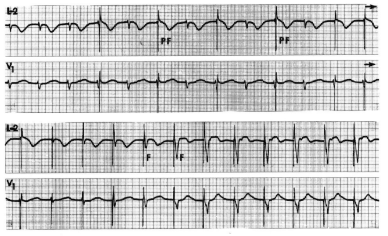

Figure 11–5. A continuous rhythm strip of both leads II and V₁ in a patient with accelerated junctional rhythm and a ventricular inhibited (VVI) pacer. The rate of the spontaneous rhythm is almost identical with the pacer rate, resulting in alternation of a paced beat and a pseudo fusion beat (PF) before consecutive discharge of the pacer occurs at the end of the upper rhythm strip. This discharge of the pacer initially results in the inscription of several pseudofusion beats in succession before the pacer spike starts to contribute to ventricular depolarization, giving rise to true fusion beats (F). In the second half of the lower rhythm strip, pure paced beats are seen. Note that in pseudo fusion beats, the large (unipolar) pacer artifact significantly distorts the spontaneous QRS complex.

POSTPACING ST CHANGES

Chatterjee and associates first described the frequent occurrence of ST–T-wave changes in the unpaced electrocardiogram subsequent to right ventricular endocardial pacing that persist for a varying length of time, depending on the duration of pacing[20] (Fig. 11–6). Similar changes were later reported with intermittent LBBB.[26] Rosenbaum and coworkers noted that postpacing T-wave changes in normally conducted beats have a direction similar to that of the QRS complex of the paced abnormally conducted beats in each of the 12 leads of the electrocardiogram.[65] The recovery time of the ST–T-wave changes seems to depend on the magnitude of the change attained during the pacing period. During continuous right ventricular pacing, marked ST–T-wave changes are induced in a gradually cumulative

fashion. After the provoking stimulus is discontinued and its effects are no longer apparent, the heart seems to keep a "memory" of the previous effect, so that reintroduction of the stimulus will result in redevelopment of the ST–T-wave changes in a much shorter time span.[65]

DIAGNOSIS OF MYOCARDIAL INFARCTION DURING VENTRICULAR PACING

Since ventricular pacing results in abnormal activation and repolarization patterns, the diagnosis of acute ischemia or infarction during pacing is often difficult. The pacing artifact, particularly with unipolar pacing, frequently distorts the initial part of the QRS complex,

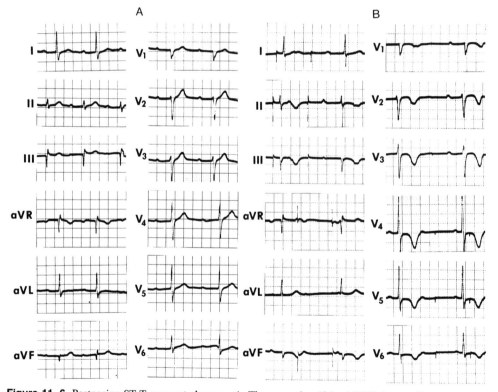

Figure 11–6. Postpacing ST-T segment changes. *A,* The prepacing 12-lead ECG from a 41-year-old man with myotonic dystrophy and both atrioventricular (AV) nodal and intra–His bundle conduction delay, as shown in an electrophysiologic study. The ECG shows normal sinus rhythm and first-degree AV block. Other records, however, showed periods of a Wenckebach-type block and 2:1 AV block. A transvenous right ventricular apical VVI pacer was implanted because of symptoms of dizziness and near-syncope that were thought to be related to the AV conduction abnormality. *B,* The patient's 12-lead ECG obtained 6 months after pacer implantation. The VVI pacer was suppressed by chest wall stimuli. The underlying spontaneous cardiac rhythm alternated between 2:1 AV block and complete AV dissociation with a supraventricular escape focus. The QRS configuration of escape beats was similar to that of conducted beats shown in *A.* There is, however, marked symmetric inversion of T waves in inferior leads and all precordial leads in the postpacing tracing compared with the prepacing recording.

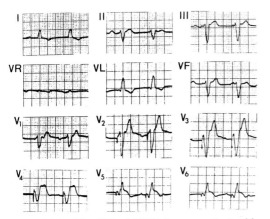

Figure 11–7. The 12-lead ECG from a patient with a permanent right ventricular endocardial VVI pacemaker. The patient presented with a clinical picture suggestive of acute myocardial infarction, with characteristic changes in cardiac enzymes. The ECG showed the development of new q waves in leads V$_5$ and V$_6$ associated with ST-segment elevation consistent with acute anteroseptal infarction in the presence of pacing-induced LBBB pattern.

making the presence of Q waves difficult to discern.

Marked ST-segment elevation, especially when associated with T-wave inversion, indicates underlying myocardial ischemia or infarction. This is true of changes seen in the anterior or inferior leads. Serial changes in the ST-T segment are very important in the diagnosis of acute ischemia. During right ventricular endocardial pacing, the initial forces due to septal activation cause initial positive deflections in leads I, aVL, V$_5$, and V$_6$. With anteroseptal infarction, these leads usually develop abnormal q waves (Fig. 11–7). Notching in the ascending limb of the QRS complex (S wave) in precordial leads V$_3$ and V$_4$ has been noted in the majority of patients with LBBB and acute anteroseptal infarction.[14] Similar findings during pacing-induced LBBB have been mentioned in the literature.[27]

Inferior wall infarction is more difficult to diagnose during pacing, since right ventricular pacing produces QS complexes in the inferior leads. Barold and colleagues have described a QR or Qr pattern in the inferior leads as being specific for inferior wall infarction.[7]

MODES OF PACING

Asynchronous Pacemaker (VOO)

The asynchronous pacemaker was the first type of pacemaker used in the early 1960s for patients with complete heart block, which was the predominant indication for pacing at that time.[83] The pacemaker generator delivers stimuli at a preset constant rate, independent of the spontaneous rhythm of the patient. The pacemaker stimuli will capture the ventricles if and when they fall outside the ventricular refractory period following spontaneous beats. At the present time, an electrocardiogram that shows asynchronous ventricular pacing is almost always caused by loss of the sensing function of a ventricular inhibited pacemaker (Fig. 11–8). Competition between the asynchronous pacemaker and the spontaneous cardiac rhythm may cause serious ventricular tachyarrhythmias, if the pacemaker stimulus interrupts the T wave of a spontaneous beat and captures the ventricles during the vulnerable period.[78] Ventricular fibrillation induced by the falling of a pacemaker stimulus in the vulnerable period has been reported.[11] However, its occurrence is much less common than theoretically anticipated. Ventricular fibrillation rarely occurs in the absence of an abnormally enhanced ventricular vulnerability. The latter may be due to myocardial ischemia (Fig. 11–9), electrolyte abnormalities, or autonomic imbalance.

Figure 11–8. Asynchronous ventricular pacing. The spontaneous cardiac rhythm is sinus with incomplete AV dissociation and slow idioventricular escape rhythm. The pacemaker stimuli appear at a constant rate regardless of the spontaneous cardiac rhythm and capture the ventricles only when they fall outside the refractory period of the preceding spontaneous beat.

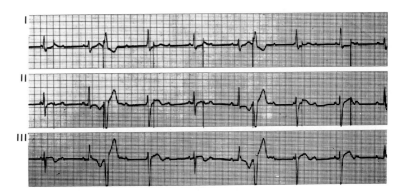

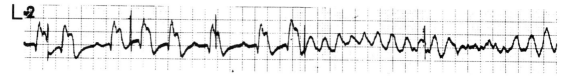

Figure 11–9. Recording obtained from a 62-year-old patient with a malfunctioning VVI pacer that was asynchronously firing at an irregular, slow rate. The patient was admitted to the coronary care unit with acute anterior wall myocardial infarction and subsequently developed RBBB and left posterior hemiblock. The tracing shows the presence of frequent atrial premature beats and the sudden onset of ventricular fibrillation that was probably related to the falling of the pacer spike on the early ST-T segment of the preceding spontaneous beat. The apparently long latency between the stimulus and the first induced ventricular beat is probably related to the occurrence of the spike during the relative refractory period. In this particular example, the fortuitous occurrence of the arrhythmia cannot be excluded.

Ventricular Triggered Pacemaker (VVT)

The ventricular triggered, or QRS triggered, pacemaker is also referred to as an "R"-wave synchronous pacemaker. It has both sensing and pacing mechanisms. Unlike VVI pacemakers, the R-wave synchronous pacemaker emits a stimulus with every sensed intrinsic ventricular depolarization. However, since the spike occurs within the QRS complex, it is ineffective, being in the absolute refractory period of the ventricle. In addition, the pacer fires when needed after an escape interval during which the patient's intrinsic ventricular depolarization is not sensed. All sensed QRS complexes with a VVT pacemaker show a spike after the onset of the QRS complex, and all paced QRS complexes show a pacer artifact preceding the complex (Fig. 11–10). Since the pulse generator emits an impulse continuously, its longevity is abbreviated.

During spontaneous cardiac rhythm, the presence of spike in the QRS complex indicates that the sensing function of the pacemaker is intact. However, whether the output of the pacemaker is effective in capturing the ventricle can be established only by placing an external magnet and converting the pacemaker to an asynchronous mode. External chest wall stimulation can also be used to check the integrity of the pacer. The external stimuli will normally capture the VVI pacer in a 1:1 fashion, until limited by the refractory period of the pacer (Fig. 11–11). The VVT pacer will sense every external stimulus and emit a spike of its own and capture the ventricle. Impending failure of the pulse generator of a VVT pacemaker usually results in slowing of the automatic rate. Concomitantly, the normal response to chest wall stimulation is frequently lost (Fig. 11–11).

Ventricular (Demand) Inhibited Pacemaker (VVI)

The ventricular inhibited pacemaker, also called the R-wave inhibited pacer, is the commonest type of pacemaker in use today (Fig. 11–12). The generator has a sensing circuitry, which senses the intrinsic R wave of the patient and inhibits the generator output. The pacer spike will be delivered on demand if no spontaneous R wave is sensed for a present interval. There are three pacing intervals that describe the pacing function of a demand R-wave inhibited pacer.

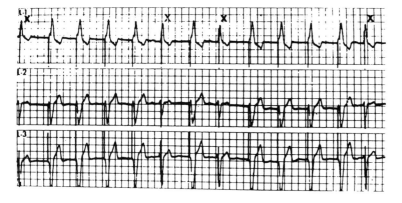

Figure 11–10. Ventricular triggered pacer (VVT). All beats are paced except those marked "X," which are spontaneous conducted beats. All spontaneous beats fall outside the refractory period of the pacer (400 msec) and trigger the pacer to fire a spike within the QRS complex.

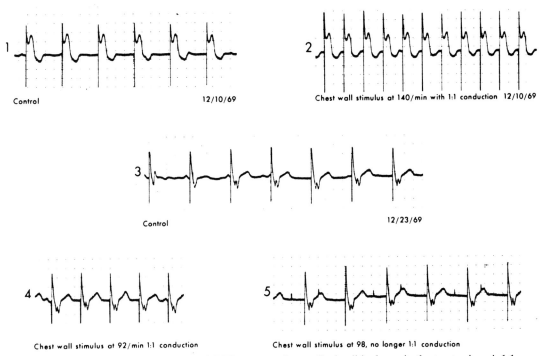

Figure 11–11. Normal response of a (VVT) pacer to chest wall stimuli is shown in the top tracing. A 1:1 response is usually maintained up to rates of 150 per minute (the pacer refractory period is 400 msec). The middle strip illustrates impending failure of the pulse generator, resulting in slowing of the automatic rate. The bottom strip shows loss of normal response to chest wall stimuli, with 1:1 response maintained only up to a rate of 92 per minute.

1. The *automatic pacing interval* is the time between two consecutive pacer stimuli during demand pacing.

2. The *pacer escape interval* is measured from a sensed spontaneous ventricular depolarization to the subsequent escape pacer spike. In most VVI pacemakers, these two intervals are identical. In the surface electrocardiogram, however, the escape interval, which is measured from the spontaneous sensed QRS complex to the next pacer spike, may be slightly longer than the automatic pacing interval. This occurs because one cannot precisely determine the moment within the QRS complex when the intrinsic ventricular depolarization at the site of the pacer sensing electrode has reached adequate voltage and slew rate (dV/dt) to activate the sensing mechanism and initiate a new escape interval. Occasionally, the pacer is built to have an escape interval longer than the automatic pacing interval. This pacer is said to have a *positive rate hysteresis*[16, 36] (Fig. 11–13). The rationale behind this design is to maintain the spontaneous

Figure 11–12. Ventricular inhibited pacer (VVI). Same patient as in Figure 11–10. The VVT pacer has been replaced by a VVI unit. In contrast to the VVT pacer, in a VVI pacer, spontaneous beats that are successfully sensed by the pacer (marked "X") inhibit the spike and recycle the pacer to discharge after a set interval.

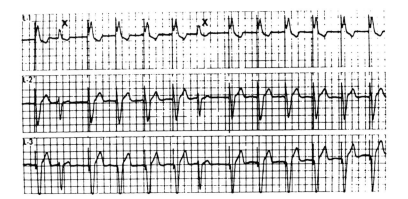

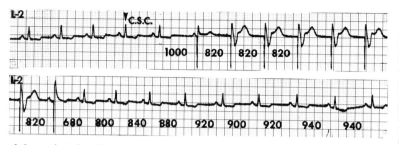

Figure 11–13. VVI pacer with positive rate hysteresis. In the upper rhythm strip, carotid sinus compression (C.S.C.) resulted in slowing of the sinus rate and escape of the pacer after an interval of 1000 msec. This activity is followed by automatic pacing at a shorter interval of 820 msec. The lower rhythm strip shows sinus arrhythmia. The relatively short sinus cycles resulted in inhibition of demand pacing. However, the sinus interval later lengthened to well beyond the pacer automatic interval without pacer escape. This occurrence illustrates a paradoxical situation in which a slower spontaneous rhythm inhibits a faster pacer rhythm.

sinus rhythm with its known hemodynamic advantage over the ventricular paced rhythm at cycle lengths longer than the pacemaker automatic cycle length, but shorter than the escape cycle length.

3. The magnet mode rate, or fixed-rate pacing interval, is the rate obtained during placement of a magnet over the implanted generator. All VVI pacers have a magnetic reed switch, which is activated by the application of a test magnet, allowing the generator to operate in a fixed-rate mode.[6, 28] This rate is the most stable and reliable pacer rate and is the recommended rate to follow for the detection of impending battery failure.[6] By contrast, the automatic or pacing interval can change by up to 40 mscc in most normally functioning pacemakers.

In some pacemakers, the magnet rate is the same as the automatic pacing rate. In this case, the function of the magnetic reed switch will be difficult to ascertain in the presence of an exclusive paced rhythm, and chest wall stimulation may be necessary to assess sensing function. In other pacers in which the magnet rate is faster than the automatic pacer rate, an increase in rate with the application of a mag-

net can be discerned in an electrocardiographic rhythm strip (Fig. 11–14). In some VVI pacers, when the magnet is waved over the pulse generator, prolonged inhibition may occur[6, 70, 74] (Fig. 11–15). A possible explanation is the changes in the electrochemical potential difference between the ground plate and the intracardiac electrode, which may be shorted out each time the reed switch is in operation. The voltage change is sensed by the pacemaker, and inhibition may occur.[6] This inhibition can occur in VVI pacemakers in which the reed switch is connected with the sensing circuit. In models in which the reed switch is isolated from the sensing circuit, magnet application or removal cannot produce inhibition. Malfunction of the reed switch as a result of mechanical failure can rarely occur.[6, 28] The reed switch may stay in either the open or the closed position, regardless of the external magnetic field. This is called a *sticky reed switch.*

Pacemaker Refractory Periods

There are two pacemaker refractory periods:

1. *The delivery (paced) refractory period:* the

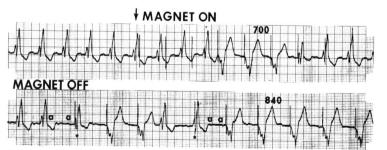

Figure 11–14. VVI pacer with the magnet fixed rate faster than the automatic pacing rate. The VVI pacer was implanted in a patient with the tachycardia-bradycardia syndrome. The spontaneous cardiac rhythm is an atrial tachycardia with AV block (a = atrial waves). The first half of the upper rhythm strip shows atrial tachycardia with 2:1 AV block simulating a regular sinus rhythm at a rate of 95 per minute and no paced beats. Application of the magnet resulted in fixed-rate pacing at an interval of 700 msec. The lower rhythm strip illustrates the occurrence of a higher degree of AV block, resulting in pacer escape at an automatic interval of 840 msec. Beats marked by asterisks are conducted supraventricular beats with RBBB configuration and a pacer spike within the QRS complex during demand pacing (pseudo fusion beats).

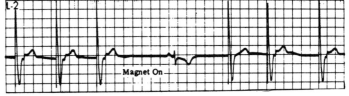

Figure 11–15. Magnet waving in front of a VVI generator, causing inhibition of the pacemaker discharge.

pacer refractory period following the emission of a pacing pulse.

2. *The sensing (sensed) refractory period:* the pacer refractory period following sensing of an electrical signal either spontaneous or paced. Although usually similar, the delivery and sensing refractory periods may differ in some VVI pacers.

The *relative refractory period* of the pacemaker is defined as the period immediately following the delivery refractory period during which the demand mechanism has not regained its full sensitivity. During the relative refractory period, some generators require a larger signal to activate the sensing mechanism; others can only be partially recycled by a signal capable of completely recycling the generator outside this period.

Chest Wall Stimulation

The VVI pacemaker functions as a demand unit by sensing the intrinsic R wave. The pacemaker can also be suppressed by an external electrical field.[8, 68] In chest wall stimulation, two suction cups are applied to the chest and connected with an external pacemaker, which is set at a rate higher than the implanted device. The implanted pacer senses the external electrical field and is inhibited (Fig. 11–16). The underlying rhythm can then be identified and can be monitored during the pacemaker follow-up. If during chest wall stimulation the patient is shown to have a markedly slow or unreliable intrinsic rhythm, more frequent monitoring may be necessary.

Atrial Demand Pacemaker (AAI)

In patients with sinus node disease and normal atrioventricular (AV) conduction, atrial demand pacing may be considered a "semiphysiologic" mode of pacing, since it ensures AV synchrony but the paced heart rate cannot vary. It is particularly effective in some patients with symptomatic sick sinus syndrome and associated myocardial disease[33, 56] because it has been amply documented that preservation of AV synchrony can improve the hemodynamic state.[69] In fact, ventricular demand (VVI) pacing in those patients may result in persistent symptoms of dizziness, lightheadedness, and episodes of hypotension induced by the onset of ventricular pacing that have been called "the pacemaker syndrome."[33] The syndrome is probably related to persistent retrograde AV conduction with unfavorable hemodynamic and reflex autonomic responses.[29] Atrial pacing is also indicated in the management of selected types of intractable supraventricular and ventricular tachyarrhythmias.[33, 56] The fixation problems of early transvenous atrial J electrodes led to a brief attempt to pace from the coronary sinus.[56] This technique has been all but abandoned following the use of tined leads. In the AAI pacer, the duration of the paced refractory period determines whether the QRS complex will be sensed after a pacemaker-induced atrial depolarization. The paced refractory period should be close to 400 msec to avoid intermittent sensing of the QRS after paced atrial beats. This inter-

Figure 11–16. Suppression of VVI pacer by external chest wall stimuli (CWS). Note the emergence of an underlying slow junctional rhythm *(A)* that gradually increased its rate *(B)*, illustrating the phenomenon of overdrive suppression by the faster pacer rhythm. The pacemaker was implanted in a patient with symptomatic sick sinus syndrome.

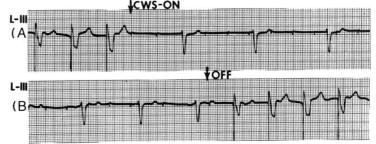

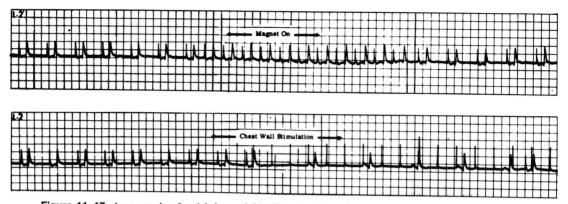

Figure 11-17. An example of atrial demand (AAI) pacing from the coronary sinus, illustrating inappropriately slower pacer rate due to abnormal sensing of the conducted QRS complex. The pacemaker was implanted for control of sinus bradycardia and complex ventricular arrhythmias, and the demand rate was set at 115 beats per minute, with the escape interval at 540 msec. The top tracing shows that the actual pacing rate was 85 per minute (spike-to-spike interval of 750 msec). The demand unit was an old model with a standard refractory period of 200 to 240 msec. Since the combined duration of the P-R interval and the conducted QRS complex was greater than the pacer refractory period, the unit sensed its own generated QRS and was recycled by the ventricular deflection. This recycling resulted in an inappropriately slower pacer rate. The top panel shows that when a magnet was applied over the demand unit, converting the pacer to asynchronous pacing mode, the pacing rate increased to the originally set rate of 115 per minute. The lower panel illustrates the effect of external chest wall stimulation, which resulted in inhibition of the demand pacer, revealing the underlying spontaneous rhythm of sinus bradycardia.

mittent sensing can result in inappropriately slower pacer rate (Fig. 11–17). The response of the AAI pacer to magnet application and to chest wall stimulation is qualitatively similar to that of the VVI pacer (Fig. 11–17).

PACEMAKER MALFUNCTION

The causes of pacemaker malfunction can be broadly classified into (1) problems related to pacemaker stimulus and capture and (2) problems related to sensing.

Problems Related to Pacemaker Stimulus and Capture

The various causes for abnormal activation or failure to capture are (1) battery failure, resulting in slow or fast rates; (2) lead displacement, perforation, or failure; (3) pacemaker exit block; and (4) changes in mode of pacing.

Changes in Rate from Battery Depletion

Small variations in the pacer's automatic rate can be seen with all pacers and are based on changes in ambient body temperature.[35] However, the magnet rate of the pacemaker is stable and is a sensitive indicator of battery depletion.[28] In earlier pacer models, battery depletion resulted in rate increase, and pacing rates of 100 to 400 per minute were occasionally seen.[12, 58] The condition was called *runaway pacemaker* and has occasionally resulted in fatal pacer tachyarrhythmias. With the current lithium-source generator, battery depletion most often leads to a decrease in pacing rate. Eventually, battery depletion will result in totally ineffective stimuli. Since rate is often a programmable parameter, magnet rate should always be checked before diagnosing battery depletion.

Lead Displacement, Perforation, or Failure

Gross displacement of a bipolar lead may be evident in the radiograph or by a change in the frontal plane axis of the electrocardiogram. Similarly, perforation of the septum may result in stimulation of the left ventricle and in a change in the QRS pattern from LBBB to RBBB.

Loss of insulation will lead to the creation of an alternate pathway for current flow. There is usually an increase in the amplitude of the pacemaker spike in the case of a bipolar lead system. Pacing and sensing may continue in the presence of insulation breaks; however, excessive current drain will result in premature battery failure. Occasionally, sensing problems and muscle stimulation can occur owing to insulation break. Serial measurements of the peak-to-peak amplitude of the intrinsic deflection of the ventricular electrogram may show diminution in size and could be used to predict lead failure months before it manifests clinically.[73]

Pacemaker Exit Block

Exit block can be defined as the failure of an impulse falling outside the refractory period of the surrounding tissue to elicit a propagated response.[32] The failure of the tissue to respond may be caused either by an alteration of the stimulus intensity or by failure of conduction from the site of the pacemaker. In the case of a cardiac artificial pacemaker, exit block describes the clinical condition in which a normal pacemaker stimulus fails to excite the heart because of an abnormally high threshold.[64] An increase in pacing threshold often occurs after initial placement of the lead. Alterations of pacemaker threshold by physiologic factors, drugs, and electrolyte changes have been extensively studied.[40, 64] Type I antiarrhythmic drugs have been shown to increase the pacing threshold.[39, 44] Although modest elevation of the serum potassium level may decrease the pacemaker threshold,[64] marked elevation of the serum potassium level is associated with significant increase in threshold[40] and pacemaker exit block[60] (Fig. 11–18).

Occasionally following cardioversion or defibrillation, the pacemaker output voltage may decrease, leading to noncapture of the pacer stimuli.[24] Levine and colleagues[49] described patients in whom a transient or chronic rise in stimulation threshold of the permanently implanted unipolar catheter resulted in loss of effective pacing after therapeutic defibrillation or cardioversion. They recommend that the defibrillator paddles be placed at least 5 inches from the generator or as far as possible in the case of implantation in the right pectoral fossa. In patients with pacers, an anteroposterior paddle placement would be ideal when defibrillation is necessary. Stimulation threshold should be checked in all patients after defibril-

lation. Similarly, after transvenous catheter countershock, the pacing threshold has been shown to increase.[81]

Changes in Pacing Mode

Changes in output and mode of operation (i.e., change from VVI to VVT) can occur if defibillation paddles are placed directly over the pacemaker generator.[24, 49] Similar problems have been noted following therapeutic radiation.[1] It is recommended that pulsed x-ray radiation be avoided even at therapeutic levels.[1]

Problems Related to Sensing in VVI Pacers

The various problems can be classified into (1) failure to sense or undersensing, (2) apparent or pseudo failure to sense, (3) oversensing, and (4) partial sensing (partial recycling).

Undersensing

Excluding both temporary reversion of a VVI pacer to the VOO mode as a result of electromagnetic interference and occurrence of a ventricular depolarization during the pacemaker refractory period, the failure of a VVI pacer to sense a spontaneous QRS results either from the delivery of an inadequate ventricular depolarization to a normally functioning pacer or from the delivery of an adequate QRS signal to a malfunctioning pacer. Analysis of both the unipolar and the bipolar electrograms recorded from the pacing electrode is sometimes essential to evaluate the adequacy of the QRS signal. Normally, a unipolar ventricular electrogram measures 5 to 15 mV,[42] which is more than adequate for a VVI pacer to sense. Most units usually need 2 to 3 mV for proper sensing. However, marked diminution of the intracardiac electrogram may occur as a result of excessive fibrosis at the tip of the lead and results in inadequate sensing as well as pacing.[52] Acute myocardial infarction

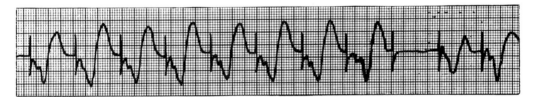

Figure 11–18. Pacemaker exit block of the Wenckebach type in a patient with marked hyperkalemia. Note the presence of a slight, but definite, gradual increase of the spike-to-QRS interval prior to failure to capture, followed by shortening of the interval in the beat subsequent to the ineffective spike.

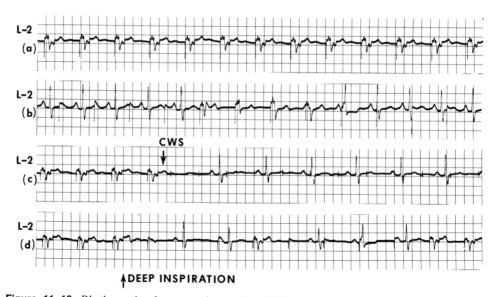

Figure 11–19. Rhythm strips from a patient with a VVI pacer implanted 6 months previously for symptomatic sick sinus syndrome. On the chest radiograph, the electrode tip was found to be displaced close to the tricuspid valve. Panel *A* was obtained during normal respiration and shows continuous pacing. Panel *B* was recorded following the administration of 0.6 mg of atropine, which resulted in modest acceleration of the sinus rate. The rhythm strip shows failure of sensing, resulting in asynchronous ventricular pacing. Panel *C* shows that the VVI pacer could be successfully inhibited by external chest wall stimulation (CWS). Panel *D* was obtained during deep inspiration and shows transient loss of both sensing and pacing.

can result in a decrease in the size of the intracardiac electrogram and predisposes to undersensing.[19] Drug toxicity with type 1A or 1C antiarrhythmic agents as well as hyperkalemia may also cause problems with sensing, although these conditions are more often associated with failure to capture. A bipolar signal may occasionally be much smaller than either of its two component unipolar signals.[4] In this case, unipolarization usually restores normal sensing.

Displacement of the pacing electrode with loss of intimate contact with the endocardium may be associated with loss of sensing or failure of both sensing and pacing. This failure is sometimes intermittent and is brought on only by deep respiratory or body movements (Fig. 11–19). Intermittent pacing and sensing failure can also result from the lead's not being properly positioned in the generator or from a loose contact. The diagnosis can be confirmed by moving the generator gently in its pocket or by movement of the shoulder, which will result in sensing failure. A normally functioning VVI pacer may occasionally be able to sense conducted supraventricular beats but may fail to sense certain ventricular ectopic beats (Fig. 11–20). This feature is usually explained by failure of the ectopic depolarization to generate an adequate voltage and slew rate (dv/dt) for proper sensing.

In some instances, an adequate signal from a ventricular depolarization may not be sensed because the signal occurred during the refractory period of the pacemaker. With the pacers currently in use, the refractory period of the pacemaker is programmable and can be modified to sense early signals.

Apparent Failure to Sense

A normally functioning pervenous VVI pacer may fail to sense late-occurring sponta-

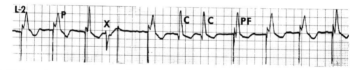

Figure 11–20. Failure to sense a ventricular ectopic beat (X) in a normally functioning VVI pacer. Note that conducted supraventricular beats (C) are normally sensed. P = paced beat; PF = pseudofusion beat.

neous ventricular beats, which results in the discharge of the pacer spike into the QRS complex, giving rise to pseudo fusion beats. This failure to sense is explained by failure of a late-occurring intrinsic ventricular depolarization to reach adequate voltage and slew rate (dV/dt) at the site of the sensing electrode to activate the sensing circuit before the time of the next pacer automatic cycle. An exaggerated form of this phenomenon occurs with right ventricular endocardial VVI pacers in the presence of an RBBB pattern of conducted supraventricular beats (Fig. 11–14) as well as in the case of left ventricular ectopic beats (Fig. 11–21). Both types of QRS complexes will be associated with delayed arrival of the ventricular depolarization at the site of the pacer sensing electrode. These cases may be misinterpreted as failure of sensing by the VVI pacer. It should be stressed, however, that a pacer spike that falls clearly outside the QRS complex would obviously indicate failure of sensing.

Another reason for apparent undersensing is the circuit designs of the pacer, as is seen with the new Activitrax rate-responsive pacemaker (Medtronic, Minneapolis, MN). In the activity modes, the pacemaker's stimulation rate is controlled by an activity-sensing detector and circuitry.[51] The sensor, a piezoelectric crystal on the inside of the pacemaker, transforms the mechanical vibrations in the body resulting from physical activity into an electrical signal that is further processed for rate control. Occasionally, a single output pulse may be emitted at the programmed maximal activity rate when a sensed ventricular event occurs within 8 msec after the pacemaker activity detection/rate circuit is triggered.[54] Such an output pulse will be noted on the electrocardiogram at intervals of 400, 480, or 600 msec after the sensed event corresponding to

the programmed maximal activity rate of 150, 125, or 100 beats per minute. This pulse, as observed clinically, can be mistaken for sensing malfunction of the device. It usually occurs following a run of sensed intrinsic rhythm and is the result of the pacemaker circuitry (Fig. 11–22).

Abnormal Sensing (Oversensing)

Oversensing should be considered in the presence of irregular lengthening of the automatic interspike interval. Abnormal sensing can occur as a result of either extrinsic or intrinsic signals.

ABNORMAL SENSING CAUSED BY EXTRINSIC SIGNALS. Both VVT and VVI pacers can be modified by external electromagnetic interference.[55, 59, 76] Although less frequent with the present generation of pacemakers, electrical appliances that emit continuous-wave energy with a frequency of 50 to 60 Hz can interfere with pacemaker function. Such interference can occur with household appliances and electrocardiographic recording equipment. Butrous and associates found that following exposure to a 50-Hz electrical field (up to a maximum of 20 kV/m), some pacers showed normal function, some reverted to a fixed-rate mode, some showed slow and irregular pacing, and others demonstrated a mixed response.[13] In general, the interference threshold depended on the magnitude and distribution of the electrical field and varied with the patient's height, build, and posture. Interference has been reported to occur if the pacemaker is in the vicinity of pulsed energy sources, such as radio[63] or television transmitters,[25] radar,[80] auto ignition systems, or arc welders,[38] or by direct contact of the patient with electric razors,[23] electric toothbrushes,[30] or other household appliances. Pulsed energy signals may

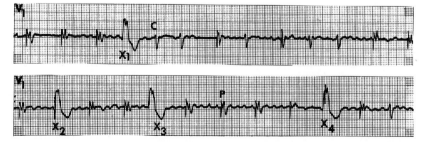

Figure 11–21. Apparent failure to sense left ventricular ectopic beats by a transvenous VVI pacer. Note the presence of atrial fibrillation, paced beats (P), conducted supraventricular beats (C), and ventricular ectopic beats (X), probably of left ventricular origin, as suggested by the RBBB configuration in lead V_1. Ectopic beats marked X_2 and X_4 have late coupling, and the pacer spike is inscribed within the QRS complex as late as 60 msec after the onset of the QRS complex in the ectopic beat marked X_4. See text for explanation.

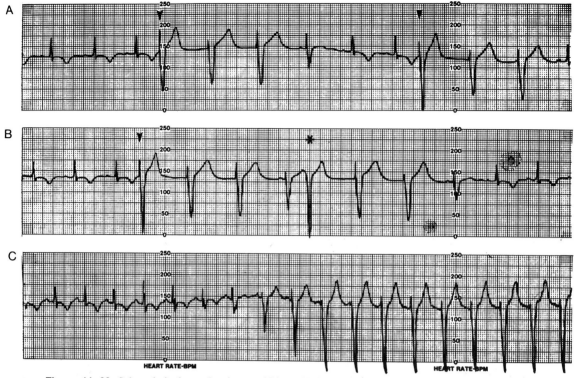

Figure 11–22. Selected rhythm strips from a 24-hour Holter recording in a patient with an Activitrax pacemaker. *A* and *B* were recorded during sleep and show sinus rhythm alternating with ventricular paced rhythm. The first paced beat follows the last sensed spontaneous beat by 480 msec (marked by *arrows*). This apparent failure to sense is the result of the pacemaker circuitry (see text for details). The sensing mechanism is intact, as shown by proper sensing of the ventricular premature contraction, marked by an asterisk. *C* was obtained during the morning hours and shows sinus tachycardia followed by ventricular pacing at a rate of 105 beats per minute. The programmed maximal activity rate was 125 beats per minute. Note several pseudo fusion and true fusion beats during the transition from sinus to paced beats.

mimic the R-wave potential and inhibit a VVI pacer. Conversion of a VVI pacer to a VOO mode in the vicinity of microwave radio-transmitters[47] or microwave ovens has been reported. Electrical interference may be caused by poor grounding or by close contact with the apparatus. Current leakage is particularly dangerous in the presence of diathermy and electrocautery equipment.[50, 75] Interference from external signals is less common with the newer pacemakers owing to better shielding of the pulse generator with a stainless steel or titanium capsule.

Another extrinsic signal commonly associated with oversensing and inhibition is myopotentials. Mypotential inhibition is common with unipolar rather than bipolar pacing systems.[43] This phenomenon, first reported in 1972,[79] has been related to the difficulty in discriminating skeletal muscle potentials from myocardial potentials. Dizziness and light-headedness during active exercise may occur owing to inhibition of the pacer in the presence of an inadequate intrinsic cardiac rhythm (Fig. 11–23). Inhibition during active exercise involving the pectoralis muscle can be reproduced in the clinic. Although abdominal implantation of the pulse generator has been reported to decrease the incidence of myopotential inhibition,[66] other studies have shown that both the rectus abdominis and pectoralis muscles can be a source of myopotentials.[41] Bipolar units, by virtue of the rejection of far-field interference and superior signal-to-noise ratio, are not modified by myopotentials. Thus, conversion of a unipolar system to a bipolar system may be a solution for myopotential inhibition. In addition, with the generators currently in use, programming the R-wave sensing to an improved value (i.e., lower sensitivity) may prevent oversensing.

ABNORMAL SENSING CAUSED BY INTRINSIC SIGNALS. Oversensing of intrinsic signals from the atrium or ventricle can result in inhibition of VVT pacemakers. P-wave sensing was described in cases of epicardial leads near the AV groove[3, 72] and displacement of a right ventricular endocardial electrode near the tri-

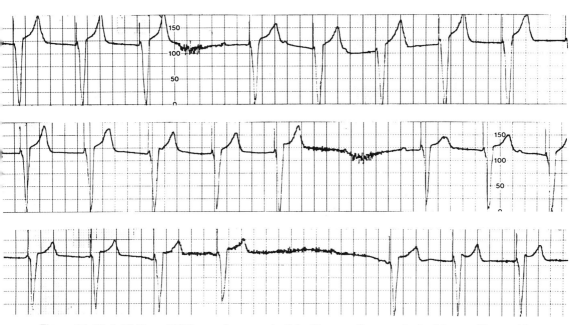

Figure 11–23. Inhibition of VVI pacer by myopotentials. The recording was obtained from a 65-year-old patient who had a unipolar transvenous VVI pacer implanted subcutaneously in the right infraclavicular region for symptomatic complete AV block. Eighteen months following implantation, he had return of symptoms in the form of dizzy spells. A routine ECG showed evidence of power source depletion (lengthening of the interspike interval from 840 to 1020 msec). The patient noted that symptoms occurred only when he used his right arm, especially when the arm maintained a forceful adduction position. The tracing was obtained while the patient was asked to exert intermittent pressure medially against resistance with the right hand, resulting in tensing of the pectoral muscle. This tensing produced intermittent inhibition of the VVI pacer with prolonged asystolic intervals. Note the occurrence of baseline artifact from interference during the maneuver.

cuspid valve or in the coronary sinus.[77] If the atrial rate is faster than the pacer automatic rate, constant P-wave sensing would result in total suppression of a VVI pacer.[77]

T-wave sensing is more common than P-wave sensing[3, 9, 21, 37, 82] and may be seen with pacers programmed to a long pulse width, especially when the refractory period is short and the sensitivity is high. Sensing of the T wave of paced ventricular beats is far more common than sensing of the T wave of spontaneous beats (Fig. 11–24), probably because the voltage contribution from the pacemaker afterpotential following a paced beat tends to generate a larger T-wave signal. Abnormal sensing of the pacemaker afterpotential has also been described.[3, 37, 46, 82] Oversensing can be corrected by using a bipolar system or by decreasing the sensing (i.e., increasing the sensitivity voltage).

Concealed extrasystole has been suggested as a possible reason for oversensing-induced inhibition,[53] although this phenomenon has not been adequately documented. Rarely, autointerference of demand generators could be due to signals originating within a pulse generator itself.[5] The absence of any visible interference on the surface electrocardiogram and the rel-

Figure 11–24. An example of probable T-wave sensing. Note that the VVI pacer escape interval following the ectopic beat marked X_2 is shorter than the pacer normal escape interval of 820 msec. This feature suggests that complete recycling occurred after sensing of the T wave of the ectopic beat marked X_1. An alternative explanation would be partial sensing of the ectopic beat X_2, resulting in partial recycling and an abbreviated escape interval.

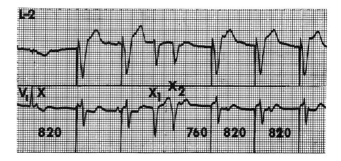

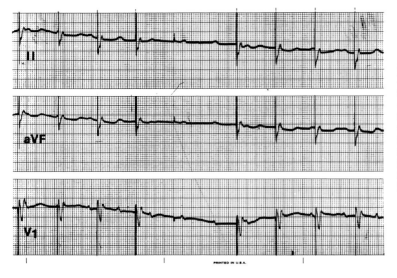

Figure 11–25. A characteristic ECG of partial lead fracture, showing sudden diminution of the amplitude of the pacer artifact associated with loss of ventricular capture. In this case, partial lead fracture also generated false signals, resulting in abnormal sensing. This explains the abnormally long pacer interval following the ineffective pacer artifact.

atively late appearance of autointerference in the life of a pulse generator may mimic insulation defect or intermittent failure.

Partial electrode fracture may generate false potentials because of changes in electrode resistance and may result in oversensing.[22, 48] The characteristic finding on a surface electrocardiogram is marked variation in the amplitude of the pacer artifact, with intermittent loss of ventricular capture (Fig. 11–25). Diagnosis of electrode fracture can be ascertained by analysis of the stimulus artifact as displayed on an oscilloscope. Distortion of the artifact may be the only sign, even in the absence of radiologic evidence for fracture of the lead.[34]

Partial Sensing

As a rule, VVI pacers respond to sensed signals in an all-or-none fashion, resulting in full recycling. Certain VVI pacer models exhibit partial sensing in response either to borderline signals falling anywhere outside their refractory period or to large signals—otherwise capable of recycling the generator completely—that fall within their short relative refractory period.[9] This partial sensing would result in partial recycling, leading to an abbreviated escape interval. Figure 11–26 illustrates an example of partial sensing of a ventricular ectopic beat that probably generated a borderline electrical signal, resulting in a shortened escape interval.

VALUE OF HOLTER MONITORING FOR FOLLOW-UP OF PACEMAKER PATIENTS

Ambulatory long-term electrocardiographic monitoring is valuable for follow-up of patients with pacemakers. The recording is well suited to document bradyarrhythmic and tachyarrhythmic events accompanied by conspicuous changes in cardiac rhythm. (Fig. 11–27). Ambulatory electrocardiograms should be analyzed with care, because of the new, uncommon occurrence of recording artifacts (Fig. 11–28). Although commercial Holter recorder/scanner systems can faithfully reproduce ordinary electrocardiographic waveforms whose major frequency components lie below 50 Hz, they severely attentuate signals of high frequency. Thus, pacing spikes, typically lasting 500 msec, with very rapid rise time, may sometimes be attentuated and slurred beyond recognition on the scanner oscilloscope or paper print-out. The ability to monitor an amplified pacemaker stimulus on a dedicated channel was first introduced by Kelen and associates.[45] This marker channel, with various degrees of sophistication, has resulted in marked improvement in the diagnosis of pacemaker problems.[31] Subtle or intermittent failure to sense (Fig. 11–29) or failure to capture (Fig. 11–30) can be easily detected. The system can also be used to evaluate AV sequential pacer program-

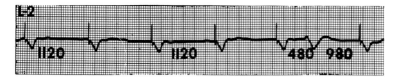

Figure 11–26. Partial sensing of a ventricular premature beat, resulting in a shortened escape interval. See text for details.

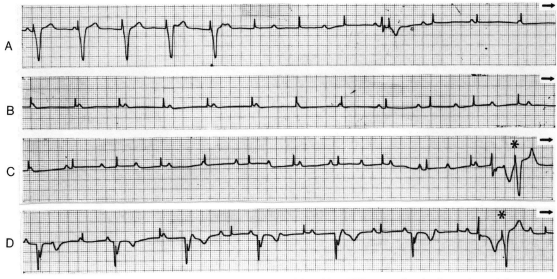

Figure 11–27. Ambulatory Holter recording from a patient with a VVI pacer, showing intermittent failure of capturing. The first half of record *A* shows a regular paced rhythm followed by abrupt loss of capturing. This loss of capturing resulted in a prolonged period of asystole (records *B* and *C*) before the escape of a fairly regular idioventricular rhythm (record *D*). Note the presence of two effective pacer stimuli (marked by asterisks). These are a manifestation of the supernormal phase of cardiac excitation and occur only when the pacer spike falls on or close to the end of the T wave of a preceding spontaneous depolarization. The presence of these two paced beats suggests that the intermittent failure to pace was caused by subthreshold pacer stimuli.

Figure 11–28. Ambulatory Holter recording from a patient with a VVI pacer, showing ECG artifact. The recording was obtained from a 69-year-old man with a VVI pacer implanted 6 months previously for symptomatic high-degree AV block. The patient presented with symptoms of light-headedness, and routine ECG examination showed normal pacing and sensing functions of the pacemaker.

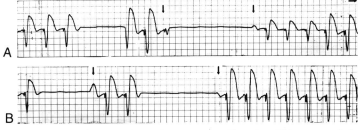

However, the 24-hour Holter recording was interpreted as indicating intermittent pacer malfunction. This prompted the change of the pulse generator. A thorough examination later failed to show any evidence of malfunction of the pulse generator, including both batteries and electronic components. A reexamination of the Holter recording clearly revealed the artifactual nature of the tracing. The representative tracings shown in the figure illustrate a paced rhythm with intermittent isoelectric pauses that are exact multiples of the pacer automatic interval. The artifact should have been readily identified by the deflections, marked by arrows, that represent partial inscription of paced QRS-T complexes and by the obvious variation in the amplitude of the recorded ECG complexes. The artifact was probably related to intermittent loss of contact between a loose electrode and the magnetic tape recorder.

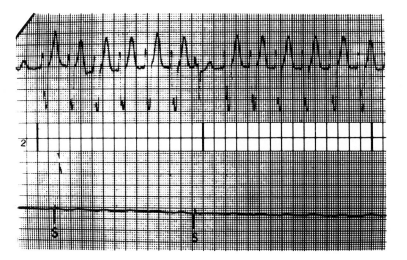

Figure 11–29. Ambulatory Holter recording using the marker channel. The intermittent inscription of pacing spike (s) clearly seen only on the marker channel represents sensing failure during supraventricular tachycardia.

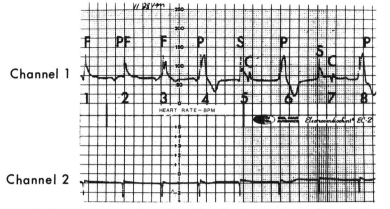

Figure 11–30. Ambulatory Holter recording using the marker channel. The recording was obtained from a 70-year-old patient with presyncopal symptoms and illustrates the problem of beat classification when multiple QRS morphologies occur. Beat 2 is a pseudo fusion beat (PF), and beats 1 and 3 are true fusion beats (F); beats 4, 6, and 8 are normally paced (P), and beats 5 and 7 are spontaneously conducted beats (C). The fifth and seventh pacemaker spikes (S) failed to capture. Sensing failure is also suggested by failure of the pacemaker to recycle after the spontaneously conducted beat 7, although this beat falls outside the known pacemaker sensing refractory period. Because of the slurring of the trailing edge of the pacing spike in channel 1, the noncapturing spikes could also be easily mistaken for QRS complexes, were the ambiguity not resolved by the marker channel 2.

ming and to assess programming efficacy of antitachycardia pacemakers.[15]

REFERENCES

1. Adamec R, Haefliger JM, Killisch JP, et al: Damaging effect of therapeutic radiation on programmable pacemakers. PACE 5:146, 1982.
2. Barold SS, Center S: Electrocardiographic diagnosis of perforation of the heart by pacing catheter electrode. Am J Cardiol 24:274, 1969.
3. Barold SS, Gaidula JJ: Evaluation of normal and abnormal sensing functions of demand pacemakers. Am J Cardiol 28:201, 1971.
4. Barold SS, Gaidula JJ: Failure of demand pacemaker from low bipolar electrograms. JAMA 215:923, 1971.
5. Barold SS, Levine PA: Auto interference of demand pulse generators. PACE 4:274, 1981.
6. Barold SS, Gaidula JJ, Castillo R: Unusual response of demand pacemakers to magnets. Br Heart J 35:353, 1973.
7. Barold SS, Ong LS, Banner RL: Diagnosis of interior wall myocardial infarction during right ventricular apical pacing. Chest 69:232, 1976.
8. Barold SS, Gaidula JJ, Castillo R, et al: Evaluation of demand pacemakers by chest wall stimulation. Chest 63:598, 1973.
9. Barold SS, Gaidula JJ, Lyon JL, et al: Irregular recycling of demand pacemakers from borderline electrographic signals. Am Heart J 82:477, 1971.
10. Bernstein AD, Camm AJ, Fletcher RD, et al: The NASPE/BPEG generic pacemaker code for anti-bradyarrhythmia and adaptive-rate pacing and antitachyarrhythmia devices. PACE 10:794, 1987.
11. Bilitch M, Cosby RS, Cafferky EA: Ventricular fibrillation and competitive pacing. N Engl J Med 276:598, 1967.
12. Bramowitz AD, Smith JW, Eber LM, et al: Runaway pacemaker: A persisting problem. JAMA 228:340, 1974.
13. Butrous GS, Male JC, Webber RS, et al: The effect of power frequency high intensity electronic field on implanted cardiac pacemakers. PACE 6:1282, 1983.
14. Cabrera E, Friedland C: La Onda de activacion ventricular en el bloqueo de rama izquierda caon infarcto: Un nuevo signo electrocardiografico. Arch Inst Cardiol Mex 23:441, 1953.
15. Casey TP, Miyasaki P, Rylaarsdam A, et al: Holter monitoring of pacemaker patients. Cardio, January 1988, pp 47–52.
16. Castellanos A Jr, Lemberg L: Pacer arrhythmias and electrocardiographic recognition of pacemakers. Circulation 47:1382, 1973.
17. Castellanos A Jr, Maytin O, Lemberg L, et al: Unusual QRS complexes produced by pacemaker stimuli. Am Heart J 77:732, 1969.
18. Castellanos A Jr, Ortiz JM, Pastis N, et al: The electrocardiogram in patients with pacemakers. Prog Cardiovasc Dis 13:190, 1970.
19. Chatterjee K, Sutton R, Davis JG: Low intracardiac potentials in myocardial infarction as a cause of failure of inhibition of demand pacemakers. Lancet 1:511, 1968.
20. Chatterjee K, Harris A, Davies G, et al: Electrocardiographic changes subsequent to artificial ventricular depolarization. Br Heart J 31:770, 1969.
21. Cheng TO, Chaithiraphan S, Baltazarn A, et al: Suppression by a prominent T-wave: An unusual cause of malfunction of a transvenous demand pacemaker. Chest 60:502, 1971.
22. Coumel P, Mugica J, Barold SS: Demand pacemaker arrhythmias caused by intermittent incomplete electrode fracture: Diagnosis with testing magnet. Am J Cardiol 39:105, 1975.
23. Crystal RG, Kastor JA, De Sanctis RW: Inhibition of discharge of an external demand pacemaker by electric razor. Am J Cardiol 28:695, 1971.
24. Das G, Eaton J: Pacemaker malfunction following transthoracic countershock. PACE 4:487, 1981.
25. D'Cunha GF, Nicoud T, Pemberton AH, et al: Syncopal attacks arising from erratic demand pacemaker function in the vicinity of a television transmitter. Am J Cardiol 31:789, 1973.
26. Denes P, Pick A, Miller RH, et al: A characteristic precordial repolarization abnormality with intermittent left bundle branch block. Ann Intern Med 89:55, 1978.

27. Dodinot B, Kubler L, Aliot E, et al: Electrocardiographic diagnosis of myocardial infarction and coronary insufficiency in the pacemaker patient. *In* Thalen HJ Th, Harthorne JW (eds): To Pace or Not to Pace: Controversial Subjects on Cardiac Pacing. Boston, Martinus Nijhoff, 1978, pp 295–301.

28. Driller J, Barold SS, Parsonnet V: Normal and abnormal function of the pacemaker magnetic reed switch. J Electrocardiol 9:283, 1976.

29. Erlbacher JA, Danner RL, Stelzer PE: Hypotension with ventricular pacing: An atrial vasodepressor reflex in human beings. J Am Coll Cardiol 4:550, 1984.

30. Escher DJW, Parker B, Furman S: Pacemaker triggering (inhibition) by electric toothbrush. Am J Cardiol 38:126, 1976.

31. Famularo MA, Kennedy HL: Ambulatory electrocardiography in the assessment of pacemaker function. Am Heart J 104:1086, 1982.

32. Fisch C, Greenspan K, Anderson GJ: Exit block. Am J Cardiol 28:402, 1971.

33. Furman S: Therapeutic uses of atrial pacing. Am Heart J 86:835, 1973.

34. Furman S: Cardiac pacing and pacemakers. VI. Analysis of pacemaker malfunction. Am Heart J 94:378, 1977.

35. Furman S: Cardiac pacing and pacemakers. VIII. The pacemaker follow-up clinic. Am Heart J 94:795, 1977.

36. Furman S, Escher DJW: Arrhythmias associated with hysteresis ventricular inhibited pacing. Chest 64:666, 1973.

37. Furman S, Huang WM: Pacemaker recycle from repolarization artefact. PACE 5:927, 1982.

38. Furman S, Parker B, Krauthamer M, et al: The influence of electromagnetic environment on the performance of artificial cardiac pacemakers. Ann Thorac Surg 6:90, 1968.

39. Gay RJ, Brown DF: Pacemaker failure due to procainamide toxicity. Am J Cardiol 34:728, 1974.

40. Gettes LS, Shabetai R, Downs TA, et al: Effect of changes in potassium and calcium concentrations on diastolic threshold and strength-interval relationship of the human heart. Ann NY Acad Sci 167:693, 1969.

41. Gialafos J, Maillis A, Kalogeropoulos C, et al: Inhibition of demand pacemakers by myopotentials. Am Heart J 109:984, 1985.

42. Gordon AJ, Vagueiro MC, Barold SS: Endocardial electrograms from pacemaker catheters. Circulation 38:82, 1968.

43. Hauser RG: Bipolar leads for cardiac pacing in the 1980's: A reappraisal provoked by skeletal muscle interference. PACE 5:34, 1982.

44. Hellestrand KH, Burnett PJ, Milne JR, et al: Effect of antiarrhythmic agent flecainide acetate on acute and chronic pacing thresholds. PACE 6:892, 1983.

45. Kelen GJ, Bloomfield DA, Hardage M, et al: Clinical evaluation of an improved Holter monitoring technique for artificial pacemaker function. PACE 3:192, 1980.

46. Keller JW, Gosselin AJ, Nathan DA, et al: Rhythm anomalies in contemporary demand pacing. Am J Cardiol 29:572, 1972.

47. King GR, Hanburger AC, Parsa F, et al: Effect of microwave oven on implanted cardiac pacemaker. JAMA 212:1213, 1970.

48. Lasseter KC, Buchanan Jr JW, Yoshonis KF: A mechanism for false inhibition of demand pacemaker. Circulation 42:1093, 1970.

49. Levine PA, Barold SS, Fletcher RD, et al: Adverse acute and chronic effects of electrical defibrillation and cardioversion on implanted unipolar cardiac pacing systems. J Am Coll Cardiol 1:1413, 1983.

50. Lichter I, Borrie J, Miller WM: Radio frequency hazards with cardiac pacemakers. Br Med J 1:513, 1965.

51. Lindemans FW, Rankin IR, Murtaugh R, et al: Clinical experience with an activity sensing pacemaker. PACE 9:978, 1986.

52. Magilligan DJ, Hakimi M, Davila JC: The sutureless electrode: Comparison with transvenous and sutured epicardial electrode placement for permanent pacing. Ann Thorac Surg 22:80, 1976.

53. Massumi RA, Mason DT, Amsterdam EA, et al: Apparent malfunction of demand pacemaker caused by nonpropagated (concealed) ventricular extrasystoles. Chest 61:426, 1972.

54. Medtronic Activitrax technical manual. Minneapolis, MN, Medtronic, p. 20.

55. Michaelson SM, Moss AJ: Environmental influences on implanted cardiac pacemakers. JAMA 216:2006, 1971.

56. Moss AJ, Rivers RJ: Atrial pacing from the coronary vein: Ten-year experience in 50 patients with implanted pervenous pacemakers. Circulation 57:103, 1978.

57. Mower MM, Aranaga CE, Tabatznik B: Unusual patterns of conduction produced by pacemaker stimuli. Am Heart J 74:24, 1967.

58. Nasrallah A, Hall RJ, Garcia E, et al: Runaway pacemaker in seven patients: A persisting problem. J Thorac Cardiovasc Surg 69:365, 1975.

59. Ohm OJ: Interference with cardiac pacemaker function. Acta Med Scand [Suppl] 86:596, 1976.

60. O'Reilley MV, Murnaghan DP, Williams MB: Transvenous pacemaker failure induced by hyperkalemia. JAMA 228:236, 1974.

61. Parsonnet V, Furman S, Smyth NPD: Implantable cardiac pacemakers: Status report and resource guidelines. Pacemaker Study Group, Intersociety Commission for Heart Disease Resources (ICHD). Circulation 50: A21, 1974.

62. Parsonnet V, Furman S, Symth NPD: Revised code for pacemaker identification. PACE 4:400 1981.

63. Pickers BA, Goldberg MJ: Inhibition of a demand pacemaker and interference with monitoring equipment by radio frequency transmission. Br Med J 2:504, 1969.

64. Preston TA, Judge RD: Alteration of pacemaker threshold by drug and physiological factors. Ann NY Acad Sci 167:686, 1969.

65. Rosenbaum MB, Blanco HH, Elizari MV, et al: Electronic modulation of the T wave and cardiac memory. Am J Cardiol 50:213, 1982.

66. Rosenqvist M, Norlander R, Andersson M, et al: Reduced incidence of myopotential pacemaker inhibition by abdominal generator implantation. PACE 9:417, 1986.

67. Saksena S: Mechanism of unusual QRS pattern associated with right ventricular pacing. Am Heart J 105:337, 1983.

68. Samet P, Abbas SZ, Hildner FJ, et al: Effect of chest wall stimulation on cardiac pacemaker function. Am J Med Sci 260:285, 1970.

69. Samet P, Castillo C, Bernstein WH: Hemodynamic consequences of atrial and ventricular pacing in subjects with normal beats. Am J Cardiol 18:522, 1966.
70. Sinnaeve A, Williams R, Stroobandt R: Inhibition of the demand pacemakers by magnet waving. PACE 5:878, 1982.
71. Sodi-Pollares D, Calder RM: New Bases of Electrocardiography. St Louis, CV Mosby, 1956.
72. Tabesh E: Intermittent P- and T-wave sensing in demand pacemakers. J Electrocardiol 5:295, 1972.
73. Van Beck GW, Den Dulk K, Lindemans FW, et al: HJJ detection of insulation failure by gradual reduction in non-invasively measured electrogram amplitudes. PACE 9:772, 1986.
74. Voukydis PC, Shulman AN, Cohen SI: Unmasking of slow intrinsic ventricular excitation by magnet inhibition of R wave inhibited demand pacemakers. Chest 67:304, 1975.
75. Wajszczuk WJ, Mowry FM, Dungan NF: De-activation of a demand pacemaker by transurethral electrocautery. N Engl J Med 230:34, 1969.
76. Walter WH, Mitchell JC, Rustan PL, et al: Cardiac pulse generators and electromagnetic interference. JAMA 224:1628, 1973.
77. Weinstock M, De Guia R, Daniell M, et al: Inhibition of transvenous pacing through the coronary sinus by the atrial P wave: Diagnosis with the aid of isoproterenol. Chest 59:563, 1971.
78. Wiggers CJ, Wegria R: Ventricular fibrillation due to single, localized induction and condensor shocks applied during the vulnerable phase of ventricular systoles. Am J Physiol 128:500, 1940.
79. Wirtzfeld A, Lampadius M, Ruprecht EO: Unterdruckung von Demand-Schritt machen durch Muskelpotentiale. Dtsch Med Wochenschr 97:61, 1972.
80. Yatteau RF: Radar-induced failure of a demand pacemaker. N Engl J Med 283:1447, 1970.
81. Yee R, Jones DL, Klein GJ: Pacing threshold changes after transvenous catheter countershock. Am J Cardiol 53:503, 1984.
82. Yokoyama M, Wada J, Barold SS: Transient early T wave sensing by implanted programmable demand pulse generator. PACE 4:68, 1981.
83. Zoll PM: Resuscitation of the heart in ventricular standstill by external electric stimulation. N Engl J Med 247:7786, 1952.

12

ELECTROCARDIOGRAPHY OF CONTEMPORARY DDD PACEMAKERS

A. Basic Concepts, Upper Rate Response, Retrograde Ventriculoatrial Conduction, and Differential Diagnosis of Pacemaker Tachycardias

S. SERGE BAROLD, MICHAEL D. FALKOFF, LING S. ONG, *and* ROBERT A. HEINLE

The large variety of commercially available DDD pulse generators with innumerable programmable functions is truly intimidating, and each new refinement of pacemaker operation creates a new layer of complexity. Electrocardiographic patterns seen with dual-chamber pacemakers may render the distinction between normal and abnormal pacemaker function quite difficult.[21, 53, 67, 84, 86, 90–92, 101, 110] It is no longer possible to analyze the electrocardiogram with only an elementary understanding of pacemaker technology. The first and probably the most important step is mastery of the basic timing cycles of DDD pulse generators.[13, 52, 53] Although some of the timing cycles may vary according to the model and manufacturer, all DDD pacemakers possess fundamental timing cycles that do not vary from device to device (Fig. 12–1). This chapter is presented in two parts. The first part deals with the basic concepts, timing cycles, upper rate response, retrograde ventriculoatrial (VA) conduction (endless loop tachycardia and atrioventricular [AV] desynchronization

arrhythmia), and the differential diagnosis of pacemaker tachycardia. The second part deals with basic troubleshooting and some of the more complex electrocardiographic manifestations of normal and abnormal DDD pacing.

DEFINITIONS

1. *Lower rate interval* (corresponding to programmed lower rate): The longest interval between consecutive ventricular stimuli without an intervening sensed P wave or from a sensed ventricular signal to the succeeding ventricular stimulus without an intervening sensed P wave. This term may also be defined as the longest interval between sensed ventricular events without a ventricular pacemaker stimulus.

2. *AV interval:* The programmed interval from the atrial stimulus to the ventricular stimulus or the interval between the point at which a P wave is sensed to the following ventricular stimulus. It is the electronic analog of the PR

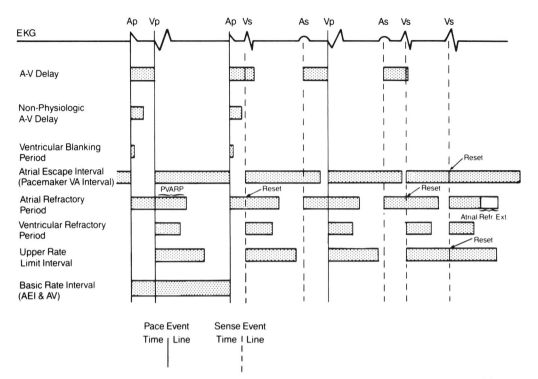

Figure 12–1. Diagrammatic representation of timing cycles of a typical DDD pulse generator with an upper rate limit interval (URI) separately programmable from the total atrial refractory period (TARP).

1. Atrial pace (Ap) event followed by a ventricular pace (Vp) event: Ap-Vp. When no events are sensed in either chamber during the atrial escape (pacemaker VA) interval, the pulse generator delivers an atrial output pulse (Ap) that initiates the following cycles: AV delay and the two crosstalk intervals, ventricular blanking period (VBP) and ventricular triggering period (VTP). The latter is also known as the ventricular "safety pacing" period or nonphysiologic AV delay. The atrial channel of all DDD pulse generators is refractory during the AV interval. If no events are sensed by the ventricular channel by the end of the programmed AV interval, an output pulse is delivered to the ventricle (Vp). This pulse in turn initiates the following timing cycles: a new lower rate interval (LRI = atrial escape interval + AV delay), a new atrial escape (pacemaker VA) interval, a ventricular refractory period (VRP), an atrial refractory period or the postventricular atrial refractory period (PVARP), and an upper rate limit interval (URI).

2. Atrial pace (Ap) event followed by a ventricular sense (Vs) event: Ap-Vs. If no atrial or ventricular events are sensed during the atrial escape (pacemaker VA) interval, an output pulse is delivered to the atrium (Ap). This pulse delivery will initiate the following timing cycles: AV delay and its atrial refractory period, VBP, and VTP. Two possibilities may then arise: (a) A ventricular event (Vs) sensed outside the VTP, but still within the programmed AV delay, will cause inhibition of the ventricular output; or (b) if the ventricular event (Vs) is sensed within the VTP (after the VBP), a ventricular output pulse (Vp) is delivered at the completion of the VTP. This would, of course, lead to abbreviation of the AV (Ap-Vp) interval. Regardless of its timing, the ventricular stimulus will always initiate the next LRI, the atrial escape (pacemaker VA) interval, the VRP, the URI, and the PVARP.

3. Atrial sense (As) event followed by a ventricular pace (Vp) event: As-Vp. A sensed atrial (As) event during the atrial escape (pacemaker VA) interval will inhibit the next atrial output pulse and will initiate an AV delay and an atrial refractory period. If no ventricular event is sensed during the programmed AV delay, a ventricular output pulse is delivered (Vp) at the end of the AV delay. The ventricular paced event (Vp) in turn initiates a new LRI, a new atrial escape (pacemaker VA) interval, VRP, URI, and PVARP.

4. Atrial sense (As) event followed by a ventricular sense (Vs) event: As-Vs. If an atrial event is sensed (As) during the atrial escape interval, it will initiate an AV delay and its accompanying atrial refractory period. A ventricular event (Vs) sensed during the programmed AV interval inhibits the ventricular output. Vs also initiates a new LRI, an atrial escape (pacemaker VA) interval, a VRP, a URI, and a PVARP.

5. Ventricular extrasystole. In the presence of a ventricular event (Vs) sensed outside the programmed AV delay, both the atrial and the ventricular outputs are inhibited and Vs initiates a new atrial escape (pacemaker VA) interval, a URI, a VRP, and a PVARP. In addition, the PVARP initiated after Vs interpreted as an extrasystole (i.e., not preceded by As or Ap) may be automatically extended in some DDD pulse generators by a value equal to the "programmed atrial refractory period extension."

Ap = atrial pace event; As = atrial sense event; Vp = ventricular pace event; Vs = ventricular sense event; AEI = atrial escape (pacemaker VA) interval; PVARP = postventricular atrial refractory period; Atrial Refr. Ext. = atrial refractory period extension. (Adapted from the technical manual for the Intermedics Cosmos pulse generator, Intermedics, Freeport, TX.)

interval. The AV interval initiated by atrial sensing is generally equal to that initiated by an atrial stimulus. In some DDD pulse generators, the AV interval initiated by atrial sensing is shorter than that initiated by an atrial stimulus.

3. *Atrial escape (pacemaker VA) interval:* The interval from a ventricular pacing stimulus or sensed ventricular signal to the following atrial stimulus. The atrial escape (pacemaker VA) interval is derived by subtracting the AV interval from the lower rate interval.

4. *Ventricular refractory period:* Traditionally, this has been defined as the interval following a paced or sensed event during which the ventricular amplifier is insensitive to incoming signals. However, contemporary pulse generators may sense signals during part of the refractory period (sometimes known as the noise-sampling period) and use them to modify some aspect of pacemaker function. In the light of these considerations, the ventricular refractory period is best defined as the period during which the lower rate interval cannot be reset (and reinitiated) by any signal, whether or not it is actually recognized by the pulse generator.

5. *Postventricular atrial refractory period (PVARP):* Pacemaker atrial refractory period occurring after the emission of a ventricular stimulus or a sensed QRS complex or other ventricular signal. This period is designed to prevent the atrial channel from sensing the ventricular pacing stimulus, the far-field QRS complex, and ectopic premature or retrograde P waves. The PVARP should be programmed to a value longer than the retrograde VA conduction time to prevent the atrial channel from sensing retrograde atrial depolarization.

6. *Total atrial refractory period (TARP):* The TARP consists of two components. The first part starts with the beginning of an atrial event (paced or sensed) and extends through the AV delay. Because it is undesirable for a second atrial event to be sensed once the AV interval has begun, the atrial sensing amplifier is always refractory for the duration of the AV interval. The second component is the PVARP, which starts with a ventricular event (paced or sensed). The total atrial refractory period equals the AV interval plus the PVARP. The duration of the TARP always defines the shortest upper rate limit interval (or the fastest ventricular tracking rate).

7. *Upper rate limit interval* (corresponding to the upper rate or maximal tracking rate): This term applies to the ventricular channel of a dual-chamber pacemaker, unless otherwise specified. This is the shortest interval between two consecutive ventricular stimuli or from a sensed ventricular event to the succeeding ventricular stimulus while maintaining 1:1 AV synchrony with sensed atrial events.

TIMING CYCLES AND BASIC BEHAVIOR OF DDD PACEMAKERS

The operational concepts and timing cycles of a representative DDD pulse generator are depicted in Figure 12–2. The key to understanding pacemaker function depends on (1) thinking in terms of intervals rather than rate, just as the pacemaker functions, and (2) know-

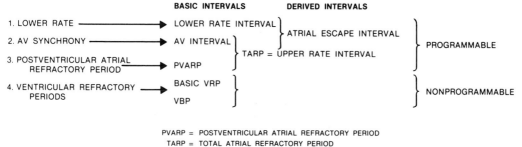

Figure 12–2. Basic and derived timing cycles of a simple DDD pulse generator. A simple DDD pulse generator requires three fundamental timing cycles, that is, LRI, AV interval, and PVARP, all of which must be programmable. The atrial escape (pacemaker VA) interval, the TARP, and the URI may be derived from these three basic intervals. As in a VVI pulse generator, the ventricular channel of a DDD pulse generator must generate a VRP. The VBP is required to prevent crosstalk. Programmability of VRP and VBP is not essential.

ing the various timing cycles initiated by paced and sensed events in either the atrium or the ventricle.

Basic Concepts

1. The atrial escape (pacemaker VA) interval is initiated by a paced or sensed ventricular event.

2. An atrial stimulus is released at the end of the atrial escape (pacemaker VA) interval.

3. Atrial sensing before the termination of the atrial escape (pacemaker VA) interval inhibits the atrial output.

4. The AV interval is started by a paced or sensed atrial event.

5. A ventricular stimulus is emitted at the end of the programmed AV interval.

6. A sensed ventricular event before termination of the AV interval inhibits the ventricular output.

7. Both atrial and ventricular outputs are inhibited by a sensed ventricular event (e.g., Ventricular premature contraction [VPC]) that occurs before the end of the atrial escape (pacemaker VA) interval.

8. A paced or sensed ventricular event starts the ventricular refractory period and the PVARP.

9. The atrial channel of a DDD pacemaker is always refractory during the entire duration of the AV interval. The TARP is equal to the sum of the AV interval plus the PVARP.

10. The delivery of the atrial stimulus (output) initiates a short ventricular refractory period (known as the ventricular blanking period) to minimize or prevent crosstalk. Crosstalk refers to sensing of the atrial stimulus by the ventricular channel, with resultant inappropriate inhibition of the ventricular output. Crosstalk may be particularly dangerous in pacemaker-dependent patients with little or no spontaneous underlying rhythm.

11. In some pulse generators, the first part of the AV interval initiated by an atrial stimulus contains a safety mechanism to prevent inhibition of the ventricular channel, should the ventricular blanking period be unsuccessful in dealing with crosstalk. This is the so-called "ventricular safety pacing period." A sensed ventricular signal during this particular period forces the pulse generator to deliver a triggered ventricular stimulus at the completion of the ventricular safety pacing period.[13, 84] The latter is also known as the nonphysiologic AV delay or crosstalk sensing window,[84] but we believe the term "ventricular triggering period" is more appropriate.[10]

12. Because atrial sensing does not interfere with the function of the ventricular channel, there is no need for ventricular blanking and ventricular triggering periods after atrial sensing.

All DDD pulse generators possess nine fundamental timing cycles, five related to the ventricular channel and four to the atrial channel (Fig. 12–3). A ventricular event (paced or sensed) initiates a lower rate interval, an upper rate interval, PVARP, ventricular refractory period, and atrial escape (pacemaker VA) interval. Although the last-named is a derived rather than a fundamental interval, it is included because of its importance in controlling the timing of the atrial stimulus. The four intervals initiated by an atrial event consist of the AV interval, atrial refractory period (encompassing the AV interval), the ventricular blanking period, and, in some pulse generators, an additional ventricular triggering period that usually occupies the first 100 to 110 msec of the

DDD TIMING CYCLES

FURTHER REFINEMENTS

1. CROSSTALK INTERVALS	ADD VTP. (AV>VTP>VBP)
	PROGRAMMABLE VBP & VTP
2. UPPER RATE	SEPARATELY PROGRAMMABLE UPPER RATE.
	URI>TARP (WENCKEBACH RESPONSE)
3. VENTRICULAR REFRACTORY PERIOD	PROGRAMMABLE

VTP = VENTRICULAR TRIGGERING PERIOD
(VENTRICULAR SAFETY PACING PERIOD)

Figure 12–3. Further refinements of DDD timing cycles. 1. Addition of the so-called ventricular safety pacing period or ventricular triggering period (VTP) to deal with crosstalk not prevented by the VBP. Note the relative duration of the timing cycles initiated by the emission of an atrial stimulus. 2. A separately programmable URI (with a Wenckebach upper rate response) can exist only when it is longer than the TARP. 3. Programmable VRP.

AV interval, beginning with the termination of the ventricular blanking period.[10, 13, 17] No ventricular blanking or triggering period occurs coincidentally with atrial sensing. The atrial intervals are best remembered in terms of decreasing duration, the longest being the AV interval, then the ventricular triggering period, and finally the ventricular blanking period. The TARP is a derived interval composed of the sum of the AV interval and PVARP.

THE MANY FACES OF DDD PACING

The DDD mode, being a universal modality, contains within itself simpler modes of pacing. The behavior of DDD pacemakers may be simplified by examining a single cycle at a time in a continuous electrocardiogram. The DDD mode incorporates the essentials of three simpler modes: DVI, AAI, and VDD[56] (Fig. 12–4). In any one pacemaker cycle, starting with either a sensed or a paced ventricular event, one of these three modes may be seen on the electrocardiogram. The descriptive mode for a single pacemaker cycle is determined only by the way the cycle terminates.

No Pacemaker Stimuli

If there are no stimuli, the pacemaker is fully inhibited and the mode for a given cycle cannot be determined. Thus, if there are no

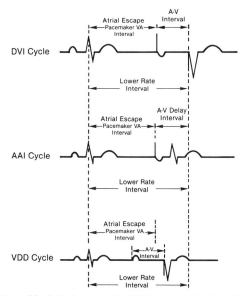

stimuli, the pacemaker could be operating in any one of its three modes for any given cycle (AAI, VDD, or DVI) or all of them together. In this situation, the RR interval is shorter than the lower rate limit interval, and the PR interval is shorter than the AV interval. However, inhibition does not always mean that the pulse generator senses both ventricular and atrial signals. Thus, during total inhibition, a DDD pulse generator may actually be working continuously in the DVI mode (e.g., if the atrial signal is too small to be sensed), and if the RR interval is shorter than the atrial escape (pacemaker VA) interval, atrial undersensing may be masked.

One Pacemaker Stimulus

If there is only one stimulus, the pacemaker could be operating in any one of three modes:

1. *AAI mode:* If there is only an atrial stimulus, the pacemaker functions in the AAI mode. This occurs if the atrial rate is slow, with intact AV conduction.

2. *VVD (VAT) mode:* If there is only a ventricular stimulus, the pacemaker functions in the VDD (VAT) mode. This occurs with a normal atrial rate, but abnormal AV conduction.

3. *VVI (VOO) mode:* If there is a single ventricular stimulus, the pacemaker may also be functioning in the VVI or VOO mode rather than the VDD mode. Automatic conversion of a DDD pulse generator to the VVI (or VOO) mode may occur as a result of sensing extraneous interference or when there is battery depletion, the reset mode being an end-of-service indicator. In addition, some pulse generators programmed to the DDD mode may be converted to the VOO (not DOO) mode upon application of the test magnet, as, for example, with the CPI Delta DDD pulse generator (Cardiac Pacemakers, Inc, St. Paul, MN). The VVI (VOO) mode can usually be ignored in the routine electrocardiographic analysis of pacemaker function because it occurs only under unusual circumstances.

Two Pacemaker Stimuli

If there are two pacemaker stimuli, three possibilities exist:

1. *DVI mode:* This is the most likely mode, and it occurs with a slow atrial rate and abnormal AV conduction. In this context, the DVI mode refers to a partially committed

Figure 12–4. Behavior of a DDD pacemaker based on examination of a single cycle. Starting with either a paced or a sensed ventricular event, DVI, AAI, or VDD may be seen. The mode described for a single pacemaker cycle is determined by the way the cycle terminates.

system, that is, the pulse generator is capable of sensing ventricular activity during part of the AV interval (after termination of the ventricular blanking period to prevent detection of the atrial stimulus or crosstalk).

2. *DOO mode:* This may occur in the presence of excessive noise or interference or upon application of the test magnet.

3. *DDT (triggered) mode:* Under certain circumstances, a DDD pulse generator may be considered to be working in the DDT mode, a code suggested by Garson and colleagues[56] to denote the ventricular safety pacing period or ventricular triggering period characteristic of some DDD pulse generators. A signal sensed by the ventricular channel during the ventricular triggering period forces the delivery of a triggered ventricular stimulus at the end of the ventricular triggering period, thereby abbreviating the AV interval.[13]

We believe that the approach of Garson and colleagues[56] is useful for analysis of DDD pacing function in terms of six pacing modes. These consist of three basic modes (AAI, DVI, and VDD), together with three less important ones (VVI, DDT, and DOO). Thus, with only one pacemaker stimulus, the pulse generator is functioning in the AAI, VDD, or VVI (VOO) mode and, with two stimuli, in the DVI, DDT, or DOO mode.

UPPER RATE RESPONSE

The value of the programmed upper rate of a DDD pulse generator depends on the patient's activity, age, left ventricular function, and propensity to endless loop tachycardia, a reentrant pacemaker tachycardia initiated by repetitive sensing of retrograde P waves secondary to VA conduction. An upper rate of 180 beats per minute does not make sense in the average patient with sick sinus syndrome because during treadmill exercise such patients rarely achieve a rate faster than 110 to 120 beats per minute,[62] whereas a relatively fast upper rate would be extremely important in a young and active individual with complete AV block and normal sinus node responsiveness to increased metabolic demands.

As a rule, an increase in heart rate during exercise is hemodynamically more beneficial than maintenance of AV synchrony without a rate increase.[107, 130] Consequently, proper understanding of the upper rate response is of crucial importance in the management of pa-

tients with DDD pulse generators. Today's DDD pulse generators offer many methods to limit the ventricular response to physiologic or pathologic atrial rates, but none is ideal. The maximal rate of a DDD pacemaker can be defined by either the duration of the TARP or a separate timing circuit controlling the ventricular output.[13, 52, 53, 84, 91] In general, a fixed-block response (2:1, 3:1, and so on) is less suitable than Wenckebach-like behavior (6:5, 5:4, and so forth). The advantages of other characteristics such as the fallback response (synchronous or asynchronous), rate smoothing, and other types of upper rate response are unclear, and their use should be individualized.[73] Holter recordings and treadmill exercise testing may be useful in evaluating the upper rate response and tailoring pacemaker parameters to the needs of the individual patient. When programming the upper rate response, several important questions should be considered. Can the programmed upper rate be tolerated by the patient? During sinus tachycardia, will the patient be able to withstand a sudden drop in ventricular rate, as in fixed-ratio block? Will the patient tolerate sustained ventricular pacing at a fast rate, particularly with loss of AV synchrony, as may occur during atrial fibrillation or flutter?

Fixed-Ratio Block

The simplest way for a DDD pulse generator to control the upper rate is by programmability of the AV delay and the PVARP. The upper rate becomes a function of the programmed TARP, which is equal to the sum of the AV interval and PVARP[73] (Fig. 12–5). The upper rate may be calculated by the following formula: upper rate (ppm) = 60,000/refractory period (in milliseconds) or 60/refractory period (in seconds).[66] As the atrial rate increases, any P wave falling within the PVARP is unsensed. The number of unsensed P waves (or degree of block) depends on the atrial rate and where the P waves occur in the pacemaker cycle. The AV interval always remains constant. As the atrial rate increases, more P waves fall within the atrial refractory period, and the degree of block increases. If the upper rate limit is 120 ppm (TARP = 500 msec) and the lower rate is 70 ppm, the pacing rate will not drop by half to 60 ppm (i.e., 2:1) when the atrial rate reaches 120 ppm because the paced ventricular rate cannot fall below the lower rate limit. This response is often called 2:1 block, though

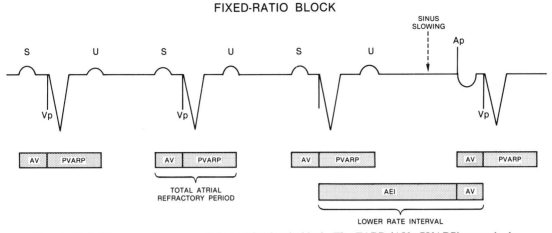

Figure 12–5. Diagrammatic representation of fixed-ratio block. The TARP (AV + PVARP) controls the URI. Every second P wave is unsensed because it falls within the PVARP (2:1 block). When sinus slowing occurs on the right, the pacemaker functions according to the programmed LRI, thereby delivering an atrial stimulus that terminates the pause. S = sensed P wave; U = unsensed P wave; Ap = atrial pace event; Vp = ventricular pace event; AEI = atrial escape interval.

it is really a misnomer. Actually, the paced ventricular rate will be exactly half the atrial rate or equal to the lower rate of the pacemaker, whichever is higher. When half the atrial rate is slower than the programmed lower rate, the pulse generator must pace AV sequentially at the lower rate, that is, an atrial stimulus rather than a sensed P wave initiates the AV interval (see Fig. 12–5). An upper rate response using fixed-ratio block may be inappropriate in young or physically active individuals because the sudden reduction of the ventricular rate with activity may be poorly tolerated.

Wenckebach Pacemaker Response

Only DDD pulse generators possessing an independently programmable upper rate capability allow a pulse generator to respond in a Wenckebach (or pseudo Wenckebach) fashion to fast atrial rates.[12, 13, 51–53, 73, 84, 91, 114] The purpose of the Wenckebach response is to avoid sudden reduction of the paced ventricular rate (as occurs with fixed-ratio block) and to maintain some degree of AV synchrony.

The Wenckebach mode of upper rate limitation depends on separate programmability of the upper rate (upper rate limit interval) and the atrial refractory period (AV interval plus the PVARP). In order for a Wenckebach response to occur with *prolongation* of the AV (atrial sense–ventricular pace) interval, the upper rate limit interval must be *longer* than the TARP (Figs. 12–6, 12–7, and 12–8). The maximal prolongation of the AV interval during a pacemaker Wenckebach sequence represents the difference between these two intervals. When the separately programmable upper rate limit interval becomes equal to the TARP, the Wenckebach response cannot occur, and the upper rate interval becomes a function of the programmed TARP, thereby creating fixed-ratio block (Figs. 12–5, 12–6, and 12–9). With a progressive increase in the atrial rate, the Wenckebach response eventually switches to 2:1 fixed-ratio block when the PP interval becomes shorter than the TARP.[1–4] When the upper rate limit interval is programmed to a shorter value than the TARP, despite the fact that the programmer and the pulse generator may seem to have accepted the command, the upper rate can be controlled only by the duration of the TARP, and the pacemaker will not exhibit Wenckebach behavior. The Wenckebach upper rate response should therefore be considered a way of providing a smoother transition from a 1:1 ventricular response to a fixed-ratio block (see Figs. 12–7 and 12–8).

During the Wenckebach response, the pacemaker will synchronize its ventricular stimulus to sensed atrial activity, but the pacemaker cannot violate its (ventricular) upper rate limit interval, so that the ventricular stimulus can be released only at the completion of the upper rate limit interval (see Figs. 12–7 and 12–8). The AV delay (initiated by a sensed P wave) becomes progressively longer as the ventricular channel waits to deliver its stimulus until the

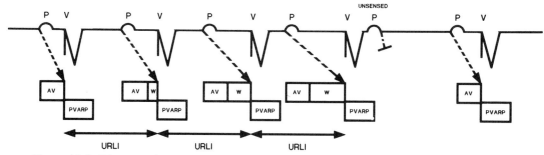

Figure 12–6. Diagrammatic representation of pacemaker Wenckebach periodicity. A slow URL interval (75 per minute or interval of 800 msec) was selected for more graphic understanding of the pacemaker Wenckebach concept. As the atrial rate increases (PP interval = 700 msec, corresponding to a rate of approximately 86 ppm), the ventricular paced rate equals the programmed URL (interval = 800 ms). The increase in atrial rate results in automatic prolongation of the AV delay by the addition of a "waiting period" (W) so as not to yield ventricular pacing before the end of the URL interval (800 msec). Subsequent P waves occur relatively earlier in relation to the paced ventricular beat, until the P wave occurs in the PVARP and is therefore unsensed. The unsensed P wave is not followed by a ventricular stimulus. Note that the URL interval is longer than the TARP (AV + PVARP). The maximal duration of the W period is the difference between the URL interval and the TARP. Adapted, with permission, from: Luceri RM, Castellanos A, Zaman L, Myerburg R: The arrhythmias of dual chamber cardiac pacemakers and their management. *Ann Intern Med* 1983: 99:354.

upper rate limit interval has timed out. The atrial channel remains refractory and therefore insensitive to incoming signals through the entire duration of the AV interval, regardless of its length. Eventually, a P wave falling within the PVARP will not be followed by a ventricular output, and a pause will occur. In other words, Wenckebach behavior limits the paced ventricular rate by extending the AV interval.

There are important differences between the artificial and the natural Wenckebach phenomenon:

1. Although a spontaneous, atypical AV nodal Wenckebach phenomenon may occasionally cause some regularization of the RR intervals, it is never associated with absolutely constant RR intervals, as seen with the pacemaker response to a rapid atrial rate. The interval between the pacemaker stimuli is constant because they are locked at the upper rate limit interval.

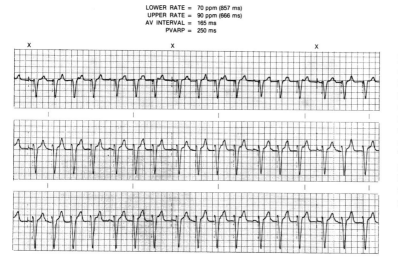

Figure 12–7. Wenckebach upper rate response of DDD pulse generator, with programmed parameters shown above the electrocardiograms (ECGs) with three leads recorded simultaneously. The URI was deliberately lengthened to demonstrate the Wenckebach sequence. The pauses after unsensed P waves (within the PVARP) are terminated by either a sensed or a paced (X) P wave. Barring the pauses, all pacemaker cycles are equal to the URI.

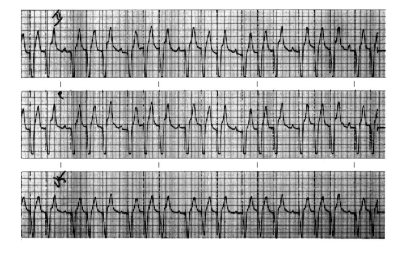

Figure 12–8. A 4:3 Wenckebach response of a DDD pulse generator during treadmill exercise test. The programmed parameters were as follows: URI = 500 msec (rate = 120 ppm), AV delay = 200 msec, PVARP = 200 msec, and LRI = 857 msec (rate = 70 ppm). When the sinus rate exceeded 120 beats per minute, pacemaker Wenckebach response occurred. Most of the sinus P waves are not discernible because they are buried in the ST–T-wave segment of the paced beats.

2. There appears to be AV dissociation during the pacemaker Wenckebach period because the P waves march through the ventricular cycle. In contrast to spontaneous AV dissociation, in which atrial and ventricular events are unrelated, in pacemaker-mediated Wenckebach-like periods there is a definite link between each P wave and its triggered ventricular stimulus.

3. The blocked P wave is not really blocked but is unsensed as it falls within the PVARP. The pacemaker then synchronizes its ventricular output to the next P wave.

The Wenckebach response is therefore characterized by variability of the AV interval, a sustained higher rate, and occasional abrupt change in the beat-to-beat ventricular rate. There are two intervals during a pacemaker Wenckebach response: (1) repeated ventricular pacing at the upper rate limit and (2) a longer interval following the undetected P wave in the PVARP. The maximal duration of this pause measured between two consecutive ventricular stimuli (after a blocked or unsensed P wave) is equal to the sum of the PVARP, PP interval, and programmed AV interval, provided the pulse generator senses the P wave that follows the unsensed one in the PVARP at the end of the Wenckebach sequence.[43] Should a P wave not occur before the end of the atrial escape (pacemaker VA) interval, the pause will be equal to the lower rate interval.

Let us consider two clinical examples of upper rate limitation. A DDD pulse generator is programmed as follows: Upper rate equals 100 ppm (upper rate limit interval = 600 msec), AV interval equals 150 msec and PVARP equals 250 msec, and TARP equals 400 msec. The pacemaker will therefore respond to an atrial rate faster than 100 beats per minute by exhibiting Wenckebach sequences, with the longest AV interval prolongation being 200 msec $(600 - 400)$; that is, the so-called "W

Figure 12–9. ECG taken after mild exercise in a patient with an Intermedics Cosmos DDD pulse generator. The patient complained of effort intolerance. The parameters are shown above the ECG: URI = 500 msec, TARP = 495 msec, and W (Wenckebach, or waiting) period = 5 msec. This set of values, in effect, produces an upper rate response with fixed-ratio block. There is an intermittent 1:1 response and 2:1 fixed-ratio block. Note that the cycles during 2:1 fixed-ratio block terminate with either a sensed P

COSMOS, LRI = 1000, URI = 500, AV = 150, PVARP = 345
TARP = 345 + 150 = 495

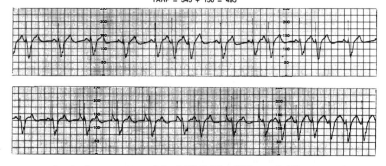

wave or a paced P wave. The latter occurs to maintain the constancy of the LRI (LRI = 1000 msec). The pacemaker was therefore reprogrammed with a shorter PVARP and correspondingly shorter URI. The new settings eradicated the patient's symptoms on exercise.

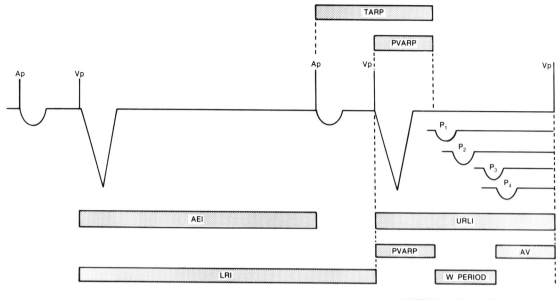

$$W\ PERIOD = URLI - (AV + PVARP)$$
$$= URLI - TARP$$

Figure 12–10. Diagrammatic representation of the mechanism of AV interval prolongation in a pulse generator with a separately programmable TARP and upper rate limit interval (URLI). The Wenckebach, or waiting, period $(W) = URLI - (AV + PVARP) = URLI - TARP$. A P wave (P_1) occurring immediately after the termination of the PVARP will exhibit the longest AV interval, that is, $AV + W$. A P wave just beyond the W period (P_4) will initiate an AV interval equal to the programmed value. P waves occurring during the W period $(P_2$ and $P_3)$ will exhibit varying degrees of AV prolongation to conform to the URLI depicted as the shortest interval between two consecutive ventricular paced beats. AEI = atrial escape interval; LRI = lower rate interval; Ap = atrial paced beat; Vp = ventricular paced beat.

period" (Wenckebach window or waiting period) is equal to 200 msec. Thus, the AV interval will vary from its programmed value of 150 msec to a maximum of 350 msec.

The response of a DDD pacemaker to a sensed atrial extrasystole may at first appear complicated. The AV interval engendered by a sensed premature atrial depolarization depends on its timing within the pacing cycle, bearing in mind that the release of a triggered ventricular stimulus must wait until the upper rate limit interval has timed out (Fig. 12–10). In the above example, the duration of the AV interval may assume any value between 150 msec and 350 msec, according to the timing of the atrial extrasystole in the cardiac cycle. The upper rate limit interval may be identified on the electrocardiogram by moving calipers from a premature ventricular stimulus back to the previous ventricular event. If this interval corresponds to the upper rate limit interval, it provides proof that an atrial sensed event occurred between the two ventricular events bracketing the upper rate limit interval. Thus, an atrial extrasystole that is invisible on the electrocardiogram may often be presumed to exist if the upper rate limitation is invoked.

In contrast, if the same DDD pulse generator were programmed with an AV interval equaling 200 msec, a PVARP equaling 250 msec, and an upper rate equaling 125 ppm (upper rate interval = 480 msec), it would be difficult to produce an actual pacemaker Wenckebach effect. The prolongation of the AV interval during Wenckebach behavior (W interval) would be only 30 msec (480 − 450). The maximal duration of the AV interval would therefore be 230 msec. In the above situation, where the TARP equals 450 msec (corresponding to a rate of 133 ppm), the pulse generator will respond with a Wenckebach response to an atrial rate higher than 125 ppm but less than 133 ppm. When the atrial rate exceeds 133 ppm, fixed-ratio block will occur without a Wenckebach response. A short W period means that the pulse generator will respond basically with fixed-ratio block (Fig. 12–10). The sudden, sharp drop in the ventricular pacing rate may not be well tolerated in patients with sinus tachycardia caused by activity or other factors.

In patients with retrograde VA conduction, progressive lengthening of the AV delay to conform to the upper rate limit interval during the pacemaker Wenckebach response may result in the atria's being "ready" to accept a retrograde impulse generated by the ventricular paced beat. Critical prolongation of the AV interval during a pacemaker Wenckebach sequence may therefore initiate endless loop tachycardia.[13, 54] Rarely, the same mechanism may also initiate endless loop tachycardia during exercise in predisposed individuals.[30, 124]

Extension of the Atrial Escape Interval at the Upper Rate Limit

Whenever an Intermedics Cosmos DDD pulse generator (Intermedics, Freeport, TX)

paces at the upper rate limit, the subsequent atrial escape (pacemaker VA) interval is extended to increase the opportunity for sensing spontaneous atrial activity (Fig. 12–11). This extension was designed to prevent atrial arrhythmias faster than the (ventricular) upper rate of the pulse generator from being artificially accelerated by a relatively early atrial paced event.[10] Consequently, if no intrinsic atrial event occurs during the extended atrial escape (pacemaker VA) interval, AV pacing will drop below the programmed "rate" for one cycle only. The extension of the atrial escape interval measures about 400 msec for some of the earlier Cosmos DDD pulse gen-

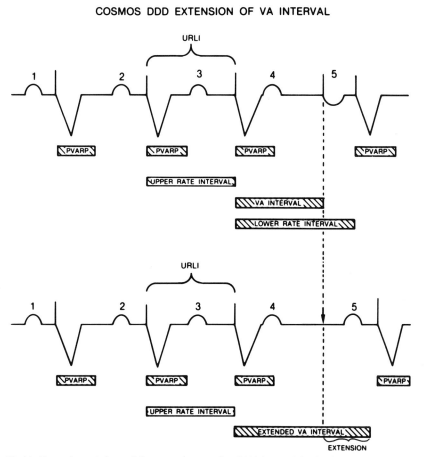

Figure 12–11. Extension of the atrial escape (pacemaker VA) interval in the Intermedics Cosmos DDD pulse generator. *Top,* Diagrammatic representation of a pacemaker exhibiting a Wenckebach upper rate response because the atrial rate is faster than the programmed upper rate. The fourth P wave falls in the PVARP and is therefore unsensed. Release of an atrial stimulus at the completion of the atrial escape (pacemaker VA) interval yields a paced P wave (5) that produces an artificial increase in the atrial rate. *Bottom,* Diagrammatic representation of the Intermedics Cosmos DDD pulse generator with the same parameters as the pulse generator depicted on top. The sequence is similar except that the atrial escape (pacemaker VA) interval initiated by the third ventricular stimulus is automatically extended because the duration of the preceding cycle was equal to the URLI. This extension of the AEI allows a spontaneous P wave (5) to initiate a new AV interval. If P$_5$ had not occurred, the pulse generator would have delivered its atrial stimulus at the completion of the extended atrial escape (pacemaker VA) interval.

erators and about 300 msec for the later models. Pacemaker VA extension may occur after only one cycle at the upper rate interval and bears no relationship to the pause seen at the end of the tachycardia termination algorithm of this particular pulse generator, where the pause is equal to the upper rate limit interval plus the atrial escape (VA) interval.

Fallback Response

The object of the fallback is to limit the time the ventricular rate remains at the programmed upper rate and may be useful in patients who cannot tolerate a sustained upper rate.[73] The fallback response is activated by the detection of an atrial rate faster than the programmed upper rate. The fallback mechanism then gradually returns the ventricular rate to more tolerable levels than the upper rate of the pulse generator. According to the model and manufacturer, AV synchrony may or may not be maintained during the fallback response. Three aspects of fallback may be programmable: (1) onset time (the ventricular rate

may fall back immediately or operate in a Wenckebach fashion for a given number of cycles before the onset of fallback); (2) fallback slope (the rate or slope of deceleration, which may be programmable [milliseconds per cardiac cycle], determines how rapidly the paced ventricular rate changes from upper rate to fallback rate or lower rate, as the case may be); and (3) fallback rate (in some pulse generators, the fallback rate is actually the lower rate limit interval).

In pacemakers with a fallback response without AV synchrony, VVI pacing will occur. During the fallback response, the pulse generator continues to monitor atrial activity but does not use it for recycling or initiation of any intervals. The ventricular pacing rate falls back gradually to the lower rate limit or other programmed value (as in the CPI Delta DDD pacemaker shown in Fig. 12–12). Therefore, the length of each VV interval progressively increases by a predetermined value until the fallback rate is reached. Pacing will then continue at the fallback rate in the VVI mode as long as the atrial rate remains faster than the

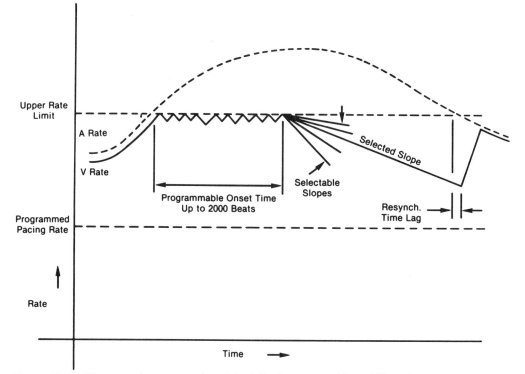

Figure 12–12. Diagrammatic representation of the fallback response without AV synchrony. 1:1 P wave–triggered ventricular pacing occurs up to the upper rate limit. The pacemaker then responds with Wenckebach upper rate limitation. After a programmed onset time, the fallback response is initiated and the ventricular rate gradually decreases (asynchronously) to the fallback rate (programmed lower rate). When the atrial rate falls below the programmed upper rate, the pacemaker restores 1:1 P wave–triggered ventricular pacing after a resynchronization time lag. A = atrial; V = ventricular. (Courtesy of Cardiac Pacemakers, Inc, St Paul, MN; with modification.)

programmed upper rate. When the detected atrial rate falls below the programmed upper rate (or another preselected rate), fallback terminates and atrial synchronous pacing resumes. This response may cause a jump from fallback—for example, 70 ppm to P-wave synchronous pacing just below the upper rate limit interval. (This abrupt transition may be avoided by using rate smoothing, an option available only in the CPI Delta DDD pulse generator.)

In some pulse generators, the maintenance of AV synchrony during the fallback period produces a Wenckebach upper rate response. AV synchrony is maintained, but a small increment is added to the upper rate limit interval after each sensed atrial event, provided the pacing cycle terminates at the upper rate limit. In other words, the pulse generator is temporarily revising its own upper rate limit, which gradually decreases by a known value in successive pacing cycles. This decrease results in a gradual slowing of the paced ventricular rate to the programmed fallback rate. Once the fallback rate has been reached, the rate will stabilize at that level. Although the ventricular rate is quite predictable, AV delays may be inconsistent in length even when there is AV

synchrony present. At the fallback rate, the rate will stabilize at that level, and the pacemaker will continue to use the Wenckebach response to limit the ventricular rate at its new lower value (or fallback rate). If at any time (either during the deceleration process or at the fallback rate) the atrial rate becomes slower than the ventricular paced rate, the system will be reset, the fallback response will terminate, and 1:1 P-wave tracking at the programmed AV delay will resume.

Rate Smoothing

Rate smoothing is a programmable option that is not specifically an upper rate response because it is designed to eliminate pronounced variations in cycle length, and therefore it functions over all rate ranges. This mode of operation is complex and available only in one pulse generator (CPI Delta), and its clinical advantages and disadvantages are not yet fully known. Rate smoothing can provide an effective ventricular response to pathologic atrial rates (Fig. 12–13). Rate smoothing is an attempt to replace abrupt changes in rate with gradual transition by limiting the maximal change in the pacing rate from cycle to cycle

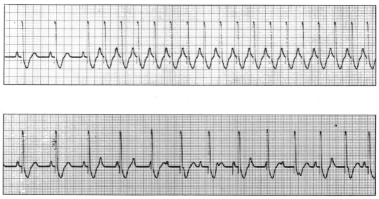

Figure 12–13. Rate smoothing with the CPI Delta 925 DDD pulse generator. The programmed parameters were as follows: lower rate = 65 per minute, upper rate = 150 per minute, AV interval = 150 msec, and PVARP = 250 msec. The top tracing shows 1:1 P-wave tracking during supraventricular tachycardia without rate-smoothing operation. The bottom strip shows the same supraventricular tachycardia with rate-smoothing operation (smoothing factor of 6 percent). The pulse generator stores in its memory the most recent R-R interval, either paced or sensed. It then calculates "rate control windows" for the next cycle based on the R-R interval and the programmed rate-smoothing value (6 percent in this example). A separate window is calculated for the atrium and the ventricle. Atrial synchronization window = (previous R-R interval ± rate-smoothing value) − AV delay. Ventricular synchronization window = previous R-R interval ± rate-smoothing value. The timing for both windows is initiated at the end of a ventricular event. For example, if the previous R-R interval is 800 msec with a 6 percent rate-smoothing factor, the ventricular window would be 800 ± 6 percent = 800 ± 48 msec. The window would therefore extend from 752 to 848 msec. Paced activity (atrial or ventricular), if it is to occur, must occur during these rate control windows. When an atrial event occurs before the atrial synchronization window, the ventricle is paced after an interval that equals the previous RR interval less the rate-smoothing value. When an atrial event occurs within the synchronization window, the programmed AV delay is initiated, and the ventricle is paced at the end of the AV delay period. When no atrial event occurs during the synchronization window, the interval becomes equal to (previous R-R interval + rate smoothing value) − AV delay, so that the atrium is paced at the end of this interval, followed by ventricular pacing at the end of the programmed AV delay. (Courtesy of Cardiac Pacemakers, Inc, St Paul, MN.)

to some percentage of the previous R-R interval (smoothing factor). Rate smoothing controls the response of a pulse generator because of increases and decreases in the intrinsic rate (see Fig. 12–13). Rate smoothing may be quite useful in patients who cannot tolerate marked fluctuations of paced rate during fixed-ratio or Wenckebach block response during the upper rate response of a DDD pulse generator.[100, 121] Rate smoothing may prevent the sudden deceleration of the ventricular rate during exercise, as with the development of 2:1 or 3:1 fixed-ratio block. During rate smoothing, the pulse generator loses effective AV synchrony and thus sacrifices optimal AV relationships to maintain pacing rates. For increasing atrial rates, rate smoothing will look similar to a Wenckebach response with prolonged AV delays and occasional unsensed P waves falling in the PVARP.

Rate smoothing modifies the onset of endless loop tachycardia by preventing abrupt variations in the paced rhythm. Actually, rate smoothing may itself precipitate endless loop tachycardia because of its propensity to induce AV dissociation.

Omission of Pacemaker Stimuli to Conform to the Upper Rate Limit

The tachycardia termination algorithms of some DDD pulse generators necessitate the periodic omission of a pacemaker stimulus. Barring this response, some pulse generators, under certain circumstances, are designed to omit either atrial or ventricular stimuli to avoid violation of the upper rate limit interval.[10, 19] For example, the Medtronic Symbios DDD pulse generator (Medtronic, Minneapolis, MN) was designed with two upper rate limit intervals, one for the atrial channel and the other for the ventricular channel. Under the appropriate circumstances, the pulse generator may omit an anticipated atrial stimulus to conform to its atrial upper rate limit interval, and this behavior should not be misinterpreted as pacemaker malfunction.

ENDLESS LOOP TACHYCARDIA: A CONTINUING CHALLENGE

Pacemaker reentrant tachycardia, or endless loop tachycardia, is a well-known complication of dual-chamber pacing with DDD (or VDD) pulse generators.[2, 13, 24, 30, 31, 54, 66, 69, 91, 92] Endless loop tachycardia usually starts with sensing of a retrograde P wave often related

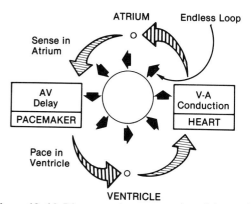

Figure 12–14. Diagrammatic representation of the mechanism of endless loop tachycardia. When the atrial channel senses a retrograde P wave, a ventricular pacing stimulus is issued at the completion of the programmed AV interval. The pulse generator itself provides the anterograde limb of the macroreentrant loop because it functions as an artificial AV junction. Retrograde VA conduction following ventricular pacing provides the retrograde limb of the reentrant loop. The pulse generator again senses the retrograde P, and the process perpetuates itself. Termination of endless loop tachycardia can be accomplished by disrupting either the anterograde limb (by eliminating atrial sensing) or the retrograde limb (by eliminating retrograde VA conduction). (From Barold SS, Falkoff MD, Ong LS, Heinle RA: Pacemaker endless loop tachycardia: Termination by simple techniques other than magnet application. Am J Med 1988, 85:817 with permission.)

to a ventricular extrasystole with retrograde VA conduction (Fig. 12–14). The sensed retrograde P wave triggers the next ventricular stimulus either at the end of the programmed AV interval or sometimes beyond it (with prolongation of the AV delay) to allow completion of the upper rate limit interval controlling the maximal or upper rate of ventricular stimulation. The paced ventricular beat engenders another retrograde P wave, again sensed by the atrial channel, and this mechanism perpetuates itself, creating a tachycardia that may continue for only several beats or become sustained. Endless loop tachycardia may be considered a macroreentrant or circus movement tachycardia, with the pacemaker itself as the anterograde limb and the conducting tissue of the heart as the retrograde limb. Despite the very sophisticated programmability of contemporary DDD pulse generators, endless loop tachycardia will probably continue to be a troublesome or potentially serious problem because of either inappropriate pacemaker programming or unpredictable variation of VA conduction that occurs spontaneously or secondary to the administration of cardiac drugs.[2, 30, 65, 102, 106]

Initiation of Endless Loop Tachycardia

Intact retrograde VA conduction occurs in approximately two-thirds or more of patients with sinus node dysfunction and 14 to 35 per cent of patients with complete AV block (if the block is in the AV node, virtually no patients exhibit VA conduction).[1, 2, 57, 88, 89, 96, 109, 120, 122, 129] This means that 35 to 50 percent of all patients receiving VDD or DDD pacemakers for any indication may be susceptible to endless loop tachycardia[80, 88] (see Fig. 12–14). Hayes and Furman[68] analyzed VA conduction in 53 patients during incremental ventricular pacing and found a mean VA conduction time of 235 ± 50 msec, with a range of 100 to 380 msec. In some patients, the VA conduction time may be longer than 400 msec.[88, 89, 122] We believe in the concept that until proven otherwise all patients should be considered capable of retrograde VA conduction, with particular emphasis on its unpredictable behavior.[21] Retrograde VA conduction is influenced by various circumstances, including the resting heart rate, level of activity, changes in autonomic tone, pacing rate, catecholamines, and concurrent drug therapy.[5, 65, 102] In some patients, measurements made at the time of pacemaker implantation may have little bearing on future VA conduction patterns because improvement in VA conduction may occur with ambulation and may indeed return when it was absent at the time of implantation. However, only a minority of patients (5 to 10 per cent) with no VA conduction at the time of implantation will subsequently develop VA conduction.[72, 106, 122] Therefore, absent retrograde VA conduction at the time of implan-

tation or even later provides no absolute guarantee of protection against endless loop tachycardia because of the dynamic nature of VA conduction. In some patients showing no VA conduction during routine testing (by ventricular pacing), VA conduction may occasionally be demonstrated only during AV sequential pacing.[94] However, testing for retrograde VA conduction during AV sequential pacing with only a single premature ventricular stimulus does not reveal the maximal VA conduction time or whether an endless loop tachycardia would be sustained.[128]

Causes of Endless Loop Tachycardia

Any circumstance capable of causing AV dissociation, coupled with the capability of retrograde VA conduction, may initiate endless loop tachycardia. The initiating mechanism is always due to AV dissociation, with separation of the sinus P wave from the QRS complex. The following are initiating mechanisms:

1. Ventricular extrasystoles with retrograde VA conduction are the most common mechanism[13, 54, 116] (Fig. 12–15).

2. Loss of atrial capture[12, 30, 31, 73] may allow VA conduction to occur after a ventricular paced beat (Figs. 12–16 and 12–17).

3. Undersensing of P waves (Fig. 12–18) may be responsible. Loss of sensing of sinus P waves may be associated with normal sensing of retrograde P waves. P-wave undersensing causes the delivery of an ineffectual atrial stimulus, with the development of AV dissociation.

4. Application and withdrawal of the mag-

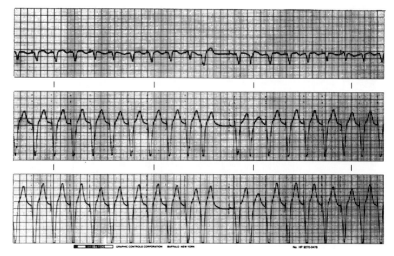

Figure 12–15. Endless loop tachycardia terminated and reinitiated by a ventricular extrasystole. The three ECG leads were recorded simultaneously. URI = 500 msec (120 ppm), LRI = 857 msec (70 ppm), and AV delay = 150 msec. The cycle length of the tachycardia is longer than the URI.

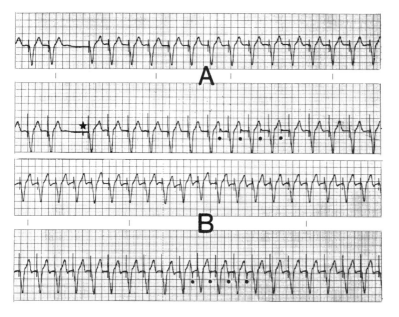

Figure 12–16. Intermedics Cosmos DDD pulse generator. In *A* (two ECG leads recorded simultaneously), the pulse generator was programmed as follows: URI = 600 msec (100 ppm), AV interval = 150 msec, and PVARP = 200 msec. The atrial pacing output was programmed to a value less than the pacing threshold (*star* in the second strip). When the sensed atrial event marker function is activated,[16] special markers are delivered for four consecutively sensed P waves *(solid black circles)*. The retrograde VA conduction time is approximately 360 msec, and the consequent AV interval measures approximately 240 msec, thereby yielding the URI of approximately 600 msec. This time value is the cycle length of the endless loop tachycardia precipitated by subthreshold atrial stimulation *(star)*.

In *B* (two ECG leads recorded simultaneously), the pacemaker parameters were identical except that the upper rate was programmed to 125 per minute. Note the presence of endless loop tachycardia at a rate less than 125 per minute (480 msec). The cycle length measured 520 msec because of delayed retrograde VA conduction. The marker channels *(solid black circles)* demonstrate a VA conduction interval of approximately 370 to 380 msec. This interval plus the AV interval of 150 msec gives approximately 520 msec, the cycle length of the endless loop tachycardia.

Figure 12–17. Subthreshold atrial stimulation leading to unsustained endless loop tachycardia in a patient with a Cosmos (Intermedics) DDD pulse generator (three-lead ECG). The programmed parameters were as follows: LRI = 880 msec, URI = 480 msec, PVARP = 200 msec, and AV interval = 180 msec. The retrograde VA conduction time is just over 200 msec, so that the retrograde P wave is sensed by the atrial channel, thereby initiating runs of nonsustained endless loop tachycardia. (From Barold SS, Falkoff MD, Ong LS, Heinle RA: Function and electrocardiography of DDD pacemakers. *In* Barold SS [ed]: Modern Cardiac Pacing. Mount Kisco, NY, Futura Publishing Co, 1985; p 645; with permission.)

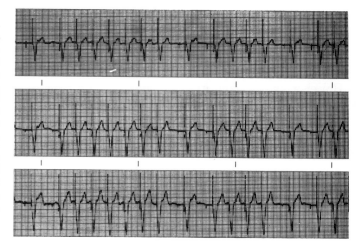

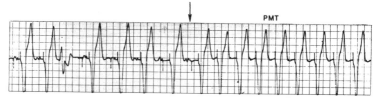

Figure 12–18. Initiation of endless loop tachycardia (PMT) due to undersensing of sinus P waves and normal sensing of retrograde P waves. The arrow points to the unsensed P wave responsible for initiation of PMT.

Figure 12–19. Initiation of endless loop tachycardia from oversensing of myopotentials in a patient with a unipolar Medtronic 7000 DDD pulse generator (two-lead ECG). The programmed upper rate was 125 per minute (URI = 480 msec), and the AV delay was 250 msec. Isometric exercise causes myopotential sensing by the atrial channel, thereby triggering a ventricular stimulus independent of atrial activity. This triggering leads to retrograde VA conduction with a retrograde P wave falling beyond the PVARP of 155 msec for this particular model. (From Barold SS, Falkoff MD, Ong LS, Heinle RA: Function and electrocardiography of DDD pacemakers. *In* Barold SS [ed]: Modern Cardiac Pacing. Mount Kisco, NY, Futura Publishing Co, 1985, p 645; with permission.)

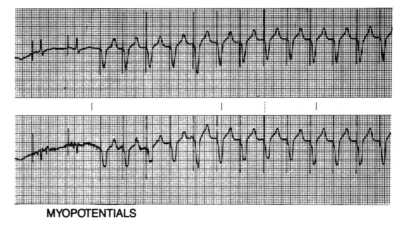

MYOPOTENTIALS

net over certain DDD pulse generators may create endless loop tachycardia.[14, 20, 30, 31, 91, 117] In the case of the Pacesetter AFP DDD pulse generator (Pacesetter-Siemens, Sylmar, California), in the "magnet off" mode, application of the programmer head or magnet may create an extraneous signal in the atrial channel and, if the signal is sensed, the pulse generator will emit a synchronized ventricular stimulus, setting the stage for retrograde VA conduction.[14] In this situation, the endless loop tachycardia cannot be terminated by the magnet unless the magnet function is restored by appropriate programming.

5. Myopotential oversensing by the atrial channel may trigger a ventricular stimulus independent of atrial activity (Fig. 12–19). Myopotential inhibition of the ventricular channel may also precipitate endless loop tachycardia.

Each of these sequences may lead to ventricular depolarization without a preceding atrial depolarization, thereby favoring retrograde VA conduction.[13, 26, 30, 31, 44, 48, 71, 104, 105, 132]

6. A long AV interval, regardless of its cause, predisposes to retrograde VA conduction because the separation between atrial and ventricular events may allow sufficient recovery of atrial and AV nodal refractoriness for VA conduction to occur.[46] This occurrence is particularly prominent in pulse generators with a separately programmable upper rate limit interval when a long electrical AV (atrial sense–ventricular pace) interval may occur. Such a long AV interval may occur during the Wenckebach upper rate response of pulse generators, sometimes demonstrable only with exercise or with atrial premature beats[13, 50, 66, 75] (Fig. 12–20).

Figure 12–20. Initiation of endless loop tachycardia by an atrial extrasystole (premature contraction = APC) sensed by a Medtronic Symbios 7006 DDD pulse generator (see marker channel). Retrograde VA conduction secondary to a relatively long paced AV interval cannot be ruled out. Real-time event markers (emanating from the pulse generator) are shown in the middle strip. The atrial sense marker is smaller than the atrial pace marker. The lower strip is a compound lead consisting of ECG and markers. The programmed parameters of the pulse generator are shown above the ECG.

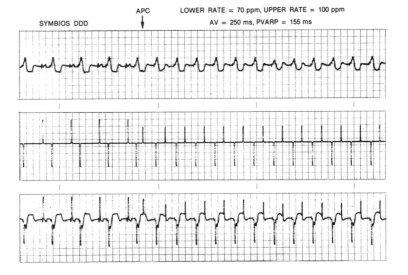

APC

SYMBIOS DDD

LOWER RATE = 70 ppm, UPPER RATE = 100 ppm
AV = 250 ms, PVARP = 155 ms

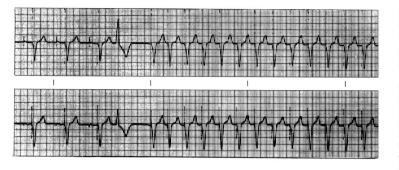

Figure 12–21. Apparent VVI pacing during DDD pacing by a Medtronic Versatrax 7000 DDD pulse generator (two-lead ECG). Programmed parameters: lower rate = 60 ppm, AV interval = 250 msec, and upper rate = 125 ppm. This pulse generator defines a ventricular premature beat as the second of two successive ventricular events that have no intervening P wave. When this circumstance exists, the device will not be able to start an AV delay if the P wave is sensed within the 340 msec (AV "disabling period") after the premature ventricular event. The initial portion of the T wave is deformed by a P wave. If no spontaneous ventricular event occurs, the device will try to pace AV sequentially, but since the atrial channel will be in a refractory state, only the ventricular stimulus will be delivered. This concept of "bigeminy protection" was incorporated to prevent atrial events from triggering the delivery of ventricular stimuli into the prolonged repolarization cycle associated with ventricular premature beats. The ventricular paced beat terminating the cycle (without preceding atrial depolarization) causes retrograde VA conduction and precipitates an endless loop tachycardia. (From Barold SS, Falkoff MD, Ong LS, Heinle RA: Function and electrocardiography of DDD pacemakers. *In* Barold SS [ed]: Modern Cardiac Pacing. Mount Kisco, NY, Futura Publishing Co, 1985, p 645; with permission.)

7. An excessively long PVARP extension or the DDX mode may paradoxically predispose to endless loop tachycardia[29] (discussed later).

8. The AV disable mechanism of the Medtronic Versatrax DDD pulse generator, with which an atrial stimulus is omitted under special circumstances,[13] may cause endless loop tachycardia (Fig. 12–21).

9. Electromagnetic interference emitted from some programmers may be sensed by the atrial channel, thereby initiating endless loop tachycardia because of AV dissociation in the same way that the sensing of myopotentials by the atrial channel does.

10. Chest wall stimulation[11, 13, 15, 30, 35, 89] (Fig. 12–22) may initiate endless loop tachycardia.

11. In the VDD (VAT) mode, a sinus rate that is slower than the programmed lower rate would effectively cause VVI pacing, leading to AV dissociation and retrograde VA conduction.[20]

12. Far-field (or cross-ventricular) sensing refers to detection of the far-field QRS electrogram by the atrial channel.[25, 36, 38, 39, 103] The far-field ventricular signal may also originate from the tail-end of the paced QRS complex (Figs. 12–23 and 12–24). Consequently, far-field endless loop tachycardia can occur only in the presence of a very short PVARP, particularly in unipolar DDD pulse generators programmed at a high atrial sensitivity. The diagnosis depends on demonstrating the absence of retrograde VA conduction or ectopic P waves at the initiation of endless loop tachy-

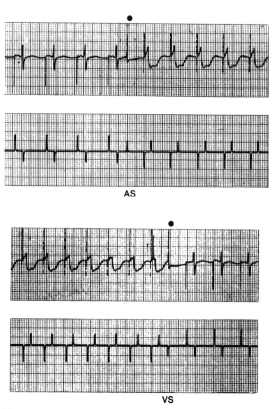

AS

VS

Figure 12–22. Effect of chest wall stimulation (CWS) on Medtronic Symbios 7005 unipolar pulse generator. Real-time event markers are shown below the ECG. *Top,* CWS *(solid black circle),* sensed only by the atrial channel, initiates endless loop tachycardia. *Bottom,* Endless loop tachycardia terminated by the second CWS *(solid black circle)* sensed by the ventricular channel. The first CWS falls within the refractory period of the ventricular channel. The markers depicting sense events are smaller than those related to pace events. As = atrial sense event; Vs = ventricular sense event.

LOWER RATE = 70 ppm
UPPER RATE INTERVAL = 180 ms
AV INTERVAL = 130 ms
PVARP = 125 ms

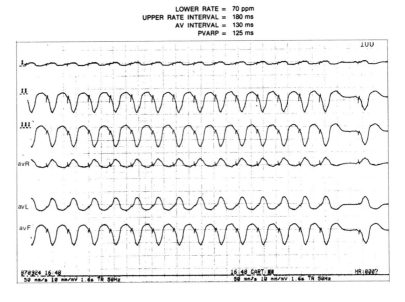

Figure 12–23. Far-field endless loop tachycardia with a CPI 925 Delta DDD pulse generator. The programmed parameters are shown above the ECG with six leads recorded simultaneously. The atrial channel senses far-field ventricular depolarization and not retrograde P waves. This diagnosis cannot be made from the surface ECG because there was no clear-cut evidence of AV dissociation during the tachycardia.

cardia and AV dissociation during the tachycardia. Event markers will label the sensed far-field signals as sensed P waves.[39] Esophageal electrocardiography may be invaluable in making this diagnosis.[25]

Spontaneous Endless Loop Tachycardia

Oseran and associates[97] recently reported five cases of "spontaneous" endless loop tachycardia, four of which were documented by Holter monitoring. All cases started after a normally timed spontaneous P wave preceding a ventricular stimulus or a paced P wave followed by a paced QRS complex. The purported retrograde P waves initiating endless loop tachycardia were not clearly seen on the surface electrocardiogram. Four of the five cases involved unipolar DDD pulse generators. One case of a slow endless loop tachycardia at a rate of 80 ppm occurred in a patient whose pulse generator was programmed to a PVARP of 100 msec, raising the possibility that endless loop tachycardia might have been initiated by far-field sensing of the QRS complex rather than retrograde P waves. The authors emphasized that in the absence of more

LOWER RATE = 70 ppm (750 ms)
UPPER RATE INTERVAL = 180 ms
AV = 130 ms
PVARP = 125 ms

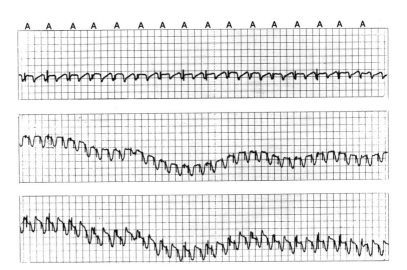

Figure 12–24. Same patient as in Figure 12–23. Three-lead ECG with bipolar esophageal recording in the upper strip and compound leads below. "A" indicates atrial depolarization. AV dissociation excludes the usual type or near-field endless loop tachycardia related to sensing of retrograde P waves. The tachycardia was terminated and prevented by lengthening the PVARP.

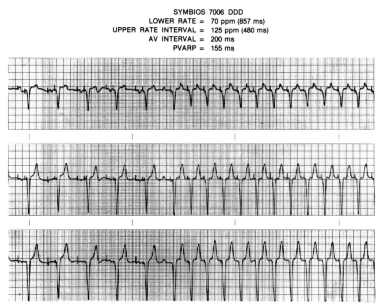

SYMBIOS 7006 DDD
LOWER RATE = 70 ppm (857 ms)
UPPER RATE INTERVAL = 125 ppm (480 ms)
AV INTERVAL = 200 ms
PVARP = 155 ms

Figure 12–25. "Spontaneous" endless loop tachycardia in a patient with a Symbios 7006 DDD pulse generator. The programmed parameters are shown above the ECG of three leads recorded simultaneously. The paced AV (Ap-Vp) interval is not associated with retrograde VA conduction. When the AV interval is initiated by a sensed sinus P wave (As-Vp), retrograde VA conduction occurs and initiates an endless loop tachycardia. This initiating mechanism was repeatedly documented in long ECG recordings. Endless loop tachycardia was prevented by programming the AV interval to 150 msec. No atrial extrasystoles were observed. The sequence of events suggests that a sinus impulse reaches the AV junction earlier than a paced atrial depolarization. Earlier recovery of the AV junction permits retrograde VA conduction only after a sinus P wave. The relatively late recovery of the AV junction after a paced atrial depolarization prevents retrograde VA conduction.

detailed electrophysiologic study the precise mechanism of the onset of endless loop tachycardia could not be elucidated. Although some instances might have been triggered by retrograde or other P-wave activity, it is possible that others might have been precipitated by myopotential triggering, because four of the five cases occurred with unipolar DDD pulse generators. We have also observed such cases of "spontaneous" endless loop tachycardia under similar circumstances, mostly on Holter recordings. Most of our cases turned out to be secondary to myopotential sensing by the atrial channel. Occasionally, such "spontaneous" endless loop tachycardia cannot be attributed to myopotential triggering, far-field sensing, or atrial extrasystoles (Figs. 12–25 and 12–26). We believe that a relatively long PR interval (such as a paced AV interval of 250 msec) may, in predisposed patients, favor retrograde VA conduction and precipitate endless loop tachycardia without any apparent reason.

Diagnosis of Endless Loop Tachycardia

Endless loop tachycardia should be suspected whenever a patient complains of palpitations, increasing angina, or even congestive heart failure. There are many ways of evaluating retrograde VA conduction and susceptibility to endless loop tachycardia when there

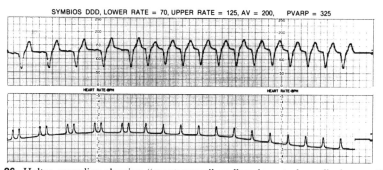

SYMBIOS DDD, LOWER RATE = 70, UPPER RATE = 125, AV = 200, PVARP = 325

Figure 12–26. Holter recording showing "spontaneous" endless loop tachycardia in a patient with a Symbios 7006 bipolar DDD pulse generator. The lower channel depicts the pacemaker stimuli. The initiating mechanism cannot be determined from the surface ECG, but myopotential triggering can be excluded with certainty because no interference could be demonstrated at high atrial sensitivities. Far-field atrial sensing of a ventricular signal is highly unlikely with a relatively long PVARP of 325 msec. The tachycardia was probably initiated by an atrial extrasystole.

LRI = 856 ms, URI = 480 ms, AV = 250 ms, PVARP = 155 ms

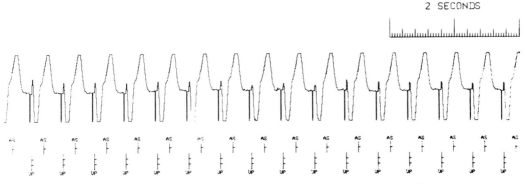

Figure 12–27. Endless loop tachycardia with Medtronic Symbios DDD pulse generator. The event markers indicate the precise timing of pacemaker operation. Vp = ventricular pace event; As = atrial sense event. (Courtesy of Medtronic, Minneapolis, MN.)

are no spontaneous ventricular extrasystoles or other disturbances likely to cause VA conduction. The identification of retrograde VA conduction may be facilitated by telemetered event markers[41, 77, 82, 87] or telemetry of the atrial electrogram[87] (Figs. 12–27 and 12–28). Some pulse generators may be permanently (Cordis Gemini, Miami, Florida) or temporarily (Intermedics Cosmos, for four cycles only) programmed to the DDT mode[16] that provides a triggered atrial output upon sensing P waves (Fig. 12–29). The atrial stimuli then function

as markers of atrial depolarization and indicate the precise time of atrial sensing. The latter cannot be determined on the surface electrocardiogram. Event markers permit accurate determination of the VA conduction time as seen by the atrial channel of the pulse generator sensing from the right atrial appendage.[41, 77]

DETERMINATION OF VENTRICULOATRIAL CONDUCTION BY PROGRAMMING THE UPPER RATE. When the rate of endless loop tachycardia is equal to the programmed upper rate, the VA conduction time cannot be determined

Figure 12–28. Telemetry of atrial electrogram in a patient with a 283 AFP Pacesetter pulse generator showing retrograde VA conduction following a paced ventricular beat (seen on the left of the recording). The P wave is in the middle of the recording. The retrograde VA conduction time is approximately 240 msec from the ventricular stimulus to the onset of the first sharp deflection of the atrial electrogram.

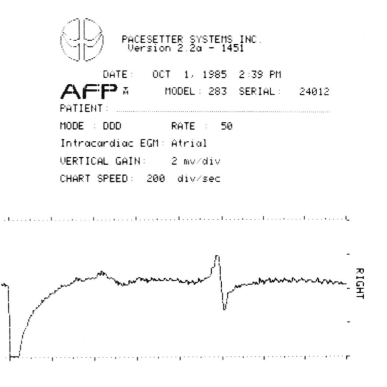

CORDIS GEMINI 415A DD $\frac{\text{T}}{1}$ MODE
LOWER RATE = 80 ppm, AV = 150 ms, PVARP = 300 ms
SUBTHRESHOLD ATRIAL STIMULATION

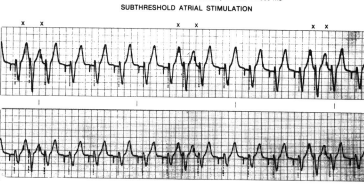

Figure 12–29. Subthreshold atrial stimulation with Cordis Gemini 415A in the DD $\frac{\text{T}}{1}$ mode, a variant of the DDD mode in which atrial sensing does not inhibit, but rather triggers, the atrial output. Triggered atrial stimuli act as markers for atrial sensing (represented by X).

precisely in pulse generators with a separately programmable upper rate because the AV interval might be prolonged so as not to violate the upper rate limit. When the rate of endless loop tachycardia is slower than the programmed upper rate, the retrograde VA conduction time is equal to the difference between the tachycardia cycle length and the AV interval, which in this case is equal to the programmed value[55, 59] (Fig. 12–30). Programming the upper rate to relatively fast values may therefore permit the measurement of VA conduction time when the rate of the endless loop tachycardia becomes slower than the programmed upper rate. However, this approach may be thwarted by the development of VA conduction block at faster ventricular rates. When the VA conduction time is measured in this fashion, it may be assumed that it is similar or shorter at slower programmed upper rates.

Techniques for the Induction of Endless Loop Tachycardia[3, 32, 58, 71]

SUBTHRESHOLD STIMULATION.[12, 30, 71] Programming the atrial output to a subthreshold level is the simplest and most useful technique for the induction of endless loop tachycardia.

To bring out retrograde VA conduction, the PVARP is programmed to its shortest value, and atrial sensitivity is increased to its maximal value (see Figs. 12–16 and 12–17). The lower rate should be faster than the spontaneous rate, and ideally the propensity to endless loop tachycardia should be evaluated at several lower rates. If VA conduction and endless loop tachycardia occur, the upper rate should be altered to determine whether the endless loop tachycardia is sustained or unsustained at various upper rates.

CHEST WALL STIMULATION.[11, 13, 15, 30, 89] In most patients, programming the atrial output to subthreshold levels will be sufficient to bring out retrograde VA conduction and endless loop tachycardia. In an occasional patient with an extremely low threshold for atrial pacing, successful atrial capture may persist even at the lowest programmable atrial output. This limitation may be circumvented by using chest wall stimulation (provided it is sensed only by the atrial channel) because it easily induces endless loop tachycardia in patients who exhibit the arrhythmia spontaneously (see Fig. 12–22). The characteristics of the endless loop tachycardia induced by chest wall stimulation (rate, sustained or unsustained) correlate well with those documented clinically.[13] Fletcher

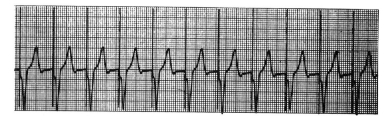

Figure 12–30. Endless loop tachycardia at a rate of 90 per minute, slower than the programmed upper rate of 100 per minute. This slower rate permits calculation of the retrograde VA conduction time because the AV interval is not prolonged to conform to the supremacy of the URI. Therefore, the VA conduction time is equal to the cycle length of the tachycardia (650 msec) minus the AV delay (250 msec), that is, approximately 400 msec. (From Barold SS, Falkoff MD, Ong LS, Heinle RA: Function and electrocardiography of DDD pacemakers. *In* Barold SS [ed]: Modern Cardiac Pacing. Mount Kisco, NY, Futura Publishing Co, 1985, p 645; with permission.)

and colleagues[45] determined the duration of VA conduction during AV sequential (DDD) pacing by the delivery of ventricular premature stimuli with a modified investigational programmer not generally available. Basically the same determination may be obtained quite simply by chest wall stimulation sensed only by the atrial channel. A single programmed chest wall stimulus may be delivered with varying prematurity just beyond the PVARP, though slower random chest wall stimulation achieves basically the same result. A chest wall stimulus sensed by the atrial channel triggers a ventricular stimulus that paces the ventricle prematurely, producing a physiologic event identical with a ventricular extrasystole preceded by a normal AV relationship. Greater prematurity of ventricular stimulation by the chest wall technique may be accomplished by shortening the AV interval.

APPLICATION AND WITHDRAWAL OF THE MAGNET.[14, 20, 30, 91, 117] Withdrawal of the magnet may occasionally precipitate endless loop tachycardia when a retrograde P wave is sensed by the pulse generator immediately upon restoration of the atrial sensing capability. However, this method often produces inconsistent results.

ISOMETRIC PECTORAL MUSCLE EXERCISE IN UNIPOLAR DDD PULSE GENERATORS.[13, 26, 30, 44, 48, 71, 104, 105, 132] Myopotentials may be interpreted as P waves by the atrial channel of a unipolar DDD pulse generator, which therefore triggers a ventricular output (see Fig. 12–19). This ventricular output may lead to retrograde VA conduction and the initiation of endless loop tachycardia. However, some patients do not exhibit myopotential interference, and this approach is obviously not applicable to patients with bipolar pulse generators.

MAXIMAL PROLONGATION OF THE AV INTERVAL. During testing, the AV interval should be programmed to its maximal value to produce the greatest separation between atrial and ventricular activity so as to favor retrograde VA conduction.[46]

TREADMILL EXERCISE TESTING.[30] In DDD pulse generators with a separately programmable upper rate interval, the pacemaker Wenckebach upper rate response comes into play whenever the sinus rate is increased by exercise or the upper rate is programmed to a value less than the sinus rate. In this situation, prolongation of the AV interval may lead to wide separation of a sinus P wave and its accompanying ventricular paced beat, a situation that may set the stage for endless loop

tachycardia by predisposing to retrograde VA conduction. However, endless loop tachycardia is rarely precipitated by exercise through this mechanism, even with a relatively slow programmed upper rate.

CHEST THUMP. Den Dulk and coworkers[30] have used this method to induce ventricular premature beats, which in turn may initiate endless loop tachycardia.

PROGRAMMING TO ANOTHER PACING MODE. In the VDD mode, the lower rate is programmed to a value 10 to 15 beats faster than the sinus rate.[122] This programming is unsuitable in the presence of a relatively fast sinus rate and impossible in pulse generators that cannot be programmed to the VDD mode. The VVI and VVT modes may demonstrate retrograde VA conduction.[122] In the VVT mode, programmed chest wall stimulation allows the determination of VA conduction following premature ventricular depolarization. However, the demonstration of retrograde VA conduction during relatively slow ventricular pacing may not always correlate with the development of sustained endless loop tachycardia in the VDD or DDD mode.

HOLTER MONITORING. This may provide the ultimate proof that the programmed parameters prevent endless loop tachycardia.

Termination of Endless Loop Tachycardia

Anterograde Limb of the Reentrant Loop

The easiest way of terminating endless loop tachycardia is by application of the testing magnet over the DDD pulse generator[13] (Fig. 12–31). This action temporarily converts the pulse generator to the asynchronous dual- or single-chamber mode (DOO or VOO according to the manufacturer). Elimination of atrial sensing abolishes endless loop tachycardia by causing block in the anterograde limb of the reentrant loop. Most of the other methods used to terminate or prevent endless loop tachycardia also eliminate atrial sensing by prolongation of the PVARP, programming to another mode without atrial sensing (e.g., DVI), or decreasing the sensitivity of the atrial channel because retrograde P waves are often of lower amplitude than anterograde ones.[79]

Retrograde Limb of the Reentrant Loop: Loss of Retrograde VA Conduction

Endless loop tachycardia may occasionally terminate spontaneously because of a block in

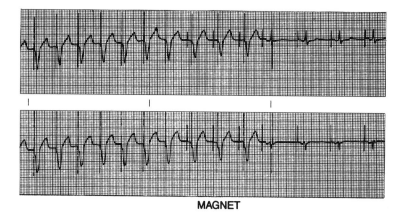

MAGNET

Figure 12–31. Endless loop tachycardia terminated by application of the magnet, with reversion to DDD pacing. (From Barold SS, Falkoff MD, Ong LS, Heinle RA: Function and electrocardiography of DDD pacemakers. *In* Barold SS [ed]: Modern Cardiac Pacing. Mount Kisco, NY, Futura Publishing Co, 1985, p 645; with permission.)

VA conduction from a fatigue phenomenon in the conducting system. Retrograde VA conduction may be deliberately abolished by direct action on the retrograde pathway either with cautious carotid sinus massage or with drugs such as verapamil or beta blockers.[2, 5, 63, 102] However, pharmacologic therapy is generally not recommended for the prevention or termination of endless loop tachycardia.[76, 91] Ventricular extrasystoles without retrograde VA conduction may also terminate endless loop tachycardia (see Fig. 12–15). Indeed, any sensed premature ventricular event (QRS or any other signal) without accompanying retrograde VA conduction inhibits the ventricular channel and disrupts VA synchrony. The separation of atrial and ventricular events, as seen by the pulse generator, terminates endless loop tachycardia and allows the return of normal AV synchrony initiated by atrial pacing or a sensed sinus P wave. The same concept is incorporated in the automatic tachycardia termination algorithm of some DDD pulse generators by the omission of a single ventricular stimulus. Separation of atrial and ventricular events may also be achieved by provoking oversensing of skeletal myopotentials of the

ventricular channel of a unipolar DDD pulse generator (Fig. 12–32). However, myopotential inhibition can be achieved in only about half the cases involving unipolar pulse generators; bipolar ones are almost invariably immune to this form of interference.[127] Chest wall stimulation from an external pulse generator may also terminate endless loop tachycardia[13] (see Fig. 12–22). Chest wall stimulation may be helpful in the rare instance of magnet-unresponsive endless loop tachycardia,[18] in the presence of a defective reed switch,[40] or when an appropriate programmer is unavailable.

Tachycardia Termination Algorithm

Some DDD pulse generators possess a tachycardia termination algorithm to terminate endless loop tachycardia automatically. After 15 paced ventricular beats (triggered by sensed P waves) at the upper rate limit interval, the sixteenth paced ventricular stimulus output is blocked by inhibiting the delivery of the sixteenth ventricular stimulus[46, 119] (Fig. 12–33). This pause aborts endless loop tachycardia by separating atrial and ventricular events. VA synchrony is disrupted, with the reestablishment of AV synchrony with the next pacing

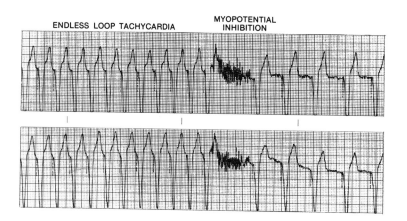

Figure 12–32. Endless loop tachycardia in a unipolar DDD pulse generator terminated by inhibition of the ventricular channel caused by oversensing of myopotentials (two-lead ECG).

Figure 12–33. Operation of the tachycardia termination algorithm of the Intermedics Cosmos DDD pulse generator. Subthreshold atrial stimulation induced endless loop tachycardia at a rate equal to the programmed upper rate. The programmed fallback deceleration of 10 msec/cycle causes a gradual lengthening of the URI by 10 msec/cycle. First cycle = 500 msec. The fifteenth cycle = 500 + (14 × 10) = 640 msec. In the fallback mechanism, this pulse generator revises its URI with each cycle. Consequently, each pacing cycle terminates at the completion of

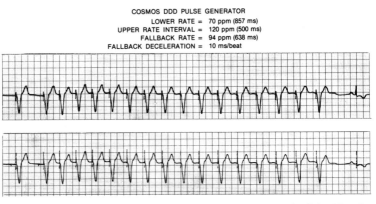

the URI, which, however, changes with each cycle according to the fallback mechanism. Because each of the 15 cycles actually terminates at its own URI, the tachycardia termination algorithm comes into operation and the sixteenth Vp is omitted. The subsequent pause should be equal to the sum of the URI (of the last cycle, i.e., 640 msec) plus the atrial escape (pacemaker VA) interval (857 msec). This is equal to 1497 msec. The actual interval between two consecutive ventricular stimuli is shorter at 1280 msec because the ventricular stimulus is triggered prematurely by a sensed P wave. The ventricular stimulus actually produces a pseudofusion beat.

cycle. This concept is based on the assumption that endless loop tachycardia always occurs at the upper rate of the pulse generator. However, the algorithm does not come into play when the cycle length of the endless loop tachycardia is longer than the upper rate limit interval of the pulse generator, that is, the sum of the retrograde VA conduction time and the programmed AV interval is longer than the upper rate limit interval. Occasionally, the

tachycardia termination algorithm comes into play during sinus tachycardia, particularly when the programmed upper rate is relatively slow (Fig. 12–34). Sinus tachycardia with a PP interval slightly shorter than the upper rate limit interval may cause Wenckebach progression without discernible prolongation of the AV delay, especially if the programmed AV interval is relatively long and the P wave is concealed within the T wave of the previous

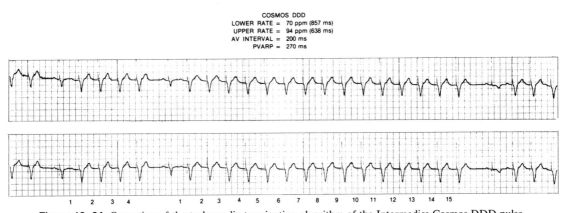

Figure 12–34. Operation of the tachycardia termination algorithm of the Intermedics Cosmos DDD pulse generator during sinus rhythm. The sinus rate is close to the programmed upper rate of 94 ppm. On the left there is a pacemaker Wenckebach sequence with four cycles (indicated by the numbers 1 to 4). The P wave following cycle 4 falls in the PVARP and is unsensed. The subsequent atrial escape (pacemaker VA) interval is equal to 657 plus the VA extension (300 msec for this particular pulse generator). This is equal to 957 msec. The extended VA interval terminates prematurely because of P-wave sensing. The next sequence is another pacemaker Wenckebach response with very small increments of the AV (As-Vp) interval, so that all the cycles occur at the URI and no P waves fall in the PVARP. The pulse generator activates the tachycardia termination algorithm after detecting 15 cycles at the URI. The pause at the end of the tachycardia termination algorithm is equal to the URI (638 msec) plus the AEI (657 msec). This is equal to 1295 msec. This interval is aborted by sensing of a P wave about 1000 msec after the previous ventricular stimulus. Note that the pause after the tachycardia termination algorithm is longer than the extended VA interval; that is, 1000 msec is greater than 957 msec, the maximal duration of the pause from the previous 6:5 Wenckebach response.

beat. This Wenckebach sequence does not terminate in the usual fashion, that is, with a P wave ultimately falling within the PVARP. Rather, after 15 cycles at the upper rate limit interval, the pulse generator activates its tachycardia termination algorithm and omits the sixteenth ventricular stimulus.

When the Intermedics Cosmos DDD pulse generator omits the release of a ventricular stimulus at the end of the tachycardia termination algorithm, the longest duration of the subsequent pause (interval from the last ventricular stimulus to the next atrial stimulus) will be equal to the upper rate limit interval (duration of pacemaker cycle if omission of the ventricular stimulus had not occurred) plus the atrial escape (pacemaker VA) interval (i.e., the cycle initiated at the time the omitted ventricular stimulus would have occurred).

Prevention of Endless Loop Tachycardia

Programmability of the Postventricular Atrial Refractory Period

With present technology, the best way to prevent endless loop tachycardia is to render the atrial amplifier refractory for a sufficient period of time after a paced or sensed ventricular event to prevent sensing of retrograde atrial depolarization. Appropriate programmability of the PVARP should prevent most cases of endless loop tachycardia.[83] In general, the PVARP should be programmed to 50 msec beyond the duration of retrograde VA conduction, as determined noninvasively during pacemaker programming.[89] As a rule of thumb, a PVARP of 300 msec offers protection against endless loop tachycardia in most patients.[122] If possible, patients without demonstrable retrograde VA conduction at the time of the implantation should have a PVARP programmed to 300 msec, provided there is no compromise of the upper rate. The availability of a programmable PVARP has virtually eliminated endless loop tachycardia with second- and third-generation DDD pulse generators.[21, 69] This elimination of endless loop tachycardia is in sharp contrast to its frequent occurrence with first-generation DDD pulse generators equipped with a short, nonprogrammable PVARP.[21] A programmable PVARP does not provide an absolute guarantee of preventing endless loop tachycardia because VA conduction may occasionally be quite variable. A contemporary DDD pulse generator rarely has

to be downgraded to another mode because of endless loop tachycardia. The problem of endless loop tachycardia cannot as yet be considered eradicated because its management really involves a compromise in the programmability of various pacemaker parameters.

MAXIMAL PACING RATE IN ENDLESS LOOP TACHYCARDIA. Patients with prolonged retrograde VA conduction may require substantial increase in PVARP duration, with a resultant marked reduction in the maximal programmable rate, which is directly correlated with the duration of the TARP (AV delay + PVARP). When preservation of the upper rate is desirable, particularly in the presence of "slow" retrograde VA conduction, some of the following options should be considered.

Shortening of the Atrioventricular Interval

Decreasing the AV delay may prevent endless loop tachycardia in the absence of an effect on the duration of the PVARP.[59] Indeed, dual-chamber pacemakers with short AV intervals have been used in the same way to prevent reentrant supraventricular tachycardia if the AV node is part of the reentry circuit.[113] When the AV interval is initiated by atrial pacing, the onset of atrial contraction is more delayed than when the same AV interval is initiated by a sensed atrial beat.[3, 4, 9, 74, 123, 131] The optimal duration of the AV interval should be individualized and may be determined by two-dimensional and Doppler echocardiography. In patients with complete AV block and normal sinus node function, a relatively short AV interval of 50 to 100 msec following sensed atrial events may be hemodynamically optimal.[4, 123] In pulse generators with AV interval hysteresis (or fallback),[74, 125] the AV interval initiated by atrial sensing may be programmed to a value shorter than that initiated by atrial pacing. The AV interval initiated by atrial sensing rather than pacing determines the atrial tracking capability of a DDD pulse generator, so that a shorter sensed AV interval without a change in PVARP will increase the upper rate of the pulse generator.

During exercise, the PR interval shortens,[27, 93] and the hemodynamically optimal AV (atrial sense–ventricular pace) interval may even be shorter than the PR interval at rest. In an active patient with relatively slow VA conduction and normal atrial chronotropic function, a very short atrial sense–ventricular pace AV interval may be programmed to allow a longer

PVARP to contain retrograde P waves without substantially compromising the upper rate limit. While a very short AV interval initiated by atrial sensing may not provide optimal hemodynamics at rest, this is probably inconsequential because the main function of atrial pacing at rest is to prevent retrograde VA conduction and the pacemaker syndrome.[8] On exercise, maintenance of AV synchrony does not contribute significantly to the increase in cardiac output, which is almost totally mediated by an increase in the ventricular pacing rate.[107, 130] A short atrial sense–ventricular pace interval (in a patient with normal atrial function) provides an adequate rate response on exercise and may also provide more advantageous AV synchrony.[95, 130] At present, only a few DDD pulse generators contain an algorithm to shorten the AV interval initiated by atrial sensing on exercise.

Pacemaker Response to Ventricular Extrasystoles

AUTOMATIC EXTENSION OF THE PVARP. Some second- and third-generation DDD pulse generators incorporate an automatic extension of the PVARP (for one cycle only) after a sensed ventricular event (outside the AV delay) that the pacemaker interprets as a ventricular extrasystole. In some pulse generators, PVARP extension after a ventricular extrasystole may be programmable.[13, 64, 83, 84] PVARP extension is based on the concept that most

episodes of endless loop tachycardia are initiated by ventricular extrasystoles with retrograde VA conduction. Another design related to PVARP extension, the so-called DDX mode, consists of conversion to the DVI mode (i.e., asynchronous atrial channel) until a subsequent atrial stimulus restores DDD pacing.[108] This conversion, in effect, functions like the automatic PVARP extension after a ventricular extrasystole, except that the atrial channel remains refractory for one complete cycle (corresponding to the programmed lower rate) and the pacemaker will continue to function in the DVI mode until delivery of an atrial stimulus restores DDD pacing (Fig. 12–35). Consequently, with activation of the DDX mode, the DVI mode need not be restricted only to one pacing cycle, and it may indeed continue indefinitely as long as the interval between two consecutive sensed ventricular events exceeds the pacemaker atrial escape (or pacemaker VA) interval[108] (Fig. 12–36). Termination of the DVI mode requires delivery of the atrial stimulus either spontaneously or after application of the magnet. Automatic PVARP extension does not sacrifice the atrial tracking capability (upper rate) because the standard PVARP remains unchanged. Automatic PVARP extension or the DDX mode may play a role in the prevention of endless loop tachycardia, but the protection does not come into play when the first retrograde P wave is engendered by a ventricular paced event. Under

PACESETTER DDX

LOWER RATE = 45 ppm
UPPER RATE = 110 ppm
AV INTERVAL = 115 ppm

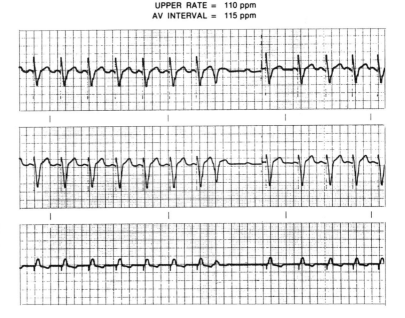

Figure 12–35. DDX mode operation of the 283 AFP Pacesetter DDD pulse generator. A sensed ventricular extrasystole initiates a pacemaker cycle in the DVI mode that is terminated by the succeeding atrial stimulus. A sinus P wave is unsensed, as the atrial channel is refractory in the DVI mode. In this way, an atrial stimulus close to the unsensed P wave may fall within the atrial myocardial refractory period and not cause atrial capture. In a patient with retrograde VA conduction, this sequence would favor retrograde VA conduction and initiation of endless loop tachycardia, as shown in Figure 12–37.

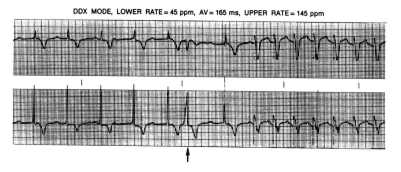

DDX MODE, LOWER RATE = 45 ppm, AV = 165 ms, UPPER RATE = 145 ppm

Figure 12–36. DDX mode of operation of the 283 AFP Pacesetter DDD pulse generator. The programmed parameters are shown above the ECG with two leads recorded simultaneously. The DDX mode of operation initiated the DVI mode after sensing of a ventricular extrasystole. The DVI mode can terminate only with the emission of an atrial stimulus. This stimulus does not occur, because the RR interval of the AV junctional escape rhythm (approximately 1000 msec) is shorter than the AEI (1333 − 165 = 1168 msec). A ventricular extrasystole *(arrow)* induces a longer pause, thereby allowing the release of an atrial stimulus at the termination of the AEI. The atrial stimulus produces a pseudo pseudofusion beat. This atrial stimulus terminates the DVI mode, with the return of P-wave tracking in the DDX (or DDD) mode.

certain circumstances, both the DDX mode and excessive extension of the PVARP may themselves paradoxically increase susceptibility to endless loop tachycardia[29] (Fig. 12–37).

Occasionally, a long PVARP (with or without extension) may cause P-wave undersensing that may be perpetuated from cycle to cycle if the pulse generator continually interprets the spontaneous supraventricular QRS complex (i.e., preceded by a P wave) as a ventricular extrasystole or premature ventricular event whenever P waves occur consistently within the relatively long PVARP and remain undetected. Apparent lack of atrial sensing may thus occur in the presence of an adequate atrial electrogram when it falls within a relatively long PVARP.[60] This form of atrial undersensing (or pseudoundersensing of P wave) disappears when the PVARP is shortened.

SYNCHRONOUS ATRIAL STIMULATION (SAS) UPON DETECTION OF A VENTRICULAR EXTRASYSTOLE. SAS works by the delivery of a triggered atrial stimulus whenever the DDD pulse generator detects a ventricular extrasystole, defined as a ventricular depolarization not preceded by a paced or sensed atrial event.[28, 32, 34, 42, 70] In this way, retrograde VA conduction engendered by a ventricular extrasystole cannot cause atrial depolarization and initiation of endless loop tachycardia because the previously released SAS renders the atrium refractory. In this design, if a ventricular extrasystole is preceded by another ventricular extrasystole with SAS, the second ventricular extrasystole is also interpreted as a premature ventricular event. This prevents pairs or runs of ventricular extrasystoles from starting endless loop tachycardia. Like PVARP extension, SAS is of limited value if endless loop tachycardia starts by another mechanism of retrograde VA conduction—for example, atrial extrasystole or pseudo P wave, such as myopotentials sensed by the atrial channel. Den Heijer and colleagues[34] recently reported a new

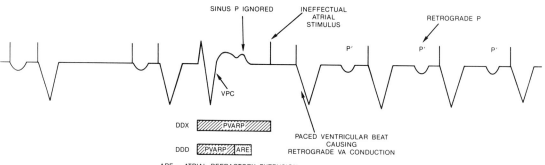

Figure 12–37. Diagrammatic representation of the mechanism of paradoxical induction of endless loop tachycardia by excessive prolongation of the PVARP with either atrial refractory period extension (ARE) or the DDX mode, in which the PVARP extends for the entire duration of the pacemaker cycle. An unsensed sinus P wave renders the succeeding atrial stimulus ineffectual because the stimulus falls within the atrial myocardial refractory period. This ineffectiveness of the atrial stimulus causes AV dissociation, followed by retrograde VA conduction and initiation of endless loop tachycardia.

form of pacemaker reentrant tachycardia related to SAS, which they called orthodromic pacemaker circus movement tachycardia. In the presence of atrial undersensing, a normally conducted QRS complex sensed by the ventricular channel of the pacemaker may be interpreted as a ventricular premature event, with the consequent delivery of SAS. The paced P wave (secondary to SAS) may then be conducted with a long PR interval. If the DDD pulse generator again interprets the conducted QRS complex as a ventricular premature event, SAS will be delivered again. This process tends to perpetuate itself in the form of an orthodromic pacemaker reentrant tachycardia. The reentrant loop is composed of an anterograde limb in the heart (AV junction), and the retrograde limb occurs via the pacemaker (sensing by the ventricular channel). This mechanism is in contrast to endless loop tachycardia in which anterograde conduction occurs via the pacemaker and retrograde VA conduction occurs via the conducting system of the heart (AV junction). The conditions responsible for orthodromic pacemaker reentrant tachycardia are SAS, atrial undersensing, and prolonged AV conduction, so that the conducted QRS complex secondary to SAS is sensed because it falls beyond the ventricular refractory period of the pulse generator. It is also theoretically possible for this reentrant tachycardia to be initiated by a sensed ventricular premature event (without preceding P wave) if SAS gives rise to a conducted QRS complex with a long PR interval. A related pacemaker tachycardia may occasionally be seen during single-chamber AAT pacing.[37] In this particular case, the far-field QRS complex is sensed in the atrium, and the pacemaker delivers an atrial stimulus synchronously with sensing of the QRS complex. This action initiates AV conduction, so that the resultant QRS complex falls beyond the refractory period of the atrial pacemaker and another atrial stimulus is then delivered, capturing the atrium, and this mechanism is perpetuated. This sequence of events has been called single-chamber endless loop tachycardia, but it is probably best called single-chamber orthodromic pacemaker reentrant tachycardia.

Differential Discrimination of Anterograde and Retrograde Atrial Depolarization

The mean amplitude of anterograde P waves generally exceeds that of retrograde P waves.[23,][79,][99] Indeed, approximately three quarters of all anterograde P waves are at least 0.5 mV larger than the corresponding retrograde P waves. Therefore, by selectively sensing anterograde-atrial depolarization and ignoring retrograde signals, endless loop tachycardia may be eliminated. This approach may be useful in pulse generators with extensive selections of atrial sensitivity settings that allow fine tuning to discriminate between the large anterograde and the smaller retrograde signals.[79] The use of lower atrial sensitivity to eliminate sensing of retrograde atrial depolarization may occasionally result in sporadic undersensing of anterograde atrial depolarization, which appears to be of no clinical significance.[79] Bernheim and associates[23] investigated the configuration and amplitude of anterograde and retrograde P waves in 130 patients who underwent implantation of a dual-chamber pulse generator. Fifty-nine patients (45 per cent) showed intact retrograde VA conduction with a mean duration of 251 msec. The electrographic amplitude of the sinus P wave averaged 3.6 mV, with a mean slew rate of 0.8 mV/sec. The corresponding retrograde P wave showed a mean amplitude of 2.3 mV with a mean slew rate of 0.5 mV/sec. The amplitude of sinus P waves exceeded that of the retrograde conducted signal, more than 0.5 mV in 48 patients (82 per cent) and more than 1.5 mV in 35 patients (59 per cent). The authors concluded that in about 60 per cent of the patients with retrograde VA conduction it could have been possible to prevent endless loop tachycardia by reprogramming atrial sensitivity to avoid the detection of retrograde P waves while maintaining a reasonably good safety margin for the detection of sinus P waves. This approach will most probably become more important in the future, when highly precise fine tuning of atrial sensitivity becomes available in all DDD pulse generators.

Prevention of Endless Loop Tachycardia by Programming a Faster Upper Rate

Klementowicz and colleagues[80] recently reported that the retrograde VA conduction time lengthens with increasing ventricular pacing rates and retrograde VA block occurs in more than half the patients with VA conduction at a ventricular rate of 120 ppm. These workers suggested that approximately 90 per cent of patients will not have endless loop tachycardia by selecting an upper rate of 140 ppm, a PVARP of 300 msec, and an AV interval of

125 msec. Programming a fast upper rate may render endless loop tachycardia unsustainable, but this approach should be used only under exceptional circumstances.[6, 35] Because of the unpredictability of retrograde VA conduction, programming a faster maximal rate may ultimately be unsuccessful and may be unsafe in patients with ischemic heart disease and in those with atrial tachyarrhythmias.

Endless Loop Tachycardia: New Engineering Considerations

We believe that the marvel of modern electronics will ultimately solve the problem of endless loop tachycardia by the design of appropriate algorithms to terminate endless loop tachycardia virtually as soon as it is initiated.[22, 32, 33, 81, 98, 126] Such algorithms would be able to discriminate between physiologic and nonphysiologic rate variations, adapt the atrial refractory period to the sensed atrial rate, or detect dissociation between atrial and ventricular events, whereupon the PVARP would be temporarily lengthened to avoid the start of endless loop tachycardia. Obviously, algorithms for the detection of endless loop tachycardia will not be based upon the upper rate of the DDD pulse generator because some endless loop tachycardias are slower than the programmed upper rate.

ATRIOVENTRICULAR DESYNCHRONIZATION ARRHYTHMIA

Endless loop tachycardia may be considered a form of VA synchrony, that is, the reverse of AV synchrony. VA synchrony may also occur in the absence of endless loop tachycardia when a paced ventricular beat engenders an *unsensed* retrograde P wave falling within the PVARP. Under certain circumstances, this form of VA synchrony may become self-perpetuating because an ineffectual atrial stimulus is continually delivered during the atrial *myocardial* refractory period generated by the preceding retrograde atrial depolarization[18, 115, 118] (Fig. 12–38). We have called this form of VA synchrony "AV desynchronization arrhythmia."[18] It represents a repetitive process similar to VA synchrony responsible for endless loop tachycardia, except that the atrial channel does not sense retrograde atrial depolarization (Fig. 12–39). Loss of atrial capture occurs despite a low atrial pacing threshold when the atrial escape (pacemaker VA) interval is shorter than the sum of the retrograde VA conduction time and the effective refractory period of the atrial myocardium.

The predisposing factors for the development of AV desynchronization arrhythmia in-

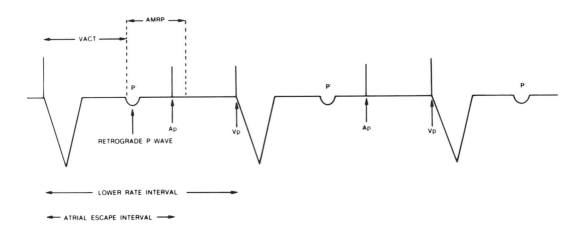

Figure 12–38. Diagrammatic representation of AV desynchronization arrhythmia. There is relatively slow retrograde VA conduction. The first ventricular paced beat causes retrograde VA conduction. The retrograde P wave (P ') is unsensed either because it falls within the PVARP or because the magnet causes asynchronous DOO pacing. At the completion of the AEI, the pacemaker delivers an atrial stimulus (Ap) falling too closely to the preceding retrograde P wave and therefore still within the atrial myocardial refractory period (AMRP) engendered by the preceding retrograde atrial depolarization. Ap is therefore ineffectual. Barring any perturbations, this process becomes self-perpetuating. VACT = retrograde VA conduction time; Vp = ventricular stimulus.

Figure 12–39. AV desynchronization arrhythmia. *A* and *B*, Intermedics Cosmos DDD pulse generator LRI = 720 msec (rate = 84 ppm), URI = 570 msec (rate = 106 ppm), AV interval = 300 msec, and PVARP = 300 msec. *A*, Application of the magnet causes DOO pacing, with the pulse width of the fifth atrial stimulus reduced by 50 percent and subthreshold (threshold margin test). Lack of atrial capture causes retrograde VA conduction, with the initiation of AV desynchronization arrhythmia. This arrhythmia persisted upon removal of the magnet. *B*, Same AV desynchronization arrhythmia as in *A*, terminated by premature ventricular stimulation due to crosstalk (CT) with extension of the VTP (from 100 to approximately 150 msec) to

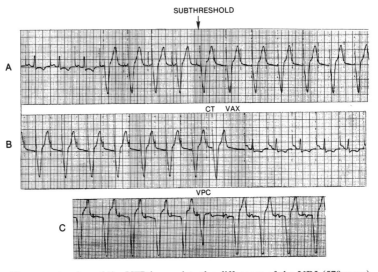

conform to the URLI of 570 msec. The 50 msec extension of the VTP is equal to the difference of the URI (570 msec) and the sum of the atrial escape (pacemaker VA) interval (420 msec) and the VTP (100 msec). There is also extension of the atrial escape (pacemaker VA) interval (VAX). Prolongation of the atrial escape (pacemaker VA) interval is unique to this pulse generator and occurs when the previous pacing cycle ends at the URLI. The relatively long pause gives the subsequent atrial stimulus the opportunity to capture the atrium, and the AV desynchronization arrhythmia is terminated. *C*, Medtronic Symbios 7006 DDD pulse generator programmed to the DDD mode and to the following parameters: LRI = 750 msec (rate = 80 ppm), URI = 600 msec (rate = 100 ppm), AV interval = 250 msec, and PVARP = 325 msec. A ventricular extrasystole (VPC) without retrograde VA conduction terminates AV desynchronization arrhythmia.

clude a prolonged retrograde VA conduction time, a relatively fast programmed lower rate, and a relatively long AV delay, so that the atrial escape (pacemaker VA) interval becomes relatively short. This shortening of the atrial escape interval produces early emission of the atrial stimulus (in relation to the preceding ventricular stimulus) and unsuccessful atrial capture if it is too close to the preceding retrograde P wave (see Fig. 12–39). When this mechanism perpetuates itself, it causes an AV desynchronization arrhythmia that is often temporary but may occasionally become sustained. When it is sustained, disruption of VA synchrony will immediately terminate the arrhythmia. This disruption may be produced by an early sensed ventricular event (extrasystole, myopotential, chest wall stimulation, and so on) without accompanying retrograde VA conduction. The absence of atrial activation permits delivery of the subsequent atrial stimulus beyond the atrial myocardial refractory period, with consequent successful atrial capture. Without the above mechanisms, termination of sustained AV desynchronization arrhythmia may require reprogramming of the DDD pulse generator to lengthen the atrial escape (pace-

maker VA) interval either by slowing the lower rate (longer lower rate interval) or by shortening the AV interval or both. The relative delay in the emission of the atrial stimulus disrupts VA synchrony by allowing the return of successful atrial capture beyond the effective refractory period of the atrial myocardium.

Application of the magnet over a DDD pulse generator generally converts it to the DOO mode, often with an increase in the pacing rate and shortening of the AV interval. Consequently, during magnet application, when there is a substantial increase in the pacing rate, AV desynchronization arrhythmia occurs frequently in patients with retrograde VA conduction. When the PVARP is relatively short, an AV desynchronization arrhythmia, produced by application of the magnet, may be converted to endless loop tachycardia upon withdrawal of the magnet. In contrast, if the PVARP is longer than the retrograde VA conduction time and the programmed atrial escape (pacemaker VA) interval is relatively short, withdrawal of the magnet may produce an AV desynchronization arrhythmia rather than endless loop tachycardia.

An AV desynchronization arrhythmia is sustained by a DDD pulse generator as its anterograde limb, with the cardiac conducting system providing the retrograde limb. In contrast to endless loop tachycardia, the loop does not really close, but the process is repeated with each pacing cycle because the retrograde P wave is unsensed and the delivery of the ventricular stimulus does not depend on the timing of the unsensed retrograde P wave. Endless loop tachycardia and AV desynchronization arrythmia are closely related because they both depend on retrograde VA conduction and both share similar mechanisms for initiation and termination.

AV desynchronization arrythmia should not be misinterpreted as primary failure of atrial capture. When sustained, AV desynchronization arrythmia represents another cause of the pacemaker syndrome[8] during normal function of a DDD pulse generator. Because the duration of the atrial escape (pacemaker VA) interval can be easily controlled, AV desynchronization arrythmia should not be an important problem with conventional DDD pulse generators. However, the forthcoming release of rate-responsive DDD pulse generators (DDDR) may induce AV desynchronization arrythmia on exercise when the sensor-driven increase in pacing rate shortens the atrial escape (pacemaker VA) interval. Conceivably, during exercise a ventricular extrasystole could precipitate AV desynchronization arrythmia, with perpetuation of retrograde VA conduction, thereby negating the potentially beneficial effects of AV synchrony. Although the hemodynamic effect of synchronized atrial activity may be negligible at relatively high levels of exercise when the cardiac output is controlled solely by the increase in the ventricular pacing rate,[107] it may be important at lesser levels of exercise, particularly in patients with significant left ventricular dysfunction and decreased left ventricular compliance, in whom retrograde VA conduction may be quite deleterious.[8]

DIFFERENTIAL DIAGNOSIS OF TACHYCARDIA DURING DDD PACING

Tachycardia during DDD pacing is a common problem, and the diagnosis is often quite simple.[13] The diagnosis of tachycardia during DDD pacing may be facilitated by telemetry of the atrial electrogram to identify atrial de-

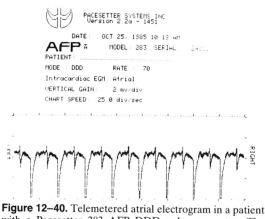

Figure 12–40. Telemetered atrial electrogram in a patient with a Pacesetter 283 AFP DDD pulse generator. The atrial electrogram shows ventricular pacing followed by a P wave compatible with the diagnosis of endless loop tachycardia. The retrograde VA conduction time is approximately 300 msec.

polarization (Fig. 12–40) and by event markers to demonstrate how the pacemaker interprets signals (Fig. 12–41), or alternatively by programming the triggered mode in the atrium—for example, DDT (or AAT in the absence of AV block), in which the atrial triggered stimuli function as atrial event markers.

Sinus Tachycardia or Supraventricular Tachycardia

Carotid sinus pressure should be applied in the usual fashion for the differential diagnosis of supraventricular tachycardia. Application of

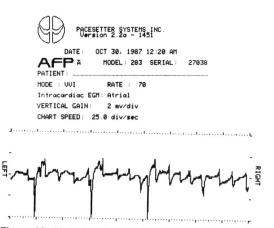

Figure 12–41. Telemetered atrial electrogram in a patient with a Pacesetter AFP 283 DDD pulse generator programmed to the VVI mode. The atrial electrogram shows irregularly occurring f waves consistent with the presence of atrial flutter-fibrillation.

Figure 12–42. Atrial fibrillation in a patient with a Pacesetter 283 AFP DDD pulse generator. The programmed parameters are shown above the ECG. The paced ventricular rate is irregular and rapid, and an occasional pacemaker cycle occurs at the URI. Upon application of the magnet, immediate slowing of the pacing rate demonstrates the typical baseline seen in atrial fibrillation.

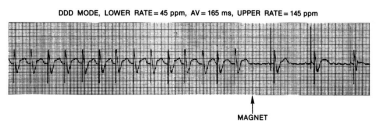

DDD MODE, LOWER RATE = 45 ppm, AV = 165 ms, UPPER RATE = 145 ppm

MAGNET

the magnet (slower DOO or VOO mode) may reveal P waves, and tachycardia returns upon withdrawal of the magnet. Programming the pulse generator to the VVI mode at a relatively slow rate may also allow analysis of atrial activity. A pacemaker Wenckebach response suggests that the atrial rate is faster than the programmed upper rate of the pacemaker, but it does not rule out sinus tachycardia, particularly if the programmed upper rate is relatively slow. In the presence of a long programmed AV interval, the P wave may be concealed in the T wave of the preceding beat. Shortening of the AV interval may reveal the morphology of the P wave in the 12-lead electrocardiogram, allowing differential diagnosis of normal sinus rhythm from supraventricular tachycardia in the usual fashion. The diagnosis of sinus tachycardia may be quickly confirmed by shortening the AV interval and increasing the upper rate. In sinus tachycardia, the ventricular pacing rate will remain unchanged after this maneuver. In contrast, with endless loop tachycardia, changing these two variables (upper rate and AV interval) will cause an obvious alteration in the ventricular pacing rate.

Atrial Fibrillation and Flutter[35, 49, 61, 78, 85]

The diagnosis of atrial fibrillation or flutter is suggested when the ventricular pacing rate is rapid and irregular (Fig. 12–42). In both atrial flutter and atrial fibrillation, varying amplitude of the atrial f waves may lead to intermittent loss of atrial sensing, with the occasional delivery of atrial stimuli at the end of the atrial escape (pacemaker VA) interval. Coupled with periods of rapid and irregular ventricular pacing, this produces a chaotic pattern virtually diagnostic of underlying flutter or fibrillation (Figs. 12–42 to 12–44). Atrial flutter may occasionally produce regular and rapid ventricular pacing, sometimes at the upper rate, thereby mimicking endless loop tachycardia with retrograde VA conduction (Fig. 12–45). In the latter, application of the magnet terminates the tachycardia, while in atrial flutter, slower pacing in the DOO mode will reveal the regular, characteristic f waves of atrial flutter, with immediate resumption of tachycardia upon withdrawal of the magnet. The diagnosis of atrial flutter and fibrillation should actually be one of exclusion, particu-

LOWER RATE = 80 ppm
UPPER RATE INTERVAL = 160 ppm (375 ms)
AV INTERVAL = 160 ms

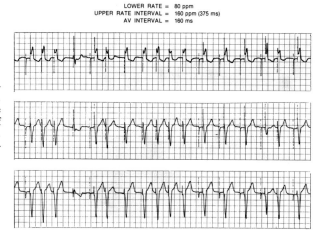

Figure 12–43. Three-lead ECG showing atrial fibrillation in a patient with a DDD pulse generator. The programmed parameters are shown above the ECG. Note the constantly changing pattern of pacing due to intermittent sensing of the f waves. When the f waves are not sensed, the AEI terminates with the delivery of an atrial stimulus.

DDD MODE
AV = 165 ms, LOWER RATE = 70 ppm, UPPER RATE = 145 ppm

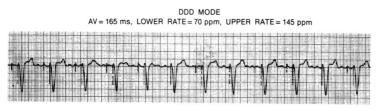

Figure 12–44. Atrial fibrillation in a patient with a Pacesetter DDD pulse generator. The programmed parameters are shown above the ECG. PVARP = 325 msec. The ventricular pacing rate remains relatively low with relatively slight variability of the pacing cycles because the f waves are sensed intermittently.

larly when telemetry of the intracardiac atrial electrogram or event markers are not available. Programming the pulse generator to the VVI mode at a relatively slow rate is always helpful in the delineation of atrial activity.

Near-Field Endless Loop Tachycardia

Near-field endless loop tachycardia related to sensing of retrograde atrial depolarization is almost always terminated upon application of the magnet (conversion to DOO or VOO mode). Rarely, when endless loop tachycardia is unresponsive to magnet application, it can be easily terminated by chest wall stimulation to inhibit the ventricular channel of the pulse generator. The diagnosis may be substantiated by the subsequent induction of a similar tachycardia by the usual methods to induce retrograde VA conduction.

Far-Field Endless Loop Tachycardia[25, 36, 38, 39, 103, 111]

This pacemaker tachycardia is rare and may pose a difficult diagnostic problem with unipolar DDD pulse generators (high sensitivity, short PVARP) when the atrial lead senses far-field phenomena. As a rule, this diagnosis is impossible without telemetry of the atrial electrogram or esophageal electrocardiography to delineate atrial activity.

Myopotential Triggering[13, 26, 30, 44, 48, 71, 104, 105, 132]

Tachycardia triggered by myopotentials sensed by the atrial channel may be regular or irregular, and the cycle length is often at the upper rate limit interval. It may also be associated with periods of myopotential inhibition of the ventricular channel and asynchronous pacing at the interference rate. This arrhythmia may be easily reproducible by isometric exercise (Figs. 12–46 and 12–47). Myopotential triggering may be reduced or eliminated by decreasing atrial sensitivity.

Crosstalk Tachycardia

In pulse generators with a ventricular safety pacing period (also known as a ventricular triggering period), tachycardia may occur during continual crosstalk. For example, with a lower rate of 80 ppm (lower rate interval = 750 msec) and an AV interval of 300 msec, the atrial escape (pacemaker VA) interval is equal to 450 msec. During crosstalk with a ventricular triggering period of 100 msec, the AV interval shortens to 100 msec. Consequently, the pacemaker interval is equal to 450 plus 100, or 550 msec, corresponding to a rate of 109 ppm. This pacemaker tachycardia is immediately recognized by the abbreviation of the AV interval, reflecting crosstalk (Fig. 12–48).

False Signals Sensed by the Atrial Channel

When the atrial channel senses false signals from a defective atrial electrode, an irregular pacemaker tachycardia may ensue. Sensing of a false signal by the atrial channel may cause AV dissociation and may initiate endless loop tachycardia, further complicating the diagnosis. In addition, the diagnosis may be difficult

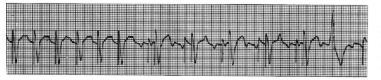

Figure 12–45. Atrial flutter causing pacemaker tachycardia in a patient with a Cordis 233F DDD pulse generator. The magnet was applied after the sixth beat. The slower magnetic rate revealed atrial flutter as the cause of the pacemaker tachycardia. (From Barold SS, Falkoff MD, Ong LS, Heinle RA: Function and electrocardiography of DDD pacemakers. *In* Barold SS [ed]: Modern Cardiac Pacing. Mount Kisco, NY, Futura Publishing Co, 1985, p 645; with permission.)

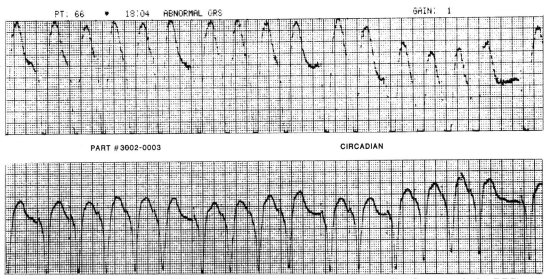

Figure 12–46. Two-channel Holter recording of a patient with an Intermedics Cosmos unipolar DDD pulse generator. The programmed parameters were as follows: lower rate = 60 ppm (1000 msec), URI = 480 msec (125 ppm), AV interval = 250 msec, PVARP = 200 msec, and atrial sensitivity = 0.8 mV. There is an irregular pacemaker tachycardia. Differential diagnosis includes myopotential triggering, atrial fibrillation, and false signals from a defective atrial electrode.

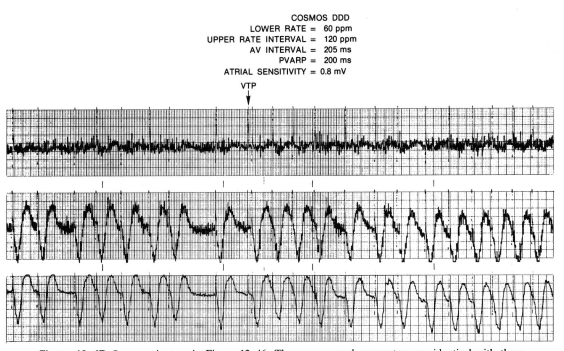

Figure 12–47. Same patient as in Figure 12–46. The programmed parameters are identical with those indicated in Figure 12–46. Three ECG leads are recorded simultaneously. Myopotential sensing was deliberately induced by appropriate pectoral muscle exercises. Myopotential sensing by the atrial channel causes ventricular triggering at a rapid and irregular rate. Myopotential is also sensed by the ventricular channel because the interval between the seventh and eighth paced beats is approximately 1120 msec and longer than the LRI (1000 msec). At the arrow, myopotential signals were sensed by the ventricular electrode within the VTP. This sensing causes the delivery of the ventricular stimulus at the end of the VTP, leading to abbreviation of the AV interval (110 msec). When the sensitivity of the atrial channel was decreased to 2.8 mV, P-wave sensing was still present. Consequently, atrial sensitivity was left at 2.4 mV. At this new setting, myopotential triggering could not be induced. A repeat Holter recording showed no myopotential triggering and normal sensing of P waves.

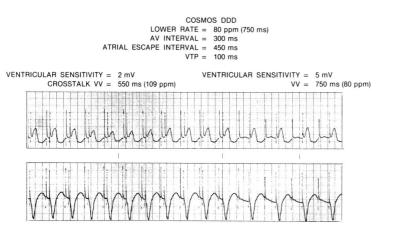

COSMOS DDD
LOWER RATE = 80 ppm (750 ms)
AV INTERVAL = 300 ms
ATRIAL ESCAPE INTERVAL = 450 ms
VTP = 100 ms

VENTRICULAR SENSITIVITY = 2 mV
CROSSTALK VV = 550 ms (109 ppm)

VENTRICULAR SENSITIVITY = 5 mV
VV = 750 ms (80 ppm)

Figure 12–48. Crosstalk tachycardia with the Cosmos DDD pulse generator. Two ECG leads were recorded simultaneously. On the left, there is crosstalk at a ventricular sensitivity of 2 mV. Crosstalk causes abbreviation of the AV interval to the duration of the VTP. The interval between two consecutive ventricular stimuli is therefore equal to 450 + 100 = 550 msec, corresponding to a rate of 109 ppm. On the right, when the ventricular sensitivity was reduced to 5 mV, crosstalk was eliminated. The interval between two consecutive ventricular stimuli now becomes equal to the LRI of 750 msec.

because the ventricular response resembles atrial fibrillation. The diagnosis is one of exclusion if telemetry of the electrogram or event markers are not available (Fig. 12–49).

Orthodromic DDD Pacemaker Reentrant Tachycardia

This tachycardia, recently reported by DenHeijer and associates,[34] was discussed above in detail under "Synchronous Atrial Stimulation (SAS) upon Detection of a Ventricular Extrasystole." This tachycardia exhibits a deformed supraventricular QRS complex by the delivery of synchronous atrial stimulation.

Vulnerable Period Tachycardia

This tachycardia is induced by the delivery of a pacemaker stimulus in the vulnerable period of the ventricle (ventricular tachycardia or fibrillation) or the atrium (atrial flutter or fibrillation).[47]

Other Pacemaker Tachycardias

Autonomous tachycardia related to idiosyncratic behavior of a pulse generator has been described.[112] Pseudo endless loop tachycardia[7] has also been described. Figure 12–50 may be considered to represent a form of pseudo endless loop tachycardia somewhat different from the arrhythmia described by the workers who coined this term.

The initiating mechanism of a pacemaker tachycardia may not necessarily be the same as the one sustaining it; that is, far-field sensing of the QRS complex may initiate an endless loop tachycardia that may then be perpetuated by continual sensing of retrograde atrial depolarization. Two mechanisms may coexist,

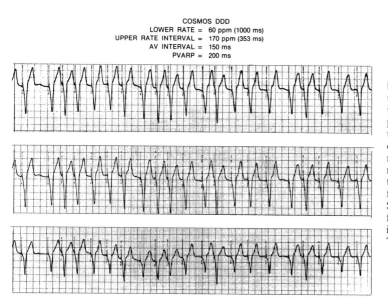

COSMOS DDD
LOWER RATE = 60 ppm (1000 ms)
UPPER RATE INTERVAL = 170 ppm (353 ms)
AV INTERVAL = 150 ms
PVARP = 200 ms

Figure 12–49. Irregular pacemaker tachycardia in a patient with an Intermedics Cosmos unipolar DDD pulse generator with a defective electrode creating false signals. This defective electrode produces an irregular pacemaker tachycardia that mimics the presence of atrial fibrillation. This patient had normal sinus function and complete AV block. Some of the paced beats appear to be followed by retrograde P waves causing notching of the ST segment and T wave.

Figure 12–50. Holter recording of pseudo endless loop tachycardia in a patient with an Intermedics Cosmos DDD pulse generator. This ECG could be interpreted as representing the spontaneous occurrence of an endless loop tachycardia possibly due to myopotential oversensing or related to an atrial extrasystole. This explanation is quite plausible because of the relatively long AV interval. The pause after the fifth ventricular paced beat could be explained in terms of loss of retrograde VA conduction with termination of endless loop tachycardia. The tachycardia would then restart after the ventricular paced beat that follows the atrial stimulus causing atrial fusion. The correct diagnosis was actually sinus tachycardia with the P waves depicted by the solid black circles. The fifth P wave falls within the PVARP. The seventh P wave also falls within the PVARP. The lower channel depicts the pacemaker stimuli.

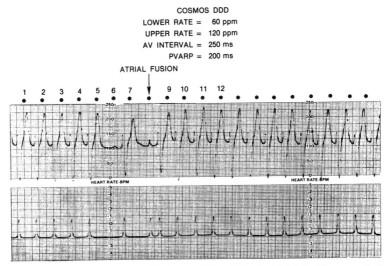

alternating from one to the other. For example, myopotential triggering may precipitate endless loop tachycardia,[13, 105] which may be terminated by myopotential sensing by the ventricular channel and again restarted by myopotential sensing by the atrial channel. Similarly, a defective atrial lead may generate false signals that may cause a chaotic paced ventricular arrhythmia that may in part be due to retrograde VA conduction. In some cases, even continuous recording of the intracardiac electrogram or event markers may be insufficient to clarify the diagnosis. With a complex problem, the clear delineation of atrial activity with an esophageal ECG is invaluable.

REFERENCES

1. Akhtar M: Retrograde conduction in man. PACE 4:548, 1981.
2. Akhtar M, Gilbert C, Mahmud R, et al: Pacemaker-mediated tachycardia: Underlying mechanism, relationship to ventriculoatrial conduction, characteristics and management. Clin Progress Pacing and Electrophysiol 3:90, 1985.
3. Alt E, Wirzfeld A, Seidel K, et al: Delayed atrial excitation following bifocal pacemaker stimulation. Z Kardiol 72:245, 1983.
4. Alt EV, von Bibra H, Blömet H: Different beneficial AV intervals with DDD pacing after sensed or paced atrial events. J Electrophysiol 1:250, 1987.
5. Altamura G, Boccadamo R, Toscano S, et al: Incidence of and drug effect on ventriculoatrial conduction in patients with bradyarrhythmias. *In* Pérez Gómez F (ed): Cardiac Pacing: Electrophysiology: Tachyarrhythmias. Mount Kisco, NY, Futura Media Services, 1985, p 735.
6. Amikam S, Furman S: Programmed upper-rate limit dependent endless loop tachycardia. Chest 85:286, 1984.
7. Amikam S, Andrews C, Furman S: "Pseudo-endless loop" tachycardia in an AV universal (DDD) pacemaker. PACE 7:129, 1984.
8. Ausubel K, Furman S: The pacemaker syndrome. Ann Intern Med 103:420, 1985.
9. Ausubel K, Klementowicz P, Furman S: Interatrial conduction during cardiac pacing. PACE 9:302, 1986.
10. Barold SS, Belott PH: Behavior of the ventricular triggering period of DDD pacemakers. PACE 10:1237, 1987.
11. Barold SS, Falkoff MD, Ong LS, Heinle RA: Clinical usefulness of chest wall stimulation in patients with implanted DDD pacemakers. PACE 6:A–44, 1983.
12. Barold SS, Falkoff MD, Ong LS, Heinle RA: Programmability in DDD pacing, PACE 7:1159, 1984.
13. Barold SS, Falkoff MD, Ong LS, Heinle RA: Function and electrocardiography of DDD pacemakers. *In* Barold SS (ed): Modern Cardiac Pacing. Mount Kisco, NY, Futura Publishing Co, 1985, p 645.
14. Barold SS, Falkoff MD, Ong LS, Heinle RA: Paradoxical induction of endless loop tachycardia by magnet application over DDD pacemaker. PACE 9:503, 1986.
15. Barold SS, Falkoff MD, Ong LS, Heinle RA: Clinical usefulness of chest wall stimulation in patients with DDD pulse generators. PACE 10:641, 1987.
16. Barold SS, Falkoff MD, Ong LS, Heinle RA: Crosstalk due to activation of atrial sense marker function of DDD pulse generators. PACE 10:293, 1987.
17. Barold SS, Ong LS, Falkoff MD, Heinle RA: Crosstalk or self-inhibition in dual-chambered pacemakers. *In* Barold SS (ed): Modern Cardiac Pacing. Mount Kisco, NY, Futura Publishing Co, 1985, p 615.
18. Barold SS, Falkoff MD, Ong LS, et al: AV desynchronization arrhythmia during DDD pacing. *In* Belhassen B, Feldman S, Copperman Y (eds): Cardiac Pacing and Electrophysiology: Proceedings of the VIIIth World Symposium on Cardiac

Pacing and Electrophysiology. Jerusalem, Keter-press Enterprises, 1987, p 177.

19. Barold SS, Falkoff MD, Ong LS, et al: Unusual consequences of upper rate limitation in DDD pulse generators. PACE 10:641, 1987.
20. Bathen J, Gunderson T, Forfang K: Tachycardia related to atrial synchronous ventricular pacing. PACE 5:471, 1982.
21. Belott PH: Clinical experience with over 250 DDD pacemakers. In Barold SS (ed): Modern Cardiac Pacing. Mount Kisco, NY, Futura Publishing Co, 1985, p 439.
22. Berkovits BV, Friedman PL, Haffajee CI: Improved DDD pacing with a new rate-limiting algorithm. In Belhassen B, Feldman S, Copperman Y (eds): Cardiac Pacing and Electrophysiology: Proceedings of the VIIIth World Symposium on Cardiac Pacing and Electrophysiology. Jerusalem, Keter-press Enterprises, 1987, p 171.
23. Bernheim C, Markewitz A, Kemkes BM: Can reprogramming of atrial sensitivity avoid an endless loop tachycardia? PACE 9:293, 1986.
24. Bertholet M, Materne P, Dubois C, et al: Artificial circus movement tachycardias: Incidence, mechanisms and prevention. PACE 8:415, 1985.
25. Brandt J, Pahlm O, Schüller H: Esophageal ECG recording—a valuable diagnostic tool in dual chamber pacing. Eur Heart J 6:342, 1985.
26. Chomka E, Edwards-Strauss L, Papp MA, Hauser RG: Myopotential oversensing in DDD pacemakers. PACE 8:295, 1985.
27. Daubert C, Ritter P, Mabo P, et al: Physiological relationship between AV interval and heart rate in healthy subjects: Applications to dual chamber pacing. PACE 9:1032, 1986.
28. DeJongste MJL, van Binsbergen EJ, Nagelkerke D, et al: Early experience with the Quintech 931 DDD pacemaker. In Pérez Gómez F (ed): Cardiac Pacing: Electrophysiology: Tachyarrhythmias. Mount Kisco, NY, Futura Media Services, 1985, p 713.
29. Den Dulk K, Wellens HJ: Failure of the post-ventricular premature beat DVI mode in preventing pacemaker circus movement tachycardia. Am J Cardiol 54:1371, 1984.
30. Den Dulk K, Lindemans FW, Wellens HJJ: Noninvasive evaluation of pacemaker circus movement tachycardia. Am J Cardiol 53:537, 1984.
31. Den Dulk K, Lindemans FW, Wellens HJJ: Management of pacemaker circus movement tachycardia. PACE 7:346, 1984.
32. Den Dulk K, Lindeman FW, Wellens HJJ: Merits of various antipacemaker circus movement tachycardia features. PACE 9:1055, 1986.
33. Den Dulk K, Hamersa M, Wellens HJJ: Role of an adaptable atrial refractory period for DDD pacemakers. PACE 10:425, 1987.
34. Den Heijer P, Crijns HJGM, van Binsbergen EJ, et al: Orthodromic pacemaker circus movement tachycardia. PACE 10:955, 1987.
35. Dodinot B, Kubler L: La Pathologie du "physiologique." Stimucoeur Med 10:220, 1982.
36. Dodinot BP, Medeiros P, Galvão SS, Godenir JP: Endless loop dual chamber pacemaker tachycardia related to R wave sensing by the atrial circuit. PACE 8:A–36, 1985.
37. Dodinot B, Medeiros P, Galvão S, Godenir JP: Single chamber endless loop pacemaker tachycardia: A possible complication of AAT pacing. PACE 8:A–19, 1985.
38. Dodinot BP, Medeiros P, Galvão SS, Godenir J:

Endless loop dual chamber pacemaker tachycardias related to R wave sensing by the atrial circuit. PACE 8:301, 1985.
39. Dodinot B, Medeiros P, Galvão S, et al: Dual chamber pacemaker sustained tachycardias related to "cross ventricular sensing." Stimucoeur Med 14:15, 1986.
40. Driller J, Barold SS, Parsonnet V: Normal and abnormal function of the pacemaker magnetic reed switch. J Electrocardiol 9:283, 1976.
41. Duffin EG: The marker channel period: A telemetric diagnostic aid. PACE 7:1165, 1984.
42. Elmqvist H: Prevention of pacemaker mediated tachycardia. PACE 6:382, 1983.
43. Fearnot NE, Smith HJ, Geddes LA: A review of pacemakers that physiologically increase rate: The DDD and rate-responsive pacemakers. Prog Cardiovasc Dis 29:145, 1986.
44. Fetter J, Hall DM, Hoff GL, Reeder JT: The effects of myopotential interference on unipolar and bipolar dual chamber pacemakers in the DDD mode. Clin Prog Electrophysiol Pacing 3:368, 1985.
45. Fletcher RD, Cohen AI, del Negro AA: Noninvasive electrophysiologic studies using implanted pacemakers. In Barold SS (ed): Modern Cardiac Pacing. Mount Kisco, NY, Futura Publishing Co, 1985, p 421.
46. Fontaine JW, Maloney JD, Castle LW, Morant VA: Noninvasive assessment of ventriculoatrial conduction and early experience with the tachycardia termination algorithm in pacemaker mediated tachycardia. PACE 9:212, 1986.
47. Freedman RA, Rothman MT, Jason JW: Recurrent ventricular tachycardia induced by an atrial synchronous ventricular inhibited pacemaker. PACE 5:490, 1982.
48. Fröhlig G, Sen S, Blank W, et al: Susceptibility of a unipolar dual chamber pacemaker to chest wall myopotentials. In Pérez Gómez F (ed): Cardiac Pacing: Electrophysiology: Tachyarrhythmias. Mount Kisco, NY, Futura Media Services, 1985, p 698.
49. Fröhlig G, Sen S, Rettig G, et al: Atrial flutter and fibrillation with DDD pacing. In Pérez Gómez (ed): Cardiac Pacing: Electrophysiology: Tachyarrhythmias. Mount Kisco, NY, Futura Publishing Co, 1985, p 685.
50. Frumin H, Furman S: Endless loop tachycardia started by an atrial premature beat in a patient with a dual chamber pacemaker. J Am Coll Cardiol 5:707, 1985.
51. Furman S: Retreat from Wenckebach. PACE 7:1, 1984.
52. Furman S: Dual-chambered pacemakers. Upper rate behavior. PACE 8:197, 1985.
53. Furman S: Comprehension of pacemaker cycles. In Furman S, Hayes DL, Holmes DR (eds): A Practice of Cardiac Pacing. Mount Kisco, NY, Futura Publishing Co, 1986, p 159.
54. Furman S, Fisher JD: Endless loop tachycardia in an AV universal (DDD) pacemaker. PACE 5:476, 1982.
55. Gabry MD, Klementowicz P, Furman S: Balanced endless loop tachycardia. PACE 9:294, 1986.
56. Garson A Jr, Coyner T, Shannon CE, Gillette PC: A systematic approach to the fully automatic (DDD) pacemaker electrocardiogram. In Gillette PC, Griffin JC (eds): Practical Cardiac Pacing. Baltimore, The Williams & Wilkins Co, 1986, p 181.

57. Gascon DA, Errazquin F, Nieto J, et al: Intra-atrial recording of ventriculoatrial conduction during pacemaker implantation. *In* Steinbach K (ed): Cardiac Pacing: Proceedings of the VIIth World Symposium on Cardiac Pacing. Darmstadt, Federal Republic of Germany, Steinkopff Verlag, 1983, p 135.

58. Gascon D, Errazquin F, Nieto J, et al: Maneuvers for induction of PMT during follow-up. PACE 8:A–100, 1985.

59. Greenspon AJ, Greenberg RM: Noninvasive evaluation of retrograde conduction times to avoid pacemaker-mediated tachycardia. J Am Coll Cardiol 5:1403, 1985.

60. Greenspon AJ, Volasin KJ: "Pseudo" loss of atrial sensing by a DDD pacemaker. PACE 10:943, 1987.

61. Greenspon AJ, Greenberg RM, Frankl WS: Tracking of DDD pacing: Another form of pacemaker mediated tachycardia. PACE 7:955, 1984.

62. Griffin JC, Spencer WH, Cashron R, et al: Exercise capability of patients receiving DDD pacemakers. PACE 7:460, 1984.

63. Guzman PA, Brinker JA: The electrophysiologic and pharmacologic management of pacemaker induced tachycardia in patients receiving a new DDD pacemaker. PACE 6:A–37, 1983.

64. Haffajee C, Murphy J, Gold R, Charos G: Automatic extension vs. programmability of the atrial refractory period in the prevention of pacemaker mediated tachycardia. PACE 8:A–56, 1985.

65. Harriman RJ, Pasquariello JL, Gomes JAC, et al: Autonomic dependence of ventriculoatrial conduction. Am J Cardiol 56:285, 1985.

66. Harthorne JW, Eisenhauer AC, Steinhaus DM: Pacemaker-mediated tachycardias: An unresolved problem. PACE 7:1140, 1984.

67. Hauser RG: The electrocardiography of AV universal DDD pacemakers. PACE 6:399, 1983.

68. Hayes DL, Furman S: Atrioventricular and ventriculo-atrial conduction times in patients undergoing pacemaker implant. PACE 6:38, 1983.

69. Hayes DL, Holmes DR, Vliestra RE, Osborn MJ: Changing experience with dual chamber (DDD) pacemakers. J Am Coll Cardiol 4:556, 1984.

70. Irnich W: The ideal pacemaker. *In* Harthorne JW, Thalen HJ (eds): Boston Colloquium on Cardiac Pacing. The Hague, Martinus Nijhoff, 1977, p 111.

71. Irwin ME, Lee TK, St Clair WR: A method for predicting the potential for pacemaker-induced reciprocating tachycardia in patients with DDD pacemakers. *In* Steinbach K (ed): Cardiac Pacing: Proceedings of the VIIth World Symposium on Cardiac Pacing. Darmstadt, Federal Republic of Germany, Steinkopff Verlag, 1983, p 519.

72. Irwin ME, Lee TK, St Clair WR: A method for predicting the potential for pacemaker-induced reciprocating tachycardia in patients with DDD pulse generators. PACE 6:A37, 1983.

73. Isicoff C: Understanding upper rate responses of DDD pacemakers. Heart Lung 14:327, 1985.

74. Janosik D, Pearson A, Redd R, et al: The importance of atrioventricular delay fallback in optimizing cardiac output during physiologic pacing. PACE 10:410, 1987.

75. Johnson CD: AV universal (DDD) pacemaker mediated reentrant endless loop tachycardia initiated by a reciprocal beat of atrial origin. PACE 7:29, 1984.

76. Jordaens L, Clement DL: The prevention of pace-

maker mediated tachycardias in double-chamber pacing. Acta Cardiol 39:449, 1984.

77. Keefe JM, Mann B, Snell J: Real-time annotated ECG event markers: Engineering aspects and clinical applications. Clin Prog Electrophysiol Pacing [Suppl] 4:52, 1986.

78. Kerr CR, Mason MA: Amplitude of atrial electrical activity during sinus rhythm and during atrial flutter-fibrillation. PACE 8:348, 1985.

79. Klementowicz PT, Furman S: Selective atrial sensing in dual chamber pacemakers eliminates endless loop tachycardia. J Am Coll Cardiol 7:590, 1986.

80. Klementowicz P, Ausubel K, Furman S: The dynamic nature of ventriculoatrial conduction. PACE 9:1050, 1986.

81. Kroiss D, Jacobson P, Limousin M, et al: Pacemaker mediated tachycardia: New engineering solutions. Clin Prog Electrophysiol Pacing [Suppl] 4:4, 1986.

82. Kruse I, Markowitz T, Ryden L: Timing markers showing pacemaker behavior to aid in the follow-up of a physiological pacemaker. PACE 6:801, 1983.

83. Levine PA: Post-ventricular atrial refractory periods in pacemaker-mediated tachycardia. Clin Prog Pacing Electrophysiol 1:394, 1983.

84. Levine PA: Normal and abnormal rhythms associated with dual-chamber pacemakers. Cardiol Clin 3:595, 1985.

85. Levine PA, Seltzer JP: AV universal (DDD) pacing and atrial fibrillation. Clin Prog Pacing Electrophysiol 1:275, 1983.

86. Levine PA, Schüller H, Lindgren A: Pacemaker ECG: An Introduction and Approach to Interpretation. Solna, Sweden, Siemens-Elema AB, 1986.

87. Levine PA, Sholder J, Duncan JL: Clinical benefits of telemetered electrograms in assessment of DDD function. PACE 7:1170, 1984.

88. Lévy S, Corbelli JL, Labrunie P, et al: Retrograde (ventriculoatrial) conduction. PACE 6:364, 1983.

89. Littleford P, Curry RC Jr, Schwartz KM, Pepine CJ: Pacemaker mediated tachycardia: A rapid bedside technique for induction and observation. Am J Cardiol 52:287, 1983.

90. Luceri RM, Hayes DL: Follow-up of DDD pacemakers. PACE 7:1187, 1984.

91. Luceri RM, Castellanos A, Zaman L, Myerburg R: The arrhythmias of dual chamber cardiac pacemakers and their management. Ann Intern Med 99:354, 1983.

92. Luceri RM, Parker M, Thurer RJ, et al: Particularities of management and followup of patients with DDD pacemakers. Clin Prog Pacing Electrophysiol 2:261, 1984.

93. Luceri RM, Smith E, Interian A, et al: Dynamic PR interval variability: Implications for autoadaptive physiologic pacemakers. PACE 9:300, 1986.

94. Mahmud R, Denker S, Lehmann MH, Akhtar M: Effect of atrioventricular sequential pacing in patients with no ventriculoatrial conduction. J Am Coll Cardiol 2:273, 1984.

95. Mehta D, Gilmour SM, Ward DE, Camm JA: Optimizing the atrio-ventricular delay at rest and during exercise with atrioventricular synchronous pacing. Circulation 76 [Suppl IV]:IV–80, 1987.

96. Morley C, Sutton R, Perrins J, Ghan SL: Importance of retrograde atrioventricular conduction in physiological pacing. PACE 4:A–60, 1981.

97. Oseran D, Ausubel K, Klementowicz PT, Furman S: Spontaneous endless loop tachycardia. PACE 9:379, 1986.

98. Pannizzo F, Furman S: Automatic discrimination of retrograde P wave for dual chamber pacemakers. J Am Coll Cardiol 5:393, 1985.

99. Pannizzo F, Akikam S, Bagwell P, Furman S: Discrimination of antegrade and retrograde atrial depolarization by electrogram analysis. Am Heart J 112:780, 1986.

100. Papp MA, Mason T, Gallastegni J: Use of rate smoothing to treat pacemaker mediated tachycardias and symptoms due to upper rate response of a DDD pacemaker. Clin Prog Pacing Electrophysiol 2:547, 1984.

101. Parsonnet V, Bernstein AD: Pseudomalfunctions of dual chamber pacemakers. PACE 6:376, 1983.

102. Perrins EJ, Morley CA, Dixey J, Sutton R: The pharmacologic blockade of retrograde atrioventricular conduction in paced patients. PACE 6:A–112, 1983.

103. Pimenta J, Soldá R, Britto Pereiva C: Tachycardia mediated by an AV universal (DDD) pacemaker triggered by a ventricular depolarization. PACE 9:105, 1986.

104. Quintal R, Dhurandhar RW, Jain RK: Myopotential interference with a DDD pacemaker: Report of a case. PACE 7:37, 1984.

105. Rozanski JJ, Blankstein RL, Lister JW: Pacemaker arrhythmias: Myopotential triggering of pacemaker mediated tachycardia. PACE 6:795, 1983.

106. Rubin JW, Frank MJ, Boineau JP, Ellison RG: Current physiologic pacemakers: A serious problem with a new device. Am J Cardiol 52:88, 1983.

107. Rydén L: The future of single chamber pacing. PACE 9:1131, 1986.

108. Satler LF, Rackley CE, Pearle DL, et al: Inhibition of a physiologic pacing system due to its anti–pacemaker-mediated tachycardia mode. PACE 8:806, 1985.

109. Schuilenburg RM: Patterns of VA conduction in the human heart in the presence of normal and abnormal conduction. In Wellens HJJ, Lie KI, Janse MJ (eds): The Conduction System of the Heart. Philadelphia, Lea & Febiger, 1976, p 485.

110. Schüller H, Fåhraeus T: Pacemaker Electrocardiograms: An Introduction to Practical Analysis. Solna, Sweden, Siemens-Elema AB, 1983, p 99.

111. Schüller H, Brandt J, Fåhraeus T: QRS-sensing via atrial lead in AAI and DDD pacing. PACE 8:A–95, 1985.

112. Seltzer JP, Levine PA, Watson WS: Patient-initiated autonomous pacemaker tachycardia. PACE 7:961, 1984.

113. Spurrell RAJ, Sowton E: An implanted atrial synchronous pacemaker with a short atrioventricular delay for the prevention of paroxysmal supraventricular tachycardias. J Electrocardiol 9:89, 1976.

114. Stoobandt R, Willems R, Holvoet G, et al: Prediction of Wenckebach behavior and block response in DDD pacemakers. PACE 9:1040, 1986.

115. Sudduth B, Goldschlager N: Retrograde ventriculoatrial conduction in atrial refractoriness: Cause of apparent failure of atrial capture. Clin Prog Electrophysiol Pacing 4:56, 1986.

116. Tolentino AO, Javier RP, Byrd C, Samet P: Pacer-induced tachycardia with an atrial synchronous ventricular-inhibited (ASVIP) pulse generator. PACE 5:251, 1982.

117. Van Gelder LM, El Gamal MIH: Magnet application, a cause of persistent arrhythmias in physiological pacemakers. PACE 5:710, 1982.

118. Van Gelder LM, El Gamal MIH: Ventriculoatrial conduction: A cause of atrial malpacing in AV universal pacemakers. A report of two cases. PACE 8:140, 1985.

119. Van Gelder LM, El Gamal MIH, Sanders RS: Tachycardia-termination algorithm: A valuable feature for interruption of pacemaker-mediated tachycardia. PACE 7:283, 1984.

120. Van Mechelen R, Hagemeijer F: Atrioventricular and ventriculoatrial conduction in patients with symptomatic sinus node dysfunction. In Steinbach K (ed): Cardiac Pacing: Proceedings of the VIIth World Symposium on Cardiac Pacing. Darmstadt, Federal Republic of Germany, Steinkopff Verlag, 1983, p 121.

121. Van Mechelen R, Ruiter J, DeBoer H: Pacemaker electrocardiography of rate smoothing during DDD pacing. PACE 8:684, 1985.

122. Van Mechelen RV, Ruiter J, Vanderkerckhove Y, et al: Prevalence of retrograde conduction in heart block after DDD pacemaker implantation. Am J Cardiol 57:797, 1986.

123. Von Bibra H, Busch V, Wirtzfeld A: The beneficial effect of short A-V intervals in VDD pacemaker patients. J Am Coll Cardiol 5:394, 1985.

124. Warren J, Falkenberg E: Wenckebach type upper rate behavior: A mixed blessing. PACE 8:A–37, 1985.

125. Warren J, Messenger J, Belott P: A-V interval hysteresis: A provision for improved tracking behavior in a DDD pacemaker. PACE 8:A–9, 1985.

126. Warren J, Baker R, Falkenberg E, et al: New developments for upper rate response in DDD pacing. PACE 9:1047, 1986.

127. Watson WS: Myopotential sensing in cardiac pacemakers. In Barold SS (ed): Modern Cardiac Pacing. Mount Kisco, NY, Futura Publishing Co, 1985, p 813.

128. Webb CR, Spielman SR, Greenspan AM, et al: Improved method for evaluating ventriculoatrial conduction before implantation of atrial-sensing dual chamber pacemakers. J Am Coll Cardiol 5:1395, 1985.

129. Westveer DC, Stewart JR, Goodfleish R, et al: Prevalence and significance of ventriculoatrial conduction. PACE 7:784, 1984.

130. Wirtzfeld A, Schmidt G, Stangl K: Physiologic pacing: Present status and future developments. PACE 10:41, 1987.

131. Wish M, Fletcher RD, Gottdiener S, Cohen AI: Importance of left atrial timing in the programming of dual chamber pacemaker. Am J Cardiol 60:596, 1987.

132. Zimmern SH, Clark MF, Austin WK, et al: Characteristics and clinical effects of myopotential signals in a unipolar DDD pacemaker population. PACE 9:1019, 1986.

B. Multiprogrammability, Follow-up, and Troubleshooting

S. SERGE BAROLD, MICHAEL D. FALKOFF,
LING S. ONG, and ROBERT A. HEINLE

The aim of DDD pacemaker follow-up is to provide optimal and safe pacing from both hemodynamic and electrophysiologic points of view. Appropriate programmability should prevent the problems of endless loop tachycardia, potentially dangerous pacemaker behavior, crosstalk, and myopotential interference, as well as optimizing parameters such as rate, pulse width, voltage output, atrioventricular (AV) interval, sensitivity, and refractory periods to provide optimal hemodynamic benefit. In this part of Chapter 12, we present our approach to follow-up and troubleshooting of DDD pacemakers, with emphasis on the diagnostic and therapeutic uses of multiprogrammability[9] (Table 12-1).

UNDERLYING RHYTHM

An attempt should be made to document the patient's spontaneous underlying rhythm. If there is continuous pacing function, the pacemaker may be reprogrammed to a lower rate to unmask the patient's rhythm. Several systems also have an inhibit mode of function. One model is programmable to the OOO mode temporarily.

TABLE 12-1. USEFULNESS OF PROGRAMMABILITY IN DDD PACING

TEST	METHOD
Atrial capture	Program to AAI (AOO) at a rate faster than spontaneous rhythm, provided there is an underlying ventricular rhythm; if AAI or AOO mode is unavailable or contraindicated, try DVI with lowest ventricular output (AVI) or DVI with the longest AV interval and program the rate faster than the spontaneous rhythm
Ventricular capture	In Cordis DDD pulse generators with application of the magnet, sensing occurs during the atrioventricular (AV) interval, and it may be impossible to obtain a ventricular stimulus; this may be resolved by shortening the AV interval or programming to the VVI mode
Atrial sensing (tracking)	Program the lower rate below the spontaneous rate; decrease the AV interval; the atrial sensing safety margin is determined by decreasing sensitivity in a stepwise fashion until tracking is lost
Myopotential interference in atrial channel	Program maximal atrial sensitivity and test in the usual fashion
Crosstalk	Program maximal atrial pulse width and voltage and maximal ventricular sensitivity; also increase the lower rate (if necessary) and decrease the AV interval to less than the spontaneous PR interval to ensure continuous ventricular pacing; also program the shortest blanking period
Retrograde ventriculoatrial (VA) conduction	Program lower rate above spontaneous rate to ensure continuous ventricular pacing, atrial output to subthreshold value, and the postventricular atrial refractory period (PVARP) to its minimal value; program the atrial sensitivity to its highest value and then adjust the PVARP to exceed the retrograde VA conduction time by about 50 msec; use automatic PVARP extension if there is prolonged retrograde VA conduction after a ventricular extrasystole
Propensity to endless loop tachycardia	As above; production of myopotential interference with maximal atrial sensitivity and lowest ventricular sensitivity, chest wall stimulation sensed only by the atrial channel
Upper rate characteristics	Set upper rate limit to lowest setting; exercise or chest wall stimulation

ATRIAL PACING

Documentation of atrial capture is mandatory, and if it is not done, follow-up is grossly incomplete.[60, 62, 96] The overshoot of the atrial stimulus in unipolar pulse generators may make the diagnosis of successful atrial depolarization difficult, and indeed we have found it impossible in about 5 to 10 per cent of our patients by standard 12-lead electrocardiography at normal sensitivity.[13]

The threshold for atrial pacing is determined at the lowest voltage and pulse width. We prefer programming the atrial output to the lowest possible voltage setting to avoid crosstalk. For example, if the atrial pacing threshold is less than 2.7 V at 0.1 msec, we would program the atrial output to 2.7 V and 0.3 or 0.4 msec. However, if the threshold for atrial pacing is less than 2.7 V at 0.3 msec, we would prefer reprogramming the pacemaker to the full output of 5.4 V with a pulse width of 0.3 msec because of the flat characteristic of the strength-duration curve for pulse-width values greater than 0.5 msec. The use of a low atrial output voltage is extremely important for the prevention of crosstalk[12] and in our experience it appears more efficacious than reduction of the pulse width alone.

Atrial capture is best documented by reprogramming the pulse generator to the AAI or AOO mode, provided the patient is not pacemaker dependent (Fig. 12–51). Several techniques may demonstrate successful atrial capture, and this is particularly important during unipolar pacing.[13, 60]

Physical Examination

The presence of intermittent or regular cannon waves in the jugular venous pulsation, as well as varying intensity of the first heart sound, suggests AV dissociation. The presence of regular A and V waves certainly suggests atrial capture.

Electrocardiogram

THE 12-LEAD ELECTROCARDIOGRAM. A 12-lead electrocardiogram recorded at double standardization may be invaluable in bringing out an otherwise undiscernible P wave or bipolar atrial stimuli.

P WAVES. A finding of retrograde P waves after a paced ventricular beat, seen as notching of the ST segment or deformity of the T wave, suggests the presence of retrograde ventriculoatrial (VA) conduction that may indicate lack of capture by the preceding atrial stimulus (Fig. 12–52).

BIPOLAR CHEST LEADS.[13] Exploring the chest (and occasionally the epigastrium or back) by means of Lewis bipolar leads almost always demonstrates atrial capture, particularly when recorded at double standardization.

ESOPHAGEAL RECORDINGS WITH UNIPOLAR AND BIPOLAR LEADS (PREFERABLY FILTERED). These recordings are easily accomplished by using a flexible Medtronic bipolar coronary sinus lead (without tines) or the pill electrode in conjunction with a three-channel electrocardiograph machine (Fig. 12–53).

Programmability

AAI OR AOO MODES. In the presence of relatively intact AV conduction, reprogramming the pulse generator to the AAI or AOO mode is the most useful and rapid technique in determining atrial capture by demonstrating a consistent relationship of the atrial pacing stimulus to a succeeding spontaneous ventricular depolarization. Atrial capture may be inferred when an increase in the atrial pacing rate causes a corresponding increase in the ventricular rate, that is, conducted supraventricular impulse. In many patients who are continuously paced, a gradual reduction of the ventricular rate in the VVI mode to 30 per

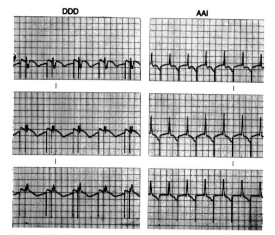

Figure 12–51. DDD pulse generator. On the left, during DDD pacing it is impossible to determine successful atrial capture. On the right, by reprogramming to the AAI mode at various pacing rates, there was a corresponding increase in the ventricular rate (conducted QRS complex), so that atrial capture may be inferred. (From Barold SS, Nanda NC, Ong LS, et al: Determination of successful atrial capture during unipolar dual-chambered pacing. *In* Barold SS [ed]: Modern Cardiac Pacing. Mount Kisco, NY, Futura Publishing Co, 1985, p 677; with permission.)

Figure 12–52. DDD pulse generator. *Top,* The atrial stimulus does not give rise to visible atrial depolarization. Notching on the ST segment suggests the presence of retrograde VA conduction, which indicates lack of atrial capture by the preceding atrial stimulus. *Bottom,* When the atrial output was increased, retrograde VA conduction disappeared, implying that there was appropriate atrial capture despite the absence of clearly visible P waves. (From Barold SS, Nanda NC, Ong LS, et al: Determination of successful atrial capture during unipolar dual-chambered pacing. *In* Barold SS [ed]: Modern Cardiac Pacing. Mount Kisco, NY, Futura Publishing Co, 1985, p 677; with permission.)

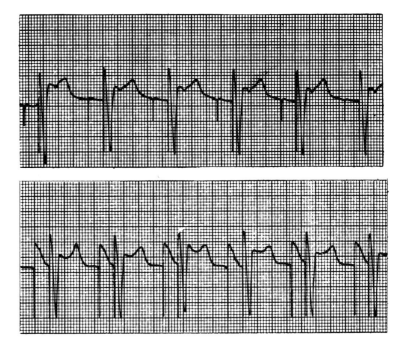

minute, if tolerated, often leads to a ventricular escape at a modest rate. This practice allows the use of the AAI or AOO mode to evaluate atrial capture (Fig. 12–54).

AVI MODE.[67] This mode may be useful in certain DDD pulse generators with limited programmability, for example, the DVI or VVI mode (Fig. 12–55). When the ventricular stimuli are subthreshold, this may be considered the AVI mode.[53, 67] By simply increasing the pacing rate, atrial capture is implied by the constant relationship of the atrial stimulus to a spontaneous QRS complex as the rate is changed. This maneuver produces a sequence composed of atrial stimulus, ineffectual ventricular stimulus (in the PR interval), and a conducted, spontaneous QRS complex. The use of the AVI mode is contraindicated in patients with a poor underlying rhythm.

AV DELAY. Programming the AV delay to its maximal value may allow spontaneous AV conduction. If that occurs, increasing the atrial rate will demonstrate atrial capture by a synchronous relationship with the spontaneous QRS complex. Occasionally, with latency (delay from the atrial stimulus to the onset of visible atrial depolarization) or considerable delay in interatrial conduction, atrial depolar-

Figure 12–53. Esophageal bipolar ECG demonstrating atrial capture by atrial stimulus. A flexible bipolar pacing catheter was positioned in the esophagus, where the largest atrial depolarization was recorded. Note how atrial depolarization is recorded after a considerable delay from the atrial stimulus, almost synchronously with the delivery of the ventricular stimulus (lead I). Leads II and III are combined esophageal and surface ECGs. (From Barold SS, Nanda NC, Ong LS, et al: Determination of successful atrial capture during unipolar dual-chambered pacing. *In* Barold SS [ed]: Modern Cardiac Pacing. Mount Kisco, NY, Futura Publishing Co, 1985, p 677; with permission.)

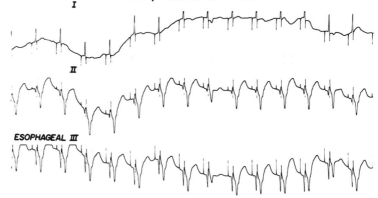

DVI ? ATRIAL CAPTURE

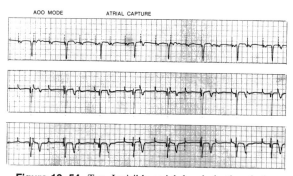

Figure 12–54. *Top,* Invisible atrial depolarization during DVI pacing. *Middle* and *bottom,* The ventricular output was programmed to its lowest amplitude, with consequent lack of ventricular capture. This may be considered the AVI mode. The large atrial stimulus is followed by a native QRS complex due to antegrade AV conduction. In the bottom strip, increasing the pacing rate maintains the constant relationship of the atrial stimulus to a spontaneous QRS complex, providing evidence of successful atrial capture. (From Barold SS, Nanda NC, Ong LS, et al: Determination of successful atrial capture during unipolar dual-chambered pacing. *In* Barold SS [ed]: Modern Cardiac Pacing. Mount Kisco, NY, Futura Publishing Co, 1985, p 677; with permission.)

ization may be invisible in all 12 electrocardiographic leads in the presence of a relatively short AV interval (e.g., 150 msec), suggesting failure of atrial capture.[2] The considerable delay from the onset of the right atrial stimulus to the relatively late paced P wave may be unmasked by programming a longer AV delay to 250 to 300 msec.

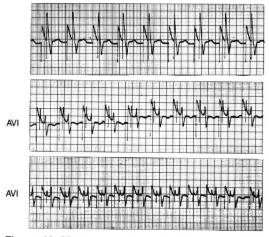

Figure 12–55. Demonstration of atrial capture in the AOO mode of a DDD pulse generator in a patient with complete AV block. The pacemaker was programmed to the slowest rate in the VVI mode to allow the emergence of an idioventricular rhythm. In this way, the pacemaker was safely reprogrammed to the AOO mode. The three ECG leads were recorded simultaneously.

Mode-Mode, Two-Dimensional, and Doppler Echocardiography[13, 60, 92]

MITRAL VALVE ECHOCARDIOGRAM. The demonstration of a properly timed A wave in normal sinus rhythm and its disappearance during VVI pacing, as well as its restoration during dual-chamber pacing, provides proof of atrial capture. In some circumstances an A wave may not be clearly seen, particularly in patients with poor ventricular compliance or congestive heart failure, and sometimes for technical reasons.

LEFT ATRIAL MOTION. This may be recorded directly, but this is less useful than right atrial motion.

RIGHT ATRIAL MOTION. This technique was originally described by Drinkovic[29] for the diagnosis of cardiac arrhythmias because right atrial motion represents a marker of atrial depolarization. The procedures of M-mode and especially two-dimensional echocardiography are relatively easy to perform from the subcostal region in the elderly patient with a permanent DDD pacemaker. The four-chamber view easily identifies the right atrium, and an appropriate M-mode recording of right atrial motion is easily obtained. Simultaneous recording of the electrocardiogram may identify hidden P waves (Fig. 12–56).

DOPPLER ECHOCARDIOGRAPHY.[92] An increase in the cardiac output from VVI to DVI (or DDD) pacing suggests atrial capture. In Doppler transmission, flow with normal AV synchrony is characterized by an early diastolic peak during rapid ventricular filling and the late diastolic peak due to flow from left atrial contraction.

Telemetry of the Atrial Electrogram

Most contemporary pulse generators are incapable of telemetering paced atrial depolarization. However, special leads have been designed to detect effective paced atrial depolarization, and this design is available from only one manufacturer.[13]

DIFFERENTIAL DIAGNOSIS OF LACK OF CAPTURE BY THE ATRIAL STIMULUS

Differential diagnosis of lack of capture includes the following:

1. High threshold situation or displacement.
2. Isoelectric P waves in all 12 electrocar-

Figure 12–56. Subcostal right atrial echogram during DVI pacing. For the first five beats, spontaneous atrial depolarization precedes the delivery of the atrial stimulus. This is clearly seen in the early onset of right atrial contraction, which causes prominent posterior right atrial movement, labeled "A." The sixth atrial stimulus falls outside the atrial myocardial refractory period (AMRP) of the preceding spontaneous P wave. Consequently, the atrial stimulus depolarizes the atrium, producing A'. The last atrial stimulus appears to depolarize the atrium . Although there is slight posterior movement of the right atrial wall during ventricular diastole, the sharp and rapid posterior movement coincident with atrial contraction is unmistakable. (From Barold SS, Nanda NC, Ong LS, et al: Determination of successful atrial capture during unipolar dual-chambered pacing. *In* Barold SS [ed]: Modern Cardiac Pacing. Mount Kisco, NY, Futura Publishing Co, 1985, p 677; with permission.)

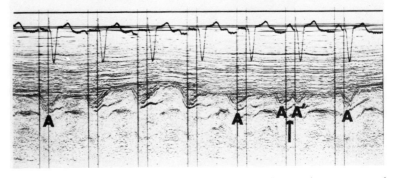

diographic leads. Double standardization to bring out the P wave, bipolar chest leads, and esophageal electrocardiography should be used.

3. Atrial fibrillation with poorly discernible f waves (Fig. 12–57).

4. Atrial fusion beats with isoelectric P waves (Fig. 12–58).

5. Latency and delayed interatrial conduction.[2, 104]

6. Invisible, unsensed atrial extrasystole preceding the atrial stimulus, which therefore falls within the refractory period of the atrial myocardium.

7. AV desynchronization arrhythmia (see part A of this chapter) or its equivalent with unsensed retrograde VA conduction or sinus P waves after ventricular extrasystoles (Fig. 12–59).

8. Hyperkalemia.[10] This should be suspected when the paced QRS complex is unduly wide. We recently reported a patient with hyperkalemia-induced failure of atrial capture and preservation of ventricular pacing in whom treatment of hyperkalemia restored atrial pacing. The atrial myocardium is more sensitive to the effect of hyperkalemia than is the ventricular myocardium.

ATRIAL SENSING

One of the commonest problems in DDD pacing is atrial undersensing.[97, 107] Atrial sensing is evaluated by making several program changes:

1. First, the lower rate should be pro-

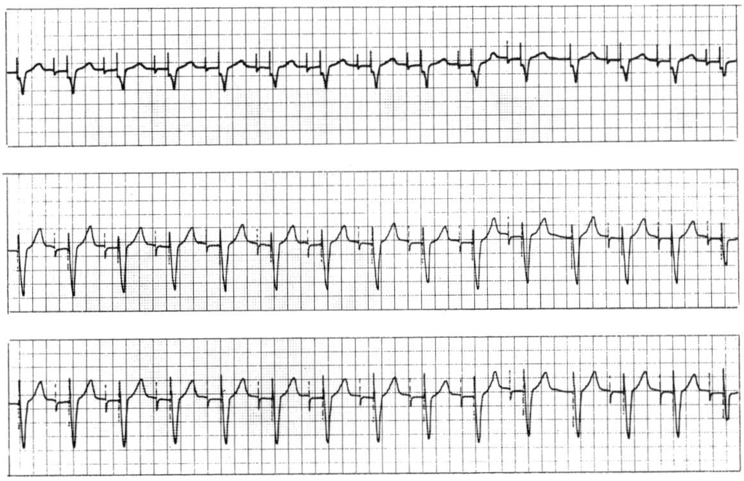

ATRIAL FIBRILLATION

Figure 12–57. DDD pacemaker with apparent failure of atrial capture during atrial fibrillation. The eleventh paced QRS complex initiates an atrial escape (pacemaker VA) interval that does not terminate with the delivery of an atrial stimulus. This is because an f wave sensed by the atrial lead initiated the AV interval. The absence of the atrial stimulus suggests the diagnosis of atrial fibrillation. The three-lead ECG was obtained during held respiration.

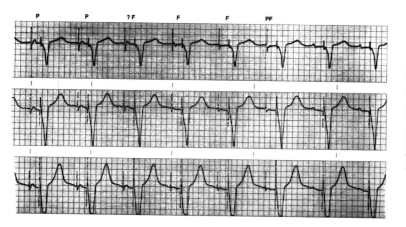

Figure 12–58. Three-lead ECG showing interplay between spontaneous and paced atrial rhythms with paced atrial beats (P), atrial fusion (F), and atrial pseudofusion beats (PF). Note that the fifth atrial stimulus associated with atrial fusion gives rise to an isoelectric P wave in the upper two leads.

grammed to a value below the patient's spontaneous atrial activity.

2. The AV delay is then shortened to 50 to 100 msec. This guarantees that any P wave, if sensed, would be coupled to a paced ventricular response.

3. Once P-wave tracking is confirmed, rate responsiveness and upper rate characteristics can be demonstrated by a third program change by lowering the upper rate limit to its lowest setting or exercising the patient. Ideally, exercise should be performed on the treadmill, but in elderly patients leg lifts and hand-grip exercises may be sufficient.

The programmable sensitivity of a DDD pulse generator also provides an indirect measurement of the amplitude of the atrial electrogram, that is, the atrial signal delivered to the pulse generator. With the outlined programming sequence to document P-wave tracking,

a semiquantitative assessment of the atrial signal is easily obtained by sequentially changing the atrial sensitivity setting from the lowest numerical value (or most sensitive) to the highest numerical value (or least sensitive) until P-wave tracking is lost (Fig. 12–60). In this respect, DDD pulse generators that allow a triggered response in the atrium may be extremely useful because the delivery of an atrial stimulus at the time of atrial sensing serves as an event marker. Atrial undersensing is often associated with the occurrence of the spontaneous QRS complex within the ventricular triggering period (also known as the ventricular safety pacing period), whereupon AV sequential pacing occurs with an abbreviated AV interval (Fig. 12–61).

Telemetry, when available, provides not only proof of atrial sensing but also its exact timing by transmitting event markers that may

CPI DELTA DDD, LOW RATE = 70 ppm, UPPER RATE = 120 ppm
AV = 250 ms, PVARP = VRP = 350 ms, RATE SMOOTHING = 6%

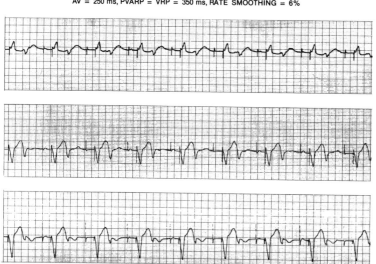

Figure 12–59. Apparent failure of atrial capture by a DDD pacemaker. Three ECG leads were recorded simultaneously. Each ineffectual atrial stimulus is preceded by a sinus P wave best discernible in the upper tracing. The sinus PP interval measures approximately 600 msec and is disturbed only because of intermittent atrial capture. There is no evidence of retrograde VA conduction. The sinus P waves preceding the ineffectual atrial stimuli fall within the relatively long 350-msec PVARP and are therefore not sensed. Ineffectual atrial stimuli fall in the atrial myocardial refractory period (AMRP) generated by the preceding spontaneous sinus P wave. VRP = ventricular refractory period.

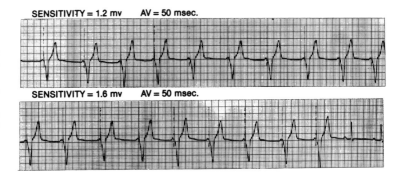

Figure 12–60. Semiquantitative assessment of atrial signal by programmability of sensitivity. *Top,* With an atrial sensitivity of 1.2 mV, all the P waves are tracked. *Bottom,* With an atrial sensitivity of 1.6 mV, there is failure to sense the last two P waves.

be recorded simultaneously with the electrocardiogram. Inhibition of the pulse generator by the patient's spontaneous rhythm does not necessarily indicate normal P-wave sensing because inhibition may result from sensing of the QRS complex. Atrial sensing may be present and remain undetected if the interval between two consecutive QRS complexes is less than the programmed atrial escape or pacemaker VA interval (Figs. 12–62 and 12–63).

Atrial sensing may be influenced by changes in body position, congestive heart failure, and exercise, the last decreasing P-wave voltage.[17, 58] Consequently, the capability of atrial sensing should be evaluated with changes in position—lying, sitting, and standing—and preferably with exercise and deep respiration[93] (Fig. 12–64). Atrial sensitivity should be programmed to approximately double the atrial sensing threshold. Furthermore, atrial sensitivity in unipolar devices should be programmed to avoid myopotential interference yet guarantee adequate P-wave sensing for normal P-wave tracking. Study of atrial sensitivity is also valuable in evaluating the importance of far-field signals, such as the QRS complex. Holter recordings should be obtained to demonstrate the efficacy of atrial sensing. In our experience,

random, infrequent loss of atrial sensing is not uncommon and rarely of any clinical significance unless the patient is susceptible to endless loop tachycardia and the atrial signal from the retrograde P wave is larger than that of the sinus P wave.

Apparent Atrial Undersensing

Atrial undersensing may occur in the presence of an adequate atrial signal that falls within an extended postventricular atrial refractory period (PVARP). This form of atrial undersensing disappears when the PVARP is shortened. Apparent atrial undersensing[46] may also occur when P waves (with an adequate electrogram) appear to be clearly beyond the PVARP. In this situation, paradoxical restoration of atrial sensing may occur by actually decreasing atrial sensitivity. This occurrence suggests elimination of an unsuspected PVARP initiated by far-field atrial sensing of the tail-end of the QRS complex. When atrial sensitivity is decreased, the far-field signal is no longer sensed and the additional PVARP initiated by the QRS complex cannot occur. A decrease in atrial sensitivity therefore leads to a return of normal P-wave sensing. In addition,

Figure 12–61. Medtronic 7000 DDD pulse generator programmed to the DVI mode with an AV interval of 200 msec to illustrate the consequences of atrial undersensing in a pulse generator with a VTP. Atrial stimuli occur coincidentally with or after a spontaneous P wave. A conducted QRS complex falls within the VTP and "triggers" a premature ventricular stimulus at the end of the VTP of 110 msec,

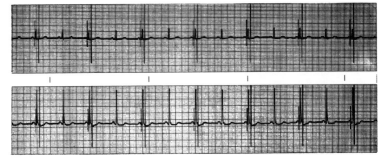

thereby abbreviating the AV interval. (From Barold SS, Ong LS, Falkoff MD, Heinle RA: Crosstalk or self-inhibition in dual-chambered pacemakers. *In* Barold SS [ed]: Modern Cardiac Pacing. Mount Kisco, NY, Futura Publishing Co, 1985, p 615; with permission.)

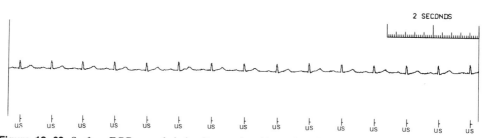

Figure 12–62. Surface ECG recorded simultaneously with marker channel showing that inhibition of a Symbios Medtronic DDD pulse generator does not necessarily imply normal atrial and ventricular sensing. The marker channel indicates that P waves are unsensed, but this is masked on the surface ECG. The interval between two consecutive QRS complexes is less than the atrial escape (or pacemaker VA) interval. P-wave undersensing is therefore masked. VS = Ventricular sense event.

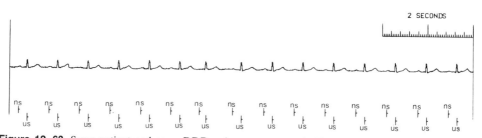

Figure 12–63. Same patient and same DDD pulse generator as in Figure 12–62. The same parameters were programmed except for an increase in atrial sensitivity to its maximal value, thereby restoring P-wave sensing. As = atrial sense event. Note that the surface ECGs for Figures 12–62 and 12–63 are identical, in contrast to the different marker functions.

undersensing may also occur when the P wave falls in the noise-sampling period of the Cordis Gemini (Miami, FL) and Sequicor series of DDD pulse generators. The noise-sampling period occupies the last 100 msec of the shorter of the atrial or ventricular refractory periods and occurs simultaneously in both channels. When P waves are detected in the noise-sampling period, the pulse generator will pace asynchronously at the lower programmed rate interval for one cycle only.[97]

VENTRICULAR PACING AND SENSING

Ventricular pacing and sensing may be easily tested by reprogramming the pulse generator to the VVI mode in the usual fashion. In the case of Cordis DDD pulse generators, sensing will occur during the AV interval upon application of the magnet (Fig. 12–65). Consequently, if the pacemaker is programmed with a relatively long AV interval, application of the magnet may produce atrial pacing followed by sensing of the conducted QRS complex if AV conduction is intact. Obviously, one must ensure that the pacemaker is capable of ventricular pacing, and this is done by reprogramming to either the VVI mode or the DDD mode with a shorter AV delay. Semiquantitative determination of the amplitude of the ventricular electrogram may be performed in the same manner as with the atrial signal. Determination of the ventricular sensing threshold is particularly important in optimizing ventricular sensitivity to avoid crosstalk or myopotential inhibition.

INSPIRATION

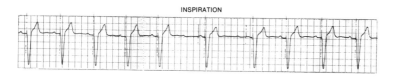

Figure 12–64. Intermittent failure of atrial sensing by a DDD pulse generator unraveled by deep inspiration.

Figure 12–65. Cordis Sequicor 233F DDD pulse generator. Programmed rate = 70 ppm (LRI = 857 msec), and AV interval = 200 msec. On top, during spontaneous pacing, the atrial stimulus captures the atrium and is followed by a conducted QRS complex. The conducted QRS complex occurs before the AV delay has timed out and is therefore sensed by the pulse generator, which initiates a new atrial escape (pacemaker VA) interval. In the bottom strip, the magnet was placed over the pulse generator.

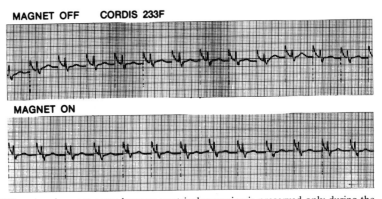

MAGNET OFF   CORDIS 233F

MAGNET ON

In this DDD pulse generator, true DOO pacing does not occur because ventricular sensing is preserved only during the AV delay. This feature should not be misinterpreted as pacemaker malfunction because it is a normal characteristic of these pulse generators.

CROSSTALK, VENTRICULAR BLANKING PERIOD, AND VENTRICULAR TRIGGERING PERIOD

Crosstalk, or self-inhibition, is unique to dual-chamber pacing systems and refers to the inappropriate detection of the atrial stimulus by the ventricular sensing amplifier.[12, 14, 19, 20, 28, 41, 43, 52, 62, 71, 81, 83] Crosstalk may be troublesome or occasionally life threatening. Apart from rapid recharge pulses and the use of bipolar sensing used to minimize crosstalk, most contemporary DDD pulse generators deal with crosstalk in the following two ways:

1. *Ventricular blanking period:* During this period, the ventricular amplifier is disabled. The blanking period starts coincidentally with the atrial stimulus and continues for a brief period after the atrial output pulse. The duration of the blanking period varies from 10 to 60 msec, according to the manufacturer, and is programmable in some pulse generators. The blanking period should be considered a very short absolute (ventricular) refractory period.

2. *Ventricular safety pacing period:* The AV delay following the emission of an atrial stimulus (and the brief blanking period) is divided into two intervals. The first interval is called the ventricular safety pacing period, or the nonphysiologic AV delay, the latter term implying that it would not be physiologically normal for a spontaneous impulse to be conducted from the atrium to the ventricle within that interval, which is usually 100 to 110 msec. Ventricular events sensed within the ventricular safety pacing period do not cause inhibition

of the pacemaker but rather initiate (or trigger) a ventricular stimulus delivered only at the completion of this interval and therefore prematurely before the end of the longer programmed AV interval. This additional safety mechanism suggests that the blanking period may not always be sufficient to prevent crosstalk. We believe that the present terminology is unwieldy. Levine aptly called this period the "crosstalk sensing window."[62] The term "ventricular triggering period" may be more suitable and its function self-evident, even in the absence of crosstalk, because other signals may be sensed by the ventricular channel during this period.[8] Although the duration of the ventricular triggering period is generally described as beginning from the atrial stimulus, it is obvious that ventricular sensing cannot occur until the brief preceding blanking period has elapsed. The ventricular triggering period is programmable in some pulse generators. If a ventricular sensed event, regardless of its origin (i.e., polarization phenomenon, QRS complexes, myopotential interference, and the like), occurs after the brief blanking period but during the ventricular triggering period, the pulse generator will deliver a ventricular stimulus at the end of the ventricular triggering period. Thus, in a pulse generator with this characteristic, crosstalk causes shortening of the AV interval to prevent inappropriate ventricular inhibition with retention of some degree of AV synchrony (Fig. 12–66). Consequently, during continual crosstalk, if the atrial escape (ventricular VA) interval remains constant and the AV interval is shortened, the AV sequential pacing rate is faster than the programmed lower rate.

In pulse generators without a ventricular

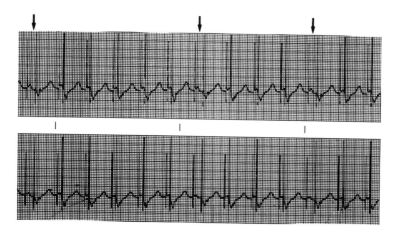

Figure 12–66. Intermedics Cosmos DDD pulse generator showing intermittent crosstalk. Because this pulse generator has a VTP, there is consequent abbreviation of the AV interval to 100 msec. The AV intervals at the arrows correspond to the programmed value of 200 msec in the absence of crosstalk. (From Barold SS, Ong LS, Falkoff MD, Heinle RA: Crosstalk or self-inhibition in dual-chambered pacemakers. *In* Barold SS [ed]: Modern Cardiac Pacing. Mount Kisco, NY, Futura Publishing Co, 1985, p 615; with permission.)

triggering period, crosstalk produces distinctive electrocardiographic manifestations:

1. Unexpected prolongation of the interval between the atrial stimulus and the succeeding conducted (spontaneous) QRS complex to a value greater than the programmed AV interval (Fig. 12–67). If there is no AV conduction, ventricular asystole will occur (Fig. 12–68). In this respect, myopotential interference sensed during the AV interval of unipolar DDD pulse generators may superficially resemble crosstalk.

2. Faster rate of atrial pacing (without a succeeding paced QRS complex). The rate of atrial pacing increases compared with the programmed free-running AV sequential (lower) rate. This is because the atrial stimulus (sensed by the ventricular channel) initiates a new atrial escape (pacemaker VA) interval (see Fig. 12–67). Consequently, the interval between the two consecutive atrial stimuli (AA interval) becomes equal to the atrial escape (pacemaker VA) interval (ignoring the negligible duration of the blanking period).

The presence of crosstalk and effective blanking is tested by reprogramming the atrial output to its maximal value and the ventricular

sensitivity to its most sensitive setting in the DDD or DVI mode. To avoid competition, the lower rate is set above the patient's own spontaneous rate, and the AV delay is shortened to less than the spontaneous PR interval. During crosstalk, a pulse generator without a ventricular triggering period will not deliver a ventricular stimulus at the end of the programmed AV interval initiated by an atrial stimulus. This failure to deliver a ventricular stimulus is obviously dangerous in pacemaker-dependent patients with AV block and no underlying rhythm. If crosstalk is observed, the atrial output should be decreased (voltage rather than pulse width), the ventricular sensitivity should be decreased, or both. If these maneuvers are unsuccessful or undesirable, the blanking period should be prolonged, but this is programmable in only a few pulse generators. Some pulse generators automatically adjust the duration of the blanking period according to the programmed atrial output and ventricular sensitivity. If this duration is insufficient, we would suggest increasing the blanking period by at least 10 to 15 msec over the longest value in which crosstalk was demonstrated. An unduly long blanking period predisposes to unsensed QRS complexes[71] (Fig.

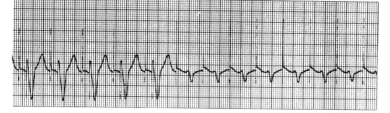

Figure 12–67. Crosstalk in a Pacesetter AFP DDD pulse generator (without a VTP) induced by deliberately increasing the voltage of the atrial stimulus. The lower rate was programmed at 100 ppm (600 msec), and the AV interval at 140 msec. Crosstalk on the right leads to prolongation of the interval between the atrial stimulus and the succeeding conducted QRS complex to a value greater than the programmed AV interval. The rate of atrial pacing increases because the sensed atrial stimulus by the ventricular lead initiates a new atrial escape (pacemaker VA) interval. The interval between two consecutive atrial stimuli becomes equal to 510 msec, representing the sum of the AEI $(600-140)=460$ plus the VBP (50 msec).

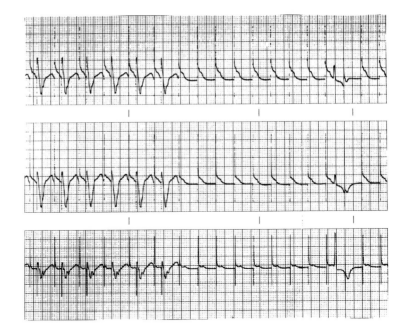

Figure 12–68. Crosstalk in a Pacesetter AFP DDD pulse generator without a VTP. Note that crosstalk causes atrial pacing at a faster rate than the free-running AV sequential rate (lower rate shown on the left) and prolonged ventricular asystole.

12–69). After successful elimination of crosstalk with what appears to be a good leeway in terms of duration of blanking period, atrial output, and ventricular sensitivity, we have occasionally observed the development of crosstalk minutes or hours later. If there is concern about the margin of sensitivity and atrial output, we recommend a Holter recording to ascertain the absence of crosstalk. Although crosstalk is an inherent design limitation of DDD pulse generators, particularly unipolar ones, it may sometimes be caused by atrial lead dislodgment or an insulation break in the ventricular electrode.

As far as the ventricular electrode is concerned, delivery of the atrial stimulus generates a signal that must be superimposed on any residual afterpotential at the ventricular electrode. The contribution of ventricular afterpotential may become substantially larger if the ventricular output (voltage or pulse width or both) is increased or the ventricular pacing rate is increased, thereby providing less time for dissipation. Therefore, crosstalk may be

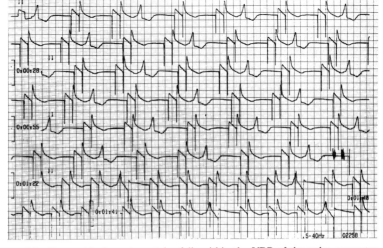

Figure 12–69. Normally functioning Cordis Gemini 415A DDD pulse generator. Lower rate = 50 ppm, and AV interval = 250 msec. In the top six rhythm strips, all ventricular extrasystoles are sensed by the pulse generator. The programmed lower rate was increased to 70 ppm (LRI = 857 msec) near the end of the sixth strip. Owing to "late sensing" of these identical ventricular extrasystoles, atrial stimuli now fall within the QRS complex ("pseudo" pseudofusion beats). Because of the relatively long blanking period (39 to 47 msec) and relatively long programmed AV delay (250 msec), the ventricular stimuli are issued at the apex of the T wave because the effective ventricular electrogram generated by the ventricular extrasystoles falls within the VBP of the pulse generator (initiated by the atrial stimulus). This tracing demonstrates that a long blanking period predisposes to undersensing of ectopic ventricular events and may lead to the delivery of a ventricular stimulus in the vulnerable period, particularly in the presence of a long programmed AV interval.

induced by an increase in either the ventricular output or the ventricular rate.[83] The forthcoming rate-responsive DDD pulse generators (DDDR), with the capability of faster AV (Ap-Vp) sequential pacing, may be more susceptible to crosstalk for this reason.

INTERPLAY OF THE VENTRICULAR TRIGGERING PERIOD AND UPPER RATE LIMIT INTERVAL

In the first part of this chapter, we underscored the importance of understanding the timing cycles and the concept of supremacy of the upper rate limit of DDD pulse generators for the appropriate electrocardiographic interpretation of pacemaker function. Theoretically, in pacemakers with a separately programmable upper rate, the upper rate limit interval should take hierarchical precedence over all other DDD timing intervals. The behavior of the Intermedics Cosmos DDD pulse generator exemplifies this concept because the delivery of a ventricular stimulus at the completion of the ventricular triggering period cannot preempt the (ventricular) upper rate limit interval before the latter has timed out[8] (Fig. 12–70). In contrast, under certain circumstances, the Medtronic Symbios pulse generator may violate its upper rate interval to maintain constancy of the ventricular triggering period.[8]

ATRIOVENTRICULAR INTERVAL

Variability of the AV interval is common during DDD pacing, and its interpretation requires a thorough understanding of pacemaker timing cycles. The differential diagnosis of variable AV intervals during DDD pacing is discussed, with the following abbreviations depicting atrial and ventricular events: Ap = atrial pacing, As = atrial sensing, Vp = ventricular pacing, and Vs = ventricular sensing (Fig. 12–71). Four combinations (As-Vs, Ap-Vp, Ap-Vs, and As-Vp), with the possibility of shortening or lengthening, yield eight possible situations for consideration. As-Vs or Ap-Vs may be short during normal

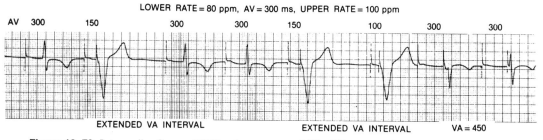

LOWER RATE = 80 ppm, AV = 300 ms, UPPER RATE = 100 ppm

AV 300   150   300   300   150   100   300   300

EXTENDED VA INTERVAL   EXTENDED VA INTERVAL   VA = 450

Figure 12–70. Intermedics Cosmos DDD pulse generator. LRI = 750 msec, and atrial escape (pacemaker VA) interval = 750 − 300 = 450 msec. The VTP was left at its nominal value of 100 msec. The first atrial stimulus captures the atrium, producing a normally conducted QRS complex. The PR interval is shorter than the programmed AV delay of 300 msec, and the ventricular output is inhibited. The first spontaneous QRS complex initiates a pacemaker VA interval that terminates 450 msec later with the delivery of the second atrial stimulus. The second atrial stimulus produces crosstalk and activates the VTP. Because the VA interval measures 450 msec, the anticipated ventricular stimulus would have occurred 550 msec from the onset of the preceding spontaneous QRS complex. This occurrence would violate the URI of 600 msec. Consequently, the pacemaker extends the VTP to 150 msec. so that the first ventricular stimulus is issued at the end of the URI initiated by the first sensed QRS complex. The subsequent pacemaker VA interval is extended by 400 msec. In this particular pacemaker model, the VA interval extension (operative only after a previous cycle equivalent to the URI) was tested and found to be approximately 400 msec (when the PVARP was equal to the VRP). The extended atrial escape (pacemaker VA) interval therefore represents the sum of the programmed atrial escape or VA interval (450 msec), and the VA interval extension (400) = approximately 850 msec. The fifth atrial stimulus again causes crosstalk and forces extension of the VTP from 100 to 150 msec by the same mechanism. The ventricular stimulus is then delivered at the completion of the URI. The subsequent pacemaker VA interval is extended by approximately another 400 msec. The atrial stimulus terminating this extended VA interval produces crosstalk. Because of the additional delay provided by the extended VA interval, the VTP is activated at the programmed duration of 100 msec. This ECG illustrates the supremacy of the URI. The AV interval assumes three different values according to circumstances (300, 150, and 100 msec). Extension of the VTP should not be confused with extension of the atrial escape (pacemaker VA) interval. (From Barold SS, Belott PH: Behavior of the ventricular triggering period of DDD pacemakers. PACE 10:1237, 1987; with permission.)

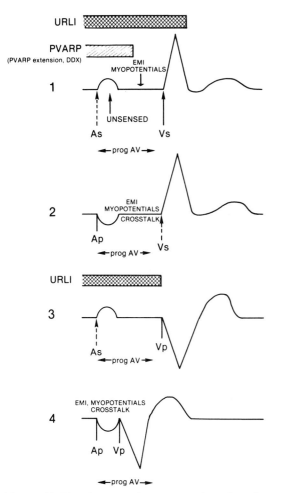

Figure 12–71. Diagrammatic representation of mechanism determining the duration of the AV interval. As = atrial sense event; Ap = atrial pace event; Vs = ventricular sense event; Vp = ventricular pace event; prog AV = programmed AV delay. 1. The As-Vs may be prolonged if the P wave is unsensed because of a small atrial electrogram. The As-Vs interval may also lengthen from oversensing of electromagnetic interference (EMI) or myopotentials. The lower bar (PVARP) demonstrates how a P wave of adequate amplitude may be unsensed when it occurs near the terminal portion of the PVARP, particularly if there is excessive PVARP extension. In the DDX mode, the PVARP extends further to the end of the pacing cycle. The top bar shows how the As-Vs interval may also be prolonged when Vs occurs within the URLI. In this situation, a ventricular stimulus cannot be delivered until the URLI has timed out. 2. Prolongation of the Ap-Vs interval may be due to crosstalk or to oversensing of EMI or myopotentials during the AV interval. 3. Prolongation of the As-Vp interval occurs in pulse generators with a separately programmable URLI, provided the URLI (bar over diagram) is longer than the TARP. 4. An abbreviated Ap-Vp is due to activation of the VTP by crosstalk, myopotentials, EMI, and so on. Note that in 2, crosstalk is shown in a pulse generator without a VTP.

function according to the status of AV conduction.

PROLONGATION OF THE INTERVAL BETWEEN AN ATRIAL SENSED EVENT AND VENTRICULAR SENSED EVENT (AS-VS) BEYOND THE PROGRAMMED AV INTERVAL (APPARENT LACK OF ATRIAL TRACKING). Prolongation of the As-Vs may occur in the presence of a normally sensed P wave whenever there is oversensing of myopotentials or electromagnetic interference during the AV interval. Prolongation of the As-Vs interval may also result from failure of delivery of the ventricular stimulus if the upper rate limit interval has not yet timed out by the time the AV interval has terminated. In the latter situation, the interval between two consecutive QRS complexes must be shorter than the upper rate limit interval of the pulse generator (Figs. 12–71, part 1, and 12–72).

Unsensed P waves may, of course, be due to a low-voltage atrial electrogram. However, in the presence of a large electrogram, P waves may be forced into the PVARP whenever it is excessively long, sometimes secondary to automatic extension. This form of atrial undersensing may occur with pulse generators that have an automatic extension of the PVARP (or DDX mode) activated by a premature ventricular event. If the patient's P-R interval is quite long and the spontaneous rate is relatively fast, there is a greater likelihood that the P wave will fall closer to the preceding QRS complex and therefore in the PVARP, which in this case need not be necessarily very long (see Fig. 12–72).

PROLONGATION OF THE Ap-Vs. This phenomenon may be due to crosstalk in pulse generators without a ventricular triggering period or sensing of myopotentials, false signals, or electromagnetic interference during the AV interval (Fig. 12–71, part 2, and 12–73).

ABBREVIATION OF THE Ap-Vp. This abbreviation is due to activation of the ventricular triggering period, which may result from crosstalk, QRS complexes, and myopotentials.

PROLONGATION OF THE Ap-Vp. Prolongation of the Ap-Vp is rare and may be seen during programming of Cordis DDD pulse generators, battery depletion in some DDD pulse generators, and pacemaker malfunction.

ABBREVIATION OF THE As-Vp. This phenomenon may be due to AV delay hysteresis—or to fallback,[50, 99] when As-Vp is less than Ap-Vp—to produce similar (mechanically) effective AV intervals (Fig. 12–74). Apparent shortening may occur if an inapparent signal

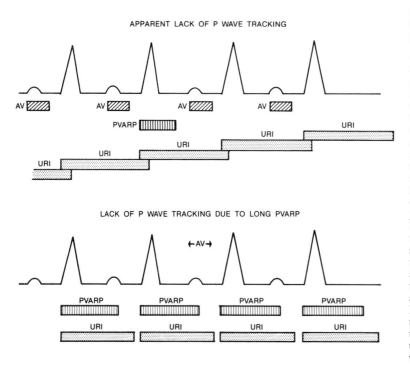

APPARENT LACK OF P WAVE TRACKING

LACK OF P WAVE TRACKING DUE TO LONG PVARP

Figure 12–72. Diagrammatic representation of mechanisms of apparent lack of P-wave tracking. *Top,* The spontaneous RR interval is shorter than the (ventricular) URI. After sensing the QRS complex, the pulse generator initiates the URI, and it cannot deliver a ventricular stimulus before the URI has timed out. Therefore, when the spontaneous rate is fast, a relatively early P wave initiates an AV interval, but at its completion the ventricular stimulus cannot be emitted as long as the URI has not yet timed out. The next QRS complex therefore occurs just before the completion of the URI; so that the process perpetuates itself. *Bottom,* An excessively long PVARP and a relatively fast spontaneous rate in association with prolongation of the P-R interval may also cause apparent lack of P-wave tracking. In this situation, the P wave is unsensed because it falls within the PVARP, so that shortening of the PVARP will restore normal P-wave tracking.

preempts sensing of the P wave, as, for example, with a myopotential or false signal sensed by the atrial channel.

PROLONGATION OF THE AS-Vp. This prolongation may be seen during the pacemaker Wenckebach response at the upper rate or in the presence of an atrial extrasystole or any premature signal sensed by the atrial lead. Only DDD pulse generators possessing an independently programmable upper rate capability allow the pulse generator to respond with a longer AV interval.

Optimization of the Atrioventricular Interval

Most DDD pacemakers have identical AV intervals after atrial pacing and sensing. The pacemaker senses on the right side of the heart, yet the timing relationships of atrial and ventricular activity on the left side of the heart determine hemodynamic performance. Thus, the constancy of the programmed AV interval may be associated with markedly different effective PR intervals during atrial pacing as opposed to atrial sensing. A great deal of work has been done to evaluate the hemodynamic benefits of DDD pacing (compared with VVI pacing) and the selection of the optimal AV interval.[3, 4, 5, 22, 50, 56, 59, 73, 82, 88, 95, 98, 99, 104, 106]

In the presence of delayed left atrial activation following right atrial pacing, the programmed AV delay may not provide adequate time for effective atrial systole before ventricular systole (Fig. 12–75). Latency is the interval from the onset of the pacemaker stimulus (excitation) to the beginning of an identifiable depolarization. The delay from the atrial stim-

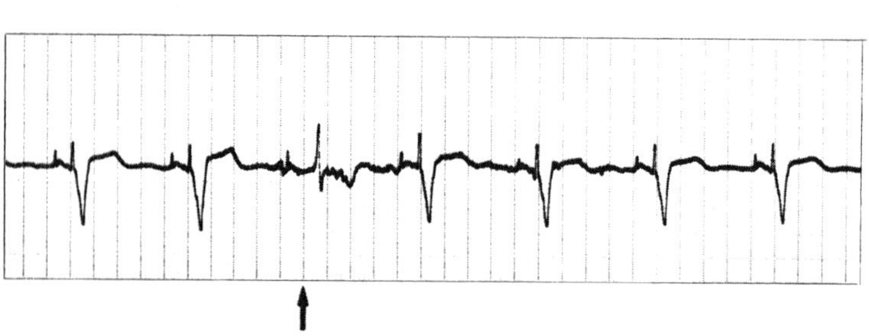

Figure 12–73. Unipolar DDD pulse generator without a VTP. The third atrial stimulus is followed by unexpected prolongation of the AV interval due to oversensing of myopotentials. This occurrence may mimic crosstalk. (From Barold SS, Ong LS, Falkoff MD, Heinle RA: Crosstalk or self-inhibition in dual-chambered pacemakers. *In* Barold SS [ed]: Modern Cardiac Pacing. Mount Kisco, NY, Futura Publishing Co, 1985, p 615; with permission.)

1.   Sensed p-wave

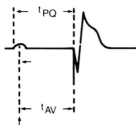

Start: AV-delay

2.   Stimulated p-wave

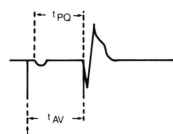

Start: AV-delay

3.   Constant PQ-interval
      by means of AV-fallback

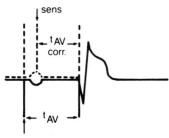

Stimulation

Figure 12–74. AV fallback or hysteresis. 1. Sensing of the P wave depends on electrode position and the configuration and amplitude of the intracardiac atrial electrogram. For this reason, the programmed AV delay starts sometime after the onset of the P wave registered on the surface ECG. Consequently, the P-Q interval is longer than the programmed AV delay. 2. Depending on the position of the electrode and the propagation of atrial depolarization, the paced P wave follows the atrial stimulus after some delay. Consequently, the P-Q interval is shorter than the programmed AV interval. 3. A constant P-Q interval after pacing and sensing occurs by means of the AV fallback mechanism. After a sensed P wave, the programmed AV delay is reduced by a programmable AV fallback time (corrected AV time). Therefore, a constant PQ interval is produced regardless of P-wave sensing or atrial stimulation. (Courtesy of Biotronik, Lake Oswegon, OR, with modification.)

ulus to the onset of atrial depolarization depends mostly on the type of atrial disease and the site of stimulation. If there is both latency and delayed interatrial conduction, the time from right atrial stimulation to the peak of the

A wave on the mitral valve echocardiogram can be considerably lengthened.[3, 104–106] The duration of the diastolic period may be easily determined with the simultaneous recording of the ECG and M-mode echocardiogram by measuring the opening of the mitral valve at the onset of diastole and the closure of the mitral valve at the end of diastole. Alt and colleagues[3] found delayed left atrial contraction of 46 ± 24 msec following paced atrial events, compared with sensed atrial events, in a small number of patients. These workers suggested that the diastolic filling period after a sensed and after a paced atrial event be more or less equalized by adjusting the duration of the AV interval initiated by pacing or sensing. They indicated that as a general rule prolongation of the AV interval after atrial pacing by 50 msec may produce basically the same effective AV interval as that initiated by atrial sensing.

Wish and associates[104] investigated the interval between the right atrial pacing artifact and left atrial depolarization and found it to be 70 to 380 msec, with a mean of 144 ± 82 msec.

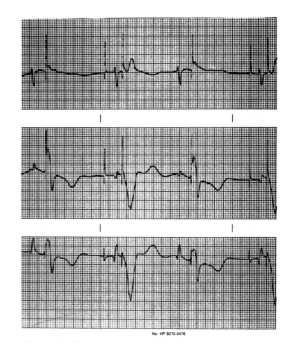

Figure 12–75. Disparity between the effective PR intervals after atrial pacing and sensing demonstrated by esophageal ECG in three simultaneously recorded leads. (Top strip shows esophageal ECG, and middle and lower strips are compound leads.) The programmed AV interval is 200 msec, and the recordings were obtained at double speed. After atrial pacing, the interval from left atrial depolarization to the ventricular stimulus is about 100 msec. When the AV interval is initiated by atrial sensing, the left atrial to ventricular stimulus interval is 180 msec.

This interval represents the intraatrial conduction delay (together with latency). In the DVI mode when the programmed AV delay was 150 msec, the average interval between left atrial depolarization (via esophageal leads) and ventricular pacing (stimulus) was only 6 ± 81 msec. Three patients demonstrated a negative left atrial to ventricular sequence when the interatrial conduction time was longer than the programmed AV delay of 150 msec. With the mode changed to VDD at the same AV delay, the left atrial to ventricular sequence increased from 6 ± 81 msec to 137 ± 50 msec, a statistically significant difference. The difference represents the left-sided AV extension due to atrial sensing. The relatively short time required to complete conduction to the left atrium after actual sensing in the right atrial appendage causes left atrial depolarization to occur earlier within the programmed AV delay and further from the ventricular stimulus than during atrial pacing. At a given AV interval, the sequence between left atrial and ventricular contraction is longer in the VDD mode compared with the DVI mode. These workers emphasized that the optimal AV delay required knowledge of the left atrial to ventricular sequence because of the marked variability of the interatrial conduction delay.

Janosik and colleagues[50] found that the optimal duration of the AV delay was 164 ± 53 msec during VDD pacing, compared with $202; \pm 40$ msec during DVI pacing at a slightly faster pacing rate. The mean difference was 39 msec, with a range of 0 to 100 msec. The greatest difference was found in patients with an enlarged, poorly contractile left ventricle. This finding underscores the importance of adjusting the AV delay in patients with poor left ventricular function.

Two-dimensional and Doppler echocardiography are therefore quite important in "fine tuning" and individualizing the hemodynamic response to pacing. Doppler echocardiography allows the determination of stroke volume cardiac dimensions and volumes and the function of the AV valves.[31, 32, 36, 92] The optimal AV interval may vary considerably from patient to patient and depends on many factors, including left ventricular compliance, left ventricular filling pressure, atrial contractility, mitral valve function, and heart rate (Fig. 12–76). Doppler echocardiography during exercise is now feasible and may allow further "fine tuning" for the individual patient.

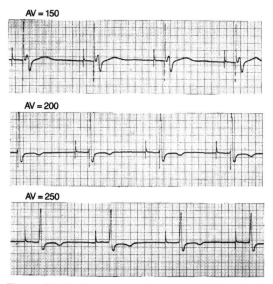

Figure 12–76. Importance of programmability of AV interval in dual-chamber pacemakers. *Top,* A relatively short AV interval of 150 msec causes ventricular depolarization by the pulse generator. *Middle,* With an AV interval of 200 msec, ventricular pseudofusion beats are produced. *Bottom,* With an AV interval of 250 msec, the conducted spontaneous QRS complex is sensed by the pulse generator, which therefore does not emit any ventricular stimuli. In this situation, a relatively long AV interval avoids the delivery of potential wasteful energy and probably optimizes cardiac function by maintaining natural ventricular depolarization. Recordings were obtained at 50 mm/sec. (From Barold SS, Mugica J, Falkoff MD, et al: Multiprogrammability in cardiac pacing. *In* Barold SS [ed]: Modern Cardiac Pacing. Mount Kisco, NY, Futura Publishing Co, 1985, p 377; with permission.)

RETRIGGERABLE VENTRICULAR REFRACTORY PERIODS

The pacemaker ventricular refractory period (VRP) was, in the past, defined as the interval during which the pulse generator is insensitive to any incoming signals, i.e., the pulse generator would be unable to respond in any way to a signal. With the advent of sophisticated pulse generators with complex circuitry, the definition of the VRP has changed, so that it has now become known as the period during which the lower rate timer cannot be reset or restarted. Therefore, a pulse generator may actually recognize ventricular signals during part of the VRP, but these detected signals are used only to reset timing intervals other than the inviolable lower rate interval. In most pulse generators, the duration of the VRP initiated by the ventricular stimulus is equal to the refractory period initiated by ventricular sensing (with or without a preceding P wave).

The VRP of the Medtronic Symbios DDD pulse generators (models 7001, 7005, and 7006)

Figure 12–77. Diagrammatic representation of the atrial and ventricular refractory periods of a Medtronic Symbios DDD pulse generator. No marker signals can be generated in either the atrial or the ventricular absolute refractory periods. A detected atrial signal in the noise-sampling period is unused by the pulse generator but is depicted as an ~~AS~~ marker. A ventricular signal sensed in the noise-sampling period is depicted by an SR marker. ARP = absolute refractory period (also called blanking period by Medtronic); VPC = ventricular premature contraction or ventricular extrasystole; Ap = atrial paced event; As = atrial sensed event; ~~AS~~ = atrial unused event; SR = sensed in the refractory period, that is, ventricular sensed event in the noise-sampling period of the VRP; Vs = ventricular sensed event; Vp = ventricular paced event. (See text for details.)

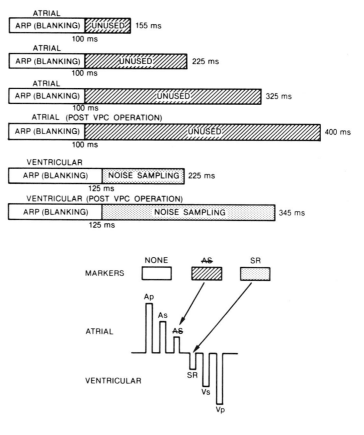

MEDTRONIC SYMBIOS DDD PULSE GENERATOR
REFRACTORY PERIODS

(Medtronic, Minneapolis, MN) lasts for 225 msec[94] (235 msec for models 7000 and 7000A) from the onset of a ventricular event, defined as a paced ventricular stimulus or a sensed QRS complex (i.e., preceded by a sensed P wave) (Fig. 12–77). The VRP of each model under these circumstances is composed of an initial 125-msec absolute refractory period (also called the ventricular blanking period by Medtronic) followed by the noise-sampling period, which constitutes the terminal part of the VRP. This terminology is potentially misleading because this particular blanking period may be confused with the brief ventricular blanking period occurring coincidentally with the atrial stimulus and designed to prevent crosstalk. When the Symbios DDD pulse generator senses a ventricular extrasystole (defined by the pacemaker as two successive ventricular events without any sensed intervening atrial activity), the noise-sampling period is automatically lengthened to 220 msec, giving a total VRP of 345 msec (340 for models 7000 and 7000A).

A signal detected during the noise-sampling period of the Symbios pulse generator is rep-resented by a telemetered marker pulse indicating a ventricular "sense refractory" (SR) event. Although such a signal does not reset the lower rate timer, it will reset (restart) other intervals in the Symbios pulse generator, as follows:

1. A new 345-msec VRP, the first 125 msec consisting of the blanking period because the signal is interpreted by the pulse generator as a sensed ventricular extrasystole (ventricular premature beat).

2. A new PVARP, together with its automatic extension. The latter occurs because the pulse generator interprets the sensed signal as a VPC, thereby automatically lengthening the duration of the PVARP to 400 msec. When the extension comes into play, the total duration of the PVARP is always increased automatically to 400 msec, and this is not programmable.

3. New upper rate limit interval. By design, the upper rate limit circuit governs only the rate of atrial triggered ventricular pacing.

These considerations have important implications. When a ventricular signal is detected during the noise-sampling period, it retriggers another complete VRP. If this triggering occurs continually, the pulse generator will eventually time out at the lower rate limit interval and will appear to be pacing asynchronously.[35] This refractory period design (also called "retriggerable") is particularly effective in preventing inhibition of the pacing output by electromagnetic or skeletal muscle interference. A relatively long noise-sampling period permits continuous resetting of the VRP in the presence of rapidly recurring signals, resulting in asynchronous DOO pacing (interference mode) (Fig. 12–78). Conceptually, this design is similar to that of the automatic antitachycardia "dual-demand" mode of pacing with overlapping refractory periods and activation of the pulse generator to pace during both bradycardia and tachycardia. The same response can also be initiated by intrinsic cardiac activity if the cycle length is short enough to allow sensing within the noise-sampling period. This response may be seen during ventricular tachycardia[26] with a cycle length less than 345 msec or during atrial fibrillation with a rapid ventricular rate and numerous RR intervals shorter than 345 msec.[39] During atrial fibrillation, asynchronous pacing may be intermittent, depending on interplay between the constantly varying RR intervals and the timing intervals of the pulse generator. Therefore, in the case of the Medtronic DDD pulse generators, undersensing due to a signal detected in the noise-sampling period should not be attributed to a low electrographic signal or misinterpreted as pulse generator malfunction.

When there is intermittent failure of ventricular capture, some of the spontaneous QRS complexes will fall intermittently in the absolute refractory period, in the noise-sampling period, or outside the refractory period. When these spontaneous QRS complexes fall within the noise-sampling period, the interpretation of the pacemaker response necessitates knowledge that the Medtronic Symbios pulse generator "uses" a sensed ventricular signal to restart all its timing cycles except the lower rate limit interval.

The timing and duration of the noise-sampling period vary from manufacturer to manufacturer. In addition, the response of the pulse generator to sensed signals within the noise-sampling period depends on the design and the manuufacturer. For example, in the Cordis series of DDD pulse generators, the noise-sampling period occupies the terminal portion of both the PVARP and the VRP. It is therefore possible for a physiologic signal, such as the P wave, to be detected within the noise-sampling period, whereupon the pulse generator will pace asynchronously for one cycle.[89]

ATRIAL REFRACTORY PERIODS

The total atrial refractory period (TARP) consists of two components. The first part starts with the beginning of an atrial event (As or Ap) and extends through the AV delay. Because it is undesirable for a second atrial event to be sensed once the AV interval has begun, the atrial sensing amplifier is always

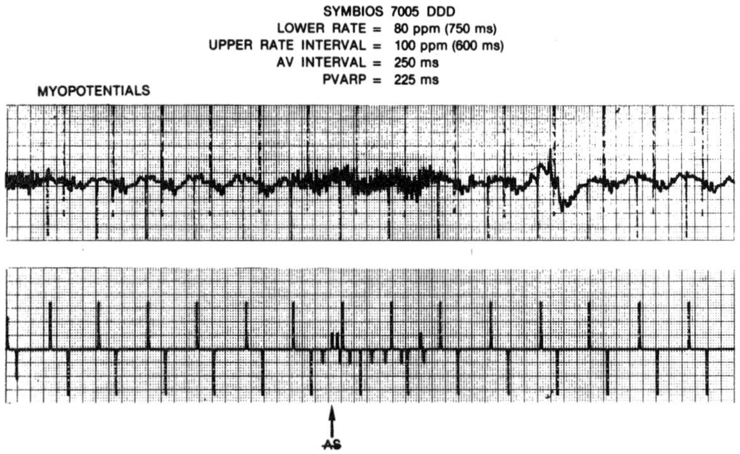

```
                    SYMBIOS 7005 DDD
             LOWER RATE = 80 ppm (750 ms)
      UPPER RATE INTERVAL = 100 ppm (600 ms)
             AV INTERVAL = 250 ms
                   PVARP = 225 ms
MYOPOTENTIALS
```

Figure 12–78. Response of the Medtronic Symbios 7005 unipolar DDD pulse generator to oversensing of myopotentials. The programmed parameters are shown above, and the lower strip represents the marker channel. The origin and size of the markers are depicted as in Figure 12–77. In the middle of the tracing, rapidly occurring myopotential signals are sensed within the noise-sampling period of the ventricular channel and therefore do not cause inhibition. Myopotential signals sensed by the ventricular channel in the noise-sampling period initiate a new VRP. In the new VRP, the absolute refractory period remains constant, but the noise-sampling period is extended whenever two ventricular events occur without an intervening sensed P wave or atrial event. Continual reinitiation of the retriggerable VRP by myopotential signals causes the pulse generator to pace asynchronously at the LRI. Myopotential signals are also detected by the atrial channel, but they are represented as unused (A̶S̶) events.

refractory for the duration of the AV interval. The second component is the PVARP, which starts with a ventricular event (Vs or Vp). Published pacemaker specifications are somewhat confusing because some manufacturers refer to the atrial refractory period as the TARP, while others refer only to the PVARP.

Factors Influencing Duration of the Total Atrial Refractory Period

The following factors influence the duration of the TARP:

1. Programmed AV interval or the entire interval from As or Ap, ending at the onset of Vp. The AV interval initiated by sensing may differ from that initiated by pacing (AV delay hysteresis).

2. Abbreviation of the AV interval that begins with As or Ap and ends prematurely with the onset of Vs.

3. Abbreviated Ap-Vp interval (usually 100 to 110 msec) according to the function of the so-called ventricular safety pacing period (or ventricular triggering period). Occasionally, the ventricular safety pacing period may lengthen beyond its programmed value to a value less than the programmed AV interval, to avoid violating the upper rate limit interval.

4. Extension of the As-Vp interval beyond the programmed AV interval imposed by upper rate limitation (Wenckebach behavior).

5. In some pulse generators, a ventricular sensing event (Vs without preceding As or Ap) is interpreted as a ventricular extrasystole and generates an automatic atrial refractory period extension that will add to the duration of the PVARP.

In the Medtronic Symbios DDD pulse generator, the first portion of the PVARP (100 msec), like the VRP, consists of an absolute refractory period (also called the ventricular blanking period by Medtronic), during which the atrial sensing function is turned off. An atrial event beyond the blanking period and within the PVARP (and its extension) does not reset any of the pacemaker intervals and is simply noted by the pulse generator as an "unused" atrial sense event in the marker channel (see Fig. 12–77). In addition, such an "unused" atrial signal is not counted as a P wave insofar as the pacemaker interpretation of a premature ventricular event (ventricular premature beat) is concerned. Therefore, the detection of P waves by the pulse generator during the AV interval, the noise-sampling period, and extension of the PVARP remains absolutely passive in that the P waves are "unused" and do not influence pacemaker electronics. The telemetry marker function of the pulse generator displays the timing of these detected "unused" P waves to simplify the overall interpretation of the electrocardiogram.

In contrast to the Symbios series of DDD pulse generators, which contain a noise-sampling period only in relation to the VRP, the Siemens 674 DDD pulse generator (Siemens-Elema, Solna, Sweden) contains a noise-sampling period in relation to both the atrial and the ventricular refractory periods. The presence of an atrial or noise-sampling period functions in the same way as the VRP of the Medtronic Symbios series of pulse generators. In other words, the Siemens 674 unit possesses a retriggerable atrial refractory period. Thus, a sensed atrial event in the noise-sampling period is actually used to restart another PVARP. Because the pulse generator has a separately programmable upper rate interval and TARP, it will therefore exhibit a Wenckebach response if the upper rate interval is longer than the TARP. When the PP interval becomes shorter than the TARP, the pulse generator reverts to asynchronous atrial pacing at the programmed lower rate. This response is similar to the behavior of the Symbios DDD pulse generator when it is presented with repetitive ventricular signals within the noise-sampling portion of the VRP. In the case of the Siemens 674 pulse generator, it then functions in the DVI mode when the PP interval is less than the TARP. For this reason, the Siemens 674 DDD pulse generator can never develop fixed-ratio block in response to a fast atrial rate if the PP interval is < TARP.

RESPONSE OF DDD PACEMAKER TO VENTRICULAR EXTRASYSTOLES

Most DDD pulse generators respond to a ventricular extrasystole (sensed ventricular event without preceding sensed atrial depolarization) by the initiation of a new lower rate interval and atrial escape (pacemaker VA) interval. In the Siemens-Elema 674 DDD pulse generator, a ventricular extrasystole is followed by a prolonged atrial escape (pacemaker VA) interval equal to the lower rate interval plus the AV delay. This response was designed to simulate the actual behavior of the heart,

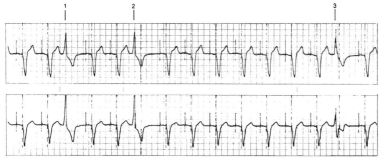

Figure 12–79. Response of DDD pulse generator to sensed ventricular extrasystoles (VPC). Lower rate = 70 ppm (LRI = 857 msec), AV interval = 200 msec, atrial escape (pacemaker VA) interval = 657 msec, and VTP = 110 msec. The first VPC is sensed and initiates a new atrial escape (pacemaker VA) interval of 657 msec. In this way, it can be determined that the VPC electrogram was sensed relatively late in relation to the surface ECG. The second VPC is unsensed because the effective electrogram falls within the VBP. The third VPC is sensed after the VBP, but within the VTP, so that the AV interval becomes abbreviated. The delivery of the atrial stimulus within the QRS complex of the second and third VPCs represents "pseudo" pseudofusion beats.

with a compensatory pause after a ventricular extrasystole. In contrast to the CPI Delta DDD pulse generator[27] (Cardiac Pacemakers, Inc, St Paul, MN), whenever rate smoothing is programmed, the pause after a sensed ventricular extrasystole is shortened. Rate smoothing eliminates abrupt changes in the RR interval, so that when a ventricular extrasystole is sensed, the rate-smoothing windows of the event preceding the ventricular extrasystole are retained and the next output pulses will occur within these intervals. The clinical importance of long or short pauses after sensed ventricular extrasystoles is unknown. The proponents of rate smoothing believe that the perpetuation of ventricular extrasystoles is favored by a preceding long R-R interval. Figures 12–79 and 12–80 illustrate the usual response of a DDD pulse generator to sensed ventricular extrasystoles.

DIFFERENTIAL DIAGNOSIS OF SINGLE ATRIAL STIMULUS DURING DDD PACING

NORMAL SITUATION. Delivery of only atrial stimuli may normally be seen during DDD pacing. This delivery occurs when spontaneous ventricular activity falls within the AV interval, so that the subsequent ventricular stimulus is inhibited. In this instance, the interval between two consecutive atrial stimuli (AA interval) shortens because the pacemaker recycles according to its atrial escape (pacemaker VA) interval. This shortening of the AA interval leads to an increase in the atrial pacing rate above the programmed lower rate. The diagnosis may be confirmed by conversion to the DOO mode, usually with the magnet, whereupon both atrial and ventricular stimuli become evident.

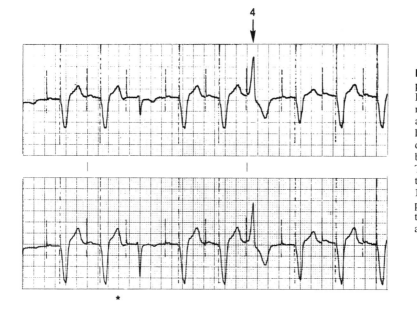

Figure 12–80. Response of DDD pulse generator to sensed VPC. Lower rate = 80 ppm (LRI = 750 msec), AV interval = 250 msec, and VTP = 110 msec. The VPC labeled "4" is sensed after the delivery of the atrial stimulus, but beyond the VBP and the VTP. This sensed VPC is in contrast to the three sensed VPCs in Figure 12–79, in which the first is not preceded by an atrial stimulus and the third is associated with atrial and ventricular stimuli.

ISOELECTRIC VENTRICULAR STIMULI IN ONE OR TWO LEADS. Obviously, the full 12-lead electrocardiogram should be examined to avoid this pitfall, especially with bipolar DDD devices. Double standardization may bring out tiny stimuli.

CONCEALED VENTRICULAR STIMULI. Ventricular stimuli are often concealed within the QRS complex, especially with bipolar pulse generators. It may be impossible to determine whether the ventricular stimulus is delivered before ventricular sensing would have occurred (pseudofusion) or whether it is inhibited by sensing the electrogram. Marker channel function is invaluable in this situation.

DISCONNECTION OF THE VENTRICULAR CIRCUIT (LOOSE CONNECTION OR FRACTURE OF THE VENTRICULAR ELECTRODE). This leads to apparent AAI pacing. The diagnosis is made by reprogramming to the VVI mode, whereupon no stimuli will be seen after application of the magnet, with conversion to the VOO mode. By reprogramming the pulse generator to the DDD mode, AAI pacing will reappear.

CROSSTALK. Crosstalk should be suspected if the interval from the atrial stimulus to the succeeding spontaneous QRS complex is greater than the programmed AV interval. The ventricular output cannot occur because it is inhibited. The diagnosis may be confirmed by conversion to the DOO mode, whereupon both atrial and ventricular stimuli should return.

OVERSENSING. During the AV interval, oversensing of, for example, myopotentials and false signals (generated by an intermittent defect in the pacing lead) may inhibit the ventricular stimulus.

PRESERVATION OF SENSING DURING THE AV INTERVAL UPON APPLICATION OF THE MAGNET. In Cordis DDD pulse generators, ventricular sensing may be preserved during the AV interval even after application of the magnet (see Fig. 12–65). The QRS complex may be sensed before the completion of the AV interval, and the ventricular stimulus is therefore inhibited. In this situation, the ventricular stimulus may be exposed by programming the AV interval to a shorter value than the spontaneous PR interval.

DIFFERENTIAL DIAGNOSIS OF VENTRICULAR (SINGLE-CHAMBER) PACING DURING DDD PACING

This differential diagnosis pertains to ventricular pacing (real or apparent) without a preceding atrial stimulus or identifiable atrial sensed event. The causes are discussed below.

APPLICATION OF THE TEST MAGNET OVER A DDD PULSE GENERATOR. This causes VOO rather than DOO pacing in some DDD pulse generators, such as the CPI Delta 925 DDD pacemaker.

DISCONNECTION OF ATRIAL CIRCUIT. This leads to VVI pacing when the pacemaker is programmed to the DDD mode. When reprogrammed to the AAI or AOO mode, no stimuli will be seen, even with magnet application. In the DDD mode, no atrial stimuli will be seen upon conversion to the DOO mode with the magnet.

INAPPARENT PROGRAMMING TO THE VVI MODE. The pacemaker should be reprogrammed to the DDD or DVI mode for diagnosis.

ISOELECTRIC ATRIAL STIMULI. The presence of two pacemaker stimuli should be determined by taking three simultaneous electrocardiographic leads or the 12-lead electrocardiogram. Low-amplitude atrial stimuli from a bipolar pulse generator may be extremely difficult to discern electrocardiographically. The paced P wave may also be inapparent. Occasionally, doubling the sensitivity of the electrocardiograph may bring out tiny atrial stimuli showing successful atrial capture.

CONCEALED ATRIAL STIMULI WITHIN THE QRS COMPLEX. These concealed stimuli may occur with a ventricular extrasystole not preceded by a P wave. Only the ventricular stimulus that falls within the terminal portion of the QRS complex or the ST segment is visible. Timing of the concealed atrial stimulus may be defined by determining the end of the atrial escape (pacemaker VA) interval initiated by the previous ventricular event. Event markers are invaluable in demonstrating the occurrence of paced and sensed events.

APPARENT VVI PACING DURING NORMAL DDD PACING. This phenomenon may occur when the atrial stimulus (occasionally because of atrial undersensing) is coincident with the onset of the spontaneous QRS complex with a left bundle branch block configuration, thereby mimicking ventricular depolarization by the transvenous pacemaker.

AV DISABLE FUNCTION. This function is a characteristic of the Medtronic 7000 and 7000A DDD pulse generators, as discussed in the first part of this chapter.

ATRIAL UPPER RATE LIMIT. The Medtronic Symbios 7001, 7005, and 7006 are designed with separate upper rate limitation for the atrial and ventricular channels.[66] Although the

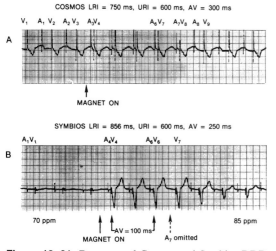

Figure 12–81. Response of Cosmos and Symbios DDD pulse generators to the testing magnet. *A,* Cosmos DDD pulse generator with parameters shown above the ECG. Application of the magnet causes DOO pacing at a rate of 90 ppm (666 msec), with an AV interval equal to 100 msec. This interval is followed by DOO pacing at the programmed lower rate and AV interval seen on the right. The (ventricular) URI is violated upon application of the magnet (V_3–V_4). The (atrial) upper URI is violated after a five-beat sequence with the magnet in place (A_7–A_8). *B,* Symbios DDD pulse generator with parameters shown above the ECG. Application of the magnet has two effects: It causes a threshold margin test at a rate 10 percent faster than the magnet rate (85 ppm + 8.5 ppm = 93.5 ppm) and an AV delay of 100 msec for three intervals. Then the magnet rate changes to 85 ppm (when the battery is functioning normally) with the programmed AV delay. This rate continues until magnet removal. Although the mode is DOO and temporary, the programmed upper rate has an implied atrial upper rate (as seen during the permanent DDD mode). This implied atrial rate is the key to understanding the magnet response. Following the threshold margin test with the magnet rate of 85 ppm and AV delay of 250 msec, the atrial escape (pacemaker VA) interval measures $700 - 250 = 450$ msec. A_6–$V_6 = 100$ msec. The succeeding AV interval (A_7–V_7) should be 250 msec. However, because of the preceding AV interval (A_6–V_6) of 100 msec, the delivery of A_7 at the broken arrow would produce an A_6–A_7 interval of $(100 + 450) = 550$ msec. This interval exceeds the programmed (or implied) atrial URI of 600 msec. Since this is not permitted, the pacemaker does not elicit an atrial stimulus (A_7) at the expected time. From then on, the usual magnet response takes place. With a programmed upper rate of 125 ppm or higher, this response would not occur because the AA interval can never be shorter than the URI. (From Barold SS, Belott PH: Behavior of the ventricular triggering period of DDD pacemakers. PACE 10:1237, 1987; with permission.)

atrial and ventricular upper rate limit intervals are identical in duration, they obviously do not occur simultaneously.[8] Under appropriate circumstances, the pulse generators may omit the delivery of an atrial stimulus to obey the atrial upper rate limit interval (Fig. 12–81).

The commonest cause is application of the magnet over a Symbios DDD pulse generator when the basic low rate varies from 40 to 90 ppm, when the AV interval is either 225 or 250 msec, and when the upper rate is 100 ppm. In the DDD mode, magnet application has the effect of causing a threshold margin test at a rate 10 per cent faster than the magnet rate (85.0 ppm + 8.5 ppm = 93.5 ppm), with an AV delay of 100 msec for three intervals. Then the magnet rate changes to 85 ppm (provided the battery voltage is adequate), with the programmed AV delay occurring until magnet removal. Although the mode is DOO and temporary, the programmed upper rate has an implied atrial upper rate (as seen during the permanent DDD mode). This implied atrial rate is the key to understanding the magnet response. There cannot be any pacing stimulus delivered faster than the upper rate limit interval in either chamber. For example, with the programmed settings of a lower rate equal to 60 ppm, an upper rate equal to 100 ppm, an AV interval equal to 250 msec, the atrial escape interval would be 450 msec (700 msec. – 250 msec) following the threshold margin test (magnet rate of 85 ppm, with a programmed AV delay of 250 msec). With a preceding AV delay of 100 msec, there would be an AA interval of 550 msec (100 msec + 450 msec). This interval would exceed the programmed (or implied) atrial upper rate limit interval of 600 msec. Since this is not permitted, the pacemaker does not elicit an atrial stimulus at the expected time. From then on, the usual magnet response takes place. With an upper rate of 125 ppm or higher, this scenario would not occur because the AA interval can never be shorter than the upper rate limit interval.

In patients with a propensity for retrograde VA conduction, the omission of an atrial stimulus under these circumstances may cause retrograde VA conduction. This may be perpetuated, and an AV desynchronization arrhythmia will occur. Because of the relatively fast magnet rate of 85 ppm, the pacemaker atrial escape interval is relatively short. The atrial stimulus (particularly in the presence of a long AV interval) may fall within the atrial myocardial refractory period generated by the preceding retrograde atrial depolarization. Upon withdrawal of the magnet, endless loop tachycardia starts immediately at the programmed upper rate of 100 ppm.

Omission of the atrial stimulus to obey the atrial upper rate limit interval may also occur

Figure 12–82. Symbios 7005 DDD pulse generator exhibiting crosstalk. Programmed parameters: URI = 600 msec (rate = 100 ppm), LRI = 666 msec (rate = 90 ppm), and AV interval = 250 msec. The upper and lower ECGs were recorded simultaneously with the telemetered marker pulses in the middle strip. The upper and lower ECGs represent compound leads with deformity of the waveform by the real-time markers generated by the Medtronic programmer 9701-A3. Each marker consists of a 20-msec pulse with a specific amplitude and polarity to designate the following pulse generator function: atrial pace (AP), atrial sense (AS), unused atrial sense (A̶S̶), ventricular pace (VP), ventricular sense (VS), and sensing during the VRP (SR).

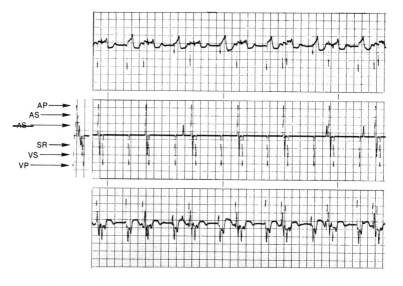

The markers confirm the presence of crosstalk by showing a VS event immediately after an atrial pace (AP) event. Delivery of a ventricular stimulus (VP) at the end of the VTP (110 msec) violates the (ventricular) URI of 600 msec. The subsequent atrial stimulus is omitted. This omission is clearly shown by the absence of any pacemaker atrial event in the 666-msec LRI separating the two ventricular paced events. The mechanism of this response is depicted diagrammatically in Figure 12–83. (From Barold SS, Belott PH: Behavior of ventricular triggering period of DDD pacemakers. PACE 10:1237, 1987; with permission.)

under other circumstances unrelated to magnet application.[8] These situations are complex and relatively rare (Figs. 12–82 to 12–84). This fact must be known in order to analyze some of the more complex arrhythmias generated by these devices.

DDI MODE. The DDI mode may resemble VVI pacing when the PVARP is short and all

Figure 12–83. Diagrammatic representation of the behavior of the Medtronic Symbios DDD pulse generator during crosstalk when programmed to the following parameters: LRI = 666 msec (rate = 90 ppm), URI = 600 msec (rate = 100 ppm), AV interval = 250 msec, and atrial escape (pacemaker VA) interval = 416 msec. The pacemaker delivers an atrial stimulus (A_1) followed 250 msec later by a ventricular stimulus (V_1). The second atrial stimulus (A_2) is delivered 666 msec after A_1 at the completion of the atrial escape (pacemaker VA) interval of 416 msec. A_2 induces crosstalk, thereby activating the VTP, and the second ventricular stimulus (V_2) is issued 110 msec after A_2. V_2 initiates another atrial escape (pacemaker VA) interval of 416 msec. Theoretically, the pulse generator should have delivered the next atrial stimulus (A_3) at the

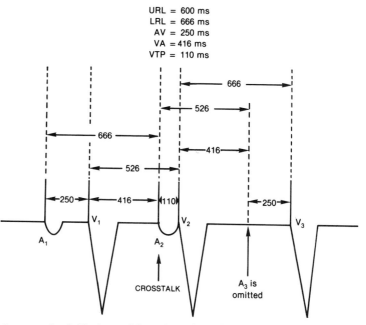

completion of the AEI of 416 msec, but A_3 was omitted. The interval from A_2 to the anticipated delivery of A_3 is equal to the sum of the AEI (416 msec) and the VTP (110 msec), that is, 526 msec. This pulse generator has been designed with a separate atrial URI. Consequently, A_2 initiates an atrial URI of 600 msec that has not yet timed out when A_3 is ready to be delivered. The pulse generator, remaining faithful to its atrial URI, therefore omits A_3. The subsequent ventricular stimulus (V_3) occurs on time, at the completion of the LRI (V_2–V_3) of 666 msec. With this particular combination of parameters, the Symbios DDD pulse generator responds to crosstalk by violating its ventricular URI, though it preserves its atrial upper rate response by the omission of an atrial stimulus. (From Barold SS, Belott PH: Behavior of the ventricular triggering period of DDD pacemakers. PACE 10:1237, 1987; with permission.)

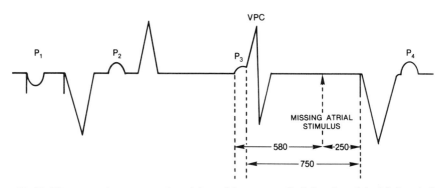

URLI = 600 ms, LRI = 750 ms, AV = 250 ms, VA = 500 ms

Figure 12–84. Diagrammatic representation of the atrial upper rate limit function of the Medtronic Symbios series of DDD pulse generators. Parameters are shown above the diagram, and the VTP was programmed off. The atrial upper rate limit interval (AURLI) is equal to the ventricular upper rate limit interval (VURLI), both being 600 msec. The third P wave (P_3) is sensed by the atrial channel and initiates an AV interval of 250 msec and the AURLI of 600 msec. A VPC is sensed by the ventricular channel 80 msec after the sensed P_3. This sensing of the VPC aborts the AV interval, and a new VURLI and atrial escape (pacemaker VA) interval are initiated. This AEI should have terminated with the delivery of the atrial stimulus at the vertical arrow, but the atrial stimulus is missing. This is because the interval from P_3 to the anticipated atrial stimulus is equal to 80 msec + 500 msec = 580 msec. The delivery of the atrial stimulus 580 msec after P_3 would have violated the AURLI. The pulse generator therefore omits the atrial stimulus.

the P waves are sensed.[7] There will be no atrial stimuli, and the P waves appear to be dissociated from the paced QRS complexes. Similarly, in the DDI mode, with atrial fibrillation and f waves continually sensed, VVI pacing may be mimicked, as no atrial stimuli are delivered because they are constantly inhibited. DDI pacing with constant retrograde VA conduction, in which the retrograde P wave falls continually beyond the PVARP, will also resemble VVI pacing because there are no atrial stimuli (to be discussed further on).

SPECIAL FUNCTIONS. Rate smoothing (CPI Delta DDD) may mimic VVI pacing.[27] In some pulse generators, the fallback upper rate response (to a predetermined level or lower rate) may actually be in the VVI mode.

DISLODGMENT OF THE ATRIAL LEAD. A dislodged atrial lead capturing the ventricle may produce complex electrocardiographic patterns that result from the interplay of several factors[6, 47, 75, 87]:

1. The ventricular electrode may sense the atrial stimulus (crosstalk) or the paced QRS complex engendered by the stimulus from the atrial channel.
2. The ventricular triggering period may be in operation.
3. Intermittent movement of the atrial leads toward the right ventricle may yield two different patterns of ventricular depolarization because ventricular stimulation by the atrial

lead does not occur at the right ventricular apex.

4. During ventricular pacing by atrial stimuli, ventricular stimuli may be buried within the QRS complex. Marker channels may be diagnostically invaluable in this situation.
5. The atrial lead may sense the spontaneous QRS complex (far-field sensing), so that the pulse generator initiates an AV interval upon sensing the QRS complex and delivers a ventricular stimulus on the ST segment or T wave (Fig. 12–85). Such far-field atrial sensing of the QRS complex is rare in a normally functioning pulse generator unless the PVARP is considerably shorter than the VRP (Fig. 12–86).

Electrocardiographic Patterns. The following electrocardiographic patterns are associated with atrial lead dislodgment (Fig. 12–87):

1. Intermittent atrial and ventricular pacing by the atrial stimulus (emanating from the atrial lead) may occur, occasionally with an alternating pattern.
2. Double ventricular stimulation by the atrial and ventricular outputs may occur when the AV interval is long and the effective ventricular (myocardial) refractory period is relatively short.
3. If a stimulus from a displaced atrial electrode is persistently sensed by the correctly positioned ventricular electrode, crosstalk exists and the VV interval (interval between two

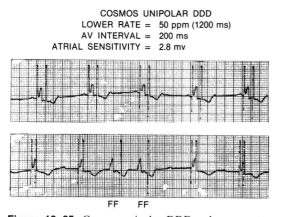

COSMOS UNIPOLAR DDD
LOWER RATE = 50 ppm (1200 ms)
AV INTERVAL = 200 ms
ATRIAL SENSITIVITY = 2.8 mv

FF   FF

Figure 12–85. Cosmos unipolar DDD pulse generator with the atrial lead displaced to the right ventricular inflow tract. VTP = 100 msec. *Top,* Apparent lack of atrial sensing and ventricular capture by the atrial stimulus (2.7 V at 0.3 msec, thereby excluding cross-stimulation). The paced QRS complex is not sensed by the ventricular lead. *Bottom,* This ECG was recorded 24 hours after the top tracing. Atrial non-sensing persists. The atrial stimulus captures the ventricle, and the resultant paced QRS complex is sensed by the ventricular electrode within the VTP, so that the AV interval is abbreviated to 100 msec. The spontaneous QRS complexes labeled FF (far-field) are sensed by the atrial electrode, which interprets them as P waves. This occurrence initiates an AV interval, and at its termination the ventricular stimulus is delivered within the ST segment. Atrial undersensing was present with an atrial sensitivity of 0.4 mV. The atrial sensitivity was decreased to 2.8 mV to reduce the possibility of far-field sensing. In the top strip, the fortuitous occurrence of the P wave before the paced QRS complex suggests AV conduction with a spontaneous QRS complex. However, AV conduction was absent. The spontaneous QRS complexes in the bottom strip resemble the paced QRS complex, suggesting that they are induced mechanically by the displaced atrial electrode.

consecutive paced ventricular beats) will be equal to the atrial escape (or pacemaker VA) interval (plus the negligible duration of the ventricular blanking period) (Fig. 12–87C).

4. If there is no crosstalk, the correctly positioned ventricular electrode may sense the signal from the paced ventricular depolarization emanating from the displaced atrial electrode. The ventricular pacing rate will be slower than in No. 3 above; that is, the VV interval will be longer than the sum of the VA (atrial escape) interval and the blanking period, but shorter than the basic VV interval or lower rate interval (Fig. 12–87D).

5. In a pulse generator with a ventricular triggering period, crosstalk or sensing (by the correctly positioned ventricular electrode) of a paced QRS complex (from the displaced atrial electrode) will abbreviate the VV interval by a value equal to the difference between the AV interval and the ventricular triggering period (Fig. 12–87E).

6. When neither the stimulus from the atrial channel nor its paced QRS complex is sensed, the VV interval will remain the same as the programmed lower rate interval (see Fig. 12–87B).

CROSS-STIMULATION.[61] Under certain circumstances, the atrial stimulus of a normally functioning DDD pacemaker with correctly positioned atrial and ventricular leads may capture the ventricle (Fig. 12–88). This may occur when the ventricular threshold is exceedingly low, as with the Intermedics Cosmos DDD pulse generator (Intermedics, Freeport, TX) upon application of the testing magnet. The atrial stimulus actually captures the atrium and ventricle simultaneously. Atrial depolarization is invisible because of the large QRS complex. The second stimulus from the ventricular channel of the pulse generator is buried within the paced QRS complex initiated by the preceding stimulus from the atrial channel. This is an idiosyncrasy of this particular pulse

Figure 12–86. Diagrammatic representation of far-field sensing by the atrial electrode of a DDD pulse generator. When the VRP is substantially longer than the PVARP, it creates a window within which a ventricular signal can be sensed by the atrial channel and ignored by the ventricular channel. Upon sensing the VPC, the atrial channel initiates an AV interval with the ultimate delivery of the ventricular stimulus on the T wave of the VPC. The likeli-

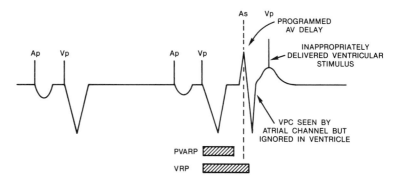

hood of delivering a ventricular stimulus at the apex of the T wave is increased by programming a relatively long AV interval. Ap = atrial paced event; As = atrial sensed event; Vp = ventricular paced event; PVARP = postventricular atrial refractory period; VRP = ventricular refractory period; VPC = ventricular premature contraction.

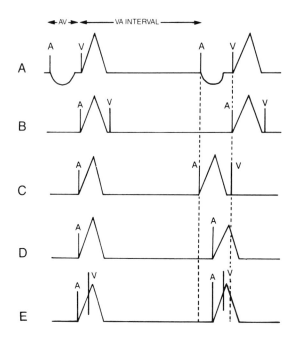

Figure 12–87. Diagrammatic representation of patterns seen with atrial lead dislodgment of a DDD pacemaker. When a dislodged atrial lead captures the ventricle, several different timing intervals or rates of ventricular pacing are possible. This occurrence is described in terms of the VV interval, or the interval between two consecutive ventricular depolarizations. In *A,* normal AV sequential pacing is shown with the programmed AV and VA (atrial escape) intervals. *B,* No change in the ventricular rate or VV interval occurs when neither the atrial stimulus nor the paced QRS complex is sensed by the nondisplaced ventricular electrode. *C,* If the stimulus from the displaced atrial electrode is sensed by the undisplaced ventricular electrode, crosstalk will occur. Assuming a negligible duration of the blanking period, the VV interval will be equal to the atrial escape (pacemaker VA) interval. The second atrial stimulus does not cause crosstalk. *D,* If there is no crosstalk (and no VTP) and the correctly positioned ventricular electrode senses a signal from the paced ventricular depolarization, the VV interval will be shorter than the basic VV interval, but longer than the atrial escape (pacemaker VA) interval. *E,* Response of a pulse generator with a VTP. Crosstalk or sensing of the paced QRS complex within the AVS will abbreviate the VV interval by a value equal to the difference of the AV interval and the VTP.

generator and does not represent malfunction or lead displacement (Fig. 12–89). Occasionally, when a Cosmos pulse generator is programmed to the AAI mode, the atrial stimulus may capture the ventricle in the presence of an exceedingly low threshold for ventricular pacing. This form of cross-stimulation necessitates a high atrial output and may occasionally occur in an alternating pattern (Fig. 12–90).

REVERSAL OF THE LEADS DUE TO INCORRECT CONNECTION. Although this situation is more theoretical than real, it has been reported.[54]

RESETTING OF DDD PACEMAKERS TO THE VVI OR VOO MODE. Pacemaker reset may be defined as the automatic conversion of the pulse generator from the programmed mode (e.g., DDD) to another preset mode (usually VVI or VOO). The phenomenon of resetting to another pacing mode is, at present, unique to DDD pulse generators.[11, 15, 16, 28, 45, 49, 57, 69] As a rule, a change in the magnet rate occurs before the reset point.[63] The end-of-service (EOS) point is triggered by a significant fall in the battery voltage (Fig. 12–91). Most EOS indicators occur in the VVI or VOO mode. When the EOS point is reached, it seems

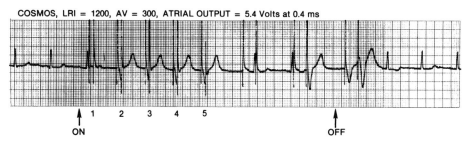

COSMOS, LRI = 1200, AV = 300, ATRIAL OUTPUT = 5.4 Volts at 0.4 ms

ON   OFF

Figure 12–88. Intermedics Cosmos DDD pulse generator programmed to the DDD mode with parameters shown above the ECG. Upon application of the magnet (at the *first arrow*), the first four pacing cycles (faster pairs of atrial and ventricular stimuli) are delivered at a rate of 90 ppm and an AV delay of 100 msec. Note that the second, third, fourth, and fifth atrial stimuli capture the ventricle. The succeeding stimulus from the ventricular channel falls in the refractory period of the ventricular myocardium and is therefore ineffectual and merely deforms the paced QRS complex. After the fifth pair, the pulse generator begins to pace asynchronously at the programmed rate and AV delay. When the magnet is removed *(second arrow),* the atrial stimulus captures the ventricle, and the stimulus from the ventricular channel (delivered 300 msec later) also causes ventricular depolarization. Cross-stimulation upon removal of the testing magnet was not described in the original report of Levine,[61] but it also represents normal function of this pulse generator. This eccentricity is seen only when the ventricular pacing threshold is exceedingly low.

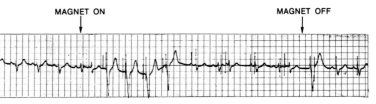

Figure 12–89. Application of magnet on Cosmos DDD pulse generator does not cause cross-stimulation, as in Figure 12–88. However, removal of the magnet causes cross-stimulation of the last atrial stimulus (with ventricular pacing) in the DOO mode. The mechanism of this response is similar to that shown in Figure 12–88. This mechanism is explained by the fact that the output of the last atrial stimulus is somewhat higher than the output of the stimuli in the initial magnet sequence. This is a normal response for this pulse generator and should not be misinterpreted as pacemaker malfunction or atrial lead dislodgment.

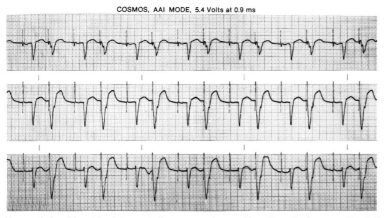

Figure 12–90. Intermedics Cosmos DDD pulse generator programmed to the AAI mode. The ventricular threshold was less than 2.7 V at a pulse width of 0.06 msec and the atrial threshold was less than 2.7 V at a pulse width of 0.10 msec. The leads were correctly positioned. When the pulse generator was programmed to the AAI mode, every alternate atrial stimulus captured the ventricle. This alternating pattern, once initiated, tends to perpetuate itself, perhaps because of cyclic variation in ventricular volume, which influences threshold. This occurrence is another form of cross-stimulation and should not be interpreted as pacemaker malfunction. Such cross-stimulation disappeared when the atrial output was reduced to 5 V at a pulse width of 0.5 msec. The pulse generator is functioning normally, and this type of response is due to a tiny current leak from the atrial to ventricular channels. Cross-stimulation occurs only in patients with an extremely low ventricular threshold for pacing.

Figure 12–91. Battery stress test performed on a 3-year-old Cosmos DDD pulse generator. The pulse generator was programmed to the DDD mode at 8.1 V and 1.0-msec pulse width for both the atrial and the ventricular channels, and the pacing rate was set at 100 ppm. Upon programming, the pulse generator is converted to the VVI mode at 65 ppm, that is, reset mode (not backup mode). Telemetry indicated that the end-of-service point had been reached. The pulse generator was reprogrammed to the DDD mode with considerably lower atrial and ventricular outputs and has remained

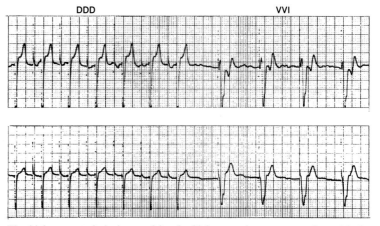

in the DDD mode for over 6 months. The high current drain imposed by the higher requirements, together with the increased current during programming, was sufficient to pull the battery voltage below the 2.4-V level, whereupon the pulse generator was reset. This sequence rules out impending battery failure and illustrates the importance of telemetered battery data in the diagnosis of pacemaker resetting.

advantageous for a pulse generator to be converted automatically to a relatively simpler and less demanding mode, such as the VVI or VOO mode. The reset mode should be considered a protective mechanism designed to conserve energy and allow basic function to continue for some time. In the simple VVI (VOO) mode, the reduced battery current drain increases available battery voltage, resulting in conservation of energy. The pulse generator may continue to function in the VVI (VOO) mode for approximately 6 months after the EOS point has been reached. In this way, the circuit voltage is prevented from falling too rapidly to the end-of-life (EOL) point, when the pacemaker can no longer function reliably, even in the VVI or VOO mode. The EOL should not be confused with the EOS indicator. In the latter state, the pulse generator functions normally, but in the reset VVI or VOO mode.

A DDD pulse generator may reset to the EOS indicator (or the backup mode in other pulse generators) when exposed to fields of high-strength electromagnetic interference (EMI). Exposure to powerful EMI causes a transient dip in battery voltage, as seen by the logic circuitry. The drop in battery voltage triggers the EOS indicator by activating a special switch in the pacemaker circuit. Once the switch is thrown, regardless of the cause, the pacemaker will remain in its EOS or backup mode until a programming command returns it to the DDD mode. In the case of DDD pulse generators with programmable polarity, the reset mode is always unipolar. In some pulse generators, such as the Intermedics Cosmos DDD pulse generator, a two-stage system responds to a transient drop in battery voltage: First, the EOS mode is triggered, and subsequently, with more drop in voltage, the backup mode becomes activated. In the reset VVI mode, some pulse generators may not respond to application of the magnet by conversion to asynchronous pacing, as in the CPI Delta in the reset mode and Intermedics Cosmos in the backup mode.[25] This failure to respond to magnet application should not be misinterpreted as no output or as component failure.

The use of electrocautery during surgery is probably the most common cause of reset. Defibrillation may also reset a DDD pulse generator. Both electrocautery and defibrillation may occasionally cause permanent damage to a pulse generator if the procedure is not performed according to suggested guidelines by the manufacturer. Rarely, the memory of the pulse generator may become scrambled, and reprogramming is ineffectual. Each DDD pulse generator has a characteristic EOS indicator (or backup mode) and reprogramming sequence to reestablish normal function. With one manufacturer, electrocautery may erase the serial and model numbers. This "loss of identity" may be corrected by a programming command only from a special programmer not generally available, but supplied by the manufacturer upon request. Resetting, as such, does not represent malfunction because the pulse generator is not damaged. The importance of the reset phenomenon lies in its recognition, so that the misdiagnosis of pacemaker malfunction or EOS state, resulting in inappropriate pacemaker removal, may be avoided. All patients with DDD pulse generators demonstrating EOS characteristics (or backup mode) should therefore be considered to have reset pacemakers from a cause other than battery depletion, until proven otherwise. Reprogramming to the desired parameters should always be attempted before considering pulse generator replacement. If the power cell is indeed depleted (battery voltage below the EOS point), a reprogramming command may be able to return the pacemaker to normal operating conditions only momentarily. Once the circuitry detects a low battery voltage, it will revert on the very next cycle to the EOS mode.

The problem of reset will become more important several years from now, when patients with DDD pulse generators will be considered for pacemaker replacement. It is important to know that the activation of the EOS of DDD pulse generators may occur during an episode of relatively high current drain. For example, during exercise the pacing rate of a DDD pulse generator may have increased from 70 to 150 ppm, thereby increasing the battery current drain, with consequent reduction in battery voltage and triggering of the EOS. When the patient is evaluated with the pacemaker in the reset mode, the low pacing rate (considerably lower than 150 ppm) will result in a battery voltage above the EOS. With a patient such as this and a 4-year-old device, does one assume that the device has truly reached the EOS point, or should one take a more conservative approach and reprogram the pulse generator out of the EOS mode and follow the patient at monthly intervals to determine whether the pulse generator resets again? Without the aid of noninvasive telemetric measurement of battery voltage (and cell impedance), it may be difficult to handle this situation. The significance of the EOS point should be evaluated by first reprogramming the pulse generator to the DDD mode. Then an attempt to provoke the EOS point should be made by reprogramming the output to maximum as well as increasing the rate. In the absence of telemetered battery voltage, this battery "stress test" gives an idea of battery reserve and optimal time for pulse generator replacement. In other words, it allows postponement of elective replacement.

With a battery voltage indicator, one can easily differentiate between the EOS indicator activated by true EOS from one activated from EMI, thereby avoiding more frequent follow-up or, worse, the early, unnecessary replacement of the device. In this respect, telemetry showing a marked increase in battery impedance corroborates the presence of a depleted lithium-iodine battery. Depletion increases the internal resistance and lowers the available voltage secondarily. Thus, at the EOS point, a pulse generator reprogrammed to a lower output and rate will require less current drain and may continue to function in the new programmed condition for hours, days, or weeks until such time that the battery voltage again drops below the EOS point.

MYOPOTENTIAL INTERFERENCE

The presence of myopotential interference in unipolar DDD pacemakers should be routinely searched for in a 24-hour Holter recording and directly tested during pacemaker follow-up. The pacemaker is first programmed to the highest ventricular sensitivity, and the lower rate is increased to ensure continuous pacing. Then an electrocardiographic strip is taken during isometric exercise. The atrial channel is programmed to the highest sensitivity that will allow continuous atrial tracking. At this sensitivity, the presence of myopotentials sensed by the atrial channel may be demonstrated by isometric exercise.

Myopotential interference may occur in as many as 30 to 50 per cent of unipolar DDD pulse generators.[23, 35, 38, 42, 48, 74, 80, 84, 100, 108] According to the programmed atrial and ventricular sensitivities, the following manifestations may occur:

1. Inhibition of the ventricular channel.
2. An increase in the ventricular pacing rate

by triggering of the ventricular output when the atrial channel senses myopotentials. The pacemaker tachycardia may be regular or irregular and often at or near the upper tracking rate of the pulse generator.

3. Mixed response of alternating ventricular triggering and ventricular inhibition.

4. Reversion to interference asynchronous pacing for one or more cycles (see Fig. 12–79).

5. Precipitation of endless loop tachycardia by myopotential sensing by the atrial channel (or inhibition of the ventricular channel, allowing ventricular escape beats to conduct retrogradely to the atrium).[84]

6. Single missing stimulus. Oversensing by the atrial channel may prevent the delivery of an atrial stimulus with apparent VVI pacing. Conversely, a ventricular stimulus may not succeed an atrial one if myopotential sensing occurs during the AV interval, a situation that may mimic crosstalk.

7. Abbreviation of the AV interval if myopotentials are sensed in the ventricular triggering period of a pulse generator possessing this characteristic (ventricular safety pacing).

TREADMILL STRESS TEST

In active individuals, a treadmill stress test is helpful in evaluating the upper rate response. In rare cases, endless loop tachycardia may actually be precipitated by pacemaker Wenckebach upper rate response during exercise. Stress testing also allows optimization of the AV interval (initiated by atrial sensing) and the selection of its shortest value to increase the maximal tracking rate. The amplitude of the atrial electrogram may also drop during exercise, so that sensitivity may have to be readjusted for optimal P-wave sensing during exercise.[17, 58] Occasionally, myopotential inhibition (especially in children with a pulse generator near the rectus abdominis muscles) may occur during exercise, with sudden lowering of the pacing rate.[18]

HOLTER RECORDINGS

The interpretation of Holter recordings in patients with DDD pulse generators may be difficult or impossible because of various pauses, apparent shortening of intervals, and missing and concealed pacemaker stimuli. A dual-channel Holter recorder, with a special

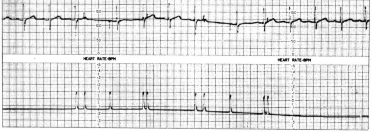

Figure 12–92. Holter recording (with pacemaker channel) in a patient with a DDD pulse generator. There is intermittent atrial undersensing. The invisible pacemaker stimuli on the ECG are clearly delineated by the pacemaker channel at the bottom. The abbreviated AV intervals represent ventricular sensing within the VTP.

channel to enhance the pacemaker stimulus, is extremely helpful[34, 51] (Fig. 12–92). However, such a system may occasionally generate electrostatic discharges that produce deflections resembling pacemaker stimuli (pseudo pacemaker spikes), occasionally arising from a loose electrode, crushed tape, or a dirty recording head. As yet, it is impossible to record pacemaker event markers on a Holter recording. If this option ever becomes available, it will be of benefit to the interpretation of Holter recordings. The difficulty in determining whether atrial capture actually occurs remains the single most important limitation of all Holter recordings, despite various levels of sophistication.

TELEMETRY

Telemetry is an indispensable feature of all sophisticated DDD pulse generators and can no longer be regarded a luxury.[21, 68] The display of programmed settings is merely a memory dump, and it may not reflect what the pacemaker is actually doing. This form of telemetry indicates how the pacemaker was instructed to perform. Thus, a pacemaker programmed to a rate of 70 ppm may generate an interstimulus interval corresponding to a rate of 90 ppm because of crosstalk and an AV interval of 110 msec (ventricular triggering period), a value considerably shorter than the programmed AV delay. In this situation, the AV delay on the surface electrocardiogram does not correspond to the programmed and telemetered AV delay. This lack of correspondence should not be misinterpreted as pacemaker malfunction.

Real-time or measured data represent information actually measured by the pacemaker itself on how it is operating at the time the information is requested, that is, self-analysis of pacemaker function. The ability to acquire real-time data varies according to the pulse generator model and manufacturer. Measured data constitute two groups: (1) rate, pulse width, pulse amplitude (volts), output current (milliamperes), pulse charge and energy delivered to the lead, and lead system impedance; and (2) battery voltage, power cell impedance, and average current drain from the battery (microamperes). The battery current drain should not be confused with the output current delivered to the pacing lead. A discrepancy between programmed data and measured data can indicate pacemaker malfunction or battery EOL. The real-time battery data are valuable in confirming battery depletion, together with other indicators, such as a slowing of the free-running rate or magnet rate or both.

Telemetry of the Electrogram and Event Markers

Transmission of the atrial and ventricular electrogram and the availability of event markers (for pacing and sensing and, in one model, the refractory periods) together constitute one of the most important functions of telemetry and provide real-time evaluation of the pacing system.[24] The transmitted electrogram becomes invaluable in determining the nature of a malfunction caused by lead displacement or fracture or by a poor signal delivered to the pulse generator.[64, 70] In particular, the telemetered atrial electrogram or event markers can be useful in documenting the existence of retrograde VA conduction and its precise duration. Telemetry of the electrogram may unravel complicated sensing problems by demonstrating sensed signals not otherwise apparent on the surface electrocardiogram.[44] Telemetry may confirm the diagnosis of myopotential oversensing in unipolar DDD pulse generators and may allow more accurate optimization of the sensitivity for prevention of oversensing and maintenance of normal P-wave and, QRS-complex sensing. Continuous recording of the electrogram (e.g., atrial) may be accomplished with modified ambulatory monitoring in one channel connected with a radiofrequency coil taped over the pulse generator. This monitoring allows continuous telemetry of the atrial electrogram on a two-channel recorder.[102, 103] This arrangement is available for the Pacesetter AFP DDD (Pacesetter, Sylmar, CA) pulse generator and utilizes a negligible amount of current with an inconsequential effect on battery longevity.

The event marker reflects how the pacemaker interprets a specific cardiac event, particularly how it deals with a sensed event.[30, 55] When recorded simultaneously with the surface electrocardiogram, this event marker provides a precise recording of timing intervals and may allow the programmed pacemaker to generate a diagnostic diagram of its function.[77, 78] Event markers as such cannot identify the actual signal sensed by the pulse generator—for example, myopotentials or false signals—particularly when the sensed event is not visible on the surface electrocardiogram. The marker function is limited to showing which channel senses a signal, regardless of its nature. The telemetered electrogram provides accurate characterization of the sensed signal[24] and is therefore complementary to the marker function. Forthcoming pulse generators will have the capacity for simultaneous recording of event markers, and electrograms with the surface electrocardiogram, a combination that will greatly enhance the evaluation of pacemaker function.

Diagnostic Data

Diagnostic data record the interaction between pulse generator and patient over an extended period and serve as a mini-Holter recording.[1, 33, 40, 65, 85, 101] In the case of one DDD pulse generator, the Intermedics Cosmos unit (models 283–01 and 284–02), a random access memory (RAM) incorporated into the device is allocated a series of counters. Every beat paced or sensed by the pacemaker is entered into these counters. Most counters count up to 17 million events and should therefore permit the accumulation of data over a period of 6 months. Each of the four DDD pacemaker cycles may be analyzed according to the way the cycle terminates, for example, inhibited (As-Vs), VDD (As-Vp), AAI (Ap-Vs), or DVI (Ap-Vp). In addition, the pulse generator interprets a Vs without a preceding atrial event as a ventricular extrasystole. A series of sequence counters can record all these events, and they can be stored for later retrieval as "diagnostic data." Thus, an apparent ventricular extrasystole may be due to other signals, such as myopotential oversensing and an atrial extrasystole conducted but not detected if it occurs during the PVARP. The system for detecting ventricular extrasystoles therefore lacks specificity. The pulse generator also provides the percentage of atrial and ventricular pacing with respect to the total number of counted paced and sensed events. In the Intermedics Cosmos DDD pulse generator, the ventricular tracking limit (VTL) diagnostic counter will increment once each time the pulse generator paces at the VTL for one or more consecutive cycles. During a sustained endless loop tachycardia at the VTL, the counter will increment only once. The same is true for a sensed atrial premature beat, which causes a VTL paced cycle. Atrial premature beats are rather common, and since this particular counter is smaller than the other counters in the pacemaker memory (a maximum of 255 counts compared with 17 million), it fills up rapidly to its maximal level. The counter is reset and is ready to increment once again following two consecutive cycles below the VTL. This feature ensures that the counter increments only once during sustained Wenckebach upper rate behavior.

A new change in the currently available Cosmos DDD pulse generator offers an additional counter that increments whenever the tachycardia termination algorithm is activated. This feature adds specificity to the upper rate diagnostic function. Activation of the tachycardia termination algorithm means that the paced rate was at the upper rate limit for 15 cycles. This situation may be due to endless loop tachycardia and may require lengthening of the PVARP. It could also be caused by a sinus tachycardia or paroxysmal atrial fibrillation. The next generation of Cosmos pulse generators will have a modified VTL counter that will increment only when VTL pacing occurs for two or more consecutive cycles, thereby preventing single atrial premature beats from incrementing the VTL counter (R. Sanders, Intermedics, Freeport, TX, Personal Communication, 1985).

In the next few years, models will be introduced with larger memories that will store rate profiles on patients. A 24-hour rate histogram with 15-minute resolution could be stored. Real-time clocks will allow correlation of recorded events with high-rate episodes with the patient's symptoms occurring in the same time frame. Future memory data will be telemetered to a computer-based program for graphic display and print-out.

PROGRAMMING OF DIFFERENT PACING MODE

A DDD pulse generator may be programmed temporarily to another mode for testing purposes or permanently to correct a problem.[72, 76, 79, 86] Some pulse generators contain a wide variety of programmable pacing modes, some with little or no clinical value. A DDD pulse generator must be programmable to at least the VVI or DVI mode to treat complications. Programmable modes should also include, at a minimum, the DVI, AAI (or AOO), and VVI modes. With separate programmability to the AAI (or AOO) as well as VVI modes, the function of each chamber can be tested individually. Conversion to the AAI or AOO mode provides the fastest and most efficient way of testing for atrial capture (in the absence of AV block).

Pacing modes such as VAT, committed DVI, DOO, DAT, DAD, and VVT are of little or no value for permanent pacing. However, programmability to the DAT, committed DVI, or VDD mode may be theoretically useful in the presence of otherwise unmanageable crosstalk. In patients with relatively normal sinus function, programming from the DDD to the VDD mode may be useful to eliminate muscle twitching at the anodal site

from a unipolar atrial channel or right phrenic nerve stimulation, which may occasionally occur with a malpositioned atrial J lead. In patients with a high atrial pacing threshold and relatively normal chronotropic function, the DDD mode may be converted to the VDD mode. The triggered mode—for example, DDT, AAT, and VVT—is useful for noninvasive electrophysiologic interventions for the diagnosis and treatment of tachyarrhythmias that occur in a small proportion of patients with DDD pulse generators. Temporary modes such as DDT may provide a way of testing for retrograde VA conduction because the triggered mode in the atrium serves as a marker for sensed P waves.

DDI Mode

The DDI mode is a potentially useful mode of pacing that has generally been considered an improved DVI mode (with atrial sensing) or a hybrid of DVI and DDD modes.[7, 37] Conceptually, the DDI mode is best regarded as a DDD pulse generator with identical upper and lower rate intervals. In both DDD and DDI modes, a sensed atrial signal may be considered to initiate the AV interval (Fig. 12–93). In the DDI mode, as in the DDD mode, an early atrial sensed event beyond the

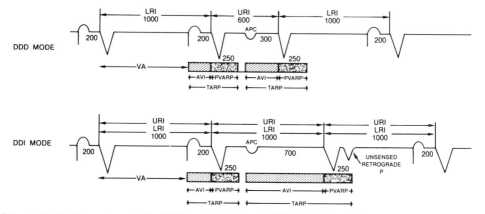

Figure 12–93. Comparison of the DDD mode *(top)* and DDI mode *(bottom)*. DDD mode: LRI = 1000 msec (60 ppm), URI = 600 msec (100 ppm), AV interval (AVI) = 200 msec, pacemaker VA (AEI) = 800 msec, PVARP = 250 msec, and TARP = 450 msec. The pulse generator senses an atrial premature beat (APC) outside the PVARP. This initiates an AV interval of 300 msec because the subsequent ventricular stimulus cannot be delivered until the URI (600 msec) has timed out. DDI mode: URI = LRI = 1000 msec (60 ppm), AV interval = 200 msec, pacemaker VA (AEI) = 800 msec, PVARP = 250 msec, and TARP = 450 msec. An APC 300 msec after the preceding ventricular stimulus falls beyond the PVARP and is therefore sensed. This APC may be considered to initiate an AV interval of 700 msec. This is because the succeeding ventricular stimulus cannot occur until the URI (1000 msec) has timed out. Note that the entire AV interval (regardless of its duration) is refractory for atrial sensing in both the DDD and the DDI modes. The third paced ventricular beat gives rise to a retrograde P wave that is unsensed because it falls within the PVARP. Consequently, an atrial stimulus is delivered at the end of the AEI, thereby avoiding the perpetuation of retrograde VA conduction illustrated in Figure 12–95. (From Barold SS: The DDI mode of cardiac pacing. PACE 10:480, 1987; with permission.)

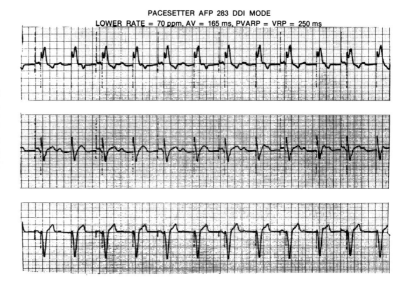

Figure 12-94. DDI mode. Note how the sinus P wave is sensed, provided it occurs beyond the 250-msec PVARP. Each sensed P wave may be considered as initiating an AV interval terminating with the delivery of the ventricular stimulus.

PVARP initiates an AV interval that cannot terminate before completion of the upper rate limit interval, which, in the DDI mode, is identical with the lower rate interval (Fig. 12–94). Therefore, the characteristic prolongation of the AV interval seen during the DDD mode (when the upper rate interval is longer than the TARP) also occurs in the DDI mode but will be more obvious because the difference between the upper rate interval and the TARP (the so-called "W interval," defined in the first section of this chapter) is considerably greater than during conventional DDD pacing. In the DDI mode, programmability of the PVARP is essential to avoid VA synchrony, that is, endless loop "tachycardia" without tachycardia

(Fig. 12–95), a situation that may lead to the pacemaker syndrome. It is often stated that in the DDI mode P waves are sensed but atrial tracking does not occur because the identical upper and lower rate intervals preclude an increase in the ventricular pacing rate above the programmed lower rate. According to the concept that the DDI mode is really a modified DDD mode, it seems preferable to characterize the DDI mode as being capable of atrial tracking, but only at the lower rate limit interval, effectively the equivalent of having no atrial tracking capability at all. Dual-chamber pacing may be denied to patients with paroxysmal supraventricular tachyarrhythmias because a DDD pulse generator tracking rapid

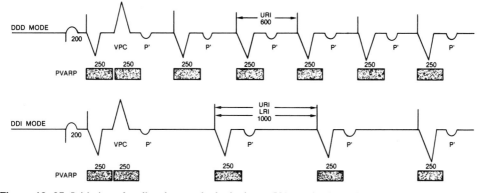

Figure 12-95. Initiation of endless loop arrhythmia due to VA conduction. The pacemaker parameters in the DDD and DDI modes are identical with those in Figure 12–93. *Top,* DDD Mode. A ventricular premature beat (VPC) causes retrograde VA conduction with a retrograde P wave (P') falling beyond the PVARP. This occurrence initiates an endless loop tachycardia with a cycle length of 600 msec, equal to the URI. *Bottom,* DDI Mode. A VPC with identical timing and retrograde VA conduction also causes an endless loop arrhythmia at the URI of 1000 msec, equal to the LRI. These examples illustrate the importance of programming the PVARP in both the DDD and the DDI modes to avoid sensing of retrograde P waves. (From Barold SS: The DDI mode of cardiac pacing. PACE 10:480, 1987; with permission.)

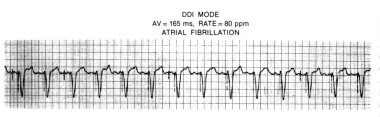

DDI MODE
AV = 165 ms, RATE = 80 ppm
ATRIAL FIBRILLATION

Figure 12–96. DDI mode and atrial fibrillation. (URI = LRI = 750 msec). Atrial fibrillation produces atrial signals occasionally sensed when they occur outside the PVARP of 325 msec. When atrial activity is unsensed, the AEI terminates with an atrial stimulus. The atrial stimuli are ineffectual because of atrial fibrillation.

atrial activity may result in rapid ventricular pacing. Dual-chamber pacing may be superior to VVI pacing because atrial pacing may also prevent supraventricular tachyarrhythmias by overdrive suppression.[90, 91] Consequently, some patients with the bradycardia-tachycardia syndrome might benefit from AV synchrony between attacks of supraventricular tachyarrhythmias when the atria will regain responsiveness to stimulation. In the DDI mode during supraventricular tachyarrhythmias, the pacing rate remains constant at the lower rate (equal to the upper rate), and upon termination, noncompetitive AV sequential pacing is automatically restored (Fig. 12–96). The fixed frequency of the DDI mode is also important in some patients with symptomatic coronary artery disease or rate-dependent ventricular arrhythmias in whom wide fluctuations of heart rate should be avoided.

Oseroff and colleagues[79] investigated the indications for permanent mode change in 423 patients with DDD pulse generators implanted over a period of 5 years. The DDD mode was abandoned in 78 patients (18.4 per cent), with 55 programmed to the VVI mode (13.0 per cent), 15 to the DVI mode (3.5 per cent), 7 to the VDD mode (1.6 per cent) and 1 to the AAI mode (0.2 per cent). The reasons were either technical or pathophysiologic. The technical reasons involved 44 patients (56.4 per cent), with a high atrial pacing threshold in 8, no atrial sensing in 20, neither atrial pacing nor sensing in 5, myopotential interference in 2, endless loop tachycardia in 6, diaphragmatic stimulation in 2, and local pectoral stimulation in 1. The pathophysiologic reasons involved 34 patients (43.5 per cent), 32 with sustained atrial arrhythmias, 22 with atrial fibrillation, 8 with atrial flutter, 2 with junctional rhythm, 1 with ventricular pseudofusion, and 1 with angina at normal atrial rates. Soler and associates[86] also reported the incidence of mode change in 150 consecutive patients followed over 1.0 to 75.0 months (average, 27.5 months). Eighty-eight of all pacer systems were still in the VDD or DDD mode. Conversion from the DDD mode to another per-

manent mode is indicated only when complications cannot be treated by the usual programming methods. Programming a pacemaker out of the DDD mode constitutes the least desirable action because a new mode may be associated with unwanted characteristics and may lack the benefits of DDD pacing. A DDD pulse generator should be programmed to the VVI mode in established atrial fibrillation, but not necessarily in the presence of paroxysmal atrial fibrillation, when it should preferably be programmed to the DDI mode in most cases.

REFERENCES

1. Adler S, Whistler S, Martin R: Advances in single chamber pacemaker diagnostic data. Clin Prog Electrophysiol Pacing [Suppl] 4:13, 1986.
2. Alt E, Wirtzfeld A, Seidl K, et al: Delayed atrial excitation following bifocal pacemaker stimulation. Z Kardiol 72:245, 1983.
3. Alt EU, von Bibra H, Blömer H: Different benefit AV intervals with DDD pacing after sensed and paced atrial events. J Electrophysiol 1:250, 1987.
4. Ausubel K, Klementowicz P, Furman S: The AV interval during DDD pacing. Clin Prog Electrophysiol Pacing 4:60, 1986.
5. Ausubel K, Klementowicz P, Furman S: Interatrial conduction during cardiac pacing. PACE 9:302, 1986.
6. Barber K, Amikam S, Furman S: Atrial lead malposition in a dual-chamber (DDD, M) pacemaker. Chest 84:766, 1983.
7. Barold SS: The DDI mode of cardiac pacing. PACE 10:480, 1987.
8. Barold SS, Belott PH: Behavior of the ventricular triggering period of DDD pacemakers. PACE 10:1237, 1987.
9. Barold SS, Falkoff MD, Ong LS, Heinle RA: Programmability in DDD pacing. PACE 7:1159, 1984.
10. Barold SS, Falkoff MD, Ong LS, Heinle RA: Hyperkalemia-induced failure of atrial capture during dual chamber cardiac pacing. J Am Coll Cardiol 10:467, 1987.
11. Barold SS, Falkoff MD, Ong LS, et al: Resetting of DDD pulse generators due to cold exposure. PACE 11:736, 1988.
12. Barold SS, Ong LS, Falkoff MD, Heinle RA: Cross talk or self-inhibition in dual-chambered pacemakers. In Barold SS (ed): Modern Cardiac Pacing. Mount Kisco, NY, Futura Publishing Co, 1985, p. 615.

13. Barold SS, Nanda NC, Ong LS, et al: Determination of successful atrial capture during unipolar dual-chambered pacing. In Barold SS (ed): Modern Cardiac Pacing. Mount Kisco, NY, Futura Publishing Co, 1985, p 677.

14. Beaver BB, Maloney JD, Castle LW, et al: Design-dependent cross-talk in a second generation DDD pacemaker. PACE 9:65, 1986.

15. Belott PH, Sands S, Warren J: Resetting of DDD pacemakers due to EMI. PACE 7:169, 1984.

16. Bourke J, Gold RG, Adams PC, Bexton RS: Diathermy-induced loss of DDD pacemaker identity. Ann Thorac Surg 40:97, 1985.

17. Bricker JT, Ward KA, Zinner A, Gilette PC: Decrease in canine endocardial and epicardial voltages with exercise: Implications for pacemaker sensing. PACE 9:282, 1986.

18. Bricker JT, Garson G, Traweek MS, et al: The use of exercise testing in children to evaluate abnormalities of pacemaker function not apparent at rest. PACE 8:656, 1985.

19. Byrd CL, Schwartz SJ, Gonzales M, et al: Crosstalk: Mechanisms and clinical significance. Clin Prog Electrophysiol Pacing [Suppl] 4:52, 1986.

20. Byrd CL, Schwartz SJ, Gonzales M, et al: Mechanisms and clinical significance of crosstalk in Cosmos and AFP pulse generators. PACE 9:279, 1986.

21. Castellanet MJ, Garza J, Shaner SP, Messenger JC: Telemetry of programmed and measured data in pacing system evaluation and follow-up. J Electrophysiol 1:360, 1987.

22. Catania SL, Maue-Dickson W: AV delay latency compensation. J Electrophysiol 1:242, 1987.

23. Chomka E, Edwards-Strauss L, Papp MA, Hauser RC: Myopotential oversensing in DDD pacemakers. PACE 8:295, 1985.

24. Clarke M, Allen A: Use of telemetered electrograms in the assessment of normal pacemaker function. J Electrophysiol 1:388, 1987.

25. Cosmos technical manual. Freeport, TX, Intermedics, 1985.

26. Del Negro A, Cohen A, Miller F, et al: Automatic extension of the ventricular refractory period: A cause of sensing failure during tachycardia in dual-chamber pacemakers. PACE 9:304, 1986.

27. Delta Model 925 technical manual, type DDD dual chamber pulse generator. St Paul, MN, Cardiac Pacemakers, Inc, 1985.

28. Den Dulk K, Lindemans TW, Bär FW, Wellens HJJ: Pacemaker related tachycardias. PACE 5:476, 1982.

29. Drinkovic N, Ferek B, Jursic M: Subcostal M-mode echocardiography of the right atrial wall in evaluation of cardiac arrhythmias and pacing. PACE 8:110, 1985.

30. Duffin EG: The marker channel period: A telemetric diagnostic aid. PACE 7:1165, 1984.

31. Faerestrand S, Ohm OJ: A time-related study of the hemodynamic benefit of atrioventricular synchronous pacing evaluated by Doppler echocardiography. PACE 8:88, 1985.

32. Faerestrand S, Oie B, Ohm OJ: Noninvasive assessment by Doppler echocardiography of hemodynamic responses to temporary AV synchronous and to ventricular pacing. PACE 9:301, 1986.

33. Falkenberg E, Baker R, Martin R: Advances in dual chamber pacemaker diagnostics. Clin Prog Electrophysiol Pacing [Suppl] 4:14, 1986.

34. Famularo MA, Kennedy HL: Ambulatory electro-cardiography in the assessment of pacemaker function. Am Heart J 104:1086, 1982.

35. Fetter J, Hall DM, Hoff GL, Reeder JT: The effects of myopotential interference on unipolar and bipolar dual chamber pacemakers in the DDD mode. Clin Prog Electrophysiol Pacing 3:368, 1985.

36. Forfang K, Otterstad JE, Ihlen H: Optimal atrioventricular delay in physiological pacing determined by Doppler echocardiography. PACE 9:17, 1986.

37. Floro J, Castellanet M, Florio J, Messenger J: DDI: A new mode for cardiac pacing. Clin Prog Pacing Electrophysiol 2:255, 1984.

38. Fröhlig G, Sen S, Blank W, et al: Susceptibility of a unipolar dual chamber pacemaker to chest wall myopotentials. In Pérez Gómez (ed): Cardiac Pacing: Electrophysiology: Tachyarrhythmias. Mount Kisco, NY, Futura Media Services, 1985, p 698.

39. Fröhlig G, Tyckmans J, Doenecke P, et al: Noise reversion of a dual-chamber pacemaker without noise. PACE 9:690, 1986.

40. Frumin H, Goldberg M, Goldman L, Beyler M: Clinical utility and limitations of a permanent cardiac pacing "event counter." PACE 8:296, 1985.

41. Furman S, Reicher-Reiss H, Escher DJW: Atrioventricular sequential pacing and pacemakers. Chest 63:783, 1973.

42. Gabry MD, Behrens M, Andrews C, et al: Myopotential interference in programmable polarity DDD pacemakers. PACE 9:279, 1986.

43. Galvao SS, Vignon MC, Godenir JP, Dodinot BP: Dual chamber pacemaker inhibition related to "crosstalk." PACE 8:A-96, 1985.

44. Gladstone PJ, Duxbury GB, Berman ND: Arrhythmia diagnosis by electrogram telemetry involving a dual chamber pacemaker. Chest 91:115, 1987.

45. Gould L, Patel C, Betzu R, et al: Pacemaker failure following electrocautery. Clin Prog Electrophysiol Pacing 4:53, 1986.

46. Greenspon AJ, Volosin KJ: "Pseudo" loss of atrial sensing by a DDD pacemaker. PACE 10:943, 1987.

47. Greenspon AJ, Cox J, Greenberg RM: Atrial lead dislodgement with a DDD pacemaker. PACE 9:436, 1986.

48. Halperin JL, Camuñas JL, Stern EH, et al: Myopotential interference with DDD pacemakers: Endocardial electrographic telemetry in the diagnosis of pacemaker related arrhythmias. Am J Cardiol 54:97, 1984.

49. Hayes DL, Trusty J, Christiansen J, et al: A prospective study of electrocautery's effect on pacemaker function. PACE 10:442, 1987.

50. Janosik D, Pearson A, Redd R, et al: The importance of atrioventricular delay fallback in optimizing cardiac output during physiologic pacing. PACE 10:410, 1987.

51. Kelen GJ, Bloomfield DA, Hardage M, et al: A clinical evaluation of an improved Holter monitoring technique for artificial pacemaker function. PACE 3:192, 1980.

52. Kersschot IE, Ortmans P, Goethals MA: Atrial pacing bigeminy: A manifestation of crosstalk. PACE 8:402, 1985.

53. Kersschot IE, Goethals MA, Vanagt EJ, et al: Temporary AVI pacing by chest wall stimulation. PACE 8:4, 1985.

54. Konz KH, Schick KD, Clausnitzer R, et al: Ungewöhnliche Rhythmusstörungen bei DDD-Schrittmacher. Z Kardiol 74:552, 1985.

55. Kruse I, Markowitz T, Ryden L: Timing markers showing pacemaker behavior to aid in the follow-up of a physiological pacemaker. PACE 6:801, 1983.

56. Labovitz AJ, Williams GA, Redd RM, Kennedy HL: Noninvasive assessment of pacemaker hemodynamics by Doppler echocardiography: Importance of left atrial size. J Am Coll Cardiol 6:260, 1985.

57. Lamas GA, Antman EM, Gold JP, et al: Pacemaker backup mode reversion and injury during cardiac surgery. Ann Thorac Surg 41:155, 1986.

58. Langenfeld H, Maisch B, Kochsiek K: Variations of the intra-atrial potential in patients with a DDD pacemaker. In Belhassen B, Feldman S, Copperman Y (eds): Cardiac Pacing and Electrophysiology: Proceedings of the VIIIth World Symposium on Cardiac Pacing and Electrophysiology. Jerusalem, Keterpress Enterprises, 1987, p 185.

59. Leman RB, Kratz JM: Radionuclide evaluation of dual chamber pacing: Comparison between variable AV intervals and ventricular pacing. PACE 8:408, 1985.

60. Levine PA: Confirmation of atrial capture and determination of atrial capture thresholds in DDD pacing systems. Clin Prog Pacing Electrophysiol 2:465, 1985.

61. Levine PA: Cross stimulation: The unexpected stimulation of the unpaced chamber. PACE 8:600, 1985.

62. Levine PA: Normal and abnormal rhythms associated with dual-chamber pacemakers. Cardiol Clin 3:595, 1985.

63. Levine PA: Magnet rates and recommended replacement time indicators of lithium pacemakers 1986.Clin Prog Electrophysiol Pacing 4:608, 1986.

64. Levine PA: The complementary role of electrogram, event marker, and measured data telemetry in the assessment of pacing system function. J Electrophysiol 1:404, 1987.

65. Levine PA, Lindenberg BS: Diagnostic data: An aid to the follow-up and assessment of the pacing system. J Electrophysiol 1:396, 1987.

66. Levine PA, Lindenberg BS: Upper rate limit circuit induced rate slowing. PACE 10:310, 1987.

67. Levine PA, Brodsky SJ, Seltzer JP: AVI pacing: A new diagnostic and therapeutic pacing modality. PACE 6:A–35, 1983.

68. Levine PA, Sholder J, Duncan JL: Clinical benefits of telemetered electrograms in assessment of DDD function. PACE 7:1170, 1984.

69. Levine PA, Balady GJ, Lazar HL, et al: Electrocautery and pacemakers: Management of the paced patient subject to electrocautery. Ann Thorac Surg 41:313, 1986.

70. Luceri RM, Castellanos A, Thurer RJ: Telemetry of intracardiac electrograms: Applications in spontaneous and induced arrhythmias. J Electrophysiol 1:417, 1987.

71. Markewitz A, Bernheim C, Kemkes BM: Clinical concerns of the blanking period. PACE 9:293, 1986.

72. Markewitz A, Hemmer W, Weinhold C: Complications in a dual chamber pacing: A six year experience. PACE 9:1014, 1986.

73. Mehta D, Gilmour SM, Ward DE, Camm JA: Optimizing the atrio-ventricular delay at rest and during exercise with atrioventricular synchronous pacing. Circulation 76 [Suppl IV]:IV–80, 1987.

74. Michalek RE, Williams WH, Hatcher CR Jr: My-opotential inhibition of unipolar pacing in children. PACE 8:25, 1985.

75. Nathan AW, Camm AJ: Double ventricular pacing in a patient with a "DDD" universal pacemaker. PACE 7:432, 1985.

76. Nyendwa P, Haffajee C, Gold R, et al: Long term experience with 158 DDD pacer implants. PACE 10:440, 1987.

77. Olson WH, Goldreyer BA, Goldreyer BN: Computer-generated diagnostic diagrams for pacemaker rhythm analysis and pacing system evaluation. J Electrophysiol 1:376, 1987.

78. Olson WH, McConnell MV, Sah RL, et al: Pacemaker diagnostic diagrams. PACE 8:691, 1985.

79. Oseroff O, Klementowicz P, Andrews C, et al: Indications for permanent mode change during DDD pacing. PACE 10:409, 1987.

80. Quintal R, Dhurandhar RW, Jain RK: Myopotential interference with a DDD pacemaker: Report of a case. PACE 7:37, 1984.

81. Quintal R, Dhurandhar RW, Jain RK: Pseudo failure of sensing in patients with universal pacemakers and junctional rhythms. J Electrocardiol 17:205, 1984.

82. Rao G, Winzelberg G, Flaherty P: What is the optimum AV interval in DDD pacing. Angiology 36:253, 1985.

83. Reynolds D, Combs W, Bennett T: "Crosstalk" in bipolar DDD pacemakers. PACE 10:413, 1987.

84. Rozanski JJ, Blankstein RL, Lister JW: Pacemaker arrhythmias: Myopotential triggering of pacemaker mediated tachycardia. PACE 6:795, 1983.

85. Sanders R, Martin R, Frumin H, Goldberg MJ: Data storage and retrieval by implantable pacemakers for diagnostic purposes. PACE 7:1228, 1984.

86. Soler M, Pfisterer M, Cueni T, Burkart F: Long term follow-up of dual chamber pacemakers: Incidence and duration of physiologic pacing. PACE 10:745, 1987.

87. Stark F, Farshidi A, Hager WD, Donaldson MC: Unusual presentation of DDD pacemaker system malfunction. PACE 8:255, 1985.

88. Stewart WJ, Dicola VC, Harthorne JW, et al: Doppler ultrasound measurement of cardiac output in patients with physiologic pacemakers: Effects of left ventricular function and retrograde ventriculoatrial conduction. Am J Cardiol 54:308, 1984.

89. Sudduth BK, Morris DL, Gertz EW: Noise mode response at peak exercise in a DDD pacemaker. PACE 8:746, 1985.

90. Sutton R, Kenny RA: The natural history of sick sinus syndrome. PACE 9:1110, 1986.

91. Sutton R, Ingram A, Kenny RA, et al: Clinical experience of DDI pacing. In Belhassen B, Feldman S, Copperman Y (eds): Cardiac Pacing and Electrophysiology: Proceedings of the VIIIth World Symposium on Cardiac Pacing and Electrophysiology. Jerusalem, Keterpress Enterprises, 1987, p 161.

92. Switzer DF, Nanda NC, Barold SS: Two-dimensional and Doppler echocardiographic techniques in cardiac pacing. In Barold SS (ed): Modern Cardiac Pacing. Mount Kisco, NY, Futura Publishing Co, 1985, p 919.

93. Sykosch HJ, Pletschen B, Thornander H, et al: Post implant evolution of detected P-wave amplitude. PACE 10:730, 1987.

94. Technical manual, Symbios 7005 and 7006 universal A-V telemetric pacemaker. Minneapolis, MN, Medtronic, 1985.

95. Torresani J, Ebagosti A, Allard-Latour G: Pacemaker syndrome with DDD pacing. PACE 7:1148, 1984.
96. Van Mechelen R, Vanderkerckhove V: Atrial capture and dual chamber pacing. PACE 9:21, 1986.
97. Van Mechelen R, Hart CT, deBoer H: Failure to sense P waves during DDD pacing. PACE 9:498, 1986.
98. Von Bibra H, Busch U, Ulm K, et al: Mitral valve closure determining left ventricular filling time in VDD pacemaker patients. Br Heart J 55:355, 1986.
99. Warren J, Messenger J, Belott P: A-V interval hysteresis: A provision for improved tracking behavior in a DDD pacemaker. PACE 8:A–9, 1985.
100. Watson WS: Myopotential sensing in cardiac pacemakers. *In* Barold SS (ed): Modern Cardiac Pacing. Mount Kisco, NY, Future Publishing Co, 1985, p. 813.
101. Westveer D, McCurley S, Stewart J, Timmis G: Reprogramming guided by telemetry of intrinsic pacemaker diagnostic data: The effect of pacemaker use. PACE 9:279, 1986.
102. Winter UJ, Hoeher M, Behrenbeck DW, et al:

Holter monitoring of the intracardiac electrogram. Clin Prog Electrophysiol Pacing [Suppl] 4:15, 1986.
103. Winter UJ, Hoeher M, Behrenbeck DW, et al: Holter recording of the intracardiac electrogram: First clinical experience. PACE 9:292, 1986.
104. Wish M, Fletcher RD, Gottdiener JS, Cohen AI: Importance of left atrial timing in the programming of dual-chamber pacemakers. Am J Cardiol 60:566, 1987.
105. Wish M, Gottdiener J, Fletcher R, Cohen A: Use of M-mode echocardiograms for determination of optimal left atrial timing in patients with dual chamber pacemakers. PACE 9:290, 1986.
106. Wish M, Gottdiener JC, Cohen AI, et al: Use of M-mode echocardiograms for determination of interatrial conduction times in dual chamber pacemaker patient. PACE 8:297, 1985.
107. Young TE, Byrd CL, Greenberg JJ, et al: Pacemaker center evaluation vs. ambulatory Holter monitoring in the detection of acute atrial malsensing. PACE 8:791, 1985.
108. Zimmern SH, Clark MF, Austin WK, et al: Characteristics and clinical effects of myopotential signals in a unipolar DDD pacemaker population. PACE 9:1019, 1986.

13

USE OF NONINVASIVE CARDIAC DIAGNOSTIC TECHNIQUES IN PATIENTS WITH CARDIAC PACEMAKERS

GILBERT J. PERRY *and* NAVIN C. NANDA

Early echocardiographic studies of pacemakers focused primarily on visualization of pacing leads and identification of complications of pacemaker insertion. However, more recently, Doppler echocardiographic techniques have been applied to the evaluation of pacemaker physiology, with particular reference to the influence of pacing parameters, such as pacing site, pacing mode, and atrioventricular (AV) interval on cardiac performance. This chapter will review both the traditional role of echocardiography in guiding pacemaker placement and identifying complications of pacemaker insertion, and the emerging research and clinical applications of Doppler echocardiography to the evaluation of pacemaker physiology.

TWO-DIMENSIONAL ECHOCARDIOGRAPHY IN THE PATIENT WITH A CARDIAC PACEMAKER

Identification and Positioning of Pacemaker Leads

Two-dimensional echocardiography can be used to identify pacing catheters and to follow their course through the venous system and heart.[34, 36, 39, 49] The ultrasound beam is strongly reflected by the pacing wire in the center of the pacing catheter. When the beam transects the pacing wires, the result is a single, bright, thick, linear echo due to reflection of the beam, often with an area of increased lucency or shadowing immediately posterior to the wire resulting from incomplete penetration of the ultrasound beam through the wire[39] (Fig. 13–1). Alternately, two linear, parallel echoes separated by an echo-free space will result if the transducer is angled slightly so that the echo beam traverses the Silastic sheath of the pacing catheter without transecting the pacing wire (Fig. 13–2). Reverberation bands radiating from the distal tip of the catheter are frequently noted; these occur as a result of the metallic ring electrode located there and are helpful in identifying the tip of the pacing catheter. Bipolar electrodes may result in two sets of reverberation bands (Fig. 13–3). These various echocardiographic features allow pacing catheters in the right side of the heart to be distinguished from other structures in the right side of the heart that may cause bright, linear echoes, such as right ventricular muscle bands or the tricuspid valve.

The pacing catheter can usually be traced through its entire course from the superior vena cava to the right ventricle by using multiple transducer positions. The superior vena cava is best visualized from the suprasternal or the right parasternal window. The right atrium is well visualized from the parasternal short

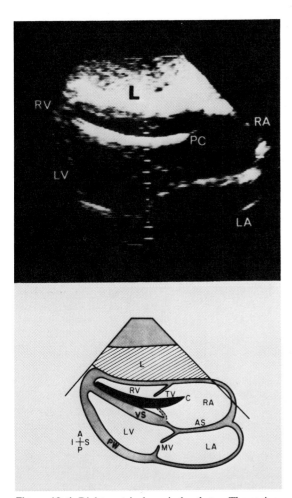

Figure 13–1. Right ventricular apical catheter. The pacing catheter in this patient appears as a dense, bright, linear echo that is easily recognized. The catheter tip is located in the right ventricular apex. This examination was performed by placing the transducer in the subcostal region. A = anterior; AS = atrial septum; I = inferior; L = liver; LA = left atrium; LV = left ventricle; MV = mitral valve; P = posterior; PW = left ventricular posterior wall; C, PC = pacing catheter; RA = right atrium; RV = right ventricle; S = superior; TV = tricuspid valve; VS = ventricular septum. (From Nanda NC, Barold SS: Usefulness of echocardiography in cardiac pacing. PACE 5:222, 1982; with permission.)

axis, the right parasternal, the right ventricular inflow, the subcostal windows. The right ventricle can be well imaged from the parasternal long axis, the apical, and the subcostal windows; the last-named usually best demonstrates the right ventricular course of the pacing wire and its termination at the right ventricular apex. These windows can be utilized to guide pacing wire placement either for electrophysiologic studies[10, 39] or for temporary or permanent pacemaker implantation.

The advantage of echocardiography over fluoroscopy in the electrophysiology laboratory is the ability of the former to identify more exactly the intracardiac position of the catheter tip. The subcostal window has been used successfully to guide the pacing catheter to the bundle of His during electrophysiologic studies (Fig. 13–4).[10, 39] Drawbacks to using echocardiography to guide placement of pacing catheters include the necessity for an extra person well trained in echocardiography to be present in the catheterization laboratory; the inability to visualize the catheter in patients with poor windows or with very large cardiac chambers; the longer time required to identify and follow the catheter by echocardiography compared with fluoroscopy; and the frequent necessity for multiple views using different windows to follow the catheter throughout its intravascular course, which generally is not practical in the catheterization laboratory. Thus, whereas echocardiography is useful and practical for following the catheter tip over small distances or for identifying the exact intracardiac location of a pacing catheter, fluoroscopy is more efficient for rapid advancement of the catheter over large distances and for guiding passage of the catheter through the tricuspid valve.

As a result of these limitations, echocardiographic guidance of pacing catheters is generally reserved for special situations, such as pregnancy, in which fluoroscopy is contraindicated, or complex congenital anomalies, in which echocardiography may more readily confirm placement of the catheter in the desired position. Echocardiography has been successfully utilized to guide catheter placement to the left ventricular apex from the inferior vena cava in a patient with tricuspid atresia and an atrial septal defect (Fig. 13–5).[39] Echocardiography is also useful in congenital anomalies of the venous circulation, such as persistent left superior vena cava with absent right superior vena cava. The presence of a dilated coronary sinus is usually the first echocardiographic clue to this diagnosis.[7] The aberrant superior vena cava can be directly visualized from the suprasternal or supraclavicular window, and its identity as a venous structure can be confirmed either by injection of agitated saline in an ipsilateral arm vein, in conjunction with two-dimensional echocardiography, or by use of pulse or color Doppler echocardiography. Placement of permanent pacing catheters in the coronary sinus has been described in this situation[52] and could be guided by echocardiography if desired.

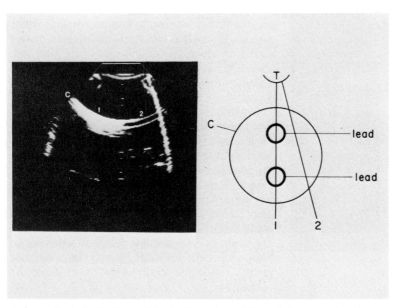

Figure 13–2. In vitro studies of a pacing catheter. A bipolar pacing catheter was immersed in a water bath, and the two-dimensional transducer (T) was placed at the water surface. The left side (1) of the catheter was manipulated so that the ultrasonic beam passed centrally through the two pacing leads, producing a dense linear image associated with posterior reverberations. The right side (2) of the catheter was slightly moved so that the beam did not pass through the pacing leads but only through the surrounding Silastic material. The resulting image demonstrates two linear echoes that represent the two interfaces of the catheter with the surrounding water medium. The echo-free space enclosed between the leading and trailing edges of the catheter is related to the homogeneous nature of the Silastic material, which has a uniform acoustic impedance. Both the leading and the trailing edges of the catheter present as linear echoes at the water interface because the acoustic impedance of water is significantly different from that of the catheter. C = catheter. (From Nanda NC, Barold SS: Usefulness of echocardiography in cardiac pacing. PACE 5:22, 1982; with permission.)

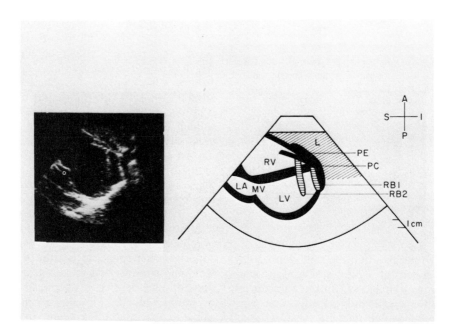

Figure 13–3. Two-dimensional echocardiogram showing perforation by a bipolar catheter (PC) through the apex of the right ventricle (RV). The tip of the pacing catheter is seen extending beyond the epicardium. The coexisting pericardial effusion (PE) facilitates identification of the tip. Prominent reverberation bands (RB1 and RB2) emanate from the two electrodes and further define the tip area. A = anterior; I = inferior; L = liver; LA = left atrium; LV = left ventricle; MV = mitral valve; P = posterior; S = superior. (From Switzer DF, Nanda NC: Doppler-echocardiographic assessment of cardiac pacemakers. Cardiol Clin 3:631, 1985.)

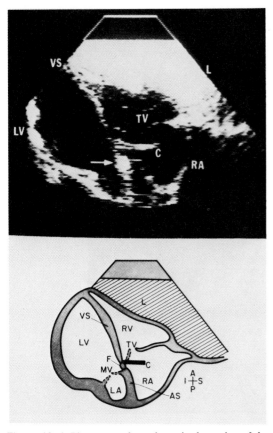

Figure 13–4. Placement of a catheter in the region of the bundle of His. In this patient, the catheter was advanced under direct echocardiographic monitoring without using fluoroscopy, and the tip was positioned just beyond the central fibrous body, touching the superior portion of the ventricular septum (*arrow*). A = anterior; AS = atrial septum; C = pacing catheter; F = central fibrous body; I = interior; L = liver; LA = left atrium; LV = left ventricle; MV = mitral valve; P = posterior; RA = right atrium; RV = right ventricle; S = superior; TV = tricuspid valve; VS = ventricular septum. (From Nanda NC, Barold SS: Usefulness of echocardiography in cardiac pacing. PACE 5:222, 1982; with permission.)

Diagnosis of Iatrogenic Complications

Anatomic complications that have been reported following pacemaker implantation include myocardial perforation, hemopericardium, pacemaker-induced thrombosis, malposition of pacing leads, and, rarely, endocarditis involving the pacemaker or tricuspid valve or both.[3–6, 8, 12, 16, 21, 22, 25, 28, 30, 32, 37, 40, 42, 45, 47] Two-dimensional echocardiography is the diagnostic tool of choice for most of these complications.

Myocardial perforation by both transvenous and epicardial pacemakers has been success-

fully diagnosed by two-dimensional echocardiography.[6, 21, 42] Myocardial perforation is rare, with an incidence of 0.7 per cent in one retrospective review of 1376 pacemaker insertions.[22] Echocardiography is indicated in patients in whom pacemaker perforation is suspected clinically owing to hemodynamic evidence of tamponade, loss of pacing, increased threshold, or electrocardiographic evidence of perforation. In these patients, echocardiography can confirm the presence of pacemaker perforation, reveal the chamber or cavity into which the perforation has occurred, and evaluate any secondary complications due to the perforation, such as pericardial effusion or tamponade. Echocardiography may at times be superior to chest radiography or even ventriculography in making this diagnosis, since the exact location of the tip of the catheter can be more readily identified echocardiographically[6, 21] (Figs. 13–3 and 13–6 to 13–8). When using echocardiography to localize the tip of the pacing catheter, caution must be taken not to confuse pacemaker reverberations, which may be visualized outside the right ventricular cavity, with the true course of the pacing catheter.

The incidence of thrombosis of the pacing wire or of the vein occupied by the pacing wire is uncertain. In series retrospectively reviewing the incidence of various pacemaker complications, the development of symptomatic occlusion of a large vein or pulmonary thromboembolism from thrombosis of a pacing wire is decidedly rare.[40] Autopsy series or prospective series in which venograms are performed on an unselected group of patients with permanent transvenous pacemakers, on the other hand, reveal a very high incidence of thrombotic complications, most of which are asymptomatic.[25, 37, 47] In one series of 100 patients, 39 per cent had an abnormal venogram, including 15 per cent with complete occlusion of the axillary or subclavian vein,[37] while in another series involving 34 consecutive patients, 44 per cent had 50 to 90 per cent stenosis of the subclavian vein and an additional 21 per cent had complete subclavian vein occlusion. The marked difference in the incidence of thrombosis between the retrospective and prospective series results from the fact that almost all of the venous thrombotic events are asymptomatic and thus will not be detected unless specifically looked for. The pacing catheter is also frequently involved in thrombosis and fibrosis. Autopsy examination of pacing catheters reveals marked thrombosis of the pacing

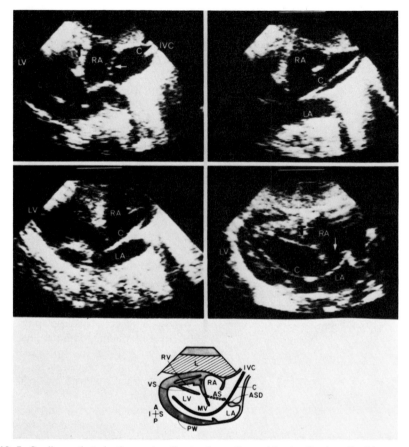

Figure 13–5. Cardiac catheterization under direct echocardiographic visualization. In this young patient with tricuspid atresia, the catheter was passed under direct two-dimensional echocardiographic monitoring (using the subcostal approach) from the inferior vena cava *(upper left)* into the right atrium toward an atrial septal defect *(upper right)*, then was moved into the left atrium through the atrial septal defect *(lower left)*, and finally was maneuvered into the left ventricle with the tip lying near the apex *(lower right)*. Fluoroscopy was not used during these manipulations. LV = left ventricle; PW = left ventricular posterior wall; RA = right atrium; RV = right ventricle; T = atretic tricuspid valve; VS = ventricular septum; arrow in upper left panel = a large eustachian valve; C = catheter; IVC = inferior vena cava; LA = left atrium; vertical arrow in lower right panel = a large atrial septal defect; ASD = atrial septal defect; AS = atrial septum; L = liver; MV = mitral valve; I = inferior; S = superior; A = anterior; P = posterior. (From Nanda NC, Barold SS: Usefulness of echocardiography in cardiac pacing. PACE 5:222, 1982; with permission.)

catheter within 4 to 5 days of implantation.[25] Subsequently, there is fibrosis and endothelialization of the pacing catheter, ultimately resulting in a fibrotic sheath covering the entire extent of the catheter. Thickening of the pacing catheter from this chronic thrombotic process is a relatively common echocardiographic finding in patients with longstanding transvenous pacing wires; at times this thickening may be quite marked. Rarely, a large, localized area of thrombosis may develop around the pacing catheter in the right atrium or right ventricle. The incidence of this complication is uncertain, but it is clear that symptomatic pulmonary thromboembolism either from a pacing catheter or from a vein thrombosed by

a pacing catheter is extremely rare. In 1979, Kinney and colleagues[30] reported a patient with recurrent pulmonary emboli secondary to a right atrial thrombus attached to a pacing catheter and, on review of the literature, could find only nine case reports of pulmonary embolism associated with pacing catheters. On the other hand, small pulmonary thromboemboli were found in two of nine patients with pacing catheters in one autopsy series, suggesting that subclinical pulmonary thromboemboli may be more common than generally suspected.[25] Pacing catheter thrombosis as a source of pulmonary emboli has been diagnosed by two-dimensional echocardiography.[45] The diagnosis by echocardiography is most

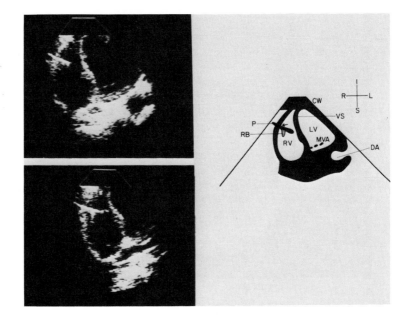

Figure 13–6. Pacing catheter perforation. The right ventricular pacing catheter (P) is seen extending outside the heart through the right ventricular free wall *(arrow)*. CW = chest wall; RB = reverberation; RV = right ventricle; LV = left ventricle; MVA = mitral valve apparatus; VS = ventricular septum; DA = descending aorta; I = inferior; S = superior; R = right; L = left. (From Nanda NC: Evaluation of pacing function by real time two-dimensional echocardiography. Impulse 17:2, 1980; with permission of Cardiac Pacemakers, Inc.)

secure when the thrombus is large, localized, and/or mobile. Smaller degrees of thrombosis are difficult to distinguish echocardiographically from the normal thrombosis and fibrosis of pacing catheters described above. The optimal management for asymptomatic patients noted to have substantial thickening of a pacing catheter on routine echocardiographic examination is uncertain, because of limited information on the natural history of this process and the inability to distinguish chronic organized fibrosis from more active thrombosis by echocardiography. Conservative management with antibiotic prophylaxis for surgical procedures and careful echocardiographic follow-up seems reasonable in almost all asymptomatic patients, given the high incidence of pacemaker-associated asymptomatic thrombosis and the low incidence of embolic or symptomatic veno-occlusive complications. Surgical removal of the pacing catheter may be indicated for symptomatic veno-occlusion, infection of the pacing wire, and recurrent thromboembolism refractory to anticoagulant therapy. Patients noted echocardiographically to have very large or mobile thrombi of the pacing catheter may be at higher risk of developing complications, and thus more aggressive management

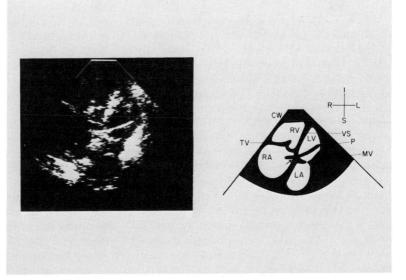

Figure 13–7. Perforation *(arrow)* of the atrioventricular (AV) septum. Two-dimensional echocardiogram in the apical four-chamber view shows the pacing catheter (P) entering the left ventricle (LV) from the right atrium (RA) through an area of the septum between the mitral (MV) and tricuspid valves (TV). The tip of the catheter is lodged against the middle portion of the left ventricular posterior wall. CW = chest wall; I = inferior; L = left; LA = left atrium; R = right; RV = right ventricle; S = superior; VS = ventricular septum. (From Gondi B, Nanda NC: Real-time two-dimensional echocardiographic features of pacemaker perforation. Circulation 64:97, 1981; by permission of the American Heart Association, Inc.)

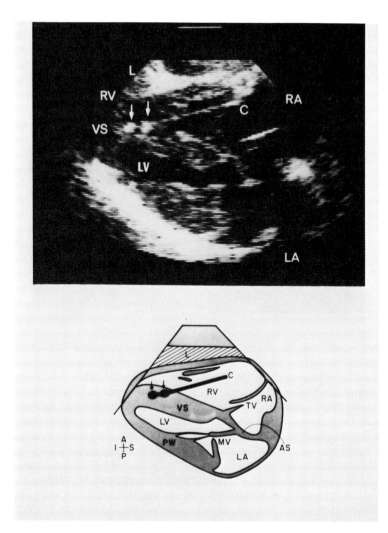

Figure 13–8. Partial perforation of the ventricular septum by pacing catheter. In this patient, the temporary pacing catheter has partially perforated the ventricular septum, so that both the tip and the proximal ring electrodes *(arrows)* lie within the septal muscle. This examination was performed by placing the transducer in the subcostal region. RV = right ventricle; VS = ventricular septum; LV = left ventricle; PW = left ventricular posterior wall; C = pacing catheter; RA = right atrium; LA = left atrium; L = liver; AS = atrial septum; MV = mitral valve; TV = tricuspid valve; I = inferior; S = superior; A = anterior; P = posterior. (From Nanda NC, Barold SS: Usefulness of echocardiography in cardiac pacing. PACE 5:222, 1982; with permission.)

of this subgroup may be indicated even if they are asymptomatic. Unfortunately, little information is available regarding the natural history in this situation.

Pacemakers have rarely been reported to cause serious damage to the tricuspid valve, including tricuspid laceration,[16] avulsion (following removal of an entrapped pacing lead),[32] and endocarditis.[3] It is not uncommon for the aforementioned catheter fibrosis to involve the tricuspid valve apparatus, but fortunately, clinically important tricuspid regurgitation as a result of this is rare.[28] A lacerated or flail tricuspid valve can be detected echocardiographically, and the degree of tricuspid regurgitation can be estimated by pulsed or color Doppler echocardiography. Less severe degrees of structural damage may not be detectable echocardiographically but may be suspected if significant, unexplained tricuspid regurgitation is observed on Doppler examination. Infection of permanent pacemakers is

estimated to involve less than 6 per cent of all units and generally is limited to subcutaneous infection of the pulse generator pocket, with *Staphylococcus aureus* the most common pathogen.[4] If pulse generator pocket infection is not diagnosed and treated early, the infection may spread to involve the pacing wire and subsequently the heart. Alternately, endocarditis in some instances may be initiated by infection of a thrombus on the pacing wire as a result of bacteremia from a distal source.[4, 42] Several authors have reported success in visualizing pacing wire vegetations echocardiographically.[5, 8, 12] However, given the common occurrence of pacemaker thickening described earlier, one would anticipate difficulty distinguishing echocardiographically a vegetation of the pacing electrode from the much more common sterile thrombosis and fibrosis of the electrode. Large, localized areas of thickening would be more suggestive of a possible vegetation, although such localized thickenings can be seen in asymptomatic patients who are clearly not infected. The echocardiographic finding of pacemaker thrombosis in the setting of septicemia should therefore not preclude a careful search for other possible etiologies of infection, particularly if the organism is atypical. Conversely, persistent septicemia is an indication for pacemaker removal regardless of the echocardiographic findings.

Evaluation of Atrial Capture

Echocardiography has been used to detect and time atrial activity in a variety of ventricular and supraventricular arrhythmias in which atrial activity is not evident on the 12-lead electrocardiogram, including atrial fibrillation and flutter, supraventricular tachycardia, and ventricular tachycardia.[11, 43] The same technique can be used to assess atrial capture in patients with atrial pacemakers when the p wave on the surface electrocardiogram is obscured by the pacing artifact or to assess retrograde AV conduction in patients with pacemaker-mediated tachycardia or pacemaker syndrome. Atrial capture can be assessed either directly by analysis of right or left atrial wall motion or indirectly by analysis of AV valvular motion or Doppler inflow through the AV valves. A normal A wave in the M-mode or Doppler trace of either the mitral or the tricuspid valve confirms the presence of normal atrial activity and, when present, obviates the need for further investigation. However, the absence of an A wave in the AV valve on the M-mode or Doppler trace can be due to a variety of conditions, ranging from sinus tachycardia (resulting from combined "A" and "E" waves) to simultaneous atrial and ventricular contraction, as is seen in AV nodal reentrant tachycardia or retrograde VA conduction, and is thus nonspecific. For this reason, direct analysis of atrial wall motion is necessary whenever a normal A wave cannot be identified by M-mode or Doppler evaluation of the AV valves.

Atrial motion is analyzed directly by passing a two-dimensional echocardiographically guided M-mode cursor through the right or left atrial wall to compare the timing of atrial wall motion with a simultaneously displayed electrocardiogram. Left atrial wall motion is best assessed from the suprasternal notch or from the right parasternal or right suprasternal window.[43] The left atrium is visualized in these views just beneath the aortic root. Right atrial wall motion is best evaluated from the subcos-

tal view near the AV groove. Right atrial motion is more reliably visualized in adults and therefore has been more extensively studied. Normal right atrial contraction visualized from the subcostal window results in a prominent posterior movement of the atrial wall coincident with the p wave on the electrocardiogram.[11] Barold and coworkers used this technique to identify the presence or absence of atrial capture in patients with unipolar pacemakers in whom this distinction could not be made on the 12-lead electrocardiogram owing to the large pacing artifact.[1] Drinkovic and colleagues used echocardiographic identification of right atrial activity to diagnose a variety of arrhythmias accurately, including atrial fibrillation, atrial flutter, and AV nodal reentry tachycardia, and have been able to recognize retrograde AV conduction in conditions such as ventricular tachycardia, junctional rhythm, and ventricular pacing.[11] Unfortunately, simultaneous AV contraction due to retrograde ventriculoatrial (VA) conduction, which is frequently the most important atrial activity to recognize echocardiographically because the p wave generally is not visible on the electrocardiogram, is also the most difficult atrial activity to identify because the atrial wall motion is small in this setting and the timing of the wall motion is only slightly different from normal. Drinkovic and colleagues were able to identify atrial activity successfully even in this situation, however. In doubtful situations, pulse or color Doppler echocardiography may be helpful in confirming the presence of retrograde VA conduction by identifying retrograde flow in the superior vena cava during ventricular systole, the Doppler equivalent of "cannon A waves."[24, 49] These techniques can potentially be used to evaluate patients with ventricular pacemakers who are suspected of having pacemaker syndrome and patients with DDD pacemakers who are suspected of having pacemaker-mediated tachycardia. Echocardiography could also conceivably be used in combination with external (transthoracic) ventricular pacing, or in combination with transvenous ventricular pacing in patients with temporary ventricular pacemakers, to screen for retrograde atrial conduction prior to pacemaker implantation.

Evaluation of Ventricular Activation Sequence

The effect of ventricular pacing on the activation sequence of the ventricles has been studied mostly by M-mode echocardiography of the interventricular septum.[20, 27, 34, 53] Normal systolic septal motion consists of brief anterior motion of the septum immediately coincident with electrical activation, followed by sustained posterior motion of the septum (toward the ventricular cavity). During diastole the septum moves gradually anteriorly, interrupted only by a brief posterior movement ("beaking") shortly after maximal mitral opening in early diastole.[15] Several abnormal patterns of septal activation have been described with right ventricular pacing. The most universal abnormality of septal activation in patients with right ventricular pacemakers is a rapid beaking of the septum occurring within 70 msec of the pacing artifact and lasting 40 to 50 msec. This abnormality during the preejection period occurs whenever right ventricular activation precedes left ventricular activation, whether from a right ventricular pacemaker, left bundle branch block, or type B Wolff-Parkinson-White syndrome, and appears to be independent of the location of the pacing catheter in the right ventricle.[20] In one study of patients with transvenous ventricular pacemakers and a right bundle branch pattern during pacing, the presence of this characteristic posterior beaking during the preejection period reliably excluded perforation into the left ventricle as the etiology of the right bundle branch pattern.[27] Septal motion during subsequent ventricular ejection is more variable, however. Some authors report that septal motion during ventricular ejection in patients with ventricular pacemakers is normal, that is, consists of septal thickening with normal systolic motion toward the left ventricular cavity.[53] This observation is in contradistinction to the most common pattern in left bundle branch block, which consists of early posterior beaking followed by either paradoxical anterior motion or flattening during ventricular ejection.[9, 15] However, posterior beaking followed by normal posterior motion has been described in left bundle branch block, while posterior beaking followed by paradoxical septal motion during ventricular ejection has been described in some patients with pacemakers.[20, 27] Gomes and colleagues found that most patients with pacing catheters at the right ventricular apex and all patients with pacing catheters in the right ventricular inflow or outflow tract had paradoxical septal motion during ventricular ejection.[20] Conversely, Zoneraich and associates studied the septal motion of 21 patients with transvenous right ventricular pacemakers and found that septal motion during ejection was abnormal only in those patients with prior septal infarction or right ventricular overload.[53] In patients with left bundle branch block, paradoxical septal motion may be more common in the presence of concomitant left-axis deviation, possibly as a result of early, unopposed activation of the posterior left ventricle.[48] If these findings in left bundle branch block are extrapolated to the case of right ventricular pacemakers, it is possible that the disparate results of various investigators regarding the presence or absence of paradoxical ventricular septal motion during ventricular pacing are attributable to variation in pacing catheter positioning, with more posterior placement of the pacing catheter resulting in paradoxical septal motion.

Two-dimensional echocardiography provides the potential for more detailed analysis of the alterations in ventricular activation that occur with ventricular pacing. Maurer and associates were able to localize the level of the pacing catheter in an open-chest dog model by the markedly decreased systolic fractional shortening in the short-axis view closest to the stimulating electrode.[35] Future studies using two-dimensional echocardiography and computer-assisted edge detection to map the sequence of right and left ventricular activation should allow detailed investigation of the effect of various pacing sites on the sequence of ventricular activation and on regional and global ventricular function.

In conclusion, late activation of the left ventricle, whether due to left bundle branch block or to right ventricular pacing, results almost universally in early posterior beaking of the interventricular septum. Subsequent septal motion during ventricular ejection is variable and appears to be influenced by several factors, which, in the case of right ventricular pacemakers, include the pacing rate, the location of the pacing catheter, and the presence or absence of concomitant septal infarction or right ventricular overload. Ventricular pacing results in altered wall motion and decreased fractional shortening near the site of the pacing electrode, which can be detected echocardiographically. Relatively little is known about the effect of ventricular pacing on global ventricular function, but preliminary studies suggest that the pacing site may influence ventricular function.[35] Echocardiographic studies of regional and global ventricular function during ventricular pacing could conceivably be combined with Doppler echocardiographic studies of cardiac output to assess the effect of different activation patterns and pacemaker locations on overall ventricular performance.

COMBINED DOPPLER AND TWO-DIMENSIONAL ECHOCARDIOGRAPHIC EVALUATION OF PACEMAKER HEMODYNAMICS

Doppler echocardiography in combination with two-dimensional echocardiography has made possible accurate estimation of flow volumes in the heart and, in particular, allows accurate estimation of changes in stroke volume on a beat-to-beat basis. This feature has permitted assessment of the change in stroke volume produced by loss of AV synchrony during ventricular pacing or the rise in stroke volume resulting from optimization of dual-chamber pacing parameters. Analyzing mitral inflow enables one to determine the contribution of atrial contraction to total stroke volume. This section will begin with a summary of the means by which stroke volume is determined by Doppler echocardiography and will then consider the applications of Doppler techniques to pacemaker evaluation.

Doppler Echocardiographic Determination of Stroke Volume

Flow through an orifice can be determined if the cross-sectional area of the orifice and the velocity of flow through the orifice are known. Flow volumes in the heart are determined by Doppler echocardiography by using Doppler to measure blood flow velocities and two-dimensional echocardiography to measure cross-sectional area. Blood flow velocity (v) is derived directly from the Doppler shift of the ultrasound pulse reflected from the moving blood cells:

$$v = cf/2F\cos\theta$$

where c is the velocity of sound in tissue, f is the Doppler frequency shift, F is the carrier frequency of the transmitted pulse, and θ is the angle between the direction of blood flow and the ultrasound beam. The mean blood flow velocity, derived from integration of the Doppler time-velocity trace, is multiplied by the echocardiographically determined cross-sectional area through which blood is flowing, to yield flow volumes:

$$Q = A \int vdt$$

where Q is stroke volume, A is the cross-sectional area where flow velocity is being measured, and $\int vdt$ is the time-velocity integral of the Doppler trace[44] (Fig. 13–9).

With this approach, cardiac flow across any of the valves can theoretically be determined. In practice, most studies have used mitral or aortic flow to derive stroke volume information, because the cross-sectional areas of these valves are most readily determined.[19, 26, 33] Determination of cross-sectional area is the major source of inaccuracy in Doppler determination of stroke volumes. Whereas Doppler velocities can be measured with an interobserver and intraobserver variability of approximately 5 per cent,[18] determination of cross-sectional area generally entails uncertainties on the order of 10 to 15 per cent. Difficulties include the changing size of the valvular or annular orifice during the cardiac cycle, the necessity to be perpendicular to the orifice being measured to define edges most precisely and avoid overestimation of orifice diameter, the need for a high-quality study to identify orifice edges confidently, and uncertainty regarding the optimal site to make the Doppler velocity and two-dimensional area measurements. These uncertainties have limited the determination of absolute stroke volume by Doppler techniques. Fortunately, the accuracy and reproducibility of Doppler flow velocities allow very accurate measurement of changes in stroke volume. Since valvular cross-sectional area does not change appreciably with alterations in stroke volume, changes in stroke volume are directly proportional to changes in the integral of Doppler flow velocity. This approach is particularly applicable to the evaluation of pacemaker physiology, in which one is concerned primarily with changes in stroke volume on a beat-to-beat basis (Fig. 13–10).

The effect of pacing on both mitral and aortic flow velocities has been studied. Aortic flow velocity can be determined from the apex, using the apical five-chamber or long-axis view; from the suprasternal notch or right suprasternal view; or from the right parasternal view (Fig. 13–11). All three views should probably be examined, and the site of highest velocity should be used for measurement of changes in velocity with interventions. However, if these studies are performed at the time of pacemaker insertion, the apical window will likely be the only view available. Mitral inflow velocities are determined from the apical four- or two-chamber view. Care needs to be taken that the

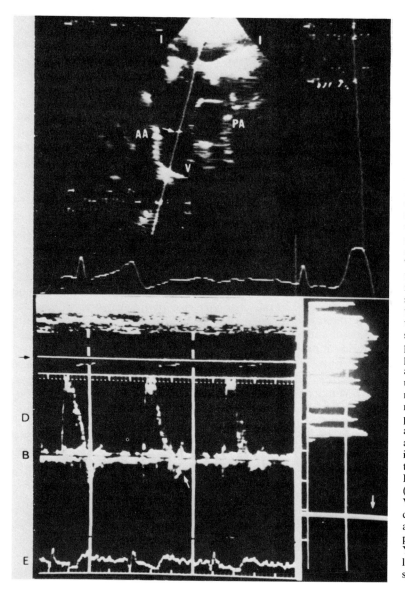

Figure 13–9. Doppler estimation of left ventricular output, suprasternal approach. *Top*, the Doppler cursor line *(arrow)* is aligned parallel to the ascending aorta (AA), imaged from the suprasternal transducer position. The sample volume and the transducer are adjusted to record the maximal Doppler frequency shift signal, which is often obtained when the Doppler cursor line is nearly, but not absolutely, parallel to the vessel walls. PA = pulmonary artery; I = innominate vein; V = ventricle. *Bottom*, Doppler time-velocity signal in the ascending aorta, with the sample volume located as above. The horizontal axis is time, and the vertical axis is velocity. The movement of red blood cells toward the transducer in systole results in the displayed Doppler shift. If the velocity profile across the aorta is assumed to be flat, then the area under the Doppler shift signal (integral of the Doppler time-velocity curve) multiplied by aortic cross-sectional area at the spot where velocity is measured will yield stroke volume. The maximal systolic aortic diameter is measured at the level of the Doppler sample volume, usually from a parasternal long-axis window, and the aortic cross-sectional area is calculated as r^2. D = Doppler time-velocity signal; B = baseline; E = electrocardiogram (ECG). (From Main J, Nanda NC, Saini VD: Clinically useful Doppler calculations and illustrative case examples. *In* Nanda NC [ed]: Doppler Echocardiography. New York, Igaku-Shoin Medical Publishers, 1985, p 511; with permission.)

Figure 13–10. Beat-to-beat changes in aortic flow velocities during VVI pacing in a patient with AV dissociation, illustrating the ability of Doppler ultrasonography to detect small changes in beat-to-beat ventricular performance. When atrial systole fortuitously precedes ventricular systole by a physiologic interval (first three QRS complexes), the flow velocity is much higher than when atrial systole coincides with ventricular systole. (From Stewart WJ, Dicola VC, Harthorne JW, et al: Doppler ultrasound measurement of cardiac output in patients with physiologic pacemakers: Effects of left ventricular function and retrograde ventriculoatrial conduction. Am J Cardiol 54:308, 1984; with permission.)

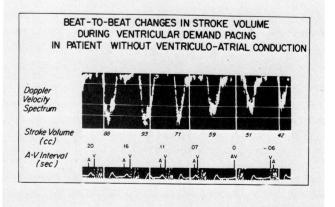

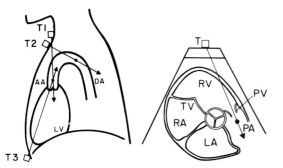

Figure 13–11. Doppler techniques for measurement of cardiac output. *Left,* The transducer is placed in the suprasternal notch and angled inferiorly to pass the ultrasonic beam through the ascending aorta (T1) or the descending aorta (T2). The transducer may also be placed over the cardiac apex and angled superiorly to obtain Doppler shifts from the proximal ascending aorta (T3). Note that the ultrasonic beam is kept nearly parallel to the walls of the aorta in all three transducer positions to obtain maximal Doppler shifts. AA = ascending aorta; DA = descending aorta; LV = left ventricle. *Right,* An alternate technique for measuring cardiac output is to pass the ultrasonic beam parallel to the long axis of the pulmonary artery (PA), which is imaged by two-dimensional echocardiography in the standard parasternal short-axis plane. The Doppler sample volume (*black dot*) is placed beyond the pulmonic valve (PV) in the midlumen of the pulmonary artery (PA). LA = left atrium; RA = right atrium; TV = tricuspid valve; T = transducer; RV = right ventricle. (From Schuster AH, Nanda NC: Doppler echocardiography. Part I: Doppler cardiac output measurements: Perspective and comparison with other methods of cardiac output determination. Echocardiography 1:46, 1984; with permission.)

position of the pulse Doppler sample volume relative to the mitral valve is standardized, as the peak velocities and the ratio of early to late filling (A/E ratio) both will vary as the sample volume is moved from the mitral annulus to the tips of the mitral leaflets.

Doppler Evaluation of the Contribution of Synchronous Atrial Contraction to Ventricular Function

A variety of factors contribute to the fall in cardiac performance that is seen with ventricular pacing. These include loss of AV synchrony and rate responsiveness, an altered ventricular activation sequence, and, rarely, the induction of significant AV valvular regurgitation.[49] The two most significant of these factors are loss of AV synchrony and loss of rate responsiveness to physiologic demand, but which of these two is generally more important is uncertain and may vary from patient to patient and under different conditions. For example, atrial contraction probably contributes significantly to resting stroke volume, but rate responsiveness is likely to be the more

important contributor to exercise tolerance.[13] Dual-chamber pacemakers, of course, provide both AV synchrony and rate responsiveness but are not without disadvantages, including higher cost, shorter pacemaker lifetime, longer insertion time, and pacemaker-mediated tachycardia. In addition, these pacemakers cannot be used in patients with atrial tachyarrhythmias, such as atrial flutter or fibrillation, and do not provide reliable rate responsiveness in patients with sinus node dysfunction. Given these disadvantages of dual-chamber pacemakers—and the likely availability in the future of ventricular pacemakers capable of rate responsiveness in response to markers of increased physiologic demand other than atrial activity, such as blood pH or temperature, right ventricular electrical impedance, QT interval, oxygen saturation, or body activity—it is likely that the contribution of synchronous atrial contraction to maintenance of cardiac output in an individual patient will increasingly influence the choice of pacing mode.

Doppler aortic flow velocities have been used to quantify the fall in stroke volume that occurs when switching from synchronous to asynchronous pacing. Various groups have reported decreases in aortic flow velocity ranging from 16 to 46 per cent upon switching from synchronous to asynchronous pacing (Table 13–1).[14, 17, 29, 31, 39, 46, 54] The improvement in resting aortic flow velocities with synchronous pacing persists over a 12-month follow-up.[14]

All of these studies have noted a marked patient-to-patient variability in the contribution of synchronous atrial contraction to stroke volume. Factors that conceivably could influence the importance of synchronous atrial contraction in the individual patient include ventricular compliance, age, heart rate, the presence of mitral stenosis, left atrial size and contractility, and left ventricular systolic function. Doppler echocardiography has proved a useful means of evaluating which of these factors is predictive of patients likely to benefit from dual-chamber pacing. For example, it has been suggested that patients with left ventricular dysfunction are especially sensitive to loss of AV synchrony.[2, 41] However, Stewart and colleagues measured the change in aortic flow velocity integral due to reprogramming DDD pacemakers from VVI to DVI pacing mode in 29 patients and found that the baseline ejection fraction was not predictive of greater improvement with dual-chamber pacing.[46] Similarly, Labovitz and associates found in a study of 26 patients that left ventricular function, as as-

TABLE 13–1. ATRIAL CONTRIBUTION TO LEFT VENTRICULAR STROKE VOLUME: EVALUATION BY DOPPLER ECHOCARDIOGRAPHY IN PATIENTS WITH DUAL-CHAMBER PACEMAKERS

		CHANGE IN SV: AV SYNCHRONOUS VERSUS ASYNCHRONOUS PACING		
AUTHORS	No.	No. of Patients Who Increased SV	Increase in SV (%)	Predictors of Increased SV
Nanda[39]	6	5/6	18	—
Zugibe[54]	10	10/10	20	—
Stewart[46]	29	—	16	Pacemaker syndrome, intact VA conduction
Labovitz[31]	26	21/26	27	Left atrial size
Faerestrand[14]	13	11/13	21	—
Forgang[17]	8	—	35	LV disease (see text)
Iwase[29]	20	20/20	46	Size of mitral "A" wave

SV = stroke volume; AV = atrioventricular; VA = ventriculoatrial; LV = left ventricular.

sessed by echocardiographic fractional shortening, was not predictive of patients more likely to benefit from AV synchronous pacing, as assessed by aortic flow velocity.[31] On the other hand, in the latter study, left atrial size determined by two-dimensional echocardiography was predictive of the response to loss of atrial synchrony, those patients with atria of normal size being significantly more sensitive to loss of atrial synchrony. The investigators attributed this result to limited atrial contribution to ventricular filling in the patients with large atria due to poor atrial contractility in this group.

Atrial function can be investigated more directly, either by M-mode evaluation of atrial wall motion, as discussed earlier, or by Doppler evaluation of the proportion of mitral inflow due to atrial contraction. Normal mitral inflow is biphasic, consisting of an early diastolic filling wave ("E" wave) and a late atrial filling wave ("A" wave), and is measured by placing the pulse Doppler sample volume at the level of the mitral annulus (Fig. 13–12). In one study, the ratio of late diastolic filling (A wave) to total diastolic filling (A + E waves) during AV sequential pacing correlated with the change in cardiac output, as measured by Doppler technique, upon switching acutely from AV sequential to VVI pacing ($r = .62$).[29] These results suggest that analysis of the ratio of atrial to total mitral inflow velocity during sinus rhythm might aid in selection of those patients for whom dual-chamber pacemakers are most likely to be of benefit. Another approach to the clinical problem of identifying those patients most likely to benefit from preservation of synchronous AV contraction is to measure the change in Doppler aortic flow velocity during synchronous versus asynchronous rhythm. Although in the clinical setting most patients will not have temporary dual-chamber pacemakers, thus precluding direct

comparison of synchronous and asynchronous pacing, many patients will have temporary ventricular pacemakers. The latter group can be studied by setting the pacemaker to asynchronous mode and measuring the change in aortic flow velocity integral during periods of relative AV concordance and discordance as the P wave marches through the cardiac cycle. This approach has been validated in a preliminary study by Halperin and coworkers, who

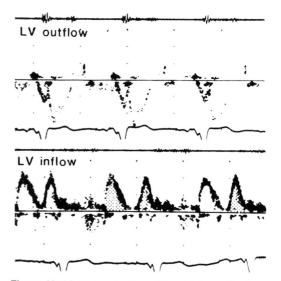

Figure 13–12. Determination of the atrial contribution to ventricular filling by Doppler evaluation of left ventricular inflow. With use of an apical window, the Doppler cursor is placed in the left ventricle just beneath the mitral valve to record mitral inflow. The second beat shows measurement of the time-velocity integral of total left ventricular inflow. The third beat measures that portion of inflow due to atrial contraction. The ratio of atrial to total inflow was found to correlate with the fall in stroke volume during asynchronous pacing in this study. Stroke volume in this study was determined from the time-velocity integral of total left ventricular inflow. (From Iwase M, Sotobata I, Yokota M, et al: Evaluation by pulsed Doppler echocardiography of the atrial contribution to left ventricular filling in patients with DDD pacemakers. Am J Cardiol 58:104, 1986; with permission.)

derived a variance index based on the variation in beat-to-beat aortic flow velocity during AV-dissociated ventricular pacing and showed that it was predictive of the benefit gained by AV sequential compared with ventricular asynchronous pacing.[23] Patients without temporary transvenous pacemakers could conceivably be studied by transthoracic ventricular pacing or by means of transvenous pacemakers at the time of permanent pacemaker insertion.

In conclusion, atrial function can be evaluated by measurement of left atrial size, by M-mode tracings of atrial wall motion, by analysis of the mitral inflow pattern, and by measurement of the effect of AV dissociation on Doppler flow velocities. Quantitation of atrial function has been of limited importance in the past because dual-chamber pacemakers provided the only means of rate-responsive pacing and were therefore often preferable regardless of atrial function. However, if the newer ventricular rate-responsive pacemakers prove to be reliable and effective, determination of atrial function will become an important factor to be considered when choosing between ventricular and dual-chamber rate-responsive pacing, particularly in patients with abnormal sinus node function.

Doppler Determination of Optimal Atrioventricular Pacing Intervals

Traditionally, pacemaker AV intervals have been chosen arbitrarily. It is known, however, that the AV interval can affect stroke volume and that the optimal AV interval varies from person to person, depending on such variables as ventricular compliance, atrial function, heart rate, and the presence of mitral valve disease. In addition, the programmed AV interval necessary to attain the optimal AV delay will vary in patients with DDD pacemakers, depending on whether the pacemaker is in atrial sensing (VDD) or atrial pacing (DVI) mode. These considerations have spurred several groups to use Doppler techniques to optimize the pacing intervals to maximize stroke volume.

Several studies have shown that reprogramming the AV interval of dual-chamber pacemakers results in measurable changes in stroke volume, which can be quantitated by Doppler measurement of flow velocities.[14, 17, 29, 54] These measurements are best made by orienting the Doppler transducer so that maximal aortic flow velocities are obtained and then, without moving the transducer sequentially, reprogramming the pacemaker to various AV intervals.

The pacemaker can be reprogrammed to each AV interval several times to eliminate the effect of small changes in transducer angulation or small random variations in stroke volume. Zugibe and colleagues measured aortic flow velocities in seven patients with dual-chamber pacemakers programmed to DVI mode at AV intervals ranging from 0 to 250 msec.[54] The difference between the best and worst flow velocity within the entire range of AV intervals ranged from 9 to 25 per cent in these patients (mean, 19.5 per cent) but was only 0 to 13 per cent (mean, 8.5 per cent) when only physiologic AV intervals of 100 to 200 msec were considered. The optimal AV interval varied from 150 to 200 msec for individual patients in this series, and in some patients there were significant differences in stroke volume within this relatively narrow physiologic range (Fig. 13–13). Faerestrand and associates studied 13 patients and found

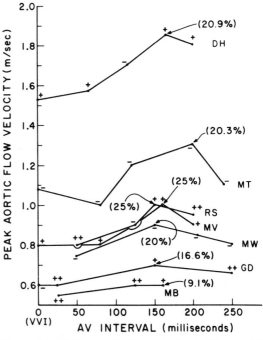

Figure 13–13. Peak aortic flow velocity at different AV intervals (seven patients). + = mitral regurgitation present; + + = increased mitral regurgitation; − = mitral regurgitation not evaluated by Doppler. The number in parentheses indicates the maximal percentage change in peak aortic flow velocity obtained in a given patient compared with the VVI value or value at the shortest AV interval (in patients in whom VVI values were not available). Note that the optimal flow velocity occurred at AV intervals between 150 and 200 msec in all patients. (From Zugibe FT Jr, Nanda NC, Barold SS, Akiyama T: Usefulness of Doppler echocardiography in cardiac pacing: Assessment of mitral regurgitation, peak aortic flow velocity and atrial capture. PACE 6:1350, 1983; with permission.)

that the optimal AV interval for a given patient ranged between 100 and 250 msec; the magnitude of the difference in benefit between the optimal AV interval and a standard AV interval of 150 msec is not mentioned, however.[14] Similar results can be demonstrated if mitral rather than aortic velocities are measured. Iwase and coworkers studied mitral inflow velocity integrals in 20 patients at AV intervals ranging from 50 to 250 msec.[29] They found a mean difference of 46 per cent in stroke volume, as measured by mitral inflow velocity integral, between the best and worst AV intervals and a mean difference of 18 per cent within the physiologic range of 100 to 200 msec. However, the optimal stroke volume as defined by Doppler techniques resulted in a 5 per cent or greater improvement in stroke volume compared with a standard AV interval of 150 msec in only 5 of 20 patients. These three studies utilizing Doppler flow velocities to investigate the effect of AV interval on stroke volume in DVI mode indicate that the optimal pacing interval in most patients lies between 150 to 200 msec. The resting stroke volume in most patients during DVI pacing will be optimal at a standard AV interval of 150 msec, but in some patients modest improvements in stroke volume on the order of 5 to 15 per cent can be expected with individual optimization of the AV interval, with more dramatic improvements in stroke volume possible in occasional patients. Clearly, patients who are most dependent on synchronous atrial contraction—for example, patients with ventricular hypertrophy or diastolic ventricular dysfunction—will be most sensitive to changes in AV interval. In these patients, as well as in patients with significant systolic ventricular dysfunction, in whom a 5 to 15 per cent improvement in stroke volume would be clinically important, it is certainly reasonable to optimize the AV interval by maximizing Doppler flow velocities. Whether routine optimization of pacing parameters in all patients will prove sufficiently beneficial to justify the time and expense involved remains to be determined.

Forfang and colleagues, in a study of eight patients, found both a more marked dependence of stroke volume on AV interval and a wider variation of optimal AV interval, with the optimal AV delay ranging from as little as 75 msec in some patients to as much as 225 msec in others.[17] Reprogramming the pacemaker from the standard AV delay of 150 msec to an AV delay of 75 msec resulted in an approximately 25 per cent improvement in Doppler aortic flow velocity in two patients. The marked sensitivity of the stroke volume to the AV delay noted by these investigators may have in part resulted from the fact that three of the patients (38 per cent) had had aortic valve replacement for aortic stenosis and thus constituted a group likely to be extremely dependent on atrial contraction. An important difference between this study and those of Zugibe, Faerestrand, and Iwase, however, is that in the study of Forfang the dual-chamber pacemakers were reprogrammed to VDD mode, as opposed to the DVI mode used in the latter studies. Wish and associates have demonstrated that the optimal AV interval is significantly shorter during VDD pacing than during DVI pacing in the same patient.[51] These investigators measured the time interval between left atrial and left ventricular activation and found that for a given programmed AV interval the measured left atrial to left ventricular delay was significantly longer (mean difference of 78 msec) when the pacemaker was in the atrial sensing (VDD) mode than when it was in the atrial pacing (DVI) mode. The increase in left atrial to left ventricular activation time due to atrial sensing resulted in optimal programmed AV intervals that were significantly shorter during VDD pacing than during DVI pacing. Other investigators have also found that patients with VDD pacemakers benefit from very short programmed AV intervals.[50] Thus, when optimizing the AV interval, the clinician needs to consider which pacing mode the patient is likely to be most dependent on. Patients who will be paced primarily in the VDD mode (e.g., those with high-grade AV block) either should be studied during VDD pacing or should empirically have 75 msec subtracted from the optimal AV interval determined during DVI pacing.[50] Newer pacemakers allow programming of separate AV intervals for DVI and VDD pacing modes, in which case Doppler echocardiography can be used to optimize both AV intervals independently. An additional problem encountered in programming an optimal AV interval for VDD pacing is the possibility that the optimal interval may be a function of heart rate. In DVI pacing, for example, Halperin and colleagues demonstrated that the optimal interval was shorter at a heart rate of 90 beats per minute than at a heart rate of 70 beats per minute.[23] It is thus unclear whether an AV interval optimized at one arbitrary heart rate (usually a resting heart rate) will be suitable for a wide range of heart rates. Studies measuring exercise stroke volumes or maximal exercise capacity at various AV intervals might help resolve this question. The relative contribution of properly timed atrial contraction to total stroke volume in Halperin's study was greater at the lower heart rate, suggesting that the atrial kick is more important at rest than during exercise and that the AV interval should be optimized at a lower heart rate.

Doppler Evaluation of Pacemaker-Induced Valvular Regurgitation

Ventricular pacing may frequently result in mild amounts of AV valvular regurgitation and, rarely, important regurgitation. Maurer and associates used agitated saline bubbles as echo contrast to study the effect of pacing site on the severity of regurgitation in a closed-chest dog model.[35] They noted severe mitral regurgitation during pacing from the right ventricular apex, compared with only mild mitral regurgitation during coronary sinus pacing. The authors felt that alteration in the timing of papillary muscle contraction, depending on the pacing site, may have been responsible for these findings.

The incidence of AV valvular regurgitation due to ventricular pacing is unknown, but hemodynamically significant regurgitation due to pacing is probably rare in the absence of preexisting valvular incompetence. Valvular regurgitation in humans is best diagnosed noninvasively by pulse or color Doppler technique. Valvular regurgitation results in a high-velocity, turbulent jet in the receiving chamber, which is readily detected by either of these Doppler techniques (Fig. 13–14). Color Doppler allows more accurate semiquantitation of the severity of regurgitation than does pulse Doppler (Fig. 13–15). We have observed one patient who had marked worsening of mitral regurgitation upon reprogramming of his AV interval from 150 to 100 msec.[36] Damage to the tricuspid valve due to trauma at the time of pacemaker insertion or subsequent adhesion of a tricuspid leaflet to the pacemaker wire as a result of fibrosis can rarely result in significant tricuspid regurgitation.[45] Tricuspid regurgitation can be semiquantitated by pulse or color Doppler echocardiography in a fashion similar to mitral regurgitation, by the magnitude of the flow disturbance in the atrium. In addition, severe tricuspid regurgitation generally results in retrograde systolic flow in the hepatic veins, which can be detected by either pulse or color Doppler technique.[38]

CONCLUSIONS

Combined Doppler echocardiographic study of patients with pacemakers can provide useful anatomic and physiologic information. Echo-

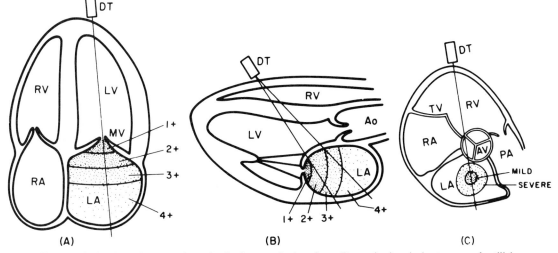

Figure 13–14. Doppler mapping of mitral regurgitation flow. Regurgitation is best assessed utilizing multiple two-dimensional planes. This approach provides a three-dimensional evaluation of the size, extent, and distribution of the regurgitant jet. With progressively more severe regurgitation, a left atrial flow disturbance can be detected over an increasingly larger area and further from the mitral valve (MV) plane. DT = Doppler transducer; 1+, 2+, 3+, 4+ = angiographic grades of severity; RV = right ventricle; LV = left ventricle; RA = right atrium; LA = left atrium; Ao = aorta; TV = tricuspid valve; PA = pulmonary artery; AV = aortic valve. (From Adhar GC, Abbasi AS, Nanda NC: Doppler echocardiography in the assessment of mitral regurgitation and mitral valve prolapse. *In* Nanda NC [ed]: Doppler Echocardiography. New York, Igaku-Shoin Medical Publishers, 1985, p 200; with permission.)

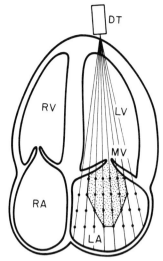

Figure 13–15. Principles of two-dimensional color Doppler flow mapping. Conventional pulse Doppler evaluates the frequency shift of an emitted ultrasound pulse, and thereby blood flow velocity, from one point in a two-dimensional plane. Color Doppler machines measure Doppler shifts at multiple points in a two-dimensional plane. The frequency shifts are analyzed for direction, magnitude, and variance, and the resulting flow information is color coded and superimposed on a standard two-dimensional echocardiographic display. Flow toward the transducer is traditionally represented by shades of red, and flow away from the transducer by shades of blue, with brighter shades of red or blue corresponding to higher blood flow velocities. The variance of the Doppler shift between adjacent pixels, which reflects disturbance of flow, is coded by shades of green. Mitral regurgitation is readily identified by the abnormally directed, frequently turbulent flow extending from the mitral valve into the left atrium during ventricular systole. The percentage of the left atrium occupied by the regurgitant flow has been shown by us to correlate with the severity of regurgitation. DT = Doppler transducer; RV = right ventricle; LV = left ventricle; MV = mitral valve; RA = right atrium; LA = left atrium. (From Adhar GC, Abbasi SS, Nanda NC: Doppler echocardiography in the assessment of mitral regurgitation and mitral valve prolapse. *In* Nanda NC [ed]: Doppler Echocardiography. New York, Igaku-Shoin Medical Publishers, 1985, p 201; with permission.)

cardiography provides data about pacemaker location and any complications of pacemaker insertion, as well as supplying useful preimplantation information regarding the patient, such as the presence of right ventricular infarction or thrombosis, or a dilated left atrium, which may alter the physician's approach. Doppler echocardiography is emerging as a useful noninvasive means of evaluating pacemaker physiology and assessing the hemodynamic consequences of altering parameters such as pacing site, pacing mode, and AV interval. Doppler echocardiography can aid in the identification of patients who would benefit from dual-chamber pacing and can be used to

optimize AV intervals in those patients who receive dual-chamber pacemakers. The clinical role of Doppler echocardiographic evaluation of atrial function may grow as rate-responsive ventricular pacemakers become perfected and more widely available in the future, as an aid in choosing the physiologically most appropriate pacemaker for an individual patient.

REFERENCES

1. Barold SS, Falkoff MD, Ong LS, et al: Determination of successful atrial capture in unipolar dual-chambered pulse generators. PACE 6:35A, 1983.
2. Benchimol A, Ellis JG, Dimond EG: Hemodynamic consequences of atrial and ventricular pacing in patients with normal and abnormal hearts: Effect of exercise at a fixed atrial and ventricular rate. Am J Med 93:911, 1965.
3. Bryan CS, Sutton JP, Saunders DE Jr, et al: Endocarditis related to transvenous pacemakers. J Thorac Cardiovasc Surg 75:758, 1978.
4. Bryan CS, Sutton JP, Saunders DE, et al: Endocarditis related to transvenous pacemakers: Syndromes and surgical implications. J Thorac Cardiovasc Surg 5:758, 1978.
5. Chan W, Ikram H: Echocardiographic demonstration of tricuspid valvulitis and right atrial thrombus complicating an infected artificial pacemaker: A case report. Angiology 29:559, 1978.
6. Chazal R, Feigenbaum H: Two-dimensional echocardiographic identification of epicardial pacemaker wire perforation. Am Heart J 107:165, 1984.
7. Cohen BE, Winer HE, Kronzon I: Echocardiographic findings in patients with left superior vena cava and dilated coronary sinus. Am J Cardiol 44:158, 1979.
8. Daelemans R, Kersschot B, Branden F, et al: Pacemaker endocarditis: Contribution of two-dimensional echocardiography. Acta Cardiol 39:293, 1984.
9. Dillon JC, Chang S, Feigenbaum H: Echocardiographic manifestations of left bundle branch block. Circulation 49:876, 1974.
10. Drinkovic N: Subcostal echocardiography to determine right ventricular pacing catheter position and control advancement of electrode catheters in intracardiac electrophysiologic studies. Am J Cardiol 47:1260, 1981.
11. Drinkovic N, Ferek B, Jursic M: Subcostal M-mode echocardiography of the right atrial wall in evaluation of cardiac arrhythmias and pacing. PACE 8:110, 1985.
12. Eichhorn EJ, Winters WL, Crawford S, et al: Bacterial endocarditis and right atrial vegetation: Detection by two-dimensional echocardiography. JAMA 246:2724, 1981.
13. Eisenhauer AC, McElroy PA, Weber KT: Chronotropic dysfunction and exercise. *In* Weber KT, Janicki JS (eds): Cardiopulmonary Exercise Testing. Philadelphia, WB Saunders Co, 1986, pp 255–271.
14. Faerestrand S, Ohm OJ: A time-related study of the hemodynamic benefit of atrioventricular synchronous pacing evaluated by Doppler echocardiography. PACE 8:838, 1985.
15. Feigenbaum H: Echocardiographic findings with altered electrical activation. *In* Feigenbaum H: Echocardiography. Philadelphia, Lea & Febiger, 1986, pp 230–248.

16. Fishenfeld J, Lamy Y: Laceration of the tricuspid valve by a pacemaker wire. Chest 61:697, 1972.
17. Forfang K, Otterstad JE, Ohlen H: Optimal atrioventricular delay in physiologic pacing determined by Doppler echocardiography. PACE 9:17, 1985.
18. Gardin JM, Dabestini A, Natin K, et al: Reproducibility of Doppler aortic blood flow velocity measurements: Studies on intra-observer, inter-observer and day-to-day variability in normal subjects. Am J Cardiol 54:1092, 1984.
19. Gardin JM, Tobis JM, Dabestini A, et al: Superiority of two-dimensional measurement of aortic vessel diameter in Doppler echocardiographic estimates of left ventricular stroke volume. J Am Coll Cardiol 6:66, 1985.
20. Gomes JAC, Damato AN, Akhtar M, et al: Ventricular septal motion and left ventricular dimensions during abnormal ventricular activation. Am J Cardiol 39:641, 1977.
21. Gondi B, Nanda NC: Real time, two-dimensional echocardiographic features of pacemaker perforation. Circulation 64:97, 1981.
22. Grogler FM, Frank G, Greven G, et al: Complications of permanent transvenous cardiac pacing. J Thorac Cardiovasc Surg 69:895, 1975.
23. Halperin JL, Teichholz LE, Steinmetz MY, et al: Selection of patients for dual-chamber pacing by noninvasive means: The VVI-variance index [abstract]. Circulation 70:II, 1984.
24. Hsiung MC, Nanda NC, Kan MN, et al: Influence of different pacing modes and ventriculo-atrial conduction on hemodynamics evaluated by color Doppler. Clin Res 35:288A, 1987.
25. Huang T, Baba N: Cardiac pathology of transvenous pacemakers. Am Heart J 83:469, 1972.
26. Huntsman LL, Stewart DK, Barnes SR, et al: Noninvasive Doppler determination of cardiac output in man. Circulation 67:593, 1983.
27. Ishikawa K, Yanagisawa A: Evaluation of unusual QRS complexes produced by pacemaker stimuli—with special reference to the vectorcardiographic and echocardiographic findings. J Electrocardiol 13:409, 1980.
28. Isner JM: The pathology of pacemakers. Intelligence Rep Cardiac Pacing Electrophysiol Vol 2, No. 2, December 1983.
29. Iwase M, Sotobata I, Yokota M, et al: Evaluation of pulsed Doppler echocardiography of the atrial contribution to left ventricular filling in patients with DDD pacemakers. Am J Cardiol 58:104, 1986.
30. Kinney EL, Allen RP, Weidner WA, et al: Recurrent pulmonary emboli secondary to right atrial thrombus around a permanent pacing catheter: A case report and review of the literature. PACE 2:196, 1979.
31. Labovitz AJ, Williams GA, Redd RM, Kennedy HL: Noninvasive assessment of pacemaker hemodynamics by Doppler echocardiography: Importance of left atrial size. J Am Coll Cardiol 6:196, 1985.
32. Lee ME, Chaux A, Matloff JM: Avulsion of a tricuspid valve leaflet during traction on an infected, entrapped endocardial pacemaker electrode. J Thorac Cardiovasc Surg 74:433, 1977.
33. Lewis JF, Kuo LL, Nelson JG, et al: Pulsed Doppler echocardiographic determination of stroke volume and cardiac output: Clinical validation of two new methods using the apical window. Circulation 70:425, 1984.
34. Liebson PR: Echocardiography in electrophysiologic studies: A review. Clin Prog Pacing Electrophysiol 2:440, 1984.

35. Maurer G, Torres MAR, Corday E, et al: Two-dimensional echocardiographic contrast assessment of pacing-induced mitral regurgitation: Relation to altered regional left ventricular function. J Am Coll Cardiol 3:986, 1984.
36. Meier B, Felner JM: Two-dimensional echocardiographic evaluation of intracardiac transvenous pacemaker leads. J Clin Ultrasound 10:421, 1982.
37. Mitrovic V, Thormann J, Schlepper M, Neuss H: Thrombotic complications with pacemakers. Int J Cardiol 2:363, 1983.
38. Miyatake K, Mitsunori O, Kinoshita N, et al: Evaluation of tricuspid regurgitation by pulsed Doppler and two-dimensional echocardiography. Circulation 66:777, 1982.
39. Nanda NC, Barold SS: Usefulness of echocardiography in cardiac pacing. PACE 5:222, 1982.
40. Phibbs B, Marriot HJL: Complications of permanent transvenous pacing. N Engl J Med 312:1428, 1985.
41. Rahimtoola SH, Ehsani A, Sinno MZ, et al: Left atrial transport function in myocardial infarction. Am J Med 59:686, 1975.
42. Reeves WC, Nanda NC, Barold SS: Echocardiographic evaluation of intracardiac pacing catheters: M-mode and two-dimensional studies. Circulation 58:1049, 1978.
43. Sasse L, Frolick CA: Suprasternal notch echocardiography and atrial arrhythmias. Cardiovasc Dis Bull Tex Ht Inst 6:61, 1979.
44. Schuster AH, Nanda NC, Maulik D, Saini VD: Doppler evaluation of cardiac output. In Nanda NC (ed): Doppler Echocardiography. New York, Igaku-Shoin Medical Publishers, 1985, pp 149–187.
45. Schuster AH, Zugibe F Jr, Nanda NC, Murphy GW: Two-dimensional echocardiographic identification of pacing catheter–induced thrombosis. PACE 5:124, 1982.
46. Stewart WJ, Dicola VC, Harthorne JW, et al: Doppler ultrasound measurement of cardiac output in patients with physiologic pacemakers: Effects of left ventricular function and retrograde ventriculoatrial conduction. Am J Cardiol 54:308, 1984.
47. Stoney W, Addlestone RB, Alford WC, et al: The incidence of venous thrombosis following long-term transvenous pacing. Ann Thorac Surg 22:166, 1976.
48. Strasberg B, Rich S, Lam W, et al: M-mode echocardiography in left bundle branch block: Significance of frontal plane QRS axis. Am Heart J 104:775, 1982.
49. Switzer DF, Nanda NC: Doppler-echocardiographic assessment of cardiac pacemakers. Cardiol Clin 3:631, 1985.
50. Von Bibra H, Busch U, Wirtzfeld A: The beneficial effect of short A-V intervals in VDD patients. J Am Coll Cardiol 5:394, 1985.
51. Wish M, Fletcher RD, Gottdiener JS, et al: Optimal left atrioventricular sequence in dual chamber pacing—limitations of programmed A-V interval [abstract]. J Am Coll Cardiol 3:507A, 1984.
52. Zardo F, Nicolosi GL, Burelli C, Zanuttini D: Dual-chamber transvenous pacemaker implantation via anomalous left superior vena cava. Am Heart J 112:621, 1986.
53. Zoneraich S, Zoneraich O, Rhee JJ: Echocardiographic evaluation of septal motion in patients with artificial pacemakers: Vectorcardiographic correlations. Am Heart J 93:596, 1977.
54. Zugibe F, Nanda NC, Barold SS, Akiyama T: Usefulness of Doppler echocardiography in cardiac pacing: Assessment of mitral regurgitation, peak aortic flow velocity and atrial capture. PACE 6:1350, 1983.

14

COMPLICATIONS OF PERMANENT PACING SYSTEMS: Diagnosis and Management

LINDA M. KALLINEN, ROBERT G. HAUSER, *and* JAY WARREN

Permanent cardiac pacing is a highly successful form of therapy that often challenges the clinician or technician with a variety of complications. Most of these problems are amenable to treatment without surgery, provided the nature of the difficulty is understood and the tools are available to correct the malfunction. Not infrequently, the problem is not a pacemaker failure but rather a lack of knowledge of the device or the lead system. Individuals who are responsible for analyzing and correcting a potential malfunction must be certain of the pacemaker's operating characteristics, and he or she must be familiar with the hardware that was designed to program or otherwise alter the functional behavior of the device.

In this chapter, we will discuss pacing malfunction in terms of the basic properties of sensing and pacing, as well as the use of programmability to correct or avoid many clinical problems. Always, the clinician should remember that hardware failures should not usually be treated by programming or other less definitive measures; rather, a pulse generator or lead defect almost always requires replacement or repair.

PACING MALFUNCTIONS: SENSING

Sensing is a fundamental property of any pacing system. A sensed event that satisfies specific electrical criteria will govern the stimulation behavior of all contemporary pacemakers. The physician can select from a variety of lead electrodes for atrial or ventricular applications. Unipolar or bipolar electrode pairs are available. A unipolar electrode configuration consists of the stimulating cathode, which is in contact with the endomyocardium, and a remote anode, usually the pulse generator's metal housing, which is outside the heart. Bipolar electrodes consist of two intracardiac electrodes. Whereas only the cathode tip electrode of an endocardial bipolar pair may be in contact with cardiac tissue, both electrodes of an epimyocardial bipolar system are contacting, and it is possible that the remote ring anode of a bipolar endocardial lead may be on or near responsive myocardium.

The difference in voltage potential registered between the two electrodes is represented on the electrogram. The voltage in unipolar systems is acquired primarily at the cathode, and the anode contributes little to the absolute amplitude of the unipolar signal. The electrogram in a bipolar system combines the signals registered at both electrodes; the result depends on the distance between the electrodes and the speed and orientation of the wave of cardiac depolarization.

It may be inferred that a change in the orientation of the depolarization wave front to the bipolar electrodes will result in a new bipolar signal. Such a reorientation may occur if the wave front travels a different pathway, for example, intraventricular conduction defect, or if a displaced lead shifts the electrodes. In most cases, it is unlikely that minor changes in the spatial orientation of the depolarization wave front to bipolar electrodes will result in undersensing. However, one may minimize the risk of such an occurrence by having the patient breathe deeply and cough while the bipolar signal is observed. If the signal changes, then the lead is probably unstable and should be repositioned. Should undersensing occur after implantation, normal sensing may be restored if the pulse generator can be programmed from a bipolar to a unipolar configuration.

According to our experience, undersensing has never occurred if the bipolar ventricular electrogram at implantation was stable and if the peak-to-peak amplitude exceeded 6 mV. It is also our impression that the use of fixation leads, principally those of the tined or screw-in design, has facilitated successful bipolar sensing by enhancing lead stability and thus preserving the optimal relationship between the electrodes and the depolarization wave front.

Another implication of the wave front pertains to interference signals from far-field sources. The clinical manifestations of interference will be discussed below, but it is convenient to consider the different effects of far-field electrical noise on unipolar and bipolar electrodes.

Figure 14–1 illustrates how pectoral myopotentials will be sensed by unipolar and bipolar pacing systems. For the unipolar configuration, the pectoral muscle signals are generated near the anode. Hence, larger myopotentials are registered earlier at the anode than at the cathode, and thus the net unipolar potential may possess the amplitude and spectral characteristics of an intracardiac QRS. Such an interference signal may be detected by the pulse generator's sensing circuit, which will respond by inhibiting (or triggering) the output circuit. Although this sensing malfunction is termed oversensing, the pacemaker is, in fact, responding appropriately to an electrical event that it considers to represent a ventricular depolarization.

The bipolar electrode configuration is relatively immune to skeletal myopotentials. In the bipolar system, the pectoral muscle signals recorded at the anode and cathode are similar in amplitude and timing. Consequently, the net bipolar myopotential is inadequate for sensing, and it does not interfere with pacemaker function. Bipolar electrodes in certain situations are susceptible to interference signals, particularly if the myopotential is generated close to the electrode. For example, dia-

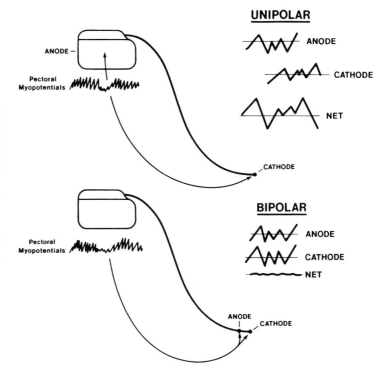

Figure 14–1. Far-field interference, that is, pectoral myopotentials, will affect unipolar and bipolar systems differently. In contrast to the unipolar configuration (*top*), bipolar electrodes (*bottom*) register a smaller net signal because the myopotentials arrive at the anode and cathode simultaneously. (From Hauser RG, Edwards LM, Stafford JL: Bipolar and unipolar sensing: Basic concepts and clinical applications. *In* Barold SS [ed]: Modern Cardiac Pacing. Mount Kisco, NY, Futura Publishing Co, 1985, p 140; with permission.)

phragmatic myopotentials may interfere with bipolar ventricular sensing. Presumably, the proximity of the diaphragm to the ventricular electrode permits the development of a wave front that travels parallel to the interelectrode axis. This parallel wave front arrives first at the cathode and then at the anode and thus creates a net signal that is larger than individual potentials recorded at each electrode. Hypothetically, at least, bipolar atrial electrodes may be subject to the same near-field effects, including not only diaphragmatic potentials but also those originating from the thoracic muscles overlying the right atrium.

Very far-field interference signals will not usually affect even unipolar pacing systems with nominal sensitivities. In fact, extracorporeal electrical noise rarely results in oversensing unless it is quite intense or is radiated from sources near the pulse generator. The more remote the source of interference, the less likely is the possibility that a significant potential will appear between either unipolar or bipolar electrodes.

The intracardiac R wave or P wave is characterized by a voltage amplitude (millivolts [mV]), slew rate (V/s), and duration (milliseconds [msec]). The R or P wave is also referred to as the intrinsic deflection that represents the depolarization wave as it passes adjacent to the electrode. Table 14–1 contains acute unipolar and bipolar R- and P-wave values for amplitude and slew rate, and Figure 14–2 illustrates the measured parameters.

Tissue-Electrode Interface

When a lead is positioned in the right ventricle or atrial appendage, the electrode contacts native endomyocardium. A current of injury may be recorded, but the acute electrogram is fairly representative of otherwise undisturbed intracardiac electrical activity. Subsequently, as the electrode-tissue interaction occurs, the electrogram is modified, and the changes may affect clinical sensing.[18, 28]

The stability of the contacting electrode will affect acute and chronic sensing performance.

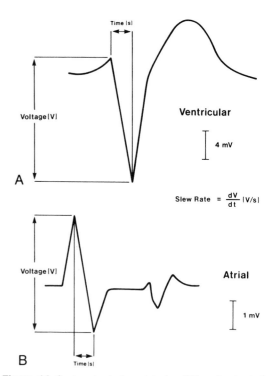

Figure 14–2. An atypical ventricular *(A)* and a typical atrial *(B)* electrogram. Atrial and ventricular electrogram morphologies actually are quite similar except in amplitude. The far-field QRS is represented by the low-amplitude complex in *B* following the atrial electrogram. (From Hauser RG, Edwards LM, Stafford JL: Bipolar and unipolar sensing: Basic concepts and clinical applications. *In* Barold SS [ed]: Modern Cardiac Pacing. Mount Kisco, NY, Futura Publishing Co, 1985, p 141; with permission.)

The resolution of conventional imaging techniques such as fluoroscopy and echocardiography limits our ability to assess motion at the electrode-tissue interface. However, a major benefit of fixation mechanisms, such as tines or screws, is to eliminate or reduce motion at the electrode-tissue interface. A secure electrode will eliminate microdisplacement, which may be manifested by intermittent failure to sense or capture or both. Further, over months or years a mechanically stable electrode-tissue interface should result in less tissue injury and fibrous capsule formation. Therefore, the effectiveness of newer electrode designs may be attributed not only to improved electrophysi-

TABLE 14–1. ELECTROGRAM CHARACTERISTICS

	VENTRICULAR (R WAVE)*		ATRIAL (P WAVE)†	
	Bipolar	Unipolar	Bipolar	Unipolar
Amplitude (mV)	11.8 ± 6.0	12.2 ± 5.2	4.3 ± 0.5	3.7 ± 0.4
Slew rate (V/sec)	2.8 ± 1.8	2.8 ± 1.7	1.2 ± 0.3	0.9 ± 0.1

*± SD.
†± SEM.

ologic characteristics but also to fixation mechanisms. In addition, leads that are compliant tend to absorb forces that may otherwise be directed to the electrode, and thus the flexible lead should produce less tissue trauma and chronic reaction.

Oversensing

Oversensing occurs when the pulse generator's sensing circuit incorrectly identifies an electrical signal as an appropriate cardiac event (R or P wave) and resets or triggers a timing circuit. Some pulse generators may also misinterpret biologic signals as extracorporeal electrical noise and may revert to their interference modes; this is a distinct form of oversensing whose manifestations are uniquely those of particular pulse generator models.

The differential diagnosis of oversensing includes the following:

I. Biologic signals

   A. Skeletal myopotentials
      1. Pectoral
      2. Abdominal
      3. Diaphragmatic
   B. Cardiac events
      1. R waves in atrium
      2. P wave in ventricle
      3. T wave
      4. Concealed extrasystoles

II. Pacemaker system

   A. Pulse generator
      1. High sensitivity or output
      2. Short refractory period
      3. Electronic malfunction
   B. Connector assembly
      1. Loose set screw
      2. Current leak
   C. Lead electrode
      1. Conductor fracture
      2. Insulation break
      3. Polarization potentials

III. Environmental interference

Skeletal Myopotentials

Only since 1972 has it been appreciated that skeletal muscle potentials may interfere with pacemaker function. One of us reported our findings in 228 patients who had unipolar pacing systems and who were evaluated for pectoral muscle myopotential oversensing during exercise or 24-hour Holter monitoring or both.[31] Myopotential inhibition was defined as inappropriate resetting of the pulse generator's automatic timing cycle with resultant prolongation of the interval between paced beats. The exercises included sustained isometrics and both pushing and pulling against a load, usually the arm of the examiner. Some patients exhibited oversensing only during one maneuver. Overall, 39 per cent of the study population developed oversensing during pectoral muscle exercises, and 14 per cent had myopotential inhibition documented on Holter monitoring. Of the 86 patients with oversensing, 12 patients, or 14 per cent, had symptoms ranging from mild dizziness to syncope during one or more episodes of myopotential inhibition. All patients who had severe symptoms became symptomatic during inhibition of their pulse generators by chest wall stimulation. More than half of the symptomatic patients required a corrective intervention, including reprogramming and pulse generator replacement. Patients who did not have suitably programmable models and who were only mildly symptomatic did not undergo pulse generator replacement. Silastic-coated pulse generators were no less prone to skeletal muscle interference than were uncoated models.

On the basis of these observations, it was concluded that (1) skeletal muscle interference with normal demand function will be observed in more than a third of patients with unipolar pacing systems; (2) nearly one in seven patients with myopotential inhibition will experience symptoms and the majority of these will require corrective intervention; (3) all unipolar pulse generators should have a wide range of programmable sensitivities; and (4) Silastic coating or boots will not eliminate myopotential interference.

Bipolar systems even at high sensitivity are practically immune to skeletal muscle interference. Further, undersensing is seen in similar proportions of unipolar and bipolar models, and thus it is not a unique side effect of the bipolar electrode configuration.

Bipolar electrodes may be susceptible to skeletal myopotentials originating from the diaphragm. Barold and colleagues[4] reported such a case. Whenever episodes of inappropriate inhibition are seen in a bipolar system, diaphragmatic muscle interference should be suspected. Most commonly, this is observed at higher sensitivities and may be provoked by a maximal inspiratory effort, coughing, or the Valsalva maneuver. Naturally, these maneuvers can also uncover a conductor fracture or insulation break, and these defects may be manifested as a pacemaker pause that cannot be differentiated from myopotential inhibition.

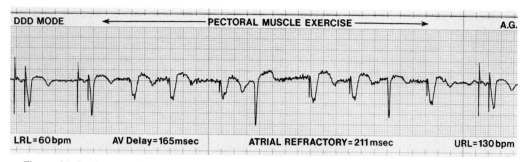

Figure 14–3. Myopotential-triggered tachycardia. Skeletal muscle signals are sensed by the atrial channel and trigger ventricular stimulation. LRL = lower rate limit; URL = upper rate limit. (From Hauser RG, Edwards LM, Stafford JL: Bipolar and unipolar sensing: Basic concepts and clinical applications. *In* Barold SS [ed]: Modern Cardiac Pacing. Mount Kisco, NY, Futura Publishing Co, 1985, p 148; with permission.)

Skeletal muscle interference also creates problems with unipolar dual-chamber DDD pacemakers. High-sensitivity settings are commonly used in the atrial channel, and these create an ideal setting for a variety of complications, including inhibition of atrial output and triggered ventricular stimulation.[29] The patient whose rhythm strip is shown in Figure 14–3 experienced palpitations that were quite troublesome and prompted her to seek the advice of her physician. During exercises that simulated those she performed in the garden, the atrial sensing circuit misinterpreted the myopotentials as P waves and triggered ventricular stimulation at or near the programmed upper rate limit of the device. Unfortunately, the atrial sensitivity could not be decreased because P-wave undersensing would occur, and thus she continues to have pacemaker-induced palpitations. This not unexpected finding was reported to occur in 15 per cent of patients who were evaluated by Jost and associates[20] during pectoral muscle exercises while their DDD pulse generators were programmed to high atrial sensitivities of 0.75 mV or 1.25 mV.

Oversensing on the ventricular channel of a DDD unit not only may confound the electrocardiographer but also may create a more hazardous situation for the patient. The resting and exercise tracings shown in Figure 14–4 are from an individual who had a DDD pulse generator that develops pure atrioventricular (AV)-block at the upper rate limit defined by the total atrial refractory period. While exercising on the treadmill, this patient increased his sinus rate normally and developed electronic AV block when the atrial rate exceeded 150 beats per minute. The resultant decrease in ventricular rate caused him to grasp the side rails of the treadmill because he felt faint. The pectoral muscle signals (bottom tracing) inhib-

ited ventricular (and atrial) output, producing a long pause and near-syncope.

In patients who have DDD, VDD, or VAT pacemakers with intact ventriculoatrial (VA) conductions, a reentrant pacemaker-mediated tachycardia (PMT) may be initiated by myopo-

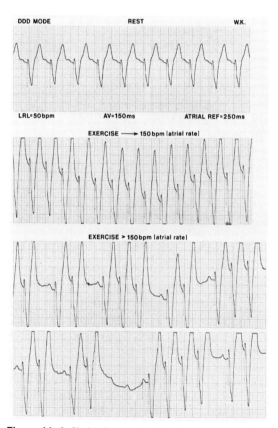

Figure 14–4. Skeletal myopotentials *(bottom tracing)* inhibit atrial and ventricular output during exercise. See text for additional discussion. (From Hauser RG, Edwards LM, Stafford JL: Bipolar and unipolar sensing: Basic concepts and clinical applications. *In* Barold SS [ed]: Modern Cardiac Pacing. Mount Kisco, NY, Futura Publishing Co, 1985, p 149; with permission.)

tential oversensing.[10] Reprogramming of atrial sensitivity, AV interval, or atrial refractory period may prevent the PMT, but the result may limit the hemodynamic benefits of dual-chamber pacemakers.

Cardiac Events

Ventricular pacing systems may detect sinus P waves when the electrode or electrodes are near the atria. Such situations exist during coronary sinus pacing and when ventricular epimyocardial leads are located in close proximity to the AV groove. We have not observed sinus P-wave oversensing in 1031 patients who had unipolar transvenous leads positioned in the right ventricular apex. As reported by Mond and Sloman,[26] P-wave oversensing may be seen when a right ventricular endocardial lead is displaced toward the tricuspid valve, and Barold and colleagues[3] described a case of ectopic P-wave oversensing by a demand pacemaker. Similarly, an atrial sensing circuit may detect the remote QRS, which may have sufficient amplitude to be sensed by pulse generators programmed to high or even nominal sensitivities.

T-wave oversensing is a rare malfunction unless the pulse generator is programmed to a high sensitivity or to a short refractory period (Fig. 14–5). It is the paced T wave that is almost always oversensed, and thus one must consider the possibility that the pacemaker stimulus afterpotential may contribute to the signal detected by the sensing circuit. T-wave oversensing is not particularly hazardous with VVI pacemakers, but when the triggered mode is used, competitive arrhythmias may be produced.

Concealed ventricular extrasystoles (premature ventricular contractions [PVCs]) can result in apparent oversensing,[25] and whether this phenomenon is the result of a combination of events—that is, afterpotential, T wave, or late potentials—is speculative.[2] The diagnosis requires the exclusion of other causes of oversensing, and post–T-wave recycling by a concealed PVC should be eradicated by antiarrhythmic therapy.[23]

The aforementioned oversensing of cardiac events occurs with both unipolar and bipolar pulse generators. A bipolar electrode pair is less likely to register a far-field signal from the opposite chamber, but any near-field signal, such as a T wave or extrasystole, may be detected by unipolar or bipolar systems. Nonstimulating, noncontacting pure sensors are not confounded by nonphysiologic signals.[14] If the source of an intracardiac electrical event is known, or at least predictable, then pulse generators may be designed to perform tasks, such as capture verification or the detection of late potentials, which are key to the development of more sophisticated bradycardia pacemakers and intelligent antitachycardia devices.

Pacemaker System

High-sensitivity, high-output, and short refractory period settings can be associated with inappropriate recycling. Available multiprogrammable pulse generators are capable of being adjusted to worst case conditions for oversensing events that normally would be ignored. Certainly, any unit that is programmed to high sensitivity will be prone to interference by biologic and environmental interference. Increasing output amplitude or pulse width may produce afterpotential oversensing by any pulse generator, and it may result in crosstalk between the channels of a dual-chamber system.

Afterpotentials are time-changing voltages at the electrode-tissue interface that dissipate following delivery of the pacemaker stimulus (Fig. 14–6). When the afterpotential persists beyond the refractory period, it may be sensed and may recycle the pulse generator's timing circuit.[16]

Afterpotential oversensing is associated with

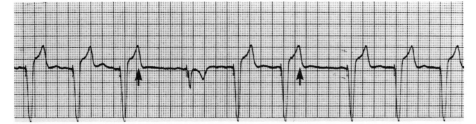

Figure 14–5. T-wave oversensing *(arrows)* by a high-sensitivity unipolar pacing system. (From Hauser RG, Edwards LM, Stafford JL: Bipolar and unipolar sensing: Basic concepts and clinical applications. *In* Barold SS [ed]: Modern Cardiac Pacing. Mount Kisco, NY, Futura Publishing Co, 1985, p 150; with permission.)

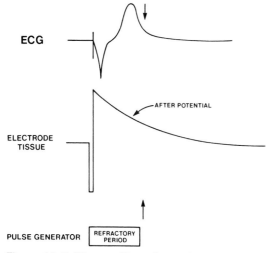

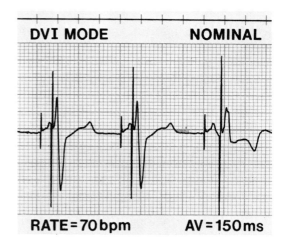

Figure 14–6. Diagram illustrating surface electrocardiogram (ECG) *(top panel)*, pacemaker pulse at electrode-tissue interface *(middle panel)*, and pulse generator's refractory period *(bottom panel)*. Vertical arrows indicate recycling because of the afterpotential signal. (From Hauser RG, Edwards LM, Stafford JL: Bipolar and unipolar sensing: Basic concepts and clinical applications. *In* Barold SS [ed]: Modern Cardiac Pacing. Mount Kisco, NY, Futura Publishing Co, 1985, p 151; with permission.)

Figure 14–8. Crosstalk in a noncommitted DVI unipolar pacing system. The first two atrial stimuli trigger ventricular safety pacing (nonphysiologic atrioventricular [AV] delay). See text for additional discussion. (From Hauser RG, Edwards LM, Stafford JL: Bipolar and unipolar sensing: Basic concepts and clinical applications. *In* Barold SS [ed]: Modern Cardiac Pacing. Mount Kisco, NY, Futura Publishing Co, 1985, p 154; with permission.)

(1) high-current or long pulse width stimuli, (2) large-capacitance electrodes, (3) close apposition of bipolar myocardial electrodes, (4) long output circuit recovering time, and (5) short refractory period. If high-output stimuli are required to preserve capture, it may be necessary to extend the duration of the refractory period to prevent afterpotential recycling. Alternatively, the relative magnitude of the afterpotentials may be reduced by decreasing the pulse width while capture is maintained with a high-current or high-voltage setting.

Crosstalk between atrial and ventricular leads is a potential problem for any pacing system, but at least theoretically it is more likely when unipolar leads are used. One manifestation of crosstalk is the inhibition of ventricular output by the afterpotentials produced by atrial stimulation. The optimal substrate for crosstalk is the combination of high atrial output, high ventricular sensitivity, and short ventricular blanking period. Figure 14–7 illustrates atrial stimuli sensed by the ventricular channel and subsequent inhibition of ventricular output.

The electrocardiographic rhythm strip shown in Figure 14–8 demonstrates crosstalk present in a unipolar, noncommitted DVI pulse generator at nominal settings. An event detected by the ventricular lead within 110 msec after an atrial stimulus triggers ventricular stimulation. This feature has been designated by various manufacturers as the ventricular safety pacing interval or nonphysiologic AV delay.[15] The first two AV-paced complexes have AV delays of 110 msec, or 40 msec shorter than the third paced P-QRS. Therefore, it is reasonable to assume that the atrial afterpotential was sensed by the ventricular channel, which in turn triggered ventricular stimulation at the end of the safety pacing interval. Crosstalk inhibition may be prevented by using minimal output settings in the atrium.

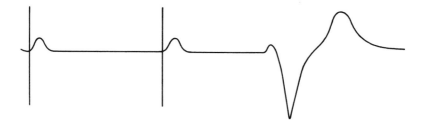

Figure 14–7. Example of crosstalk inhibition. The atrial stimulus is sensed by the ventricular channel, and the ventricular output is inhibited. The QRS complex is a ventricular escape beat.

If high or even nominal outputs result in cross-talk, the availability of the blanking period or the AV-triggered response will facilitate management; however, such safety features may interfere with optimal pacing electrophysiology and hemodynamics.

Electromagnetic Interference (EMI)

The sources of EMI and their impact on pacing systems have been reviewed by War-nowicz-Papp.[36] In addition to false inhibition or triggering of the output circuit, EMI may result in asynchronous stimulation when the pulse generator reverts to its interference mode.[12] Reversion to the interference mode occurs when the pulse generator's electronic circuit detects continuous 60-cycle electrical noise over a specific interval of time; subsequently, the demand function is disabled, and a stimulus is delivered at the end of the timing cycle. The interference or reversion rate is the asynchronous pacing rate that will be observed in the presence of noise, and different models will exhibit a variety of reversion rates. For example, the electrocardiogram shown in Figure 14–9 demonstrates false inhibition and reversion to the interference mode in the presence of 60-cycle noise; for this unit, the reversion rate (I) is about 85 beats per minute and allows the electrocardiographer to distinguish between it and the demand rate (70 beats per minute).

The interference mode was designed to prevent asystole in the presence of EMI. Its obvious application is for unipolar systems, since bipolar models are not affected by commonly encountered field strengths.[6] Unfortunately, asynchronous pacing, even for brief periods, may be hazardous, especially in patients who may be susceptible to ventricular tachyarrhythmias. The potential for harmful competitive pacing is demonstrated by the patient whose electrocardiogram is shown in Figure 14–10. This tracing was obtained in the intensive care unit 2 hours after insertion of an epimyocardial lead and a unipolar pulse generator that had been programmed to high sensitivity intraoperatively because of failure to sense at the nominal setting. Ventricular fibrillation was induced by a competitive stimulus (S3), which was delivered on the T wave of a spontaneous beat that was not sensed by the pacemaker. The interval between S2 and S3 is 660 msec, or 90 beats per minute, which is this pacemaker's reversion rate. Since the programmed automatic rate was 72 beats per minute, this finding was consistent with interference mode pacing. Thus, 60-cycle noise in the intensive care unit caused the pulse generator to function asynchronously. After successful defibrillation, the pulse generator was reprogrammed to the VVT mode, which disabled the interference mode circuit, and no further sensing problems occurred.

Sensitivity Programming

Most permanent sensitivity programming is done for undersensing. Increasing sensitivity often corrects this malfunction, provided it is not due to lead dislodgment or a defective pacing system. However, increasing sensitivity is not a benign maneuver, especially if the pacemaker is unipolar and consequently susceptible to interference. Even at nominal sensitivities, unipolar pacing systems are prone to oversensing, and the most common source of interference is the skeletal myopotential.[30] High sensitivities, therefore, may relieve undersensing, but for unipolar pacemakers the

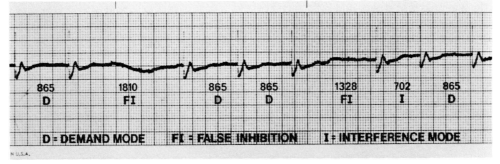

Figure 14–9. Two effects of excessive 60-cycle electrical noise on a unipolar VVI pacing system. The interference mode interval (I) of 702 msec serves as a marker for asynchronous pacing in the presence of noise detected by the pulse generator. In this case, however, 60-cycle noise was also misinterpreted as an actual ventricular event, resulting in false inhibition (FI). (From Hauser RG, Edwards LM, Stafford JL: Bipolar and unipolar sensing: Basic concepts and clinical applications. *In* Barold SS [ed]: Modern Cardiac Pacing. Mount Kisco, NY, Futura Publishing Co, 1985, p 157; with permission.)

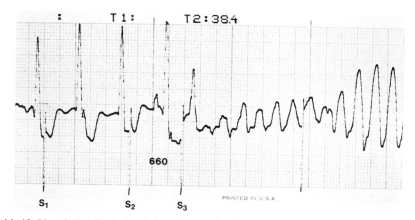

Figure 14–10. Ventricular fibrillation induced by a unipolar VVI pulse generator that had reverted to its noise mode, as indicated by the 660-msec interval between S2 and S3. (From Hauser RG, Edwards LM, Stafford JL: Bipolar and unipolar sensing: Basic concepts and clinical applications. *In* Barold SS [ed]: Modern Cardiac Pacing. Mount Kisco, NY, Futura Publishing Co, 1985, p 157; with permission.)

result may be as unacceptable as the original problem. One difficult situation involves the patient who is dependent (e.g., one who has no underlying sinus rhythm) and whose unipolar VVI pacemaker is not sensing his or her ventricular ectopy. After sensitivity is programmed to 0.8 mV, the PVCs are sensed, but now the pulse generator detects the pectoral muscle signals whenever he or she pushes or pulls with the arm on the same side as the implanted pulse generator. The most satisfactory option at this juncture is to program the unit to the VVT mode so that the pectoral myopotentials trigger rather than inhibit the pacemaker. Fortunately, most pulse generators have rate-limiting circuitry that prevents triggering at rates faster than 120 to 130 beats per minute, but the patient may complain of palpitations during muscular exercise.

High sensitivities are frequently needed for atrial applications. Sensitivity settings of 0.5 to 1.0 mV are not unusual, and, again, the side effects may be undesirable. Oversensing myopotentials by the atrial channel of a DDD pulse generator will trigger ventricular pacing, and it may induce a PMT.[11] There is no satisfactory solution because the only option is to decrease atrial sensitivity or to program the pacemaker to another mode. A lower sensitivity may result in undersensing, and a mode that does not provide P-wave–triggered ventricular pacing removes the major physiologic benefit of dual-chamber pacing.

Another distressing complication of high-sensitivity unipolar pacing is asynchronous pacing caused by oversensing. This phenomenon is seen when the pulse generator has an interference mode that initiates asynchronous pacing in the presence of continuous electrical noise. This intermittent or continuous fixed-rate pacing may mimic typical undersensing. The interference mode of some models results in asynchronous pacing at a rate that is measurably different from the automatic rate. This asynchronous pacing may be the physician's only clue that he or she is confronted not by an inadequate electrogram but rather by excessive noise. By decreasing sensitivity, the sensing of electrical noise or myopotential interference may be eliminated. Alternatively, the interference mode circuit may be disabled by programming the unit to a triggered mode.

The major advantage of programmability is the opportunity it offers the physician to change the characteristics of the pulse generator during or after implantation. The selection of a unipolar pacing system clearly limits such flexibility without, in turn, providing any significant electrophysiologic advantage over bipolar models. High-sensitivity and high-output settings are compatible with bipolar systems, but often they cannot be applied safely or comfortably with unipolar pacemakers. DDD pulse generators should be bipolar for the additional reasons that ultrahigh sensitivities are beneficial in patients who have very low-amplitude P waves and that the incidence of crosstalk may be reduced. Moreover, all automatic antitachycardia pacemakers should be bipolar because interference could trigger a burst of rapid pacing with potentially catastrophic results.

Experience with polarity programmability is limited, but certain benefits are implicit. Temporary programming from bipolar to unipolar can aid in the electrocardiographic interpretation of paced rhythms by providing a larger and hence more visible artifact. Similarly, temporary unipolar sensing is beneficial when using chest wall stimulation to inhibit or trigger the implanted pacemaker. Permanent programming from bipolar to unipolar may be warranted to correct undersensing when high-sensitivity settings are unsuccessful.

PACING MALFUNCTIONS: PACING

The second principle of complete pacing involves the successful firing of the pacemaker stimulus and the subsequent depolarization and repolarization of the cardiac tissue. A specific current density is required to stimulate myocardial tissue. The minimal energy level required to consistently cause rhythmic contraction of the heart is the stimulation threshold. This threshold is extremely dependent upon lead position, and even microdisplacements can affect these threshold values and thus affect the ability of the pacemaker stimulus to capture the heart.

At the time of initial implantation, the stimulation threshold must be accurately measured and the pulse generator output programmed accordingly. This stimulation threshold rises acutely (during the first several weeks) owing to the physiologic response of the heart tissue to the electrode. As illustrated in Figure 14–11, the output required to capture the heart changes during the acute phase and then stabilizes to a chronic level after the first several weeks. Once the threshold stabilizes, it remains relatively steady.

In addition to the electrode-tissue interface, other factors that affect the stimulation threshold include the maturity of the electrode, the electrode surface area, the polarity of the pacing system, lead conductor material, conductor or insulation breaks, pulse duration, myocardial injury or infarction, and drug or electrolyte balance.

The output, or the amount of energy in a pulse generator's stimulus pulse, is the product of the voltage amplitude and the pulse width. These are both programmable variables in the majority of today's pulse generators. Once the stimulation threshold has been ascertained, the output (both amplitude and pulse width) needs to be programmed, allowing an adequate safety margin. At implantation, if the capture threshold is less than 1 V at 0.5 msec, then the output can be left at the nominal setting, or at 5 V and 0.5 msec. Higher acute thresholds require correspondingly higher output settings because the threshold may increase fivefold during the first 2 weeks after lead insertion. Additional safety margin may be provided by programming the pulse width to 1.5 or 2.0 msec. The safety margin should be especially generous in the dependent patient, who may become symptomatic or may develop ventricular escape rhythms when capture is lost.

Threshold evolution may continue for months, but most leads will exhibit stable threshold values after 6 to 8 weeks. At that time, further output programming should be done to conserve energy and prolong battery life.

Failure to Capture

When evaluating an electrocardiographic rhythm strip, such as the one shown in Figure

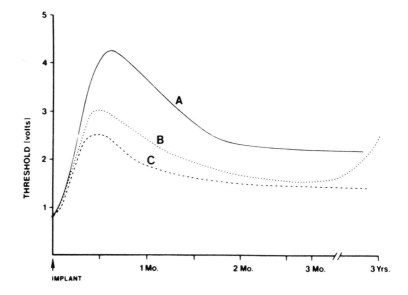

Figure 14–11. Acute and chronic stimulation thresholds. *A, B,* and *C* demonstrate stimulation thresholds from 3 different patients. See text for additional discussion.

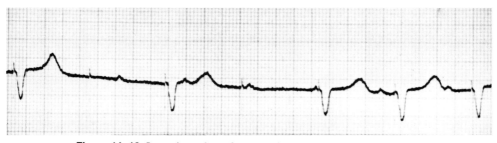

Figure 14–12. Intermittent loss of capture demonstrated on a rhythm strip.

14–12, it is important to determine whether the pacemaker is truly failing to capture or whether the pacemaker artifacts are falling within the refractory period, indicating a sensing malfunction. A pacemaker programmed to an asynchronous mode or the application of a magnet during the recording could also produce pacing artifacts that fall within the refractory period and thus appropriately do not capture the heart.

When capture is truly absent or intermittent, the cause may be due to the following:

I. Improper lead position

    A. Displacement due to dislodgment, perforation, or retraction from endocardium

    B. Incorrect placement at implantation

II. Output of the pulse generator below pacing threshold

    A. Power source failure

    B. Voltage programmed too low

    C. Component failure—output circuit

III. Increased pacing threshold

    A. Exit block

        1. Early—4 to 6 weeks

        2. Late—fibrosis

    B. Myocardial infarction

    C. Metabolic, toxic, or electrical event

IV. High resistance in the lead system

    A. Lead design

    B. Lead fracture

If the failure is due to a hardware problem, such as a fracture in the lead system, random component failure, or power source failure, appropriate operative intervention to replace the component at fault should be performed.

If the failure is related to the tissue-electrode interface, programming of the output to higher levels should be attempted. Thresholds should be measured and an adequate safety margin maintained. If the energy required to safely and consistently stimulate the cardiac tissue is not available with the implanted pacemaker system, then operative intervention is required.

Lack of Output

Lack of output occurs when pacemaker artifacts are absent on the electrocardiogram and pauses occur that are longer than the escape interval of the pulse generator. These pauses can be due to (1) inhibition of the pacemaker secondary to oversensing, (2) firing of the stimulus with interruption of the current before depolarization of the tissue-electrode interface secondary to a lead fracture, or (3) failure to fire secondary to component failure or battery depletion. Occasionally, this apparent lack of output can be due to electrocardiographic monitoring equipment that is undersensitive or an electrocardiographic lead that does not clearly identify the pacing artifact. An unknown programming change of the rate of hysteresis can also demonstrate apparent inappropriate intervals.

Placing the generator in the asynchronous mode with a magnet helps to identify whether the lack of output is due to a component failure or to oversensing of other voltage signals. If the asynchronous mode does not produce pacemaker activity, the problem is caused by either pulse generator component failure, including battery exhaustion, or an incomplete conduction system.

Evaluation of other indicators for battery depletion, such as rate and pulse width, can help identify the likelihood of component failure secondary to battery depletion and the need for generator replacement. An overpenetrated chest film may detect a fracture in the lead system, although lead fractures are not always apparent on radiographs. Operative intervention should then be undertaken to replace the depleted pulse generator or the fractured lead.

Output Programming

The rationale for output programming is illustrated by the three hypothetical patient stimulation threshold curves shown in Figure 14–11. At the time of implantation, patients A, B, and C had thresholds of about 0.75 V. However, following implantation, the stimulation threshold requirements of the three patients varied significantly. Patient A developed a rather high acute threshold rise exceeding 4 V, but the threshold declined thereafter to a chronic stable level. In contrast, patient C peaked at 2.5 V about 2.5 weeks after implantation, when the chronic threshold was approximately twice the acute threshold value. Patient B exhibited a modest acute threshold rise, which then declined to a lower level; subsequently, however, the threshold of stimulation for patient B gradually increased over a period of months. Thus, for any given patient, early and long-term threshold behavior cannot be predicted by the threshold value obtained at implantation.

Because of early and possibly late threshold elevation, nonprogrammable pacemakers had to be designed with sufficient energy to protect patients A and B from loss of capture or exit block during the early and late postimplantation periods. The majority of patients, however, require less energy than the nominal output provided by these nonprogrammable units. By programming the output to an efficient but safe level, we have increased projected battery life by 30 to 50 per cent.

The availability of output programming is also extremely beneficial in the patient who develops high thresholds or exit block. By increasing the programmed output energy, operative intervention to replace the lead or pulse generator or both has been avoided. Output programming is also useful for reducing and possibly eliminating extracardiac muscle stimulation.

Programmability, however, is no substitute for careful lead placement and must not be used to manage a defective pulse generator or lead. Further, whenever the programmed output energy is reduced, the patient should return every 6 months so that threshold requirements may be reassessed.

DDD Output Programming

The thresholds of chronic atrial and ventricular leads are very similar. For DDD systems, it may be unnecessary or unwise to provide the atrial lead with the same safety margin as the ventricular lead. If atrial capture is lost, then ventricular pacing protects the patient against asystole. Considerable energy savings can be gained by programming the output to values that approximate the chronic threshold. This approach can be adopted at the 6- to 8-week follow-up visit or later if appropriate. Reducing atrial output to near threshold levels may be contraindicated in patients who are prone to PMT or who experience disabling symptoms when atrial or AV sequential pacing is lost. Although intermittent or sustained loss of atrial capture may be of little consequence for most individuals, AV dissociation may produce hemodynamic embarrassment, and it is an excellent electrophysiologic substrate for inducing PMT. Nevertheless, lowering atrial output energy not only conserves battery capacity but also reduces the possibility of crosstalk interference wherein the atrial stimulus is sensed by the ventricular channel.[22]

PACEMAKER LEAD COMPLICATIONS

Pacemaker lead fractures and lead insulation failures have become a relatively infrequent complication of current pacemaker implantation procedures. However infrequent, lead failure presents a potentially serious clinical problem, almost always requiring surgical intervention for resolution.

Lead Fracture

Permanent cardiac pacing leads flex tens of millions of times yearly, imposing tremendous stresses on the materials used in the construction of both the conductor and the insulator. Lead conductor fracture has been reported in the early literature to be between 1 and 7 per cent,[1, 5, 8, 21] and conductor survival has continued to improve with the evolution of pacing leads.

Early conductors were composed of a single wire wound like a spring and bonded at the proximal end to a connector mechanism, designed to mate with the implantable pulse generator. The distal end of the spring conductor was bonded to a stimulating electrode to be placed in or on the heart. By adding multiple conductors lying side by side and wound in a similar spring configuration, which is known as multifilar construction, pacing conductor reliability has been significantly improved.[19]

Lead conductor failure can frequently be identified noninvasively through the use of the electrocardiogram and radiograph.

A complete conductor fracture, one that lacks continuity altogether, will manifest as no pacing artifact on the electrogram. A more frequent occurrence is a lead fracture that demonstrates intermittent function as it "makes and breaks" electrical contact (Fig. 14–12).

The type of fracture that makes intermittent contact frequently demonstrates aberrant system behavior, including both inappropriate sensing and erratic pacing. An intermittent conductor in the ventricular lead of a single- or dual-chamber pacemaker is likely to result in prolonged pacing intervals or total inhibition because of inappropriate sensing of the artifact generated by the contacting of the conductor. The same lead malady occurring in the atrial lead of a DDD type of pacemaker would most likely result in high-rate ventricular tracking of the noise from the atrial lead. Manual manipulation of the pacemaker pocket and lead insertion site while monitoring the electrocardiogram for inappropriate pacer function will help confirm the diagnosis of lead fracture.

Radiographic examination of the defective lead will frequently reveal a conductor fracture.[9] Distortion of the lead body at the anchoring ligature site and the bifurcation of the lead conductor at the connector end of a bipolar lead should not be misinterpreted as conductor fracture.[37] Coaxial bipolar leads must be carefully inspected, since an intact outer conductor can easily mask a damaged inner conductor.[34, 35]

Pacemaker programming will not resolve the problems associated with a broken conductor. Reoperation with pacing lead replacement provides the only effective long-term solution.

Lead Insulation Failure

Early experience with leads and reliability data were almost exclusively discussed in terms of lead conductor fracture, dislodgment rate, exit block, and so forth, with little attention given to the insulating material. In the late 1970s, polyurethane was commercially introduced as a pacemaker lead insulating material. The introduction of polyurethane as an insulating material brought attention to lead insulation, owing to the high failure rates of early designs.[32]

Lead insulation failure may be the result of different processes. The most common is a nick made by a needle during the closure of the incision site or damage caused by a scalpel when opening an existing pacemaker pocket at device replacement time. A less frequent but much more serious problem is lead insulation degradation through design-related failures, which in certain lead designs have approached 30 per cent.[27, 32, 33]

The failure of lead insulation, in many instances, may be diagnosed electrocardiographically. A small break in the insulation may result in inappropriate sensing, mimicking oversensing. If the damage to the insulation is severe, the patient may demonstrate lack of capture because of current shunting, as well as inappropriate sensing.

If the patient is the recipient of a unipolar pacemaker and has severe damage to the insulation of a pacing lead, it is not unusual to see the onset of pocket stimulation. This pocket stimulation, occurring late after implantation, is reason to suspect insulation failure. The stimulation is the result of increased current delivered by a constant-voltage pacemaker to the low impedance presented by the damaged lead.

Device programming will not, in most instances, provide a permanent solution to lead insulation damage. The problem of oversensing may be temporarily resolvable through adjusting the sensitivity of the implanted device, and lack of capture may be circumvented by increasing the pacing output at the expense of longevity. Repairing the lead insulation or replacement of the lead is the most reliable solution.

Intraoperative testing provides the final piece of information required to confirm the diagnosis. In the case of a fractured conductor in which there is no electrical contact whatsoever, a pacing system analyzer will read an infinite impedance. Where electrical contact is intermittent, the analyzer will show erratic impedance readings ranging anywhere from normal to infinite impedance.

A simple nick in the pacing electrode insulation may be apparent upon visual examination during reoperation but will probably not show an abnormal impedance reading on an analyzer. A major insulation failure, such as one caused by stress cracking or metal-catalyzed autooxidation, will show a lead impedance far below the range of normal.

PACEMAKER INFECTION AND WOUND COMPLICATION

Pacemaker infection is one of the least common but most serious complications of permanent pacing. It has replaced electronic malfunction as the complication most likely to cause death or debility, and pacemaker infection remains a controversial patient management issue.

Pacemaker infection may be manifested by a variety of signs and symptoms. For this discussion, it will be defined as inflammation or erosion (or both) of the pacemaker pocket, accompanied by fever and a positive blood culture. Infection that occurs early after pacemaker implantation is usually associated with *Staphylococcus aureus,* while late infection is most often due to *Staphylococcus epidermidis.*[7] In either case, complete removal of the entire pacing system has produced the most satisfactory results.[13, 24] Indeed, many of these patients are in a septic state and have stigmata of bacterial endocarditis. Vigorous treatment should include (1) culture-guided antibiotic therapy; (2) total removal of the pulse generator and lead; (3) local wound management, including drainage and secondary closure; and (4) implantation of a new pacing system in a different site. The timing of the reinsertion procedure remains controversial. Although a successful one-stage surgical approach—removal of the infected hardware and insertion of a new system—has been reported,[13, 24] it may be prudent to effect a bacteriologic cure before reimplanting a permanent lead and pulse generator. This requires a two-stage approach with an interim need for temporary rate support using either pharmacologic or electrical means in patients who are pacemaker dependent.

Pacemaker pocket erosion may occur without bacteremia. Such erosion often occurs late after implantation and is frequently seen when a pacemaker is located laterally in a thin, elderly patient. Erosion or ulceration may also occur after trauma to the skin overlying the pulse generator. So-called dry erosions may yield negative cultures, and the physician may elect simply to relocate the pocket and pulse generator. Occasionally, it may be necessary to divide the pacing lead above the eroded pocket and splice a new terminal pin and tunnel it to a new pocket where a replacement pulse generator is connected.[13]

REFERENCES

1. Alt E, Volker R, Blomer H: Lead fracture in pacemaker patients. Thorac Cardiovasc Surg 35:101, 1987.
2. Barold SS: Can a demand pacemaker really sense concealed ventricular extrasystoles? PACE 4:226, 1981.
3. Barold SS, Gaidula JJ, Banner RL, et al: Interpretation of complex demand pacemaker arrhythmias. Br Heart J 34:312, 1972.
4. Barold SS, Ong LS, Falkoff MD, et al: Inhibition of bipolar demand pacemaker by diaphragmatic myopotentials. Circulation 56:679, 1977.
5. Bernstein S, Van Natta B, Ellestad M: Experiences with atrial pacing. Am J Cardiol 61:113–116, 1988.
6. Bridges JD, Frazier MJ, Hauser RG: Effects of 60 Hz electrical fields and current on implanted cardiac pacemakers. Proceedings of the International Symposium on Electromagnetic Compatibility. New York, IEEE, 1978, p 258.
7. Choo MH, Holmes DR Jr, Gersh BJ, et al: Permanent pacemaker infections: Characterization and management. Am J Cardiol 48:559, 1981.
8. Conklin E, Giannelli S, Nealon T: Four hundred consecutive patients with permanent transvenous pacemakers. J Thorac Cardiovasc Surg 69:1–7, 1975.
9. De la Llana R, Munoz D, Sanz R: Letter to the Editor. PACE 10:1387, 1987.
10. Den Dulk K, Lindemans F, Wellens HJJ: Management of pacemaker circus movement tachycardias. PACE 7:346, 1984.
11. Den Dulk K, Lindemans FW, Wellens HJJ: Noninvasive evaluation of pacemaker circus movement tachycardias. Am J Cardiol 53:537, 1984.
12. Falkoff M, Ong LS, Heinle RA, et al: The noise sampling period: A new cause of apparent sensing malfunction of demand pacemakers. PACE 1:250, 1978.
13. Goldman BS, MacGregor DC: Management of infected pacemaker systems. Clin Prog Electrophysiol Pacing 2:220, 1984.
14. Goldreyer BN, Bruske R, Knudson MB, et al: Orthogonal ventricular electrogram sensing. PACE 6:761, 1983.
15. Hauser RG: The electrocardiography of AV universal DDD pacemakers. PACE 6:399, 1983.
16. Hauser RG, Susmano A: After potential oversensing by a programmable pulse generator. PACE 4:391, 1981.
17. Hauser RG, Edwards LM, Stafford JL: Bipolar and unipolar sensing: Basic concepts and clinical applications. *In* Barold SS (ed): Modern Cardiac Pacing. Mount Kisco, NY, Futura Publishing Co, 1985.
18. Irnich W: Comparison of pacing electrodes of different shape and material—recommendations. PACE 6:422, 1983.
19. Jaschke W, Hoellen I: Lead fracture—a still frequent cardiac pacemaker complication? Zentralbl Chir 109:1066, 1984.
20. Jost M, Pfisterer M, Schelker D, et al: Incidence and significance of muscle potential interference in patients with dual chamber pacemakers. *In* Steinbach K (ed): Cardiac Pacing: Proceedings of the VIIth World Symposium on Cardiac Pacing. Darmstadt, Federal Republic of Germany, Steinkopf, 1983, p 549.
21. Lagegren H, Levander-Lindgren M: Ten-year follow-up on 1000 patients with transvenous electrodes. PACE 7:1017, 1984.
22. Levine PA, Mace RG: Pacing Therapy: A Guide to Cardiac Pacing for Optimum Hemodynamic Benefit. Mount Kisco, NY, Futura Publishing Co, 1983, p 239.
23. Levine PA, Pirzada FA: Pacemaker oversensing: A possible example of concealed ventricular extrasystoles. PACE 4:199, 1981.

24. Lewis AB, Hayes DL, Holmes DR Jr, et al: Update on infections involving permanent pacemakers. J Thorac Cardiovasc Surg 89:758, 1985.
25. Massumi RA, Mason DT, Amsterdam EA, et al: Apparent malfunction of demand pacemaker caused by nonpropagated (concealed) ventricular extrasystoles. Chest 61:426, 1972.
26. Mond HG, Sloman JG: The malfunctioning pacemaker system: Part II. PACE 4:168, 1981.
27. Phillips R, Frey R, Martin R: Long-term performance of polyurethane pacing leads: Mechanisms of design-related failures. PACE 9:1166, 1986.
28. Ripart A, Mugica J: Electrode-heart interface: Definition of the ideal electrode. PACE 6:410, 1983.
29. Rozanski JJ, Blankstein RL, Lister JW: Pacer arrhythmias: Myopotential triggering of pacemaker mediated tachycardia. PACE 6:795, 1983.
30. Secemsky S, Hauser RG, Denes P, Edwards LM: Unipolar sensing abnormalities: Incidence and clinical significance of skeletal muscle interference and undersensing in 228 patients. PACE 5:5, 1982.
31. Secemsky SI, Hauser RG, Denes P, et al: Unipolar sensing abnormalities: Incidence and clinical significance of skeletal muscle interference and undersensing in 228 patients. PACE 5:10, 1982.
32. Stokes K: Recent advances in lead technology. In Barold SS, Mugica J (eds): New Perspectives in Cardiac Pacing. Mount Kisco, NY, Futura Publishing Co, 1988, pp 217–228.
33. Stokes K, Church T: Ten-year experience with implanted polyurethane lead insulation. PACE 9:1160, 1986.
34. Stokes K, Staffenson D, Lessar J, et al: A possible new complication of subclavian stick: Conductor fracture [abstract 476]. PACE 10:748, 1987.
35. Suzuki Y, Fujimori S, Sakai M: A case of pacemaker lead fracture associated with thoracic outlet syndrome. PACE 11:326, 1988.
36. Warnowicz-Papp MA: The pacemaker patient and the electromagnetic environment. Clin Prog Electrophysiol Pacing 1:166, 1983.
37. Witte AA: Pseudo-fracture of pacemaker lead due to securing suture: A case report. PACE 4:716, 1981.

15

PEDIATRIC CARDIAC PACING

PAUL C. GILLETTE, BERTRAND A. ROSS,
and VICKI ZEIGLER

Cardiac pacing is being used with increasing frequency in children with both bradycardias and tachycardias. This increased use is due not only to a better understanding of the mechanisms and prognosis of certain dysrhythmias but also to major improvements in the size, technology, and reliability of cardiac pacemakers and leads. The use of transvenous subpectoral implantation technique and the ability of pacemakers to sense the atrial rate to provide both atrioventricular (AV) synchrony and rate increase during exercise have improved the utility of pacemakers in children.

INDICATIONS

The indications for cardiac pacing in children are varied. They are presented in the joint American College of Cardiology (ACC) and American Heart Association (AHA) Task Force report.[1] Most children who need pacemakers are symptomatic. The symptoms range from syncope to excessive fatigue and inability to keep up with peers. One syncopal episode in a child with significant bradycardia is an indication for pacing.

Congenital complete AV block is one of the most common conduction disturbances that require a pacemaker. If the ventricular rate is less than 55 beats per minute in a neonate, a pacemaker is indicated.[8] A ventricular rate of 65 beats per minute in a neonate with significant congenital heart disease is considered an indication for a pacemaker. Most deaths in patients with congenital complete AV block occur in infants with significant congenital heart defects in the first year of life. In older

children with congenital complete AV block, one syncopal spell or near-syncopal spell should indicate a permanent pacemaker. It is not necessary to correlate an excessively slow rate with the symptoms. A ventricular rate less than 45 beats per minute has been strongly correlated with early syncope in older children with congenital complete AV block and thus is considered to be a pacemaker indication.[6] Frequent or complex premature ventricular contractions at rest or with exercise in a patient with complete AV block also indicate a permanent pacemaker.

Excessive fatigue, poor school performance, of new onset or an inability to keep up with peers may be pacemaker indications. We are often told by patients and parents about great improvements in lifestyle after DDD pacemaker implantation in patients with congenital complete AV block. We are probably waiting too long to implant pacemakers in many patients.

Surgery-related complete AV block that persists for more than 10 to 14 days is an indication for permanent pacing in children. The ventricular rate is often surprisingly fast early in this period but will usually decrease later after surgery. The repaired heart does better with a faster rate, AV synchrony, and rate variability.

Surgery-related sinus bradycardia associated with tachycardias often requires pacing. In the bradycardia-tachycardia syndrome, the use of an antiarrhythmic drug other than digoxin requires the implantation of a pacemaker. Often an atrial antitachycardia pacemaker is useful in this situation. Any syncope, near-syncope, or excessive fatigue in a patient in the postoperative period who has sinus bradycardia or

335

junctional rhythm may be effectively treated by pacing. Clinically evident congestive heart failure or increasing cardiac size on chest radiography or echocardiography will respond to cardiac pacing.

Sinus node dysfunction rarely causes symptoms in patients with normal hearts, but when it does, pacing results in symptomatic improvement. Other situations will occur rarely and are covered in the ACC/AHA report.

PACING MODE

The decision of pacing mode (Table 15–1) is as important as the decision to implant a pacemaker. The restoration of normal physiology should always be our goal, although it is not yet possible in every case. In patients with AV block, the use of an atrial synchronous pacemaker will nearly restore normality in most patients. Some patients with either congenital or surgery-related AV block will later develop chronotropic incompetence and will not be able to increase their sinus rate to normal during exercise. In patients with sinus bradycardia and intact AV conduction, an atrial pacemaker will be significantly more physiologic than ventricular pacing. If AV conduction is intact clinically and if AV conduction is maintained 1:1 at rates of 100 beats per minute or greater during atrial pacing, we have found no incidence of progression to AV block. If AV conduction is inappropriate or if the patient has had repair of a ventricular septal defect, then a dual-chamber pacemaker is used. In the postoperative period for patients who have had atrial surgery (atrial septal defect, atrial repair of transposition, or a Fontan operation), an atrial automatic antitachycardia pacemaker should be used.

As sensor-driven pacemakers become more available and have more appropriate parameters for atrial pacing, they will be used more frequently for both atrial and dual-chamber applications. Ventricular pacemakers are reserved for extremely small premature infants and patients with very infrequent bradycardia.

IMPLANTATION TECHNIQUE

Most pacemakers in children are implanted by the transvenous technique.[3] Pacemakers in infants as small as 8 kg are now routinely implanted transvenously. Indications for epicardial pacing are (1) right-to-left shunt, (2) lack of access from the superior vena cava to the chamber to be paced, (3) inexcitable right atrium, and (4) newborn or premature infants.[9]

The technique of implanting a pacemaker in a child is not dissimilar to the technique used in adults. It should be performed by an operator familiar with pediatric catheterization techniques who performs an adequate number of implantations to keep his or her technical skills honed. The left infraclavicular area is the preferred site for venous access. Lead manipulations seem to be easier from this site. The subclavian puncture technique is used with a retained guide wire to avoid a second puncture.

Screw-in leads are used in increasing numbers of pediatric patients owing to their security and their removability. This latter feature is significant, considering the theoretically greater likelihood that the pacemaker lead in pediatric patients will be removed at some later time.

The ventricular lead is not placed in the apex of the right ventricle (Fig. 15–1) but, rather, one third to one half of the way up the septum (Fig. 15–2) to avoid diaphragmatic pacing. The atrial lead is placed anywhere in the right atrium except the lateral wall near the phrenic nerve (Figs. 15–3 and 15–4). In patients who have had venous repair of transposition of the great arteries (a Senning or Mustard procedure), the atrial lead should be positioned in the roof of the anatomic left atrium away from the radiographic border of the left side of the heart to avoid the left phrenic nerve. High-output (10 V, 2 msec) pacing should be performed on both leads during implantation to predict stimulation of noncardiac structures.

The pulse generator is positioned under the pectoralis major muscle. The muscle is spread by blunt dissection and resutured with 2–0 absorbable suture.

TABLE 15–1. INDICATIONS FOR PACING MODE

CLINICAL SITUATION	PACING MODE
CCAVB	DDDCO
SCAVB	DDDCO
SSSS with tachycardia	AAICP
SSSS with impaired AV conduction	DDDCO
SSSS without tachycardia	AAICP
SSS	AAICO
Transient, infrequent AVB	VVICO
Premature infant	VVICO
Atrial fibrillation with bradycardia	VVIRO

CCAVB = congenital complete AVB; SCAVB = surgical complete AVB; SSSS = severe sick sinus syndrome; AV = atrioventricular; SSS = sick sinus syndrome; AVB = atrioventricular block.

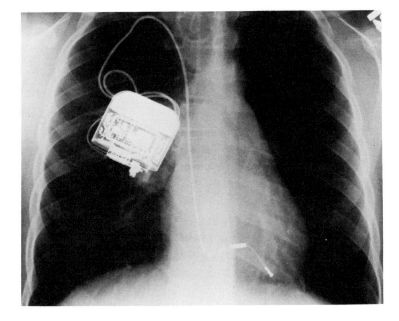

Figure 15–1. Posteroanterior (PA) chest radiograph of a 12-year-old patient with a transvenous VVI pacemaker. The lead has been introduced from the right subclavian puncture and positioned in the apex of the right ventricle. This is not the optimal lead position in a pediatric patient, since the right ventricular wall in pediatric patients with normal hearts is so thin that pacing of the diaphragm may occur. Diaphragmatic pacing was more common with unipolar than with bipolar leads but has occurred also with bipolar ventricular leads.

PHYSIOLOGY

We now have a variety of ways to attempt to maintain as normal a physiologic response with a pacemaker as possible. Pacemakers that sense the atrium and pace the ventricle after a programmable AV delay have been available for several years (Fig. 15–5).[2] These pacemakers require that the patient's sinus node have a normal or acceptable response to ex-

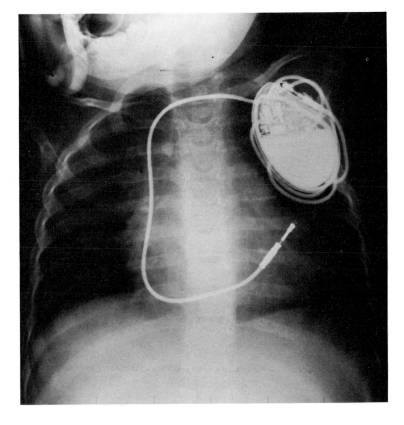

Figure 15–2. PA chest radiograph of a 2-year-old child with an implanted transvenous pacemaker. The bipolar screw-in lead has been introduced into the left subclavian vein, and the lead tip has been positioned approximately one third to one half of the way up the ventricular septum. This is the optimal lead position for a pediatric patient, since diaphragmatic pacing may result from right ventricular apex positioning. The extra lead has been left in the right atrium to permit growth without traction of the lead.

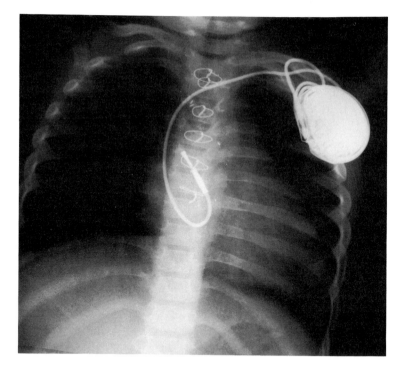

Figure 15–3. PA chest radiograph of a patient who had removal of a right atrial tumor, with subsequent destruction of the sinus node. A transvenous bipolar pacing lead has been introduced into the left subclavian vein and positioned in the stump of the right atrial appendage attached to the right atrial wall with a small screw. The **J** has been formed in the right atrium to allow for growth of the patient.

ercise and other stresses that require a response in heart rate. Alternatively, we now have single-chamber devices that sense a body function such as activity and increase their pacing rate in response. It is proved that atrial synchronous pacemakers will improve cardiac performance and the sense of well-being in adults and probably children. It is not sure yet how closely ventricular pacemakers that increase their rate will come to achieving this

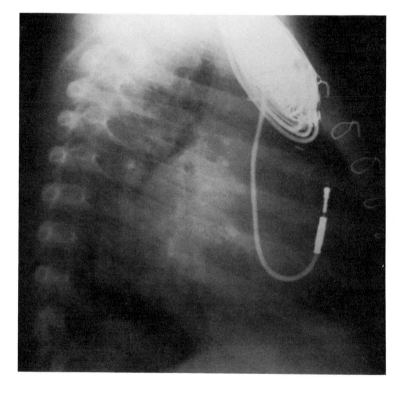

Figure 15–4. Lateral chest radiograph showing the position of a bipolar screw-in lead in the stump of the right atrial appendage in a patient who had removal of a right atrial tumor. The lead has been positioned from the left subclavian vein and screwed into the stump of the right atrial appendage.

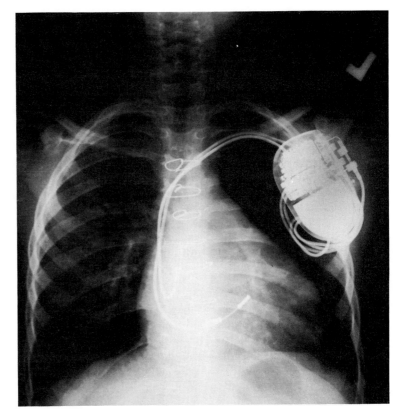

Figure 15–5. PA chest radiograph showing a dual-chamber in-line, bipolar DDD pacemaker. The leads have been positioned by percutaneous puncture of the left subclavian vein. The ventricular lead is positioned approximately one third of the way up the ventricular septum. The atrial lead has been positioned in the stump of the right atrial appendage. The ventricular lead is a tined target tip lead, and the atrial lead is a porous-tipped screw-in lead.

response. Clearly, they allow a greater exercise performance for adults than does a single-rate ventricular pacemaker.

Since our experience with dual-chamber, atrial synchronous pacemakers has been excellent, and since we have not seen a significant number of problems in children resulting from a two-lead system, we continue to use DDD pacemakers in most children. The advent of dual-chamber, rate-modulated pacemakers will allow us to test exercise responses in the same patient in two modes.

Atrial pacing is a viable option in children with sinus node dysfunction and intact AV conduction, as occurs frequently after the Senning, Mustard, and Fontan operations.[4] In this setting, there are often isolated sinus node abnormalities, while the AV node is spared. There does not seem to be a significant amount of progression to AV block in these patients. Thus, a simpler, smaller, less expensive pacing system can be used. In patients who have undergone a Fontan procedure, this allows a transvenous approach, whereas ventricular or dual-chamber pacing would require an epicardial approach.[5] The early postoperative period of a patient who has had a Fontan operation presents a special challenge, since thresholds are often higher than in other clinical settings.

LEADS

The pacing lead has evolved tremendously in the past decade. A major advance from the pediatric perspective is size. The size of either bipolar or unipolar leads is now acceptable for children of all sizes. Polyurethane insulation may help prevent thrombosis, although this has not been a problem in pediatric transvenous pacing. Noninvasive screening for subclavian thrombosis has failed to reveal any abnormalities.

Although tined leads have prevented almost all lead dislodgments for ventricular leads and for atrial leads, when an appendage is present, screw-in leads are preferred in children who have had previous heart surgery. They may also be easier to remove after many years, which is an important consideration in children. The advantage is partially lost if the entire lead is not isodiametric, since sheaths that develop where the lead touches the vascular wall may impede removal.

The in-line bipolar connector has been a major advance as well, since it saves bulk not only on the lead but also on the pulse generator header. Some of this advantage is currently lost, since there is not yet standardization of the in-line connectors, which require bulky adapters in some situations.

The use of a small quantity of steroid released from the lead tip has been beneficial in patients with repeated high stimulation thresholds.[7] It also improves stimulation thresholds and flattens the acute peak in thresholds. Other innovations, such as "porous" tips and grooved, platinized tips, have also resulted in improved stimulation and sensing thresholds.

We currently use bipolar, porous-tipped, screw-in or grooved, platinized electrodes with in-line bipolar connectors. Our average stimulation threshold at 6 months is 0.07 msec at 5 V. We then usually set the pulse generators at 2.7 V at 0.2 or 0.3 msec, resulting in a large saving in energy when compared with nominal settings.

Bipolar leads offer many advantages over unipolar leads, more than outweighing their size disadvantage. Bipolar atrial leads have a smaller far-field "R" wave than do unipolar leads. They are less sensitive to pectoral muscle sensing and other unwanted sensing. Their insertion allows creation of a subpectoral pocket, which improves the cosmetic result and may minimize erosion and trauma. The use of two bipolar leads has never led to a clinical problem with venous thrombosis or embolus in children as small as 12 kg. No damage to the tricuspid valve has been noted.

It is now clearly proved that epicardial leads are less desirable than endocardial leads. This is especially true in atrial applications, but it is also true for ventricular pacemakers. The incidence of fracture is clearly higher, chronic stimulation thresholds are higher, and the incidence of excessively high thresholds is greater. In addition, postpericardiotomy syndrome, with the need for pericardiocentesis, is a not uncommon problem with epicardial leads. We reserve epicardial leads for patients without venous access, tiny newborn babies, and those with right-to-left shunts.

PULSE GENERATORS

We currently use bipolar, multiprogrammable, telemetric DDD (atrial synchronous) pulse generators (Fig. 15–6). For children, we believe each pulse generator should have an upper rate limit of 175 beats per minute. The upper rate response should probably be gradual second-degree AV block, not 2:1 AV block. The atrial refractory period must be

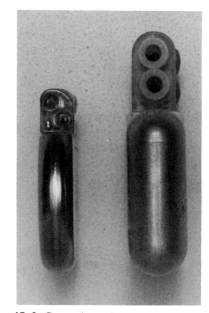

Figure 15–6. Comparison of pacemaker size with a 10-year period between pacemakers. The pacemaker on the left is a bipolar, in-line DDD pacemaker. The pacemaker on the right is a bipolar, single-chamber, rechargeable pacemaker manufactured 10 years ago. The pacemaker on the left is multiprogrammable and multitelemetric, whereas the pacemaker on the right had no programmability or telemetry functions. Thus, a major decrease in size has occurred at the same time as a major increase in functional capabilities of pacemakers. This aspect is particularly important in pediatric patients.

programmable to prevent pacemaker-mediated tachycardia. The maximal atrial sensitivity should be at least 0.6 mV. With bipolar units, these high sensitivities are usable. Telemetry is essential. It allows confirmation and documentation of programmed settings at the beginning and end of noninvasive pacemaker evaluations. In many units, measurement of lead and battery parameters is possible. Telemetry can also be used to confirm programming changes. Event counters have also proved useful but are not essential.

Single-chamber pulse generators should be capable of all the appropriate programming of which dual-chamber generators are capable. When single-chamber generators are used in an atrial application, as we usually do, high sensitivity and programmable refractory periods are very useful.

The degree of programmability available in current pulse generators has obviated the need for "special order" pediatric pulse generators, since one can program any pulse generator to pediatric specifications.

ANTITACHYCARDIA PACING

Atrial antitachycardia pacing is a useful modality in children. The two most frequent clinical situations are the postoperative bradycardia-tachycardia syndrome and atrial reentry. The fact that antiarrhythmic drugs often worsen sinus bradycardia is particularly important in patients in the postoperative period. The additive negative effect of AV dissociation on cardiac output due to junctional escape rhythm is also important. Each of these problems is addressed by atrial antitachycardia pacing. Marked improvement in symptoms and in objective indices of cardiac performance is the rule after implantation of these pacemakers. The transvenous bipolar route of implantation is particularly important in these patients because of the marginal size of atrial electrograms both in sinus rhythm and during tachycardia.

The most common tachycardia we have treated is atrial flutter. Aggressive tachycardia reduction algorithms are sometimes necessary. For example, one patient required 32 beats, beginning at 85 per cent of the tachycardia cycle length and decreasing by 2 msec with each beat. On the other hand, one patient has repeatedly had successful tachycardia termination with two beats at 70 per cent of the tachycardia cycle length.

In patients who have had repair of atrial septal defect or transposition of the great arteries, digoxin is usually the only drug necessary after antitachycardia pacing. During the postoperative period in patients who have had the Fontan procedure, other powerful antiarrhythmic drugs must often be used.

Tachycardia is recognized by setting a recognition rate and a rate of change of rate. Using these two criteria, we have not been able to "fool" the second-generation antitachycardia pacemaker with sinus tachycardia.

FOLLOW-UP

The aim of follow-up is to detect pacing system malfunction or normal battery depletion while it is in the asymptomatic stage, without giving the patient or family pacemaker psychosis or neurosis.[10] The techniques are essentially the same as in adults. To these ends, we use transtelephonic and "hands on" follow-up. We see patients at 6 weeks, 6 months, and then yearly. Transtelephonic follow-up is performed monthly for the first year

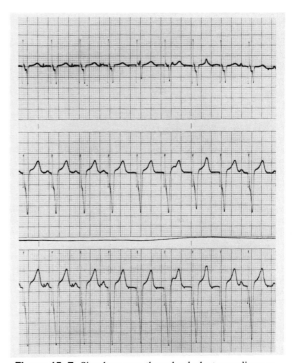

Figure 15–7. Simultaneous three-lead electrocardiogram (ECG) showing loss of atrial capture. DDD pacing is occurring. At the left for the first three beats, both the atrium and the ventricle are being paced and captured. The fourth atrial pacemaker spike does not capture the atrium, and no atrial depolarization is seen on the surface ECG leads. Ventricular capture occurs normally, and the p wave can be seen to march through the t wave and, on the last beat, appear before the QRS. A low output was being used on the atrial lead in this pacemaker, and the threshold was very close to the output of the pacemaker.

and then every 3 months. The threshold is tested within 25 per cent of output energy automaticity at each telephone check by decreasing the output energy on the fourth magnet beat. Atrial sensing can usually be seen in DDD and atrial antitachycardia units, but atrial capture is hard to detect transtelephonically in DDD units (Fig. 15–7).

At the first (6 weeks) "hands on" visit, we test capture thresholds and adjust pulse generator output to two times the threshold value for the atrial channel and three times the threshold value for the ventricle. The absence of pacemaker dependence, if such is the case, is demonstrated to the patient at each visit by completely inhibiting the pulse generator for 2 to 3 minutes. This demonstration results in a significant improvement in the patient's and family's feeling of well-being. The use of the subpectoral pocket, with its improvement in cosmetic results, also makes the patient feel better about the pacemaker (Fig. 15–8). In the

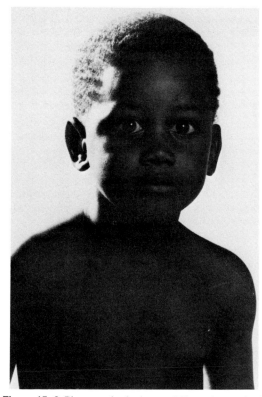

Figure 15–8. Photograph of a 4-year-old boy who received a transvenous DDD pacemaker implant in his left subpectoral region for congenital atrioventricular (AV) block with syncope. It can be seen from this back-lighted photograph that only a small bulge is made in his chest because the pacemaker is implanted beneath the pectoralis major muscle.

past 4 years, we have not detected a pulse generator malfunction. Lead problems are still encountered. These are almost exclusively found in the atrial lead of patients in the postoperative period.

The effect of growth on lead position is of great importance in pediatric pacing. As much extra lead as possible is left in the right atrium at implantation. The lead is sutured at the subclavian vein entrance with an absorbable suture in the hope that lead may be "played out" of the pocket. Periodic advancements of the lead may be necessary, but this has rarely been the case.

The patients are encouraged to lead a normal life. Only tackle football and hockey are proscribed. Very little psychopathology is noted in patients treated in this manner.

REFERENCES

1. Fry R, Collins JJ, DeSanctis RW, et al: Guidelines for permanent cardiac pacemaker implantation: A report of the Joint American College of Cardiology/ American Heart Association Task Force on Assessment of Cardiovascular Procedures (Subcommittee on Pacemaker Implantation). Circulation 70:331A–339A, 1984.
2. Gillette PC: Atrial sensing pacemakers. *In* Gillette PC, Griffin JC (eds): Practical Cardiac Pacing. Baltimore, Williams & Wilkins, 1986, pp 87–103.
3. Gillette PC: Transvenous implantation technique. *In* Gillette PC, Griffin JC (eds): Practical Cardiac Pacing. Baltimore, Williams & Wilkins, 1986, pp 45–62.
4. Gillette PC, Wampler DG, Shannon C, Ott D: Use of atrial pacing in a young population. PACE 8:94–100, 1985.
5. Hayes DL, Holmes DR Jr, Maloney JD, et al: Permanent endocardial pacing in pediatric patients. J Thorac Cardiovasc Surg 85:618–624, 1983.
6. Karpawich PP, Garson A, Gillette PC, et al: Congenital complete atrioventricular block: Clinical and electrophysiologic prediction of need for pacemaker insertion. Am J Cardiol 48:1098–1102, 1981.
7. King DH, Gillette PC, Shannon C, Cuddy T: A steroid eluting endocardial pacing lead for treatment of exit block. Am Heart J 106:1438–1440, 1983.
8. Michaelsson M, Engle MA: Congenital complete heart block: An international study of the natural history. Cardiovasc Clin 4:86–101, 1972.
9. Ott DA: The epicardial approach to cardiac pacing. *In* Gillette PC, Griffin JC (eds): Practical Cardiac Pacing. Baltimore, Williams & Wilkins, 1986, pp 63–75.
10. Shannon CE: Pacing system follow-up. *In* Gillette PC, Griffin JC (eds): Practical Cardiac Pacing. Baltimore, Williams & Wilkins, 1986, pp 137–160.

16

RATE-RESPONSIVE PACING AND SENSORS

DAVID WARD *and* CLIFFORD GARRATT

Devices for long-term cardiac stimulation have undergone many developments since the first single-chamber pacemaker was implanted 30 years ago. The main limitation of single-chamber devices is the lack of a rate response to exercise or other causes of increased energy demand. The VAT pacing system introduced by Nathan and colleagues[28] in 1963 provided an increased heart rate on exercise by linking the ventricular response to atrial sensing. These systems did not gain acceptance because epicardial leads and thoracotomy were required. With the improvement in both atrial and ventricular endocardial lead technology in the 1970s, and the development of DDD or universal pacing systems, dual-chamber pacing became established. By tracking the atrial electrogram, such systems are able to provide changes in heart rate determined by the sinus node. The integrity of the sinus node is central to the effective operation of such a system. In most patients with sinoatrial disorders, the sinus rate increases in response to exercise. Only a minority have so-called chronotropic incompetence. In patients with complete atrioventricular (AV) block, however, there is a high prevalence of an inadequate sinus node response to exertion.[14, 38] In terms of exercise ability, these patients may not benefit from simple dual-chamber pacing systems. Dual-chamber devices may not be suitable in patients with frequent atrial arrhythmias, which may result in inappropriate pacing tachycardias.

In the normal human, cardiac output increases on maximal exercise by approximately three to four times. This effect is the result of increases in stroke volume, due to greater venous return, and a rise in heart rate. AV synchrony contributes about 20 per cent of the stroke volume at rest, but as heart rate rises on exertion, this contribution becomes less and less important.[34] Given the above, a single- or dual-chamber pacemaker that increases the rate of stimulation in response to exercise and other physiologic stimuli is appropriate for a large number of patients with bradycardia. Such pacemakers have been termed "rate responsive," that is, they modulate heart rate in response to changing circumstances. A better term is "rate-adaptive" pacemakers. Clinical settings in which such pacemakers might be considered are summarized in Table 16–1. Increasing use of these devices is being considered in specific iatrogenic conditions, e.g., after catheter ablation of the atrioventricular junction.

Indicators and Sensors

The distinguishing feature of a rate-adaptive pacemaker is a sensor that detects an indicator of metabolic demand that can then be used to modulate the rate of myocardial stimulation. Several indicators and sensors have been proposed, and some have been successfully incorporated into pacemakers (Table 16–2). There is, as yet, no perfect indicator of metabolic demand under all circumstances, but most are sensitive to changes induced by exercise.

TABLE 16–1. INDICATIONS FOR RATE-ADAPTIVE PACING

Ventricular
  Complete or high-grade atrioventricular (AV) block
    plus:
    Established atrial arrhythmias
    Frequent atrial arrhythmias
    "Silent" atrium (unable to pace or sense)
    "Giant atrium" (difficult to fix an atrial lead)

Atrial
  Normal AV conduction *plus:*
    Frequent sinus pauses even during exercise
    Inadequate sinus response to exercise

Dual-chamber
  Complete or high-grade AV block plus inadequate
    sinus response to exercise

TABLE 16–2. SENSORS INCORPORATED INTO RATE-ADAPTIVE PACEMAKERS

1. Ventricular repolarization
    Stimulus-T sensing (TX, Quintech, Rhythmyx—Vitatron, Dieren, Netherlands)
2. Ventricular depolarization
    Ventricular depolarization gradient (Prism—Telectronics, Englewood, CO)
3. Activity and vibration
    Activitrax (Medtronic, Minneapolis, MN) and Sensolog (Siemens, Solna, Sweden)
4. Respiration
    Respiratory rate (Biorate, RDP3, MB 1—Biotec Alpha, Bologna, Italy)
    Minute ventilation (Meta MV—Telectronics, Englewood, CO)
5. Temperature
    Nova MR (Intermedics, Freeport, TX), Kelvin 500 (Cook, Leechburg, PA), and Thermos (Biotronik, Berlin, West Germany)
6. Myocardial contractility
    Rate of change of right ventricular pressure (Deltatrax, DPDT—Medtronic, Minneapolis, MN)
    Stroke volume, rate of change of stroke volume, and preejection interval (Precept—Cardiac Pacemakers, Inc, St. Paul, MN)

Ideally, the sensor of a rate-adaptive pacemaker should have the following properties:

1. It should be sensitive to exercise and other physical states resulting in a physiologic change in heart rate (sleep, stress, posture, and so on).

2. The output from the sensor should respond specifically, appropriately, and predictably to predetermined signals and should be insensitive to inputs (intrinsic and extrinsic) not normally associated with significant changes in heart rate (e.g., extraneous vibration, normal respiratory modulation).

3. It should respond as promptly as the normal sinus node.

4. It should be durable and robust.

5. It should have low power consumption.

6. It should operate with conventional pacing leads (i.e., the sensor either is inside the pacemaker can, as in activity sensing, or is processed information from a conventional lead, as in the evoked-response sensing systems).

As yet, no single sensor exists that satisfies all of these criteria.

The Interrelationship Between Sensor and the Pacing System: Open- and Closed-Loop Systems

Most of the rate-adaptive pacemakers currently available operate as an "open-loop" system, whereby the rate-responsive "slope"

(ratio of the change in sensor signal to pacemaker output) has to be estimated for each individual patient by means of trial and error. In contrast, in a "closed-loop" system, increased metabolic demand and increased pacing rate affect the sensor in opposite directions; the pacemaker output operates to keep the sensor signal at a fixed reference value. For instance, if the sensor signal decreases as a response to exercise, the pacemaker will increase its rate sufficient to maintain the sensor signal at the reference value. For any individual patient, the amount of sensor change induced by a given degree of exercise does not matter, as long as it is proportional to the pacing rate change required to produce an equal but opposite change in the sensor. The pacemaker that uses the ventricular depolarization gradient (VDG) as an indicator of metabolic demand (see below) operates as a closed-loop system; there is no need for programmable slope or sensitivity settings. It should be noted that a closed-loop system is different from a pacing system with an "automatic slope." The latter term refers to a system whereby the "trial-and-error" approach to slope programming is performed automatically and does not require repeated manual checking by the physician.

RATE-RESPONSIVE PACING SYSTEMS

Ventricular Repolarization

Principle

One of the earliest rate-responsive pacing systems utilized the known effects of exercise on the duration of ventricular repolarization. During exercise, the QT interval on the surface electrocardiogram shortens, as recognized by Bazett.[4] Initially, it was thought that this shortening was solely a result of increases in heart rate (hence the many attempts to correct, normalize, or predict the QT interval for a given heart rate). It is now recognized that exercise may shorten the QT interval independently of the changes in heart rate[12, 25, 30] (Fig. 16–1), probably as a result of changes in the levels of sympathetic tone and circulating catecholamines. The duration of the QT interval or its equivalent may therefore be used to modulate the frequency of a pacing system. Donaldson and Rickards[10] (1983) devised an endocardial sensing system (using a standard unipolar electrode) that measured and monitored the duration of the local endocardial

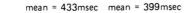

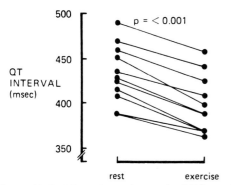

Figure 16–1. Effect of exercise on the QT interval at a fixed pacing rate. Shortening of the QT interval with exercise is independent of heart rate. (Modified from Milne JR, Ward DE, Spurrell RAJ, Camm AJ: The ventricular paced QT interval—effects of rate and exercise. PACE 5:352–358, 1982.)

equivalent of the QT interval, known as the paced evoked response.

Clinical Experience

The duration of the stimulus-T interval of the paced evoked response varies according to the level of exercise, in an analogous way to the QT interval. In the system devised by Rickards and coworkers,[30] shortening of the interval results in an increase in pacing rate and lengthening results in a decrease in rate. In the original system, these changes were linearly related.

Although a simple and attractive concept, several technical and physiologic problems were identified with the early devices.

1. T-wave sensing was unreliable.[13] The rate response is disabled by loss of T-wave sensing, with the unpleasant consequence of this effect at high-paced rates being a precipitous fall in rate to the basic rate. T-wave oversensing also occurred, with resultant inappropriate rate ac-

celeration. High slope settings could result in oscillations of the pacing rate thought to be due to variable T-wave sensing or variations in QT duration. Measurements of the size of the evoked T wave had to be made at implantation to assess suitability. Several patients were described who had very small paced evoked QT response to exercise and, as a consequence, suffered from minimal rate response to exercise.[40]

2. The response of the pacing system was slow, leading to a long latency between the onset of exercise and increase in rate,[24] together with inappropriate postexercise tachycardia with short periods of exercise (such as climbing a flight of stairs). The principal reason for this response is inherent in the indicator of metabolic demand: There is a delay in the onset of QT shortening with exercise (approximately 60 seconds).

3. The system was cumbersome and difficult to program. The rate-responsive slope required frequent reprogramming.

4. Drugs that affect the QT interval may also change the modulated response. For example, beta blockers may completely abolish rate modulation.[13]

Some of these problems have been overcome in the latest models, in which many of the adjustments have been automated.

1. T-wave sensing has been improved.

2. The rate of change of pacing is determined by the absolute rate at which the unit is operating. For example, a given change in the QT interval near the lower rate will result in a more rapid change in the pacing rate than will the same change at higher rates. This modification has been brought about in the light of studies that have shown a nonlinear relationship between pacing rate and QT duration[3] (Fig. 16–2). The dynamic slope has

Figure 16–2. Nonlinear relationship between the QT interval and the pacing interval. At high pacing rates (short pacing interval), the rate of change of the QT interval is greater than that at lower rates.

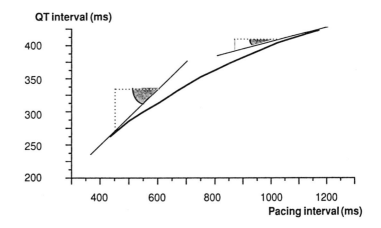

resulted in a more rapid onset of a pacing rate increase at the start of exercise, with shallower increases at rates near the upper limit. Oscillations due to high upper rate slopes are also less common.

3. The slope value can be adjusted automatically and can be continually updated by the pacemaker. The lower rate relationship is measured while the patient is resting at night. The low rate slope is derived from the QT interval at the low rate and a higher rate equivalent to shortening the pacing interval by 102 msec. A new slope value is set if the new value deviates from the existing value.

These rate-adaptive pacemakers have not achieved the popularity of the vibration-sensing devices (see below), principally because of the problems outlined above. Although the problems related to the relative complexity of the device and the requirement for reprogramming are much diminished in the latest models, problems with slow response time are, to a large extent, inherent in the use of the stimulus-T interval as an indicator of metabolic demand. The potential advantage with this form of pacing lies in the good correlation between magnitude of pacing rate increase and magnitude of metabolic demand. QT pacemakers are capable of responding to physiologic stimuli other than isotonic exercise, such as isometric exercise and mental activity (Fig. 16–3).

Ventricular Depolarization Gradient (VDG)

Principle

Another experimental device utilizes the ventricular evoked response to control pacing rate. The ventricular depolarization gradient or VDG is derived from the electronic integration of a paced evoked QRS complex. At a constant pacing rate, performance of exercise leads to a decrease in the VDG (as well as the "QT" duration).[7] Conversely, an increase in pacing rate leads to an *increase* in the VDG (unlike the "QT" interval). The output of the pacemaker is modulated by changes in the VDG, the principle of operation of the pacing system being to maintain the value of the VDG constant. The reference value, or target VDG, is measured at rest over a 20-cycle period. Subsequently, the measured value (sampled every fourth beat) is compared with the target value. Measured values less than the target value result in an increase in rate of 1.25 ppm per cycle. If the measured value exceeds the target value, there is a similar decrease in rate. This process continues until the values are equivalent. Thus, this system is automatic and closed-loop. At present, devices are being implanted as part of an initial evaluation, but clinical results are not yet published. Early results suggest that the system responds reasonably promptly to exercise and to nonexercise stimuli (Fig. 16–4).

Mixed Venous Oxygen Saturation

Principle

The input for this type of device is generated by an optical sensor that measures the oxygen saturation of hemoglobin in mixed venous blood (So_2). The So_2 falls rapidly with the onset of exercise and reaches a new plateau level within 1 minute.[42] The extent of the fall is proportionate to the stable exercise load. The decline in So_2 is almost linearly related to oxygen consumption and workload, providing a potentially highly physiologic rate-adaptive pacing system. In any individual subject, a given workload corresponds to a particular level of So_2, which is determined by both cardiac output and oxygen extraction. Increasing the cardiac output will diminish the AV oxygen difference and reduce the rate of fall of So_2 during exercise.

In the system devised by Wirtzfeld and associates,[42] the sensor is mounted in the stimulation electrode about 8.5 cm from the tip. The So_2 is measured once during each cycle

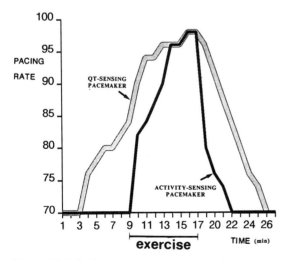

Figure 16–3. Pacing rate response to exercise in a patient with a QT-sensing pacemaker (Vitatron 919) and an external Activitrax device. Anticipation of the activity resulted in an increase in the pacing rate of the QT-sensing pacemaker. Mental activity and emotional stress increase pacing rate in most patients with QT-sensing pacemakers.

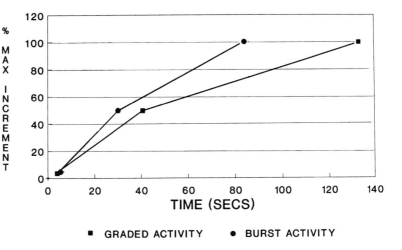

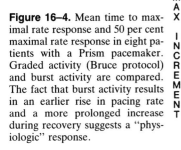

Figure 16–4. Mean time to maximal rate response and 50 per cent maximal rate response in eight patients with a Prism pacemaker. Graded activity (Bruce protocol) and burst activity are compared. The fact that burst activity results in an earlier rise in pacing rate and a more prolonged increase during recovery suggests a "physiologic" response.

(in diastole). Sampling is synchronized to the QRS complex to minimize the variations in the signal resulting from changes in electrode position. The signal from the sensor is noisy and requires processing before it can be used by a microprocessor to modulate the stimulation frequency. The actual So_2 value is normalized to a range of values known to occur in any particular patient. This value is then used to control the pacing output according to a set of exponential curves relating the value to pacing rate. The major problem with the development of the device has been that related to the incorporation of a reliable sensor of So_2 into the pacing lead. Coating of the surface of the sensor with fibrin or endothelium has been a major difficulty.

The first clinical experience with such a device was reported in November 1988 by Stangl and colleagues (two patients).[36] In this system, the sensor is placed some way back from the tip of the pacing lead, so that it rests in the right atrium. There is thought to be a smaller chance of tissue growth, and hence attenuation of the signal, in the atrium as opposed to the ventricle. Another advantage of this position is that artifacts caused by valve leaflet and trabecular contact are avoided. The reported follow-up of these two patients has been 5 and 3 months, and more extensive data are awaited.

Activity and Vibration

Principle

Body motion may be detected as vibrations by a piezoelectric crystal that acts as a simple accelerometer or other form of mechanical sensor. The output of such a crystal can be used to modulate pacing frequency. The first

system of this type was devised and marketed by Medtronic (Activitrax) (Minneapolis, MN). The crystal is bonded to the inside of the pulse generator casing. The threshold for detecting the output of the crystal is programmable to low, medium, and high sensitivities. A choice of rate response slopes of between 1 and 10 is available. Similarly, the Sensolog device (Siemens, Solna, Sweden) has programmable threshold and slope functions; in addition, histograms of pacing output can be obtained by telemetry, eliminating the requirement for exercise testing and Holter monitoring during programming.

Clinical Experience

Several studies have shown the Activitrax system to be clinically effective, that is, to provide an appropriate increase in heart rate during normal daily activities, such as walking and running. Faerestrand and associates[11] showed a 29 per cent increase in exercise duration with rate-responsive ventricular pacing compared with standard VVI pacing. Similar results were reported by Lipkin and colleagues[22] and Benditt and coworkers.[6]

However, the response to increasing gradients,[20] swimming, and cycling is inappropriate, as the amplitude of body vibrations during these forms of exercise is not commensurate with the level of energy expenditure. It is not surprising that vibration-responsive pacing systems do not respond to physiologic stimuli other than isotonic exercise, such as isometric exercise, postural changes, mental activity, or emotional stress. Conversely, inappropriate symptomatic tachycardias can result from train and air travel, particularly in helicopters[39] (Fig. 16–5). Recently, we attempted to determine the reasons for the limitation in proportionality of response of vibra-

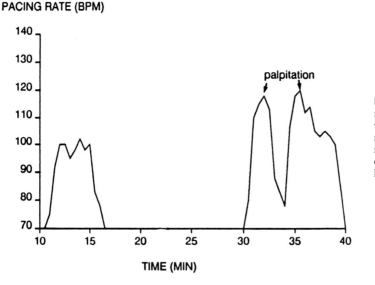

Figure 16–5. Inappropriate pacing rates during train travel in a patient with an Activitrax pacemaker. Pacemaker settings: threshold = medium; response = 7. The patient experienced "palpitations" during these high pacing rates.

tion-sensing pacemakers. We found that in 20 normal subjects fitted with an external Activitrax pacemaker the number of "counts" registered simply reflects the number of acceleration peaks and therefore the number of steps taken by the subjects. With the use of accelerometers attached to the pacemaker casing, acceleration changes during walking were measured in three planes. It was found that the total root mean square value of acceleration in either the anteroposterior or the vertical axis had a better correlation with sinus rate ($r = 0.8$) than the pacemaker rate ($r = 0.51$). This finding suggests that selective sensing of the acceleration level may provide a more "physiologic" means of rate-adaptive pacing.

The major advantages of vibration-sensing rate-adaptive pacing are fast response time (almost immediate) and the robust nature of the sensor. It is sealed within the pulse generator casing with no exposure to body fluids. No special lead is required, and the implantation procedure is uncomplicated. The fact that the magnitude of rate response is not always "physiologic" in terms of the metabolic demand has not significantly diminished its popularity with implanting physicians: The Activitrax system is the largest-selling rate-adaptive pacemaker worldwide.

Respiration-Controlled Pacemakers

Principle

The idea of a pacemaker controlled by respiratory rate was first proposed by Krasner in 1966.[17] During increasing exercise, it is well established that the minute ventilation in-

creases linearly with oxygen consumption up to the anaerobic threshold.[2] At the onset of exercise (during the first seconds), the major determinant of minute ventilation is an elevation in instantaneous breath rate followed by increases in tidal volume.[9] Instantaneous cardiac output (measured by the Doppler method) increases mainly by rises in rate with smaller changes in stroke volume. Heart rate increases correlate closely with minute ventilation[23] and, predictably, so too does the increase in beat-to-beat cardiac output. Thus, the notion of a respiration-driven pacemaker is based on sound physiologic principles.

The development of a clinically operational system using respiratory rate to modulate pacing rate was undertaken by Rossi and colleagues.[31] These investigators reported a linear relationship between heart rate and respiratory rate during increasing exercise. The implantable device (RDP3 and its successor, MB-1) (Biotec Alpha, Bologna, Italy) monitors breathing rate by monitoring changes in thoracic impedance measured by injecting current through an auxiliary sensing electrode placed subcutaneously across the anterior chest wall.[32]

Another device developed by Nappholz[27] monitors changes in transthoracic impedance using a single bipolar electrode in the right ventricle. Impedance is measured by injecting a small current (0.5 μA at 20 Hz) between the ring electrode and the pacemaker casing. Transthoracic electrical impedance rises with expiration and falls with inspiration. The amplitude of these changes is closely related to tidal volume; thus, an estimation of minute ventilation is easily obtained (tidal volume × respiratory rate). Minute ventilation shows a

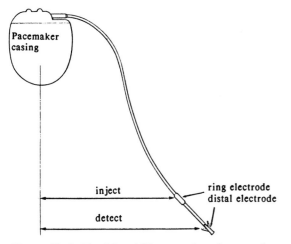

Figure 16–6. The Meta MV pacemaker. See text for mode of operation.

better correlation with heart rate and oxygen consumption than respiratory rate alone.[23] The Meta MV pacemaker (Telectronics, Englewood, CO) (Fig. 16–6) uses measurements of minute ventilation made in this manner to modulate heart rate. The relationship between minute ventilation and paced rate is determined by programming any one of a family of 60 nonlinear curves (Fig. 16–7).

When set to the adaptive mode, the device continually monitors the changes in thoracic impedance and updates two memories that store a time integral of impedance. The long-term measurement is averaged over a period of 60 minutes and provides a baseline value. The short-term memory is averaged over 60 seconds. When this latter value deviates from the baseline, a rate response is initiated. Thus, the device is programmed by allowing at least 1 hour at rest in the adaptive mode to set the baseline. A symptom-limited exercise test is then performed, and the maximal level of change of minute ventilation is recorded. This measurement is then programmed into the pacemaker, and a slope is selected automatically so that the maximal pacing rate (when switched to the rate-responsive mode) is reached at this peak level of change of minute ventilation. In theory, therefore, programming requires only a single exercise test.

Clinical Experience

The long-term follow-up in 143 patients paced (121 ventricular and 22 atrial) with the RDP3 or its successors has been reported by Rossi and associates.[32] As in the preliminary reports, exercise tolerance, oxygen uptake, and anaerobic threshold were increased in the rate-responsive mode. Pacing rate and oxygen uptake were well correlated in 90 per cent of patients (even beyond the anaerobic threshold in 70 per cent). However, in 10 per cent of patients, there appeared to be no relationship between one and the other variable. Malfunctions of the pacemaker occurred in fewer than 8 per cent of patients. These included oversensing of respiratory impedance changes, leading to suppression of the pacing output (3.5 per cent), and undersensing of respiration (3.5 per cent). Myopotential inhibition occurred in 38 per cent of patients but in none of the cases was it sufficient to lead to symptoms. Rossi and coworkers make no mention of erosion of the auxiliary lead. This erosion occurred in 20 per cent of our patients[18] and has been a major limitation of this device.

In a clinical study of 10 patients reported by Lau and associates,[18] both treadmill exercise duration and Doppler-measured minute distance, a measure of cardiac output, were significantly increased by pacing in the rate-adaptive mode compared with the constant-rate VVI mode. Simple daily activities were also assessed. Ascending and descending four flights of stairs resulted in appropriate in-

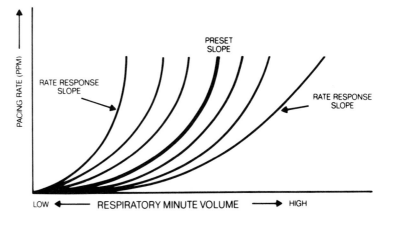

Figure 16–7. A family of rate response curves for the Meta MV pacemaker. Following the exercise test in the adaptive mode, an appropriate curve is selected automatically.

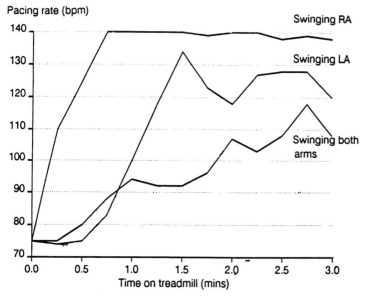

Figure 16–8. Effect of swinging arm movement in a patient with an RDP3 pacemaker. The pacemaker was in the left prepectoral area, and the tip of the auxiliary lead was in the right second intercostal space lateral to the midclavicular line. A higher pacing rate was achieved when the arm on the side of the auxiliary lead was swung.

creases in rate, which peaked after the end of exercise. Similar results were obtained with on-the-spot jogging. Arm swinging has also been observed to result in an increase in pacing rate,[21, 41] even during breath holding. When only one arm was swung, the effect was most marked with swinging of the arm closest to the tip of the auxiliary electrode (which could be either ipsilateral or contralateral with respect to the pacemaker) (Fig. 16–8). These changes in rate are mediated by changes in thoracic impedance.

Widespread experience has been gained with the Meta MV pacemaker.[19, 26] Rate response is well correlated with the degree of exertion, during both graded and burst exercise. The onset of rate response is intermediate between that of vibration-sensing and QT-sensing pacemakers. No complications specific to minute ventilation sensing have been identified. The combination of the highly physiologic nature of the sensor and the reliable nature of the system makes this device one of the most promising of the recently developed rate-adaptive pacemakers.

Temperature-Controlled Pacemakers

Principle

The changes in inferior vena cava blood temperature with exercise were demonstrated by Bazett in 1951.[5] The use of blood temperature to modulate pacing rate was suggested by Weisswange in 1978 and subsequently by Griffin and associates in 1983.[15] Detailed studies by Alt and colleagues in 1986[1] confirmed

the findings of Bazett. At the onset of exertion, the temperature in the right ventricle falls and is followed by a gradual, smooth increase as exercise progresses. The increase in temperature has been shown to correlate with an increase in sinus rate,[1] particularly at high levels of exercise. Other workers, however,[23] have shown that temperature changes correlate less well with heart rate than other physiologic parameters.

Currently, there are three temperature-sensing rate-adaptive pacemakers undergoing clinical trials (Nova MR [Intermedics, Freeport, TX], Thermos [Biotronik, Berlin, West Germany], and Kelvin 500 [Cook, Leechburg, PA]), each using a different algorithm for processing temperature signals. The Nova MR and Kelvin systems use the initial dip in temperature at the onset of exercise to trigger a rate response (arbitrarily set at 85 beats per minute). In the case of the Thermos device, the initial temperature dip is used to set up a "start interval," and rate response occurs when subsequent temperature changes confirm the beginning of exercise.

Clinical Experience

Early clinical results by Alt and colleagues[1a] and Sellers and associates[34a] suggest that a response time of 20 to 30 seconds is achievable with temperature-sensing pacemakers. Improvements in oxygen consumption, exercise performance, and subjective well-being in the rate-adaptive compared with the fixed-rate mode have all been demonstrated. Only early clinical results are available with these units, but no major problems have been reported.

Potential difficulties relate to problems inherent in the use of temperature as an indicator of metabolic demand. The initiation of exercise in a patient who is recovering from previous exercise may not cause an initial dip in temperature.[34b] In addition, the temperature response to submaximal exercise may not be appropriate to the degree of exercise being performed.

Pacemakers Using Indices of Myocardial Contractility

Although there is no variable that is a perfect indicator of metabolic demand under all circumstances, it is likely that indicators related to catecholamine level may be particularly "physiologic"; recent attention has focused on indices of ventricular "contractility" that are affected by sympathetic and vagal influences in a similar way to the normal sinus node. Such variables include right ventricular stroke volume (dependent on venous return as well as "contractility"), right ventricular preejection interval, and right ventricular rate of change of pressure (dp/dt).

Right Ventricular Stroke Volume

Stroke volume increases in response to exercise and is linearly related to heart rate. Stroke volume changes may be estimated by means of changes in intraventricular impedance, calculated from the voltage detected by an intracavitary electrode following a current delivered from a second intracavitary electrode.[29] Beat-to-beat changes in stroke volume (such as those generated by extrasystoles) can be detected by changes in intravascular impedance. In patients with temporary bipolar leads, intracardiac impedance changes vary directly with the right ventricular stroke volume, as measured by two-dimensional echocardiography.

Right Ventricular Preejection Period

The right ventricular preejection period is the time between the onset of ventricular depolarization and the opening of the pulmonic valve. It is determined by the time required for excitation-contraction coupling, together with the isovolumetric contraction time of the ventricle. It is the latter variable that is thought to reflect the inotropic state of the ventricular muscle. On exercise there is significant shortening of the right ventricular preejection period, which has been described as correlating well with the increase in sinus rate.[8] With use

of a multipolar pacing lead, the right ventricular preejection period can be derived from the timing of the electrogram and the onset of volume reduction, as indicated in the previous paragraph. Other workers, however,[35, 37] have shown that the preejection interval is not well correlated with heart rate, and further confirmation of the reliability of the system is awaited.

Rate of Change of Right Ventricular Systolic Pressure

The rate of change of pressure in the right ventricle can be detected by means of an intracavitary piezoelectric crystal, similar to that used to measure body vibration. Right ventricular dp/dt is a variable that rapidly responds to the onset of exercise and is linearly related to the severity of exercise. A unipolar implantable system has been developed;[38a] the pressure waveform is measured 200 msec following a pacing stimulus or spontaneous R wave. The system has been demonstrated to respond rapidly to exercise and to postural changes.

Although all three variables are potentially useful sensors, little is known about long-term reliability or the effects of atrial arrhythmias, pulmonary vascular disease, or right ventricular disease. Measurement of right ventricular stroke volume, preejection interval, and dp/dt has recently been incorporated into a single implantable rate-adaptive system, and clinical evaluation is awaited.

Sensors: Comparisons and Combinations

The important differences between the various sensors can be placed into four categories: speed of rate response, proportionality of rate response, response to nonexercise stimuli, and reliability (Table 16–3). As discussed above, no rate-adaptive pacemaker currently available is superior to the others in all four categories. The vibration sensors are prompt in response, simple to manage, and reliable, and these are no doubt the reasons for the worldwide popularity of activity sensors. It has been suggested that proportionality of response and response to physiologic stimuli other than isotonic exercise are not clinically important requirements and that "inappropriate" tachycardias, such as those experienced in aircraft,[39] are rare and may not be that inappropriate. Although the value of a rate response closely related to physiologic requirements has yet to

TABLE 16–3. COMPARISON OF RATE-ADAPTIVE PACEMAKERS

	SPEED OF RESPONSE	PROPORTIONALITY	NONEXERCISE STIMULI	RELIABILITY
Stimulus-T	+	+ + +	+ + +	+ +
Ventricular depolarization gradient (VDG)	+ +	+ + +	+ +	?
Activity	+ + +	+	0	+ + +
Respiration	+ +	+ + +	0	+ +
Temperature	+ +	+ +	+	+ +
Contractility	+ +	?	+ +	?

be proved to be more beneficial than the response to simple vibration, it is reasonable to assume that "physiologic" rate responses to isometric exercise and postural changes are advantageous. Consequently, it is a logical step to attempt to combine two types of sensor: one with a rapid onset of rate response and one that is more closely linked to metabolic demand (e.g., vibration and evoked response, vibration and rate of change of right ventricular systolic pressure). Several such devices are currently under development, but, as yet, none are undergoing clinical trials.

Dual-Chamber Rate-Adaptive Pacing

Dual-chamber pacing has been considered to be more "physiologic" than ventricular rate-adaptive pacing because AV synchrony is maintained. In addition, there is evidence that long-term ventricular pacing is more likely to lead to atrial arrhythmias than is atrial pacing, perhaps by means of asynchronous retrograde stimulation of the atrium. However, the fact that as many as 40 per cent of patients with AV block have poor sinus node response to exercise[38] limits the usefulness of this form of pacing. In such patients, the combination of dual-chamber pacing with rate responsiveness would appear to be the ideal option. Two DDDR units are currently under clinical evaluation, both using vibration sensing to determine pacing rate in the absence of "adequate" atrial response. In some respects, it would be expected that one of the more "physiologic" sensors would be more useful in this setting, as most patients with sinoatrial disease have some rate response at the immediate onset of exercise.

The Future of Rate-Adaptive Pacing

It is clear that the current abundance of sensors and rate-adaptive pacemakers undergoing clinical evaluation is evidence of a transitional period in pacing technology. With the further refinement of current devices, or the development of sensor combinations, ventricular rate-adaptive pacing is likely to be used in increasing numbers of patients. The most reliable devices will declare themselves once follow-up extends to several years.

Conversely, it could be argued that the parallel development of dual-chamber rate-adaptive pacing will lead to diminishing numbers of VVIR implants. It has been suggested that all the current devices are merely stepping stones to rate-adaptive dual-chamber systems. Certainly, dual-chamber rate-adaptive pacing can be considered more "physiologic" than VVIR pacing in that AV synchrony is provided. However, in certain pathologic conditions, restoration of a normal AV relationship is not possible; the presence of permanent atrial arrhythmias or "silent atrium" will remain a contraindication to dual-chamber pacing. In summary, it is likely that all future pacemakers will have the capacity for rate response: AAIR or DDDR in the majority, and VVIR when the atrium cannot be paced or sensed.

REFERENCES

1. Alt E, Hirgstetter C, Heinz M, Blomer H: Rate control of physiological pacemakers by central venous blood temperature. Circulation 73:1206–1212, 1986.
1a. Alt E, Volker R, Hogl B, Blomer H: Function of the temperature controlled Nova MR pacemaker in everyday life: Preliminary clinical results. PACE 10:1206, 1987.
2. Asmussen E: Muscular exercise. *In* Handbook of Physiology and Respiration. Washington, DC, American Physiological Society, 1965, pp 939–953.
3. Baig MW, Boute W, Begemann M, Perrins EJ: Nonlinear relationship between pacing and evoked QT intervals. PACE 11:753–759, 1988.
4. Bazett HC: An analysis of the time relationships of the heart. Heart 7:353–370, 1920.
5. Bazett HC: Theory of reflex controls to explain regulation of temperature at rest and during exercise. J Appl Physiol 4:245, 1951.
6. Benditt DG, Mianulli M, Fetterr J, et al: Single-chamber cardiac pacing with activity-initiated

chronotropic response: Evaluation by cardiopulmonary exercise testing. Circulation 75:184–191, 1987.

7. Callaghan F, Camerlo J, Livingston AR: Wilson's ventricular gradient: Theoretical foundations for closed-loop pacing rate control. PACE 11:532, 1988.
8. Chirife P: Physiological principles of a new method for rate responsive pacing using the pre-ejection interval. PACE 11:1545–1554, 1988.
9. Cummin ARC, Iyarve VI, Mehta N, Saunders KB: Ventilation and cardiac output during the onset of exercise, and during voluntary hyperventilation in humans. J Physiol 370:567–583, 1986.
10. Donaldson RM, Rickards AF: The ventricular endocardial paced evoked response. PACE 6:253, 1983.
11. Faerestrand S, Breivik K, Ohm OJ: Assessment of the work capacity and relationship between rate response and exercise tolerance associated with activity-sensing rate responsive ventricular pacing. PACE 10:1277–1290, 1987.
12. Fananapazir L, Bennett DH, Faragher EB: Contribution of heart rate to QT interval shortening during exercise. Eur Heart J 4:265–271, 1983.
13. Fananapazir L, Rodemaker M, Bennett DH: Reliability of the evoked response in determining the paced ventricular rate and performance of the QT or rate-responsive (TX) pacemaker. PACE 8:701–714, 1985.
14. Fromer M, Kappenberger L, Steinbrunn W: Binodal disease: Diseased sinus node and atrioventricular block. Z Kardiol 72:410–413, 1983.
15. Griffin JC, Jutzy KR, Claude JP, et al: Central body temperature as a guide to optimal heart rate. PACE 6:498–501, 1983.
16. Kappenberger LJ, Herpers L: Rate-responsive dual chamber pacing. PACE 9:987–991, 1986.
17. Krasner JL, Voukydis PC, Nardella PC: A physiologically controlled cardiac pacemaker. JAAMI 1:14–20, 1966.
18. Lau CP, Ward DE, Camm AJ: Rate-responsive pacing with a pacemaker that detects respiratory rate (Biorate): Clinical advantages and complications. Clin Cardiol 11:318–324, 1988.
19. Lau CP, Antoniou A, Ward DE, Camm AJ: Initial clinical experience with a minute-ventilation sensing rate modulated pacemaker: Improvements in exercise capacity and symptomatology. PACE 11:1815–1822, 1988.
20. Lau CP, Mehta D, Toff WD, et al: Limitation of rate response of activity-sensing rate-responsive pacing to different forms of activity. PACE 11:141–150, 1988.
21. Lau CP, Ritchie D, Butrous GS, et al: Rate modulation by arm movements of the respiratory dependent rate responsive pacemaker. PACE 11:744–752, 1988.
22. Lipkin DP, Buller N, Frenneaux M, et al: Randomised crossover trial of rate-responsive Activitrax and conventional fixed rate ventricular pacing. Br Heart J 58:613–616, 1987.
23. McElroy PA, Janicki JS, Weber KT: Physiologic correlates of the heart rate response to upright isotonic exercise: Relevance to rate-responsive pacemakers. J Am Coll Cardiol 11:94–99, 1988.
24. Mehta D, Lau CP, Ward DE, Camm AJ: Comparative evaluation of chronotropic responses of QT sensing and activity sensing rate-responsive pacemakers. PACE 11:1405–1412, 1988.
25. Milne JR, Ward DE, Spurrell RAJ, Camm AJ: The

ventricular paced QT interval—effects of rate and exercise. PACE 5:352–358, 1982.
26. Mond H, Strathmore N, Kertes P, et al: Rate responsive pacing using a minute ventilation sensor. PACE 11:1866–1874, 1988.
27. Nappholz T, Valenta H, Maloney J, Simmons T: Electrode configurations for a respiratory impedance measurement suitable for rate responsive pacing. PACE 9:960–964, 1986.
28. Nathan D, Center S, Wu C, Keller W: An implantable synchronous pacemaker for the long term correction of complete heart block. Am J Cardiol 11:362–367, 1963.
29. Neumann G, Niederan C, Bakels N: Intracardiac impedance as stroke volume sensor [abstract]. PACE 8:A–38, 1985.
30. Rickards AF, Norman J: Relation between QT interval and heart rate: New design of physiological adaptive cardiac pacemaker. Br Heart J 45:56–61, 1981.
31. Rossi P, Plicchi G, Canducci G, et al: Respiration as a reliable physiological sensor for controlling cardiac pacing rate. Br Heart J 51:7–14, 1984.
32. Rossi P, Prando MD, Magnani A, et al: Physiological sensitivity of respiratory dependent cardiac pacing: 4 year follow up. PACE 11:1267–1278, 1988.
33. Salo RW, Pederson BD, Olive AL, et al: Continuous ventricular volume assessment for diagnosis and pacemaker control. PACE 7:1267, 1984.
34. Samet P, Castillo C, Bernstein WH: Haemodynamic sequelae of atrial, ventricular and sequential atrioventricular pacing in cardiac patients. Am Heart J 72:725–729, 1966.
34a. Sellers TD, Fearnot N, Boal B, et al: Clinical experience and follow up of a temperature-based rate modulating pacemaker. A multicenter experience of the US Kelvin implants. PACE 10:1227, 1987.
34b. Sellers TD, Fearnot NE, Smith HJ, et al: Right ventricular blood temperature profiles for rate responsive pacing. PACE 10:467, 1987.
35. Spodick DH, Doi YL, Bishop RL, Hashimoto T: Systolic time intervals reconsidered: Reevaluation of the pre-ejection period: Absence of relation to heart rate. Am J Cardiol 53:1667–1670, 1984.
36. Stangl K, Wirtsfeld A, Heinz R, Laule M: First clinical experience with an oxygen saturation controlled pacemaker in man. PACE 11:1882–1887, 1988.
37. Sundberg S: Influence of heart rate on systolic time intervals. Am J Cardiol 58:1144–1145, 1986.
38. Sutton R: Physiological cardiac pacing. In World Symposium on Cardiac Pacing, Montreal, PACE-SYMP, 1979, p 16.
38a. Sutton R, Sharma A, Ingram A, et al: First derivative of right ventricular pressure as a sensor for an implantable rate response VVI pacemaker. PACE 10:1230, 1987.
39. Toff WD, Leeks C, Joy M, et al: The effect of aircraft vibration on the function of an activity-sensing pacemaker [abstract]. Br Heart J 57:573, 1987.
40. Travill C, Ingram A, Vardas P, Sutton R: Inadequate rate response of a stimulus-T sensing pacemaker [abstract]. PACE 10:1231, 1987.
41. Webb SC, Lewis LM, Morris-Thurgood J-A, et al: Respiratory dependent pacing: A dual response from a single sensor. PACE 11:730–735, 1988.
42. Wirtzfeld A, Heinze R, Liess HD, et al: An active optical sensor for monitoring mixed venous oxygen saturation for an implantable rate-regulating pacing system. PACE 6:494–497, 1983.

III

ELECTRICAL THERAPY FOR TACHY-ARRHYTHMIAS: ANTITACHYCARDIA DEVICES

17

PHYSIOLOGIC EFFECTS OF ELECTRICAL STIMULATION IN CARDIAC MUSCLE

RAYMOND E. IDEKER, DAVID W. FRAZIER,
WANDA KRASSOWSKA, PENG-SHENG CHEN,
and J. MARCUS WHARTON

An electrical impulse stimulates myocardium by altering the transmembrane potential. Much has been learned about this phenomenon for intracellular stimulation. It is known that stimulation occurs when an intracellular electrical pulse raises the transmembrane potential above a particular threshold value, that this threshold value is different for different types of cardiac cells, and that the threshold can be changed by altering the cellular milieu.[14, 28] It is known that this threshold value is a function of the length of the stimulus pulse, as described by the strength-duration curve, and that the change in transmembrane potential decreases with distance from the site of stimulation, as described by the space constant.[17] It is also known that the mechanism and threshold of anodal stimulation may differ from that of cathodal stimulation.[9, 11, 21, 28] Finally, it is known that the underlying basis for all of these effects is the molecular structure and ion-selective channels of the cardiac membrane.[26]

In contrast, little is known about extracellular stimulation, even though the electrodes for cardiac pacemakers, cardioverters, and defibrillators are all extracellular. The reason for this apparent anomaly is that it has not been possible to measure the distribution of transmembrane potentials created by an extracellular stimulus in sufficient detail to describe and understand this type of stimulation. In the absence of this information, stimulation is characterized by specifying the voltage, current, or energy of the stimulus pulse delivered through the electrodes. The electrical field established by the electrodes causes the movement of charged particles, which changes the concentration of ions within cardiac cells and the surrounding interstitial fluid and, in turn, changes the transmembrane potential. It is thought that excitation occurs when the transmembrane potential is elevated above the same threshold as determined by intracellular stimulation.

When stimulation slightly above diastolic threshold is performed with a cardiac pacemaker, the transmembrane stimulation threshold is exceeded for a few cell layers around the pacing electrode, that is, the liminal area.[40, 41] Only these cells are directly excited by the electrical field of the stimulus pulse; the remainder of the myocardium is activated by conduction of a depolarization front away from the electrode site, similar to the spread of depolarization during a spontaneous premature contraction arising from the same site. The situation is different for cardioversion and defibrillation. The electrical field of the stimulus is much larger, so that instead of a few cells being raised above threshold, most of the nonrefractory myocardium is raised above threshold and is activated directly by the field of the stimulus rather than by the conduction of activation fronts.[8]

Supported in part by National Institutes of Health research grants HL-28429, HL-33637, and SCOR grant HL-17670, National Science Foundation Engineering Research Center CDR-8622201, and by gifts from the AMP Foundation and the Burr-Brown Corporation. Mr. Frazier was supported in part by an American Heart Association Medical Student Research Scholarship.

Thresholds for pacing, cardioversion, and defibrillation vary widely when specified in terms of the total voltage, current, or energy delivered through the stimulating electrodes. This variation may have two causes. First, a stimulus of given strength and waveform may create different changes in the transmembrane potential from case to case because of differences in the size and structure of the electrode as well as in the structure of the myocardium and because of differences in the position of the electrode with respect to the myocardium. Second, the excitation threshold of the transmembrane potential may differ from case to case. Determination of the relative importance of these two causes requires knowledge of the extracellular and intracellular potentials created by the stimulus, so that the distribution of transmembrane potentials can be determined and knowledge can be gained regarding which cardiac cells are directly activated by the electrical field of the stimulus.

EXTRACELLULAR POTENTIALS AROUND A PACING SITE

Recent advances in digital electronics have made it possible to obtain part of this information. With the use of computer-assisted cardiac mapping techniques, it is now feasible to determine the extracellular distribution of potentials generated by a stimulus.[19, 50] The extracellular potentials are obtained by recording simultaneously from many electrodes placed throughout the ventricular myocardium around the stimulating electrode. The examples shown in Figure 17–1 were obtained from a dog in which simultaneous recordings of potential were made from 120 electrodes located on forty 21-gauge needles that were inserted transmurally in a 35-mm × 20-mm portion of the right ventricular outflow tract.[19] The needles were held in place by an apparatus that spaced them evenly at 5-mm intervals. Each needle contained three recording electrodes, 2 mm apart. Thus, three planes of potentials were recorded in the thin right ventricular outflow tract: subendocardial, midmyocardial, and subepicardial. Potentials were recorded during 1-mA stimulation from the epicardium (panel *A*) and from the endocardium (panel *B*). Fiber orientation was determined histologically for each of the three planes.

In the local region close to the pacing site (10 to 12 mm along fibers and 5 to 7 mm across fibers), potentials generated by the stimuli are highest in the recording plane closest to the pacing site, that is, in the subepicardial

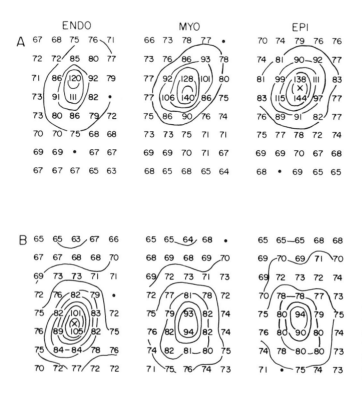

Figure 17–1. Transmural potentials during epicardial and endocardial pacing. The distribution of stimulus potentials for epicardial and endocardial pacing is shown for the subendocardial (ENDO), midmyocardial (MYO), and subepicardial (EPI) planes of recording electrodes for a dog. Numbers placed at the location of each recording electrode give the potential in millivolts. Solid circles represent sites of inadequate recordings. Isopotential lines are at 15-mV intervals in panel *A* and at 5-mV intervals in panel *B*. The lack of isopotential lines in the center of the regions of highest potential is an artifact because of the absence of recording electrodes in the region. Panel *A* represents epicardial stimulation at 1 mA from the epicardium overlying the "X" shown in the subepicardial plane. Panel *B* represents endocardial stimulation at 1 mA from the endocardium beneath the "X" shown in the subendocardial plane. The 1-mA stimuli were three to five times the diastolic pacing threshold. The isopotential lines are more circular than expected for an anisotropic medium, possibly owing to the continuous variation in fiber orientation throughout the tissue under the plaque. (From Frazier DW, Krassowska W, Chen P-S, et al: Transmural activations and stimulus potentials in three-dimensional anisotropic canine myocardium. Circ Res 63:135–146, 1988. Reprinted by permission of the American Heart Association, Inc.)

plane for epicardial pacing and in the subendocardial plane for endocardial pacing. Outside this local region, the highest values of potential appear in the subepicardial plane for both pacing sites. The reason that subepicardial potentials are larger than subendocardial potentials away from the pacing site, even for endocardial pacing, can probably be explained by differences in conductivity inside and outside the heart. The conductivity of the blood within the ventricular chamber is greater than that of the cardiac muscle. Conversely, the conductivity of the region just outside the epicardium is lower than that of cardiac muscle, whether it contains air, when the chest is open, or lung tissue, when the chest is closed.[51] Compared with the situation when the conductivities of all regions are identical, the effect of high conductivity within the ventricular cavity is to decrease the endocardial potentials and the effect of low conductivity outside the epicardium is to increase the epicardial potentials.[19]

Neither extracellular nor intracellular conductivity is uniform. Extracellular conductivity is approximately three times higher in the direction along than across the long axis of the myocardial cells,[7, 49, 51, 57] which causes the isopotential lines in some planes to be elliptical (Fig. 17–1). However, this elliptical effect of tissue anisotropy is decreased by the variation in fiber orientation between the pacing site and the recording electrodes, so that the isopotential lines are nearly circular.

SPREAD OF ACTIVATION AWAY FROM THE PACING SITE

Anisotropy has a larger effect on the conduction of activation fronts away from the stimulus site.[50, 55] The spread of activation through the tissue can be determined using the same computer-assisted cardiac mapping techniques that are used to record the potential distribution.[19] In Figure 17–2, the activation maps are shown following stimulation at twice the diastolic threshold current from the same two pacing sites and in the same animal as for Figure 17–1. During epicardial pacing, the

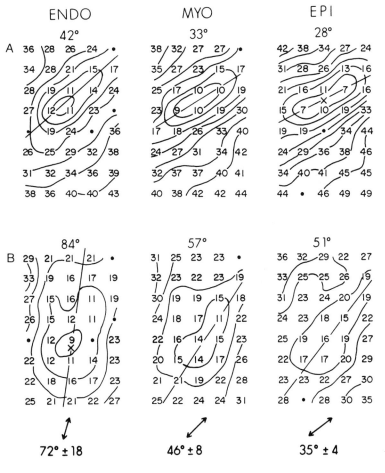

Figure 17–2. Patterns of transmural activation. Activation maps are shown for the same animal as in Figure 17–1 for epicardial (panel *A*) and endocardial (panel *B*) pacing. Numbers show the activation times at each recording electrode location, measured in milliseconds from the beginning of the stimulus. The isochrones are at 5-msec intervals. Panel *A* illustrates the activation sequence during pacing at 0.6 mA from the epicardium overlying the "X" shown in the subepicardial plane. Panel *B* illustrates the activation sequence during pacing at 0.2 mA from the endocardium beneath the "X" shown in the subendocardial plane. The major axes for ellipses of activation wave fronts are shown, and their angles, measured from the horizontal axis of the plate, are given above each map. The double-headed arrows at the bottom of the figure indicate the average direction of the long axis of the myocardial fibers in the three recording planes, with the mean angle from the horizontal given below. (From Frazier DW, Krassowska W, Chen P-S, et al: Transmural activations and stimulus potentials in three-dimensional anisotropic canine myocardium. Circ Res 63:135–146, 1988. Reprinted by permission of the American Heart Association, Inc.)

spread of activation : elliptical within the subepicardial plane of recording electrodes, with the major axis of the ellipse approximately parallel to local fiber orientation. This is consistent with the finding that conduction velocity is greater along than across myocardial fibers.[50, 55] Within the midmyocardial and subendocardial planes of recording electrodes, the activation patterns remain elliptical but are not parallel to local fiber orientation. The deviation between local fiber orientation and the major axis of the activation ellipse increases with increasing transmural distance from the pacing site. Thus, in Figure 17–2A, the degree of deviation between the major axis of each activation ellipse and fiber orientation within the recording plane is 7, 13, and 30 degrees for the subepicardial, midmyocardial, and subendocardial planes of recording electrodes, respectively. The major axis of the activation ellipse in each plane is approximately equal to the average fiber orientation throughout the myocardial wall between the pacing site and the plane of recording electrodes. The differences between these values are only 5, 2, and 3 degrees for the subendocardial, midmyocardial, and subepicardial planes, respectively, shown in Figure 17–2A.

Similar findings are observed for most pacing sites through the myocardial wall, except for those near the endocardium. Thus, the spread of activation depends on local fiber orientation between the recording plane and the pacing site. This dependence is prominent only within a local region extending approximately 5 to 7 mm across the fibers and 10 to 12 mm along the fibers from the pacing site. Outside this local region (Fig. 17–2A), the subendocardial plane of recording electrodes activates earlier than the subepicardial plane because of rapid endocardial spread of activation. The rapid endocardial conduction velocity is consistent with conduction through subjacent Purkinje tissue. Thus, outside the local region the spread of activation is predominantly first through the endocardium, with epicardial activation occurring later via wave fronts from the endocardium.

The spread of activation during endocardial pacing is rapid in all directions (Fig. 17–2B), although slightly faster along the long axis of the myofibers in the subendocardial plane. This conduction velocity is similar to that reported for Purkinje tissue.[48] Nearly circular activation patterns of this type are thought to be caused by spread through Purkinje tissue; more elliptical patterns are seen in endocardial

regions devoid of Purkinje cells.[42] The progression of activation front isochronal ellipses from subendocardial to subepicardial planes rotates in the same general direction as the transmural fiber rotation, similar to that following epicardial or midwall stimulation. Following endocardial pacing, subendocardial activation occurs earlier than subepicardial activation for all recording sites.

EXTRACELLULAR THRESHOLD FOR STIMULATION

Although computer-assisted cardiac mapping techniques can be used to record the extracellular potential distribution generated by a stimulus and the resulting spread of activation, they cannot measure the distribution of intracellular and, hence, transmembrane potentials. Present techniques do not permit recording from many intracellular electrodes placed simultaneously within a beating heart, although it may soon be feasible to determine changes in transmembrane potentials caused by the stimulus with voltage-sensitive dyes attached to the cell membrane.[12, 52] In the meantime, indirect evidence, theoretical models, and simulation studies must be relied on to determine the relationship between experimentally measurable parameters, such as the extracellular potential gradient and current density, and the transmembrane potential, which decides the course of activation. If a certain value of extracellular potential gradient or current density always gives rise to the same value of transmembrane potential throughout most of the heart, then the potential gradient or current density can express the stimulation threshold nearly as accurately as can the transmembrane potential.[38]

The bidomain model of cardiac tissue, in which extracellular and intracellular spaces are represented by two continuous overlapping three-dimensional domains, gives an indication of the relationship between potential gradient and transmembrane potential. Computer simulations based on this model demonstrate that the change in transmembrane potential caused by a uniform potential gradient field is not constant but, because of anisotropic conductivities of the intracellular and extracellular spaces, varies with location away from the stimulation site.[60] As discussed more fully below, other models that treat cardiac muscle as composed of discrete cells suggest the existence of a linear relationship between the potential gradient or current density and the amplitude of the changes in the transmembrane potential. These other models predict that a given value of extracellular potential gradient or current density should cause approximately the same change in transmembrane potential throughout most of the myocardium, so that the extracellular field parameters can be used to express the stimulation threshold.[37]

These extracellular thresholds have been estimated using computer-assisted cardiac mapping techniques for normal canine ventricular myocardium.[18] The data were obtained using the same configuration of recording electrodes shown in Figures 17–1 and 17–2. Stimuli lasting 3 msec and ranging from 5 to 70 mA in strength were given during electrical diastole from a unipolar electrode at one side of the array of recording electrodes (Fig. 17–3). Extracellular potentials generated by each stimulus were recorded at the 120 electrode sites, and the potential gradient and current density at each recording electrode were calculated. Values of potential gradients were estimated using a finite element method. To compute current density, conductivities of 0.756 ohm^{-1}m^{-1} along

myocardial fibers and 0.250 ohm^{-1}m^{-1} transverse to myocardial fibers were used.[18]

For stimuli of low strength (less than 5 mA), most of the volume of tissue containing the recording electrodes was excited after the stimulus by an activation front that conducted away from the stimulus site. As the stimulus strength was increased, the location at which the activation front after the stimulus could first be detected moved progressively farther away from the stimulus site. All recordings were divided into two groups: those not directly excited and those directly excited by the field of the stimulus. Those classified as not directly excited exhibited activation complexes following the stimulus. Sites were classified as directly excited by the stimulus if no activation complexes were detected after the stimulus and if the earliest activation fronts after the stimulus were first detected at recording sites farther away from the pacing site than the recording site in question (Fig. 17–3). The border between the directly excited and not directly excited regions should furnish an estimate of the locus of points where the transmembrane potential, and hence the extracel-

Figure 17–3. Activation map and electrode recordings. Panel *A* shows an activation map following a 40-mA anodal stimulus with a pulse duration of 3 msec. The pacing site is marked with an "X." Numbers give activation times in milliseconds at the electrode sites, with the beginning of the stimulus as time zero. The isochrones are at 5-msec intervals. Electrode sites considered to be directly excited by the stimulus are represented by triangles, and missing sites are indicated by solid circles.

Panel *B* shows the bipolar recordings from the electrodes labeled *a* to *d* in the midmyocardial level of panel *A*. The first activation in each channel is the last atrial-paced activation preceding the ventricular stimulus. The amplifier gains were automatically lowered 10 msec prior to and during the 3-msec stimulus (13 msec total) to prevent saturation. The beginning of the 40-mA stimulus is indicated by an arrow. The stimulus is not seen because of the low gains and because the recordings were made in the bipolar mode. Gain-switching artifacts occur at the beginning and end of the 13-msec time period, the latter being most apparent. Tracings *b*, *c*, and *d* exhibit postshock activations and thus are considered not directly excited by the field of the stimulus. Tracing *a* exhibits no postshock activation and so is considered to be directly excited by the stimulus field.

(From Frazier DW, Krassowska W, Chen P-S, et al: Extracellular field required for excitation in three-dimensional anisotropic canine myocardium. Circ Res 63:147–164, 1988. Reprinted by permission of the American Heart Association, Inc.)

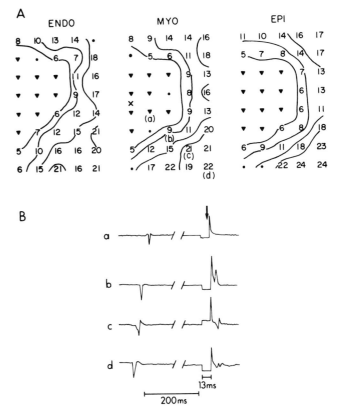

lular potential gradient or current density, is at the threshold for stimulation.

Threshold values of potential gradient and current density were found, so that a minimal and equal number of sites from the two groups were incorrectly classified as either directly excited or not directly excited by the stimulus field. A potential gradient of 804 mV/cm and a current density of 3.66 mA/cm² yielded misclassifications of 17 per cent and 8 per cent, respectively, when sites with values greater than these thresholds were considered directly excited by the stimulus field. Errors for the potential gradient are reduced if the components of the gradient along and across fibers are considered individually. Linear bivariate combinations of the components longitudinal and transverse to the long axis of the myocardial fibers yielded misclassification of 7 per cent when the potential gradient was used and 8 per cent when the current density was used. The linear function identifying the region of direct excitation for the potential gradient in millivolts per centimenter is

$$\frac{G_m}{640} + \frac{G_t}{1840} \geq 1$$

where g_l and g_t denote the gradient components in the longitudinal and transverse direction. These values are consistent with the thresholds of 1.2 to 1.3 V/cm estimated for stimulating cultures of randomly oriented myocardial cells.[31] The linear function for current density in milliamperes per square centimeter is

$$\frac{j_l}{4.6} + \frac{j_t}{4.8} \geq 1$$

where j_l and j_t are the longitudinal and transverse components of the current density. Thus, the transverse-to-longitudinal threshold ratios are 2.88:1.00 for potential gradient and 1.04:1.00 for current density.

If the cardiac cell cross-section is modeled by an elongated ellipse, a potential gradient applied across the cell produces a smaller maximal change in the transmembrane potential than the same potential gradient applied along the cell.[34] This finding may explain why a linear combination of the potential gradient components longitudinal and transverse to the cell fibers is a more accurate and sensitive predictor of the threshold for direct excitation than is the gradient magnitude alone. On the other hand, bivariate combinations of the transverse and longitudinal components of the current density may furnish no better estimate of the

excitation threshold than does the single variable of the magnitude of the current density. This is because the thresholds are almost identical for the components of the current density transverse and longitudinal to the long axis of the fibers.

The thresholds given above were computed for monophasic stimuli lasting 3 msec. Just as for stimulation thresholds expressed in terms of stimulus current, thresholds expressed as extracellular potential gradient and current density are a function of stimulus duration and can be described by a strength-duration curve.[18] The strength-duration curves for the magnitudes of potential gradient and current density in the open-chest, anesthetized dog are shown in Figure 17–4. The shape of these curves closely approximates a standard

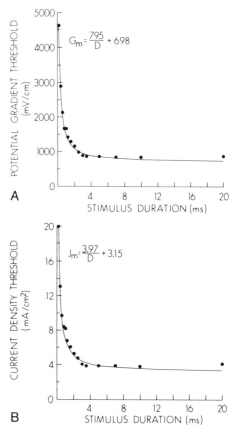

Figure 17–4. Strength-duration curves in terms of the extracellular field. The relationship between stimulus duration and excitation threshold is shown for potential gradient (panel *A*) and current density (panel *B*). The solid lines represent the best-fit curves of strength as a hyperbolic function of pulse duration, *D*. The equation is given above each strength-duration curve. (From Frazier DW, Krassowska W, Chen P-S, et al: Extracellular field required for excitation in three-dimensional anisotropic canine myocardium. Circ Res 63:147–164, 1988. Reprinted by permission of the American Heart Association, Inc.)

strength-duration curve expressed in terms of extracellular stimulus current,[27] although in the latter case the actual current values depend upon electrode size and tissue type.

COMPARISON OF ANODAL AND CATHODAL STIMULATION

The mechanisms of anodal and cathodal stimulation may be similar or different, depending on the strength of stimulation. When stimulus strength is at the smallest value that will capture the heart, so that only the liminal area around the pacing site is directly excited, the stimulus threshold for fully repolarized cells is higher for anodal pacing than for cathodal pacing.[11, 21] In contrast, when the stimulus current is stronger, so that the border of the directly excited region is at least a few millimeters from the pacing site, extracellular potential and current density stimulation thresholds are not significantly different for unipolar

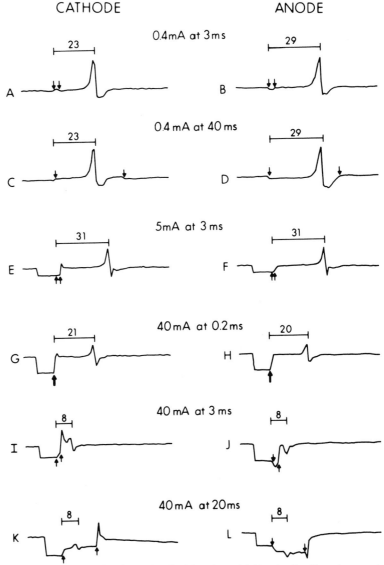

CATHODE   ANODE

Figure 17–5. Anodal and cathodal excitation. *Abbreviations and symbols:* Arrows mark initiation and termination of stimulus pulses, except for the 0.2-msec pulses in panels G and H that are marked with a single bold arrow because they are so short. The stimulus pulses are often not seen owing to the bipolar recording and low gains necessary to record activations without saturation. The bracketed line indicates the latency in milliseconds from stimulus initiation to time of activation. All panels are at the same time scale. The stimulus polarity, stimulus current in milliamperes, and pulse duration in milliseconds are shown in the panels.

Panels A and B are consistent with cathodal make and anodal break excitation. The anodal latency is approximately 6 msec greater than the cathodal latency at an identical pulse duration and stimulus current. Panels C and D show, however, that break excitation is not the mechanism for either cathodal or anodal stimulation, as the activations occur prior to the break of both 40-msec pulses. The respective latencies remain the same as for the 3-msec pulses in panels A and B. Pacing currents in panels A to D are at twice the minimal anodal pacing threshold (0.4 mA).

Panels E and F demonstrate the disappearance of the difference in cathodal and anodal latencies for 5-mA stimuli at 3-msec pulse durations. Recordings are taken from a different electrode than is used in panels A to D.

Panels G to J represent decreasing latencies as the pulse durations of cathodal and anodal 40-mA stimuli are increased from 0.2 to 3.0 msec. An increase to 20-msec pulse durations in panels K and L shows identical latency with the 3-msec stimuli, suggesting no difference in the area directly excited, assuming conduction velocity is unchanged. For both polarities at this recording site, activation occurred prior to the break of the 20-msec, 40-mA pulse. The decreasing latency for increasing pulse durations up to 3 msec indirectly demonstrates the increasing area that was directly excited.

(From Frazier DW, Krassowska W, Chen P-S, et al: Extracellular field required for excitation in three-dimensional anisotropic canine myocardium. Circ Res 63:147–164, 1988. Reprinted by permission of the American Heart Association, Inc.)

anodal or cathodal stimulation.[18] The latency, that is, the time from the onset of the stimulus to the time of activation at the recording site, is also not different for anodal or cathodal pacing when the stimulus current is at least this strong (5 mA in Fig. 17–5). The results are different for stimuli of smaller strength. For example, at twice the diastolic pacing threshold for anodal stimulation (0.4 mA in Fig. 17–5), the latency following anodal stimulation is longer than that following cathodal stimulation, even though extracellular field strengths are identical.

It was suggested many years ago that the reason for the difference in latency for anodal and cathodal unipolar stimulation is that cathodal excitation begins at the "make" of the stimulus, when depolarization starts, while anodal excitation does not begin until the "break" of the stimulus, when the hyperpolarization is removed.[9] This hypothesis was challenged by Goto and Brooks,[21] as well as by Dekker,[11] who demonstrated that both make and break excitations can occur for either polarity of stimulation, depending on the phase of the cardiac cycle. In particular, Dekker showed that whereas anodal excitation during repolarization occurs on the break of the stimulus, during electrical diastole it occurs on the make of the stimulus but is followed by a longer latency than occurs in cathodal excitation. His conclusions were based on stimulation at twice the diastolic threshold levels and are supported by the data in Figure 17–5 for this same stimulus strength (panels *A* to *D*). When the current is increased to at least 5 mA, causing the border of the directly excited region to be distant from the stimulation site, the difference in latency disappears (Fig. 17–5, panels *E* to *L*).

The explanation for some of these results can be found in simulation models of cells in an impressed extracellular electrical field. The potential of an isolated spheroidal cell, in which the extracellular and intracellular conductivities are isotropic and much higher than the conductivity of the cell membrane, varies much less within the cell than outside the cell (Fig. 17–6*A*).[34] Therefore, the change in transmembrane potential is positive in one half of the cell and negative in the other, depolarizing the portion of the cell toward the cathode and hyperpolarizing the portion toward the anode (Fig. 17–6*B*).

More recent models include multiple cells and take into account the existence of the junctions between them.[36, 37, 46, 47] One-dimen-

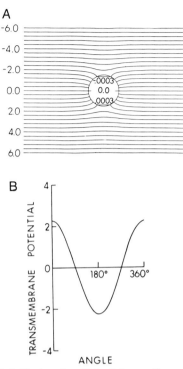

Figure 17–6. Single spheroidal cell in a uniform extracellular field. Panel *A*, The cell is exposed to a uniform electrical field created by the cathode at the top and the anode at the bottom. Extracellular potentials are given in millivolts at the left, with isopotential lines spaced every 0.4 mV. As indicated by the isopotential lines spaced every 0.00003 mV, the potential within the cell changes much less than the extracellular potential. Panel *B*, The transmembrane potential in millivolts, which is equal to the difference between the intracellular and extracellular potentials in panel *A*, is shown as a function of the location on the surface of the cell, as expressed by the polar angle, with 0 degrees at the top of the cell and 180 degrees at the bottom. The top half of the cell toward the cathode is depolarized, and the bottom half toward the anode is hyperpolarized. (Adapted from Klee M, Plonsey R: Stimulation of spheroidal cells—the role of cell shape. IEEE Trans Biomed Eng BME-23:347–354, 1976.)

sional models of a discrete cardiac strand reveal the presence of a periodic component of the transmembrane potential, which is caused by local changes in conductivity and whose amplitude is a function of the potential gradient established by the stimulus. The total change in transmembrane potential is composed of two terms: first, an aperiodic component similar to the transmembrane potential of the continuous fiber, and second, a periodic component similar to that of the isolated cell shown in Figure 17–6, which oscillates with a spatial wavelength equal to the distance between intracellular junctions (Fig. 17–7). The aperiodic component causes depolarization of the entire cell in the region very near the cathode and hyperpolarization of the entire

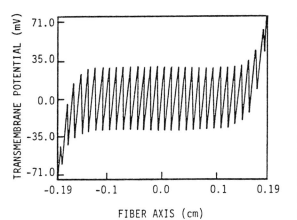

Figure 17-7. Transmembrane potential in a periodic core-conductor model. The transmembrane potential along a one-dimensional cylindrical strand of cardiac muscle, generated by an extracellular cathode at the right and an extracellular anode at the left, has two components: an aperiodic component, which causes hyperpolarization near the anode and depolarization near the cathode, and a periodic component, which oscillates with a period equal to the length of the individual cells of the strand. The aperiodic component has a significant value only close to the electrodes, while the periodic component dominates the transmembrane potential everywhere else. For increased visibility, the periodic component has been exaggerated by making the junctional resistance between cells 17 times larger than its physiologic value. (Adapted from Krassowska W, Pilkington TC, Ideker RE: Asymptotic analysis for periodic cardiac muscle. Proceedings of the Annual Conference of IEEE Engineering. Med Biol Soc 8:255–258, 1986.)

cell very near the anode. Since the magnitude of the transmembrane potential change caused by the aperiodic component falls off very rapidly with distance from the electrodes, the periodic component is probably responsible for direct excitation more than a few cells away from the electrodes. As one moves away from either source, the periodic component dominates, causing depolarization of the portion of each cell toward the cathode and hyperpolarization of the other portion toward the anode. Direct excitation of cells away from the electrodes probably occurs when the stimulus strength is sufficient to establish periodic oscillations of the transmembrane potential that exceed the stimulation threshold. This interpretation explains why the latency and extracellular stimulation threshold for anodal or cathodal stimuli of at least 5 mA are not different; changing the polarity only changes which half of the cell is depolarized.

In contrast, the latency and the diastolic threshold for pacing, during which stimulus strengths much less than 5 mA are delivered, differ for anodal and cathodal stimulation. The traditional explanation of the observed differences is based on analyzing only the aperiodic

component of the transmembrane potential, which causes depolarization of the cells in the immediate vicinity of the electrode for cathodal pacing and hyperpolarization of these cells for anodal pacing. It has been postulated, therefore, that the mechanism of anodal activation is different from that of cathodal activation and that a hyperpolarizing current can activate the membrane by an accommodation process[1] or break excitation.[9] These hypotheses are not supported by experimental data from cells in electrical diastole; first, intracellular recordings have shown the presence of depolarizing membrane current across some portions of cells during anodal stimulation, and second, activation is not possible when the membrane is hyperpolarized by intracellular rather than extracellular stimulation.[28]

An alternative hypothesis explaining the differences in stimulation threshold between cathodal and anodal pacing takes into account the periodic component of the transmembrane potential arising from the discrete structure of the myocardium. According to this explanation, the cells immediately adjacent to the anode cannot activate because of the hyperpolarization caused by the aperiodic term of the transmembrane potential; however, cells slightly farther away can activate because the amplitude of the aperiodic term is smaller and the oscillatory term causes one end of the cell to depolarize. Since for anodal pacing the aperiodic term counteracts depolarization instead of assisting it, the latency and threshold are higher than for cathodal pacing. According to this explanation, stimulation with a cathodal electrode occurs when the stimulus strength is sufficiently strong that the additive effects of the aperiodic and oscillatory terms raise the transmembrane potential of the cells immediately around the electrode to threshold. Therefore, the anodal threshold is higher than the cathodal because the stimulus field must be strong enough for the depolarizing portion of the oscillatory term to overcome the opposing hyperpolarizing effect of the aperiodic term. The increased latency associated with anodal stimulation compared with that of cathodal stimulation of the same strength (Fig. 17–5A and B) is not known but may occur because the hyperpolarizing effect of the aperiodic term near the anode slows conduction velocity.

This hypothesis explains the presence of a depolarizing current in some portions of the cell membranes during anodal stimulation. In addition, the inability to achieve activation during electrical diastole by hyperpolarizing the membrane with intracellular electrodes is explained by the finding that the periodic oscillations are practically negligible for intracellular stimulation.[37] This experimental and theoretical evidence indicates that analysis of the mechanism of extracellular stimulation should take into account the discrete structure of the cardiac tissue, as has been done for propagation.[54]

STIMULATION DURING THE RELATIVE REFRACTORY PERIOD

Up to this point, the discussion has been limited to cells that are fully recovered and in electrical diastole. Stimulation may also be performed when the myocardium is relatively refractory, either inadvertently during cardiac pacing or intentionally during programmed electrical stimulation and, with larger stimuli, during cardioversion and defibrillation.

To date, the strength-interval relationship has been expressed in terms of transmembrane potential or stimulus current, and in the latter case quantitative differences have been observed in various experimental settings.[26] By analogy to the strength-duration curve (Fig. 17–4), the strength-interval curve should be less dependent upon the experimental setting if the stimulus strength is expressed by the extracellular potential gradient or current density. However, such a curve has not yet been determined experimentally. Traditional strength-interval curves expressed in terms of stimulus current have demonstrated complex relationships between anodal, cathodal, and bipolar stimulation. Anodal stimulation in fully recovered cells apparently occurs on the make of the pulse and is due to a "virtual cathode effect," while stimulation during the relative refractory period is on the break of the pulse.[28] A virtual cathode is a region distant from the real cathode in which cells are directly activated because stimulus current flow depolarizes the cell membrane in this region. In addition, strength-interval curves for bipolar stimulation are probably a composite of anodal and cathodal excitation curves, with cathodal predominance during electrical diastole and anodal predominance during the relative refractory period.[9] The existence of a "no response" region in which no excitation occurs at suprathreshold levels of stimulation during the relative refractory period has also been demonstrated and appears to begin at stimulus levels slightly above the anodal curve.[9, 43] The reason for the "no response" phenomenon is not definitely known.

A complication affecting the interpretation of strength-interval curves determined by extracellular stimulation is that the site of capture by the premature stimulus may not always be in the same location for the entire curve. This fact has been demonstrated when the site of basic drive stimulation (S1) is given at a different site than the premature stimulation (S2).[6] As the stimulus is given more prematurely, the site of earliest excitation moves toward the site of S1 stimulation, where the cells have had more time to recover and are thus less refractory at the time of S2 stimulation (Fig. 17–8). The site of capture may remain near the site of stimulation if S1 and S2 are given from the same location, since the cells that will be most recovered at the time of premature stimulation will be those adjacent to the stimulating electrode.

If a sufficiently strong stimulus is given during a certain portion of the relative refractory period, that is, the vulnerable period, fibrillation may be induced. Evidence suggests that fibrillation induced by stimulation during the vulnerable period arises by reentry.[4, 6, 25] Most types of reentry are thought to be caused by a nonuniform dispersion of refractoriness. Until recently, nonuniform dispersion of refractoriness was thought to be responsible for reentry, initiating fibrillation by stimulation during the vulnerable period.[22, 23] The degree of temporal dispersion of recovery of excitability in ventricular muscle is minimal after basic drive beats but becomes greater after premature stimulation at 1.5 times the cathodal diastolic threshold.[24] According to the nonuniform dispersion of refractoriness hypothesis, premature stimulation causes unidirectional block in regions of inhomogeneous dispersion of recovery of excitability because activation fronts cannot conduct from the less refractory to the more refractory tissue. The more refractory tissue is activated later via conduction along other pathways. If this activation is so late that tissue proximal to the region of unidirectional block has had time to recover, reentry occurs.

Recent evidence coming from several different sources suggests that a nonuniform dispersion of refractoriness is not necessary for the initiation of reentry by a premature stimulus. Spach and colleagues[55] have shown experimentally that the safety factor for conduction along the long axis of myocardial fibers is lower than that across the fibers. They demonstrated that an appropriately timed premature stimulus can block along fibers but can conduct slowly across fibers to cause reentry. A second piece

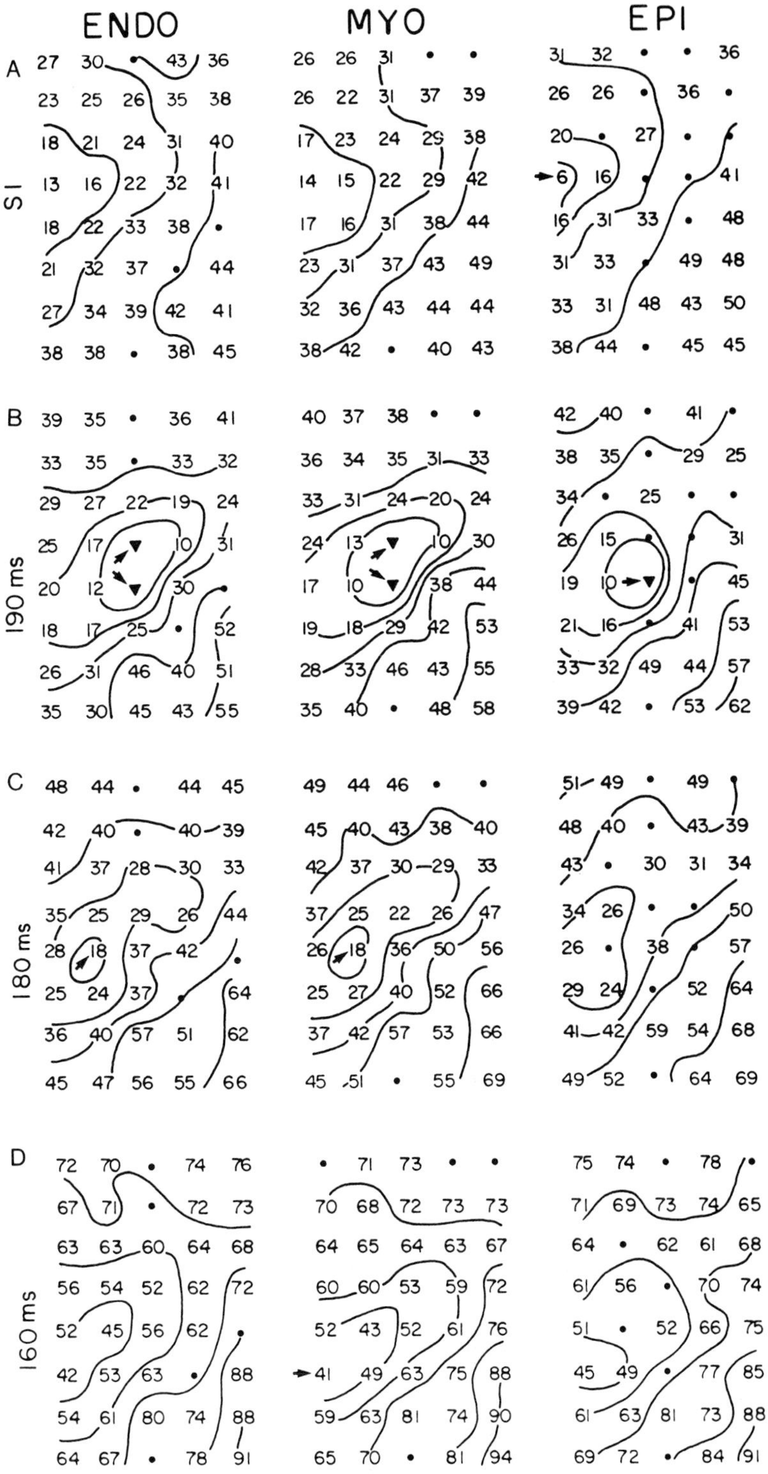

Figure 17–8. Activation maps following premature stimulation, demonstrating that the location of earliest capture is not always at the site of stimulation. The array of recording electrodes is the same as in Figures 17–1 to 17–3. Activation times are given at each recording location, with time zero taken as the time of stimulation and the site of earliest activation marked by an arrow. Small closed circles indicate recording sites where adequate recordings were not obtained. Isochronal lines are spaced 10 msec apart.

Panel A shows the activation sequence following the last of 10 basic drive (S1) stimuli given at a cycle length of 400 msec to the subendocardium near the site labeled S1. Activation first occurred near the site of S1 stimulation and then spread across the mapped region. Panel B shows activation following a premature stimulus of 10 mA delivered to the subendocardium beneath the center of the mapped region 190 msec after the last S1 stimulus. Triangles indicate recording electrodes for which the surrounding tissue was directly activated by the S2 stimulation field. Thus, at this coupling interval the site of capture was adjacent to the stimulating electrode. Panel C shows activation following a premature stimulus given 180 msec after the last S1 stimulus. The site of earliest activation has moved toward the site of S1 stimulation. Panel D shows activation following a premature stimulus given 160 msec after the last S1 stimulus, which was the shortest coupling interval that captured a 10-mA S2 stimulus. The site of earliest activation has moved to or past the edge of the mapped region and is near the site of S1 stimulation.

(Adapted from Chen P-S, Wolf PD, Dixon EG, et al: Mechanism of ventricular vulnerability to single premature stimuli in open chest dogs. Circ Res 62:1191–1209, 1988. Reprinted by permission of the American Heart Association, Inc.)

of evidence is from computer simulations in which all properties, including the refractory period, are identical for all cells.[56, 62] A properly timed premature stimulus in this model can conduct in one direction but block in the opposite direction, leading to reentry; therefore, a nonuniform dispersion of refractoriness is not required.

The third piece of evidence makes use of topologic theorems and phase-resetting phenomena of pacemaker cells to show that if an extracellular potential gradient field has a component transverse to a uniform dispersion of refractoriness, a singularity point of undefined phase must be present.[62] An activation front spirals out from a rotor source centered at the singular point. This rotor constitutes a leading-circle type of reentry pattern.[2] If the gradient field is not orthogonal to the dispersion of refractoriness, but decreases with distance from a point source, a pair of singularity points will be present and two mirror-image rotors will form.[62] This pattern, called a figure-of-eight reentry pattern,[15] has been observed experimentally.[6]

The fourth piece of evidence is based on the same experimental model as shown in Figure 17–2. The experiment suggests that reentry can begin distant from the site of premature stimulation, at the border of the directly excited region.[20] Reentry leading to fibrillation begins at the border of the directly excited tissue, in which a particular combination of refractoriness and extracellular potential gradient is present. If a monophasic square-wave stimulus of 3 msec duration is delivered to the canine right ventricle during its relative refractory phase, a leading-circle reentry circuit originates at a point where the extracellular potential gradient is approximately 5 V/cm and where the refractoriness is approximately equal to the effective refractory period for a 2-mA cathodal stimulus. When the potential gradient is greater than approximately 5 V/cm, activation fronts are not conducted away from the border of the directly excited region, suggesting that if the potential gradient through the entire myocardium were above this level, reentry and hence fibrillation would not be induced. This consideration may explain why there is an upper limit to the strength of stimuli that will induce fibrillation during the vulnerable period.[5, 16, 39] The potential gradient at which the upper limit of vulnerability occurs may be important for determining the minimal shock strength at which cardioversion may be performed without inadvertently inducing fibrillation.

This postulated minimal extracellular potential gradient has been determined for defibrillation in the dog with another waveform, a 14-msec monophasic, low-tilt, truncated, exponential shock and has been shown to be approximately 6 V/cm.[59] This finding is consistent with the hypothesis that defibrillation requires a potential gradient strong enough (1) to halt the activation fronts of fibrillation and (2) to exceed the upper limit of vulnerability so that the shock does not reinitiate fibrillation.[5]

These particular values of potential gradients will probably not hold for other durations and types of stimulation waveforms. For example, some biphasic waveforms can defibrillate at much lower energy than monophasic waveforms of the same total duration.[13, 30, 53] The minimal potential gradients necessary for defibrillation with these waveforms are still to be determined. In addition, the defibrillation threshold expressed as a potential gradient may depend upon the direction of the gradient with respect to fiber orientation, as has been demonstrated for the stimulation threshold.[18]

Other findings reported in the literature concerning the interaction of electrical stimuli and partially refractory cells may or may not be related to the above concepts. The phenomenon of a graded response, with its associated prolongation of refractoriness,[33] may explain the finding that for certain combinations of potential gradient and degree of refractoriness an activation front does not propagate away from the border of the directly excited region.[20] The graded response may be responsible for the "no response" phenomenon mentioned previously. A second stimulus given soon after a premature stimulus may prevent the initiation of an arrhythmia. This phenomenon has been called "stimulation during the protective zone"[58] as well as "inhibition."[61] The mechanism of this prevention is unknown but may also be caused by the graded response.

PATHOLOGIC EFFECTS OF STIMULATION

If a very strong shock is given, so that the stimulus potential gradient field is much greater than the upper limit of vulnerability, fibrillation can again be induced.[16, 29] This type of fibrillation can be induced by shocks given any time during the cardiac cycle, not just during the vulnerable period. Thus, this response probably represents a type of damage induced by the shock. Strong shocks can cause loss of potassium from myocytes, decreased conduction velocity, and neurostimulation with both cholinergic and adrenergic effects.[3, 35, 45] Other effects at slightly higher levels of stimulation are decreased cardiac function, absence of conduction, and inhibition of pacemaker cells.[31, 35, 44] At yet higher-strength stimulation, frank necrosis of myocardium may occur.[10]

The strengths of the stimulus field at which most of these effects occur are not yet known. Jones and associates[31] have shown that inhibition of pacemaker cells in clusters of isolated chick embryo cells can occur with fields of 80 V/cm. In particular, fields of this strength inhibit pacemaker cells for approximately 4 seconds, and during this period small holes are present in the cell membranes. Ventricular tachycardia has been shown to arise from regions with potential gradients of approximately 100 to 200 V/cm for 14-msec monophasic shocks (J.M. Wharton and colleagues, unpublished data, 1987). Voltage gradients of 200 V/cm applied to *in vitro* cardiac cells cause multiple ultrastructural changes consistent with the production of an osmotic imbalance, leading to prolonged postshock membrane depolarization, a possible cause for these high-voltage postshock arrhythmias.[32]

As research continues, it should be possible to define more precisely the ranges of potential gradient and current density field strength over which different physiologic and pathologic effects of electrical stimulation occur, such as pacing, defibrillation, induction of arrhythmias, and necrosis. These ranges will probably be affected by the stimulation waveform and by the presence of abnormal conditions such as ischemia. Determination of the therapeutic ranges of extracellular stimulation, cardioversion, and defibrillation fields, together with experimental measurements and simulation, should lead to the development of better electrode configurations for these modalities of cardiac stimulation.

ACKNOWLEDGMENT: The authors wish to thank Dr. Art Winfree and Mr. Clif Alferness for their comments about this chapter.

REFERENCES

1. Aidley DJ: The Physiology of Excitable Cells. Cambridge, England, Syndics of the Cambridge University Press, 1971.
2. Allessie MA, Bonke FIM, Schopman FJG: Circus movement in rabbit atrial muscle as a mechanism of tachycardia. III. The "leading circle" concept: A new model of circus movement in cardiac tissue without the involvement of an anatomical obstacle. Circ Res 41:9–18, 1977.
3. Arnsdorf MF, Rothbaum DA, Childers RW: Effect of direct current countershock on atrial and ventricular electrophysiological properties and myocardial potassium efflux in the thoracotomised dog. Cardiovasc Res 11:324–333, 1977.
4. Bakker JMT, Henning B, Merx W: Circus movement in canine right ventricle. Circ Res 45:374–378, 1979.
5. Chen P-S, Shibata N, Dixon EG, et al: Comparison of the defibrillation threshold and the upper limit of ventricular vulnerability. Circulation 73:1022–1028, 1986.
6. Chen P-S, Wolf PD, Dixon EG, et al: Mechanism of ventricular vulnerability to single premature stimuli in open chest dogs. Circ Res 62:1191–1209, 1988.
7. Clerc L: Directional differences of impulse spread in trabecular muscle from mammalian heart. J Physiol 255:335–346, 1976.
8. Colavita PG, Wolf P, Smith WM, et al: Determination of effects of internal countershock by direct cardiac recordings during normal rhythm. Am J Physiol 250:H736–H740, 1986.
9. Cranefield PF, Hoffman BF, Siebens AA: Anodal excitation of cardiac muscle. Am J Physiol 190:383, 1957.
10. Dahl CF, Ewy GA, Warner ED, et al: Myocardial necrosis from direct current countershock: Effect of paddle size and time interval between discharge. Circulation 50:956–961, 1974.
11. Dekker E: Direct current make and break thresholds for pacemaker electrodes on the canine ventricle. Circ Res 27:811, 1970.
12. Dillon S, Morad M: A new laser scanning system for measuring action potential propagation in the heart. Science 214:453–456, 1981.
13. Dixon EG, Tang ASL, Wolf PD, et al: Improved defibrillation thresholds with large contoured epicardial electrodes and biphasic waveforms. Circulation 76:1176–1184, 1987.
14. Dominguez G, Fozzard HA: Influence of extracellular K^+ concentration on cable properties and excitability of sheep cardiac Purkinje fibers. Circ Res 26:565–574, 1970.
15. El-Sherif N, Mehar R, Gough WB, et al: Ventricular activation patterns of spontaneous and induced ventricular rhythms in canine one-day-old myocardial infarction: Evidence for focal and reentrant mechanisms. Circ Res 51:152–166, 1982.
16. Fabiato A, Coumel P, Gourgon R, et al: Le seuil de réponse synchrone des fibres myocardiques: Application à la comparaison expérimentale de l'efficacité des différentes formes de chocs électriques de défibrillation. Arch Mal Coeur 60:527–544, 1967.
17. Fozzard HA, Schoenberg M: Strength-duration curves in cardiac Purkinje fibres: Effects of liminal length and charge distribution. J Physiol 226:593–618, 1972.
18. Frazier DW, Krassowska W, Chen P-S, et al: Extracellular field required for excitation in three-dimensional anisotropic canine myocardium. Circ Res 63:147–164, 1988.
19. Frazier DW, Krassowska W, Chen P-S, et al: Transmural activations and stimulus potentials in three-dimensional anisotropic canine myocardium. Circ Res 63:135–146, 1988.
20. Frazier DW, Wolf PD, Wharton JM, et al: A stimulus induced critical point: The mechanism for electrical induction of reentry in normal canine myocardium. J Clin Invest [in press].
21. Goto M, Brooks CM: Membrane excitability of the frog ventricle examined by long pulses. Am J Physiol 217:1236–1245, 1969.
22. Han J: Ventricular vulnerability to fibrillation. *In* Dreifus LS, Likoff W (eds): Cardiac Arrhythmias. New York, Grune and Stratton, 1973, pp 87–95.
23. Han J, Goel BG: Electrophysiologic precursors of ventricular tachyarrhythmias. Arch Intern Med 129:749–755, 1972.
24. Han J, Moe GK: Nonuniform recovery of excitability in ventricular muscle. Circ Res 14:44–60, 1964.
25. Harumi K, Smith CR, Abildskov JA, et al: Detailed activation sequence in the region of electrically

induced ventricular fibrillation in dogs. Jpn Heart J 21:533–544, 1980.

26. Hoffman BF, Cranefield PF: Electrophysiology of the Heart. Mount Kisco, NY, Futura Publishing Co, 1960.

27. Hoffman BF, Gorin EF, Wax FS, et al: Vulnerability to fibrillation and the ventricular-excitability curve. Am J Physiol 167:88–94, 1951.

28. Hoshi T, Matsuda K: Excitability cycle of cardiac muscle examined by intracellular stimulation. Jpn J Physiol 12:433–446, 1962.

29. Jones JL, Jones RE: Postshock arrhythmias—a possible cause of unsuccessful defibrillation. Crit Care Med 8:167, 1980.

30. Jones JL, Jones RE: Improved defibrillator waveform safety factor with biphasic waveforms. Am J Physiol 245:H60, 1983.

31. Jones JL, Lepeschkin E, Jones RE, et al: Response of cultured myocardial cells to countershock-type electric field stimulation. Am J Physiol 235:H214, 1978.

32. Jones JL, Proskauer CC, Paull WK, et al: Ultrastructural injury to chick myocardial cells in vitro following "electric countershock." Circ Res 46:387–394, 1980.

33. Kao CY, Hoffman BF: Graded and decremental response in heart muscle fibers. Am J Physiol 194:187–196, 1958.

34. Klee M, Plonsey R: Stimulation of spheroidal cells—the role of cell shape. IEEE Trans Biomed Eng BME-23:347–354, 1976.

35. Koning G, Veefkind AH, Schneider H: Cardiac damage caused by direct application of defibrillation shock to isolated Langendorff-perfused rabbit heart. Am Heart J 100:473, 1980.

36. Krassowska W, Pilkington TC, Ideker RE: The closed form solution to the periodic core-conductor model using asymptotic analysis. IEEE Trans Biomed Eng BME-34:519–531, 1987.

37. Krassowska W, Pilkington TC, Ideker RE: Periodic conductivity as a mechanism for cardiac stimulation and defibrillation. IEEE Trans Biomed Eng BME-34:555–560, 1987.

38. Lepeschkin E, Jones JL, Rush S, et al: Local potential gradients as a unifying measure for thresholds of stimulation, standstill, tachyarrhythmia and fibrillation appearing after strong capacitor discharges. Adv Cardiol 21:268–278, 1978.

39. Lesigne C, Levy B, Saumont R, et al: An energy-time analysis of ventricular fibrillation and defibrillation thresholds with internal electrodes. Med Biol Eng 14:617, 1976.

40. Lindemans FW, van der Gon JJD: Current thresholds and liminal size in excitation of heart muscle. Cardiovasc Res 12:477–485, 1978.

41. Lindemans FW, Heethaar RM, van der Gon JJD, et al: Site of initial excitation and current threshold as a function of electrode radius in heart muscle. Cardiovasc Res 9:95–104, 1975.

42. Myerburg RJ, Gelband H, Nilsson K, et al: The role of canine superficial ventricular muscle fibers in endocardial impulse distribution. Circ Res 42:27–35, 1978.

43. Orias O, Gilbert JL, Siebens AA, et al: Effectiveness of single rectangular electrical pulses of known duration and strength in evoking auricular fibrillation. Am J Physiol 162:219–225, 1950.

44. Pansegrau DG, Abboud FM: Hemodynamic effects of ventricular defibrillation. J Clin Invest 49:282–297, 1970.

45. Peleska B: Cardiac arrhythmias following condenser discharges and their dependence upon strength of current and phase of cardiac cycle. Circ Res 13:21–32, 1963.

46. Plonsey R, Barr RC: Effect of microscopic and macroscopic discontinuities on the response of cardiac tissue to defibrillating (stimulating) currents. Med Biol Eng Comp 24:130–137, 1986.

47. Plonsey R, Barr RC: Inclusion of junction elements in a linear cardiac model through secondary sources: Application to defibrillation. Med Biol Eng Comp 24:137–144, 1986.

48. Rawling DA, Joyner RW, Overholt ED: Variations in the functional electrical coupling between the subendocardial Purkinje and ventricular layers of the canine left ventricle. Circ Res 57:252–261, 1985.

49. Roberts DE, Scher AM: Effect of tissue anisotropy on extracellular potential fields in canine myocardium in situ. Circ Res 50:342–351, 1982.

50. Roberts DE, Hersh LT, Scher AM: Influence of cardiac fiber orientation on wavefront voltage, conduction velocity, and tissue resistivity in the dog. Circ Res 44:701–712, 1979.

51. Rush S, Abildskov JA, McFee R: Resistivity of body tissues at low frequencies. Circ Res 12:40–50, 1963.

52. Sawanobori T, Hirota A, Fujii S, et al: Optical recording of conducted action potential in heart muscle using a voltage-sensitive dye. Jpn J Physiol 31:369–380, 1981.

53. Schuder JC, Gold JH, Stoeckle H, et al: Transthoracic ventricular defibrillation in the 100 kg calf with symmetrical one-cycle bidirectional rectangular wave stimuli. IEEE Trans Biomed Eng BME-30:415, 1983.

54. Spach MS, Dolber PC: Relating extracellular potentials and their derivatives to anisotropic propagation at a microscopic level in human cardiac muscle: Evidence for electrical uncoupling of side-to-side fiber connections with increasing age. Circ Res 58:356–371, 1986.

55. Spach MS, Miller WT III, Geselowitz DB, et al: The discontinuous nature of propagation in normal canine cardiac muscle: Evidence for recurrent discontinuities of intracellular resistance that affect the membrane currents. Circ Res 48:39–54, 1981.

56. Van Capelle FJL, Durrer D: Computer simulation of arrhythmias in a network of coupled excitable elements. Circ Res 47:454–466, 1980.

57. Van Oosterom A, Boer RW, van Dam RT: Intramural resistivity of cardiac tissue. Med Biol Eng Comp 17:337–343, 1979.

58. Verrier RL, Brooks WW, Lown B: Protective zone and the determination of vulnerability to ventricular fibrillation. Am J Physiol 234:H592–H596, 1978.

59. Wharton JM, Wolf PD, Chen P-S, et al: Is an absolute minimum potential gradient required for ventricular defibrillation [abstract]? Circulation 74:II–342, 1986.

60. Wikswo JP Jr, Echt DS, Sepulveda NG: Finite element models for cardiac defibrillation. In Proceedings of the 40th Annual Conference on Engineering in Medicine and Biology, Boston, 1987.

61. Windle JR, Miles WM, Zipes DP, et al: Subthreshold conditioning stimuli prolong human ventricular refractoriness. Am J Cardiol 57:381–386, 1986.

62. Winfree AT: When Time Breaks Down: The Three-Dimensional Dynamics of Electrochemical Waves and Cardiac Arrhythmias. Princeton, NJ, Princeton University Press, 1987.

18

ENGINEERING ASPECTS OF IMPLANTABLE DEFIBRILLATORS

STANLEY M. BACH, JR. *and* J. EDWARD SHAPLAND

Early development of an implantable device to treat ventricular tachyarrhythmia focused on the automatic diagnosis and electrical termination of ventricular fibrillation. Subsequently, additional attention was given to ventricular tachycardia, which is amenable to treatment by less aggressive means (e.g., pacing, 2-J shocks). Engineering efforts of various groups were then directed down three different pathways. Some pacemaker companies worked on pace termination, while others evaluated low-energy cardioversion. Another company continued development of an implantable defibrillator.[9] Today, electrical treatment of ventricular tachyarrhythmia by implantable devices is being directed toward both ventricular tachycardia and ventricular fibrillation. As of this time, the automatic implantable cardioverter/defibrillator is viewed as the safest automatic implantable device for use in the ventricle because it rapidly and aggressively (25- to 30-J shocks) treats both ventricular tachycardia and ventricular fibrillation.

TACHYARRHYTHMIA DETECTION

One of the most fundamental requirements for an accurate diagnosis of a ventricular tachyarrhythmia is the correct interpretation of cardiac rate. The device and its leads are inextricably related. Signals provided by a set of leads must be properly matched to internal device circuitry, since their characteristics change with electrode size, spacing, and location. Performance requirements for the rate-sensing system are greater in an antitachycardia device than in a pacemaker. It must correctly interpret heart rate over a nearly 10:1 range (40 to 400 beats per minute) and cannot simply ignore, by use of refractory periods, signals faster than the usual physiologic range.

In general, cardiac rate is most easily obtained by observing a small, localized area of healthy ventricular myocardium. This practice tends to minimize the repolarization phenomena (T-wave sensing), maximize the depolarization signal time rate of change (slew rate), reduce the duration of the depolarization signal, and minimize the sensing of atrial activity. These signal characteristics reduce filtering problems, enabling a single electronic count per cardiac depolarization to be obtained. The features are often maintained during ventricular fibrillation, particularly on the endocardium.[19] On the other hand, some pattern (morphologic) recognition schemes require a more global look at the heart from a pair of electrodes that are larger in surface area and more widely separated. The signals obtained from such electrodes often have the appearance of a body-surface electrocardiogram. Recently, approaches that make a morphologic diagnosis of a local electrogram have been explored.[3]

Lead Systems

The initial clinical model of an implantable defibrillator (automatic implantable defibrillator, or AID) utilized a single pair of electrodes for both shocking and sensing. The detection scheme was directed at ventricular fibrillation. Two facts became quickly apparent during

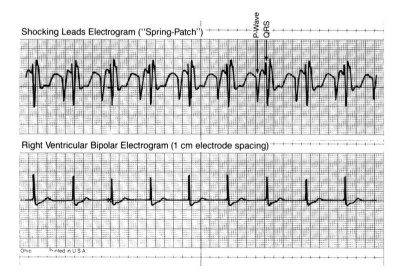

Figure 18–1. An example of simultaneous shocking leads and rate-sensing leads electrograms obtained during automatic implantable cardioverter/defibrillator (AICD) replacement. Note the size and slew rate of the P wave and ST-T portions in the top trace. The patient previously had a myocardial infarction; however, his atria were not enlarged. Implantable electronic circuitry has difficulty accurately determining cardiac rate from this signal, whereas signal processing of the local bipolar electrogram (*lower trace*) is straightforward. Paper speed is 25 mm/sec.

implantation of the first devices. First, ventricular tachycardia was common and was not always detectable by a global, morphologic fibrillation detector. Second, accurate cardiac rate was often difficult to obtain from a pair of shocking electrodes.

Circuit changes directed at correctly diagnosing ventricular tachycardia by morphologic means, based on signals from the shocking electrodes, did not improve rate counting. The challenges were as follows: (1) ability to distinguish P-wave, QRS-complex, and T-wave activity in a diseased heart with previous infarction, bundle branch block, and slowed intraventricular conduction (due to pathology or antiarrhythmic drugs); and (2) electrogram changes induced by a "current of injury" resulting from the 700-V defibrillation discharge (Figs. 18–1 and 18–2). A single-lead system and implantable circuit were unable to interpret rate optimally when the nature of the input signal was sometimes pulsatile, sometimes sinusoidal, and often a combination of these two.

Improved reliability in cardiac rate determination during a wide range of ventricular and supraventricular rhythms was obtained, in part, by utilizing a separate rate-sensing lead with a 1-cm interelectrode spacing. This took the form of an endocardial lead or a pair of epicardial leads. The endocardial lead was otherwise identical with a standard pacemaker lead (Fig. 18–1, bottom trace).

In Figure 18–3, local bipolar (endocardial) activity is compared during sinus rhythm and ventricular fibrillation. The rapid rising and falling nature of the signal, with little repolarization activity, allows a simple filtering scheme. The essential signal feature is the high

ratio of the slew rate during depolarization to that during repolarization. When this ratio is high, a circuit designed to count pulsatile activity accurately has no difficulty in counting cardiac rate. When the ratio is low, miscounting may occur.

Local bipolar electrograms often vary widely in their magnitude and slew rate. This variability probably occurs because the sensing electrode is unidirectional and the cardiac depolarization approaches the electrode from a variety of directions during different ventricular rhythms and during fibrillation. Because of the variability, addition of some kind of automatic level-adjusting circuitry was necessary. Such a system amplifies small signals more than large ones. For instance, if the desired

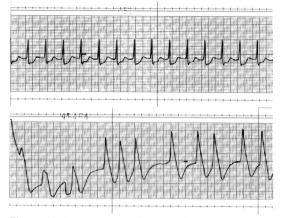

Figure 18–2. Comparison of automatic implantable cardioverter/defibrillator shocking lead electrograms before (*top trace*) and after (*bottom trace*) a 25-J discharge, which terminated ventricular fibrillation. Note the wide ventricular tachycardia–like depolarizations post shock. The patient was, in fact, in atrial fibrillation after the discharge. Paper speed is 25 mm/sec.

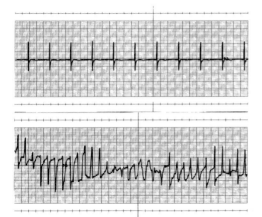

Figure 18–3. Local 1-cm bipolar electrograms during sinus rhythm (*top trace*) and ventricular fibrillation (*bottom trace*). Maintenance of a rapidly changing depolarization during fibrillation is an important characteristic, enabling electronic circuitry to obtain a reasonable approximation of "cardiac rate" during this rhythm disturbance. Paper speed is 25 mm/sec.

output is a 1-V signal, a 1-mV input signal will result in the amplifier's multiplying the signal strength by 1000. If a 10-mV input signal is applied to the amplifier, its amplification is reduced to 100.

The nature of the electrical signal obtained from large device shocking leads is similar to a body-surface electrocardiogram. Two exceptions are noteworthy. First, the signal is generally larger, nominally about 5 mV from peak to peak. In addition, as previously noted, the signal changes resulting from the device shock may be significant. This "postshock signal distortion" can confound attempts to make a morphologic diagnosis of the rhythm (Fig. 18–2, bottom trace). An additional limitation of using device shocking leads as an electrogram sensor is the inability to change their location independently to improve signal characteris-

tics, without potentially compromising their defibrillating capability.

As yet, hemodynamic monitoring has not been incorporated into an implantable cardioverter/defibrillator. Two approaches being investigated are continuous stroke volume monitoring by intracardiac impedance, and continuous pressure monitoring. Both of these techniques are likely to be confined to the right ventricle. The impedance stroke volume technique is attractive, since it does not require a special transducer and its electrodes can be used for electrogram sensing. The basic scheme is illustrated in Figure 18–4. A constant microampere alternating current (AC) is passed between two intracavitary right ventricular electrodes. The intracavitary resistance is computed by measuring the voltage drop across another electrode pair interposed between the first two. The instantaneous ventricular volume is then computed as illustrated. Since the blood resistivity is less than myocardial wall resistivity, the scheme is capable of a fairly accurate measurement of the cavity volume.[12] Such a technique gives a time-varying volume signal, which has been correlated with right ventricular pressure.[4]

Attempts at long-term right ventricular pressure monitoring have not had optimal results, partially because of biocompatibility problems. Transducer destruction by moisture penetration from the blood pool, as well as transducer fibrous encapsulation, has been noted.[2]

DETECTION CIRCUITRY

Input Protection

Implantable defibrillators/cardioverters and antitachycardia pacemaker amplifiers may be

Figure 18–4. Schematic illustration of the impedance technique used to obtain continuous ventricular volume (V). The volume is calculated based on the measured resistance, R, the electrode separation, L, and the blood resistivity, P. P is a function of the hematocrit (Hct.). A relatively uniform current distribution over the cross-section, A, is assumed. Accuracy is improved by using multiple pairs of sensing electrodes, effectively dividing the ventricle into segmental volumes. (Courtesy of Cardiac Pacemakers, Inc, St. Paul, MN.)

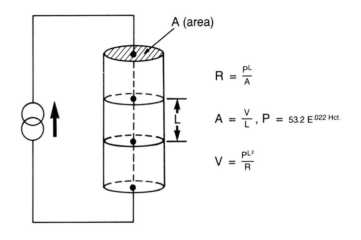

$$R = \frac{PL}{A}$$

$$A = \frac{V}{L}, \quad P = 53.2\, E^{.022\,Hct.}$$

$$V = \frac{PL^2}{R}$$

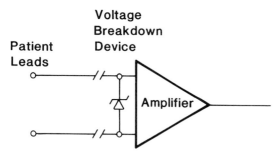

Figure 18–5. Illustration of a pacemaker sense amplifier high-voltage protection scheme. When the breakdown device conducts as a result of high input potential on the patient's leads, current becomes limited only by the lead resistance. This current may be on the order of amperes during defibrillation and may result in signal distortion and pacing threshold elevation because of localized tissue damage.

repeatedly exposed to high-voltage shocks from implanted leads, from internal defibrillation paddles placed on the heart during implantation, or from transchest defibrillation. The potentials to which these amplifiers are exposed may exceed an implantable defibrillator output capability, especially when internal defibrillation paddles are placed in proximity to device leads during implantation. These pace/sense signal amplifiers should be protected against the effects of repeated shocks. Maintenance of high input impedance during the shock and quick postshock recovery are desirable features for monitoring amplifiers (Fig. 18–5).

AUTOMATIC GAIN AND LEVEL CONTROL

Pacemakers have a programmable fixed gain (sensitivity) setting and cannot automatically adapt to a wide range of signal magnitudes, which are seen in a patient with multiple-morphology ventricular tachycardia or during ventricular fibrillation. Amplitudes of electrogram depolarization can vary over a range of 10:1 during ventricular arrhythmias. Signal rates of change (slew rate) during fibrillation vary more than 5:1 (Fig. 18–3). To count rate or make morphologic measurements during these signal changes, methods of automatic adaptability have been incorporated into sense amplifiers. This "adjustment on the fly" allows the amplifier gain, or sensitivity, to increase during times of low signal magnitude and to decrease during times of high signal, continuously attempting to maintain the sensed signal output constant (Fig. 18–6).

RATE PROCESSING

One of the simplest ways to compute cardiac rate is with an analog averaging circuit, whose output voltage is proportional to the input pulse rate. The averaging circuit time constants (response times to increases or decreases in rate) are important for proper detection of tachyarrhythmia rate. Too long a time constant does not allow rapid response to rate changes; too short a time constant does not provide enough averaging, resulting in a highly variable analog voltage.

Digital methods of handling rate range include computation of a running average over the preceding 2, 4, 8, or 16 beats or the requirement that a consecutive number of depolarizations less than a certain cycle length must exist before a tachyarrhythmia is declared. Problems exist with requiring a consecutive number of beats during attempts to declare

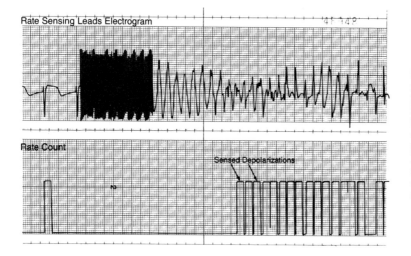

Figure 18–6. Rate counting during the onset of ventricular fibrillation. The automatic gain control has momentarily been suppressed by the very large fibrillating signal, and no rate counting could take place until amplifier recovery. Most, but not all, local depolarizations are sensed, requiring rate averaging to be utilized. Paper speed is 25 mm/sec.

fibrillation, since not all local depolarizations may be detected. Designers have, therefore, incorporated the concept of requiring only a certain percentage of these depolarizations to exceed a rate limit during a specified interval.

MORPHOLOGY DETECTION

A simplified circuit implementation of the probability density function concept was the first morphology detection scheme to be employed in an implanted device.[6] The circuit operation is depicted in Figure 18–7, using the idealized pulse to simulate a normal electrogram and a sinusoid to represent tachycardia or fibrillation. It should be noted that this scheme is used with electrodes of large surface area, which tend to average the heart's electrical activity.

After the input signal (pulse or sine wave, top tracing) is amplified and its derivative (dv/dt) obtained (second tracing from the top), the signal is passed through an absolute value circuit (third tracing from top). The absolute value circuit causes a positive polarity output when its input is either positive or negative. Therefore, polarity of the cardiac signal is usually unimportant. It may be observed that

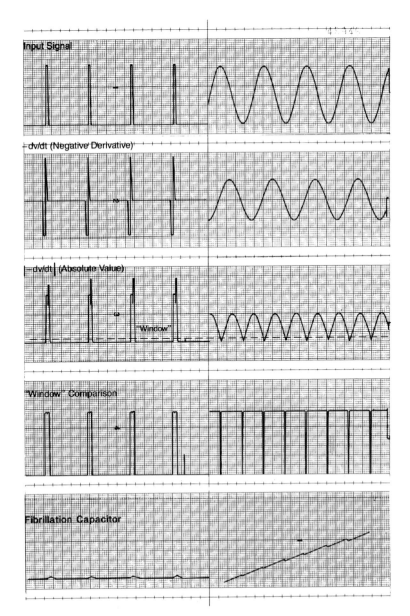

Figure 18–7. Waveforms from a probability density function circuit. The dashed line in the third tracing is the "window" reference level. See text for discussion.

in the case of a sine wave the resulting differentiated waveform is morphologically identical with the original signal but shifted in phase (cosine). The differentiated, absolute value signal is then compared with a fixed level (dashed line) in a comparison circuit, which makes an all- or-none decision about the signal magnitude. This fixed level is known as the "window." A signal magnitude less than the fixed level is considered to be baseline, resulting in no output signal; a magnitude exceeding the fixed level is considered to be nonbaseline, resulting in a high output signal (see fourth tracing labeled "window" comparison). The series of window pulses are then averaged, using the "fibrillation capacitor" (fifth tracing). When this average exceeds another level, an arrhythmia is declared. It may be noted that in the left panel the processed idealized normal electrogram spends little time above the threshold and the average value of its window pulse series is low; however, with a sine wave, the window pulses are wide and frequent, resulting in a large average value and arrhythmia declaration. Electrograms from patients obviously are only approximated by these two idealized cases. The distinction between fibrillation and normal rhythm is relatively easy by this method. However, since ventricular tachycardia may have rapidly deflecting depolarizations, it may occasionally be treated as normal by the technique. On the other hand, sinus tachycardia may be treated as abnormal because of bundle branch block, large P and T waves, and postshock signal distortion.

Autocorrelation is another technique that has been used to diagnose abnormal ventricular rhythms. It is only truly useful for diagnosis of ventricular fibrillation, since it involves looking for repeated patterns in ventricular activity by shifting in time, multiplication, and integration. It is computationally intensive, which causes difficulty for incorporation into an implantable system.

Various types of pattern recognition schemes are now being developed. A benefit of these techniques is that the implanted device learns a normal electrocardiographic morphology for each particular patient, rather than relying on some absolute criteria applicable to all patients.

INTERFERENCE CONSIDERATIONS

Interference protection for implantable devices designed to treat ventricular arrhythmias

is, in some cases, more difficult than that for a pacemaker. A notable exception is muscle noise interference, which is virtually eliminated in the device and lead system owing to closely spaced bipolar rate sensing. Signals induced into the patient's leads from a variety of electrical and magnetic fields can have fundamental frequencies that exceed the normal physiologic rate but that may still represent a ventricular arrhythmia. Such signals may come from demodulated radar pulses or magnetic resonance imaging scanners. Even more difficult sources to handle are strong fields from arc welders and electrocautery units. Many pacemaker circuits handle this problem by reverting to fixed-rate pacing during the noise. Since an antitachycardia device is designed to be silent unless an arrhythmia occurs, its circuitry must inhibit function in the presence of demodulated, conducted, or induced signals that are faster than a human tachyarrhythmia. The detection circuitry of the cardioverter/defibrillator has been demonstrated to detect arrhythmias reliably and not be falsely triggered in the presence of strong high-frequency radio sources (radar) of 450 and 3100 MHz, pulsed at rates and pulse widths comparable to human tachyarrhythmia (270 V/m; 5, 10, 20, and 50 pulses per second; 1-msec pulse widths).[10] Normal operation has also been demonstrated in the presence of a 2450-MHz microwave field averaging 15 mV/cm^2 at the device case.

Since reliable implantable defibrillation is still used with leads of large surface area placed on opposite sides of the heart, a large, nearly complete coil turn is effectively attached to the device. Because Faraday's law dictates that a magnetically induced voltage is proportional to frequency, intensity, and area of the coil, signals induced into these shocking leads will be much greater than those induced into rate-sensing (pacemaker-like) leads. Interfering magnetic field strengths causing inhibition also vary with the detected signal level in the patient, as was the case for injected power frequencies. Another important variable is the orientation of the effective coil with respect to the interfering magnetic field. Since fibrillation signal magnitudes may periodically vary over a ratio of 10:1 during a given arrhythmia, at the present time (in many environments) it is nearly impossible to predict the effect of a low-frequency magnetic field on the detection circuit.

What is not open to question is the interaction of the cardioverter/defibrillator and magnetic resonance imaging devices. As is true for other implantable devices, approaching the strong, static magnetic field will activate the cardioverter/defibrillator reed relay. Closure of this relay initiates a high-voltage capacitor-charging sequence. The energy is dissipated internally instead of being delivered to the patient. This can occur as far away as 13 feet from the isocenter of a 0.6-tesla unit (1 tesla = 10,000 gauss). In the first device models, inadvertent charging of internal capacitors or permanent inactivation of the device may be the result. Strong forces inside the scanning device can cause significant rotational forces on an implanted generator of any kind. Since a device capable of high-voltage delivery is more complicated and larger than a pacemaker, the forces are greater as a result of the ferromagnetic shielding of hybrid circuitry. For instance, inside a 1.5-tesla magnetic resonance imaging device, it was difficult to maintain an implantable cardioverter/defibrillator in a horizontal position when held in one hand. The force required to do this was estimated to be 30 pounds. With a magnetic resonance imaging device, the gaussian-shaped megahertz pulses can induce significant signals in the patient's leads. Up to 100 V of induced signal and resulting false arrhythmia detection by the device (with 10-mV normal input signals) have been observed. It is clear, at the present time, that patients with antitachyarrhythmia devices should remain well away from magnetic resonance imaging units.

Additional testing with the cardioverter/defibrillator includes potential interaction with electric blankets and radiofrequency-controlled model airplane transmitters. Neither of these was shown to have an effect on cardio-

verter/defibrillator operation. However, electrocautery, especially of the spark gap type, can cause false arrhythmia detection if a cardioverter/defibrillator is activated. To protect against this, devices are typically turned off if electrocautery is used. However, occasionally, large signals from an electrocautery may reactivate and cause false detection in a cardioverter/defibrillator (S.M. Bach, personal observations, 1982). This is especially true if the return pad is located so that much of the radiofrequency current passes through device leads. It is best to locate this pad on the patient's thigh and deactivate the device if electrocautery must be used after a cardioverter/defibrillator is attached to the patient's leads.

ELECTRICAL ARRHYTHMIA TERMINATION THERAPY

Lead Systems

From a hardware engineering point of view, pacing with antitachycardia pacemakers is not much different from pacing with bradyarrhythmia devices. The pacing rates are faster and the pulse patterns more complicated. Since a combination antitachycardia pacemaker and defibrillator is not widely available, some physicians have utilized separate implantable units to treat patients with bradycardia or relatively frequent, slow ventricular tachycardia. This practice requires utilization of a bipolar pacemaker, preferably one with closely spaced electrodes. Electrodes for the pacemaker must be located as remotely as possible from the defibrillator rate-sensing leads. This remote loca-

Figure 18–8. DVI pacing during ventricular tachycardia. The fixed sensitivity level of the pacemaker resulted in its inability to sense the rhythm continually. *Upper trace,* Defibrillating leads. *Lower trace,* Rate-sensing leads. Note the unipolar pacemaker deflections, comparable in size to the local electrogram, in the lower trace (*arrow*). Such signals can cause an incorrect rate determination. (From Bach SM: AID^{R}Cardioverter-Defibrillator: Possible Interaction with Pacemakers. Intec Systems Technical Communication, Pittsburgh, PA, August 1983; with permission.)

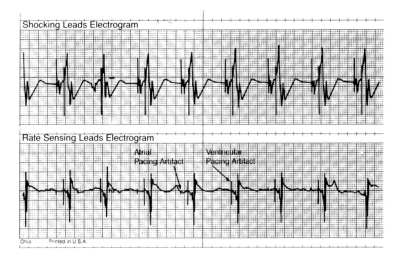

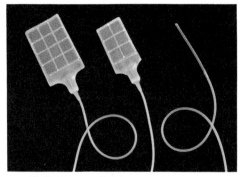

Figure 18–9. Transcardiac (shocking) electrodes for the automatic implantable cardioverter/defibrillator. CPI model Nos. 0041, 0040, and 0020 (respectively, left to right). Model No. 0020 is intravascular, and model Nos. 0040 and 0041 are epicardial, placed either inside or outside the pericardium. The active electrode surface is titanium mesh or ribbon wire.

be detected. This phenomenon results from the defibrillator's automatic gain control circuit finding the largest, fastest depolarizing signal and then referencing all others in proportion. Adverse interactions include incorrect heart rate determination, false defibrillator pulsing, and simultaneous detection by the antitachycardia pacer and defibrillator.[1]

Shocking electrodes for an implantable cardioverter/defibrillator consist of a 7-cm² intravascular spring and two sizes of patch, 13.5 and 27.0 cm² (Fig. 18–9). Typical electrode placement is illustrated in Figure 18–10. All electrodes are constructed of titanium. The lead conductors are drawn-brazed-strand (dbs) stainless steel and silver insulated with Silastic. The advantages of titanium for electrode construction are its inert properties, and the significantly low material cost. A totally transvenous lead placement has been a goal from the inception of the implantable defibrillator.[8] Locating an electrode in the right ventricular apex and one in the right atrium may cause nonuniform current distribution during the shock. Some of this current fails to pass through the fibrillating left ventricular free wall but is instead concentrated in the blood between the electrodes and in the septum. Figure 18–11

tion prevents the pacemaker stimulus from being interpreted as a cardiac depolarization by the defibrillator. Should the pacemaker stimulus occur during a ventricular tachyarrhythmia, the pacemaker may not sense the arrhythmia and may continue to pace (Fig. 18–8). The defibrillator will count the pacing stimuli instead of any local cardiac depolarization, and the ventricular tachyarrhythmia may not

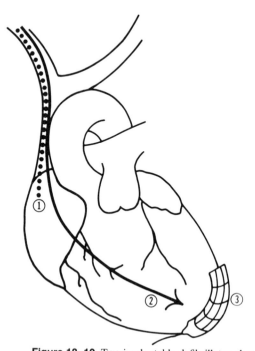

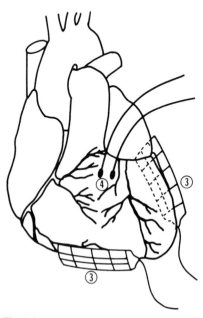

Figure 18–10. Two implantable defibrillator electrode configurations. The left panel illustrates the superior vena cava "spring" electrode (1) paired with a left ventricular patch (3) for shock delivery. Rate sensing is provided by a right ventricular bipolar sensing electrode (2) with 1-cm spacing. In the right panel, shock delivery is provided by two epicardial patch electrodes (3). Rate sensing is accomplished by two closely spaced epicardial screw-in electrodes (4).

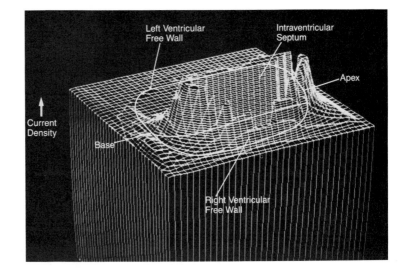

Figure 18–11. A computer-generated finite-difference model demonstrates current distribution during high-energy shock. This model represents the current density generated during a shock between electrodes in the apical (cathode) and basal (anode) regions of the right side of the heart (current in the blood has been removed for this display). Note that the highest current density is in the septal and right ventricular regions, with little current in the left ventricular free wall. (Courtesy of Cardiac Pacemakers, Inc, St. Paul, MN.)

illustrates this effect with a computer model of two electrodes placed in the right side of the heart. Figure 18–12 shows the improved current distribution obtained when a patch is located subcutaneously and shocks are delivered between it and the intravascular electrodes. This configuration appears promising as a nonthoracotomy system, as demonstrated in animal testing and initial clinical studies.[11, 14, 18] The model is also consistent with the clinical experience of using the implantable cardioverter/defibrillator, in which the lead configuration has expanded from a right atrial spring and patch to two patches. In most cases, less energy to defibrillate is required with two patches, since the current between the electrodes is more uniformly distributed through the ventricular mass.[16]

POWER SOURCES

Batteries

Power sources for commercial implantable cardioverter/defibrillators should be capable of supplying microampere current levels for long periods, as well as ampere level currents to charge high-voltage storage capacitors quickly. The previously developed lithium-iodine chemistry, used since 1972 in pacemakers, is not optimal for delivery of the high currents required. The lithium–vanadium pentoxide technology used in the first implantable defibrillator was originally developed for a National Aeronautics and Space Administration (NASA) application. Produced by Honeywell[5] (Horsham, PA), it has been clinically

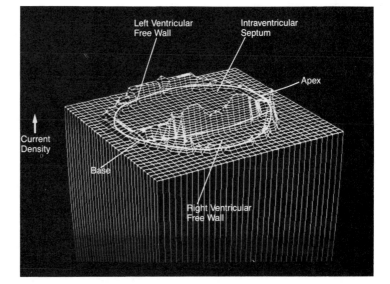

Figure 18–12. The model reflects current density using a three-electrode system, with the two catheter electrodes in Figure 18–11 connected now as cathodes and a left subcutaneous patch serving as anode. Although the initial potential was the same as with a two-electrode system (Fig. 18–11), the current distribution is more uniform, especially in the left ventricular free wall. (Courtesy of Cardiac Pacemakers, Inc, St. Paul, MN.)

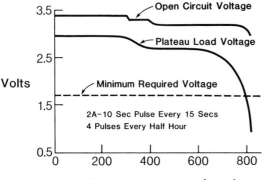

Figure 18–13. Honeywell G3061B cell discharge characteristic. mAH = milliampere-hour. (From Horning RJ, Viswanathan S: High rate lithium cell for medical application. *In* Proceedings of the 29th Power Source Symposium, Atlantic City, NJ, 1981, p 64; with permission.)

used in implantable defibrillator technology since 1980. The battery has performed well but has presented a problem in regard to determining its end-of-life characteristics. The nonuniform discharge characteristic (Fig. 18–13) shows a precipitous fall in terminal voltage near the end of the battery's life. Attempts to monitor this condition with high-voltage capacitor charge times have not always been as successful as desired because of storage capacitor variability and the variability associated with the high-voltage circuitry.

A chemistry that offers improvements in energy capacity as well as discharge characteristics is the lithium/silver–vanadium pentoxide combination. This has recently been developed by Wilson Greatbatch, Ltd.[15] (Clarence, NY). This cell has a gradual reduction in its terminal voltage throughout its usable life (Fig. 18–14). Its ampere-hour (energy storage) capacity per cubic centimeter is greater than that of the lithium–vanadium pentoxide cell. Before any cell capable of delivering such high-output currents is accepted for use in an implantable product, it must undergo a series of rigorous tests, including shock and vibration, regular electrical, short-circuit, and shelf-life evaluations.

HIGH-VOLTAGE GENERATING CIRCUITS

To provide effective voltages for defibrillation, a low battery potential must be converted to hundreds of volts. The circuit that does this is called a direct current–direct current (DC-DC) converter. A simplified diagram for such

a circuit is found in Figure 18–15. An oscillator circuit provides a series of pulses to an electronic switch, which alternately turns on and off. This provides a changing magnetic field in the primary coil of a transformer, which causes an increase in voltage in the secondary coil resulting from a relatively high turns ratio. This alternating secondary voltage is rectified (converted to unidirectional) and maintained by the high-voltage storage capacitor. The changing magnetic field can be detected when a wire coil is placed on the skin surface next to the implanted device, enabling the charge time to be measured. This charge time is a function of the condition of the device battery. It is also a function of several other parameters, the most important of which is the condition of the high-voltage storage capacitor.

High-voltage storage capacitors used for defibrillation are of the aluminum electrolytic type. The basic construction is illustrated in Figure 18–16. The material that gives the capacitors ability to store charge is the dielectric aluminum oxide (Al_2O_3) formed on the surface of the foil after it has been "etched" to increase the effective surface area (capacitance = $\epsilon A/d$, where ϵ = permittivity, A = plate surface area, and d = distance between the plates). The capacitor is constructed like a "jelly roll" of anode and cathode aluminum coils (each anodized or formed with an oxide coating) and a separator, which then prevents them from shorting (Fig. 18–17).[17] After its construction,

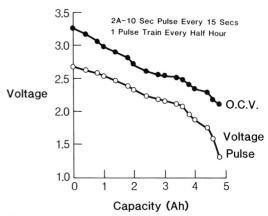

Figure 18–14. Wilson Greatbatch, Ltd., 8512 cell discharge characteristic. Ah = ampere-hour; OCV = open circuit voltage. (From Takeuchi ES, Muffoletto BC, Greenwood JM, Holmes CF: Recent advances in the development of a power source for the implantable defibrillator/cardioverter. VIIIth World Symposium on Cardiac Pacing and Electrophysiology, Jerusalem, June 7–11, 1987; with permission.)

Figure 18–15. Functional diagram of the direc current–direct current (DC-DC) converter. An interrupted DC from the battery results in an expanding and diminishing magnetic field in the transformer "primary," which induces an increased voltage in the transformer "secondary." The alternating secondary voltage is converted to direct by a rectifier, which conducts in only one direction. This "DC" voltage is stored by the high-voltage capacitor.

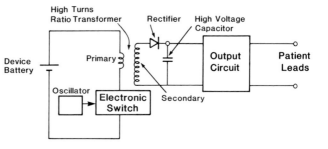

the capacitor is impregnated with an electrolytic material. This electrolyte will, with voltage applied, react with the aluminum to generate more oxide and seal imperfections in the plates. These imperfections are a result of manufacturing and a tendency for the aluminum oxide to "deform" or thin out during the time the capacitor is not under high-voltage bias, which is most of the time in an implantable defibrillator. Thus, while the implanted device spends its time monitoring the cardiac rhythm, this natural decay in oxide coating causes an increase in capacitance (thinner

plates) and initial leakage current (wasted energy) and longer charge times. These changes will result in a capacitor charge time that is a function of how recently the capacitor was charged. It is important for these high-voltage capacitors to be periodically exercised to maintain the defibrillator in a good state of readiness for an arrhythmic event. Under these conditions, the energy so drawn from the battery is delivered to an internal test load instead of to the patient.

IMPLANTABLE DEFIBRILLATOR OUTPUT CIRCUIT

The high-voltage waveform used for implantable defibrillation to date is a truncated exponential, also known as Schuder's pulse (Fig. 18–18).[13] The source for this waveform is the high-voltage capacitor previously discussed. The critical pulse parameters are the leading and trailing edge voltages, V_i and V_f, respectively; 1 minus the ratio of the final to the initial voltage (tilt); and the pulse width. Since the implantable device has a high-efficiency electronic switch to connect the high-voltage capacitor to the patient, the stored voltage and the initial voltage delivered to the patient, V_i, are very nearly equal. Because the patient's heart looks almost purely resistive,[17] the capacitor voltage falls according to the following equation

$$v(t) = V_i \exp^{(-t/RC)}$$

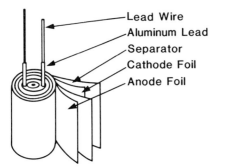

Figure 18–16. Basic aluminum electrolytic capacitor construction. The "jelly roll" configuration results in large cathode and anode areas, which increase the capacitance. (Courtesy of United Chemi-Con, Inc., Rosemont, IL.)

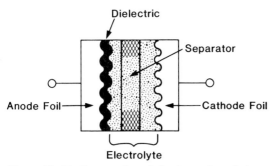

Figure 18–17. Cross-section of aluminum electrolytic capacitor. The foil areas are increased by etching. The separator prevents the foils from shorting. The electrolyte allows the capacitor to heal itself by forming more oxide, should the dielectric film (Al_2O_3) be damaged. (Courtesy of United Chemi-Con, Inc., Rosemont, IL.)

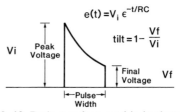

Figure 18–18. Basic waveform used in implantable defibrillation. It results from discharge of a large capacitor into the essentially purely resistive heart. See text for explanation.

where R is the heart resistance and V_i is the initial capacitor voltage. R may vary from 20 to more than 100 ohms, depending upon the surface area of the defibrillating electrode or electrodes and the bulk resistance of the tissue between them. When the capacitor voltage falls to approximately one third of the initial voltage, the output is abruptly terminated. This sharp fall in final voltage is thought to remove stimulation simultaneously from all areas of the heart so that defibrillation is effected.[13] Termination of the pulse at voltages higher than one third of the initial voltage results in more wasted energy and in the requirement for higher peak voltages. Termination at voltages much less than one third of peak can result in higher initial voltage requirements, along with more postshock arrhythmias. This pulse waveform transfers stored energy to the patient's heart with low energy loss. External defibrillators that deliver a sinusoidal Lown-type waveform utilize a magnetic material core inductor. This inductor is physically large and has significant resistance and energy losses, which are undesirable for an implanted device.

Figure 18–19 depicts a functional diagram of a truncated exponential circuit. When silicon-controlled rectifiers are used, switch A turns on, causing the capacitor to discharge into the heart. It remains on until switch B is activated, short-circuiting the capacitor and removing the current from switch A. This action turns switch A off. When using a power field effect transistor (FET) as switch A, switch B is not required, since switch A may be turned off by changing the low-voltage drive to it. However, the technology for these FETs is new. In terms of their voltage rating, current capability, and on resistance, they are not yet equal to silicon-controlled rectifiers.

As can be seen from Figure 18–19, voltages applied to the heart that have the same polarity as the implanted generator do not interfere with the device because of the output diode, which prevents current from passing the wrong direction through the implanted device. However, voltages of opposite polarity applied to the heart in parallel with the implanted device may result in the turning on of switch A. This occurrence can damage the device and shunt energy, preventing defibrillation. Typically, this is only a problem when using internal defibrillation paddles.

Recently, much attention has been paid to biphasic pulse, which reverses the voltage to the heart with a second, smaller truncated exponential shock. Conceptually, this waveform is similar to a damped sine wave. It appears to improve the efficacy of defibrillation.

CONCLUSIONS

Automatic electrical treatment of ventricular arrhythmias by implantable devices is in the early stage of technologic development. The technical challenges of the anticipated pacer-defibrillator device will be in arrhythmia detection, software algorithms for treatment, and nonthoracotomy defibrillation. At the present time, there is no good method by which an implantable device can separate ventricular from supraventricular rhythms. The solution may result from additional electrodes and better algorithms. Algorithms for treatment will likely be derived from the previous experience physicians have gained in electrophysiology laboratories. This being the case, designers face the dilemma of having to provide a more sophisticated device while keeping it simple

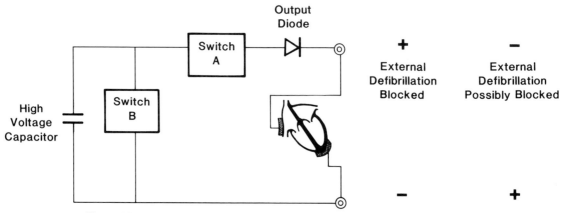

Figure 18–19. Output circuit for implantable defibrillation. See text for description.

enough for use in clinical medicine. Development of a more reliable nonthoracotomy electrode system for defibrillation has the greatest set of unknowns ahead of it. A better understanding of defibrillating current distributions and activation patterns during fibrillation may lead to success in developing such a system.

REFERENCES

1. Bach SM: AID^{R}B Cardioverter-Defibrillator: Possible Interaction with Pacemakers. Intec Systems Technical Communication, Pittsburgh, PA, August 1983.
2. Bowman L, Meindl JD: The packaging of implantable integrated sensors. IEEE Trans Biomed Eng BME-33:248, 1986.
3. Davies DW, Wainwright RJ, Tooley MA, et al: Detection of pathological tachycardia by analysis of electrogram morphology. PACE 9:200, 1986.
4. Geddes LA, Hoff HE, Mello A, et al: Continuous measurement of ventricular volume by electrical impedance. Cardiac Res Center Bull 4:118, 1966.
5. Horning RJ, Viswanathan S: High rate lithium cell for medical application. In Proceedings of the 29th Power Source Symposium, Atlantic City, NJ, 1981, p 64.
6. Langer A, Heilman MS, Mower M, Mirowski M: Considerations in the development of the automatic implantable defibrillator. Med Instrum 10:163, 1976.
7. Lawrence JH, Brin KP, Halperin HR, et al: The characterization of human transmyocardial impedance during implantation of the automatic internal cardioverter defibrillator. PACE 9:745, 1986.
8. Mirowski M, Mower MM, Gott VL, Brawley RK: Feasibility and effectiveness of low energy catheter defibrillation in man. Circulation 47:79–85, 1973.
9. Mirowski M, Mower MM, Bhagavan BS, et al: Chronic animal and bench testing of the implantable automatic defibrillator. VIth World Symposium on Cardiac Pacing, Montreal, October 2–5, 1979.
10. Pulse Generator Qualification—EMI Testing. Atlanta, Georgia Institute of Technology Report IV-106, 1986.
11. Saksena S, Parsonnet V: Implantation of a cardioverter/defibrillator without thoracotomy using a triple electrode system. JAMA 259:69, 1988.
12. Salo RW, Wallner TG, Pederson BD: Measurement of ventricular volume by intracardiac impedance: Theoretical and empirical approaches. IEEE Trans Biomed Eng BME-33:189, 1986.
13. Schuder JC, Rahmoeller GA, Stoeckle H: Transthoracic ventricular defibrillation with triangular and trapezoidal waveforms. Circ Res 19:689, 1966.
14. Shapland JE, Dawson AK, Bach SB Jr, Lang DJ: Improved defibrillation efficacy in the dog with an equipotential transvenous electrode configuration. Circulation 76 [Suppl IV]:462, 1987.
15. Takeuchi ES, Muffoletto BC, Greenwood JM, Holmes CF: Recent advances in the development of a power source for the implantable defibrillator/cardioverter. VIIIth World Symposium on Cardiac Pacing and Electrophysiology, Jerusalem, June 7–11, 1987.
16. Troup PJ, Chapman PD, Olinger GN, Kleinman LH: The implanted defibrillator: Relation of defibrillating lead configuration and clinical variables to defibrillation threshold. J Am Coll Cardiol 6:1315, 1985.
17. Understanding Aluminum Electrolytic Capacitors. United Chemi-Con, Rosemont, IL.
18. Wetherbee JN, Chapman PD, Bach SB Jr, Troup PA: "Split" single versus sequential pulse defibrillation: Are two pulses better than one? Circulation 74:111, 1986.
19. Worley SJ, Swain JL, Colavita PG, et al: Development of an endocardial-epicardial gradient of activation rate during electrically induced, sustained ventricular fibrillation in dogs. Am J Cardiol 55:813, 1985.

19

ELECTROPHYSIOLOGIC MECHANISMS UNDERLYING MANAGEMENT OF SUPRAVENTRICULAR TACHYCARDIA BY ELECTRICAL STIMULATION

SANJEEV SAKSENA *and* HUANLIN AN

The management of recurrent paroxysmal supraventricular tachycardia (SVT) by electrical stimulation techniques has been conceptually considered for over two decades. Analysis of the mechanisms of SVT has been undertaken for an even greater period. Electrophysiologic study of the mechanisms of paroxysmal SVT was greatly advanced by the early experimental studies of Moe and associates and the clinical studies of Durrer, Wellens, and colleagues on the Wolff-Parkinson-White syndrome.[12, 28, 45] Subsequent investigations clarified the physiologic basis for other types of paroxysmal SVT, including atrioventricular (AV) nodal reentrant tachycardia and atrial flutter.[6, 10, 14, 47] Correlation of the physiologic mechanisms with the anatomic substrate for paroxysmal SVT continues to generate discussion and investigation. Although the anatomic pathways for most types of reentrant SVT remain only partially defined, enough information on the interaction of these arrhythmias with electrical stimulation techniques exists to warrant presentation as the basis for tachycardia management with electrical devices. Early empirical attempts demonstrated the feasibility of this therapeutic approach, and a subsequent chapter (Chapter 26) in this text will describe its current clinical status.[7, 15, 30] The general electrophysiologic concepts underlying this therapy will be examined in this chapter.

GENERAL ELECTROPHYSIOLOGIC CONCEPTS

Paroxysmal SVT can be generated by reentrant or automatic mechanisms. Reentry requires the presence of two or more physiologically distinct conduction pathways with the capability of transient or permanent differences in electrophysiologic properties. These differences permit the development of circus movement. Specific physiologic events preceding reentrant excitation usually include the need for functional unidirectional block in one or more pathways and the presence of slow conduction in at least one other pathway. Antegrade unidirectional block results in preferential engagement of the slowly conducting link and potential retrograde penetration of the antegradely blocked pathway. Under ideal electrophysiologic circumstances, the excitation wave will traverse the retrograde pathway slowly with sufficient delay for the antegradely conducting limb to recover excitability. Maintenance of reentry requires continuation of this delicate electrophysiologic balance. These general conditions can be met by a variety of anatomic substrates that can provide two or more electrophysiologically distinct pathways. In paroxysmal SVT associated with the Wolff-Parkinson-White syndrome, this can be provided by the normal AV conduction system and one or more accessory bypass tracts. In paroxysmal SVT due to AV nodal reentry, longitudinal dissociation of the AV node and perinodal tissues into two or more distinct electrophysiologic entities has been incriminated. In recurrent atrial flutter, intraatrial dissociation, with the reentrant wave circulating around the orifices of the great veins, has been suggested. In each instance, the reentrant circuit has rapidly and slowly conducting segments. The excitation wave leaves a trail of refractoriness, the duration of which is determined by the effective and functional refractory periods of the tissue. The total revolution time is largely determined by the anatomic size of the circuit and the conduction velocity. The disparity between the total revolution time and the duration of refractoriness defines the major component of the remaining excitable tissue in the circuit, the so-called excitable gap. Continuing propagation of reentry is dependent on the availability of excitable tissue for the advancing circulating wave front. Partial or total elimination of this excitable gap by electrical stimulation methods interrupts continuing propagation of this wave front (Fig. 19–1). The collision of two wave fronts initially results in refractoriness of this tissue (*A*). For successful tachycardia termination, however, the electrical stimulation wave front not only should collide with the spontaneous tachycardia wave front but also should not initiate another wave of reentrant excitation (*B*). In many instances, this is not achieved, and the reentrant circuit continues to be inscribed but is now reset (*C*). However, the revolution time for one or more beats is now also determined by coupling interval and frequency of the electrical stimulation. As an extension to this, the reentrant circuit can be driven at different rates by pacing stimuli and is considered to be "entrained" in this circumstance.

Specific criteria have been developed by Waldo and Henthorn for defining transient entrainment by electrical pacing techniques.[40] The presence of any of these criteria suggests the existence of this phenomenon (Table 19–1). Demonstration of entrainment can be a prelude to development of therapeutic strategies. Engagement of the reentrant pathways by electrical stimulation sequences can be used as a guide to develop specific tachycardia-

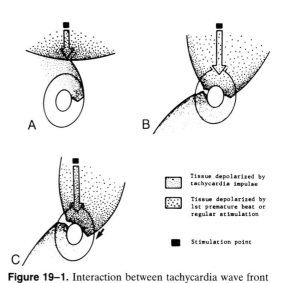

Figure 19–1. Interaction between tachycardia wave front and pacing stimulation. *A,* The tachycardia wave front propagates, demonstrating circus movement. The advancing edge of the wave front leaves behind it completely depolarized and refractory tissue followed by a tail of relative refractoriness. Pacing stimulation initiates a second wave front that collides with the refractoriness left behind by this circulating circus movement tachycardia. This results in an extinction of the pacing wave front without penetration of the tachycardia circuit. *B,* The tachycardia wave front has now advanced to another portion of the tachycardia circuit. The pacing stimulation is applied later in the tachycardia cycle, and the stimulated wave front now encounters excitable tissue. It penetrates the tachycardia circuit, and this results in antegrade and retrograde penetration of the tachycardia circuit. Collision between the retrogradely penetrating pacing wave front and the antegradely advancing tachycardia wave front results in extinction of the primary tachycardia wave front. The antegradely advancing pacing wave front encounters refractory tissue and fails to propagate. This results in termination of the reentrant tachycardia. *C,* The tachycardia wave front has advanced further into the circuit. The pacing wave front enters the circuit still later in the cycle and again results in antegrade and retrograde wave fronts. The retrograde wave front collides with the advancing tachycardia wave front. The antegradely advancing pacing wave front continues to encounter excitable tissue and follows the inscription of the tachycardia circuit. This results in the establishment of a second tachycardia wave front. Thus, the tachycardia continues, now established by the pacing wave front. However, changes in tachycardia cycle interval length for one or more beats can be noticed owing to timing differences between the two wave fronts, and this is seen as the resetting phenomenon. (Modified from Pacing for Tachycardia Control. Englewood, CO, Telectronics, 1983, p 29; with permission.)

terminating therapies. Increasing pacing stimulus prematurity, train length, or rate can be used to achieve this goal. Specific examples are illustrated in Chapter 21. Electrocardiographic criteria (Nos. 1 and 2 in Table 19–1) and recordings are adequate for this purpose.

TABLE 19–1. SUGGESTED ELECTROCARDIOGRAPHIC AND INTRACARDIAC ELECTROGRAM CRITERIA FOR TRANSIENT ENTRAINMENT OF A REENTRANT TACHYCARDIA*

1. Electrocardiographic (ECG) demonstration of constant fusion beats during pacing except for the last captured beat, which is only entrained.
2. Presence of progressive ECG fusion during differential rate pacing.
3. Tachycardia interruption coincident with localized intracardiac conduction block and subsequent morphologic and rate changes in the tachycardia with a different activation sequence of the blocked site.
4. Altered intracardiac electrogram morphology and conduction time at two or more rapid pacing rates that exceed the tachycardia rate but fail to interrupt it.

*Although suggested initially for ventricular tachycardia, these can be considered for other reentrant tachycardias.
Adapted from Waldo AL, Henthorn RW: Use of transient entrainment during ventricular tachycardia to localize a critical area in the reentry circuit for ablation. Pacing Clin Electrophysiol 12:231, 1989.

Identification of the arrhythmogenic substrate is made feasible by the combined electrocardiogram and intracardiac electrogram criteria and demonstration of "slow conduction" or a "weak link" in the tachycardia circuit. In addition to the above-mentioned manipulations, increasing the proximity of the stimulation electrodes to this site, elevating the stimulation current strength, or the use of multiple electrodes may increase the likelihood of penetrating this site.[4, 25, 43] Modification of the electrophysiologic properties of such critical areas, making genesis of reentrant circuits untenable, is also the basis for electrical strategies for tachycardia prevention. This can be accomplished by electrical methods alone or in combination with antiarrhythmic drugs. Other potential mechanisms for SVT termination include induction of another unstable SVT, especially atrial flutter-fibrillation. In the absence of atrial disease or dilatation, these rhythms are unstable and spontaneously terminate. Alternatively, this target tissue can be subjected to ablative intervention (see Chapter 34).[29]

SPECIFIC ELECTROPHYSIOLOGIC INTERACTIONS

Atrioventricular Reentrant Tachycardia

Atrioventricular reciprocating tachycardia has several components to the reentrant circuit. The atrium, normal AV conduction system, ventricle, and accessory AV connection participate together in a single chain. Electrical stimulation at several sites can thus be employed for tachycardia termination. Atrial or ventricular pacing using single or multiple extrastimuli in burst pacing is effective in these rhythms. Single extrastimuli can fail to penetrate and reset the tachycardia (Fig. 19–2A). Increasing prematurity results in antegrade and retrograde penetration and tachycardia reset (Fig. 19–2B). Reciprocating tachycardia is easily interrupted by a single extrastimulus, particularly if it is delivered near the accessory pathway. Reciprocating tachycardia is easily terminated by an early single atrial stimulus by three mechanisms: (1) production of conduction block in the AV node or His-Purkinje system; (2) depolarization of both atria to render them refractory to the returning reentrant impulse via the accessory pathway, thereby creating a form of retrograde ventriculoatrial block; and (3) antegrade penetration of the bypass tract, resulting in collision with the returning impulse or making the bypass tract refractory to the impulse as it reaches its ventricular insertion. The first mechanism is by far the most common mode of termination. The second and third mechanisms, which are most likely to occur when stimulation is performed at or near the site of the bypass tract, are difficult to distinguish from each other by currently available techniques. Multiple atrial extrastimuli and burst pacing are more effective owing to shortening of atrial refractoriness produced by the initial pacing stimuli, permitting penetration of the circuit by subsequent stimuli.

Reciprocating tachycardia may also be promptly terminated by a single ventricular stimulus by one of the following mechanisms: (1) most commonly, preexciting the atrium with subsequent block of the retrograde atrial impulse in the AV node or the His-Purkinje system; preexcitation of the atrium may not always be possible with right ventricular stimulation if the bypass tract is located on the contralateral side; (2) block in the accessory pathway;[17, 46] and (3) collision with the antegradely conducting wave front due to retrograde penetration of the normal pathway. The likelihood of achieving tachycardia termination is increased by the use of multiple extrastimuli or pacing bursts (Fig. 19–3). Information on the use of other electrical techniques, such as intracavitary shocks for the same purpose, is limited.[11] External transthoracic shocks achieve tachycardia cardioversion at relatively low

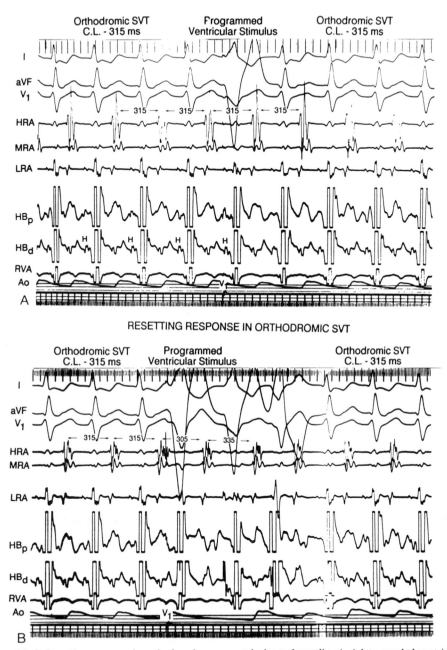

Figure 19–2. Resetting response in orthodromic supraventricular tachycardia. *A,* A late coupled ventricular extrastimulus (V_1) fails to reset the tachycardia cycle, which continues unchanged, analogous to Figure 19–1*A. B,* An earlier coupled ventricular extrastimulus now penetrates, advances, and resets the tachycardia, with the postextrastimulus beat showing a change in cycle length. Standard electrocardiographic (ECG) leads are shown in the upper three panels. HRA = high right atrium; MRA = mid right atrium; LRA = low right atrium; HB_p = proximal His bundle electrogram; HB_d = distal His bundle electrogram; RVA = right ventricular apex; Ao = aorta; C.L. = cycle length; SVT = supraventricular tachycardia; V_1 = ventricular extrastimulus.

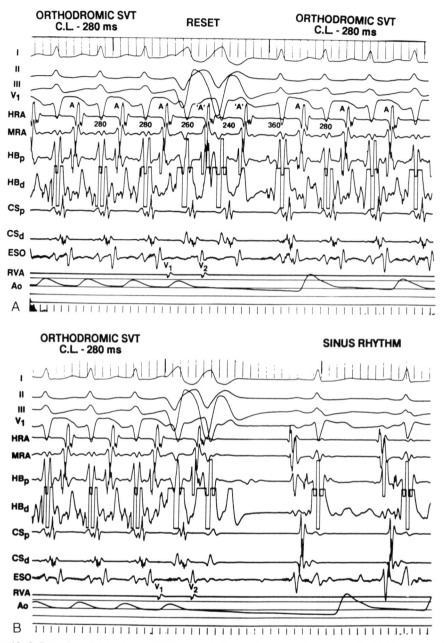

Figure 19–3. Resetting of orthodromic SVT by coupled premature ventricular extrastimulation using paired stimuli. *A,* The resetting response is observed during the orthodromic SVT with a cycle length of 280 msec in a patient with Wolff-Parkinson-White syndrome. Two ventricular extrastimuli (V_1, V_2) are applied. V_1 advances the retrograde atrial potential by 20 msec, and V_2 advances it further by another 20 msec (shown as 'A'). Despite advancing the retrograde atrial potential with the stimulus being delivered at a time when the antegrade His bundle activation results in refractoriness of the His bundle, resetting and continuation of the tachycardia are noted. The postextrastimulus beat has an atrial cycle interval of 360 msec and then reverts to the original tachycardia cycle at 280 msec. This recording also demonstrates the presence of an accessory pathway, with earliest retrograde activation being noted in the proximal coronary sinus. The postextrasystolic potentiation of aortic pressure in the reset tachycardia beat is apparent. *B,* Termination of orthodromic SVT by paired ventricular extrastimuli. The same patient with the same tachycardia as in *A* is again exposed to two ventricular extrastimuli at closer coupling intervals (V_1, V_2). V_1 results in retrograde atrial activation, which is advanced, and V_2 results in retrograde ventriculoatrial (VA) block. This results in interruption of the tachycardia. In this instance, resetting precedes termination. Abbreviations are as in Figure 19–2. CS_p = proximal coronary sinus electrogram; CS_d = distal coronary sinus electrogram; ESO = esophageal electrogram; V_1, V_2 = ventricular extrastimuli.

energies. Although the exact electrophysiologic mechanisms are unknown, conduction block is presumed, and sustained tachycardia can be interrupted in nearly all instances by this approach. Determinants of efficacy can include tachycardia rate and several specific electrophysiologic variables, such as the presence of retrograde or antegrade preexcitation or both, spontaneous degeneration into atrial fibrillation, and the presence of single or multiple accessory tracts. Formal controlled studies are lacking, but tachycardia termination with pacing techniques may be less effective in patients with wide tachycardia induction zones or extremely rapid rates. This observation may be related to repeated resetting and reinitiation in the former case and a reduced or nearly absent "excitable gap" in the latter instance. The presence of multiple bypass tracts also provides a number of options for reentry. Pacing modes can convert one form of reentrant SVT to another in this situation, for example, from orthodromic SVT to antedromic SVT. Simultaneous capture of both atria and ventricles may be considered for SVT termination in some patients. This capture results in simultaneous alterations of refractoriness and conduction in multiple areas in the reentrant circuit, thus widely disturbing the electrophysiologic balance needed for reentry. Induction of atrial fibrillation by attempts at SVT termination by rapid atrial and ventricular pacing has also been reported. Rapid atrial pacing or rapid retrograde atrial activation during ventricular pacing may encroach on atrial repolarization in the relative refractory period and may induce fibrillation. Rapid pacing techniques are thus contraindicated in patients with antegradely conducting accessory pathways with short effective refractory periods. Sudden death due to ventricular fibrillation (VF) has been reported.[23] An effective refractory period of 300 msec has been suggested as a cut-off in selecting the appropriateness of pacing therapy.[8, 22]

Tachycardia prevention by pacing techniques has been employed for temporary or permanent treatment of drug-resistant AV reentrant tachycardia. Fixed-rate atrial or ventricular pacing is occasionally employed for this purpose in patients with concomitant sinus node disease and bradycardia-dependent SVT. Dual-chamber pacing has been employed with greater success. In this approach, simultaneous atrial and ventricular pacing or sequential AV pacing with a short AV delay is employed. This method results in simultaneous atrial and ventricular activation without conduction over the specialized AV conduction system. Antegrade and retrograde invasion of the normal and anomalous AV pathways is achieved simultaneously or in close sequence by the two paced wave fronts. This results in diffuse depolarization of most components of the AV reentry substrate and eliminates the possibility of sequential activation necessary for a circulating reentrant wave front. Akhtar and coworkers noted abolition or narrowing of the tachycardia induction zone in two patients with type B Wolff-Parkinson-White syndrome with simultaneous atrial and ventricular pacing.[1] In contrast, there was no effect in one patient with type A Wolff-Parkinson-White syndrome. Sequential AV premature stimulation was effective in all three patients. The concept of simultaneous atrial and ventricular stimulation has, as alluded to above, been used for tachycardia termination as well. Implantable permanent pacing devices based on these principles have been successfully used for short- and intermediate-term SVT control in selected patients.[19, 33] Figure 19–4 shows an example of such stimulation in a patient with frequent, drug-resistant, recurrent SVT due to concealed Wolff-Parkinson-White syndrome. Orthodromic AV reentry utilized a right-sided accessory tract with an antegrade refractory period of 280 msec. A Medtronic (Minneapolis, MN) 7006 Symbios pacemaker was placed in the DVI mode to achieve permanent paced preexcitation (A). This markedly reduced the number of SVT episodes. Infrequent spontaneous SVT episodes were terminated by atrial burst pacing (B).

Prevention of AV reentrant tachycardia induction by introducing an atrial premature beat after the SVT initiating beat has also been reported.[20] The coupling intervals of this programmed extrastimulus delivered after a premature beat capable of inciting the tachycardia define a preventive zone for tachycardia initiation. Typically this zone begins 10 msec outside the effective refractory period and averages 50 msec in duration. Although the prevention of SVT was always possible with a single stimulus in this study, termination required at least two atrial extrastimuli or right ventricular stimulation. This preventive zone is independent of initial tachycardia interval or cycle length. This finding is consistent with electrophysiologic concepts requiring reduction or abolition of the excitable gap for prevention of sustained reentry. Chronic data on this technique are unavailable at present. Ex-

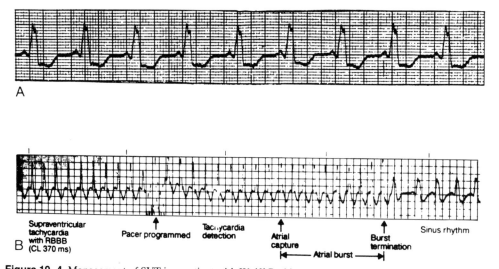

Figure 19–4. Management of SVT in a patient with Wolff-Parkinson-White syndrome using a dual-chamber antitachycardia pacemaker. *A,* In this patient with incessant SVT, a Medtronic (Minneapolis, MN) Model 7008 Symbios pacemaker was inserted, and bipolar stimulation was used to achieve permanent paced preexcitation. Atrioventricular (AV) sequential pacing was established in the DVI mode with an AV interval of 100 msec. This resulted in a marked decrease in the frequency of SVT episodes. *B,* Recurrent paroxysmal SVT was occasionally observed, and the same antitachycardia device as shown in *A* is now programmed to the automatic mode using atrial burst pacing for tachycardia termination. SVT with a right bundle branch block configuration with a cycle length of 370 msec occurred spontaneously. The pacemaker is programmed to the predetermined antitachycardia device termination mode. Automatic tachycardia detection ensues within the next 2 seconds and is followed by the delivery of an atrial burst that resets the tachycardia, results in antegrade AV nodal block with penetration of the accessory pathway antegradely, and failure of maintenance of the tachycardia wave front. The patient subsequently reverts to sinus rhythm with antegrade preexcitation.

perimental studies have suggested that sub-threshold stimuli delivered close to a threshold stimulus may also prolong atrial refractoriness.[35] The use of this stimulation mode to prevent initiation of reentrant SVT has been suggested. Early clinical studies, however, suggest that the effects of subthreshold stimuli are very local and are unlikely to be of clinical value unless applied directly at a critical site in the reentrant circuit.[39] Thus, application in ventricular or atrial regions distant from the site of bypass tract insertion is unlikely to be efficacious. Other techniques, such as over-drive pacing, have been considered for tachycardia prevention. Although increasing the heart rate beyond the resting sinus rate may prevent reentry by decreasing dispersion of refractoriness in components of the AV reentrant circuit, analogous to suggestions for ventricular tachycardia, the long-term value of this technique remains to be established. Alterations in AV nodal or bypass tract refractoriness may also be achieved by this technique. This mode may decrease the incidence of atrial or ventricular ectopic beats that may trigger SVT,[13] but reduction in sustained SVT episodes remains to be formally confirmed in controlled studies.

The role of autonomic tone in modulating the response of AV reentrant tachycardia to electrical stimulation methods has been examined. Changing autonomic tone can be instrumental in the initiation of AV reentrant SVT.[2] Further alterations in sympathetic tone after the onset of SVT may produce changing SVT rates and tachycardia-terminating zones, resulting in failure of previously effective modes.[44] Similar observations may be made with changes in posture or concomitant antiarrhythmic drug therapy. Changing autonomic tone can also be expected to influence pacing modes used for tachycardia prevention in the same fashion. This factor may be particularly applicable to dual-demand pacing modes and programmed extrastimuli.

Atrioventricular Nodal Reentrant Tachycardia

The reentrant circuit in AV nodal reentrant tachycardia utilizes electrophysiologic pathways in the AV junction. These may be intranodal or perinodal in location.[26] Thus, neither the atrium nor the ventricle is a necessary link for tachycardia generation or maintenance. Atrial stimulation can terminate this type of

SVT if the paced impulse (or impulses) penetrates the excitable gap in the AV junctional circuit and then fails to propagate because of prematurity, inducing antegrade and retrograde conduction block. This critical timing is vital to its success. The outcome of attempts at termination using single paced atrial stimuli is determined by the native cycle length of the SVT, the distance between the pacing electrode and the AV nodal region, and the refractoriness and conduction velocity of this intervening tissue. Rapid SVT (cycle lengths below 325 msec) has been infrequently terminated by this technique.[18] For rapid SVT, stimulation at a site adjoining the AV node is often required for successful results. Prolonged atrial refractory periods and slow conduction velocities observed in patients with atrial disease interfere with impulse penetration and SVT interruption. Similar observations are applicable to single ventricular extrastimuli. In unresponsive tachycardias, two or more stimuli are often successful when a single stimulus is ineffective. This finding is due to shortening of atrial refractoriness induced by the first stimulated beat, which permits the second stimulus to reach the reentrant circuit early enough to interrupt the circulating wave front. Burst atrial pacing is nearly always successful in this situation owing to similar mechanisms. However, train length is important, since excessively prolonged stimulation may reinduce SVT or atrial fibrillation. In many instances, atrial fibrillation is transient and converts to sinus rhythm.

Simultaneous AV pacing can be more effective than atrial pacing alone in many patients. This is achieved by abolishing or narrowing the paroxysmal SVT induction zone. Paradoxically, occasional patients may experience facilitation of SVT induction because of facilitation of retrograde conduction.[19, 24] Significant shortening of retrograde AV nodal refractoriness is observed during this type of stimulation. Several workers have also observed higher success rates with sequential AV pacing using very short AV intervals in comparison to underdrive atrial or ventricular pacing.[23, 27] Implantable pacemakers used for chronic therapy in this disorder have employed these principles. Burst atrial pacing has usually been the favored approach.[36, 37] This type of pacing has been accomplished by manual or automated devices. Less frequently, scanning pacemakers have been used with both manual and automated systems. In general, short-term results have been encouraging (see Chapter 26), but

long-term application reveals a significant incidence of changing SVT termination intervals and atrial fibrillation.[36] The former may also be related to changing autonomic tone and electrophysiologic properties of the circuit.[2] Automated intelligent pacemakers with memory for tachycardia termination windows are employed in this situation.[31, 38] Alternatively, other options, such as concomitant antiarrhythmic therapy or catheter ablation of the AV junction, can be considered in resistant patients. Dunbar and coworkers have demonstrated catheter cardioversion of SVT with intracavitary low-energy shocks.[11] In this method, cardioversion of experimentally induced atrial tachycardia was achieved at energies lower than 0.5 J, with the cathode being located in the right atrial appendage. The anode position in the right atrium was not critical to the results. Ventricular fibrillation was occasionally observed with asynchronous shock delivery. All VF episodes occurred with energies higher than 0.25 J. Further clinical evaluation of this method is awaited.

Paroxysmal Atrial Flutter

Atrial flutter is a common and symptomatic SVT in many patients. Paroxysmal atrial flutter is particularly difficult to control with antiarrhythmic drug therapy. Increasing interest in the mechanisms of atrial flutter has developed in the past decade.[32, 41, 42] Cardiac mapping studies performed with multiple atrial endocardial and epicardial recordings suggest a reentrant mechanism.[41] Zones of slow conduction and fragmented electrograms with periodicity have been recorded (Fig. 19–5). The reentrant loop has been reported to involve the right atrium and orifices of the great veins. Interruption with pacing techniques has also been reported.[42] Single or multiple extrastimuli are usually ineffective in this regard, though occasional reports do exist. Burst pacing from several seconds to minutes can terminate classic (type I) atrial flutter, defined as flutter with inverted "P" waves in leads II, III, and aV_F and rates of 240 to 338 beats per minute. The pacing rate typically is 10 to 30 per cent faster than the flutter rate. This faster rate results in entrainment of the flutter with a change of "P"-wave morphology ("fusion") preceding termination, which usually occurs after abrupt cessation or gradual slowing of pacing. Conversion is achieved directly into sinus rhythm or is preceded by transient atrial fibrillation. Type II, or atypical, atrial flutter is more

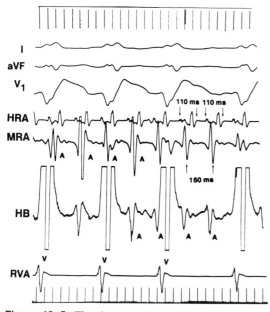

Figure 19–5. The demonstration of slowly conducting segments in an atrial flutter circuit in a patient with recurrent and refractory atrial flutter. The atrial flutter cycle length is 160 msec. Atrial endocardial recordings are obtained from the high right atrium, mid right atrium, and His bundle region. Bipolar recordings from the high right atrium show diastolic atrial potentials that precede the major atrial depolarization. These are reproducible and represent the slowly conducting segment in the tachycardia circuit.

resistant to atrial pacing and has faster rates (range from 340 to 433 beats per minute). Several factors influence success rates with pacing. These include the pacing rate, time duration of pacing, pacing threshold, and the pacing site.[34] A minimal duration of 20 to 30 seconds of pacing has been suggested. The use of high-energy output (10 to 20 mA) is often necessary. Temporary pacing for termination of atrial flutter is most commonly used after open heart surgery or in the electrophysiology

laboratory. A similar approach as detailed above can be considered for intraatrial reentrant tachycardia (Fig. 19–6).[16] Implantable pacemakers have been occasionally used for chronic management of these patients. More commonly, catheter AV junctional ablation has been preferred for this purpose, with implantable pacemakers being used for rate support on demand.

Prevention of atrial flutter by electrical stimulation techniques has been considered. Atrial flutter may coexist as part of the bradycardia-tachycardia syndrome. Atrial rate support by pacing may be useful in tachycardia prevention in selected instances. In addition, reduction in atrial ectopy by atrial overdrive pacing could theoretically reduce the trigger mechanism for atrial flutter. More commonly, atrial flutter persists despite atrial pacing to prevent these episodes. Antiarrhythmic drug therapy is usually required for prolongation of atrial refractoriness and suppression of atrial ectopic activity. Pacing may be required for rate support owing to the sinus bradycardia induced by the drug therapy, particularly if there is preexisting sinus node disease. These preventive approaches are also used in patients with paroxysmal atrial fibrillation or chronic atrial fibrillation after electrical conversion attempts, and success rates are relatively low. Electrical stimulation is occasionally effective for overdriving or preventing ectopic atrial tachycardia or intraatrial reentrant tachycardia.[3] Drug or ablative therapy remains the mainstay of treatment in these disorders.

A variety of electrophysiologic mechanisms are operative in supraventricular arrhythmias and influence the interaction with implantable antiarrhythmic devices for tachyarrhythmia management. Definition of the mechanism and interaction during an electrophysiologic study is of more than research or academic interest.

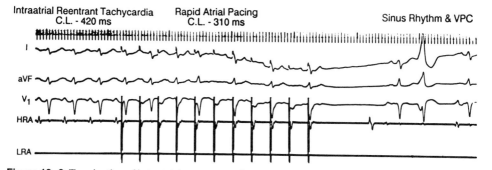

Figure 19–6. Termination of intraatrial reentrant tachycardia by rapid atrial pacing bursts. Atrial tachycardia is interrupted by a pacing train of 11 beats at 73 per cent of tachycardia cycle length. This was reproducibly demonstrated in this patient.

It is of value in the selection of patients, the optimal programming of devices, and the selection of concomitant antiarrhythmic therapy. This consideration of the electrophysiologic mechanism enhances the therapeutic efficacy and safety of this approach and improves symptomatic relief and the patient's quality of life.

REFERENCES

1. Akhtar M, Gilbert CJ, Al-Nouri M, Schmidt DH: Electrophysiologic mechanisms for modification and abolition of atrioventricular junctional tachycardia with simultaneous and sequential atrial and ventricular pacing. Circulation 60:1443, 1979.
2. Akhtar M, Damato AN, Batsford WP, et al: Induction of A-V nodal reentrant tachycardia after atropine: A report of five cases. Am J Cardiol 36:286, 1975.
3. Arbel ER, Cohen CH, Langendorf R, Glick G: Successful treatment of drug-resistant atrial tachycardia and intractable congestive heart failure with permanent coupled atrial pacing. Am J Cardiol 41:336, 1978.
4. Berkovits B, Castellanos A, Dreifus LS, et al: Double-demand sequential pacing for treatment of paroxysmal reentry tachycardias. Pacing Clin Electrophysiol 3:364, 1980.
5. Bertholet M, Demonlin JC, Waleffe A, Kulbertus H: Programmable extrastimulus pacing for long term management of supraventricular and ventricular tachycardias: Clinical experience in 16 patients. Am Heart J 110:582, 1985.
6. Bigger JT Jr, Goldreyer BN: The mechanism of supraventricular tachycardia. Circulation 42:673, 1970.
7. Coumel P, Cabot C, Fabiato A, et al: Tachycardie permanente par rhythme réciproque. I. Preuves du diagnostic par stimulation auriculaire et ventriculaire. II. Traitement par l'implantation intracorporelle d'un stimulateur cardiaque avec entraînement simultane de l'oneillette et du ventricule. Arch Mal Coeur 60:1830, 1967.
8. Curry PVL, Rowland E, Krikler DM: Dual demand pacing for refractory atrioventricular reentry tachycardia. PACE 2:137, 1979.
9. Curry PVL, Rowland E, Fox KM, et al: The relationship between posture, blood pressure and electrophysiological properties in patients with paroxysmal supraventricular tachycardia. Arch Mal Coeur 71:293, 1977.
10. Denes P, Wu D, Dhingra RC, et al: Demonstration of dual A-V nodal pathways with paroxysmal supraventricular tachycardias. Circulation 48:549, 1973.
11. Dunbar DN, Tobler HG, Fetter J, et al: Low energy transvenous cardioversion of atrial tachyarrhythmias in the dog [abstract]. J Am Coll Cardiol 5:457, 1985.
12. Durrer D, Schoo L, Scheilenberg RM, Wellens HJJ: The role of premature beats in the initiation and termination of supraventricular tachycardia in the Wolff-Parkinson-White syndrome. Circulation 36:644, 1967.
13. Fisher JD, Teichman SL, Ferrick A, et al: Antiarrhythmic effects of VVI pacing at physiologic rates:

A crossover controlled evaluation. Pacing Clin Electrophysiol 10:822, 1987.
14. Frame LH, Page RL, Hoffman BF: Atrial reentry around an anatomic barrier with a partially refractory excitable gap: A canine model of atrial flutter. Circ Res 58:495, 1986.
15. Goyal SL, Lichstein EL, Gupta PK, Chadda KD: Refractory reentrant atrial tachycardia: Successful treatment with a permanent radiofrequency triggered atrial pacemaker. Am J Med 58:586, 1975.
16. Henthorn RW, Plumb VJ, Arciniegas JG, et al: Entrainment of "ectopic atrial tachycardia": Evidence for reentry [abstract]. Am J Cardiol 59:920, 1982.
17. Jackman WM, Friday KJ, Scherlag BJ, et al: Direct endocardial recording from an accessory atrioventricular pathway: Realization of the site of block, effect of antiarrhythmic drugs and attempt at nonsurgical ablation. Circulation 68:906, 1983.
18. Josephson ME, Seides SF: Supraventricular tachycardias. In Clinical Cardiac Electrophysiology. Philadelphia, Lea & Febiger, 1979, pp 147–190.
19. Krikler DM, Curry PVL, Buffet J: Dual demand pacing for reciprocating atrioventricular tachycardia. Br Med J 1:1114, 1979.
20. Kuck KH, Kunze KP, Schluter M, Bleifeld W: Tachycardia prevention by programmed stimulation. Am J Cardiol 54:550, 1984.
21. Lau CP, Cornu E, Camm AJ: Fatal and nonfatal cardiac arrest in patients with an implanted antitachycardia device for the treatment of supraventricular tachycardia. Am J Cardiol 61:919, 1988.
22. Levy S: Role of pacing in treatment of supraventricular tachycardia. In Josephson ME, Wellens HJJ (eds): Tachycardias: Mechanisms, Diagnosis, Treatment. Philadelphia, Lea & Febiger, 1984, pp 223–240.
23. Levy S, Berkovits B, Mandel W, et al: Refractory supraventricular tachycardias: Successful therapy with double-demand sequential pacing. Am J Cardiol 45:457, 1980.
24. Mahmud R, Denker S, Lehmann MH, et al: Effect of atrioventricular sequential pacing in patients with no ventriculoatrial conduction. J Am Coll Cardiol 4:273, 1984.
25. Mann DE, Lawrie GM, Luck JC, et al: Importance of pacing site in entrainment of ventricular tachycardia. J Am Coll Cardiol 5:781, 1985.
26. McKinnie J, Avitall B, Caceres J, et al: Retrograde pathway in atrioventricular nodal tachycardias: Nodal tissue or extranodal accessory pathway [abstract]? J Am Coll Cardiol 13:175A, 1989.
27. Medina-Rowell V, Castellanos A, Portello-Acosta C, et al: Management of tachyarrhythmia with dual chamber pacemakers. Pacing Clin Electrophysiol 6:333, 1983.
28. Moe GK, Preston JB, Burlington H: Physiologic evidence for a dual A-V transmission system. Circ Res 4:357, 1956.
29. Morady F, Frank R, Kou WH, et al: Identification and catheter ablation of a zone of slow conduction in the reentrant circuit of ventricular tachycardia in humans. J Am Coll Cardiol 11:775, 1988.
30. Moss AJ, Rivers RJ: Termination and inhibition of recurrent tachycardias by implanted pervenous pacemakers. Circulation 50:942, 1974.
31. Nathan AW, Camm AJ, Bexton RS, et al: Initial experience with a fully implantable scanning extrastimulus pacemaker for tachycardia termination. Clin Cardiol 5:22, 1982.

32. Okamura K, Plumb VJ, Waldo AL: Entrainment of experimental atrial flutter and its use to localize the slow conduction area in the reentrant loop. Circulation 72:III–382, 1985.

33. O'Keefe DB, Curry PVL, Sowton E: Treatment of paroxysmal nodal tachycardia by dual demand pacemaker in the coronary sinus. Br Heart J 45:105–108, 1981.

34. Preston TA: Atrial pacing to convert atrial flutter. Am J Cardiol 32:737, 1973.

35. Prystowsky EN, Zipes DP: Inhibition in the human heart. Circulation 68:707, 1983.

36. Saksena S, Heselmeyer T, Batsford W, et al: Long-term clinical experience with a versatile antitachycardia pacemaker for tachycardia termination, induction and monitoring: A multicenter study [abstract]. Pacing Clin Electrophysiol 11:493, 1988.

37. Saksena S, Pantopoulos D, Parsonnet V, et al: Usefulness of an implantable antitachycardia pacemaker system for supraventricular or ventricular tachycardia. Am J Cardiol 58:70, 1986.

38. Sowton E, Elmquist H, Segerstad C: Two years' clinical experience with a self-searching tachycardia terminating pacemaker. Am J Cardiol 47:476, 1981.

39. Stevenson WG, Wiener I, Weiss J, et al: Limitations of bipolar and unipolar conditioning stimuli for inhibition in the human heart. Am Heart J 114:303, 1987.

40. Waldo AL, Henthorn RW: Use of transient entrainment during ventricular tachycardia to localize a critical area in the reentry circuit for ablation. Pacing Clin Electrophysiol 12:231, 1989.

41. Waldo AL, Henthorn RW, Plumb VJ: Atrial flutter—recent observations in man. *In* Josephson ME, Wellens HJJ (eds): Tachycardias: Mechanisms, Diagnosis, Treatment. Philadelphia, Lea & Febiger, 1984, pp 113–136.

42. Waldo AL, Maclean WAH, Karp RB, et al: Entrainment and interruption of atrial flutter with atrial pacing: Studies in man following open heart surgery. Circulation 56:737, 1977.

43. Waxman HL, Cain ME, Greenspan AM, Josephson ME: Termination of ventricular tachycardia with ventricular stimulation: Salutary effect of increased current strength. Circulation 65:800, 1982.

44. Waxman MB, Sharma AD, Cameron DA, et al: Reflex mechanisms responsible for early spontaneous termination of paroxysmal supraventricular tachycardia. Am J Cardiol 19:259, 1980.

45. Wellens HJJ, Durrer D: The role of an accessory atrioventricular pathway in reciprocating tachycardia: Observations in patients with and without the Wolff-Parkinson-White syndrome. Circulation 52:58, 1975.

46. Winters SL, Gomes JA: Intracardiac electrode catheter recordings of atrioventricular bypass tracts in Wolff-Parkinson-White syndrome: Techniques, electrophysiologic characteristics and demonstration of concealed and decremental propagation. J Am Coll Cardiol 7:1392, 1986.

47. Wu D, Denes P, Wyndham CRC, et al: Demonstration of dual atrioventricular nodal pathways utilizing a ventricular extrastimulus in patients with atrioventricular nodal reentrant paroxysmal supraventricular tachycardia. Circulation 52:789, 1975.

20

ELECTROPHYSIOLOGIC MECHANISMS IN ELECTRICAL THERAPY OF VENTRICULAR TACHYCARDIA

NABIL EL-SHERIF

Electrical therapy of ventricular tachycardia could be accomplished by high-energy transthoracic electrical shocks, by low-energy transvenous shocks delivered through catheter electrodes,[11, 27] or by one or more paced beats, also delivered through catheter electrodes and utilizing energy as low as twice the threshold for stimulation.[8] A pacing stimulus captures locally and generates an activation wave front that propagates to the rest of the ventricles, including the "site" of ventricular tachycardia. Experimental[3] and clinical observations[21] have recently shown that very low energy transvenous shocks may resemble a pacing stimulus by inducing a relatively localized depolarization while the rest of the ventricles will be activated by a propagating depolarization wave front. A high transvenous energy shock, however, usually results in immediate depolarization of all or major portions of both ventricles and thus resembles a high-energy transthoracic electrical shock.

To understand the electrophysiologic mechanisms for electrical therapy of ventricular tachycardia, one must analyze the mechanism by which a paced wave front interacts with the tachycardia "site." These data may also explain the mechanism of action of low-energy transvenous shocks. Detailed analysis of ventricular activation patterns requires extensive mapping techniques, which are more suitably applied to experimental models of ventricular tachycardia. This chapter will describe the effects of programmed electrical stimulation on reentrant ventricular tachycardia in the canine postinfarction model. It is generally believed that a majority of recurrent, sustained, monomorphic ventricular tachycardias in the clinical setting are due to reentrant excitation rather than abnormal pacemaker activity. The role of cycle length of stimulation, number of stimulated beats, and site of stimulation, as well as the mechanisms of termination, resetting, entrainment, and acceleration of reentrant ventricular tachycardia, will be critically analyzed.[4]

EXPERIMENTAL MODELS OF REENTRANT VENTRICULAR TACHYCARDIA

The electrophysiologic characteristics of the reentrant circuit in clinical ventricular tachycardia are not yet well defined. Experimentally, three types of circus movement reentry have been described:

1. *The ring model of reentry:* In this model,

This work was supported by Grant HL-36680 from the National Institutes of Health and by the Veterans Administration Medical Research Funds.

originally described in rings of cardiac and other tissue cut from a variety of animals, a fixed anatomic obstacle is required around which the activation wave front circulates.[15] The only two proven examples of a ring model reentry in the intact mammalian heart are circus movements involving the atrioventricular (AV) node and AV nodal accessory pathways and those involving both bundle branches. Clinical ventricular tachycardia due to bundle branch reentry, however, is rare.

2. *The figure-of-eight model of reentry:* In this model, a functional rather than a fixed anatomic obstacle is necessary for the occurrence of circus movement. This model was originally described in the surviving electrophysiologically abnormal ischemic epicardial layer overlying myocardial infarction in the dog's heart.[6, 14] Ischemia results in nonhomogeneous lengthening of refractoriness, with graded increase in refractoriness going from the border zone toward the center of the ischemic zone.[10] A critically timed premature beat that succeeds in inducing reentry results in a functional arc of unidirectional conduction block around which the reentrant wave front circulates. The arc of conduction block occurs between adjacent sites of short and long refractoriness, with the sites of longer refractoriness distal to the arc of block. Reentrant activation continues as a figure-of-eight activation pattern, whereby two circulating wave fronts advance in clockwise and counterclockwise directions, respectively, around two zones (arcs) of functional conduction block. The two wave fronts coalesce into a common reentrant wave front that conducts slowly between the two arcs of functional conduction block. This wave front represents the slow zone of the figure-of-eight reentrant circuit (Fig. 20–1). During a monomorphic reentrant tachycardia, the two arcs of block and the two circulating wave fronts remain fairly stable. During a polymorphic reentrant rhythm, however, both arcs of block and the circulating wave fronts change their geometric configuration while maintaining their synchrony.

3. *The leading-circle model of reentry:* In this model, originally described in small pieces of atrial myocardium of the rabbit,[1] the center of the circuit, or the vortex, is made of excitable tissue that is rendered functionally inexcitable by invasion of the center by multiple centripetal wavelets from the leading circuit outside the vortex. The leading-circle model of reentry may represent a special modification of the figure-of-eight model.[5]

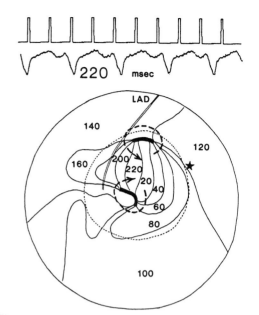

Figure 20–1. A lead II electrocardiographic (ECG) recording and a polar projection of epicardial activation during reentrant ventricular tachycardia in the canine postinfarction heart. In this and subsequent maps, the heart is viewed from the cardiac apex located at the center of the circular map, and the perimeter of the circuit represents the atrioventricular (AV) junction. The dotted line represents the epicardial outline of the ischemic zone. The isochronal lines are drawn at 20-msec intervals. The time lines represent 100-msec intervals. The reentrant circuit has a characteristic figure-of-eight configuration in the form of clockwise and counterclockwise circulating wave fronts around two arcs of functional conduction block (*heavy solid lines*). The two wave fronts coalesce into a common reentrant wave front that conducts slowly between the two arcs of block. This wave front represents the slow part of the reentrant circuit. (From El-Sherif N, Gough WB, Restivo M: Reentrant ventricular arrhythmias in the late myocardial infarction period. 14. Mechanisms of resetting, entrainment, acceleration or termination of reentrant tachycardia by programmed electrical stimulation. PACE 10:341, 1987; with permission.)

In this chapter, the effects of programmed electrical stimulation on the figure-of-eight reentrant circuit in the canine postinfarction heart will be discussed. We have recently argued that the figure-of-eight model of reentry may be more representative of reentry in the human ventricle.[5]

MECHANISMS OF TERMINATION OF REENTRANT TACHYCARDIA BY PROGRAMMED ELECTRICAL STIMULATION (Fig. 20–2)

In the figure-of-eight reentrant circuit, the two arcs of conduction block and the slow common reentrant wave front are functionally

Figure 20–2. Tachycardia termination by programmed electrical stimulation. The figure shows epicardial activation maps from the same experiment shown in Figure 20–1 during termination of reentrant ventricular tachycardia by two stimulated beats at a cycle length of 155 msec. The reentrant tachycardia has a cycle length of 220 msec. Control maps are labeled 1 and 2, and the maps of the first and second stimulated beats, 3 and 4, respectively. In this experiment, the reexcitation site was in the lower anterolateral portion of the left ventricle, with activation proceeding in an apical to basal direction, which explains the negative QRS configuration in surface lead II. Electrical stimulation was applied to the normal zone close to the border of the ischemic zone and distal (downstream) to the slow common reentrant wave front. The first stimulated beat preexcited normal myocardium and resulted in extension of the basal arc of functional conduction block. However, the slower common reentrant wave front could still conduct and reexcite normal myocardium. Thus, a single stimulated beat at a cycle length of 155 msec failed to terminate reentry. On the other hand, the second stimulated beat resulted in a shift of the arc of functional conduction block to the border between the normal and ischemic zones close to the stimulated site. The two activation wave fronts around this arc of block invaded the distal part of the original site of the

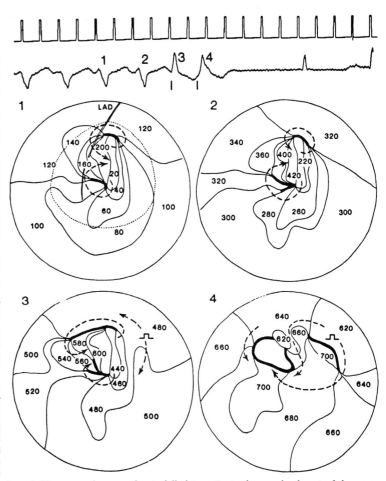

common reentrant wave front and coalesced. However, the wave fronts failed to activate the proximal part of the zone of slow conduction, creating an island of functional conduction block. The last activation isochrone at 700 msec blocked at the proximal side of the original site of the common reentrant wave front. (From El-Sherif N, Gough WB, Restivo M: Reentrant ventricular arrhythmias in the late myocardial infarction period. 14. Mechanisms of resetting, entrainment, acceleration or termination of reentrant tachycardia by programmed electrical stimulation. PACE 10:341, 1987; with permission.)

determined and cycle length is dependent. A tight fit exists during the reentrant tachycardia, with the circulating wave front closely following the refractory tail of the previous revolution. This factor is particularly significant in the zone of the slow common reentrant wave front. The reentrant circuit conduction time is determined by the area with the longest refractoriness in the zone of the slow common reentrant wave front. Myocardial refractoriness tends to shorten gradually to a new steady level in response to successive short cardiac cycles.[13] A sustained reentrant tachycardia represents a succession of short cardiac cycles. It is safe to assume that the duration of refractoriness in the zone with the longest refractoriness probably cannot shorten any further.

This is not the case, however, with the rest of the reentrant pathway, including both the normal zone and the remainder of the ischemic zone. A stimulated wave front at a cycle length shorter than the tachycardia cycle length can still conduct in these zones. In other words, these zones have a window of excitability, particularly so in the normal zone. Normal myocardium shows more shortening of refractoriness in response to successive short cardiac cycles than does ischemic myocardium.[10] In fact, certain zones of ischemic myocardium may fail to show shortening of refractoriness in response to shorter cycle lengths.

For stimulated termination of the reentrant tachycardia, the stimulated wave front must arrive at the area with the longest refractori-

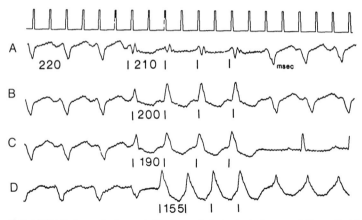

Figure 20–3. Effects of the cycle length of stimulation. Selected ECG recordings from the same experiment shown in Figures 20–1 and 20–2 that illustrate the effects of varying the cycle length of stimulation while the number of beats in the stimulated train was kept constant at 4. Record *A* shows pacing at a cycle length 10 msec shorter than the tachycardia cycle, resulting in fusion complexes. The tachycardia resumed at the control cycle length on cessation of pacing. A similar effect occurred when the cycle length of pacing was 20 msec shorter than the tachycardia cycle (record *B*). When the same train of stimulation was applied at a cycle length 30 msec shorter than the tachycardia cycle, it resulted in termination of the tachycardia (record *C*). A much faster train in record *D* resulted in tachycardia acceleration. The numbers in the figure are in milliseconds, and the time lines represent 100 msec. (From El-Sherif N, Gough WB, Restivo M: Reentrant ventricular arrhythmias in the late myocardial infarction period. 14. Mechanisms of resetting, entrainment, acceleration or termination of reentrant tachycardia by programmed electrical stimulation. PACE 10:341, 1987; with permission.)

ness in the zone of the slow common reentrant wave front before refractoriness expires, thus resulting in conduction block. If this area is strategically located between the two arcs of functional conduction block, reentrant excitation will be terminated. Otherwise, conduction block in this area may result only in a narrowing of the zone of the slow common reentrant wave front or a change of its configuration or both. The strategic zone for conduction block was found to be consistently located at the proximal part of the slow zone and never at its distal side.[4]

The three variables that determine, singly or in combination, if the stimulated wave front can reach the strategic zone for conduction block and terminate reentry are (1) the degree of premature stimulation, that is, the coupling interval of the first stimulated beat as well as the cycle length of a stimulated train (Fig. 20–3); (2) the number of stimulated beats (Fig. 20–4); and (3) the site of stimulation. When a single premature stimulated wave front fails to reach the strategic zone with the longest refractoriness early enough, a subsequent stimulated wave front may succeed. Successive premature stimulated wave fronts can conduct, probably at a control speed or only slightly

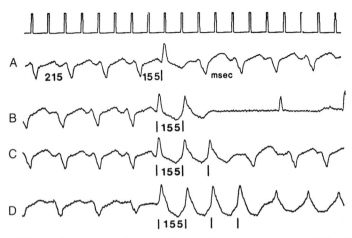

Figure 20–4. Effects of the number of stimulated beats. Selected ECG recordings from the same experiment shown in Figures 20–1 to 20–3 that illustrate the effects of the number of stimulated beats. Record *A* shows that during the reentrant tachycardia a single stimulated beat at a coupling interval of 155 msec resulted in resetting of the tachycardia by 20 msec. Record *B* shows that the tachycardia could be terminated by a train of two stimulated beats at a cycle length of 155 msec. Record *C* illustrates that a train of three stimulated beats at the same cycle length again resulted in resetting of the tachycardia. On the other hand, in record *D*, a train of four stimulated beats induced a new tachycardia (positive QRS in lead II) at a shorter cycle length (170 to 180 msec) compared with the original tachycardia cycle length (205 to 230 msec). (From El-Sherif N, Gough WB, Restivo M: Reentrant ventricular arrhythmias in the late myocardial infarction period. 14. Mechanisms of resetting, entrainment, acceleration or termination of reentrant tachycardia by programmed electrical stimulation. PACE 10:341, 1987; with permission.)

slower, in the normal zone and part of the ischemic zone but still arrive early enough at the strategic zone with the longest refractoriness to result in conduction block.

MECHANISMS OF TACHYCARDIA RESETTING

Reentrant excitation can be advanced or reset by one or two premature stimuli (Fig. 20–5) or by a train of stimulated beats. A single premature stimulated beat can arrive earlier at the proximal side of the zone of the slow common reentrant wave front, results in further slowing of conduction in this zone, but still succeeds in transversing the zone to perpetuate the reentrant process. If the degree of prematurity outweighs the further slowing of conduction in the slow zone, the next reentrant cycle will be reset. On the other hand, there are two different mechanisms for resetting of reentrant tachycardia by a train of stimulated beats at a cycle length shorter than the tachycardia cycle length, that is, overdrive stimulation: (1) tachycardia termination followed by reinitiation and (2) entrainment.

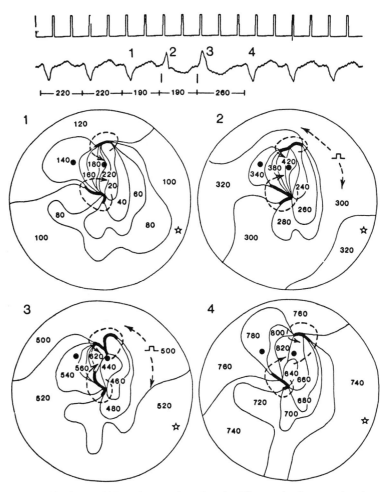

Figure 20–5. Resetting of reentrant tachycardia. Epicardial maps from the same experiment shown in Figures 20–1 to 20–4 that illustrate resetting of the tachycardia by two stimulated beats at a cycle length 30 msec shorter than the tachycardia cycle. The control map is labeled 1, and the maps of the two stimulated beats are labeled 2 and 3, respectively. The first stimulated beat preexcited normal myocardium, and the stimulated wave front arrived approximately 20 msec earlier to the proximal side of the zone of slow conduction. This resulted in relatively slower conduction in this zone. However, the stimulated wave front could still traverse this zone to reexcite normal myocardium at the distal side of the zone of slow conduction. The second stimulated wave front also arrived earlier to the proximal side of the zone of slow conduction. This earlier arrival resulted in extension of the arcs of functional conduction block into this zone, with narrowing of the slow common reentrant pathway. The stimulated wave front also showed further slowing at the proximal side of the slow zone before it could successfully traverse the zone to reexcite normal myocardium and perpetuate the reentrant excitation, as shown in map 4. The asterisk in the four maps represents the same epicardial site in the posterobasal portion of the left ventricle. If the reentrant tachycardia had continued unperturbed by the two stimulated beats at the original cycle length of 220 msec, this site would have been activated at the 760-msec isochrone rather than at the 740-msec isochrone as shown in map 4. Thus, the two premature stimulated beats resulted in advancing or resetting of the tachycardia cycle by 20 msec. The two stimulated wave fronts were each introduced at a cycle length 30 msec shorter than the intrinsic tachycardia cycle. However, the tachycardia was reset only by 20 msec. This occurred because the stimulated wave fronts that arrived earlier to the proximal side of the slow zone showed relatively slow conduction in this zone compared with control. However, the degree of prematurity of the two stimulated beats still outweighed the further slowing of conduction and resulted in advancing the tachycardia cycle by 20 msec. (From El-Sherif N, Gough WB, Restivo M: Reentrant ventricular arrhythmias in the late myocardial infarction period. 14. Mechanisms of resetting, entrainment, acceleration or termination of reentrant tachycardia by programmed electrical stimulation. PACE 10:341, 1987; with permission.)

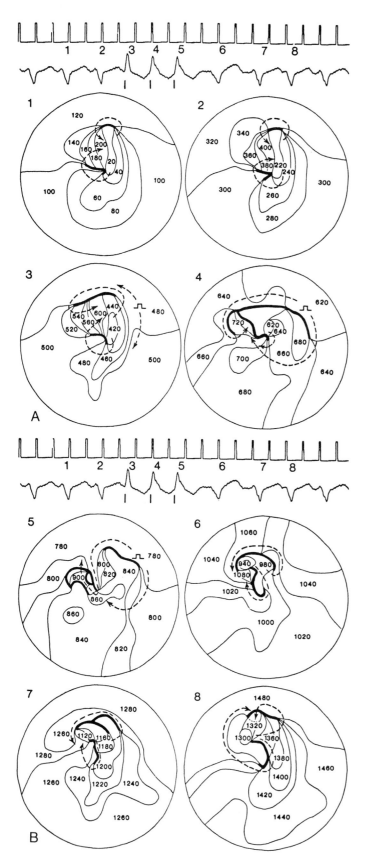

Figure 20–6. *A* and *B,* Tachycardia termination followed by reinitiation. Recordings were obtained from the same experiment shown in Figures 20–1 to 20–5. The figure shows that a train of three stimulated beats at a cycle length of 155 msec failed to terminate the tachycardia but resulted in resetting of the tachycardia cycle. The epicardial activation maps illustrate that the tachycardia was actually terminated by the second stimulated beat, as in Figure 20–2, but was reinitiated by the third stimulated beat. Control maps are labeled 1 and 2. As shown in Figure 20–2, the first stimulated beat (map 3) preexcited normal myocardium, which resulted in extension of the basal arc of conduction block and in slower conduction of the common reentrant wave front. The second stimulated beat (map 4) resulted in marked extension of the basal arc of block in lateral and septal directions. The two circulating wave fronts coalesced with the lingering wave front of the first stimulated beat. On the other hand, the last isochrone of the second stimulated beat at 740 msec arrived much earlier to the proximal side of the zone of slow conduction, resulting in conduction block and termination of reentry. The site of conduction block in the proximal part of the slow zone of reentry was slightly different from that shown in Figure 20–2. Following termination of reentry at the 740-msec isochrone, the third stimulated beat (map 5) activated normal myocardium at the 780-msec isochrone. The new activation wave front reinitiated reentrant excitation in the ischemic zone. With the exception of the first beat, the QRS configuration of the tachycardia following the stimulated train was similar to that of control, reflecting a similar pattern of activation of the normal zone. However, the activation pattern in the ischemic zone and the configuration of the arcs of functional conduction block differed from control for the first few beats following stimulation (see maps 6 and 7). Only the activation pattern in map 8 started to resemble the control reentrant circuit. Following the stimulated train, reentrant excitation was advanced (reset) by 100 msec. (From El-Sherif N, Gough WB, Restivo M: Reentrant ventricular arrhythmias in the late myocardial infarction period. 14. Mechanisms of resetting, entrainment, acceleration, or termination of reentrant tachycardia by programmed electrical stimulation. PACE 10:341, 1987; with permission.)

TACHYCARDIA TERMINATION FOLLOWED BY REINITIATION
(Fig. 20–6)

When a train of two or more stimulated beats is required to terminate reentry, the stimulated train must end following the beat that interrupts reentry. Otherwise, a subsequent stimulated beat may reinitiate the same reentrant circuit (one form of resetting) or induce a different and possibly faster circuit (tachycardia acceleration). Similar observations have been previously reported during the initiation of reentrant excitation by burst pacing.[7]

OVERDRIVE ENTRAINMENT AND TERMINATION OF TACHYCARDIA
(Figs. 20–7 and 20–8)

Entrainment represents another mechanism for resetting of the tachycardia. During entrainment, the stimulated wave front collides with the reentrant wave front distal to the slow zone. The site of collision varies according to the site of stimulation in relation to the slow zone. The stimulated wave front will also arrive earlier to the proximal part of the slow zone. This earlier arrival is consistently associated with a change in the conduction pattern in this zone, with the development of new functional arcs of conduction block and slower conduction in parts of the slow zone (see Fig. 20–7). A new balance of refractoriness and conduction velocity could develop in the different zones along the reentrant pathway; this new balance would perpetuate the reentrant process at the shorter cycle length of the stimulated train. Following termination of the stimulated train, reentrant excitation continues, and the first post-overdrive reentrant cycle is usually shorter than the control reentrant cycle. As shown in Figure 20–7, this phenomenon is explained by improvement of conduction at the zone that was showing the slowest conduction during the stimulated train.

If a number of stimulated beats entrain the reentrant tachycardia, as described above, the same number of beats at a critically shorter cycle length would terminate the tachycardia. This termination would occur if a new balance of refractoriness and conduction velocity in the different parts of the reentrant pathway could not be established. In this case, the stimulated wave front could arrive early enough at the strategic zone with the longest refractoriness, resulting in conduction block and termination of reentry (see Fig. 20–8).

The term "entrainment" denotes any stable condition with definable periodicity resulting from the interaction of two rhythms. The term has usually been utilized to denote interaction between automatic pacemakers.[12, 26] However, some authors have used it to describe the increase in the rate of a reentrant tachycardia with rapid pacing, with resumption of the control rate on cessation of pacing.[22, 23] When overdrive stimulation succeeds in perpetuating the reentrant process, some modification of the activation pattern of the common reentrant pathway always takes place. In other words, there is a change in the reentrant pathway. The modifications in the common reentrant pathway will not be detected in the absence of detailed mapping, which is not available in clinical studies of entrainment. The use of the term "entrainment" in this situation raises at least two questions: First, could the term be applied if there is a subtle but definite change in part of the reentrant circuit? (the control reentrant circuit and the entrained circuit in Fig. 20–7 can be compared). Second, assuming a reentrant circuit with a tight fit and possibly no gap of excitability at the sections with the longest refractoriness in the slow zone, could this circuit be entrained at a shorter cycle length without causing conduction block at these sections, with redirecting, and thus changing, the reentrant pathway?

MECHANISMS OF TACHYCARDIA ACCELERATION AND PRECIPITATION OF VENTRICULAR FIBRILLATION BY ELECTRICAL STIMULATION (Fig. 20–9)

Tachycardia acceleration, with precipitation of ventricular fibrillation, is considered a major limiting factor of stimulated termination of reentrant tachycardia.[8, 9, 16, 18] Our recent studies have shown that tachycardia acceleration by overdrive stimulation is always due to interruption of the original reentrant circuit by the first one or few stimulated beats followed by initiation of a different circuit by subsequent stimulated beats.[4] If the new circuit has a shorter revolution time, tachycardia acceleration is said to have been induced. The new circuit may last for one or more cycles before it spontaneously terminates, or it may become sustained. The induction of a new reentrant

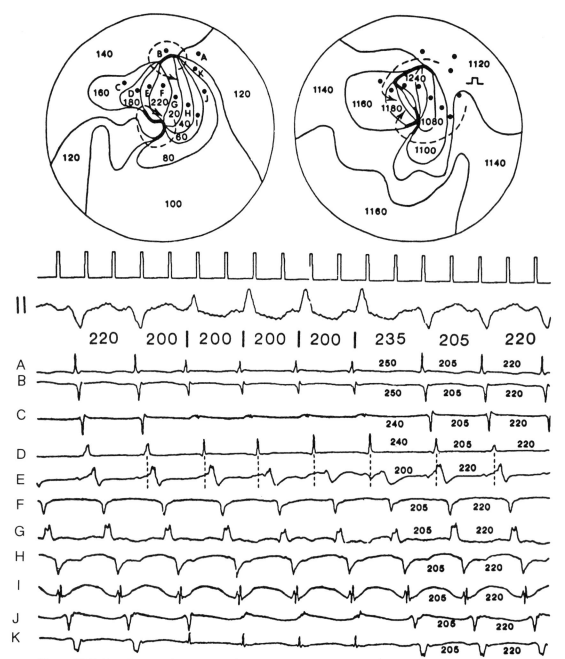

Figure 20–7. Entrainment of reentrant tachycardia by a run of four stimulated beats (marked by *vertical bars* in the lead II ECG). The cycle length of stimulation was 20 msec shorter than the tachycardia cycle. Recordings were obtained from the same experiment shown in Figures 20–1 to 20–6. The control reentrant circuit is shown on the top left panel and the map of the last stimulated beat on the top right panel. The electrograms labeled *A* to *K* represent each of the eleven 20-msec isochrones in the control reentrant circuit, and their sites on the maps are marked by solid circles. During the four-beat stimulated train, electrograms *J*, *K*, *A*, *B*, *C*, and *D*, which represented activation of the normal and border zones, had changed their configuration, denoting that these sites were activated by the stimulated wave fronts. On the other hand, electrograms *F* to *I*, which represented conduction in the middle and distal parts of the slow zone, did not change their configuration, denoting that the pathway of the activation wave fronts in these zones was similar to that of the control reentrant wave front. The collision of the stimulated and reentrant wave fronts probably occurred between sites *I* and *J*. Electrograms *D* and *E* were recorded from the proximal part of the slow zone and represented the sites where most of the conduction delay during the stimulated run took place (highlighted by the *vertical interrupted lines*). The degree of conduction delay between these two sites gradually increased during the first three stimulated beats but remained constant

Legend continued on opposite page

circuit that fails to be sustained for more than one or a few cycles is not uncommonly observed following overdrive stimulation.[4] In a recent study that correlated activation and refractory maps, we have shown that an induced reentrant circuit can terminate after one cycle and block if the circulating wave front encounters a gradient of refractoriness that provides a sufficient barrier to cause conduction block.[10] This gradient of refractoriness was usually caused by nonuniform shortening of refractory periods in the pathway of the circulating wave front.

Analysis of the ischemic zone activation pattern during the fast reentrant circuit induced by overdrive pacing in Figure 20–9 illustrates why fast reentrant excitation can rapidly degenerate into ventricular fibrillation. During a fast reentrant excitation pattern, several parts of the ischemic zone may fail to activate in a 1:1 fashion. This can result in the fractionation of a regular figure-of-eight reentrant pattern into multiple asynchronous wave fronts circulating around changing functional arcs of conduction block. A pattern akin to ventricular fibrillation may be confined briefly to the ischemic zone before the involvement of the normal zone.[15] However, as shown in Figure 20–9, a similar complex activation pattern may remain confined to the ischemic zone during a fast regular reentrant circuit without degenerating into ventricular fibrillation.

Figure 20–10 is a diagrammatic illustration of the various effects of overdrive stimulation on reentrant tachycardia. Overdrive stimulation can result in entrainment, termination, or acceleration of reentrant tachycardia, depending on the length of the drive and the cycle length of stimulation.

ROLE OF SITE OF STIMULATION
(Fig. 20–11)

Our recent studies have shown that reentry could be terminated by fewer stimulated beats when stimulation was applied to the normal zone closer to the proximal side of the slow zone (Fig. 20–11B) than to its distal side (Fig. 20–11A). When stimulation was applied closer to the distal side of the slow zone, the prematurely stimulated wave front frequently induced extension of the functional arcs of conduction block, resulting in lengthening of the reentrant pathway. In this case, one or more stimulated beats may fail to reach the strategic zone with the longest refractoriness early enough to result in conduction block. There is thus a better chance for entrainment of the reentrant tachycardia from sites closer to the distal side of the slow zone. On the other hand, the optimal site for stimulated termination of reentrant tachycardia was in the ischemic zone close to the proximal side of the slow zone (Fig. 20–11C). At this site, a critically coupled stimulus could capture locally and conduct prematurely to the proximal side of the slow zone, resulting in conduction block and termination of reentry. The site of stimulation in the ischemic zone does not have to be very close to the proximal side of the slow zone. However, it has to be able to conduct slightly prematurely to the strategic zone with the longest refractory period. The stimulus does not have to capture the normal zone, and therefore, the QRS configuration of the last reentrant beat will not change. The altered activation pattern in the ischemic zone has a negligible effect on the surface QRS configuration.

---

during the third and fourth stimulated wave fronts. On cessation of the stimulated train, conduction between sites D and E improved to a degree better than control for the first post-overdrive reentrant cycle before returning to control values during the second post-overdrive cycle. The changes in the conduction pattern in the proximal part of the slow zone both during and following overdrive stimulation resulted in characteristic changes in the cycle length of the first two post-overdrive reentrant cycles. At sites distal to the zone of marked conduction delay (electrograms E to I), the first post-overdrive cycle was shorter than the control cycle at 200 to 205 msec. On the other hand, at sites proximal to this zone (A to D and site K), as well as in the surface ECG, the cycle was longer than the control cycle at 235 to 350 msec. At these sites, however, the second post-overdrive reentrant cycle was shorter at 205 msec. Analysis of the surface ECG also reveals that the four-beat overdrive train advanced (reset) the reentrant tachycardia by approximately 65 msec (measured from the pre-overdrive to the first post-overdrive QRS complexes) or by 80 msec (measured from the pre-overdrive to the second post-overdrive QRS complexes). (From El-Sherif N, Gough WB, Restivo M: Reentrant ventricular arrhythmias in the late myocardial infarction period. 14. Mechanisms of resetting, entrainment, acceleration or termination of reentrant tachycardia by programmed electrical stimulation. PACE 10:341, 1987; with permission.)

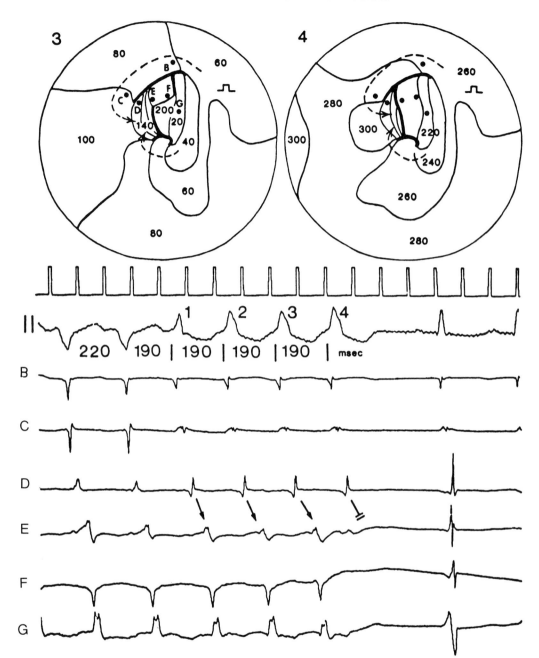

Figure 20–8. Overdrive termination of reentrant tachycardia. The figure illustrates the mechanism of overdrive termination of reentrant tachycardia by a train of four stimulated beats at a cycle length of 190 msec (30 msec shorter than the tachycardia cycle). Recordings were obtained from the same experiment shown in Figures 20–1 to 20–7. The maps of the third and fourth stimulated beats are shown on the top. Selected electrograms along the activation wave front are shown on the bottom and are labeled the same as in Figure 20–7. As was shown during the entraining train in Figure 20–7, the major conduction delay of the stimulated wave fronts occurred between sites D and E. However, in contrast to the entraining train in which conduction delay between the two sites remained constant after the second stimulated beat, here the conduction delay gradually increased during successive stimulated beats until conduction block between the two sites developed following the fourth stimulated beat. This development resulted in extension of the arc of functional conduction block across the proximal part of the slow zone and in termination of reentrant excitation. Note the electrotonic deflection in electrogram E during conduction block. (From El-Sherif N, Gough WB, Restivo M: Reentrant ventricular arrhythmias in the late myocardial infarction period. 14. Mechanisms of resetting, entrainment, acceleration or termination of reentrant tachycardia by programmed electrical stimulation. PACE 10:341, 1987; with permission.)

Figure 20–9. *A* and *B*, Tachycardia acceleration. Recordings obtained from the same experiment shown in Figures 20–1 to 20–8 that illustrate acceleration of reentrant tachycardia by a train of four stimulated beats at a short cycle length of 155 msec. Control map is shown in panel 1. As shown in Figures 20–2 and 20–5, the first two stimulated beats (maps 2 and 3) resulted in termination of the original reentrant tachycardia. The last isochrone of the second stimulated beat arrived relatively early at the proximal side of the common reentrant wave front, resulting in conduction block and termination of reentry. The activation pattern in the ischemic zone of the second stimulated beat and the exact site of conduction block were different in Figures 20–2, 20–5, and 20–8. However, in all instances, reentry terminated due to conduction block in the proximal portion of the zone of slow conduction and never at its distal side. Following termination of the original reentrant circuit, the third and fourth stimulated beats (maps 4 and 5) initiated a different reentrant circuit. The new circuit was located close to the lateral border of the ischemic zone at the 2 o'clock position on the polar map. The circuit had a shorter pathway and a faster circulation time (170 to 180 msec). The new reentrant wave front circulated in an opposite direction to the original reentrant wave front, resulting in positive QRS configuration in surface lead II. Because of the faster circulation time of the new reentrant circuit, several parts of the ischemic zone failed to activate in a 1:1 fashion. Instead, a Wenckebach-type conduction or a 2:1 block, or both, developed, resulting in a complex activation pattern for the rest of the ischemic zone that varied from beat to beat (see maps 6 to 8). Because of this complex activation pattern, the classic figure-of-eight reentrant pattern could not be established. In spite of the complex activation pattern in the ischemic zone, the reentrant pathway remained stable and ventricular fibrillation did not develop. However, in other experiments, a train of stimulated beats could induce a different faster reentrant excitation that could rapidly degenerate into ventricular fibrillation because of fractionation of activation in the ischemic zone into multiple asynchronous reentrant circuits. (From El-Sherif N, Gough WB, Restivo M: Reentrant ventricular arrhythmias in the late myocardial infarction period. 14. Mechanisms of resetting, entrainment, acceleration or termination of reentrant tachycardia by programmed electrical stimulation. PACE 10:341, 1987; with permission.)

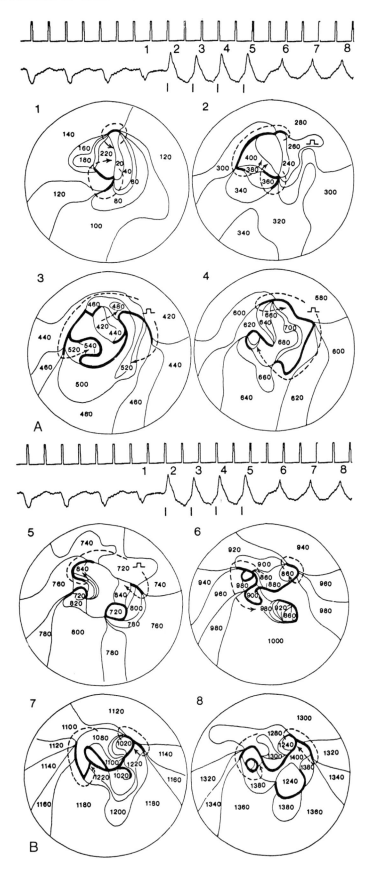

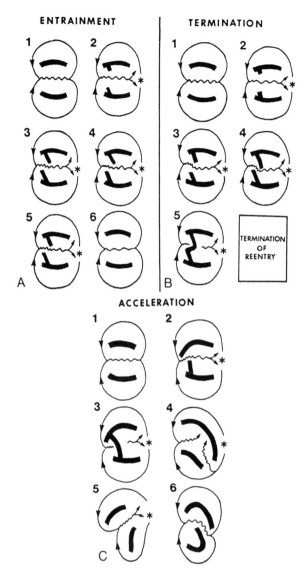

Figure 20–10. Diagrammatic illustration of the mechanisms of entrainment, termination, and acceleration of reentrant tachycardia by overdrive stimulation. In each of the three panels, the control reentrant circuit is labeled 1, and the four beats of the stimulated train are labeled 2 to 5. The control circuit has a figure-of-eight configuration, and conduction in the slow zone of reentry proceeds from left to right. The heavy solid lines represent arcs of functional conduction block. Stimulation is applied at the distal side of the slow zone, as shown by the asterisks. During entrainment, the stimulated wave front collides with the emerging slow reentrant wave front. It then circulates and arrives earlier to the proximal part of the slow zone of reentry. This earlier arrival is consistently associated with a change in the slow zone, with the development of new functional arcs of block and much slower conduction in parts of this zone. However, a new equilibrium quickly develops in which successive stimulated beats, represented by cycles 3, 4, and 5, maintain the same new conduction pattern at the shortest cycle length of stimulation, thus entraining the tachycardia. On cessation of stimulation, reentry will resume, as shown in cycle 6. For termination of reentry, on the other hand (panel B), successive stimulated beats, now applied at a relatively shorter cycle compared with the entraining train, will result in gradually more conduction delay. Eventually, conduction block develops at the proximal part of the slow zone of reentry, as shown in cycle 5. In panel C, the same four-beat stimulated train is applied at a still shorter cycle length. In this case, and because of the short cycle length of stimulation, the second stimulated beat represented by cycle 3 has already blocked in the proximal part of the slow zone of reentry. If stimulation is stopped at this point, the reentrant tachycardia would terminate. However, if stimulation is continued, the third and fourth stimulated beats, represented by cycles 4 and 5, will initiate new arcs of block and different reentrant pathways, so that on termination of the stimulated train, a new and possibly faster reentrant circuit will occur. (From El-Sherif N, Gough WB, Restivo M: Reentrant ventricular arrhythmias in the late myocardial infarction period. 14. Mechanisms of resetting, entrainment, acceleration or termination of reentrant tachycardia by programmed electrical stimulation. PACE 10:341, 1987; with permission.)

In the figure-of-eight reentrant circuit in the canine postinfarction heart, one or more sites could usually be identified in the ischemic zone where a premature stimulus could terminate the reentrant tachycardia by capturing locally and conducting prematurely to the proximal side of the common reentrant wave front.[4] On the other hand, only two clinical examples of ventricular tachycardia have been reported in which the arrhythmia could be terminated by a single stimulus that did not seem to capture the ventricles.[19, 25] This observation underscores the fact that the site for stimulated termination is less than optimal in the overwhelming majority of clinical cases.

COMPARISON BETWEEN PACED STIMULATION AND LOW-ENERGY TRANSVENOUS SHOCKS

Intracardiac shocks differ from paced stimuli quantitatively in the magnitude of electrical energy and qualitatively in that only single or very closely coupled successive shocks have been studied. The electrophysiologic effects of single intracavitary shocks delivered in electrical diastole during sinus rhythm have been examined.[3, 20, 21] Shocks with energies less than 0.05 J delivered through right ventricular catheter electrodes produce immediate local depolarization followed by propagated depolari-

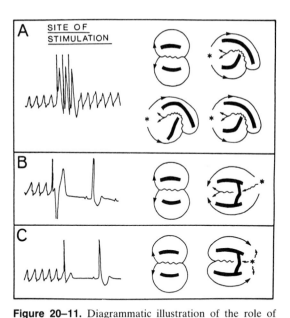

Figure 20–11. Diagrammatic illustration of the role of the site of stimulation in relation to the slow zone of reentry on termination of reentrant tachycardia by programmed stimulation. The control reentrant circuit shows conduction in the slow zone moving in the right-to-left direction. Panel *A* shows that three stimulated beats applied at a site distal to the slow zone of reentry, as represented by the asterisk, failed to terminate reentry. The stimulated wave front collided with the reentrant wave front as it emerged from the slow zone. It then circulated around much longer functional arcs of block compared with control. This resulted in lengthening of the stimulated wave front pathway. Thus, even though the stimulated wave front still arrived earlier to the proximal part of the slow zone, it failed to arrive early enough to result in conduction block and to terminate reentry. In other words, the stimulated run resulted in entrainment of the tachycardia. In panels *B* and *C*, on the other hand, reentry terminated when stimulation was applied at sites proximal to the slow zone of reentry. In *B*, stimulation was applied to the border of the ischemic zone at some distance from the proximal part of the slow zone. The stimulated wave front arrived early enough to this site, resulting in conduction block and termination of reentry. The stimulated wave front also activated most of the ventricles and collided with the emerging wave front of the last reentrant cycle at the distal side of the slow zone. In panel *C*, stimulation was applied in the ischemic zone, much closer to the proximal part of the slow zone. The stimulated wave front arrived prematurely to the slow zone, resulting in conduction block, but failed to conduct outside the ischemic zone. In this case, the ventricles were activated by the last reentrant cycle. The ECG shows what could be misinterpreted as the stimulus artifact's failure to capture and the spontaneous termination of the reentrant tachycardia, while in fact the stimulus artifact did capture locally, resulting in concealed conduction. (From El-Sherif N, Gough WB, Restivo M: Reentrant ventricular arrhythmias in the late myocardial infarction period. 14. Mechanisms of resetting, entrainment, acceleration or termination of reentrant tachycardia by programmed electrical stimulation. PACE 10:341, 1987; with permission.)

zation of distant ventricular myocardium akin to a paced stimulus.[21] The extent of immediate local depolarization is determined by the energy, with increasing energies producing wider effects. Energies higher than 0.5 J produce instantaneous depolarization of distant left ventricular myocardium.[21] Thus, immediate global depolarization of available responsive myocardium can be achieved at modest shock energy levels.

The variable efficacy of intracavitary shocks can be related to alterations in available responsive tissue. QRS-synchronized shocks in ventricular tachycardia are typically delivered when a varying proportion of both ventricles has already been activated. Thus, the shock exerts its major electrophysiologic effects on the tissue remaining to be activated, particularly that constituting the diastolic limb of the VT circuit. Alterations in the pattern of diastolic electrical activity have been observed experimentally and clinically with single or successive shocks using single or dual current pathways.[21] These alterations typically precede acceleration or termination of the ventricular tachycardia. Acceleration has been observed in conjunction with modification of diastolic electrical activity, which may change activation timing as well as location (Fig. 20–12).[21] Termination has been observed when modification of diastolic electrical activity results in immediate conduction block or instability of the ventricular tachycardia circuit, which culminates in conduction block. It is reasonable to expect that intracavitary shocks producing ventricular tachycardia acceleration at a particular energy level will produce ventricular tachycardia termination at a higher energy level.[20]

CONCLUSIONS AND CLINICAL IMPLICATIONS

Pacing termination of reentrant tachycardia occurs when a stimulated wave front arrives earlier to a strategically located area in the proximal portion of the zone of slow conduction before refractoriness expires distally, resulting in conduction block. The three factors that determine if the stimulated wave front can reach this zone in time for conduction block are (1) the cycle length of stimulation, (2) the number of stimulated beats, and (3) the site of stimulation. The optimal situation for stimulated termination of reentry is a critically coupled single stimulus applied close to the proximal side of the zone of slow conduc-

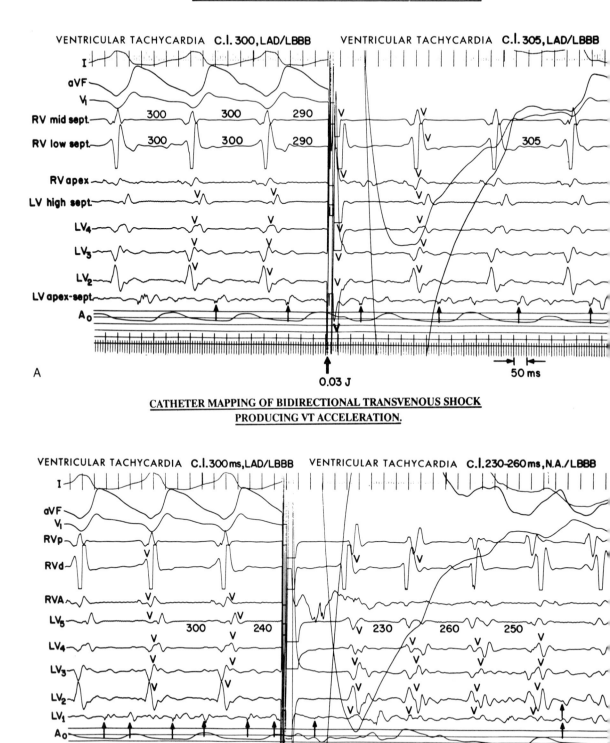

**CATHETER MAPPING OF BIDIRECTIONAL TRANSVENOUS SHOCK
FAILING TO TERMINATE VENTRICULAR TACHYCARDIA**

**CATHETER MAPPING OF BIDIRECTIONAL TRANSVENOUS SHOCK
PRODUCING VT ACCELERATION.**

Figure 20–12 *See legend on opposite page*

tion that captures locally and conducts prematurely to the strategic zone for conduction block. When a single stimulated wave front fails to terminate reentry, one or more subsequent wave fronts could succeed. However, the stimulated train has to be terminated following the beat that interrupts reentry. If not, a subsequent stimulated beat could reinitiate the same reentrant circuit or induce a different circuit. The new circuit could have a shorter revolution time, resulting in tachycardia acceleration, and could occasionally degenerate into ventricular fibrillation. Overdrive termination of reentry requires both a critical cycle length of stimulation and a critical number of beats in a stimulated train. Otherwise, the stimulated train could establish a new balance of refractoriness and conduction velocity in the reentrant pathway. This situation could perpetuate the reentrant process at the shorter cycle length of the stimulated train, and spontaneous reentry would resume on termination of the train (entrainment).

The relevance of studies of electrophysiologic mechanisms of programmed electrical stimulation in an experimental model of reentrant ventricular tachycardia depends on whether the figure-of-eight model is representative of reentry in the human ventricle. However, the experimental data provide at least two guidelines: (1) the role of the site of stimulation cannot be overemphasized; innovative techniques for more precise localization of the reentrant circuit, particularly the slow zone of reentry and the direction of the activation front in this zone, should be sought; and (2) protocols for pacing termination of reentrant tachycardias should utilize a stepwise increase in the number of paced beats, a step-

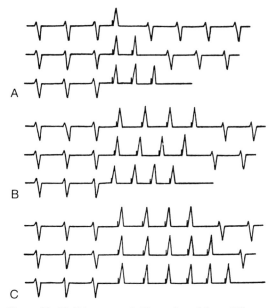

Figure 20–13. Diagrammatic illustration of three different stimulation protocols for termination of reentrant ventricular tachycardia. In diagram *A,* the extrastimulus technique is utilized, with the first stimulated beat falling just outside the refractory period at the site of stimulation. Additional stimuli are added, as required, in a stepwise fashion at a cycle length equal to the coupling interval of the first stimulated beat. In diagram *B,* a fixed train of stimuli is utilized. The cycle length of the first train is only slightly shorter than the tachycardia cycle. The cycle length of subsequent trains is shortened in a stepwise fashion until the tachycardia is terminated. Diagram *C* shows autodecremental pacing. In this protocol, the coupling interval of the first stimulated beat is only slightly shorter than the tachycardia cycle, and both a stepwise decrement of consecutive cycle lengths and a stepwise increase in the number of stimulated beats are utilized as required. (From El-Sherif N, Gough WB, Restivo M: Reentrant ventricular arrhythmias in the late myocardial infarction period. 14. Mechanisms of resetting, entrainment, acceleration or termination of reentrant tachycardia by programmed electrical stimulation. PACE 10:341, 1987; with permission.)

Figure 20–12. *A,* Catheter endocardial map of a 0.03-J bidirectional transvenous shock during ventricular tachycardia (VT). Surface ECG leads I, aV$_F$, and V$_1$, along with right ventricular apical and right and left ventricular septal electrograms, are shown. The left ventricular electrograms are obtained from the high septum (LV high sept.) and progressively inferiorly (LV$_4$, LV$_3$, and LV$_2$) 1 cm apart till the LV apex-septal recording (LV apex-sept.). Note the pattern of repetitive diastolic activity at the LV apex-septal site and the fragmented but single electrograms at the other sites. After shock delivery, there is no change in the activation time or sequence of any early systolic or diastolic electrical activity, and there is no alteration in the VT. *B,* Catheter endocardial map of a 0.14-J transvenous shock during VT. Note the persistence of the diastolic electrical activity in the LV apex-septal (LV$_1$) electrogram prior to the shock. After the shock is delivered, the pattern of diastolic electrical activity is markedly altered in LV$_1$ and LV$_2$. New areas of diastolic activity and splitting of the electrogram are observed in LV$_2$. The shock produces VT acceleration, with a change in the VT morphology. Abbreviations: RV = right ventricle; RVP = proximal right ventricle; RVd = distal right ventricle; RVA = right ventricular apex; LV = left ventricle; A$_0$ = aortic pressure recording; LAD = left-axis deviation; LBBB = left bundle branch block. (From Saksena S, Pantopoulos D, Hussain M, Gielchinsky I: Mechanisms of ventricular tachycardia termination and acceleration during transvenous cardioversion as determined by cardiac mapping in man. Am Heart J 113:1495, 1987; with permission.)

wise decrease in the cycle length of stimulation, or a combination (Fig. 20–13). The combination approach is best exemplified by the technique of autodecremental pacing.[2, 17, 24] In this technique, the coupling interval of the first stimulated beat is only slightly shorter than the tachycardia cycle, and both a stepwise decrement of consecutive cycle lengths and a stepwise increase in the number of stimulated beats are introduced as required.

REFERENCES

1. Allessie MA, Bonke FIM, Schopman FJG: Circus movement in rabbit atrial muscle as a mechanism of tachycardia. III. The "leading circle" concept: A new model of circus movement in cardiac tissue without the involvement of an anatomical obstacle. Circ Res 41:9, 1977.
2. Charos GS, Haffajee CI, Gold RL, et al: A theoretically and practically more effective method for interruption of ventricular tachycardia: Self-adapting autodecremental overdrive pacing. Circulation 73:307, 1986.
3. Colavita PG, Wolf P, Smith WM, et al: Determination of the effects of interval countershock by direct cardiac recordings during normal rhythm. Am J Physiol 250:H736, 1986.
4. El-Sherif N, Gough WB, Restivo M: Reentrant ventricular arrhythmias in the late myocardial infarction period. 14. Mechanisms of resetting, entrainment, acceleration or termination of reentrant tachycardia by programmed electrical stimulation. PACE 10:341, 1987.
5. El-Sherif N, Gough WB, Zeiler RH, Hariman R: Reentrant ventricular arrhythmias in the late myocardial infarction period. 12. Spontaneous versus induced reentry and intramural versus epicardial circuits. J Am Coll Cardiol 6:124, 1985.
6. El-Sherif N, Mehra R, Gough WB, Zeiler RH: Ventricular activation pattern of spontaneous and induced ventricular rhythms in canine one-day-old myocardial infarction: Evidence for focal and reentrant mechanisms. Circ Res 51:152, 1982.
7. El-Sherif N, Mehra R, Gough WB, Zeiler RH: Reentrant ventricular arrhythmias in the late myocardial infarction period. 11. Burst pacing versus multiple premature stimulation in the induction of reentry. J Am Coll Cardiol 4:295, 1984.
8. Fisher JD, Mehra R, Furman S: Termination of ventricular tachycardia with bursts of rapid ventricular pacing. Am J Cardiol 41:94, 1978.
9. Fisher JD, Kim SG, Matos JA, Ostrow E: Comparative effectiveness of pacing techniques for termination of well-tolerated sustained ventricular tachycardia. PACE 6:915, 1983.
10. Gough WB, Mehra R, Restivo M, El-Sherif N: Reentrant ventricular arrhythmias in the late myocardial infarction period in the dog. 13. Correlation of activation and refractory maps. Circ Res 57:432, 1985.
11. Jackman WM, Zipes DP: Low-energy synchronous cardioversion of ventricular tachycardia using a cath-

eter electrode in a canine model of subacute myocardial infarction. Circulation 66:187, 1982.
12. Jalife J, Moe GK: Effect of electrotonic potentials on pacemaker activity of canine Purkinje fibers in relation to parasystole. Circ Res 39:801, 1976.
13. Janse MJ, Van der Steen ABM, Van Dam RT, Durrer D: Refractory period of dog's ventricular myocardium following sudden changes in frequency. Circ Res 24:251, 1969.
14. Mehra R, Zeiler RH, Gough WB, El-Sherif N: Reentrant ventricular arrhythmias in the late myocardial infarction period. 9. Electrophysiologic-anatomic correlation of reentrant circuits. Circulation 67:11, 1983.
15. Mines GR: On circulating excitations in heart muscles and their possible relation to tachycardia and fibrillation. Trans R Soc Can (Ser 3, Sect IV) 8:43, 1914.
16. Naccarelli GV, Zipes DP, Rahilly TG: Influence of tachycardia cycle length and antiarrhythmic drugs on pacing terminations and accelerations of ventricular tachycardia. Am Heart J 105:1, 1983.
17. Nathan A, Hellestrand K, Ward DE, et al: Rate-related accelerating (autodecremental) atrial pacing. J Electrocardiol 15:77, 1982.
18. Roy D, Waxman HL, Buxton AE, et al: Termination of ventricular tachycardias: Role of tachycardia cycle length. Am J Cardiol 50:1346, 1982.
19. Ruffy R, Friday KJ, Southworth WP: Termination of ventricular tachycardia by single extrastimulation during the ventricular effective refractory period. Circulation 67:457, 1983.
20. Saksena S, Lindsay BD, Parsonnet V: Developments for future implantable cardioverters and defibrillators. PACE 10:1342, 1987.
21. Saksena S, Pantopoulos D, Hussain SM, Gielchinsky I: Mechanisms of ventricular tachycardia termination and acceleration during transvenous cardioversion as determined by cardiac mapping in man. Am Heart J 113:1495, 1987.
22. Waldo AL, Henthorn RW, Plumb VJ, MacLean WAH: Demonstration of the mechanism of transient entrainment and interruption of ventricular tachycardia with rapid atrial pacing. J Am Coll Cardiol 3:422, 1984.
23. Waldo AL, MacLean WAH, Karp RB, et al: Entrainment and interruption of atrial flutter with atrial pacing: Studies in man following open heart surgery. Circulation 56:737, 1977.
24. Ward DE, Camm AJ, Gainsborough J, Spurrell RAJ: Autodecremental pacing—a microprocessor base modality for termination of tachycardia. Pacing Clin Electrophysiol 3:178, 1980.
25. Wellens HJJ, Lie KI, Durrer D: Further observations on ventricular tachycardia as studied by electrical stimulation of the heart: Chronic recurrent ventricular tachycardia and ventricular tachycardia during acute myocardial infarction. Circulation 49:647, 1974.
26. Ypey DL, Van Meerwijk WPM, Ince C, Gross G: Mutual entrainment of two pacemaker cells: A study with an electronic parallel conductance model. J Theor Biol 86:731, 1980.
27. Zipes DP, Jackman WM, Heger JJ, et al: Clinical transvenous cardioversion of recurrent life threatening ventricular tachyarrhythmias: Low energy synchronized cardioversion of ventricular tachycardia and termination of ventricular fibrillation in patients using a catheter electrode. Am Heart J 103:789, 1982.

21

ELECTRICAL THERAPY IN THE ACUTE CONTROL OF TACHYCARDIAS

A. Antitachycardia Pacing in the Acute Care Setting

JOHN D. FISHER

There is a wealth of information on the use of implantable or potentially implantable antitachycardia pacemakers in patients with recurrent tachycardias. The literature abounds with case reports, institutional series involving several pacemaker models, multicenter studies of a single model, new pacing techniques, and technical details of newly introduced antitachycardia pacemakers. Much of this literature is reviewed in an accompanying chapter in this volume. Antitachycardia pacing in the acute setting, using temporary pacers, has received less attention. In contrast to Chapter 26 on long-term antitachycardia pacing, readers will find this one to be more anecdotal and advisory in nature.

This section of Chapter 21 starts with a general discussion of candidates for antitachycardia pacing in the acute setting, followed by a review of pacing techniques for prevention, hemodynamic improvement, and termination of tachycardia, along with an outline of relevant electrophysiologic concepts and a summary of the type of equipment needed for temporary antitachycardia pacing.

The Acute Setting

"Acute" antitachycardia pacing should be considered when patients present with tachycardias in the recovery room, the emergency room, intensive and coronary care units, and some office and general ward settings. Acute antitachycardia pacing is employed routinely during electrophysiologic studies.

CANDIDATES FOR ACUTE ANTITACHYCARDIA PACING

Patients with Postoperative Supraventricular Arrhythmias

Following open heart surgery, atrial arrhythmias are quite common, occurring in more than half of patients in the first several postoperative days.[44] Atrial tachycardia, fibrillation, or flutter occurs in some 20 per cent of patients.[44] Pharmacologic therapy, including digitalis, can be used to suppress atrial premature complexes, but in a milieu of rapidly changing hemodynamic metabolic status, risks of drug toxicity are considerable. In most institutions, it is now routine to leave temporary epicardial ventricular pacing wires in place after open heart surgery. Leaving an atrial wire in place provides the option of atrial pacing. If two epicardial atrial wires are used,[44] there are several advantages, including the following: (1) During pacing, the stimulus artifacts will cause less distortion on the electrocardiogram when bipolar rather than unipolar pacing is employed; and (2) diagnosis is often far easier with bipolar atrial recordings. When unipolar atrial recordings are made, interpretation is sometimes difficult if atrial activity is obscured by high-amplitude ventricular deflections. The large electrocardiographic artifacts associated with unipolar pacing may make tracings uninterpretable. Both the passive and the paced recordings are easier to read with a bipolar system. Although bipolar recordings can be made with fancy equipment, a simple bedside approach is to clip the right and left arm leads of an ordinary electrocardiograph to the two atrial wires and then to record electrocardiographic lead I. Techniques useful for terminating atrial flutter or atrial tachycardia, or for controlling the ventricular response to these rhythms, will be discussed at a later point in this chapter.

Several methods are commonly employed by cardiovascular surgeons in placing temporary epicardial leads. The experience of the University of Alabama in Birmingham suggests that the best results are achieved by placing a loop of wire on *but not through* the myocardium, held in place by a suture arranged so as to allow the temporary lead to be removed by gentle traction on the portion inside the skin.[44] Other specially designed leads may also provide reliable postoperative pacing, such as the Medtronic 6500 (Medtronic, Minneapolis, MN), which is held to the myocardium by a pull-through plastic coil.

Ventricular arrhythmias are less common than atrial tachycardias in patients in the postoperative period. The physician taking care of patients who have had surgery should nevertheless keep in mind the potential use of atrial and ventricular epicardial wires in the control of these rhythms.

Patients in the Emergency Room, Intensive Care Unit, and Coronary Care Unit

ATRIAL ARRHYTHMIAS. Most atrial tachycardias are treated pharmacologically, except for atrial flutter, which should be treated with direct-current cardioversion (DCCV). Occasionally, a patient will be encountered for whom atrial pacing is indicated. An example would be a patient with atrial flutter and a possibility of digitalis excess, in whom both drug therapy and electrical countershock can be associated with a higher than usual incidence of complications. Atrial pacing can be quite useful in such patients and can often be accomplished noninvasively by using esophageal[38] or transthoracic[28] pacing (see

"Equipment for Antitachycardia Pacing," below).

In the intensive care unit and coronary care unit, pacing for tachycardia termination or effective rate reduction (see further on) should be considered for patients with frequently recurrent supraventricular tachycardia (SVT). Pharmacologic control may be difficult in patients with other acute cardiac, pulmonary, or metabolic problems. Repeated "chemical" or electrical cardioversions may prove trying for patient and physician alike. Such crises can deflect the attention of physicians from the patient's more fundamental problems, and temporary antitachycardia pacing can defuse these situations.

VENTRICULAR TACHYCARDIA (VT). Transthoracic pacing can be used to terminate relatively slow, well-tolerated VT, without the need for general anesthesia.[28, 35] Some patients present with VT in the setting of complete heart block that becomes apparent only after termination of the VT, precipitating another crisis. Use of pacing techniques to terminate VT obviates this problem by providing antibradycardia support as well.

Pacing should be considered for recurrent VT in the intensive care unit and coronary care unit, particularly in the setting of an acute myocardial infarction. These patients do not tolerate sustained VTs well, and the sequence of multiple intravenous drugs and cardioversions can be traumatic. Rapid VTs that quickly degenerate to ventricular flutter or fibrillation can rarely be terminated by pacing techniques. However, patients with monomorphic VTs at moderate rates (generally below 200 beats per minute) should be considered by antitachycardia pacing. An approach that we have found useful at our institution is as follows. The first episode of VT is treated with drugs if needed, and electrical countershock. If a similar episode recurs, it is terminated in a similar fashion, but a temporary pacemaker is then inserted. Pacing is then used as the first modality for subsequent episodes of VT. In patients with acute myocardial infarction, the likelihood of terminating the VT is lower than in more stable patients undergoing electrophysiologic testing, and the incidence of acceleration is higher.[17] Nevertheless, termination by pacing is so much more quick and comfortable than the alternatives that most patients are very appreciative. Specific antitachycardia pacing techniques are described in a later portion of this chapter. Once a useful technique has been identified for a patient, subsequent episodes can be terminated semiroutinely. In our unit, this means an automatic antitachycardia pacemaker for some patients and prompt manual intervention by house staff or nurses for others.

Torsades de pointes is a swirling VT with a continually changing axis that seems to spiral around a central spindle. It may be sustained but is more often unsustained, though it occurs in a succession of flurries. *Torsades de pointes* occurs in a setting of inhomogeneity of ventricular refractoriness. The most frequently encountered clinical cause is the use of an antiarrhythmic drug (particularly type IA drugs, but others as well), especially with hypokalemia; patients with profound bradycardias may also have episodes of *torsades de pointes*. Least frequent are patients with the congenital prolonged QT interval syndromes. These rhythms do not respond well to most antiarrhythmic drugs and may in fact be worsened by type IA drugs. Isoproterenol or propranolol may be helpful in homogenizing refractory periods and terminating the arrhythmia; pacing, particularly in the ventricle, at rates of 90 to 120 beats per minute is usually immediately effective in preventing further episodes (Fig. 21–1).

Patients with Antitachycardia Pacemakers

As an increasing number of patients receive the implantable antitachycardia pacemakers, emergency room physicians can expect to encounter some of these.[16, 23]

Patients with *automatic* antitachycardia pacemakers usually appear in the emergency room for one or two reasons: (1) Some may have had several interventions by their pacemaker and have come to the emergency room to make sure that there are no acute ischemic, hemodynamic, or metabolic problems; and (2) others may come because of real or apparent pacemaker malfunction. In addition to the history, physical examination, and, sometimes, blood tests, an electrocardiogram with a long rhythm strip is key. In the absence of tachycardia, most automatic antitachycardia pacers either are inert or behave like antibradycardia pacemakers. Therefore, bursts of rapid stimuli during normal sinus rhythm or other anomalies should be sought. The physician should be aware that some automatic antitachycardia pacemakers will deliver a burst of rapid pacing or other therapy in response to a magnet. Patients will generally be familiar with the features of their pacemaker, and many will carry detailed information with them. The physician should not apply a magnet without asking the patient whether this will provoke an antitachycardia response from the pacemaker. In spite of this warning, the majority of antitachycardia pacers respond in a conventional way to the application of a magnet: Sensing is turned off, and pacing ensues at an ordinary rate; thus, a unit that is delivering inappropriate antitachycardia pacing can often be "tamed" by application of a magnet.

Some patients have *manually activated* antitachycardia pacemakers. Most physicians implanting such devices provide their patients with an instruction sheet to guide emergency room physicians in the use of the implanted device. Many patients know their arrhythmias

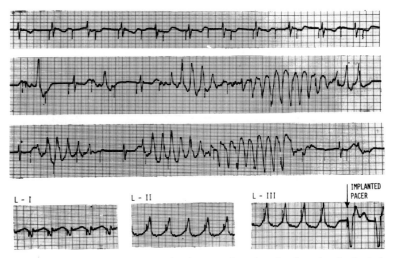

Figure 21–1. *Torsades de pointes* and prevention by VVI pacing. The rhythm strip in the top panel shows a QTc of 0.48 in this patient receiving quinidine in the presence of hypokalemia. She had had a VVI pacemaker implanted previously, which malfunctioned after multiple countershocks in the emergency room for sustained runs of *torsades de pointes*. The pacer stimuli visible on the top three rhythm strips are from an external pacer performing chest wall stimulation to inhibit the implanted pacer. In the second and third panels, there are typical runs of *torsades de pointes*. In the bottom panel, a temporary VVI pacer has been inserted. Pacing at a cycle length of 570 msec prevents further episodes of *torsades de pointes*, even though the QTc remains prolonged. At the bottom right, temporary pacing is stopped, and pacing from her implanted unit resumes.

and pacers well, and the physician should listen carefully; in many instances, the patient is the most informed person present. Some devices are activated by small "boxes" kept by the patient; others are operated by magnets; and others require sophisticated programmers. Emergency rooms are well advised to keep in a handy location the names and addresses of the major pacemaker companies as well as of the physicians on the hospital staff who are experts in antitachycardia pacemakers. There is always the possibility that a patient who received an implant in another city may require emergency room services while on a business trip or vacation.

PACING TECHNIQUES AND CONCEPTS

Pacing for Prevention of Tachycardia

RATE SUPPORT.[13, 42, 43, 45] In the prepacing era, many patients with heart block and other forms of bradycardia ultimately died of VT or ventricular fibrillation. This type of "bradycardia-dependent" tachycardia can be prevented in almost all instances by pacing at physiologic rates.

TORSADES DE POINTES.[31] This type of spiraling VT, discussed above, can usually be prevented by atrial or ventricular pacing at moderately elevated rates, for example, 90 to 120 beats per minute.

EXTRASYSTOLE/OVERDRIVE SUPPRESSION.[6–8, 10–12, 24, 25, 29, 30, 33, 34, 37, 52] Both atrial and ventricular premature complexes can often be suppressed by pacing at rates in the range of 10 to 15 beats per minute faster than the spontaneous rate. However, chronic pacing at rates in excess of 90 to 100 beats per minute is usually not well tolerated. In many patients, this type of extrasystole or overdrive suppression is more effective in reducing couplets and salvos of tachycardia than it is in suppressing individual ventricular premature complexes. In the acute setting, overdrive suppression can be invaluable in the management of patients with frequent extrasystoles leading to repetitive episodes of sustained tachycardia.

Overdrive suppression is not universally effective. In rare patients, the mere presence of a pacing wire exacerbates the tachyarrhythmias. In others, pacing at even moderately elevated rates worsens the arrhythmias by producing ischemia, hemodynamic deficits, or other mechanisms. For example, absence of

retrograde conduction is a normal variation. This condition means that ventricular stimuli are not conducted back to the atrium. The sinus node is thus unaffected by ventricular pacing, and sinus beats may be conducted to the ventricle, even though the ventricular pacing rate may be somewhat higher than the sinus rate. This situation creates an irregular ventricular response that may be arrhythmogenic. It is not uncommon for pacing rates of 100 to 125 beats per minute to be required to overcome this phenomenon. In other subjects, there is an apparent tachyphylaxis effect with overdrive suppression. Pacing at 85 beats per minute may suppress extrasystoles for a period, after which they may reemerge. Stepwise increases in pacing rate may prove futile, as intolerable rates are reached.

ABORTIVE PACING.[3, 27, 51] There are patients in whom characteristic patterns of atrial or ventricular premature complexes presage the development of a sustained tachycardia. Some temporary pacemakers can be programmed to recognize such warning arrhythmias and to intervene with extrastimuli or other brief interventions.

INHIBITION.[41] The effective refractory period at a given site in the heart can be prolonged by administering extrastimuli during the refractory period. It is possible that such extrastimuli—when delivered at strategic points, such as the beginning of known conduction pathways—could prevent tachycardias by prolonging refractoriness at "choke points" within the circuit. Although theoretically applicable in both the acute and the chronic settings, such inhibition techniques have been studied primarily in the electrophysiology laboratory.

Hemodynamic Improvement During Continuing Tachycardia[2, 18, 23, 26, 32, 40, 46, 47]

CONTINUOUS RAPID PACING.[40, 47] Atrial pacing at rates fast enough to cause atrioventricular (AV) block can achieve a reduction in the ventricular rate in patients with incessant SVTs. The technique is not readily adaptable to VT. The technique should be used cautiously, if at all, in patients with a short PR interval, sinus tachycardia, or rapid natural or drug-enhanced AV conduction.

PAIRED AND COUPLED PACING.[2, 32, 46] In paired pacing, an initial stimulus (S_1) is followed by a second stimulus (S_2), with the S_1-S_2 interval shorter than the S_2-S_1 interval. In coupled pacing, the patient's natural depolarization acts as the S_1 and a pacemaker stimulus as S_2. In the ventricle, the S_2 is timed to produce an electrical but not a mechanical response. The electrical rate may therefore be unchanged, but the mechanical or pulse rate is halved, resulting in improved hemodynamic function. The optimal time for S_2 is usually just at the end of the refractory period of S_1, that is, at the vulnerable period, if present. The risk of precipitating ventricular fibrillation or accelerating tachycardia always exists. The stimulus should be limited to 2 msec and twice the diastolic threshold. The electrode should be in stable contact with the myocardium, and the system should be isolated. The premature stimulus (S_2) should be late initially, gradually becoming more premature until satisfactory hemodynamic changes occur. The metabolic costs of paired and coupled pacing are high, and implantable pacemakers based on these principles are not likely to have a high rate of success.

AVT PACING.[18] During VT at moderate rates, hemodynamic function may be improved by AV synchrony. Additional time may then be available for assessing the effects of medication or pacing techniques designed for the termination of tachycardia. AV synchrony may be achieved by pacing the atrium at selected intervals after sensing in the ventricle (AVT). This approach is almost exclusively for temporary applications (Fig. 21–2).

Pacing for Termination of Tachycardias

ELECTROPHYSIOLOGIC CONCEPTS.[15, 16, 20–22] For details of electrophysiologic concepts related to tachycardia termination, the reader is referred to other chapters in this book and to recent publications. The following is a brief summary for the sake of continuity.

The majority of clinical tachycardias are due to a reentrant mechanism. The reentry circuit can be large or small. If the refractory period within the circuit is just equal to the time taken by the wave front to complete a cycle, the circuit will be continuously refractory to outside stimuli. An "excitable gap" will exist if the refractory period is shorter than the cycle length. The objective of pacemaker therapy is to insert a stimulated wave front into this gap, timed so that antegrade conduction is no longer possible owing to refractoriness; retrograde conduction in the circuit will collide with the oncoming antegrade wave front already in the circuit, extinguishing it. Factors affecting termination of tachycardias (most of the following factors being related to reentry) are as follows: relationships between refractory periods and conduction velocities at the stimulation site, tachycardia circuit, and intervening myocardium; effective and relative refractory periods; inhomogeneity within and between various sites; the number of pathways to and

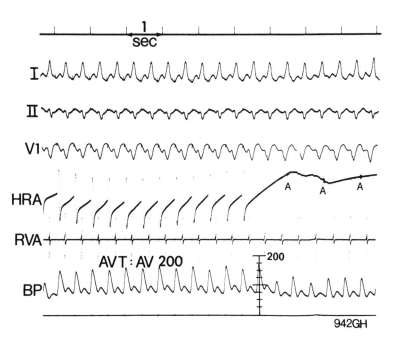

Figure 21–2. AVT pacing. In this patient with slow ventricular tachycardia (VT) at a rate of 120, surface leads I, II, and V_1 are displayed, along with tracings from the high right atrium (HRA), right ventricular apex (RVA), and an arterial blood pressure scale (BP). At the left-hand portion of the panel, AVT pacing is initiated to produce an atrioventricular (AV) interval of 200 msec and a systolic blood pressure of approximately 160 mm Hg. At the right, AVT pacing is stopped, with consequent AV dissociation and a drop in systolic blood pressure to an average of 125 mm Hg. A = atrial depolarization.

942GH

entry routes into the circuit; the distance between the stimulus and the circuit or focus; the size of the circuit; the rate of the tachycardia; stimulus strength; metabolic, neurohumoral, and pharmacologic factors; "protection"; and the disease process or substrate.

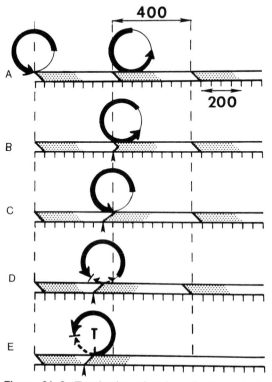

Figure 21–3. Termination of tachycardia by a single extrastimulus. The tachycardia circuit is represented by a circle, with the arrowhead representing the leading edge of the wave front and the heavy line the refractory period. The tachycardia has a cycle length of 400 msec, so that one quarter of the way through the cycle, the arrowhead will be at the "3 o'clock" position, as shown in panel A. Beneath the circles are two parallel lines, the first representing the myocardium at the exit point of the circuit and the lower representing the myocardium at the point of the pacing stimulus, with myocardium between. The stippled area represents the refractory period of this intervening myocardium. In panel B, a late extrastimulus fails to reach the tachycardia circuit before it has emitted its next wave front into the intervening myocardium. In panels C and D, the effects of successively earlier extrastimuli are shown. Finally, in panel E, an extrastimulus reaches the circuit at a point when antegrade conduction is no longer possible; only retrograde conduction can occur, and this collides with the antegrade wave front, extinguishing the tachycardia. This termination is emphasized by the capital "T" within the circuit. When termination by single extrastimuli is possible, the zone of termination within the tachycardia cycle begins just after the refractory period in nearly all instances. (Adapted from Fisher JD, Kim SG, Waspe LE, Matos JA: Mechanisms for the success and failure of pacing for termination of ventricular tachycardia: Clinical and hypothetical considerations. PACE 6:1094–1105, 1983; with permission.)

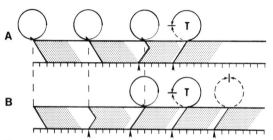

Figure 21–4. Multiple extrastimuli and burst pacing. Conventions are the same as for Figure 21–3. In panel A, an extrastimulus delivered at the end of the refractory period cannot reach the tachycardia circuit before the next wave front is emitted. However, the "peeling back" of refractoriness in the myocardium allows a second extrastimulus to reach the tachycardia circuit, resulting in termination. In panel B, four stimuli are shown, less tightly coupled than in panel A. The process of peeling back the refractoriness of the intervening myocardium begins with the first stimulus, but termination (T) is not achieved until the third. The fourth extrastimulus is irrelevant. (Adapted from Fisher JD, Kim SG, Waspe LE, Matos JA: Mechanisms for the success and failure of pacing for termination of ventricular tachycardia: Clinical and hypothetical considerations. PACE 6:1094–1105, 1983; with permission.)

Relationships between the site of programmed extrastimuli, the tachycardia circuit, and the intervening myocardium are outlined schematically in Figure 21–3.

The multiple relationships just described may conspire to prevent termination of tachycardia by single-capture techniques. In such instances, multiple extrastimuli or rapid pacing may be effective. This approach is illustrated in Figure 21–4. More than two extrastimuli may be required for the stimulation wave front to arrive at the circuit at the proper time. Other phenomena such as resetting of the tachycardia may occur, so that termination is never achieved. Because each extrastimulus can be brought progressively closer, ultimately reaching the effective refractory periods of its predecessor, the possibility of extremely rapid stimulation and acceleration of tachycardia exists. Burst pacing is shown in panel B of Figure 21–4. As with the extrastimulus technique, the refractoriness of the intervening myocardium is gradually "peeled back," until stimulated wave fronts can reach the circuit. In this illustration, the third stimulus achieves a termination, and the fourth stimulus is irrelevant.

Equipment for Antitachycardia Pacing

The following list proceeds from basic to sophisticated, with the more sophisticated equipment usually found in institutions that also perform detailed electrophysiologic studies.

LEADS, ELECTRODES, AND PATCHES. Special leads are available for temporary epicardial postoperative pacing, described in a prior section. These are placed superficially on or in the epicardium and emerge from the skin in the upper abdomen. They are designed to be removed with gentle tugging. Thresholds may be low at the time of placement but tend to rise rather rapidly, often becoming effective within a few days.

There are multitudes of temporary transvenous pacing wires, and it is beyond the scope of this chapter to describe them all or to detail the types of electrograms sought during the insertion of these wires. Some wires are flow directed and use a balloon similar to that found on a Swan-Ganz catheter, but many physicians find conventional wires without a balloon to be just as convenient. For access, we prefer the jugular or subclavian routes. Local skills permit these approaches to be done with a low complication rate; further, there is greater lead stability and freedom of motion for the patient with these approaches than with femoral or antecubital ones. The femoral approach may be more prone to thrombosis and infection, as well as generally restricting the patient to bed. The antecubital approach is associated with a high incidence of phlebitis within a few days. Strict attention to sterile technique is essential. Conventional dressings are best and should be nonocclusive. Plastic membrane bandages have a higher rate of infections, and there is a tendency not to change them daily. Bandages should be removed daily, and the insertion site should be examined for signs of local infection. In our institution, this site is then daubed with sequential solutions of hydrogen peroxide and povidone-iodine (Betadine), tapped dry with a sterile gauze, and covered with a povidone-iodine (Betadine) ointment and a loose bandage; the nonocclusive bandage is then reapplied. Wires are likely to remain most stable if a loop is made at the point of exit from the skin and is sutured to the skin, with the suture a minimum of 0.5 cm from the insertion site, so that any infection related to the suture will not automatically be transmitted into the blood stream. With the use of the approach just described, ordinary wires can remain stable for weeks or even months (in the case of some patients with serious arrhythmias who are undergoing lengthy antiarrhythmic drug trials). With the type of dressings described above, bacteremia is extremely rare, even after weeks of pacing. The incidence of bacteremia at Montefiore Medical Center in the Bronx, New York, is well under 1 per cent (even for patients who have pacemaker wires inserted for long periods so that serial electrophysiologic studies may be done).

Ventricular Pacing. For ventricular pacing, the most stable location is in the right ventricular apex. The paced QRS complex is generally of a left bundle–left axis morphology. In some instances, particularly if the tip is pointed slightly posteriorly, or in some patients with myocardial infarctions, the paced morphology will be right bundle–left axis. Left bundle–inferior axis morphology implies pacing at the right ventricular outflow tract. Although initial thresholds may be good, this position is generally unstable and should be avoided if possible. The best long-term results are obtained when the pacing threshold is well below 1 mA and when the passive electrogram reveals a "current of injury" pattern. In the trabeculated right ventricle, such patterns may be seen when the tip of the wire is actually perched precariously on a trabecula. Stability should therefore be assessed by having the patient take deep breaths and cough a few times, before the position is considered satisfactory and the wire is secured in place.

Temporary Transvenous Atrial Pacing. For temporary transvenous atrial pacing, a number of different wires are available. The classic Berkovitz hexapolar wire provides two distal poles for ventricular pacing and four more proximal poles for atrial pacing. Since the atrial poles brush by the atrium, rather than being placed in firm contact, atrial thresholds tend to be variable and to rise quickly with time. Many physicians have had good results using electrodes with fronds designed to contact the atrium or with temporary wires in a J form for placement in the right atrial appendage. We have generally found that the best long-term results have been obtained with wires inserted at least 4 to 5 cm into the coronary sinus (deeper insertion may result in excessive ventricular sensing or stimulation, and more proximal positions may displace).

Esophageal Pacing of the Atrium.[38] For esophageal pacing of the atrium, standard transvenous electrodes can be used but are less satisfactory than specially designed wires with electrodes having larger surface areas. Some esophageal wires are composed of relatively large distal electrodes encapsulated in a gelatin pill with a long strand of fine wires. The patient swallows the gelatin pill, washing it down with large amounts of water, while the proximal end is held outside the mouth. After the capsule has had time to dissolve, the electrode is pulled back under electrocardiographic control until the largest atrial deflection is observed, and this point is chosen for pacing. If the electrode is pulled up too far, it can be washed down again with more water. Although best from the viewpoint of acceptance by the patient, this type of wire cannot be used in all clinical situations. Other wires are designed for insertion in the same way as nasogastric tubes; many have multiple electrodes, and again the position is altered until the maximal atrial deflection is observed. With esophageal pacing, initial thresholds tend to be high, well above limits of conventional pacemakers designed for transvenous use. In a carefully conducted study,[38] best results and most comfort to the patient were obtained with outputs averaging 27 mA with a wide pulse duration of 8 msec, about 35 cm from the incisors. These settings are generally obtainable with devices designed for transthoracic pacing. Esophageal pacing is most appropriate for diagnostic purposes (AV relationship) or for acute use for one or two episodes of tachycardia. This approach is generally not suitable for pacing that extends over several days.

Transthoracic Ventricular Pacing.[28, 35] The ability to provide "instant pacing" has been a boon to many emergency rooms, intensive care units, and coronary care units. Large stick-on patch electrodes are used, positioned as for transthoracic countershock. Thresholds tend to be higher than with esophageal pacing, often 50 to 60 mA at pulse durations of 30 to 50 msec, and this may produce considerable chest wall stimulation. Careful adjustment of patch electrode position can minimize the patient's discomfort. In ideal situations, pacing can be accomplished with minimal unpleasantness for the patient.

Many of the devices also contain some capability for rapid pacing. Models with a continuous rate dial are preferable to those that provide only preselected rates. For tachycardias, these devices are most useful for single, acute episodes. Many patients find the sensation associated with transthoracic pacing to be unpleasant, especially when prolonged or repeated. For such patients, temporary transvenous pacing should be instituted after the acute episode has been resolved.

RAPID PACERS. These devices look similar to standard temporary antibradycardia pacemakers. Some, such as the Medtronic 5320, are asynchronous, with a dial that allows pacing rates up to 800 beats per minute. Others,

such as the Cordis Chronocor V (Cordis and Telectronics, Miami, FL), can operate as standard asynchronous or inhibited antibradycardia pacemakers, with a rapid pacing option accessible via additional controls. These devices are extremely portable. Designed for use with a temporary transvenous pacing wire, they can also be used to activate certain implanted antitachycardia pacers using the chest wall stimulation technique. Programmed extrastimuli are beyond the capabilities of these devices, but they can perform underdrive pacing, as well as the various burst and ramp techniques described in this chapter.

ELECTROPHYSIOLOGIC STIMULATORS. The flexibility of devices designed for programmed electrical stimulation makes them useful in some patients for bedside work. Programmed stimulation, coupled and paired pacing, and AVT pacing, described elsewhere in this text, can be performed using these devices.

AUTOMATIC ANTITACHYCARDIA DEVICES. There are a few commercial devices, such as the Savita Orthorhythmic pacer (Savita, Paris, France), that are designed for automatic antitachycardia interventions at the bedside, using relatively simple adjustment dials. Other devices are nonimplantable versions of sophisticated implantable antitachycardia devices, most of them requiring complex programmers. These pacemakers are useful in patients with frequently recurring tachycardias who have been found to respond reliably to certain pacing patterns.

Pacing Techniques

This section will emphasize techniques useful in emergency rooms, intensive care units, and recovery rooms. More complex techniques are covered in Chapter 26.

STIMULUS AMPLITUDE.[50] For antitachycardia pacing, the stimulus amplitude should be higher than for antibradycardia pacing. At faster rates, the threshold rises. In addition, at any given pacing rate, there is a greater likelihood of terminating the tachycardia with higher stimulus amplitudes. For transvenous pacers with a threshold of 1 mA, amplitudes of 10 to 15 mA should be used for antitachycardia pacing. With esophageal and transthoracic pacing, such excesses of stimulation over threshold amplitudes usually cannot be achieved, owing to either limitations of the pacing device or discomfort to the patient, but attempts should be made to exceed the threshold by as much as clinically appropriate or tolerated.

UNDERDRIVE.[39] Slow competitive (underdrive) pacing is sometimes useful in terminating slow, well-tolerated SVT or VT. For tachycardias at a rate of about 150 beats per minute or less, asynchronous pacing at even slower rates will result in "scanning" of the cardiac cycle. Care must be taken to ensure that the pacing rate is not exactly an even fraction of the tachycardia rate (e.g., one half, one third, one quarter, and so forth) because in such situations the stimulus falls at the same place in the cardiac cycle of every second, third, or fourth tachycardia beat. Termination of tachycardia with a single stimulus is dependent on the presence of a substantial "excitable gap" in the tachycardia circuit and often on proximity of the pacing stimulus to the tachycardia circuit. Stimuli should be delivered to the atrium for SVT and to the ventricle for VT. Patients with reciprocating tachycardias related to the Wolff-Parkinson-White syndrome may respond to either atrial or ventricular stimuli, since the tachycardia circuit involves both the atrium and the ventricle. As a general rule, atrial pacing is preferable to ventricular pacing in patients with Wolff-Parkinson-White syndrome, but there are patients in whom ventricular pacing is more effective and others in whom atrial pacing results in atrial fibrillation with an extremely rapid ventricular response.

With the underdrive method, as with other single-capture techniques, about 55 per cent of slow, well-tolerated tachycardias can be terminated, and about 0.5 per cent will be accelerated.[19] Rapid tachycardias and flutter rarely respond to single-capture stimulation techniques.

ENTRAINMENT.[1, 4, 36, 48, 49] This concept originated with Waldo and was initially employed in patients with atrial flutter in the postoperative period.[48] It is one way of identifying the slowest possible rapid pacing rate that will both interrupt the tachycardia and minimize the incidence of acceleration. In patients with type I atrial flutter (sawtooth) morphology, pacing at rates above the flutter rate can result in atrial depolarizations on electrocardiographic strips that are morphologically quite similar to the unpaced flutter waves. As the pacing rate is increased, the flutter waves may assume a morphology that is a fusion between flutter-type complexes and those that would be observed with pacing at a given site, such as the high right atrium. At a critical rate, the fusion or flutter-like morphology is suddenly lost, and this indicates interruption of the flutter and termination of the arrhythmia.

The diagnostic features of transient entrainment with final interruption of tachycardia are as follows[4, 45] (Fig. 21–5): (1) During the period of entrainment, pacing appears to accelerate the tachycardia to the same rate as the pacemaker; (2) when pacing is stopped, the tachycardia rate reverts to its previous rate; (3) at any pacing rate, there is a constant degree of fusion between the paced and the spontaneous tachycardia morphologies; and (4) as the pacing rate is increased, there is a progression in the fusion toward the morphology that occurs with pacing.

The end of the period of transient entrainment occurs when pacer-stimulated wave fronts are no longer able to enter the tachycardia circuit in an anterograde direction (i.e., the excitable gap in the anterograde direction has been "used up"). Fusion no longer exists, and in many cases the tachycardia will be found to have been terminated if the pacemaker is turned off.

In many subjects, pacing at a constant rate will produce progressive fusion as more of the surrounding myocardium is recruited by the pacing wave front; this is *not* consistent with entrainment, in which the degree of fusion is constant at a constant pacing rate (at least after a few initial beats).

Entrainment is best demonstrated with stepwise incremental pacing rates, since this approach will show the progressive fusion at constant rates. Rate-incremental ramp pacing can produce the same result, but interpretation may be difficult, since it may not be possible to distinguish whether the progressive fusion is related to entrainment or to recruitment, as distinguished above.

The technique of entrainment has proved most useful in patients who have atrial flutter postoperatively. In these patients, pacing rates approximately 125 per cent above the baseline flutter rate have been optimal. At these rates, the period of entrainment is passed, and the circuit is interrupted, achieving termination with the slowest possible pacing rate and the lowest possible risk of acceleration. Although the potential efficacy of the train technique has now been demonstrated for many supraventricular and ventricular arrhythmias, success rates are lower.

TUNE-DOWN (RATE-DECREMENTAL) RAMP PACING.[14, 18] Tune-down pacing (Fig. 21–6) represents another attempt to minimize the risk of acceleration. It is most applicable in patients with SVTs and in those with slower and well-tolerated VT. Pacing is initiated at a rate

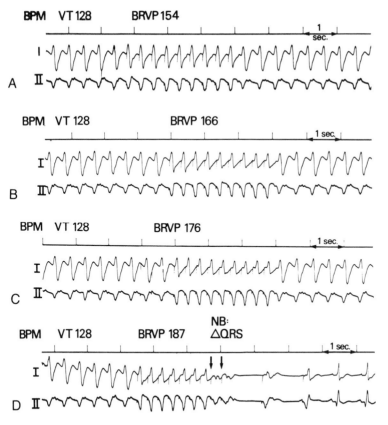

Figure 21–5. Entrainment and termination of ventricular tachycardia (VT). Surface leads I and II are displayed. In panel *A,* VT at a rate of 128 beats per minute (BPM) is treated with a burst of rapid ventricular pacing (BRVP) at a rate of 154, with minimal change in the QRS morphology and without termination of the VT. In panels *B* and *C,* an increase in the burst rate to rates of 166 and 176, respectively, produces changes in QRS morphology that are constant at each pacing rate, but again with failure to terminate the VT. In panel *D,* BRVP at a rate of 187 produces additional changes in the QRS initially, followed by two captures resulting in distinctly different QRS morphologies, indicating the end of entrainment and termination of the tachycardia. See text for details.

moderately faster than the tachycardia (10 to 20 beats per minute) and is continued for 5 to 10 seconds, after which the pacer rate is very slowly reduced to rates well below that of the tachycardia. Failure is heralded by the appearance of fusion beats as the pacer rate approaches that of the tachycardia. In other instances, the pacing rate can be brought well below that of the tachycardia, with consequent hemodynamic improvement, even though the tachycardia resumes when pacing is stopped. Success may be attributed to the long period during which stimulated wave fronts "peel

back" intervening refractoriness in the myocardium between the site of stimulation and the circuit; fatigue in the circuit, when driven for a relatively long period at a faster rate; or neurohumoral adaptations and hemodynamic changes brought about both by the rapid pacing and finally by pacing at lower rates.

"**RAMP-UP**" **PACING (CYCLE LENGTH–DECREMENTAL).**[5, 9] This type of pacing is the opposite of the tune-down technique. Pacing is started at a rate just faster than that of the tachycardia and is gradually increased. With successive attempts at termination, both the

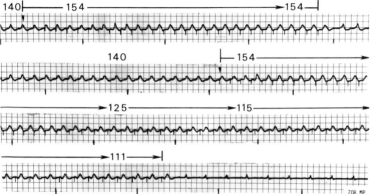

Figure 21–6. Rate decremental (tune-down) pacing for termination of VT. In the uppermost panel, VT at a rate of 140 is treated with overdrive pacing at a rate of 154, which fails to terminate the arrhythmia. Pacing at this rate for up to 2 minutes failed to terminate the VT. In the second panel, pacing is again initiated at a rate of 154, and in the third and fourth panels (which are continuous with the second), the pacing rate is gradually reduced to 111, with termination of the tachycardia. Three-second time lines are provided at the bottom of the tracings in each panel.

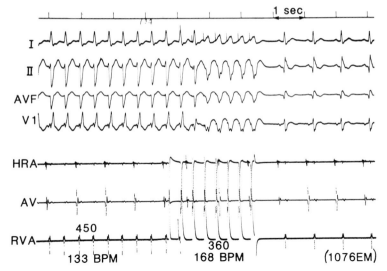

Figure 21–7. Termination of VT by burst rapid ventricular pacing. Surface leads I, II, aV$_F$ and V$_1$ are displayed, along with tracings from the high right atrium (HRA), atrioventricular junctional area (AV), and right ventricular apex (RVA). At the left, VT exists at a rate of 133 beats per minute (BPM) (450-msec cycle length), with evidence of AV dissociation. At the center, a burst at a rate of 168 (360 msec) is delivered, the eight stimuli resulting in a fusion and five captures, with termination of the VT. This is the ideal response to burst pacing.

number of stimuli and the pacing rate may be increased. This technique can be performed in its simplest version using any of the rapid temporary pacers. More sophisticated versions, requiring more complex equipment (e.g., the Medtronic SP 3056), include "autodecremental pacing"[5] (i.e., decremental cycle lengths) and "universal" pacing,[9] in which the cycle length decrements for the first several stimuli and then levels off.

BURST PACING.[16, 17, 19] Burst pacing (Fig. 21–7) implies a limited number of stimuli, usually 5 to 15, delivered at rates faster than that of the tachycardia. One protocol is to begin with five to seven captures at a rate 25 beats per minute above the tachycardia. If termination is not achieved, the rate is held constant, but the duration of the burst is increased to produce 10 to 15 captures. If the tachycardia persists, the pacer rate is increased by 10 to 25 beats per minute, depending on the urgency of the situation, and the process is repeated in as many steps as are needed either to produce termination of the tachycardia or to end in acceleration requiring countershock. In cases of VT with hemodynamic instability, in which electrical countershock would be the alternative to pacing in any case, such an endpoint is appropriate. In patients with well-tolerated VT, it may be prudent to stop at an arbitrary upper pacing rate and administer drugs to slow the tachycardia or achieve chemical conversion, before returning to pacing.

In a series of 390 episodes of well-tolerated VT,[19] burst pacing proved far superior to single-, double-, and triple-capture techniques, achieving termination of tachycardia in some 94 per cent of cases; however, the 4.4 per cent

incidence of acceleration was substantially higher than the 0.5 per cent acceleration observed with single-capture techniques. In most acute settings, burst pacing is the simplest efficacious method and is the one with which the relevant personnel should be most familiar.

CONCLUSIONS

Antitachycardia pacing in the acute setting is an efficacious (Table 21–1) but underutilized modality. Confronted with recurrent tachycardias, many physicians persist in using drugs to remedy the situation and then, failing that, try countershock. In the acute setting that is well

TABLE 21–1. PACING FOR TACHYCARDIA TERMINATION

RHYTHM/SETTING	TERMINATION BY PACING: LIKELIHOOD OF SUCCESS
1. Postoperative atrial flutter (type I)	≥ 90%
2. Other type I atrial flutter	70–90% (often after transient conversion to atrial fibrillation)
3. Type II atrial flutter	Rare unless via conversion to atrial fibrillation, thence to sinus
4. SVT	≥ 90%
5. VT (chronic substrate)	
a. Well tolerated, rate < 200	≥ 90%
b. Poorly tolerated, rate > 200	30–50%
6. VT (unstable acute infarction patients)	40–50%

SVT = supraventricular tachycardia; VT = ventricular tachycardia.

monitored, with backup countershock and other resuscitative measures available, the most serious risks associated with implantable antitachycardia pacemakers are eliminated. Esophageal and transthoracic techniques provide noninvasive pacing options for SVT and VT, respectively.

REFERENCES

1. Anderson KP, Swerdlow CD, Mason JW: Entrainment of ventricular tachycardia. Am J Cardiol 53:335, 1983.
2. Arbel ER, Cohen HC, Langendorf R, Glick G: Successful treatment of drug-resistant atrial tachycardia and intractable congestive heart failure with permanent coupled atrial pacing. Am J Cardiol 41:336, 1978.
3. Behrenbeck DW, Winter UJ, Hoher M, et al: Dynamic overdrive pacing for suppression of ventricular ectopic activity. *In* Proceedings of the International Symposium on Invasive CV Therapy: Recent Advances and Future Developments, Köln, Federal Republic of Germany, 1985, 47–47A.
4. Brugada P, Wellens HJJ: Entrainment as an electrophysiologic phenomenon. J Am Coll Cardiol 3:451, 1984.
5. Charos GS, Haffajee CI, Gold RL, et al: A theoretically and practically more effective method for interruption of ventricular tachycardia: Self-adapting autodecremental overdrive pacing. Circulation 73:309, 1986.
6. Cooper TB, Maclean WAH, Waldo A: Overdrive pacing for supraventricular tachycardias: A review of theoretical implications and therapeutic techniques. PACE 1:196, 1978.
7. Crick JCP, Way B, Sowton E: Successful treatment of ventricular tachycardia by physiological pacing. PACE 7:949, 1984.
8. DeFrancis NA, Giordano RP: Permanent epicardial atrial pacing in the treatment of refractory ventricular tachycardia. Am J Cardiol 22:742, 1968.
9. Den Dulk K, Kersschot IE, Brugada P, Wellens HJJ: Is there a universal antitachycardia pacing mode? Am J Cardiol 57:950, 1986.
10. DeSanctis RW, Kastor JA: Rapid intracardiac pacing for treatment of recurrent ventricular tachyarrhythmias in the absence of heart block. Am Heart J 76:168, 1968.
11. Dreifus LS, Berkovits BV, Kimibiris D, et al: Use of atrial and bifocal cardiac pacemakers for treating resistant dysrhythmias. Eur J Cardiol 3:257, 1975.
12. Ector H, Brabandt HV, De Geest H: Treatment of life-threatening ventricular arrhythmias by a combination of antiarrhythmic drugs and right ventricular pacing. PACE 7:622, 1984.
13. Escher DJW: The treatment of tachyarrhythmias by artificial pacing. Am Heart J 78:829, 1969.
14. Escher DJW, Furman S: Emergency treatment of cardiac arrhythmias: Emphasis on use of electrical pacing. JAMA 214:2028, 1970.
15. Fisher JD: Electrical devices for the treatment of tachyarrhythmias. Cardiol Clin 4:527, 1986.
16. Fisher JD, Kim SG, Mercando AD: Electrical devices for treatment of arrhythmias. Am J Cardiol 61:45A, 1988.
17. Fisher JD, Mehra R, Furman S: Termination of ventricular tachycardia with bursts of ventricular pacing. Am J Cardiol 41:94, 1978.
18. Fisher JD, Kim SG, Furman S, Matos JA: Role of implantable pacemakers in control of recurrent ventricular arrhythmias. J Am Coll Cardiol 3:472, 1984.
19. Fisher JD, Kim SG, Matos JA, Ostrow E: Comparative effectiveness of pacing techniques for termination of well-tolerated sustained ventricular tachycardia. PACE 6:915, 1983.
20. Fisher JD, Kim SG, Matos JA, Waspe LE: Pacing for ventricular tachycardia. PACE 7:1278, 1984.
21. Fisher JD, Kim SG, Matos JA, Waspe LE: Pacing for tachycardias: Clinical translations. *In* Zipes D, Jalife J (eds): Electrophysiology and Arrhythmias. Orlando, FL, Grune and Stratton, 1985, pp 507–511.
22. Fisher JD, Ostrow E, Kim SG, Matos JA: Ultrarapid single-capture train stimulation for termination of ventricular tachycardia. Am J Cardiol 51:1334, 1983.
23. Fisher JD, Johnston D, Furman S, et al: Long-term efficacy of antitachycardia pacing for supraventricular and ventricular tachycardias. Am J Cardiol 60:1311, 1987.
24. Fisher JD, Teichman S, Ferrick A, et al: Antiarrhythmic effects of VVI pacing at physiologic rates: A crossover controlled evaluation. PACE 10:822, 1987.
25. Friedberg CK, Lyon LJ, Donoso E: Suppression of refractory recurrent ventricular tachycardia by transvenous rapid pacing and antiarrhythmic drugs. Am Heart J 79:44, 1970.
26. Furman S: Therapeutic uses of atrial pacing. Am Heart J 86:835, 1973.
27. Gurtner HP, Gertsch M, Zacouto F: Orthorhythmischer Herzschrittmacher und salvenförmige Herzstimulation. Schweiz Med Wochenschr 105:33, 1975.
28. Heges JR, Syverud SA, Dalsey WC, et al: Prehospital trial of emergency transcutaneous cardiac pacing. Circulation 76:1337, 1987.
29. Heiman DF, Helwig J Jr: Suppression of ventricular arrhythmias by transvenous intracardiac pacing. JAMA 195:172, 1966.
30. Johnson RA, Hutter AM, DeSanctis RW, et al: Chronic overdrive pacing in the control of refractory ventricular arrhythmias. Ann Intern Med 80:380, 1974.
31. Khan MM, Logan KR, McComb JM, Adgey AAJ: Management of recurrent ventricular tachyarrhythmias associated with Q-T prolongation. Am J Cardiol 47:1301, 1981.
32. Langendorf R, Pick A: Observations on the clinical use of paired electrical stimulation of the heart. Bull NY Acad Med 41:535, 1965.
33. Lew HT, March HW: Control of recurrent ventricular fibrillation by transvenous pacing in the absence of heart block. Am Heart J 73:794, 1967.
34. Lichstein E, Chadda K, Fenig S: Atrial pacing in the treatment of refractory ventricular tachycardia associated with hypokalemia. Am J Cardiol 30:550, 1972.
35. Luck JC, Davis D: Termination of sustained tachycardia by external noninvasive pacing. PACE 10:1125, 1987.
36. MacLean WAH, Plumb VJ, Waldo AL: Transient entrainment and interruption of ventricular tachycardia. PACE 4:358, 1981.
37. Moss AJ, Rivers RJ: Termination and inhibition of recurrent tachycardias by implanted pervenous pacemakers. Circulation 50:942, 1974.

38. Nishimura M, Katoh T, Hanai S, Watanabe Y: Optimal mode of transesophageal atrial pacing. Am J Cardiol 57:791, 1986.

39. Portillo B, Medina-Ravell V, Portillo-Leon N, et al: Treatment of drug resistant A-V reciprocating tachycardias with multiprogrammable dual demand A-V sequential (DVI, MN) pacemakers. PACE 5:814, 1982.

40. Preston TA, Haynes RE, Gavin WA, Hessel EA: Permanent rapid atrial pacing to control supraventricular tachycardia. PACE 2:331, 1979.

41. Prystowsky EN, Zipes D: Inhibition in the human heart. Circulation 68:707, 1983.

42. Schwedel JB, Furman S, Escher DJW: Use of an intracardiac pacemaker in the treatment of Stokes-Adams seizures. Prog Cardiovasc Dis 3:170, 1960.

43. Sowton E, Leatham A, Carson P: The suppression of arrhythmias by artificial pacing. Lancet 2:1098, 1964.

44. Waldo LA, MacLean WAH: Diagnosis and Treatment of Cardiac Arrhythmias Following Open Heart Surgery. Mount Kisco, NY, Futura Publishing Co, 1980.

45. Waldo AL, Henthorn RW, Plumb VJ, MacLean WAH: Demonstration of the mechanism of transient entrainment and interruption of ventricular tachycardia with rapid atrial pacing. J Am Coll Cardiol 3:422, 1984.

46. Waldo AL, Krongrad E, Kupersmith J, et al: Ventricular paired pacing to control rapid ventricular heart rate following open heart surgery. Circulation 53:177, 1976.

47. Waldo AL, MacLean WAH, Karp RB, et al: Continuous rapid atrial pacing to control recurrent or sustained supraventricular tachycardias following open heart surgery. Circulation 54:245, 1976.

48. Waldo AL, MacLean WAH, Karp RB, et al: Entrainment and interruption of atrial flutter with atrial pacing: Studies in man following open heart surgery. Circulation 56:737, 1977.

49. Waldo AL, Plumb VJ, Arciniegas JG, et al: Transient entrainment and interruption of A-V bypass pathway type paroxysmal atrial tachycardia: A model for understanding and identifying reentrant arrhythmias in man. Circulation 67:73, 1982.

50. Waxman HL, Cain ME, Greenspan AM, Josephson ME: Termination of ventricular tachycardia with ventricular stimulation: Salutary effect of increased current strength. Circulation 65:800, 1982.

51. Zacouto F, Juillard A, Gerbaux A: Prevention of ventricular tachycardias by automatic rate pacing. Rean Art Org 8:3, 1982.

52. Zipes DP, Festoff B, Schaal SF, et al: Treatment of ventricular arrhythmia by permanent atrial pacemaker and cardiac sympathectomy. Ann Intern Med 68:591, 1968.

53. Zoll PM, Linenthal AJ: External and internal cardiac pacemakers. Circulation 8:455, 1963.

B. Programmed Stimulation and Transvenous Cardioversion-Defibrillation

BRUCE D. LINDSAY
and SANJEEV SAKSENA

The use of electrical therapy delivered by transvenous catheters has assumed an important role in the management of tachyarrhythmias that are not prevented by antiarrhythmic medications. This approach employs programmed ventricular stimulation or the delivery of shocks as the mode of therapy. Standard percutaneous electrode catheters can be used in the intensive care setting for overdrive pacing of recurrent reentrant supraventricular tachycardia (SVT) or ventricular tachycardia (VT). When this method is ineffective, specially designed catheters are available to deliver shocks of selected energy for the termination of sustained VT as an alternative to transthoracic direct-current cardioversion. The

application of these techniques has grown to encompass the preoperative evaluation of candidates for implantation of antitachycardia pacemakers or cardioverter/defibrillators. The automatic implantable cardioverter/defibrillator (AICD) markedly reduces the mortality of patients whose arrhythmias are refractory to medical therapy and provides an alternative for those who are not good candidates for catheter or surgical ablation of the arrhythmogenic substrate.[17, 46] Acceptance of the AICD, however, has been limited by the mortality and morbidity of implantation and the discomfort caused by high-energy shocks. The advent of implantable cardioverter/defibrillators that have the capacity to deliver programmed ventricular stimuli in addition to selected shocks will enable the implanting physician to designate an arrhythmia termination algorithm that incorporates a prescribed sequence of ventricular pacing and specified shock intensities. This approach will reduce exposure of the patient to high-intensity shocks, and the development of effective non-epicardial lead systems will facilitate implantation. The optimal pacing sequence, shock intensity, or lead configuration required for arrhythmia termination varies from one individual to another and necessitates extensive preoperative testing to identify electrical interventions that terminate VT promptly with a low risk of accelerating the rhythm to ventricular fibrillation. Failure to observe these principles may lead to the selection of electrode configurations that are ineffective or therapeutic interventions that accelerate VT to ventricular fibrillation, which ultimately increases the energy consumption of the device and reduces its longevity. This section of Chapter 21 reviews the technical aspects, efficacy, safety, and reproducibility of transvenous electrical therapy for sustained SVT and VT.

THE CARDIOVERSION SYSTEM

The requirements of conventional pacing catheters that deliver stimuli in the range of 25 µJ differ from those of catheters that deliver shocks of 1 to 40 J for transvenous cardioversion. Conventional pacing catheters emit impulses of short duration (< 1 msec) and incorporate electrodes with geometric surface areas of 8 to 12 mm^2 to generate a stimulus of optimal field intensity (lower threshold) and minimize lead polarization. The relatively high impedance (250 to 1200 ohms) of conventional lead systems, which depends on the electrode design, the resistance of the lead conductor, and the electrode-tissue interface, prevents excessive current drain from the pulse generator. In contrast, the electrodes of cardioversion catheters have larger surface areas (2.5 to 8.0 cm^2) to reduce tissue damage caused by the high field intensity of shocks and to lower impedance for high current flow. Moreover, the insulation of cardioverter/defibrillator catheters must withstand repeated shocks without loss of integrity, which could result in shunting of energy away from the electrodes. Two temporary catheters that incorporate these characteristics have been designed by Medtronic, Inc. (Minneapolis, MN), and Cardiac Pacemakers, Inc. (CPI, St. Paul, MN), for transvenous cardioversion and defibrillation (Fig. 21–8).

The Medtronic 6880 tripolar 9.5 French 100-cm catheter is composed of three coiled-wound multifilar, low-impedance, drawn-brazed-strand wire electrical conductors in a

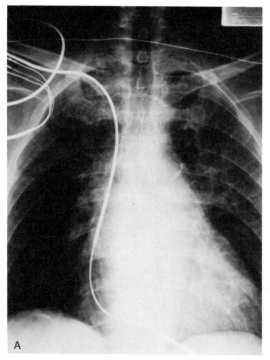

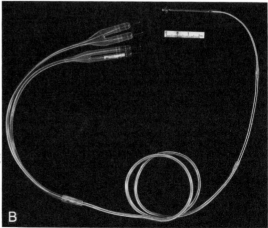

Figure 21–8. Transvenous cardioversion/defibrillation catheters. *A,* Medtronic, Minneapolis, MN. *B,* Cardiac Pacemakers, Inc, St Paul, MN, Endotak-C cardioversion/defibrillation catheter.

coaxial configuration insulated by sleeves of polyurethane. A pair of electrodes, separated by 5 mm, forms a bipole at the distal end that is used for electrogram sensing and ventricular pacing. The surface area of each electrode is 1.25 cm^2. During cardioversion these electrodes become electrically common and form the cathode. The anode comprises two electrically common electrodes, separated by 13 mm, which have a combined surface area of 2.5 cm^2. Spacing between proximal and distal electrodes of 100, 125, and 150 mm is available. The catheter is introduced via the subclavian vein, and the distal electrode pair is positioned in the right ventricular apex. This approach usually aligns the proximal pair at the junction of the high right atrium and superior vena cava. A stylet is inserted into the lumen of the inner coil via the connector pin to facilitate lead placement. The catheter may be anchored and left in position for serial testing, but it is not intended for resterilization.

Endotak-C, manufactured by CPI, is a 10 French tripolar catheter consisting of three drawn-brazed-strand conductors insulated by Silastic. A 16-mm^2 platinum-iridium–tip electrode is used for pacing. A spring electrode, 3 cm^2 in surface area, is located 4 cm from the tip, and a second spring electrode with a surface area of 6 cm^2 is located 10 or 12 cm from the proximal end of the distal spring. Pacing and sensing are performed using a bipole composed of the tip electrode and the distal spring electrode. During cardioversion, the distal spring electrode forms the cathode and the proximal spring electrode forms the anode. The catheter is designed to be introduced through a 12 French sheath, and a stylet can be inserted through the connector of the distal electrode to facilitate positioning of the tip in the right ventricular apex.

The efficacy of unidirectional and bidirectional shocks is discussed elsewhere in this chapter (pp. 430–434). As shown in Figure 21–9, unidirectional shocks can be delivered using the distal electrodes of the catheter as the cathode and the proximal pair of electrodes or a cutaneous R$_2$ patch (R$_2$ Corporation, Skokie, IL) as the anode.[55] Bidirectional shocks are generally delivered by using the distal catheter electrode pair as the cathode, and the anodes consist of the proximal catheter electrode pair and the cutaneous patch. Dual current pathways are obtained by alternating the anodes with sequential shocks or by using single shocks in which the catheter anode and R$_2$ patch are connected by a common cable with the terminal of the external cardioverter/defibrillator.[32, 41]

Several temporary transvenous bipolar and quadripolar catheters are available for atrial or ventricular pacing. Atrial catheters constructed with a J configuration facilitate lead stabilization in the atrial appendage when the catheter is inserted via the subclavian or internal jugular vein. The advantage of quadripolar catheters is that the proximal electrode pair can be used to record intracardiac electrograms during pacing from the distal pair, which often facilitates recognition of atrial or ventricular capture. The delivery of stimuli for overdrive pacing is performed in the intensive care unit by manual activation of a portable temporary pacemaker designed with extended upper rates for overdrive pacing. A programmable stimulator is used in the electrophysiology laboratory and allows for more precise selection of coupling intervals. Some units synchronize the onset of pacing to the QRS. More sophisticated pacing algorithms employ microprocessor systems to adjust coupling intervals automatically.[14, 28]

Non-Epicardial Electrode System for ICD's

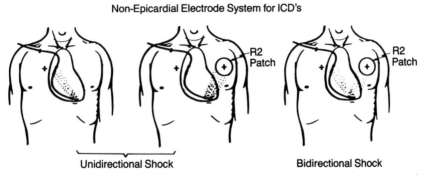

Unidirectional Shock   Bidirectional Shock

Figure 21–9. Schematic illustration of unidirectional and bidirectional current pathways using an endocardial catheter and a cutaneous R$_2$ patch. The respective defibrillation thresholds of these lead systems can be obtained preoperatively to determine the efficacy of nonepicardial leads used in conjunction with an implantable cardioverter/defibrillator (ICD).

Several external cardioverter/defibrillators have been designed for clinical use. The electrical parameter used to select shocks, the waveform, and pulse width (5 to 12 msec) may vary according to the manufacturer. The morphologies of three representative defibrillation pulses are shown in Figure 21–10. The pulse of most commercially available units is a monophasic truncated exponential or damped half-sinusoidal waveform; these appear to have comparable efficacy for cardioversion and defibrillation.[27] Preliminary results suggest that selected biphasic waveforms reduce the energy required for defibrillation. Phase duration and amplitude affect the efficacy of biphasic shocks. Waveforms in which the phases are equal in duration and the amplitude of the second phase is approximately half the amplitude of the first phase are more effective than monomorphic waveforms or biphasic morphologies in which the leading phase is of shorter duration or lower magnitude than the second phase.[9, 16, 47, 59]

Electrical parameters used to define cardioversion/defibrillation thresholds include energy (joules), voltage, and current (amperes). Energy is a somewhat ambiguous definition of threshold because the energy delivered is dependent on pulse parameters and impedance. There is a divergence of opinion over whether current or the transmembrane voltage gradient is responsible for cell depolarization.[10, 39, 40] Pulse generators available for implantation, however, use truncated exponential waveforms, for which voltage is the determinant of output. Accordingly, most preoperative and intraoperative testing is performed with an external cardioverter/defibrillator that emits a pulse with this waveform. The external cardioverter/defibrillator manufactured by CPI is a commercial unit that is readily available. The storage capacitors are designed to deliver single synchronous or asynchronous 60 per cent tilt truncated exponential pulses at 12 selected energy settings ranging from 1 to 40 J. The Medtronic 2376 external cardioverter/defibrillator has been designed for delivery of sequential shocks separated by 0.1 to 9.9 msec (0.1-msec increments), with output selections of 0 to 1090 V (leading edge) in 10 V steps. The HSV-02 (Ventritex, Sunnyvale, CA), a cardioverter/defibrillator undergoing clinical trials, can deliver monophasic or biphasic shock morphologies. The output voltage is 50 to 990 V, adjustable in 10-V increments. Two output channels allow for the delivery of sequential shocks separated by 0 to 99 msec, adjustable in 1-msec increments.

INSERTION OF CARDIOVERSION CATHETER

Percutaneous subclavian cannulation is used for placement of the Medtronic and CPI cardioversion/defibrillation catheters. The operative field is painted with povidine-iodine (Betadine). Local anesthesia is obtained with 1 per cent lidocaine or bupivacaine (Marcaine). A 5-cm 14-gauge needle is used to puncture the subclavian vein using a modified Seldinger technique, and a guide wire is advanced into the right atrium.[42, 45] It is advisable to verify the position of the guide wire fluoroscopically before proceeding further. A vein dilator introducer system, consisting of a 20-cm Teflon vessel dilator and a 13-cm peel-away Teflon sheath, is then introduced over the guide wire. While the patient holds his or her breath, the dilator and wire are removed, and the cardioversion lead is advanced through the sheath. The tip of the stylet is bent to form a smooth curve and is inserted through the connector. The resulting bend in the lead facilitates passage across the tricuspid valve. The lead is then passed into the pulmonary outflow tract to ensure that the coronary sinus has not been cannulated. The bent stylet is replaced by a straight stylet, and the lead is withdrawn until the catheter tip drops into the right ventricular apex. The tip is then advanced and should point slightly downward to ensure stability. Current thresholds less than 2 mA are generally obtained with a pulse width of 1 msec.

PATHOPHYSIOLOGIC MECHANISMS INFLUENCING THE EFFICACY OF ELECTRICAL INTERVENTIONS

The development of effective electrical interventions that terminate SVTs and VTs is

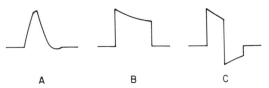

Figure 21–10. Representative defibrillating pulse morphologies are shown schematically: *A*, damped half-sinusoidal; *B*, monophasic truncated exponential; and *C*, biphasic.

predicated on the pathophysiology of these arrhythmias. Several lines of evidence indicate that reentrant mechanisms are responsible for the majority of SVTs and VTs.[2, 4, 12, 13, 15, 23, 29, 31, 34–37, 66, 68–71, 74] The conditions required for reentry are (1) the presence of two functionally discrete pathways that join proximally and distally to form a circuit of conduction; (2) selective conduction block in one limb of the circuit, with unidirectional slow conduction over the unblocked pathway; and (3) a circulating conduction time exceeding the refractory period of the initially blocked pathway. The difference between the time required for a wave front of activation to complete its circuit and the longest refractory period of the circuit's components provides an excitable gap, which may permit an extrastimulus to penetrate the circuit. By capturing part of the reentrant circuit, the stimulus may render a portion refractory to the circulating wave front and terminate the tachycardia.

Several common SVTs have been shown to depend on reentry. Evidence of dual atrioventricular (AV) nodal pathways constituting a microreentrant circuit has been accepted as the model of AV nodal reentrant tachycardia, and the reentrant circuit of AV reciprocating tachycardias in the preexcitation syndrome has been well delineated.[4, 12, 15, 23, 74] In both AV nodal and AV reciprocating tachycardia, delayed conduction occurs within the AV node and reentry depends on the refractory properties of the remaining limb of the circuit. There is also evidence that intraatrial reentry accounts for atrial flutter in humans.[31, 66, 68] The response to programmed stimuli is consistent with regions of conduction delay within the atrium, and results of atrial mapping in animals during experimentally induced atrial flutter support this hypothesis.[6] In each of these arrhythmias, programmed stimulation has been used successfully in clinical practice to penetrate the reentrant circuit and terminate the tachycardia by rendering one limb refractory to the circulating wave front of activation.

In the setting of remote myocardial infarction, areas of anatomic or functional conduction block and slow conduction provide the substrate for reentry. Anisotropic conduction within the circuit may be affected by transmembrane potential characteristics but appears to be highly dependent on fiber orientation.[61, 62] Conduction transverse to the axis of parallel muscle fibers is slow because of the high effective resistivity caused by ingrowth of connective tissue and the relative paucity of

gap junctions. In contrast, conduction velocity along the length of muscle fibers is more rapid, which correlates with the increased distribution of gap junctions.[30] These observations suggest that the cycle length of VT depends on anatomic features of the reentrant circuit, while the morphology of the tachycardia reflects the exit site and subsequent wave front of activation. Penetration of the circuit by programmed electrical extrastimuli may result in greater conduction delay, entrainment or resetting of the tachycardia, or conduction block that terminates or modifies the reentrant circuit.[2, 22, 49]

Intracardiac shocks differ from paced stimuli quantitatively in the magnitude of electrical energy and qualitatively in that only single or very closely coupled successive shocks have been studied. Their efficacy appears to depend on the ability to depolarize elements of the reentrant circuit.[57] Shocks with energies less than 0.05 J delivered by right ventricular catheter electrodes produce immediate local depolarization, which propagates to distant myocardium as a wave front of activation that may or may not penetrate the reentrant circuit. As shown in Figure 21–11, shocks of intermediate energy depolarize a larger mass of myocardium, which may include elements of the reentrant circuit, thereby terminating subsequent wave fronts of activation within the circuit. We hypothesize that in other cases a shock may depolarize components of the circuit but alternative pathways remain capable of conduction. The rate of the tachycardia may accelerate or decelerate, depending on changes in the length of the circuit and the conduction velocity of its elements. Thus, reliable termination of VT may require high-energy shocks that reproducibly depolarize a larger mass of myocardium, including a critical portion of the reentrant circuit.

The rate of the tachycardia and the anatomic location of the reentrant circuit could be expected to influence the efficacy of QRS-synchronized shocks. Shocks of lower energy are less likely to penetrate distant elements of the reentrant circuit, and the timing of shocks may be especially critical to penetrate a "narrow gap" in VT of shorter cycle length. These factors may become less critical when shocks of high energy are employed because a larger mass of myocardium is depolarized.

The reliability of cardioversion is a difficult issue to resolve during clinical evaluations. Although cardioversion thresholds tend to remain relatively stable, energies that successfully terminate several episodes of VT may

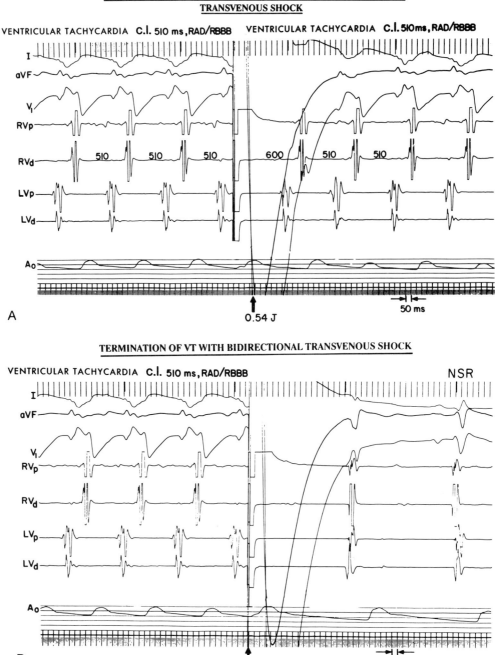

Figure 21–11. *A,* Catheter endocardial map of a 0.54-J bidirectional shock during VT. Surface electrocardiographic (ECG) recordings, along with right and left ventricular electrograms, are shown. Earliest activation of the left ventricular sites preceding the QRS complex is noted and precedes shock delivery. The subsequent QRS complex is delayed by 90 msec, with no change in the activation sequence. The following complexes show a return to the preshock rate and activation sequence. *B,* Catheter endocardial map of a 1.08-J bidirectional shock during VT. The recordings are identical with those in panel *A,* and the earliest site is unchanged. The shock produced immediate termination of VT with an escape ventricular beat and a return to sinus rhythm. RAD = right-axis deviation; RBBB = right bundle branch block; c.l. = cycle length; NSR = normal sinus rhythm; RVp = proximal right ventricle; RVd = distal right ventricle; LVp = proximal left ventricle; LVd = distal left ventricle; A = aortic pressure recording. (From Saksena S, Pantopoulos D, Hussain SM, et al: Mechanisms of ventricular tachycardia termination and acceleration during transvenous cardioversion as determined by cardiac mapping in man. Am Heart J 113:1495, 1987; with permission.)

subsequently fail and accelerate the arrhythmia to ventricular fibrillation.[44] The energy required for reproducible defibrillation has also been difficult to predict. The transition from ineffective to effective shock intensities is gradual, precluding definition of an absolute defibrillation threshold. The percentage of successful shocks as a function of shock energy forms a steep sigmoidal curve, for which the energy required for 100 per cent success is approximately twice that required for 50 per cent success.[52] If these principles are applicable to the termination of VT, it is likely that reliable cardioversion of VT over a wide range of cycle lengths will require shocks of relatively high energy.

EFFICACY OF PROGRAMMED STIMULATION AND RAPID PACING FOR TERMINATION OF TACHYARRHYTHMIAS

The use of programmed stimulation has been evaluated extensively for the treatment of sustained atrial and ventricular arrhythmias. Several modes of stimulation have been advocated. Figure 21–12 illustrates a few techniques, which can be further modified by programmable stimulators. Five fundamental pacing modalities or their variants are commonly used:

1. *Programmed extrastimuli (PES).* One or more PES are synchronized to the QRS complex, and the coupling interval of subsequent stimuli is automatically adjusted in programmed increments.

2. *Rapid burst pacing.* Bursts of extrastimuli are delivered at a fixed coupling interval. This is the most common mode employed in intensive care units or the electrophysiology laboratory for overdrive pacing of supraventricular or ventricular arrhythmias. Available temporary overdrive pacemakers or programmable stimulators may deliver these impulses asynchronously, but more sophisticated stimulators are highly programmable and synchronize the burst to the QRS complex.

3. *Burst plus PES.* A burst is followed by one or more PES. The coupling interval of the PES is adjusted incrementally.

4. *Adaptive burst.* The rate of stimulation is defined as a percentage of the tachycardia cycle length.

5. *Ramp pacing.* The coupling interval of extrastimuli is generally programmed from short to longer intervals.

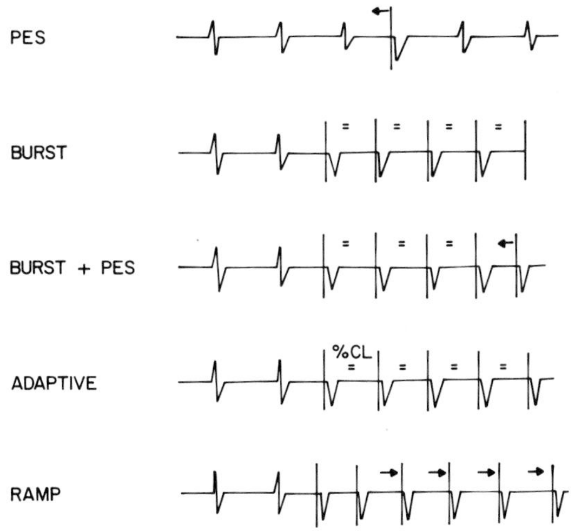

Rapid ventricular pacing terminates approximately 75 per cent of episodes of VT, but its efficacy diminishes for rapid tachycardias (cycle length < 300 msec), and the incidence of sustained acceleration is 3 to 15 per cent.[20, 21, 56, 65, 67, 76] There are few controlled data to compare the efficacy of one pacing mode with another, but available evidence indicates that burst pacing is more effective than the introduction of single PES.[67] Pacing at cycle lengths that are 75 to 80 per cent of the tachycardia cycle length is generally successful; however, the risk of accelerating the arrhythmia increases with more rapid pacing. The time required to terminate VT by burst pacing is in the range of 10 to 20 seconds. Because some patients may experience symptoms during this interval, it is desirable to identify more effective algorithms. An autoincremental algorithm has been described that delivers a synchronous burst of five pulses followed by pulses at increasing intervals. The initial intervals are automatically adjusted to the effective refractory period, which in turn is related in a nonlinear function to the cycle length of the tachycardia. The efficacy of this algorithm for termination of VT did not differ from burst pacing, but the time required to terminate VT was much shorter with autoincremental stimulation.[28]

Rapid atrial pacing is frequently used in the intensive care setting for the termination of atrial flutter. The pacing threshold is often high during the tachycardia, so stimuli of 10 to 20 mA may be required. The termination of atrial flutter is nearly always achieved by

Figure 21–12. Pacing modalities for termination of VT (see text). Vertical lines represent pacing stimuli. PES = programmed extrastimuli; CL = cycle length.

pacing for 5 to 20 seconds at rates 110 to 130 per cent of the spontaneous atrial flutter rate. Pacing at rates greater than 135 per cent of the atrial flutter rate generally precipitates atrial fibrillation. When pacing is performed from the high right atrium, successful interruption of atrial flutter is associated with a change from negative to positive polarity of atrial complexes in electrocardiographic leads II, III, and aV_F and distinguishes transient entrainment from successful overdrive suppression.[66]

Overdrive atrial pacing is also highly effective for the termination of AV nodal reentry and AV reentry.[21] Rapid atrial pacing, however, may induce atrial fibrillation and is contraindicated in patients with Wolff-Parkinson-White syndrome who are at risk of a malignant ventricular rate during episodes of atrial fibrillation. Burst or adaptive atrial pacing is generally successful for episodes of reentrant SVT, but sophisticated termination algorithms should be evaluated extensively in the electrophysiology laboratory or the telemetry unit before an antitachycardia device is implanted. Although burst ventricular pacing is very effective for terminating reentrant rhythms that require the AV node, it is not advised for a permanently implanted device because of the potential risk of inducing a sustained ventricular arrhythmia.

EFFICACY AND SAFETY OF TRANSVENOUS UNIDIRECTIONAL SHOCKS

Experience with the AICD has consistently demonstrated reliable termination of VT or ventricular fibrillation by 20- to 30-J shocks delivered by lead systems that incorporate one or more epicardial patches. This success with the AICD raises the issue of whether some ventricular arrhythmias can be terminated by low-energy shocks with nonepicardial lead systems. Potential advantages of this approach are that nonepicardial leads would facilitate implantation and reduce surgical morbidity and that low-energy shocks would be more easily tolerated by the patient and reduce demands on the capacitance of the pulse generator. Initial human studies confirmed that sustained VT could be terminated by transvenous shocks of widely ranging energies, and in selected individuals unidirectional shocks of less than 2 J delivered by an endocardial catheter were highly efficacious.[76] The first of a series of subsequent investigations compared the results of unidirectional shocks of low to intermediate energy using an endocardial catheter.[11] The percentage of episodes of sustained VT terminated by shocks with energies in the range of 0.03 to 2.20 J was 56 per cent, compared with 72 per cent for shocks of 0.5 to 10.0 J. Episodes of rapid VT were found to be more resistant to cardioversion, and a relatively high incidence of sustained acceleration (31 per cent) raised concerns about the long-term safety of low-to-intermediate energy shocks. Concurrent with these investigations, a clinical trial was conducted with the low-energy (0.2 to 2.0 J) Medtronic 7210 implantable transvenous cardioverter. Although the device was restricted to 29 patients with histories of stable episodes of relatively slow VT, four sudden deaths occurred during follow-up, and acceleration of VT was observed after a synchronized shock in two additional patients.[44, 77] Results of these studies suggested that shocks of higher energy or more effective current pathways were needed, especially in patients with rapid VT.

COMPARISON OF PACING AND LOW-ENERGY TRANSVENOUS CARDIOVERSION

The efficacy of rapid ventricular pacing and low-energy cardioversion for the termination of VT has been established in the laboratory and by long-term follow-up of patients with implanted antitachycardia devices. The advantage of pacing algorithms is that they are generally well tolerated, but they often require substantially more time than do transvenous shocks to terminate VT. The obvious disadvantage of shocks, however, is that they are painful and place greater demands on the capacitance of the pulse generator. Two studies have demonstrated comparable efficacy for termination of VT by rapid ventricular pacing and transvenous unidirectional shocks with energies of 0.01 to 5 J.[56, 67] A prospective, randomized, crossover study demonstrated rates of successful termination of VT of 83 per cent for low-energy (0.5 to 2.7 J) transvenous cardioversion and 80 per cent for rapid ventricular pacing using six asynchronous sequential bursts (10 and 15 paced stimuli at 90 per cent, 75 per cent, and 65 per cent of the VT cycle length). The concordance of these responses for similar episodes of VT was 78 per cent. Moreover, there was no difference in the incidence of sustained acceleration by cardioversion and rapid ventricular pacing (11 per cent versus 6 per cent). Subjective discomfort on the part of the patient was reported to be moderate to severe in 57 per cent of episodes treated by low-energy shocks. Patients seem to be particularly intolerant of shocks above 1 J. In comparison, rapid ventricular pacing was painless in all instances.[56] These results demonstrate comparable and concordant efficacy for rapid ventricular pacing and low-energy transvenous cardioversion; however, each may accelerate VT and thus requires the capability for high-energy cardioversion/defibrillation. Although both techniques are applicable to patients with slow VT, rapid ventricular pacing has the distinct advantage of being tolerated by the patient.

Transvenous cardioversion of supraventricular arrhythmias has attracted little interest. Limited experience in the treatment of atrial flutter, AV nodal reentry, and AV reentry indicates that pacing algorithms are more effective than transvenous shocks, engender less pain, and are less likely to induce atrial fibrillation. Moreover, once atrial fibrillation is induced, the energy required for cardioversion causes undue pain.[48] Thus, until there is further evidence to support the use of transvenous shocks, conventional transthoracic shocks are advised for the treatment of SVT that is refractory to medical therapy and pacing.

USE OF BIDIRECTIONAL SHOCKS FOR TERMINATION OF SUSTAINED VENTRICULAR ARRHYTHMIAS

The limitations of transvenous cardioversion and defibrillation by undirectional shocks have prompted investigators to examine the efficacy of bidirectional shocks using single or sequential pulses. Results of studies in animals and humans have shown a reduction in energy required for defibrillation when two current pathways are employed with epicardial lead configurations.[32, 33] A comparison of single with sequential bidirectional shocks in dogs demonstrated no significant difference in defibrillation thresholds. Of greater importance, electrode combinations with current pathways that included the interventricular septum required less energy to defibrillate than did shocks that did not include the septum.[7]

The hypothesis that a single transvenous shock with two current pathways (bidirectional) could increase the mass of myocardium depolarized and enhance the efficacy of cardioversion/defibrillation was recently evaluated

prospectively in patients with rapid VT (cycle length < 300 msec).[55] Unidirectional shocks were delivered by a Medtronic 6880 transvenous catheter, using the distal electrodes as the cathode and the proximal electrodes as the anode. Single bidirectional shocks were delivered by a triple electrode system composed of the Medtronic catheter and an R_2 cutaneous patch electrode with an area of 50 cm². The distal electrodes of the catheter formed the cathode, and the proximal catheter electrodes and R_2 patch were connected to form the anodes for bidirectional shocks. Energies of 2.7, 5.0, and 10.0 J were delivered with each lead system. When bidirectional shocks were administered, approximately 45 per cent of the total current was delivered through the right ventricular apex and R_2 patch electrodes. The mean energy required for successful cardioversion was lower in patients treated with bidirectional shocks than in those treated with unidirectional shocks; however, the overall success of cardioversion for rapid VT remained low, suggesting that higher energies were required.

Results of the preceding study led to the prospective evaluation of an algorithm that incorporated bidirectional shocks of higher energy.[41] Episodes of slow VT (cycle length > 300 msec) were first treated by bursts of asynchronous pacing. Episodes that were not terminated by pacing were exposed to three incremental bidirectional shocks (5, 15, and 25 J) synchronized to the right ventricular apical electrogram. The treatment algorithm for rapid VT (cycle length ≤ 300 msec), which omitted pacing, employed two incremental bidirectional shocks (15 J and 25 J) sequentially. This algorithm was successful in 96 per cent of episodes of slow VT and 83 per cent of episodes of rapid VT. Results at each step of the algorithm are summarized in Table 21–2. Of some concern, however, is that the incidence of VT acceleration or degeneration into ventricular fibrillation was 30 per cent with low (5 J) or intermediate (15 J) shocks. As shown in Figure 21–13, when similar episodes of VT were reinduced in these patients, the immediate delivery of a single 25-J bidirectional shock uniformly and reproducibly terminated the arrhythmia without acceleration. These results suggest that intermediate-energy shocks modify conduction, resulting in a substantial incidence of acceleration, but that shocks of higher energy prevent this complication by producing widespread high-degree conduction block within the reentrant circuit.

The limited efficacy of transvenous lead sys-

TABLE 21–2. CLINICAL EFFICACY AND SAFETY OF PRIMARY AND MODIFIED ELECTRICAL ALGORITHMS FOR VT TERMINATION*

TREATMENT MODE	N	SUCCESSFUL TERMINATIONS	FAILURES	ACCELERATION
Slow VT				
RVP	54	34 (63%)	20 (37%)	3 (5%)
5 J	15	7 (47%)	8 (53%)	7 (39%)
15 J	5	3 (60%)	2 (40%)	1 (13%)
25 J	2	2 (100%)	0 (0%)	0
25 J†	4	4 (100%)	0	0
Rapid VT				
15 J	40	30 (75%)	10 (25%)	10 (25%)
25 J	1	1 (100%)	0 (0%)	0
25 J†	8	8 (100%)	0	0
VF				
15 J	3	0 (0%)	3 (100%)	0
25 J	13	4 (31%)	9 (69%)	0

*Extent of efficacy for each therapeutic mode is shown in relation to the number of episodes of VT or VF for which termination was attempted.

†Designated secondary algorithm modified to eliminate accelerating shocks.

N = number of VT episodes to therapeutic mode; VF = ventricular fibrillation; RVP = rapid ventricular pacing.

From Lindsay BD, Saksena S, Rothbart S, et al: Prospective evaluation of a sequential pacing and high-energy shock algorithm for transvenous cardioversion in patients with ventricular tachycardia. Circulation 76:601, 1987; by permission of the American Heart Association, Inc.

tems for defibrillation remains problematic. In our experience, the success of bidirectional 25-J shocks for defibrillation is less than 40 per cent when the Medtronic 6880 catheter is used.[41, 54] Efforts are under way to improve the efficacy of transvenous defibrillation with alternative catheter electrode configurations and surface areas. Preliminary results with the Endotak-C (CPI) catheter offer promise for improved efficacy of defibrillation,[54, 58] and reliable long-term defibrillation thresholds (≤ 10 J) have been reported in one patient who had a nonepicardial lead system implanted.[53] In this individual, preoperative testing demon-

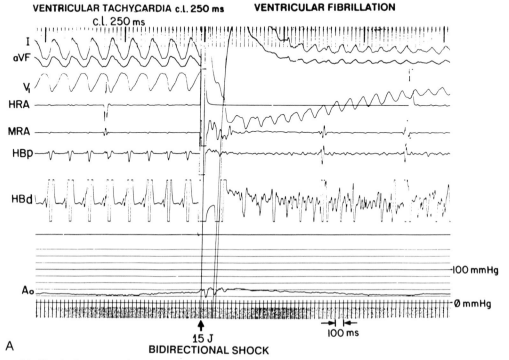

Figure 21–13. A, Representative electrograms from a patient with rapid VT (cycle length of 250 msec) in whom bidirectional 15-J shock induced ventricular fibrillation.

strated a defibrillation threshold of 20 J or less using single bidirectional shocks. At the time of implantation, the distal spring electrode of the catheter formed the cathode, and the anodes comprised the proximal spring and a submuscular patch (surface area of 28 cm^2). This lead system was used to deliver single bidirectional shocks and provided successful cardioversion over a period of 5 months. Although this approach requires further evalua-

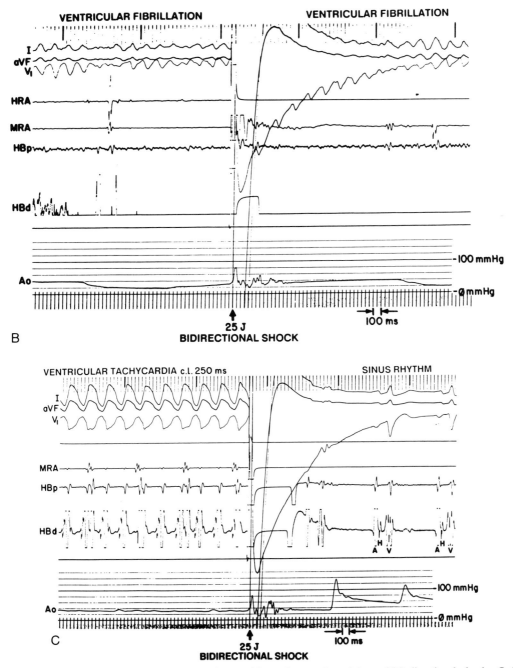

Figure 21–13 *Continued B,* Ventricular fibrillation could not be terminated by a 25-J directional shock. *C,* The termination algorithm was modified to eliminate the 15-J shock, and VT was reinduced; the arrhythmia was terminated with a single 25-J bidirectional shock. HRA = high right atrium; MRA = mid right atrium; HBd = distal His bundle; HBp = proximal His bundle; A = aorta; C.L. = cycle length. (From Lindsay BD, Saksena S, Rothbart ST, et al: Prospective evaluation of a sequential pacing and high-energy bidirectional shock algorithm for transvenous cardioversion in patients with ventricular tachycardia. Circulation 76:601, 1987; by permission of the American Heart Association, Inc.)

tion, it is likely that selected patients with low defibrillation thresholds will be candidates for transvenous cardioversion/defibrillation lead systems but that in others reliable defibrillation will necessitate implantation of one or more epicardial patches.

LONG-TERM SAFETY OF HIGH-ENERGY TRANSVENOUS SHOCKS

The long-term safety of a nonepicardial lead system depends not only on its efficacy for transvenous cardioversion/defibrillation but also on the direct cardiovascular effects of repeated discharges and the thrombogenic potential of an indwelling electrode catheter. These factors are particularly germane to systems that deliver high-energy shocks because the tissue response might adversely affect pacing or cardioversion/defibrillation thresholds. A recent study described the pathologic findings of 23 patients in whom the spring-patch electrode configuration was used with the AICD.[60] A large intravascular thrombus was associated with the spring electrode in four patients, and asymptomatic pulmonary emboli were discovered in two patients. An electrical injury resulting in fibrosis was observed in the superior vena cava of one patient who had undergone multiple defibrillations. Other patients who had undergone repeated defibrillation exhibited varying degrees of subepicardial fibrosis and myocyte necrosis beneath the epicardial patch. The myocardial mass affected was small (< 2 per cent), indicating that hemodynamic function would not be impaired by these changes. Other studies, which have shown that defibrillation thresholds of chronically implanted leads remain stable,[18, 38] suggest that the pathologic responses to high-energy shocks do not significantly affect the efficacy of arrhythmia termination.

Pathologic findings associated with nonepicardial lead systems are limited to a small number of patients observed over an interval of less than 2 weeks. Changes referable to the catheter have consisted of mural thrombi and a small region of subendocardial hemorrhage or myocardial necrosis at the cathode.[51, 76] Overall, the extent of myocardial damage produced by the catheter was minor and did not appear to be related to the number of shocks delivered. These changes would not be expected to have any hemodynamic sequelae. Similar cardiac alterations have been observed in animals subjected to repeated high-energy

shocks over several months. Myocardial necrosis and postnecrotic fibrosis induced by multiple shocks were mild. The damage was concentrated in the ventricular septum and right ventricular endocardium adjacent to the electrode. In some animals, fibrosis extended into the epicardium. There was no evidence of extracardiac damage, lead perforation, or pulmonary embolism.[64]

A twofold increase in the pacing threshold and a decrease in the amplitude of the ventricular electrogram have been observed immediately following cardioversion, with return to control values within 10 minutes.[75] Transient pacing threshold changes of this nature might compromise the patient's safety if the cardioversion/defibrillation system also served to provide chronotropic support for postcardioversion bradyarrhythmias, which occur with an incidence of approximately 3 per cent.[54] Recent clinical trials of the Endotak-C (CPI) catheter, however, demonstrated that within 2 minutes of the final defibrillation threshold testing, pacing thresholds, the amplitude of the ventricular electrogram, and impedance were unchanged from baseline values.[72] Differences in catheter design may account for these results. The Endotak-C catheter employs a cathode that is 4 mm proximal to the distal tip pacing electrode. Moreover, unidirectional shocks were delivered with the proximal catheter spring electrode serving as the anode. Therefore, the current of the defibrillating shock did not directly include the pacing or sensing electrode. An additional concern is that a chronic rise in pacing threshold might adversely affect the efficacy of pacing algorithms. Further study is required to determine the extent to which myocardial necrosis and fibrosis occur in the region of the cathode, whether this can be avoided by catheter design, or whether such changes affect chronic pacing and sensing thresholds.

The direct effects of shocks on cardiac function have been evaluated primarily in animals. When ventricular fibrillation is terminated within 15 to 30 seconds, two major responses are observed: (1) Cholinergic mechanisms mediate a chronotropic response characterized by periods of sinus node arrest and sinus bradycardia that are maximal within 20 seconds immediately after defibrillation, but sinus bradycardia may persist for several minutes; (2) an adrenergic response mediates an increase in blood pressure and cardiac output that returns to baseline within 5 minutes. These effects are more transient and of smaller magnitude when shocks are delivered during sinus rhythm, suggesting that parasympathetic and sympathetic reflexes are activated by hemodynamic changes associated with ventricular fibrillation.[50]

The response to defibrillation is affected by the intensity of shocks and the duration of ventricular fibrillation. Postdefibrillation bradyarrhythmias are more pronounced, ventricular arrhythmias are more commonly observed, and hemodynamic function is adversely affected by episodes of ventricular fibrillation that last longer than 45 seconds.[24, 25] Whether defibrillation thresholds are affected by episodes of shorter duration requires further study. Preliminary results in animals indicate that the energy required for successful defibrillation is higher at 15 to 30 seconds than at 5 seconds after the onset of ventricular fibrilltion,[5] but human studies have not confirmed this observation.[73]

Several considerations limit the intensity of shocks employed for defibrillation. The size of an implantable device is a practical constraint. Moreover, there is a range of optimal shock intensities beyond which the success of defibrillation is reduced and adverse effects such as sinus arrest and AV block become more pronounced.[26] Although many factors may affect the optimal intensity of shocks, the major determinants appear to be the pulse waveform, the lead configuration, and ventricular mass.[3, 7–9, 16, 47, 59, 63, 72]

In summary, shock intensities employed for transvenous cardioversion and defibrillation evoke mild tissue responses and rarely have major chronotropic or inotropic effects when energies in the range of 20 to 40 J are employed. The efficacy of cardioversion/defibrillation is not greatly affected by delays of 15 to 30 seconds, but longer episodes increase the defibrillation threshold and the incidence of adverse sequelae. The use of extremely high intensity shocks does not necessarily increase efficacy and is likely to exacerbate negative chronotropic and inotropic responses.

TRANSVENOUS CARDIOVERSION/ DEFIBRILLATION IN PERSPECTIVE

Pacing algorithms and transvenous cardioversion have established efficacy in the acute management of tachyarrhythmias and are applicable to selected patients with sustained ventricular arrhythmias who require implantable cardioverter/defibrillators. In such patients, electrophysiology studies can be used to delineate optimal lead systems and effective modes of electrical intervention. The selection of an arrhythmia termination algorithm ultimately depends on its efficacy, safety, and tolerance by the patient. Ideally, it will terminate VT of widely ranging cycle lengths promptly and reliably with low risk of acceleration. It should also be designed to conserve energy and extend the life of the pulse generator.

Results of laboratory and clinical investigations demonstrate that most episodes of relatively slow VT can be reliably terminated by pacing algorithms. The efficacy of low-energy shocks is comparable to that of pacing but requires more energy and is painful if more than 0.5 J is employed. It seems advisable to avoid the use of intermediate-energy shocks because of their limited efficacy, the risk of VT acceleration, and poor tolerance by the patient. Moreover, the acceleration of VT to ventricular fibrillation jeopardizes the safety of the patient and may require several high-energy shocks for defibrillation, which ultimately consumes more of the pulse generator's reserves. Whether protracted ventricular arrhythmias affect the defibrillation threshold requires further study.

High-energy single or sequential bidirectional shocks are safe and very effective for the termination of both slow and rapid VT, but they are painful and require a pulse generator with greater capacitance. The feasibility of transvenous defibrillation by high-energy bidirectional shocks has been demonstrated, but this approach will be limited to patients in whom reliable defibrillation has been confirmed by extensive preoperative testing. The effect of antiarrhythmic medications must also be considered prior to selecting a permanent lead system. In our experience, the use of concomitant antiarrhythmic medications often prolongs the cycle length of VT and facilitates its termination by rapid ventricular pacing,[41] but the effects of medications on defibrillation thresholds are diverse.[43] Accordingly, if an antiarrhythmic medication is required, defibrillation thresholds should be evaluated during treatment to determine which lead system provides an adequate margin of safety. This approach is particularly important for patients who receive amiodarone or encainide, which have been shown to increase the energy required for defibrillation.[19, 16]

Table 21–3 outlines an approach for the termination of VT that incorporates the preceding considerations. Relatively slow epi-

TABLE 21–3. APPROACH TO SELECTION OF TACHYCARDIA TERMINATION ALGORITHMS

I. Characterize spontaneous and induced ventricular tachyarrhythmias as slow VT (cycle length > 300 msec), rapid VT (cycle length ≤ 300 msec), or VF.
II. Determine hemodynamic stability during tachycardia.
III. Selection of algorithm:
    A. Slow VT
        1. Hemodynamically stable: adaptive burst or scanning pacing with high-energy (25 J), bidirectional shock backup.
        2. Hemodynamically unstable: limit adaptive pacing and follow sequentially with high-energy, bidirectional shocks.
    B. Rapid VT
        1. One or more high-energy, bidirectional shocks.
        2. Chronic therapy with antiarrhythmic medication may slow the rate of the tachycardia and facilitate termination by pacing.
    C. Ventricular fibrillation
        1. One or more high-energy, bidirectional shocks.

sodes of VT can often be terminated without discomfort by rapid ventricular pacing. The use of concomitant antiarrhythmic therapy may decrease the rate of more rapid episodes of VT and enhance the effect of pacing, thereby reducing the patient's exposure to high-energy shocks. Episodes of rapid VT or slow VT that are refractory to rapid ventricular pacing should be treated by a high-energy bidirectional shock, which is extremely effective and rarely accelerates VT. At the present, implantation of a cardioverter/defibrillator with nonepicardial leads is restricted to selected patients in whom reliable defibrillation has been demonstrated preoperatively. Ultimately, technical interventions are likely to reduce defibrillation thresholds and extend the applicability of this approach.

REFERENCES

1. Almendral JM, Gottlieb CD, Rosenthal ME, et al: Entrainment of ventricular tachycardia: Explanation for surface electrocardiographic phenomena by analysis of electrograms recorded within the tachycardia circuit. Circulation 77:569, 1988.
2. Almendral JM, Stamato NJ, Rosenthal ME, et al: Resetting response patterns during sustained ventricular tachycardia: Relationship to the excitable gap. Circulation 74:722, 1986.
3. Bardy GH, Steward RB, Ivey TD, et al: Intraoperative comparison of sequential-pulse and single-pulse defibrillation in candidates for automatic implantable defibrillators. Am J Cardiol 60:618, 1987.
4. Bigger JT, Goldreyer BN: The mechanism of supraventricular tachycardia. Circulation 42:673, 1970.
5. Black JN, Barbey JT, Echt DS: Ventricular fibrillation affects defibrillation [abstract]. J Am Coll Cardiol 9:142A, 1987.
6. Boineau JP, Schuessler RB, Mooney CR: Natural and evoked atrial flutter due to circus movement in dogs. Am J Cardiol 45:1167, 1980.
7. Chang MS, Inoue H, Kallok MJ, et al: Double and triple sequential shocks reduce ventricular defibrillation threshold in dogs with and without myocardial infarction. J Am Coll Cardiol 8:1393, 1986.
8. Chapman PD, Sagar KB, Wetherbee JN, et al: Relationship of left ventricular mass to defibrillation threshold for the implantable defibrillator: A combined clinical and animal study. Am Heart J 114:274, 1987.
9. Chapman PD, Vetter JW, Souza JJ, et al: Comparative efficacy of monophasic and biphasic waveforms for non-thoracotomy canine defibrillation [abstract]. PACE 11:497, 1988.
10. Chen PS, Wolf PD, Claydon FJ, et al: The potential gradient field created by epicardial defibrillation electrodes in dogs. Circulation 74:626, 1986.
11. Ciccone JM, Saksena S, Shah Y, et al: A prospective randomized study of the clinical efficacy and safety of transvenous cardioversion for termination of ventricular tachycardia. Circulation 71:571, 1985.
12. Coumel P: Junctional reciprocating tachycardias: The permanent and paroxysmal forms of A-V nodal reciprocating tachycardias. J Electrocardiol 8:79, 1975.
13. DeBakker JMT, van Capella FJJ, Janse MJ, et al: Reentry as a cause of ventricular tachycardia in patients with chronic ischemic heart disease: Electrophysiologic and anatomic correlation. Circulation 77:589, 1988.
14. Den Dulk K, Kersschot IE, Brugada P, et al: Is there a universal antitachycardia pacing mode? Am J Cardiol 57:950, 1986.
15. Denes P, Wu D, Dhingra RC, et al: Demonstration of dual A-V nodal pathways in patients with supraventricular tachycardia. Circulation 48:549, 1973.
16. Dixon EG, Tang ASL, Wolf PD, et al: Improved defibrillation thresholds with large contoured epicardial electrodes and biphasic waveforms. Circulation 76:1176, 1987.
17. Echt DS, Armstrong K, Schmidt P, et al: Clinical experience, complications, and survival in 70 patients with the automatic implantable cardioverter/defibrillator. Circulation 71:289, 1985.
18. Fain ES, Billingham M, Winkle RA: Internal cardiac defibrillation: Histopathology and temporal stability of defibrillation energy requirements. J Am Coll Cardiol 9:631, 1987.
19. Fain ES, Dorian P, Davy JM, et al: Effects of encainide and its metabolites on energy requirements for defibrillation. Circulation 73:1334, 1986.
20. Fisher JD, Mehra R, Furman S: Termination of ventricular tachycardia with bursts of rapid ventricular pacing. Am J Cardiol 41:94, 1978.
21. Fisher JD, Johnston DR, Kim SG, et al: Implantable pacers for tachycardia termination: Stimulation techniques and long-term efficacy. PACE 9:1325, 1986.
22. Fisher JD, Kim SG, Matas JA, et al: Pacing for ventricular tachycardia. PACE 7:1278, 1984.
23. Gallagher JJ, Pritchett ELC, Sealy WC, et al: The pre-excitation syndrome. Prog Cardiovasc Dis 20:285, 1978.
24. Geuze RH, de Vente J: Arrhythmias and left ventricular function after defibrillation during acute myocardial infarction in the intact dog. Am Heart J 106:292, 1983.
25. Geuze RH, de Vente J: Effects of duration of ventricular fibrillation and heart massage on hemodynamic responses after defibrillation in dogs. Cardiovasc Res 17:282, 1983.

26. Gold JH, Schuder JC, Stoeckle H, et al: Transthoracic ventricular defibrillation in the 100 kg calf with unidirectional rectangular pulses. Circulation 56:745, 1977.
27. Hinds M, Ayers GM, Bourland JD, et al: Comparison of the efficacy of defibrillation with the damped sine and constant-tilt current waveforms in the intact animal. Med Instrum 21:92, 1987.
28. Holley LK, Cooper M, Uther JB, et al: Safety and efficacy of pacing for ventricular tachycardia. PACE 9:1316, 1986.
29. Horowitz LN, Josephson ME, Harken AM: Epicardial and endocardial activation during sustained ventricular tachycardia in man. Circulation 61:1227, 1980.
30. Hoyt RH, Cohen HL, Saffitz JE: Structural basis for anisotropic conduction in myocardium [abstract]. Circulation 76 [Suppl IV]:241, 1987.
31. Inoue H, Matsuo H, Takayanagi K, et al: Clinical and experimental studies of the effects of atrial extrastimulation and rapid pacing on atrial flutter cycle: Evidence of macroreentry with an excitable gap. Am J Cardiol 48:623, 1981.
32. Jones DL, Klein GJ, Guiraudon GM, et al: Internal cardiac defibrillation in man: Pronounced improvement with sequential pulse delivery to two different lead orientations. Circulation 73:484, 1986.
33. Jones DL, Sohla A, Bourland JD, et al: Internal ventricular defibrillation with sequential pulse countershock in pigs: Comparison with single pulse and effects of pulse separation. PACE 10:497, 1987.
34. Josephson ME, Horowitz LN, Farshidi A: Continuous local electrical activity: A mechanism of recurrent ventricular tachycardia. Circulation 57:659, 1978.
35. Josephson ME, Horowitz LN, Farshidi A, et al: Recurrent sustained ventricular tachycardia. 1. Mechanisms. Circulation 57:431, 1978.
36. Josephson ME, Horowitz LN, Farshidi A, et al: Recurrent sustained ventricular tachycardia. 2. Endocardial mapping. Circulation 57:440, 1978.
37. Josephson ME, Horowitz LN, Farshidi A, et al: Sustained ventricular tachycardia: Evidence for protected localized reentry. Am J Cardiol 42:416, 1978.
38. Kallok MJ, Olson WH, Marcaccini SJ, et al: Temporal stability of sequential pulse defibrillation threshold. PACE 9:1361, 1986.
39. Lepeschkin E, Jones JL, Rush S, et al: Local potential gradients as a unifying measure for thresholds of stimulation, standstill, tachyarrhythmia and fibrillation appearing after strong capacitor discharges. Adv Cardiol 21:268, 1978.
40. Lerman BB, Halperin HR, Tsitlik JE, et al: Relationship between canine transthoracic impedance and defibrillation threshold: Evidence for current-based defibrillation. J Clin Invest 80:797, 1987.
41. Lindsay BD, Saksena S, Rothbart ST, et al: Prospective evaluation of a sequential pacing and high-energy bidirectional shock algorithm for transvenous cardioversion in patients with ventricular tachycardia. Circulation 76:601, 1987.
42. Linos DA, Mucha P, van Heerden JA: Subclavian vein. Mayo Clin Proc 55:315, 1980.
43. Marinchak RA, Friehling TD, Kline RA, et al: Effect of antiarrhythmic drugs on defibrillation threshold: Case report of an adverse effect on mexiletine and review of the literature. PACE 11:7, 1988.
44. Miles WM, Prystowsky EN, Heger JJ, et al: The implantable transvenous cardioverter: Long-term efficacy and reproducible induction of ventricular tachycardia. Circulation 74:518, 1986.
45. Miller FA, Holmes DR, Gersh BJ, et al: Permanent

transvenous pacemaker implantation via the subclavian vein. Mayo Clin Proc 55:309, 1980.
46. Mirowski M, Reid PR, Winkle RA, et al: Mortality in patients with implanted automatic defibrillators. Ann Intern Med 98:585, 1983.
47. Nathan AW, Barin ES, Elstob JE, et al: Defibrillation thresholds using biphasic waveforms and contoured epicardial patches in man [abstract]. PACE 11:498, 1988.
48. Nathan AW, Bexton RS, Spurrell RAJ, et al: Internal transvenous low energy cardioversion for the treatment of cardiac arrhythmias. Br Heart J 52:377, 1984.
49. Okumura K, Olshansky B, Henthorn RW, et al: Demonstration of the presence of slow conduction during sustained ventricular tachycardia in man: Use of transient entrainment of the tachycardia. Circulation 75:369, 1987.
50. Pansegran DG, Abboud FM: Hemodynamic effects of ventricular defibrillation. J Clin Invest 49:282, 1970.
51. Perkins GD, Klein GJ, Silver MD, et al: Cardioversion and defibrillation using a catheter electrode: Myocardial damage assessed at autopsy. PACE 10:800, 1987.
52. Rattes MF, Jones DL, Sharma AD, et al: Defibrillation threshold: A simple and quantitative estimate of the ability to defibrillate. PACE 10:70, 1987.
53. Saksena S, Parsonnet V: Implantation of a cardioverter/defibrillator without thoracotomy using a triple electrode system. JAMA 259:69, 1988.
54. Saksena S, Lindsay BD, Parsonnet V: Developments for future implantable cardioverters and defibrillators. PACE 10:1342, 1987.
55. Saksena S, Calvo RA, Pantopoulos D, et al: A prospective evaluation of single and dual current pathways for transvenous cardioversion in rapid ventricular tachycardia. PACE 10:1130, 1987.
56. Saksena S, Chandran P, Shah Y, et al: Comparative efficacy of transvenous cardioversion and pacing in patients with sustained ventricular tachycardia: A prospective, randomized, crossover study. Circulation 72:153, 1985.
57. Saksena S, Pantopoulos, D, Hussain SM et al: Mechanisms of ventricular tachycardia termination and acceleration during transvenous cardioversion as determined by cardiac mapping in man. Am Heart J 113:1495, 1987.
58. Saksena S, Parsonnet V, Pantopoulos D, et al: Transvenous cardioversion and defibrillation of ventricular tachyarrhythmias using bidirectional shocks: Acute feasibility studies and chronic device implant [abstract]. Circulation 76 [Suppl IV]:311, 1987.
59. Schuder JC, McDaniel WC, Stoeckle H: Defibrillation of 100 kg calves with asymmetrical, bidirectional, rectangular pulses. Cardiovasc Res 18:419, 1984.
60. Singer I, Hutchins GM, Mirowski M, et al: Pathologic findings related to the lead system and repeated defibrillations in patients with the automatic implantable cardioverter-defibrillator. J Am Coll Cardiol 10:382, 1987.
61. Spach MS, Miller WT, Dolber PC, et al: The functional role of structural complexities in the propagation of depolarization in the atrium of the dog: Cardiac conduction disturbances due to discontinuities of effective axial resistivity. Circ Res 50:175, 1982.
62. Spach MS, Miller WT, Geslowitz DB, et al: The discontinuous nature of propagation in normal canine cardiac muscle: Evidence of recurrent discontinuities of intracellular resistance that affect membrane currents. Circ Res 48:39, 1981.

63. Troup PJ, Chapman DP, Olinger GN, et al: The implanted defibrillator: Relation of defibrillating lead configuration and clinical variables to defibrillation threshold. J Am Coll Cardiol 6:1315, 1985.

64. Van Vleet JF, Tacker WA, Bourland JD, et al: Cardiac damage in dogs with chronically implanted automatic defibrillator electrode catheters and given four episodes of multiple shocks. Am Heart J 106:300, 1983.

65. Waldecker B, Brugada P, Zehender M, et al: Importance of modes of electrical termination of ventricular tachycardia for the selection of implantable antitachycardia devices. Am J Cardiol 57:150, 1986.

66. Waldo AL, MacLean WAH, Karp RB, et al: Entrainment and interruption of atrial flutter with atrial pacing: Studies in man following open heart surgery. Circulation 56:737, 1977.

67. Waspe LE, Kim SG, Matos JA, et al: Role of a catheter lead system for transvenous countershock and pacing during electrophysiologic tests: An assessment of the usefulness of catheter shocks for terminating ventricular tachyarrhythmias. Am J Cardiol 52:477, 1983.

68. Watson RM, Josephson ME: Atrial flutter. I. Electrophysiologic substrates and modes of initiation and termination. Am J Cardiol 45:732, 1980.

69. Wellens HJJ, Düren DR, Lie KI: Observations on mechanisms of ventricular tachycardia in man. Circulation 54:237, 1976.

70. Wellens HJJ, Lie KI, Düren DR: Further observations on ventricular tachycardia as studied by electrical stimulation of the heart. Circulation 39:647, 1974.

71. Wellens HJJ, Bar FHWM, Farre J, et al: Initiation and termination of ventricular tachycardia by supraventricular stimuli. Am J Cardiol 46:567, 1980.

72. Winkle RA, Bach SM, Mead RH, et al: Comparison of defibrillation efficacy in humans using a new catheter and superior vena cava spring–left ventricular patch electrodes. J Am Coll Cardiol 11:365, 1988.

73. Winkle RA, Mead HR, Ruder MA, et al: Defibrillation efficacy in man after 5 vs 15 seconds of ventricular fibrillation [abstract]. J Am Coll Cardiol 11:18A, 1988.

74. Wu D, Denes P: Mechanisms of paroxysmal supraventricular tachycardia. Arch Intern Med 135:437, 1975.

75. Yee R, Jones DL, Klein GJ: Pacing threshold changes after transvenous catheter countershock. Am J Cardiol 53:503, 1984.

76. Yee R, Zipes DP, Gulamhusein S, et al: Low energy countershock using an intravascular catheter in an acute cardiac care setting. Am J Cardiol 50:1124, 1982.

77. Zipes DP: Electrical treatment of tachycardia. Circulation 75[Suppl III]:190, 1987.

22

DIAGNOSTIC EVALUATION OF THE PROSPECTIVE ANTITACHYCARDIA DEVICE PATIENT

HELMUT KLEIN *and* SANJEEV SAKSENA

Management of patients with tachyarrhythmias can be a difficult and delicate task. These patients undergo prolonged diagnostic procedures, decision making for selecting the optimal therapeutic approach is difficult, and assessment of an effective treatment often remains debatable. It is not uncommon that two patients who demonstrate the identical type of electrophysiologic disorder might need completely different therapeutic approaches owing to a different underlying cardiac disease, different physical or psychologic condition, and—most important—a different prognosis. There is continuing progress in the field of pharmacologic as well as nonpharmacologic treatment modalities. However, the risk of the uncontrolled electrical disorder has to be compared with the risk and disability involved in a certain treatment, especially when the invasive and nonpharmacologic approaches are recommended. Advances in electronic engineering currently have resulted in new treatment modalities that require specialized knowledge and training of the treating physician. Within individual health care systems, the treating physician has to perform a cost-benefit and risk analysis, including considerations limited not only to the selection of the optimal device but also to the preliminary diagnostic procedures and clinical follow-up needs of these implanted electronic devices. When choosing a therapeutic approach, the physician must always consider the possibility of inefficacy and prospectively discuss alternative therapies with the patient. Alternatives could include a completely different treatment

option or a combination of treatment modalities.

Major objectives for an initial diagnostic evaluation of a prospective patient who may receive an antitachycardia device include rational selection of diagnostic procedures for the specific arrhythmia under evaluation (e.g., the electrophysiologic evaluation), as well as other relevant techniques and procedures that are needed to assess the underlying disease process. The major link between both routes of investigation is the clinical history and physical examination of the patient. The following text will initially discuss the various steps necessary for the diagnostic evaluation of a patient leading to the implantation of an antitachycardia device. These steps include assessment of clinical signs and symptoms, description of the noninvasive and invasive studies to document the status of the underlying disease, and, finally, discussion of the various methods of electrophysiologic evaluation necessary for the type, programming, and correct function of an implanted electrical device.[21] Diagnostic evaluation of problems during the follow-up of an implantable antitachycardia device will be largely addressed in subsequent chapters (see Chapters 24 and 25) but will be alluded to in relevant sections of this chapter.

CLINICAL EVALUATION

Clinical evaluation of a patient who is being considered for an antitachycardia device commences with a detailed history of the patient

439

and a careful physical examination. Information related to functional status and underlying heart disease and presence of heart failure must be elicited. The majority of patients with supraventricular tachyarrhythmias have no organic heart disease, whereas episodes of sustained ventricular tachycardia (VT) or ventricular fibrillation (VF) rarely occur in this setting. Therefore, in supraventricular tachycardia (SVT) the clinical history is often free of any specific symptoms related to chronic disease and generally commences with the onset of paroxysmal episodes of tachycardia.

These episodes occur from childhood and often remain undetected during youth sometimes, even if they exist as an incessant form. They become overt when the individual starts to complain of palpitations, presyncope, syncope, dyspnea, chest discomfort, or sometimes even angina pectoris. It is important for the physician to listen to and carefully interpret the wide variation of clinical symptoms associated with these tachycardia episodes. Although it is generally accepted that SVT is hemodynamically better tolerated than tachycardias originating in the ventricle, distinction between

TYPE I A-V NODAL REENTRY

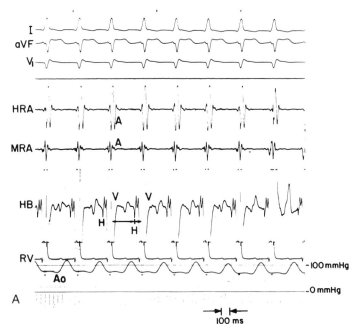

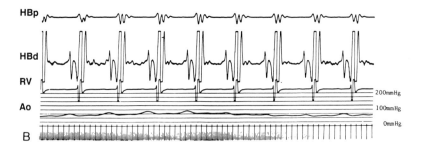

Figure 22–1. Hemodynamic status of two patients during identical supraventricular tachycardias (SVTs). *A* shows atrioventricular (AV) nodal reentrant tachycardia with a rate of 155 beats per minute of the common type (type I), with normal arterial blood pressure (Ao) during the episode. This patient had no hypotensive symptoms and no organic heart disease. *B* shows type I AV nodal reentrant tachycardia at a rate of 160 beats per minute, with hypotension and near-syncope. This patient had frequent symptomatic tachycardia episodes and underlying dilated cardiomyopathy. Note that the paper speed differs in each panel but that each elongated bar represents 50-msec intervals. Electrocardiographic (ECG) leads = standard leads I, aV_F; HRA = high right atrium; MRA = mid right atrium; HB = His bundle; p = proximal; d = distal; RV = right ventricular electrogram; Ao = aortic pressure; CL = cycle length; AV = atrioventricular.

SVT and VT exclusively by means of hemo-dynamic tolerance of the tachycardia is impossible. Tolerance of a tachycardia episode depends upon ventricular rate and preexisting ventricular function (see Chapter 23B). Similar tachycardia episodes can have markedly different hemodynamic consequences (Fig. 22–1). Several other important questions concerning the tachycardia episodes have to be answered. How often does the tachycardia occur? How long does the tachycardia usually last? Which of the symptoms that accompany the tachycardia initiate the arrhythmia? Often, patients with tachycardia feel chest discomfort or anginal symptoms during the tachycardia, suggesting concomitant ischemia. However, coronary angiography may still show normal coronary arteries without evidence of spasm. It is of further importance to know the clinical events triggering the episodes of tachycardia. Does the tachycardia occur during the day or night, with exercise or at rest? A circadian variation in the frequency of sudden cardiac death has been suggested, with a high frequency in early morning hours. Unfortunately, in the majority of cases the onset of the tachycardia remains unpredictable, so that protective or prophylactic limitations in activity or behavior will not be effective. SVTs can be accompanied by other symptoms, such as polyuria.

In more than two thirds of patients with VT, a history of coronary artery disease and prior myocardial infarction can be elicited. The time interval between the acute infarction and the first episode of tachycardia shows great variability. However, after a second infarction, the likelihood of future VT episodes will increase enormously. It has been demonstrated that 15 per cent of patients with prior myocardial infarctions will develop VT within a 5-year

period after infarction.[2] Empirically, it appears that extensive myocardial injury results in a higher likelihood of inducing sustained VT in the electrophysiology laboratory or manifesting a spontaneous episode of VT. Another frequent clinical finding is the observation that VT associated with coronary artery disease often occurs independently of physical exercise, whereas VT without coronary disease—for example, VT in arrhythmogenic dysplasia of either the right or the left ventricle—can be provoked by vigorous exercise. The role of ischemia as a trigger mechanism for VT needs diagnostic evaluation. Occasionally, one can elicit signs or symptoms of ischemia at the beginning of an arrhythmogenic event.[9] However, when the patient complains of angina or chest pain immediately preceding the tachycardia, due consideration should be given to evaluate the status of the coronary arteries and to abolish ischemia by appropriate means prior to or at the same time as antitachycardia device implantation. Figure 22–2 shows an example of ischemia-induced ventricular tachyarrhythmia documented in a patient with Prinzmetal's angina during cardiac catheterization. Treatment of ischemia with calcium channel antagonists resolved this arrhythmia.

It is also obvious that the autonomic nervous system plays an important role in the development of SVT and VT. The exact mechanism of its influence either on the arrhythmogenic substrate or on the trigger mechanism of the arrhythmia is still a matter of some debate. It is particularly difficult for the clinician to understand why some patients in a particular phase of their disease may have frequent episodes of VT and thereafter—even without antiarrhythmic treatment—will be free of tachycardia episodes for months or years before they have frequent and recurrent tachycardia

Figure 22–2. Ischemia-induced ventricular tachycardia (VT) is demonstrated in this patient with documented Prinzmetal's angina and coronary spasm recorded at cardiac catheterization. Two telemetric ECG recordings that are not continuous are shown. The top panel shows development of progressive ST elevation followed by the appearance of nonsustained VT. The lower panel recorded a few seconds later shows development of monomorphic sustained VT in the same patient associated with anginal symptoms followed by cardiac arrest. VT = ventricular tachycardia; V_2 = standard ECG lead.

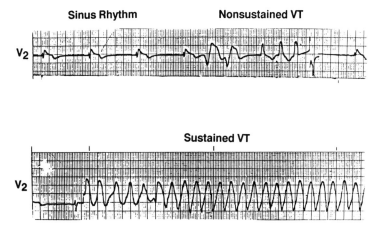

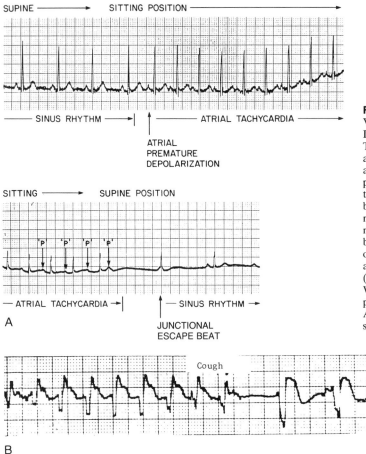

Figure 22–3. Termination of SVT and VT by unusual physical maneuvers. *A,* Initiation of SVT with change in posture. The sitting position results in a premature atrial depolarization with the onset of atrial tachycardia. Resumption of the supine posture results in termination of the tachycardia with an escape junctional beat. Note that termination of the atrial mechanism occurs at this time. *B,* Termination of monomorphic sustained VT by a cough. This was reproducibly demonstrated in this patient. Both maneuvers are associated with autonomic reflexes. (*A* from Saksena S, Siegel P, Rathyen W.: Electrophysiologic mechanisms in postural supraventricular tachycardia. Am Heart J 106:152, 1983; with permission.)

episodes. There is little doubt that psychologic stress can mediate the onset of ventricular arrhythmias or may turn solitary benign ventricular ectopic beats into life-threatening trigger mechanisms for sustained tachyarrhythmias. On occasion, specific autonomic stimuli or physical maneuvers with reflex autonomic effects will interrupt tachycardia, especially SVT. Figure 22–3 shows two uncommon observations of physical maneuvers with reflex autonomic consequences. Clinical evaluation should seek out modes of onset and termination of spontaneous tachycardia.

Modes of therapy selected for a tachycardia can be greatly influenced by the clinical situation during the tachycardia episode. Therefore, thorough assessment of the clinical status during tachycardia, as well as at its onset, is of great value. Patients who feel faint or demonstrate loss of consciousness at the very beginning of a tachycardia are poor candidates for patient- or physician-activated antitachycardia devices. These patients need immediate arrhythmia termination by an automatic defi-

brillating or cardioverting device. Yet another major clinical problem for a patient with an implanted antitachycardia device can be the hemodynamic status immediately after termination of the arrhythmia. Patients with poor ventricular function or bradyarrhythmias can have persistent hypotension after termination of the tachycardia. This may lead to further electrical instability and may result in recurrent tachycardia episodes. Another issue is the stability of the cardiac rhythm that appears after shock delivery. Some patients may need pacing for rate support during postconversion bradyarrhythmias. Finally, the psychologic impact of electrical therapy and permanent device implantation must be assessed in each patient.

Thus, assessment of the clinical history and a thorough physical examination are important elements in selecting appropriate antitachycardia device therapy. These considerations, taken together with other noninvasive and invasive diagnostic procedures, bear on the question of prognosis. The prognosis of the patient and his or her expected quality of life must guide the decision for a prospective recipient of an antitachycardia device and selection of therapeutic approach. Younger patients with severe ventricular dysfunction and an expected long-term survival of less than 2 years are candidates for future cardiac transplantation. If this is not feasible for a variety of reasons, antitachycardia device therapy may or may not be an appropriate substitute in all patients. Such therapy in an inappropriately selected patient may prolong suffering without significantly improving long-term survival or quality of life.

NONINVASIVE LABORATORY EVALUATIONS

Resting Electrocardiogram

Intracardiac recordings during electrophysiologic studies are widely used to analyze the type and origin of a tachycardia. However, the standard 12-lead electrocardiogram at rest as well as during tachycardia episodes is still the most important clinical tool for the noninvasive evaluation of the patient with tachycardia. The clinical usefulness of the standard resting electrocardiogram for patients with SVT, especially the Wolff-Parkinson-White syndrome, has been demonstrated by many authors.[18] In addition to the presence of a delta wave during sinus rhythm, which indicates an antegradely conducting accessory pathway, an algorithm for accessory pathway localization, based on division of accessory pathway locations into left lateral, right lateral, posteroseptal, and anteroseptal, has been reported (Fig. 22–4A).[10, 23, 24] Its clinical usefulness still needs to be proved and cannot replace a thorough electrophysiologic study, particularly when a surgical approach is indicated. However, it may well be helpful to assess the preoperative risk of the surgical approach, especially when combined with additional underlying diseases or malformations of the heart. For example, a significantly higher risk of complete atrioventricular (AV) block exists with resection of septal pathways. Such an algorithm has its limitations, especially with multiple accessory pathways and when a preexisting bundle branch block configuration of the QRS complex is present. Electrocardiographic recordings in the Wolff-Parkinson-White syndrome demonstrating atrial fibrillation or intermittent preexcitation can be used for identification of the patient at high or low risk of sudden death,

respectively (Fig. 22–4B). Development of bundle branch block configuration during SVT can lead to further assessment of the location of the accessory pathway. Prolongation of the tachycardia cycle length with functional bundle branch block suggests the presence of an accessory pathway ipsilateral to the site of bundle branch block (Fig. 22–5). Accessory pathway location is of particular importance when initiating SVT in the laboratory or defining the site of electrode placement for electrical termination of SVT by implantable devices.

The standard electrocardiogram is also extremely helpful in defining the underlying disease in a patient with VT. Large Q waves in the inferior limb leads will point to a scar in the inferior part of the left ventricle. Deep and broad Q waves within the precordial leads and a complete or partial loss of the R wave indicate a large anterolateral infarction, which is frequently accompanied by poor ventricular function and easily inducible VT. In patients with unexplained recurrent syncope but electrocardiographic patterns suggestive of a cardiomyopathy of either the hypertrophic or the dilated type, the cause of syncope might still be VT or VF, despite failure to induce ventricular arrhythmias with programmed stimulation in the catheterization laboratory.

Patients with sustained VT in the presence of normal coronary arteries and normal regional wall motion in the left ventricle can demonstrate intermittent or permanent T-wave inversions in the right precordial leads. These findings are highly suspicious for arrhythmogenic right ventricular disease with lipofibromatosis in the right ventricle. Catheter mapping and intraoperative mapping procedures have demonstrated that circumscribed areas of lipofibromatosis represent the arrhythmogenic milieu for the VT. The standard electrocardiographic recordings of these patients sometimes show tiny late deflections at the end of the QRS complex (Fig. 22–6). They were called epsilon waves by Fontaine and most likely represent the area of slow conduction. T-wave inversions can also be found in patients with VT and mitral valve prolapse, indicating similar myocardial alterations with lipofibromatosis of the inferobasal part of the left ventricle. This finding could explain why patients with mitral valve prolapse can develop sustained VT originating at the inferobasal ventricle. Malformation of the mitral valve alone cannot explain these episodes of sustained VT.

CONTROL

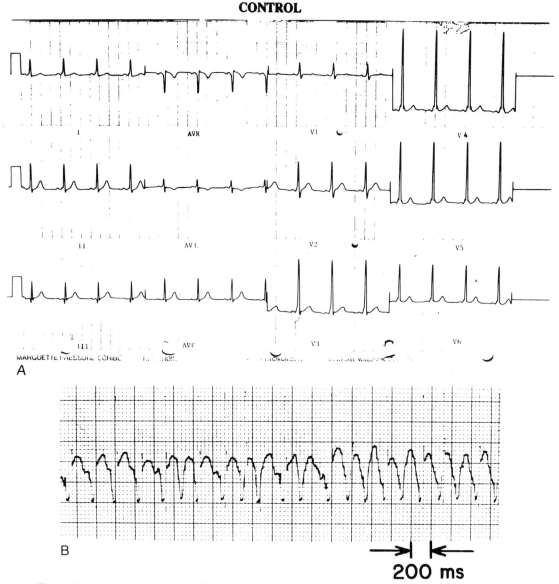

Figure 22–4. *A,* Resting 12-lead ECG recorded from a patient with Wolff-Parkinson-White syndrome. An abbreviated PR interval with a prominent delta wave is noted. ECG criteria suggest the presence of a left lateral accessory pathway. This was subsequently confirmed intraoperatively. *B,* Recording of atrial fibrillation (AF) in the patient referred to in *A*. Rapid antegrade accessory bypass tract conduction results in rapid ventricular rates and hemodynamic collapse with a cardiac arrest.

Evaluation of the QT interval in the standard electrocardiogram is important in cases of rapid polymorphic tachycardia, that is, the type referred to as *torsades de pointes*. The QT interval is significantly prolonged in the idiopathic long QT syndrome and is accompanied by life-threatening tachycardia episodes, which are provoked by mental or physical stress. QT interval prolongation can also be encountered during antiarrhythmic drug therapy, especially with quinidine or other type

I drugs, and may be associated with an increased risk of VF. Recent data have demonstrated that left ventricular dysfunction, together with the antiarrhythmic drug treatment, may predispose to such fibrillation episodes.[16] In rare instances of patients with cardiac arrest and documented and refractory *torsades de pointes* tachycardia without reversible predisposing factors, implantation of an automatic cardioverter/defibrillator may be indicated and has been performed. However, a precise and

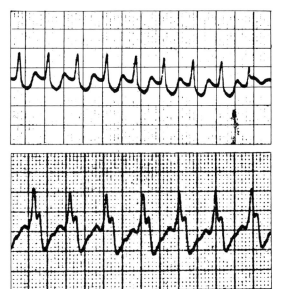

Figure 22–5. Standard ECG lead II recording in a patient with known Wolff-Parkinson-White syndrome and documented AV reentrant tachycardia. The top panel shows reciprocating tachycardia with a narrow QRS complex and a cycle length of 320 msec. The lower panel shows an ECG recording taken at another time during the same tachycardia episode that is now associated with a wide QRS complex with a cycle length of 390 msec. Electrocardiographically, this was documented to have a QRS pattern of left bundle branch block. This increase in tachycardia cycle length with left bundle branch block was ascribed to the presence of a left lateral accessory pathway involved in the retrograde limb of the AV reentrant tachycardia. Ipsilateral bundle branch block resulted in prolongation of the tachycardia circuit with slowing of the tachycardia cycle length.

thorough analysis of the tachycardia event is mandatory, since invasive electrophysiologic testing in these cases is not normally helpful. The potential for a proarrhythmic effect of drug therapy has to be considered carefully when a combination of device and drug therapy is attempted. Frequent high-energy discharges of an implantable cardioverter/defibrillator might actually be caused by the proarrhythmic effect of the drug and might not occur in its absence despite the inherent electrical disorder.

The 12-lead electrocardiogram is of great diagnostic value when recorded during an actual tachycardia episode. Several findings help to distinguish between SVT with a widened QRS complex (Fig. 22–7) and VT.[35] Heart rate and regularity of the tachycardia are not reliable parameters to distinguish these rhythms. However, capture and fusion beats, as well as a QRS duration of more than 0.14 second, strongly support the diagnosis of VT. Other important signs are the QRS axis in the frontal plane, which often shows a superior axis in

patients with VT. Left bundle branch block pattern complexes have also been reported to support a diagnosis of VT. Despite careful electrocardiographic examination, distinguishing between VT and SVT remains difficult.[1] Furthermore, the mechanism of SVT may be difficult to elucidate from electrocardiographic recordings, as QRS complex configurations and modes of initiation and termination may be identical with different reentrant rhythms (Fig. 22–8). It has even been suggested that a history of myocardial infarction may be of greater value in making this distinction.[1]

The configuration of the QRS in leads V_1 and V_6 may help to localize the origin of VT. A concordant positive QRS complex from V_1 to V_6 points to an origin at the posterobasal area of the left ventricle, whereas a concordant negative QRS pattern in V_1 to V_6 indicates that the origin of the tachycardia is at the anteroapical part of the left ventricle. Tachycardias with right bundle branch block configuration, monophasic or biphasic QRS complexes in lead V_1, and an R/S ratio of less than 1 in lead V_6 indicate VT. Left bundle branch block tachycardia with a notching of the slowly descending limb (>70 msec) of the S wave in lead V_1 favors VT.[15] In general, it can be stated that in patients with coronary disease and VT with right bundle branch block configuration the tachycardia origin is localized more often

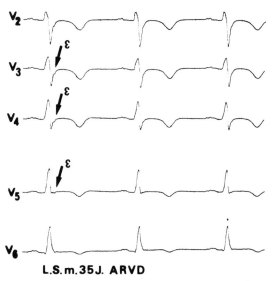

L.S. m. 35 J. ARVD

Figure 22–6. Resting 12-lead ECG (precordial leads) of a patient with arrhythmogenic right ventricular dysplasia. Note the T-wave inversions, which are especially visible over the right precordial leads. Immediately at the end of the QRS complex, small epsilon waves (ε) are visible. J ARVD = juvenile arrhythmogenic right ventricular dysplasia. ε = epsilon waves.

PREOPERATIVE ECG

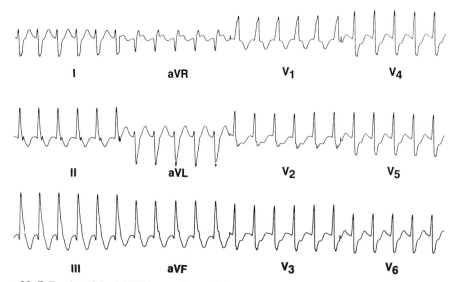

Figure 22–7. Resting 12-lead ECG in a patient with incessant wide QRS tachycardia. The tachycardia rate is 140 beats per minute, and the QRS complexes have a right bundle branch block configuration. Retrograde P waves are clearly visible in ECG leads II and V$_2$. The differential diagnosis between sustained VT and SVT with aberration cannot be clearly made.

in the anterolateral segment of the left ventricle, whereas a left bundle branch block configuration in 50 per cent of the instances points to a septal origin of tachycardia. The origin of the tachycardia has to be precisely localized by invasive endocardial catheter mapping. However, in a few instances, especially when the tachycardia is inducible by stimulation techniques, determination of the arrhythmogenic area may be useful when a surgical approach is considered, and the risk of endocardial resection has to be compared with that of an antitachycardia device.

Exercise Testing

All patients with significant arrhythmias and especially those for whom implantation of an antitachycardia device is considered should undergo exercise testing. Physical stress—that is, increase of sympathetic activity or decrease of vagal tone—can enhance ectopic activity or suppress preexisting arrhythmias. There are a variety of mechanisms during exercise that can influence the status of the arrhythmia. In no case, however, is the effect of physical stress on the arrhythmic milieu predictable, and each individual can react differently on different occasions. In patients with coronary artery disease, ischemia provoked by exercise can produce heterogeneity of impulse conduction

within an area of infarction. This may facilitate the onset of VT or VF. In patients who have arrhythmogenic right or left ventricular disease but normal coronary arteries, VT is often inducible by exercise testing. The mechanism for this phenomenon is not well established (Fig. 22–9). The role of catecholamines released in this situation may be arrhythmogenic. Isoproterenol infusion may achieve the same situation in the electrophysiology laboratory. Reproducibility and sensitivity of exercise testing for induction of VT remains low and limits its usefulness.

Exercise responses influence sensing algorithms for implantable antitachycardia devices. In patients with SVT or VT who are candidates for an antitachycardia device, it is also of great interest to know the maximal sinus rate during exercise so that the device will not be triggered inappropriately or activated by normal sinus tachycardia. It is also important to know if physical exercise provokes nonsustained episodes of tachycardia or the extent of rapid AV nodal conduction achieved with exercise in patients with atrial fibrillation. Ventricular rate increases under exercise conditions need to be studied carefully in patients with atrial fibrillation and an implanted defibrillator. Due consideration should be given to therapies to slow AV conduction to avoid interference with the programmed cut-off rate of the device. It is

PAROXYSMAL SUPRAVENTRICULAR TACHYCARDIA (PSVT)

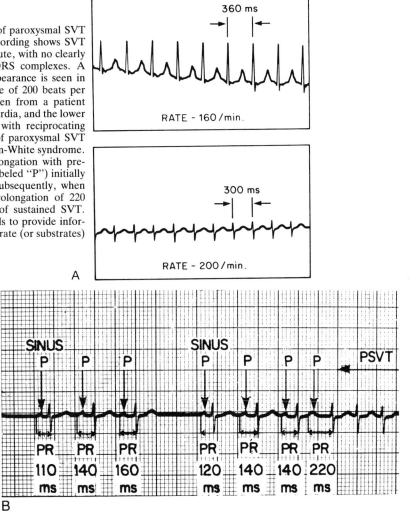

Figure 22–8. ECG recordings of paroxysmal SVT in two patients. *A,* The top recording shows SVT with a rate of 160 beats per minute, with no clearly visible P waves and regular QRS complexes. A tachycardia similar in ECG appearance is seen in the lower recording, with a rate of 200 beats per minute. The top tracing is taken from a patient with AV nodal reentrant tachycardia, and the lower panel is taken from an infant with reciprocating AV tachycardia. *B,* Initiation of paroxysmal SVT in an infant with Wolff-Parkinson-White syndrome. Note that the gradual PR prolongation with premature atrial depolarizations (labeled "P") initially fails to induce SVT and then subsequently, when accompanied by critical PR prolongation of 220 msec, results in the initiation of sustained SVT. This mechanism of initiation fails to provide information regarding the exact substrate (or substrates) for the tachycardia.

also well established that the pacing mode determined to be effective for tachycardia termination may fail to interrupt the tachycardia under exercise conditions. Often, even changing of body position from the supine to the standing posture may need a different stimulation pattern for successful termination of the tachycardia.

Signal-Averaged Electrocardiogram

Low-amplitude, high-frequency waveforms have been detected in the ST segment using various signal-averaging techniques in patients with myocardial infarction and episodes of VT. These waveforms reflect areas of slow, desynchronized impulse conduction in the area of infarction and most likely represent the arrhythmogenic substrate, where reentry can develop.

Recording of these low-level, high-frequency late potentials from the surface electrocardiogram has been used to identify patients at risk for sudden death or at risk of developing sustained VT after myocardial infarction (Fig. 22–10).[3] They correspond to the delayed deflections recorded with bipolar intracardiac electrograms during sinus rhythm or VT while performing intraoperative or catheter endocardial mapping (Fig. 22–11). It has been demonstrated that these late potentials represent an independent risk factor for VT and sudden death.[3, 30] However, the diagnostic value—that is, sensitivity and specificity—of these record-

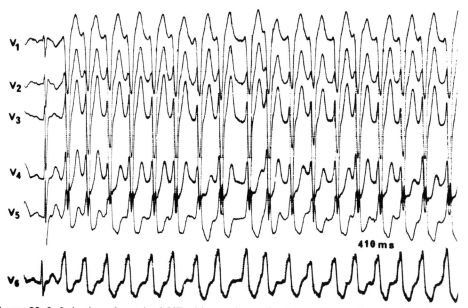

Figure 22–9. Induction of sustained VT with exercise testing in a patient undergoing bicycle exercise. Precordial ECG leads are shown. VT with a left bundle branch block configuration and changing RR intervals is noted. This patient had right and left ventricular dysplasia.

ings needs to be established in controlled studies. Assuming that it might be possible to predict that a particular patient is at risk of developing sustained VT, therapeutic approaches are unlikely to be selected only on this basis. Thus, at the present time, signal-averaged electrocardiographic recordings do not form an essential part of our protocol for evaluating the patient who is being considered for an antitachycardia device.

Holter Monitoring

The diagnostic workup of the patient who will need an antitachycardia device is incomplete without ambulatory electrocardiographic monitoring. Continuous ambulatory electrocardiographic recording over at least one 24-hour period is valuable and provides a better insight into the dynamic process of the electrical disorder. It helps to evaluate the patient's symptoms, especially when there are complaints of syncope or palpitations. It elucidates circadian heart rate variability during daily life activity and can be used to detect the mechanism of onset or termination of a tachycardia episode. Frequency and characterization of arrhythmic events, sustained or nonsustained, is feasible, with symptom-arrhythmia correlation. However, one must not forget that because of the enormous variability of such electrical events, absence of a specific finding on a single 24-hour Holter monitor recording does

not imply arrhythmia suppression or elimination.[9, 18] This is especially true for patients with infrequent symptoms.

There has been tremendous technical progress in the ambulatory electrocardiographic recording techniques over the past few years. Continuous two-channel recordings on magnetic tape with relatively light-weight recording devices are offered by many manufacturers. Event markers may help to improve assessment of the patient's symptoms. Besides continuous recordings, there are devices that perform intermittent event-triggered recordings, therefore allowing for a recording of longer than 24 hours. This feature is important for paroxysmal tachycardias. These devices are more useful for qualitative analysis than for exact quantitative assessment of electrical instability. Today, most Holter analysis systems operate on a microcomputer-based analysis system that transforms analog electrocardiographic recordings into digital signals. Analysis of these signs can be fully automated, with a complete quantitative print-out of the individual electrical events within 30 minutes or less. This feature is of great importance when a large number of patients need to be screened for potential arrhythmias. However, a well-trained technician is essential for individual tape analysis of special problems and distinction between artifacts and real events. The final report of an automated print-out needs critical and careful restudy by a knowledgeable

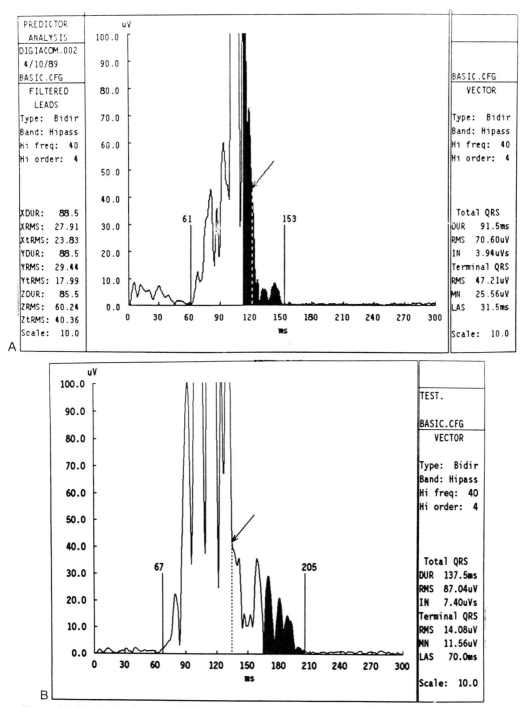

Figure 22–10. *A,* Signal-averaged ECG recording a normal record with a QRS duration of 120 msec or less and root mean square (RMS) voltage in the terminal 40 msec of 20 mV or more with no late potentials. *B,* Signal-averaged ECG showing a prolonged QRS duration, low root mean square (RMS) voltage, and late potentials.

technician or physician. For the routine evaluation of an arrhythmia of a patient being considered for an implantable device, we still prefer a fast-working, compressed 24-hour data print-out system. In the miniaturized print-outs, one can miss important informa-

tion. In most systems of this type, however, enlargement of areas of special interest is possible. Many of the currently available devices also offer ST-segment analysis programs to detect ischemic events. There are many technical problems that remain to be resolved with

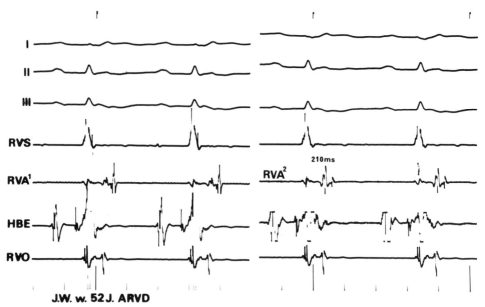

J.W. w. 52 J. ARVD

Figure 22–11. Surface and intracardiac ECG recordings during electrophysiologic study in a patient with arrhythmogenic right ventricular dysplasia and episode of sustained VT. Standard ECG leads I, II, and III are shown in addition to bipolar recordings from the right ventricular septum (RVS), right ventricular outflow tract (RVO), right ventricular apex (RVA), and the His bundle region (HBE). Note that in the left panel the right ventricular apical recording (labeled "RVA¹") shows a clearly visible delayed intracardiac potential falling after the termination of the surface QRS complex. In the right panel, at another site in the right ventricular apex, the same potential is now recorded with a change in amplitude and configuration.

ST-segment analysis. Currently, we believe that this particular analysis is useful but not essential for the evaluation and management of patients with arrhythmias. We recommend a minimum of 24 hours of ambulatory electrocardiographic recording, but recordings over 36 or 48 hours may be desirable in certain instances of infrequent arrhythmic events. Holter recordings in patients with pacemakers, for example, for detection of pacemaker stimuli or implantable cardioverter/defibrillator discharges can be helpful (Fig. 22–12). They are still not completely satisfactory, especially when using computerized print-outs of electrocardiographic recordings. Further technical improvement will be necessary to distinguish implantable device function from artifacts. The role of Holter recordings in patients with supraventricular tachyarrhythmias is relatively limited. P-wave analysis is still limited, and a study of tachycardia mechanisms is very difficult with a two-channel electrocardiographic recording. Ambulatory recordings can be of help in patients who suffer from bradycardia-tachycardia syndrome with intermittent atrial flutter or fibrillation, sinus pauses, or intermittent AV block. For example, detection of episodes of atrial fibrillation in patients with antitachycardia pacemakers for paroxysmal SVT can explain failure of the pacing termi-

nation mode. In general, with greater frequency of SVT episodes, the yield of information from ambulatory monitoring also increases.

Holter recordings should be performed prior to and after implantation of an automatic defibrillator. Intermittent episodes of atrial tachyarrhythmias with rapid ventricular response, which can cause frequent defibrillator discharges, can be documented. Detection and appropriate treatment of these arrhythmias can avoid such unpleasant events. Alternatively, selection of device detection criteria can be altered, for example, by increasing the rate cut-off to obviate such discharges. Another important use of ambulatory monitoring lies in the analysis of spontaneous ventricular arrhythmias, for both diagnostic purposes and selection of device therapy. There have been many attempts to correlate the incidence of arrhythmias with ventricular dysfunction and prognosis.[2] Progressive ventricular dysfunction is associated with an increased incidence of complex ventricular arrhythmias—that is, pairs, salvos, and nonsustained VT—and a higher incidence of sudden cardiac death.[2] Patients who have survived sudden cardiac death or who suffer from recurrent episodes of sustained VT also have a high incidence of complex ventricular arrhythmias that can be

ORTHOCOR II PACEMAKER SYSTEM

(BURST SCANNING MECHANISM)

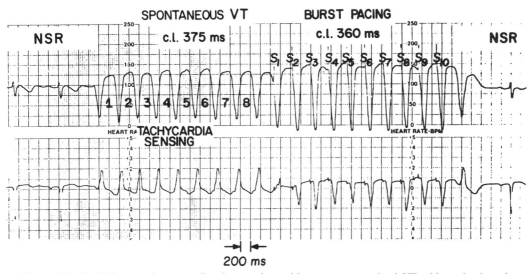

Figure 22–12. Holter monitor recording in a patient with recurrent sustained VT with an implanted antitachycardia pacemaker (Cordis Corporation, Miami, FL; model 284A–Orthocor 2). This two-channel ECG recording shows spontaneous sustained VT, which is sensed for 8 beats and then terminated by the delivery of 10 paced ventricular beats using the burst scanning mechanism of the pacemaker. In this mechanism, the interval between successive paced beats is shortened, starting initially at a cycle length of 360 msec. c.l. = cycle length; VT = ventricular tachycardia; NSR = normal sinus rhythm.

detected with Holter monitoring. When these patients undergo implantation of an automatic cardioverter/defibrillator, Holter analysis is mandatory prior to implantation. Long episodes of self-terminating VT can trigger the currently approved device (Fig. 22–13). In such patients, these complex arrhythmias have to be suppressed by antiarrhythmic drugs so that the risk of receiving inappropriate shocks can be diminished. Newer devices, such as Telectronics Guardian model 4201 or 4202 (Telectronics, Englewood, CO), reconfirm the presence of the arrhythmia and eliminate such

shock delivery. However, charging sequences are still initiated and result in shock dumping and reduction in pulse generator longevity. The probability of recording of sustained VT or the onset of VF with a single Holter recording is relatively small. However, short, nonsustained episodes of VT can provide important information for the programming of an antitachycardia device such as an automatic defibrillator. Recent studies of patients who had a Holter recording at the moment of sudden cardiac death have shown that the majority of recorded cases of sudden cardiac

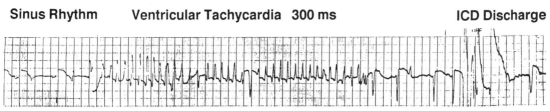

Figure 22–13. Spontaneous implantable cardioverter/defibrillator discharge in a patient with nonsustained VT. This telemetric recording is taken from a patient with an implanted automatic cardioverter/defibrillator (Ventak model 1520, Cardiac Pacemakers, Inc, St. Paul, MN). Spontaneous, nonsustained VT at a rate of 300 beats per minute that lasts for approximately 7.2 seconds is observed. This duration is sufficient to initiate a charging sequence and is followed by committed shock delivery shown on the right of the panel. At the time of shock delivery, the patient is back in sinus rhythm.

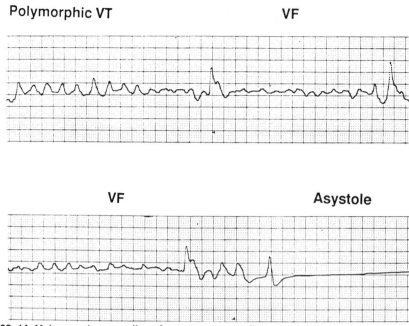

Figure 22–14. Holter monitor recording of a spontaneous cardiac arrest in a patient with inducible VT on amiodarone who refused implantation of an automatic cardioverter/defibrillator. The cardiac arrest commences as monomorphic VT and degenerates into polymorphic VT tachycardia and ventricular fibrillation (VF).

death start with VT that subsequently degenerates into VF and asystole (Fig. 22–14).[9, 19] Only a small number of patients died because of primary bradycardiac events. However, detection of bradyarrhythmias is an important element of such recordings. The need for pacemaker therapy for rate support should be assessed, particularly as the currently approved implantable cardioverter/defibrillator lacks this therapy. Bradycardiac events can also trigger ventricular arrhythmias. In addition, combination drug therapy can also depress sinus rate. Pacing therapy is of great value in this situation. Heart rate and arrhythmia monitoring through ambulatory electrocardiographic recordings should also be performed regularly during follow-up in all patients with implantable antitachycardia devices. This monitoring permits study of the interaction between the native cardiac rhythm and the sensing and therapeutic algorithms in the device. In summary, Holter recordings should be an essential element of diagnostic procedures for the prospective patient who is to receive an antitachycardia device and should be performed periodically after device implantation.

Echocardiography

Echocardiography has become a very important noninvasive method to evaluate the anatomic and physiologic status of the patient with SVT or VT. Patients with episodes of SVT—especially with the Wolff-Parkinson-White syndrome—occasionally demonstrate coexisting abnormalities like atrial or ventricular septal defect, hypertrophic cardiomyopathy, mitral valve prolapse, or Ebstein's anomaly. Two-dimensional echocardiography in patients with VT is extremely helpful to define and quantify the size and contraction pattern of both ventricles.[5] This observation has an enormous impact on the selection of nonpharmacologic therapy. Ventricles with globally poor contractility or diffuse hypertrophy are suboptimal candidates for electrophysiologically guided surgery (Fig. 22–15). Detection of the degree of abnormal regional wall motion, identification of circumscribed aneurysms that could also contain thrombus, or assessment of a dilated cardiomyopathy can be performed more easily by echocardiography than by conventional angiography. This information will be necessary in all patients with VT to evaluate the potential surgical risk. Echocardiography can easily detect these abnormalities and should be performed in all patients prior to invasive electrophysiologic studies and angiographic studies.

Echocardiography has also proved to be extremely helpful for the serial follow-up of patients with the implantable cardioverter/de-

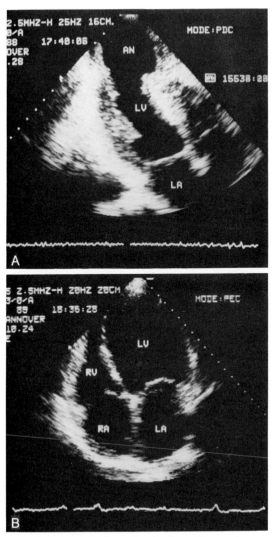

A

B

Figure 22–15. Two-dimensional echocardiogram in a patient with refractory VT and coronary artery disease. *A* shows the presence of a large anteroapical left ventricular aneurysm. *B* shows global dilatation of the left ventricle with thinning of the interventricular septum and the lateral left ventricular wall.

fibrillator. For example, we have studied left ventricular function by means of this technique in patients with epicardially glued patch electrodes in patients with implanted devices. We observed that the patch electrodes did not impair global or regional ventricular function in systole or diastole. Alternatively, problems such as pericardial effusions surrounding epicardial electrode systems can be detected by these means. However, defibrillator lead fracture or displacement is not easily diagnosed by these means. Guidance of electrode catheters during electrophysiologic studies by means of echocardiography has been attempted. This approach was advocated for evaluation of in-

tracardiac catheter electrodes (see Chapter 13). However, this approach cannot be generally recommended, since it is less reliable than standard biplane fluoroscopy for this particular application. In the patient with an antitachycardia device, echocardiographic studies are most useful to assess the status of the native cardiac disease.

Magnetic Resonance Imaging

Better noninvasive techniques for the precise diagnosis and evaluation of myocardial disorders that provide substrates for tachyarrhythmias are still awaited. It has been generally believed that sustained ventricular tachyarrhythmias do not usually arise in normal myocardium. In some patients, abnormal myocardial tissue can remain undetected with conventional angiography, and magnetic resonance imaging techniques can be used in an attempt to identify these areas. There is some evidence that magnetic resonance imaging techniques can provide us with better recognition of myocardial abnormalities in patients with arrhythmogenic ventricular disease. The amount of lipoid tissue within myocardium remains unknown with conventional angiographic techniques. However, magnetic resonance imaging can visualize this tissue scattered throughout the myocardium (Fig. 22–16). We have recently learned that in patients with so-called right ventricular dysplasia abnormal lipoid tissue accumulates not only in some parts of the right ventricle but also very often in the interventricular septum and the

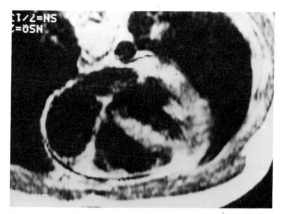

Figure 22–16. Magnetic resonance imaging of the heart in a patient with arrhythmogenic right ventricular dysplasia. Infiltration of the interventricular septum and left ventricle with fibrolipomatosis, seen as areas of reduced image density, can be seen in the interventricular septum as well as parts of the left ventricle. This finding was confirmed intraoperatively prior to ablation of the arrhythmogenic tissues.

left ventricle. The amount of fatty tissue is much larger than expected from right ventricular angiography. This is important information when a surgical approach is considered. Incomplete resection of this tissue can result in a failure to suppress the arrhythmia. These magnetic resonance imaging findings have been confirmed during the surgical exploration of patients with arrhythmogenic ventricular dysplasia. Therefore, we recommend magnetic resonance imaging in all patients with VT but with otherwise "normal" hearts. Alternative approaches, such as myocardial biopsies, provide information on a very limited tissue sample, and diseased tissue may not be selected for study.

HEMODYNAMIC EVALUATION

We have stated earlier in this chapter that electrical disorders such as VT and VF are most often based on myocardial disease. The prognosis of the patient directly depends on the degree of ventricular dysfunction. It is therefore important to evaluate the hemodynamic status of the patient before a specific therapeutic regimen is recommended. For each therapeutic approach, the physician has to consider its hemodynamic consequences and the potential need for additional procedures that improve ventricular function. The hemodynamic aspects are often the major factors that influence application of a certain therapeutic approach. The chest radiograph allows some degree of estimation of ventricular function. A large cardiac silhouette, pulmonary congestion, and pleural effusion suggest left ventricular dysfunction. However, life-threatening VT may exist in disorders in which cardiac size and shape appear normal. Invasive studies, however, can show that either ventricle may contain large areas of abnormally contracting myocardium. This finding is common in young patients who have hypertrophic cardiomyopathy or arrhythmogenic right or left ventricular dysplasia. The clinical value of noninvasive studies such as radionuclide gated cardiac blood pool scintigraphy to evaluate ventricular function—that is, by global ejection fraction and regional wall motion—has decreased with continuing improvements in two-dimensional echocardiography. The latter procedure provides detailed anatomic and physiologic information. However, in some patients, echocardiographic images of poor quality are obtained owing to technical problems. Gated cardiac blood pool scintigraphy has considerable value for noninvasive estimation of left ventricular ejection fraction and wall motion in these patients. This technique can also be applied to quantify hemodynamic status before and after implantation of antitachycardia devices.

INVASIVE LABORATORY EVALUATION

Ventricular Angiography and Coronary Angiography

A complete invasive hemodynamic evaluation of the prospective recipient of an antitachycardia device has to be performed in all cases. This evaluation includes biplane left ventricular and most often also right ventricular angiography as well as coronary angiography. The results of the hemodynamic evaluation will decide if endocardial resection, implantable defibrillator, or conservative medical therapy is appropriate for an individual patient. Accurate assessment of ventricular function through calculation of the left ventricular ejection fraction is often difficult. The ejection fraction of the left ventricle is normally calculated in the right anterior oblique projection. However, wall motion of the septal, posterior, and lateral walls of the left ventricle is ignored in this view. It is therefore necessary to evaluate the left ventricular ejection fraction using right and left anterior oblique projections. Unfortunately, many reports in the world literature mention the global left ventricular ejection fraction, measured in a single projection, as their major parameter for assessing left ventricular performance. In addition, the presence of a ventricular aneurysm may affect this parameter, lowering global ejection fraction (Fig. 22–17). This finding can be misleading if there is no other information on the clinical status and functional class of heart failure. In general, there is a consensus that a global left ventricular ejection fraction of less than 20 to 25 per cent, even when measured only in a single projection, predicts poor results of surgical ablation methods for abolition of VT. It is our belief that patients with poor ventricular function and left ventricular ejection fractions below 20 to 25 per cent, as measured in both standard projections, should undergo implantation of an automatic cardioverter/defibrillator, provided the expected survival and functional status of the patient is reasonable (e.g., New

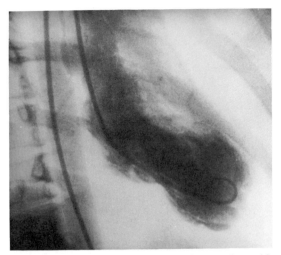

Figure 22–17. Left ventriculography in a patient with refractory VT and normal coronary arteries. The left ventricular angiogram is visualized in the right anterior oblique position in this 20-year-old patient. A large apical aneurysm is noted. Intraoperatively, extensive lipoid tissue was noted at the apex of the left ventricle, with dyskinesis of this area.

York Heart Association [NYHA] Class IV patients would be excluded).

There is general clinical agreement that selective coronary angiography is also useful in defining the recipient of an antitachycardia device. Many patients with coronary artery disease and life-threatening episodes of VT or VF will have advanced coronary disease. Coronary artery bypass surgery has been shown to prolong survival in these patients, particularly when considerable left ventricular dysfunction is present. We estimate that 25 per cent of these patients need concomitant coronary bypass surgery in addition to the potential implantation of a cardioverter/defibrillator. The presence of critical coronary artery disease, such as subtotal left main or proximal left anterior descending artery obstruction, modifies the diagnostic and therapeutic approach. Extensive electrophysiologic procedures, especially mapping, should probably be avoided in this instance. Although it has not been proved that ischemia plays an essential role in the initiation of sustained VT, we do know that coronary bypass surgery alone cannot totally eliminate recurrent episodes of sustained VT.[6] However, it remains an important adjunctive factor and requires angiographic and physiologic assessment.

Electrophysiologic Study

Implantation of an antitachycardia device in patients with SVT or VT is mainly based on extensive preimplantation and intraoperative invasive electrophysiologic studies. The indication for the study will be derived from the patient's clinical presentation, prior noninvasive evaluation, and hemodynamic and angiographic data. The baseline electrophysiologic study must provide information relevant to tachyarrhythmia diagnosis and potential treatment modalities. The decision for selecting one-device treatment or treatment combinations has to involve all aspects of the noninvasive and invasive evaluations. The electrophysiologic study has to address carefully the special needs for antitachycardia device selection. If such information is unavailable, as, for example, when a patient is referred from another center, it may be necessary to repeat the electrophysiologic study or perform it differently. In all patients, however, another intraoperative study that will test the efficacy of the implanted antitachycardia pacemaker or an automatic cardioverter/defibrillator is necessary. Finally, we would recommend a postoperative electrophysiologic study prior to patient discharge to assess chronic implantable device function. Such electrophysiologic studies should be performed only by well-trained, knowledgeable physicians to maintain quality and performance standards. The catheterization laboratory used for these procedures has to be fully equipped with fluoroscopic imaging, a multichannel amplifier and recording system, a cardiac stimulator, multielectrode catheters, equipment for cardiopulmonary resuscitation, and a defibrillator for external defibrillation. The study protocol has to be designed prior to commencement of the procedure, and it is important for the study to follow the selected protocol, which should be changed only for unforeseen events or emergent problems. Guidelines for complete electrophysiologic studies in patients with SVT as well as VT have been established and contain important information on basic principles, necessary elements, and potential risks of these studies.[32, 33]

The attempt to achieve consensus on a common stimulation protocol to be used in all electrophysiologic centers has involved intensive debate.[12, 13, 33, 36] There is agreement that pacing during such procedures should be performed at two to four times diastolic pacing threshold and that the paced impulse duration should not exceed 5 msec. Extrastimuli should be delivered during sinus rhythm and during rhythms with cycle lengths ranging between 60 and 350 msec. The number of extrastimuli at a single site should not usually exceed three.

There are a number of preferred stimulation sites for patients with SVT and VT, depending on the individual patient. Recording sites vary according to the underlying electrophysiologic mechanism of the tachycardia, and optimal filtering of the bipolar signals lies between 30 and 500 Hz. In some cases, unipolar recordings might be more helpful, as, for example, during activation mapping in SVT. Measurement of baseline conduction intervals and electrophysiologic properties of different parts of the conduction system and myocardium—that is, refractory periods of the atrium, AV node, His-Purkinje system, and ventricular myocardium—is also performed.[11] Endocardial activation mapping during induced sustained tachycardia determines the earliest endocardial site of activation. This site is believed to be close to the site of arrhythmogenesis. Recently, it has become obvious that one of the most important areas to examine is probably the area of maximal slowing of conduction during the tachycardia.[20] This zone of slow conduction may be the critical element for maintenance of the tachycardia, and manipulation of this region by electrical stimulation or elimination by ablative techniques is a key element in these nonpharmacologic therapies. Electrophysiologic studies in the operating room use the same criteria applied in the catheterization laboratory. These studies, however, address the very specific question of combining device or ablative therapy with the surgical procedure.

Electrophysiologic Evaluation of the Patient with Supraventricular Tachycardias

Indications for electrophysiologic study in a patient who may be a candidate for an antitachycardia device are present when there is a documented recurrent SVT or major symptoms due to such an arrhythmia. The tachycardia can be automatic (e.g., ectopic atrial tachycardia) or reentrant in nature (e.g., reciprocating tachycardia with an involvement of an accessory pathway). This latter arrhythmia can be found in patients with the classic type of Wolff-Parkinson-White syndrome with overt or concealed accessory pathways; other preexcitation syndromes, such as the Lown-Ganong-Levine syndrome; and accessory pathways of the Mahaim type with nodoventricular or fasciculoventricular pathways. There are various forms of AV nodal reentrant tachycardias. Less frequently, we deal with ectopic forms of SVT, that is, ectopic atrial tachycardia.

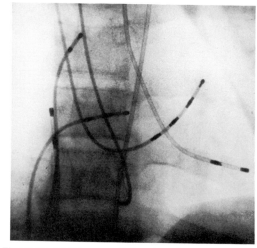

Figure 22–18. Fluoroscopic imaging of electrode catheter positions during electrophysiologic study in a patient with refractory SVT. Electrode catheters are placed in the high and low right atrium, in the His bundle region, and in the right and left ventricles.

A detailed list of clinical situations warranting electrophysiologic study has been developed. Irrespective of the suspected underlying mechanism of the tachycardia, electrode catheters are placed in the right atrium, in the coronary sinus, at the AV junction to record His bundle, and in the right ventricle (Fig. 22–18). Programmed atrial and ventricular stimulation is performed, and the tachycardia is induced. After induction, several questions have to be answered: (1) Is an accessory pathway present, and where is it located? (2) Are we dealing with only one pathway or multiple pathways? (3) How does the tachycardia propagate? Is it an orthodromic or antedromic type of tachycardia? (4) What are the electrophysiologic properties of the accessory pathway, the AV node, or His bundle? (5) Is the induced form of tachycardia identical with the spontaneous form? (6) What is the fastest rate of tachycardia? (7) What is the effect of the induced atrial fibrillation? (8) What are the effects of individual drugs or of autonomic nervous system manipulation? These questions are addressed during the baseline electrophysiologic evaluation.

The *specific* electrophysiologic study has to answer even more precisely where the accessory pathway or the ectopic focus is located and if there are other anatomic anomalies of importance present when a surgical ablative procedure is considered. When we are testing the patient who may possibly receive an antitachycardia device, we are more interested in knowing the following: (1) Where is the most

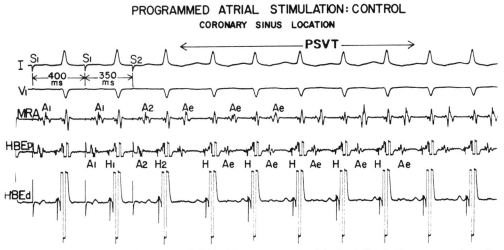

Figure 22–19. Induction of paroxysmal SVT with programmed atrial stimulation in the coronary sinus. In this patient with refractory SVT, reciprocating AV tachycardia could not be initiated with stimulation from the high right atrium. Programmed atrial stimulation from the distal coronary sinus resulted in induction of SVT with a single atrial extrastimulus that had a coupling interval of 350 msec. Shown are two surface ECG leads (I and V_1) and intracardiac electrogram recordings from the right atrium and His bundle region. MRA = mid right atrium; HBE = His bundle electrogram; p = proximal; d = distal; A_1 = atrial depolarization from pacing train; A_2 = atrial extrastimulus; Ae = atrial echo; H = His bundle electrogram.

appropriate pacing site for tachycardia induction and termination (Fig. 22–19)? (2) What is the reproducibility of the tachycardia induction and termination? (3) What is the most reliable stimulation mode for tachycardia termination? (4) Can permanent electrodes be placed at the chosen stimulation site for tachycardia termination? (5) What is the risk of acceleration or induction of unwanted forms of tachycardia with the chosen stimulation protocol? (6) Do we need additional procedures or drugs to achieve successful and reliable termination of the tachycardia? It is important to mention that the clinical data, the electrophysiologic parameters, and the patient's psychologic and social situation have to be summarized to decide that an antitachycardia device will be superior to catheter or surgical ablation or an antiarrhythmic drug treatment.

Once the device is selected, electrophysiologic evaluation is done preoperatively and intraoperatively to assess the efficacy of the implanted antitachycardia devices (Fig. 22–20). The tachycardia is induced repeatedly (a figure of up to 100 inductions before discharge has been suggested), and the device's ability to terminate SVT is documented on each occurrence.

Electrophysiologic Evaluation of the Patient with Ventricular Tachycardia

The exact basis for the electrophysiologic selection of a prospective patient for an antitachycardia device is currently debated. Electrophysiologic studies assist in defining such device recipients by providing significant additional information relevant to device func-

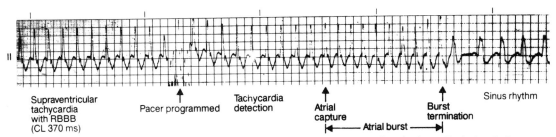

Figure 22–20. Documentation of successful SVT termination by implanted antitachycardia device during postoperative evaluation. Spontaneous SVT occurs in this patient with Wolff-Parkinson-White syndrome. The tachycardia rate is 160 beats per minute, with a right bundle branch block. The implanted pacemaker is programmed. Tachycardia detection ensues, followed by delivery of an atrial burst with atrial capture. Termination of the burst results in tachycardia termination and resumption of sinus rhythm.

tion. For example, the classic antitachycardia pacemaker is being replaced by new implantable cardioverter/defibrillator devices that have programmable sensing and pacing features for tachycardia detection and termination as well as bradycardia backup pacing (Table 22–1). Selection of appropriate pacing algorithms requires electrophysiologic study. More recently, selection of sequential pacing and shock algorithms has been possible in the same study.[11] Finally, selection of sensing parameters is often based on a combination of clinical and laboratory data. Table 22–2 shows a proposed scheme for selecting termination algorithms for implantable cardioversion/defibrillation devices for ventricular tachyarrhythmias.

In general, the vast majority of patients studied for spontaneous sustained VT are the patients who demonstrated recurrent episodes of sustained monomorphic VT and who have organic heart disease. Heart disease is most often coronary artery disease with old myocardial infarction. The area of infarction is large, and there is often severe ventricular dysfunction involved. The other forms of organic heart disease associated with ventricular tachyarrhythmias are cardiomyopathies of the dilated or hypertrophic type and structural myocardial disorders associated with valve disease.[15] Yet another type of patient with VT is one who is apparently healthy and rarely has heart failure but who is repeatedly admitted to the hospital with sustained monomorphic tachycardia. This is the clinical presentation of arrhythmogenic disease of the right or left ventricle (or both), initially referred to as right ventricular dysplasia. This entity is a form of peculiar fibrolipomatosis of one or both ventricles in multiple areas. The pathophysiologic mechanism of this form of organic disorder is still unclear. All the patients mentioned above are referred to in the following discussion as Group I.

TABLE 22–1. PROGRAMMABLE CARDIOVERTER/DEFIBRILLATORS

Programmed Parameters
1. Sensing criteria
   Electrogram rate
   Morphology
2. Electrical therapy
   Pacing
      Bradycardia
      ATP
   Sequential shocks
3. Monitoring
   Event counter
   Electrogram telemetry
   Marker channel

ATP = antitachycardia pacing

TABLE 22–2. SELECTION OF SHOCKS IN ELECTRICAL THERAPY*

1. Tachycardia rate and morphology
   Monomorphic
      Slow = sequential treatment
      Rapid = high-energy shock
   Polymorphic VT/VF = high-energy shocks
2. Hemodynamic status
   Stable = sequential
   Unstable = high-energy shock
3. Lead system
   Epicardial = unidirectional
   Endocardial = bidirectional

*With programmable devices. Suggested guidelines are based on hemodynamic stability and lead systems.
Abbreviations: VT = ventricular tachycardia; VF = ventricular fibrillation.

The second type (Group II) of patient in whom electrophysiologic evaluation has to be performed is the patient with aborted sudden cardiac death. These patients generally also have organic heart disease, and the circulatory arrest was induced by either rapid VT or VF, which may not be documented at the moment of cardiac arrest. A proposed scheme for evaluation of the patients is shown in Figure 22–21. Note that clinical information both at the time of arrest and related to the underlying cardiac disease influences the extent of electrophysiologic and device therapy, particularly implantation of a cardioverter/defibrillator.

There is a third group of patients with syncope of unknown origin associated with organic heart disease giving reason to suspect that the etiology for loss of consciousness is a paroxysmal ventricular tachyarrhythmia. Rarely, patients who have only a "primary electrical disease" will be studied for evaluation of a specific therapeutic approach. It is suspected that they also have a myocardial disease, which is, however, currently undetectable with conventional diagnostic procedures. The role of myocardial biopsy in these patients is still unclear.

Again, irrespective of the underlying organic disease or clinical symptoms, the basic electrophysiologic study will be performed with electrode catheters placed in the right atrium, at the His bundle region, and in the right and left ventricles. The ventricular catheters should contain at least four electrodes so that two bipolar recordings from each ventricle can be obtained. Programmed ventricular stimulation is performed to induce the clinical form of sustained VT using a standard stimulation protocol. Such a protocol includes diastolic scanning of the RR interval with one or two extrastimuli in steps of 10 to 20 msec. This

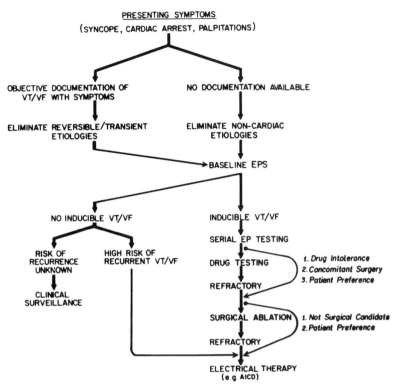

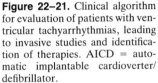

Figure 22–21. Clinical algorithm for evaluation of patients with ventricular tachyarrhythmias, leading to invasive studies and identification of therapies. AICD = automatic implantable cardioverter/defibrillator.

scanning is performed during sinus rhythm and subsequently during two or more ventricular paced cycle lengths. The premature stimuli are initially delivered into the right ventricle, usually at an apical site. The ventricular pacing drive train can have cycle lengths ranging from 600 to 400 and, rarely, 350 msec.[7, 14, 17] The more aggressive stimulation protocol delivers a third extra stimulus at the same right ventricular site until the ventricular refractory period is reached. We recommend use of this step in all patients with cardiac arrest or sustained VT. If VT is not induced, the next step usually includes stimulation at the right ventricular outflow tract, beginning with one extrastimulus, followed by two and three extrastimuli. Use of the third extra stimulus and two pacing drive cycle lengths and a minimum of two right ventricular stimulation sites is considered essential for VT-VF induction to achieve adequate sensitivity with the stimulation protocol. Rarely, in about 8 to 10 per cent of the cases, the stimulation protocol will include stimulation of the left ventricle. Ventricular burst pacing with high rates (up to 250 msec) or burst pacing with rapidly increasing rates is still performed by some centers. The reproducibility of this stimulation mode is debatable.[22] In general, it must also be emphasized that the more aggressive the stimulation protocol, the greater the likelihood of induction of nonclinical forms of VT.[17] After induction of monomorphic sustained VT, the hemodynamic status during the arrhythmia has to be assessed to determine if endocardial activation mapping will be possible. Hemodynamic stability is required to localize the earliest site of endocardial activation (Fig. 22–22) or the critical area of maximal slowing of conduction during the tachycardia.[20] The latter is considered to be an area where low amplitude or fractioned potentials or both can be recorded in the middiastole. Earliest endocardial activation has to be recorded at least 40 msec prior to the onset of the QRS complex in the standard electrocardiographic recording. Further evaluation of the critical area of the tachycardia genesis includes "pace mapping." Pace mapping attempts to reproduce the identical QRS complex by ventricular pacing, as observed during spontaneous VT. Stimulation of tachycardia results in so-called pseudoentrainment without fusion complexes (see Chapter 19) and is associated typically with an extremely long interval between the stimulus artifact and the paced QRS complex from this stimulus.

VT mapping from the left and right ventri-

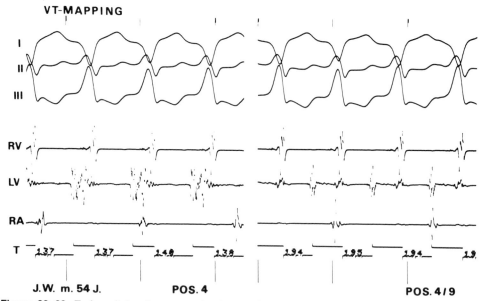

VT-MAPPING

J.W. m. 54 J.   **POS. 4**   **POS. 4 / 9**

Figure 22–22. Endocardial catheter mapping in a patient with coronary artery disease and sustained monomorphic VT. Shown are standard ECG leads I, II, and III and intracardiac electrograms from the right ventricle (RV), left ventricle (LV), and right atrium (RA). The left ventricular catheter electrode records a presystolic potential in the panel on the left and is subsequently positioned in the apicolateral region of the left ventricle in the right panel. A large middiastolic potential is clearly noted and precedes the QRS complex by more than 100 msec. The position of the electrode catheter at this site is recorded and noted for subsequent intraoperative confirmation.

cles is an essential part of the specific evaluation study to examine the possibility of an electrophysiologically guided surgical approach, that is, endocardial resection cryoablation or laser ablation of the arrhythmogenic area responsible for the maintenance of the tachycardia.[27, 28] The electrophysiologic evaluation to identify the candidate for an antitachycardia device has to provide specific information. For example, rapid pacing techniques are evaluated in the electrophysiology laboratory for efficacy, as for the patient with SVT (Fig. 22–23). In addition, the patient evaluated for an implantable cardioverter/defibrillator has to undergo another study during implantation of the device, primarily for determination of optimal electrode location to obtain the lowest reliable defibrillation or cardioversion threshold (Fig. 22–24). During follow-up, noninvasive or invasive electrophysiologic studies can be performed to assess the efficacy of the implanted device's termination modes (Fig. 22–25).

The responses to programmed stimulation in the three different groups of patients mentioned above are often quite different from each other. This difference is directly related to the underlying disease, extent of ventricular dysfunction, and probably the underlying elec-

trical mechanism of tachycardia generation. In our experience, patients with documented monomorphic sustained VT have the same clinical tachycardia inducible in 85 to 90 per cent of the cases, whereas in patients with cardiac arrest, a monomorphic sustained VT is inducible in approximately 50 per cent of patients. In approximately 10 per cent of Group I patients and 30 per cent of Group II patients, VF will be induced, requiring immediate termination. In fewer than 5 per cent of Group I patients and 20 per cent of Group II patients, we can elicit either no or only a few ventricular repetitive responses. Finally, in patients with organic heart disease who are studied for syncope, approximately 20 per cent will demonstrate inducible VT and 20 per cent will have inducible VF. It is important to emphasize that these estimates of inducible VT and VF are at best generalizations and will vary directly with an individual center's population of patients and stimulation protocol. In general, one must also emphasize that induction of a polymorphic sustained or nonsustained VT can also be the consequence of an aggressive stimulation protocol. However, in some patients, this type of VT can be the clinical disorder and cannot be dismissed as a nonspecific report. Correlation of induced and spon-

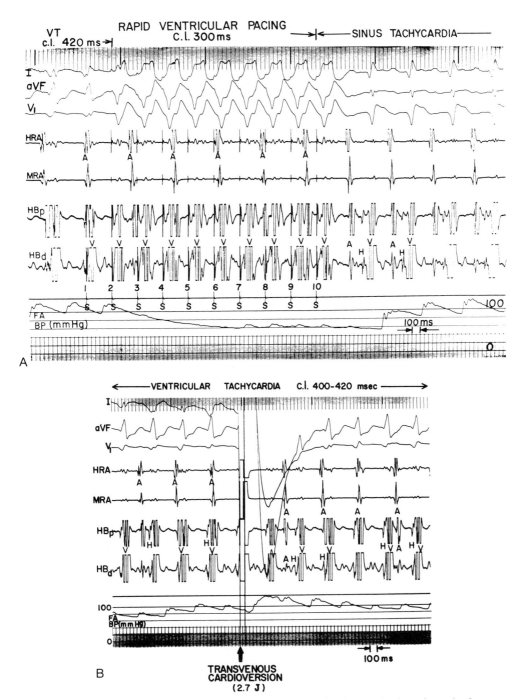

Figure 22–23. Evaluation of different therapeutic electrical modes for termination of sustained mono-morphic VT. *A* shows termination of sustained VT with a cycle length of 420 msec by a burst of rapid ventricular pacing at a cycle length of 300 msec in the electrophysiology laboratory. Conversion to sinus tachycardia was reproducibly demonstrated. *B* shows attempted termination of the same tachycardia with transvenous shocks. A transvenous cardioversion shock of 2.7 J using a dual-electrode system is unable to terminate the tachycardia. This information can be used in programming implanted devices and for selection of appropriate tachycardia termination algorithms.

PROGRAMMABLE CARDIOVERTER-DEFIBRILLATOR

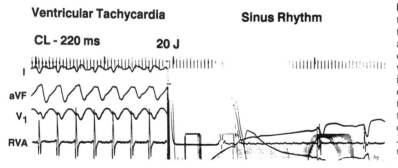

Figure 22–24. Intraoperative testing of programmed termination algorithms in a patient with an implantable programmable cardioverter/defibrillator. Rapid VT with a cycle length of 220 msec is induced, and a 20-J shock is delivered through two epicardial electrodes. Successful termination of the arrhythmia is noted. CL = cycle length; ms = milliseconds; J = joules; RVA = right ventricular apex.

taneous ventricular tachyarrhythmias is an important aspect of evaluating the information elicited from an electrophysiologic study.

CONCLUSIONS

Patients with recurrent, sustained episodes of SVT are candidates for an antitachycardia device if conventional drug treatment fails, drugs produce intolerable side effects, lifelong drug treatment is unwanted, and surgical or catheter ablation is either impossible—owing to anatomic reasons or other underlying disease—or refused. As such, it represents a tertiary therapy for this disorder. Careful and thorough noninvasive and invasive evaluation, discussed earlier, will decide if effective treatment is possible with an antitachycardia device. Common clinical dilemmas include comparison of implantable device therapy with lifelong continuous or intermittent drug therapy. It has been recognized that SVT recurrences can also occur in clusters. This phenomenon can permit periodic therapy. The majority of these patients are young and have special considerations related to an active and vigorous lifestyle, pregnancy in female patients, and employment. Drug therapy is generally avoided in pregnant patients, but because of the limited nature of this stress, this is not an indication for nonpharmacologic therapy. Implantable device therapy may limit employment opportunities and lifestyle in some instances. The psychologic impact of an implantable device should be carefully assessed. In general, we have used these devices in older patients with SVT, often with concomitant cardiac and noncardiac disorders, or when ablative therapy is unsuccessful or declined by the patient. Current utilization trends

do not suggest the application of this therapy to be increased.

In patients with VT, evaluation of the hemodynamic status during the arrhythmia and the underlying disease process will influence any prospective antitachycardia approach. Poor ventricular function and inducible rapid VT are particularly associated with a high incidence of sudden cardiac death. Serial drug testing has been conventionally advocated for the initial therapy (Fig. 22–26). Antiarrhythmic drugs, even when tested with repeated electropharmacologic testing, have a high failure rate with increasingly poor yield, as additional drugs are tested (Fig. 22–27).[26] In selected patients, successful surgical ablation of the arrhythmogenic area is feasible. The majority of the patients with impaired ventricular function and ventricular tachyarrhythmias are, however, candidates for implantation of an automatic cardioverter/defibrillator. The major elements of an algorithm for selection of these different therapies in patients with VT and VF are shown in Figure 22–28. Although surgical ablation is shown to be considered prior to device implantation, increasing concern with respect to surgical risk and endocardial lead systems for implantable defibrillators now being available reduce the selected population of surgical patients. Major clinical considerations in the selection of therapeutic alternatives are shown in Table 22–3. This table identifies ideal candidates for each form of therapy. Other issues to be considered include the individual patient's lifestyle and quality of life on the selected therapy. These issues should be discussed prospectively with the patient. However, many patients are potential candidates for more than one form of therapy or poor candidates for all current therapeutic approaches. Careful selection of

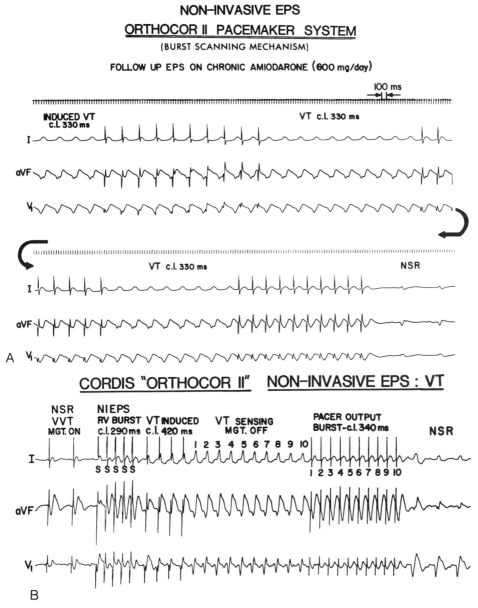

Figure 22–25. Postoperative evaluation of an implanted antitachycardia device function. *A* shows induced VT on chronic electrophysiologic study in a patient with refractory VT and an implanted antitachycardia pacemaker (Cordis model 284A–Orthocor 2). The antitachycardia pacemaker system is used for noninvasive induction of VT, and the burst scanning mechanism for tachycardia termination is evaluated. The first pacing burst on the top panel does not terminate the tachycardia. The second pacing burst also fails to terminate the tachycardia. The third pacing burst *(lower panel)* finally successfully terminates the tachycardia. Reprogramming of the termination algorithm to the last pacing burst mode that successfully terminated the tachycardia occurs automatically in this device. *B* shows noninvasive electrophysiologic study during follow-up in another patient with refractory VT and an implanted antitachycardia pacemaker. Noninvasive induction of VT by right ventricular burst pacing is shown in the left panel of the recording. VT is induced with a cycle length of 420 msec, and the magnet is removed. It is sensed for 10 beats, and the pacemaker delivers a burst at a cycle length of 340 msec for 10 beats. Termination to sinus rhythm is noted. In this patient, the first electrical therapy is successful for tachycardia termination. NSR = normal sinus rhythm; MGT. = magnet; VVT = triggered ventricular mode; NIEPS = noninvasive electrophysiologic study; RV = right ventricle; VT = ventricular tachycardia; c.l. = cycle length.

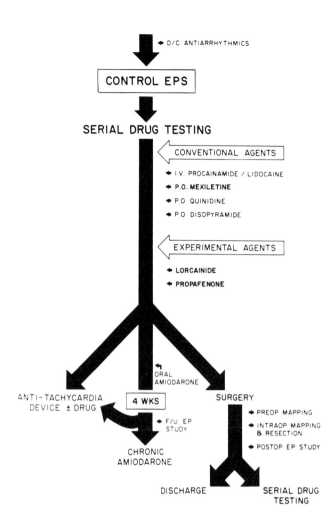

Figure 22–26. Algorithm for electrophysiologic testing in patients with sustained VT or cardiac arrest. Serial drug testing is employed after the initial diagnostic evaluation. Serial electropharmacologic testing can be used to evaluate a number of commercial and experimental antiarrhythmic drugs. Patients who fail to respond to these agents are triaged to surgical ablation, antitachycardia device alone, or antitachycardia device with chronic amiodarone therapy. Follow-up electrophysiologic testing on amiodarone is employed. Patients who continue to demonstrate inducible rapid VT on amiodarone undergo implantation of a cardioverter/defibrillator. Surgical ablation is guided by preoperative and intraoperative mapping and postoperative electrophysiologic study. (Reproduced with permission from Saksena S: Nonpharmacologic therapy for tachycardias. PACE 11:93, 1988.)

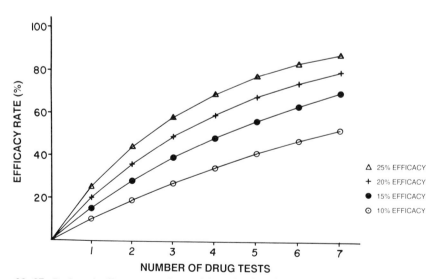

Figure 22–27. Projected efficacy rates for serial testing based on statistical assumptions, suggesting independent efficacy of each agent and efficacy rates ranging from 10 to 25 per cent per drug, as determined by electropharmacologic testing. Note that after multiple drug tests the condition in a substantial number of patients still remains uncontrolled according to electropharmacologic testing. (Reproduced with permission from Saksena S: Nonpharmacologic therapy for tachycardias. PACE 11:93, 1988.)

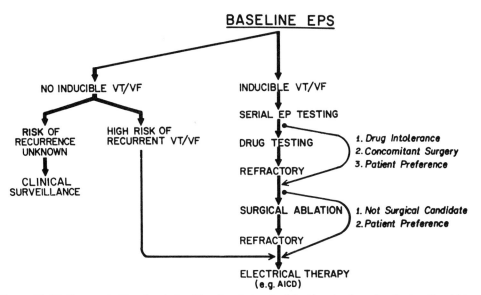

Figure 22–28. Proposed abbreviated algorithm for electrophysiologic evaluation of patients with a history of cardiac arrest or sustained ventricular tachyarrhythmias or syncope. Note that the presence of inducibility in a baseline study permits evaluation of drug therapy and consideration of mapping-guided surgery. Absence of inducibility excludes these therapeutic options. Clinical and noninvasive evaluation is used to stratify noninducible patients to determine the risk of recurrent VT or VF. In patients at high risk, electrical therapy in the form of an implantable cardioverter/defibrillator is the sole option recommended. Empiric use of drug therapy can be considered, or Holter-guided approaches may also be used in selected patients. (Reproduced with permission from Saksena S: Nonpharmacologic therapy for tachyarrhythmias. PACE 11:93, 1988.)

patients is essential to optimize the clinical outcome of electrophysiologically guided antiarrhythmic therapy in this population of patients.

TABLE 22–3. SELECTION OF PATIENTS IN THERAPY FOR VENTRICULAR TACHYCARDIA AND VENTRICULAR FIBRILLATION*

Drug Therapy	
Indications	*Contraindications*
Frequent VT/VF	Refractory VT
LVEF > 30–35%	LVEF < 20%
CAD with RWMA	CAD with aneurysm
Cardiomyopathy	

Implantable Cardioverter/Defibrillator	
Indications	*Contraindications*
Paroxysmal VT/VF	Frequent VT/VF
Prior cardiac surgery	Severe CHF
Cardiomyopathy	Anatomic abnormalities
Advanced noncardiac	requiring cardiac
disease	surgery

Intraoperative Ablation	
Indications	*Contraindications*
Frequent or paroxysmal	Polymorphic VT/VF
VT, mapping feasible	LVEF < 20%
LVEF > 20–40%	Cardiomyopathy
CAD with RWMA	

*Optimal selection of individual therapies in patients with sustained ventricular tachycardia or a history of cardiac arrest and inducible sustained ventricular tachyarrhythmias at electrophysiologic study. General guidelines are indicated.

Abbreviations: VT = ventricular tachycardia; VF = ventricular fibrillation; LVEF = left ventricular ejection fraction; RWMA = regional wall motion abnormalities; CAD = coronary artery disease; CHF = congestive heart failure.

REFERENCES

1. Akhtar M, Shenasa M, Jazayeri M, et al: Wide QRS complex tachycardia: Reappraisal of a common clinical problem. Ann Intern Med 109:905–912, 1988.
2. Bigger JT Jr, Weld FM, Rolnitzky LM: The prevalence and significance of ventricular tachycardia detected by ambulatory ECG recording in the late hospital phase of acute myocardial infarction. Am J Cardiol 48:815–822, 1981.
3. Breithardt G, Borggrefe M, Haerten K: Ventricular late potentials and inducible ventricular tachyarrhythmias as a marker for ventricular tachycardia after myocardial infarction. Eur Heart J 7[Suppl A]:127–134, 1986.
4. De Busk RF: Exercise testing in the diagnosis and management of cardiac arrhythmias. *In* Winkle R (ed): Cardiac Arrhythmias. Menlo Park, CA, Addison-Wesley, 1984, p 148.
5. Erbel R, Schweizer P, Krebs W, et al: Sensitivity and specificity of two dimensional echocardiography in detection of impaired left ventricular function. Eur Heart J 5:477–489, 1984.
6. Garan H, Ruskin JN, DiMarco JP, et al: Electrophysiologic studies before and after myocardial revascularization in patients with life-threatening ventricular arrhythmias. Am J Cardiol 51:519–524, 1983.
7. Herre JM, Mann DE, Luck JC, et al: Effect of increased current, multiple pacing sites and number of extrastimuli on induction of ventricular tachycardia. Am J Cardiol 57:102–107, 1986.
8. Kim SG, Seiden SW, Felder SD, et al: Is programmed stimulation of value in predicting the long-term success of antiarrhythmic therapy for ventricular arrhythmias? N Engl J Med 315:356–361, 1986.
9. Leclerque JF, Maisonblanche P, Couchemez B, Cou-

mel P: Respective role of sympathetic tone and of cardiac pauses in the genesis of 62 cases of ventricular fibrillation recorded during Holter Monitoring. Eur Heart J 9:1276–1283, 1988.

10. Lindsay BD, Crossen KJ, Cain ME: Concordance of distinguishing electrocardiographic features during sinus rhythm with the location of accessory pathways in the Wolff-Parkinson-White syndrome. Am J Cardiol 59:1093–1102, 1987.

11. Lindsay BD, Saksena S, Rothbart ST, et al: Prospective evaluation of a sequential pacing and high-energy bidirectional shock algorithm for transvenous cardioversion in patients with ventricular tachycardia. Circulation 76:601–609, 1987.

12. Livelli FD, Bigger JT, Reiffel JA: Response to programmed ventricular stimulation: Sensitivity, specificity and relation to heart disease. Am J Cardiol 50:452–457, 1982.

13. Lombardi F, Stein J, Podrid P, et al: Daily reproducibility of electrophysiologic test results in malignant ventricular arrhythmias. Am J Cardiol 57:96–101, 1986.

14. Mason JW: Intracardiac electrophysiologic studies: Techniques and indications. *In* Winkle RA (ed): Cardiac Arrhythmias: Current Diagnosis and Practical Management. Menlo Park, CA, Addison-Wesley, 1983, p 20.

15. Milner PG, Di Marco JP, Lerman BB: Electrophysiological evaluation of sustained ventricular tachyarrhythmias in idiopathic dilated cardiomyopathy. PACE 11:562–568, 1988.

16. Minardo JD, Heger JJ, Miles WM, et al: Clinical characteristics of patients with ventricular fibrillation during antiarrhythmic drug therapy. N Engl J Med 319:257–262, 1988.

17. Morady F, Di Carlo LA, Baerman JM, de Buitleir M: Comparison of coupling intervals that induce clinical and non-clinical forms of ventricular tachycardia during programmed stimulation. Am J Cardiol 57:1269–1273, 1986.

18. Morganroth J, Michelson EL, Horowitz LN, et al: Limitations of routine long-term electrocardiographic monitoring to assess ventricular ectopic frequency. Circulation 58:408–424, 1978.

19. Muller JE, Ludmer PL, Willich SN, et al: Circadian variation in the frequency of sudden cardiac death. Circulation 75:131–138, 1987.

20. Okumura K, Olshansky B, Henthorn RW, et al: Demonstration of the presence of slow conduction during sustained ventricular tachycardia in man: Use of transient entrainment of the tachycardia. Circulation 75:369–378, 1987.

21. Platia EV (ed): Management of Cardiac Arrhythmias: The Nonpharmacologic Approach. Philadelphia, JB Lippincott, 1987.

22. Prystowsky EN: Electrophysiologic-electropharmacologic testing in patients with ventricular arrhythmias. PACE 11:225–251, 1988.

23. Reddy GV, Schamroth L: The localization of bypass tracts in the Wolff-Parkinson-White syndrome from the surface electrocardiogram. Am Heart J 113:984–993, 1987.

24. Rinne C, Klein GJ, Sharma A, Yee R: Clinical usefulness of the 12 lead electrocardiogram in the Wolff-Parkinson-White syndrome. Cardiol Clin 5:499–509, 1987.

25. Saksena S: Non-pharmacologic therapy for tachyarrhythmias: The tower of Babel revisited [editorial]? PACE 11:93–97, 1988.

26. Saksena S, An HL, Pantopoulos D: Rapid transvenous cardioversion of sustained ventricular tachycardia by programmable implantable cardioverters/defibrillators [abstract]. J Am Coll Cardiol 11:209A, 1988.

27. Saksena S, Hussain SM, Gielchinsky I: Surgical ablation of tachyarrhythmias: Reflections for the third decade [editorial]. PACE 11:103–108, 1988.

28. Saksena S, Hussain SM, Gielchinsky I, et al: Intraoperative mapping-guided argon laser ablation of malignant ventricular tachycardia. Am J Cardiol 59:78–83, 1987.

29. Saksena S, Pantopoulos D, Parsonnet V, et al: Usefulness of an implantable antitachycardia pacemaker system for supraventricular or ventricular tachycardia. Am J Cardiol 58:70–74, 1986.

30. Simson MB: Use of signals in the terminal QRS complex to identify patients with ventricular tachycardia after myocardial infarction. Circulation 64:235–242, 1981.

31. Vandepol CJ, Farshidi A, Spielman SR, et al: Incidence and clinical significance of induced ventricular tachycardia. Am J Cardiol 45:725–733, 1980.

32. Waldo AL, Akhtar M, Benditt DG, et al: Appropriate electrophysiologic study and treatment of patients with the Wolff-Parkinson-White syndrome. PACE 11:536–544, 1988.

33. Waldo AL, Akhtar M, Brugada P, et al: The minimally appropriate electrophysiologic study for the initial assessment of patients with documented sustained monomorphic ventricular tachycardia. J Am Coll Cardiol 6:1174–1177, 1985.

34. Weaver W, Cobb L, Hallstrom A: Characteristics of survivors of exertion- and non–exertion-related cardiac arrest: Value of subsequent exercise testing. Am J Cardiol 50:671–678, 1982.

35. Wellens HJJ, Brugada P: Diagnosis of ventricular tachycardia from the 12 lead electrocardiogram. Cardiol Clin 5:511–525, 1987.

36. Wellens HJJ, Brugada P, Stevenson WG: Programmed electrical stimulation: Its role in the management of ventricular arrhythmias in coronary heart disease. Prog Cardiovasc Dis 29:165–180, 1986.

37. Wyndham CRC: Role of invasive electrophysiologic testing in the management of life-threatening ventricular arrhythmias. Am J Cardiol 62:13–17, 1988.

23

HEMODYNAMIC EFFECTS OF TACHYCARDIAS

A. Supraventricular Tachycardia

DONALD F. SWITZER, ALBERT L. WALDO,
and RICHARD W. HENTHORN

It has long been observed that comparable supraventricular tachycardias may induce an intriguing spectrum of hemodynamic responses. A tachycardia of a given mechanism and rate may be relatively asymptomatic in one patient yet induce hemodynamic collapse or syncope in another. As reviewed in other chapters of this text, the electrophysiologic mechanisms of most arrhythmias are now fairly well understood. However, the clinical relevance of any arrhythmia is determined in significant measure by the associated hemodynamic response, of which electrophysiologic aspects are but one determinant. Thus, the objectives of this chapter are to examine the central and peripheral, anatomic, and neurohumoral factors that together interact with electrophysiologic properties to determine collectively the global hemodynamic response to a given supraventricular tachycardia. This perspective should provide clinically useful insights for the management of patients with supraventricular tachycardias.

ELECTROPHYSIOLOGIC DETERMINANTS OF THE HEMODYNAMIC PROFILE

Certain electrophysiologic aspects of supraventricular tachycardias are major determi-

nants of the hemodynamic state associated with the tachycardia. In addition, there is a dynamic and reciprocating interaction between the tachycardia and hemodynamic alterations, as compensatory autonomic and neurohumoral mechanisms are stimulated that will, in turn, modify the electrophysiologic properties of the tachycardia. The electrophysiologic parameters of supraventricular tachycardias that are most relevant to the hemodynamic state include the ventricular rate, the regularity of the rhythm, the relative sequence of ventricular and atrial activation, and the atrioventricular (AV) relationship.

Increased Ventricular Rate: Acute Changes

The ventricular rate is one of the most critical determinants of the hemodynamic response to a supraventricular tachycardia. This observation has been well characterized with invasive monitoring during atrial pacing at various rates and AV intervals. If the heart rate is slowed to a bradycardiac range, left ventricular stroke volume progressively increases so that cardiac output is maintained at a constant level.[43] The maximal stroke volume is determined largely by ventricular dimensions and compliance as well as by preload and afterload. Conversely, in the resting metabolic state, during incremental right atrial pacing with preserved 1:1 AV conduction, the cardiac output will initially increase as the rate rises incrementally from 60 to 90 beats per

Supported in part by The American Heart Association Northeast Ohio Affiliate Research Initiative Award Grant and by the U.S. Public Health Service NIH-NHLBI Grant RO1 HL 38408.

minute,[64, 65] since rate increases in this range primarily diminish the period of diastolic diastasis but do not compromise ventricular filling or stroke volume. With atrial pacing rates of 90 to 140 beats per minute, diastolic filling does begin to become compromised, and thus there is no further augmentation in cardiac output,[6, 63] despite a constant ejection fraction.[35] Ross and colleagues demonstrated this plateau in the cardiac index during right atrial pacing at rates of 80 beats per minute (3.67 L/m/m^2) and 120 beats per minute (3.72 L/m/m^2).[61] DeMaria and associates used two-dimensional echocardiography in 25 normal patients during atrial pacing at rates of 50 to 150 beats per minute and demonstrated a linear decrease in both end-diastolic and end-systolic ventricular dimensions, while maintaining a constant fractional shortening.[21]

Therefore, in the normal heart, there is a relatively linear inverse relationship between heart rate and stroke volume, with maintenance of a fairly constant ejection fraction and cardiac output (if AV synchrony is preserved) up to a maximal rate of approximately 140 beats per minute. The cardiac output remains fairly constant (in the absence of organic heart disease), since the reduced stroke volume is compensated for by the increased heart rate.[25, 35, 54] With greater increments in heart rate, the cardiac output will progressively decline, since the diastolic phase of rapid ventricular filling will then be foreshortened[6, 67] and end-diastolic volume will be further compromised. The detrimental influence of rapid rate on hemodynamics is most pronounced in the setting of cardiomyopathies, ischemic heart disease, and valvular disease (especially aortic or mitral

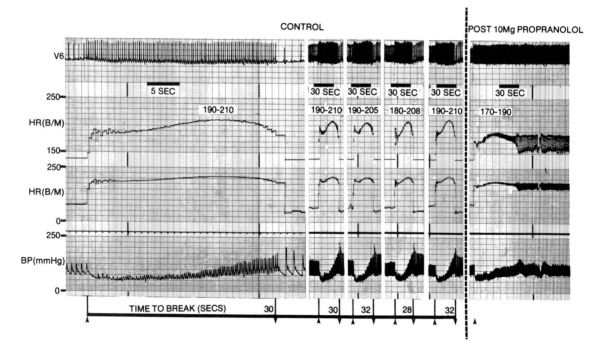

Figure 23–1. Simultaneous recording of V6, beat-to-beat heart rate (HR) on two scales and blood pressure (BP) during control conditions and after administration of 10 mg of propranolol. The arrow pointing up denotes the onset of tachycardia induced in each case by a premature atrial stimulus. The arrow pointing down signals the moment of spontaneous termination, and the numbers denote the time duration of tachycardia in seconds. Each episode of tachycardia is accompanied by a large decrease in blood pressure, which quickly begins to recover. While the pressure recovery is taking place, the rate of the tachycardia accelerates and the numbers in each panel denote the initial and maximal rate during each episode. When the blood pressure exceeds its control value, the rate slows and the tachycardia terminates. As the control panel indicates, the abrupt onset of tachycardia and associated marked decline in blood pressure and subsequent recovery is reproducible. After administration of propranolol (last panel), the decrease in blood pressure at the onset of the tachycardia is equal to that during the control episodes of tachycardia; however, the recovery of pressure is slower even though it eventually exceeds the baseline value. Thus, this example demonstrates the interaction between the hemodynamics and peripheral reflex adaptation on the electrophysiologic properties as reflected in rate. (From Waxman MB, Sharma AO, Cameron DA, et al: Reflex mechanisms responsible for early spontaneous termination of paroxysmal supraventricular tachycardia. Am J Cardiol 49:259, 1982.)

stenosis), as well as during some supraventricular tachycardias, with loss of AV synchrony or initiation of ventriculoatrial (VA) conduction.

This inverse relationship between heart rate and stroke volume, which occurs during tachycardias, does not apply to exercise-induced sinus tachycardia. Although the predominance of the increased cardiac output during exercise is related to the increased heart rate,[8] in contrast to supraventricular tachycardias (or rapid atrial pacing), ventricular stroke volume is maintained, and cardiac output therefore increases substantially.[10, 28, 61, 72, 73] Stroke volume is preserved by a combination of peripheral flow and resistance adaptations, as well as by a catecholamine-mediated inotropic augmentation in response to increased metabolic demand.

Besides cardiac output decline in response to increased rate, blood pressure can also be substantially reduced. The abrupt onset of increased rates are known to reduce blood pressure with a typical pattern of maximal decline initially, subsequent rise, and sometimes an overshoot of blood pressure compared to baseline (Fig. 23–1).[75] The response of the blood pressure depends on peripheral adaptation. In patients, the initial decline in blood pressure after the onset of a tachycardia can be associated with presyncope and even syncope in some cases. As seen in Figure 23–1, depending on the reflex response, a paroxysmal supraventricular tachycardia could terminate as a result of an overshoot of the blood pressure or stabilize at a lower, equal, or higher level of blood pressure than baseline after the initial decline. Thus, not surprisingly, blood pressure as well as cardiac output is also quite dependent on heart rate, with maximal changes associated with an abrupt increment in rate.

There is also a significant reduction in coronary blood flow during supraventricular tachycardias and a rate-related increment of myocardial oxygen consumption despite maintenance of the baseline cardiac output. Corday and coworkers demonstrated a 33 to 35 per cent mean reduction in coronary artery flow during AV reciprocating tachycardia (AVRT) or atrial fibrillation.[17] The reduction in coronary artery flow is inversely proportional to heart rate and decreases progressively to a maximum of 60 per cent of baseline. During supraventricular tachycardias, this reduction in coronary flow is induced by changes in both systolic and diastolic function. First, the diastolic interval is significantly abbreviated,

thereby limiting the time for coronary flow. Second, as mean aortic pressure declines, coronary artery perfusion pressure is reduced. Third, if there is associated ischemia[4, 69] or diastolic dysfunction, then left ventricular end-diastolic pressure rises as the supraventricular tachycardia continues. Furthermore, the decrease in coronary artery flow occurs in the face of an increase in myocardial oxygen consumption resulting from the enhanced rate of contraction. This combination of factors explains the frequent association of symptomatic ischemia with supraventricular tachycardias.

Increased Ventricular Rate: Chronic Changes (Tachycardia-Induced Cardiomyopathy)

Despite preservation of nearly baseline cardiac output during acute supraventricular tachycardias in patients without organic heart disease, it has been often observed that chronic tachycardias may induce a dilated cardiomyopathy in the absence of clinical or echocardiographic evidence of primary myocardial disease prior to the onset of the chronic tachycardia. There is now impressive clinical and laboratory support for the hypothesis that chronic tachycardia can induce significant left ventricular dysfunction.[11, 16, 19, 25, 53, 54, 56, 79] However, as cautioned by Gallagher,[25] it is often difficult to exclude the possibility that a tachycardia is a manifestation of an occult cardiomyopathy. In the latter instance, the supraventricular tachycardia is not the primary cause of subsequent progression of congestive heart failure.

Laboratory support for substantial systolic dysfunction induced by chronic supraventricular tachycardia is available from studies involving persistent atrial pacing in dogs. For example, in 13 dogs paced at a rate of 190 beats per minute for 3 months, Damiano and colleagues found a secondary reduction in ejection fraction from a baseline of 49 ± 1 per cent to 29 ± 2 per cent, associated with an increased end-diastolic volume.[19] Coleman and associates[16] noted new congestive heart failure in six dogs following 2 to 4 weeks of rapid atrial pacing. Myocardial adenosine triphosphate (ATP) and creatine phosphokinase stores were found to be significantly depleted in these dogs. However, during tachycardia at the rates used to induce a cardiomyopathy in these canine studies, there was no evidence of acute ischemia, since there was no detectable change in lactate extraction or myocardial oxygen extraction, and at postmortem evaluation, histologic examination revealed no evidence of infarction, fiber hypertrophy, or fibrosis.[79] Thus, depletion of myocardial energy stores has been the favored hypothesis explaining the reversible left ventricular dysfunction induced by chronic tachycardia.

Additional support for the potential of chronic tachycardia to induce a dilated cardiomyopathy comes from observations of patients.[11, 25, 53, 54, 56] In 1949, Phillips and Levine[56] reported on 84 patients having chronic atrial fibrillation without apparent cardiovascular disease. In those who developed congestive heart failure, there was no association with the duration of the rhythm, but there was a significant association with a fast ventricular response in those patients developing congestive heart failure. Packer and associates[54] reported on eight patients with left ventricular dysfunction in the absence of organic heart disease, in whom the left ventricular dysfunction was attributed to incessant chronic tachycardias (2 to 41 years' duration). After ablation or surgical interruption of these tachycardias, the mean left ventricular ejection fraction rose from 19 ± 9 per cent to 33 ± 17 per cent at 8 days and to 45 ± 15 per cent at 22 months.

In summary, chronic supraventricular tachycardias of any mechanism can induce a dilated cardiomyopathy and congestive heart failure. The risk is proportional to the mean ventricular rate. This left ventricular dilatation is associated with a normal myocardial histology in canine models. The mechanism of the induced ventricular dysfunction is likely related to a chronic depletion of myocardial energy stores and is mostly reversible if the tachycardia is controlled.

Atrial Contribution to Ventricular Stroke Volume

The relative importance of the atrial contribution to ventricular stroke volume varies considerably among patients. Atrial systole may contribute up to 35 per cent of the stroke volume in some circumstances.[57] Many factors determine the relative value of normal atrial function, including the ventricular rate, the relative timing of atrial and ventricular systole, and the completeness of passive ventricular filling at the time of atrial systole. The extent of this passive ventricular filling is, in turn, dependent on ventricular compliance, the left ventricular end-diastolic pressure, and the presence of AV valvular disease.

The consequences of loss of the atrial contribution to ventricular stroke volume are largely dependent on ventricular rate. For example, at a rate of 100 beats per minute with nearly normal left ventricular filling pressures, atrial systole contributes little to left ventricular stroke volume, whereas at a rate of 160 beats per minute, the left ventricular end-diastolic volume is reduced by one third if the atrial contribution is lost.[14] This effect will be exaggerated in the setting of mitral valve disease, poor left ventricular compliance, or any other preload-sensitive condition.

Furthermore, if the left ventricular end-diastolic pressure is reduced or maintained at nearly normal values during a supraventricular tachycardia, then the curvilinear relationship between stroke volume and left ventricular end-diastolic pressure is steepest and atrial systole will have a profound impact on stroke volume. Alternatively, if the left ventricular end-diastolic pressure is significantly elevated, then the flat portion of the Starling curve is in effect and any further increase in ventricular filling pressure will have little impact on stroke volume.[29] Therefore, loss of the atrial contribution to ventricular stroke volume is most deleterious during supraventricular tachycardias in the setting of inadequate left ventricular filling pressures, rapid rates, or noncompliant ventricles.

Regularity of Rate

Regularity of heart rate is a relatively minor determinant of the global hemodynamic response to a supraventricular tachycardia, but beat-to-beat variability is frequently associated with symptoms, primarily palpitations. Irregularity in any rhythm will often induce symptoms, mainly owing to variations in the beat-to-beat ventricular stroke volume, which result from several mechanisms. First, premature beats result in postventricular extrasystolic potentiation, that is, augmentation of the force of contraction (the presumed cause of a palpitation) of the subsequent beat; the earlier the premature beat, the greater the extent of potentiation of the next beat. In addition, the effects of potentiation can last for several beats. By the Starling mechanisms, the longer the preceding RR interval, the greater are the end-diastolic volume and sarcomere stretch, resulting in both a greater volume and a greater force of contraction. This beat-to-beat variation in volume and contractile force is often symptomatic. Abrupt rate changes are generally more symptomatic, since compensatory mechanisms do not occur immediately. This observation is most dramatically demonstrated in patients with the tachycardia-bradycardia syndrome.

Irregularity may also influence the hemodynamic state. Atrial fibrillation is the most frequent irregular supraventricular tachycardia. Atrial fibrillation has been found to impose a 9 per cent further reduction in cardiac output over that associated with loss of AV synchrony at a comparable rate.[45] Quantitative evaluation of the hemodynamic changes induced by supraventricular tachycardias began in the 1960s, primarily with observations on the hemodynamic changes following conversion of atrial fibrillation to sinus rhythm.[7, 26, 34, 59, 68] A minimal increment in cardiac output (6 to 10 per cent) was generally noted acutely after conversion of atrial fibrillation to sinus rhythm.[7, 59, 68] This increment in cardiac output is associated with a slower mean heart rate and therefore involves an augmentation of stroke volume. Initial hemodynamic improvements generally become more pronounced with time after cardioversion. This finding has been attributed to resolution of anesthesia effects and improved atrial contractility with time but may also reflect improvement in both atrial and ventricular function after interruption of the chronic tachycardiac state as previously discussed under "Increased Ventricular Rate: Chronic Changes (Tachycardiac-Induced Cardiomyopathy)." The cardiac output may increase up to 30 per cent 3 days after cardioversion.[68] Therefore, following cardioversion from atrial fibrillation to sinus rhythm, a modest increase in cardiac output, ranging from 6 to 30 per cent, is generally noted and is associated with a decrease in systemic vascular resistance,[7] a reduction in left ventricular end-diastolic pressure[59] and myocardial oxygen consumption, and an increased exercise performance[7, 26] and stroke index during exercise.[7]

Sequence of Ventricular Activation

The importance of the sequence of ventricular activation is generally minimal in regard to the hemodynamic state. During a supraventricular tachycardia, the sequence of ventricular activation may be altered by two mechanisms: Antegrade activation may occur over an accessory AV connection, or a functional bundle branch block may develop during the tachycardia. There is a reduction in cardiac output with abnormal ventricular activation. The significance of this reduction is inversely proportional to the amount of myocardial muscle mass that is activated slowly via myocardial conduction compared with that activated normally via the His-Purkinje system. The former is associated with a reduction in the rate of rise of the left ventricular systolic pressure and a small decrease in cardiac output, which is rarely of clinical consequence.

Atrioventricular Synchrony

The relative timing of both atrial and ventricular systole can have profound influences on the hemodynamic state during a supraventricular tachycardia. The most relevant factors are preservation of normal AV synchrony and the adverse reflex mechanisms (discussed later) resulting from atrial activation against closed AV valves.

The relative timing of atrial and ventricular systole (the AV interval) has been best quantitated in canine models. For example, Naito and coworkers utilized variable AV dual-chamber pacing intervals in 20 open-chest dogs with complete heart block and found the maximal cardiac output to occur at an AV interval of 100 msec.[45] During regular ventricular pacing at nontachycardiac rates, there was a nearly identical reduction in cardiac output (18 per cent) with either atrial fibrillation or AV dissociation. With fixed-rate AV pacing, as the AV interval was reduced from 100 to 0 msec, there was an associated reduction in left ventricular end-diastolic volume, stroke volume, cardiac output, and aortic systolic pressure.[46] This reduction in left ventricular end-diastolic volume was associated with an echocardiographically demonstrable increase in left atrial end-diastolic volume.[47]

When the AV interval was further reduced to −100 msec (simulating VA conduction), there was noted an additional acute reduction in cardiac output by 25 per cent of baseline.[45, 46] With an AV interval of −100 msec, atrial systole occurs against closed AV valves, inducing retrograde flow into the pulmonary and systemic central veins. Similarly, during rapid atrial pacing (cycle length, 400 msec), as the AV interval was reduced from +100 msec to 0 msec to −100 msec, there was a significant decline in both systolic blood pressure and cardiac output (Fig. 23–2).[52] For reasons reviewed later, this inverse AV relationship is less well tolerated hemodynamically than is atrial fibrillation or AV dissociation.

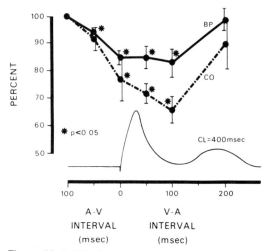

Figure 23–2. This figure demonstrates the effect of the AV and VA relationship on blood pressure and cardiac output. The above figure plots the average percentage of blood pressure (BP) and cardiac output (CO) change in relationship to various AV and VA intervals from seven dogs. Constant ventricular pacing was performed from the RV apex at 400 msec. The AV or VA interval was varied by constantly pacing the atrium using a programmable pulse generator. Cardiac output and blood pressure fall at AV intervals of <50 msec and are most marked at VA intervals of 100 msec. (From Ogawa S, Dreifus LS, Shendy PN et al: Hemodynamics of atrioventricular and ventriculoatrial pacing. PACE 1:8, 1978.)

Ogawa and associates studied the effects of the relative timing of atrial and ventricular activation on hemodynamic parameters as a function of the rate of tachycardia.[52] In instrumented dogs with complete heart block, pacing at a 400-msec cycle length with a physiologic AV interval (100 msec) was associated with an end-diastolic gradient across the AV valve favorable for ventricular filling as well as completion of atrial systole prior to the ventricular preejection period, thereby facilitating AV valve closure. Reduction of the AV interval to 0 msec was associated with a decrease in aortic pressure but without a loss of cardiac output, as atrial systole occurred at the onset of the ventricular preejection period. A further reduction of the AV interval to −50 msec (i.e., VA = 50 msec) was accompanied by a significant loss of aortic pressure and cardiac output, with cannon A waves appearing within the ventricular ejection period. Repetition of these AV intervals at a faster pacing rate (300-msec cycle length) was associated with a further hypotensive response and marked mechanical alternans, thereby demonstrating that the detrimental effects of VA conduction during supraventricular tachycardias are exaggerated with shorter cycle lengths of the tachycardia.

The number of times that the atria are activated for each ventricular systole is also relevant. For example, at a comparable ventricular rate, atrial flutter will induce a greater reduction in left ventricular stroke volume than an AV synchronous ectopic atrial tachycardia with an identical ventricular response rate. In atrial flutter, every other atrial activation occurs against a closed AV valve.[31] Therefore, a 1:1 relationship between atrial and ventricular activation is hemodynamically superior, provided that atrial systole does not occur during ventricular contraction.

AV synchrony also reverses the AV pressure gradient immediately before ventricular systole to facilitate presystolic closure of the AV valves. With the use of pulsed Doppler techniques, minimal late diastolic mitral incompetence can be demonstrated in more than 50 per cent of patients when atrial activation occurs in early diastole. This mitral incompetence is associated with the development of a left ventricular–left atrial pressure gradient at the end of diastole[55] prior to the rapid increase in left ventricular pressure at the preejection period, which normally ensures abrupt closure of the valves.

In summary, during supraventricular tachycardias, the most important electrophysiologic determinants of hemodynamics are rate, most pronounced at the initiation of an arrhythmia, and the AV relationship, which is most deleterious when the atria contract against closed AV valves. Sequence of activation and irregularity of rhythm have considerably less impact on hemodynamics. Finally, chronic increments of rate can lead to loss of myocardial energy stores, with consequent chronic, but largely reversible, loss of myocardial function.

ANATOMIC DETERMINANTS OF THE HEMODYNAMIC PROFILE

During any given supraventricular tachycardia, patients with organic heart disease are generally more symptomatic than those patients without structural heart disease. There exist a number of mechanical factors that contribute to the determination of the severity of presenting symptoms during a supraventricular tachycardia. Patients with significant organic heart disease maintain their systolic function (ejection fraction) at the expense of chronic adaptations in end-diastolic volume (preload) and end-systolic wall stress (afterload). If a supraventricular tachycardia intervenes, it is often poorly tolerated, since chronic utilization of these manipulations of preload and afterload leaves little functional reserve to improve systolic function acutely during the tachycardia. We will elaborate on how organic heart disease influences the hemodynamic response of supraventricular tachycardia by highlighting atrial fibrillation with different disease states.

During atrial fibrillation, patients with a normal heart and normal peripheral reflexes will generally have minimal or no symptoms at rest owing to the prompt recruitment of compensatory mechanisms, but there will be impairment of exercise capacity, since further functional reserve is then limited. However, patients with significant left ventricular dysfunction can become symptomatic at rest with atrial fibrillation, since they have already optimized their hemodynamic adaptive reserves.[32, 51] The influence of tachycardia on ejection fraction was reviewed earlier. In patients with compromised left ventricular systolic function at rest, there can be a further decline in ventricular ejection fraction during tachycardia related to a significant reduction in end-diastolic volume and stroke volume.[71]

In addition to impairment of systolic function imposed by rapid rates and the loss of AV synchrony, alterations in diastolic function also frequently contribute to the compromised hemodynamic state during a supraventricular tachycardia.[44] During sinus rhythm, left ventricular filling is biphasic at rest. Initial passive rapid inflow is distinguished from late diastolic flow (due to atrial systole) by a period of diastasis. Unimpaired ventricular isovolumetric relaxation is an energy-consuming process. Exercise and other methods of catecholamine exposure both enhance systolic function and reduce the time constant for isovolumetric relaxation (rapid filling phase). This augmentation of diastolic filling does not occur following postextrasystolic potentiation.[48] During atrial fibrillation, there is little beat-to-beat variation in relaxation despite considerable variability in systolic function related to potentiation. Therefore, the regulation of contractility and that of energy-dependent relaxation are independent.[48]

During tachycardia, the period of diastasis is progressively abbreviated until there is fusion of early and late flow peaks.[15, 51] In patients with moderate hypertension, there is a reduction in rapid left ventricular filling rates,[70] which becomes more pronounced during tachycardias. In patients with coronary artery disease, during sinus tachycardia there

is an additional decrease in late diastolic filling rates.[15] The decline in stroke volume during tachycardias in patients with diastolic dysfunction will be most pronounced if the left ventricular filling pressures are normal or diminished.

Patients with valvular disease, particularly aortic stenosis or mitral stenosis, often have profound deterioration in their hemodynamic and functional states with the onset of a supraventricular tachycardia. In aortic stenosis, the impaired ventricular compliance associated with the hypertrophied ventricle imposes a significant reduction in early diastolic filling rates. The severity of imposed diastolic function is inversely proportional to age, left ventricular end-systolic pressure, and left ventricular wall thickness.[23] Similar impairment occurs in patients with hypertrophic cardiomyopathy and, to a lesser extent, in patients with hypertension. Thus, every effort should be made to maintain sinus rhythm in patients with left-sided stenotic valvular lesions or those with diastolic dysfunction, including hypertrophy or hypertrophic cardiomyopathy.

Optimal diastolic filling parameters are essential if systolic stroke volume is to be maintained. With the onset of atrial fibrillation and a rapid ventricular response rate, both the abbreviated diastolic filling period and the reduced filling pressures related to loss of AV synchrony contribute to an inability to overcome adequately the exaggerated left ventricular wall stress.[30] Left ventricular end-diastolic volume is reduced, and sacromere length is not adequately lengthened to maintain resting stroke volume, resulting in symptomatic pulmonary venous hypertension. In aortic stenosis, loss of AV synchrony, even at physiologic rates, has been shown to be associated with a 31 per cent reduction in resting stroke volume.[33] Heidenreich and colleagues dissociated the booster pump atrial function from its reservoir-conduit function in patients with aortic and mitral stenosis and determined that the booster pump function is the primary determinant of this increased stroke volume with AV synchrony.[33] The mechanism of syncope and sudden death in patients with aortic stenosis is likely multifactorial, but new onset of atrial fibrillation with a rapid ventricular rate can be one contributor.

In patients with mitral stenosis, the development of atrial fibrillation is associated with substantial exaggeration of symptoms and at least a twofold increase in mortality,[24, 36] as well as a 10 to 17 per cent increase in the incidence of embolic strokes. The symptoms associated with the onset of atrial fibrillation in mitral stenosis are proportional to the ventricular rate and the severity of the valvular stenosis. Hemodynamic consequences range from new exertional dyspnea to acute pulmonary edema. This impairment is attributable to both loss of atrial booster pump function[33] and the abbreviated time for diastolic flow through the stenotic mitral valve orifice.[3]

NEUROHUMORAL DETERMINANTS OF THE HEMODYNAMIC PROFILE

We have reviewed many of the electrophysiologic and mechanical determinants of potential hemodynamic profiles during supraventricular tachycardias. However, these factors collectively do not sufficiently explain the significant hypotension associated with some supraventricular tachycardias. This exaggerated hypotensive response is often related to an inappropriate loss of systemic vascular resistance, primarily induced by neurohumoral mediators of atrial stretch reflexes.

Atrial Vasodepressor Reflex

Systolic and mean atrial pressures generally rise during supraventricular tachycardias owing to one or more of the following: The diastolic time for atrial drainage is abbreviated; atrial contraction may occur against closed AV valves; AV valvular incompetence may develop or increase; and the left ventricular end-diastolic pressure generally increases if ischemia is induced by the tachycardia.

It was recognized in 1962[66] that atrial pressure rises most dramatically during those supraventricular tachycardias that involve atrial stimulation during ventricular systole. The atria therefore contract against closed AV valves, and the atrial pressure rises substantially until the AV valves are able to reopen during ventricular relaxation. The resultant atrial distention stimulates atrial stretch receptors, which is followed by an inappropriate reflex peripheral vasodilation. The resultant loss of systemic vascular resistance antagonizes the ability of aortic and carotid baroreceptors to mediate restoration of aortic pressure. The same atrial vasodepressor reflex is largely responsible for the relative hypotension during VVI pacing in those patients with intact VA conduction and the pacemaker syndrome.[1, 2, 5, 22]

Atrial Natriuretic Peptide

Atrial natriuretic peptide (ANP) is released from specific atrial granules in response to elevation of atrial pressure and facilitates regulation of intravascular tone and volume by effecting natriuresis, vasodilation, and inhibition of aldosterone.[9, 50] It has also been well documented that ANP levels substantially increase during AVRTs.[49, 50] This ANP response can be mimicked during simultaneous atrial and ventricular pacing. The rise in ANP level observed during supraventricular tachycardias does not occur during sinus tachycardia at comparable heart rates.[49, 58] ANP levels during supraventricular tachycardias of any mechanism have a strong relationship to mean atrial pressure,[37, 58] but not directly to the heart rate.[49, 58]

Polyuria associated with paroxysmal supraventricular tachycardias was described by Wenkebach and Winteberg in 1927[78] and subsequently was further characterized by Paul Wood.[80] This polyuria does not accompany episodes of ventricular tachycardia, yet with supraventricular tachycardias, "urina spastica" occurs with a 20 to 50 per cent incidence[37, 40, 58] and has been most frequently described with atrial fibrillation.[37] It was observed by Wood that this polyuria is not dependent on the tachycardia rate but is a function of its duration, requiring episodes longer than 10 minutes before it appears.[80] This diuresis occurs despite a reduction in renal blood flow and often despite a compromised aortic pressure[38] and is now recognized to be associated with ANP release.[13, 37, 49, 62] The release of ANP and subsequent diuresis will generally be greatest when there is a significant, abrupt elevation in atrial distention during tachycardia. A comparable polyuria has also been observed in normal volunteers given an ANP extract during sinus rhythm.[60]

In summary, ANP is a potent mediator of the endocrine regulation of both vasodilation and natriuresis. Thus, during supraventricular arrhythmias associated with abrupt atrial distention, particularly noted during tachycardias with simultaneous atrial and ventricular activation, ANP plays an important role in determining the overall hemodynamic response.

Autonomic Tone

There are immediate alterations in the sympathetic and vagal tone during tachycardias of any mechanism, largely induced by primary hemodynamic alterations but also influenced by emotion and the patient's global cardiac reserve. These autonomic adaptations are most pronounced immediately after the onset of tachycardia.

As outlined by Curry[18] and Waxman and associates,[75, 77] there is an immediate interplay between the hemodynamic profile imposed by a supraventricular tachycardia and the neurohumoral reflexes compensatory for these hemodynamic alterations. These neurohumoral changes may then modify primary electrophysiologic properties of the tachycardia. The electrophysiologic consequences of this interplay between hemodynamics and neurohumoral properties may include changes in the rate of tachycardia, its duration, and its vulnerability to termination (see Fig. 23–1).[18, 27, 75]

Variations in heart rate during AVRTs (during one sustained episode or variations between recurrences) are primarily determined at the level of the AV node in any individual patient. Alternate mechanisms for rate variability include rate changes after incorporation of a second accessory AV connection in a tachycardia circuit or after the development of bundle branch block ipsilateral to the location of the accessory AV connection in those reciprocating tachycardias involving ventricular preexcitation syndromes. The temporal variability in AV node conduction, and therefore the variability in the rate of AVRTs, is largely determined by changes in the instantaneous autonomic tone. These changes, in turn, are primarily a function of changes in the afferent input from baroreceptors. Physiologically, the negative dromotropic influence of a rapid rate of stimulation on AV node response is usually overcome during ambulatory supraventricular tachycardias by a corresponding increased sympathetic tone.[12, 20, 39, 41, 42, 74, 76]

Spontaneous termination of supraventricular tachycardias, particularly reciprocating tachycardias, is also dependent on the interaction of autonomic tone with components of the tachycardia circuit. Waxman and colleagues[74–77] demonstrated that those supraventricular tachycardias that spontaneously terminate within 1 minute of initiation are consistently associated with an initial hypotension at the onset of the rhythm, followed by recovery of aortic pressure to a level above that prior to the tachycardia (overshoot), which is then followed by termination. The overshoot reflex is a sympathetic response to the initial hypotension. Termination at the level of the AV node occurs with an associated rise in vagal tone in response to baroreceptor stimulation during the aortic pressure overshoot. Waxman further noted that this sequence of events leading to spontaneous, vagally mediated termination of supraventricular tachycardia at the AV node occurred most frequently when the patient was in the supine position (45 per cent of 20 patients studied) compared with 8 per cent of patients in a Trendelenburg position (which blunts the initial hypotension) and 6 per cent of patients studied in a head-up tilt position (which blunts the sympathetic-mediated pressure overshoot).

The influences of such neurohumoral feedback on the electrophysiologic milieu should be carefully considered when selecting therapy for any individual patient. For example, beta blockade may reduce the recurrence rate of reciprocating tachycardias involving the AV node by increasing the likelihood of conduction block in the AV node during premature atrial contractions and by blunting catecholamine-induced shortening of AV node refractoriness. However, beta blockade may also blunt the sympathetic overshoot response during reciprocating tachycardia, therefore reducing the chances for spontaneous termination, should AVRT occur (see Fig. 23–1).

CONCLUSIONS

There is a complex interplay of electrophysiologic, anatomic, and neurohumoral factors that collectively determine the global hemodynamic profile during a specific supraventricular tachycardia. We have discussed their major components and reviewed their potential contributions to the hemodynamic manifestations of various supraventricular tachycardias. Because in a given patient the mechanical, electrical, autonomic, and neurohumoral systems may vary considerably, it is difficult to predict the hemodynamic response of a given supraventricular tachycardia in a given patient a priori. Furthermore, the dynamic response is complicated not only by the interaction of several of these factors but also by the variability of each of these factors from patient to patient and by the temporal variability of the magnitude of these factors at the initiation and maintenance phases of supraventricular arrhythmias. Despite these limitations in predicting the overall hemodynamic response in a given patient, knowledge of these determinants of the hemodynamic profile and their interactions should provide an enlightened framework within which the physician can tailor therapies in any given patient and thus provide for a more favorable hemodynamic outcome, should a supraventricular tachycardia not be controlled.

REFERENCES

1. Abata K, Yasue H, Horao Y, et al: Increase in atrial natriuretic polypeptide in response to cardiac pacing. Am Heart J 113:845, 1987.
2. Alicandri C, Fouad FM, Tarazi RC, et al: Three cases of hypotension and syncope with ventricular pacing: Possible role of atrial reflexes. Am J Cardiol 42:137, 1978.
3. Arani DT, Carleton RA: The deleterious role of tachycardia in mitral stenosis. Circulation 36:511, 1967.
4. Aroesty JM, McKay RG, Heller GV, et al: Simultaneous assessment of left ventricular systolic and diastolic dysfunction during pacing-induced ischemia. Circulation 71:889, 1985.
5. Ausubel K, Furman S: The pacemaker syndrome. Ann Intern Med 103:420, 1985.
6. Benchimol A, Liggett MS: Cardiac hemodynamics during stimulation of the right atrium, right ventricle and left ventricle in normal and abnormal hearts. Circulation 33:933, 1966.
7. Benchimol A, Lowe HM, Akre PR: Cardiovascular response to exercise during atrial fibrillation and after conversion to sinus rhythm. Am J Cardiol 16:31, 1965.
8. Bevegard S, Jonsson B, Karlof I, et al: Effect of changes in ventricular rate on cardiac output and central pressures at rest and during exercise in patients with artificial pacemakers. Cardiovasc Res 1:21, 1967.
9. Bolli P, Muller FB, Linder L, et al: The vasodilator potency of atrial natriuretic peptide in man. Circulation 75:221, 1987.
10. Braunwald E, Goldblatt A, Harrison DC, Mason DT: Studies on cardiac dimensions in intact unanesthetized man. III. Effects of muscular exercise. Circ Res 13:460, 1963.
11. Brill IC: Congestive heart failure arising from uncontrolled auricular fibrillation in the otherwise normal heart. Am J Med 2:544, 1947.
12. Butrous GS, Cochrane T, Camm AJ: Rapid autonomic tone regulation of atrioventricular nodal conduction in man. Am Heart J 113:934, 1987.
13. Canepa-Anson R, Williams M, Marshall J, et al: Mechanism of polyuria and natriuresis in atrioventricular nodal tachycardia. Br Med J 289:866, 1984.
14. Carleton RA, Graettinger JS: Hemodynamic role of the atria with and without mitral stenosis. Am J Med 42:532, 1967.
15. Carroll JD, Hess OM, Hirzel HO, Krayenbuehl HP: Dynamics of left ventricular filling at rest and during exercise. Circulation 68:59, 1983.
16. Coleman HN, Taylor RR, Pool PE, et al: Congestive heart failure following chronic tachycardia. Am Heart J 81:790, 1971.
17. Corday E, Gold H, De Vera LB, et al: Effect of the cardiac arrhythmias on the coronary circulation. Ann Intern Med 50:535, 1959.
18. Curry PVL: The hemodynamic and electrophysiological effects of paroxysmal tachycardia. In Narula OS (ed): Cardiac Arrhythmias: Electrophysiology, Diagnosis and Management. Baltimore, The Williams & Wilkins Co, 1979, p 364.
19. Damiano RJ, Pripp HS, Small KW, et al: The functional consequences of prolonged supraventricular tachycardia [abstract]. J Am Coll Cardiol 5:541, 1985.
20. De Beer EL, Boom HBK, Naafs B: The combined influence of the stimulus frequency of the vagal nerves and the atrial stimulus interval on the atrioventricular conduction time. Cardiovasc Res 11:47, 1977.
21. DeMaria AN, Neumann A, Schubart PJ, et al: Systematic correlation of cardiac chamber size and ventricular performance determined with echocardiography and alterations in heart rate in normal persons. Am J Cardiol 43:1, 1979.
22. Erlebacher JA, Danner RL, Stelzer PE: Hypotension with ventricular pacing: An atrial vasodepressor reflex in human beings. J Am Coll Cardiol 4:550, 1984.
23. Fifer MA, Borow KM, Colan SD, Lorell B: Early diastolic left ventricular function in children and adults with aortic stenosis. J Am Coll Cardiol 5:1147, 1985.
24. Gajewski J, Singer RB: Mortality in an insured population with atrial fibrillation. JAMA 245:1540, 1981.
25. Gallagher JJ: Tachycardia and cardiomyopathy: The chicken-egg dilemma revisited. J Am Coll Cardiol 6:1172, 1985.
26. Gilbert R, Eich RH, Smulyan H, et al: Effect on circulation of conversion of atrial fibrillation to sinus rhythm. Circulation 27:1079, 1963.
27. Goldreyer BN, Kastor JA, Kershbaum KL: The hemodynamic effects of induced supraventricular tachycardia in man. Circulation 54:783, 1976.
28. Gorlin R, Cohen LS, Elliott WC, et al: Effect of supine exercise on left ventricular volume and oxygen consumption in man. Circulation 32:361, 1965.
29. Greenberg B, Chatterjee K, Parmley WW, et al: The influence of left ventricular filling pressure on atrial contribution to cardiac output. Am Heart J 98:742, 1979.
30. Grossman W, McLaurin BP: Diastolic properties of the left ventricle. Ann Intern Med 84:316, 1976.
31. Harvey RM, Ferrer MI, Richards DW, Cournand A: Cardiocirculatory performance in atrial flutter. Circulation 12:507, 1955.
32. Hecht HH, Osher WJ, Samuels AJ: Cardiovascular adjustments in subjects with organic heart disease before and after conversion of atrial fibrillation to normal sinus rhythm. J Clin Invest 30:647, 1951.
33. Heidenreich FP, Shaver JA, Thompson ME, Leonard JJ: Left atrial booster function in valvular heart disease. J Clin Invest 49:1605, 1970.
34. Hornsten TR, Bruce RA: Effects of atrial fibrillation on exercise performance in patients with cardiac disease. Circulation 37:543, 1968.
35. Hung J, Kelly DT, Hutton BF, et al: Influence of heart rate and atrial transport on left ventricular volume and function: Relation to hemodynamic changes produced by supraventricular arrhythmia. Am J Cardiol 48:632, 1981.
36. Kannel WB, Abbott RP, Savage DD, McNamara PM: Epidemiologic features of chronic atrial fibrillation: The Framingham Study. N Engl J Med 306:1018, 1982.
37. Kaye GC, Nathan AW, Camm AJ: Polyuria associated with paroxysmal tachycardia. Clin Prog Electrophysiol Pacing 2:349, 1984.
38. Laragh JH: Atrial natriuretic hormone, the renin-aldosterone axis, and blood pressure–electrolyte homeostasis. N Engl J Med 313:1330, 1985.
39. Levy M, Martin PJ: Neural control of the heart. In Berne RM, Sperelakis N, Geiger SR (eds): Handbook of Physiology, Section 2: The Cardiovascular System. Vol 1, The Heart. Bethesda, MD, American Physiology Society, 1979, p 581.
40. Luria M: Selected clinical features of paroxysmal

tachycardia: A prospective study in 120 patients. Br Heart J 33:351, 1971.

41. Mancia G, Bonazzi O, Pozzoni L: Baroreceptor control of atrioventricular conduction in man. Circ Res 44:752, 1979.

42. Martin PJ: Paradoxical dynamic interaction of heart period and vagal activity or atrioventricular conduction in the dog. Circ Res 40:81, 1977.

43. McIntosh HD, Morris JJ Jr: The hemodynamic consequences of arrhythmias. Prog Cardiovasc Dis 8:330, 1966.

44. Mitchell JH, Shapiro W: Atrial function and the hemodynamic consequences of atrial fibrillation in man. Am J Cardiol 23:556, 1979.

45. Naito M, David D, Michelson EL, et al: The hemodynamic consequences of cardiac arrhythmias: Evaluation of the relative roles of abnormal atrioventricular sequencing, irregularity of ventricular rhythm and atrial fibrillation in a canine model. Am Heart J 106:284, 1983.

46. Naito M, Dreifus LS, David D, et al: Reevaluation of the role of atrial systole to cardiac hemodynamics: Evidence for pulmonary venous regurgitation during abnormal atrioventricular sequencing. Am Heart J 105:295, 1983.

47. Naito M, Dreifus LS, Mardelli TJ, et al: Echocardiographic features of atrioventricular and ventriculoatrial conduction. Am J Cardiol 46:625, 1980.

48. Nakamura Y, Konishi T, Nonogi H, et al: Myocardial relaxation in atrial fibrillation. J Am Coll Cardiol 7:68, 1986.

49. Nicklas JM, DiCarlo LA, Koller PT, et al: Plasma levels of immunoreactive atrial natriuretic factor increase during supraventricular tachycardia. Am Heart J 112:923, 1986.

50. Nilsson G, Pettersson A, Hedner J, Hedner T: Increased plasma levels of atrial natriuretic peptide (ANP) in patients with paroxysmal supraventricular tachyarrhythmias. Acta Med Scand 221:15, 1987.

51. Nolan SP, Dixon SH, Fisher RD, Morrow AG: The influence of atrial contraction and mitral valve mechanics on ventricular filling. Am Heart J 77:784, 1969.

52. Ogawa S, Dreifus LS, Shenoy PN, et al: Hemodynamics of atrioventricular and ventriculoatrial pacing. PACE 1:8, 1978.

53. Packer DL, Bardy GH, Gallagher JJ, et al: Tachycardia induced cardiomyopathy: A reversible form of left ventricular dysfunction [abstract]. J Am Coll Cardiol 3:521, 1984.

54. Packer DL, Bardy GH, Worley SJ, et al: Tachycardia-induced cardiomyopathy: A reversible form of left ventricular dysfunction. Am J Cardiol 57:563, 1986.

55. Panidis IP, Ross J, Munley B, et al: Diastolic mitral regurgitation in patients with atrioventricular conduction abnormalities: A common finding by Doppler echocardiography. J Am Coll Cardiol 7:768, 1986.

56. Phillips E, Levine SA: Auricular fibrillation without other evidence of heart disease: A cause of reversible heart failure. Am J Med 7:478, 1949.

57. Rahimtoola SH, Ehsani A, Sinno MZ, et al: Importance of atrial contraction to left ventricular function after myocardial infarction. Am J Cardiol 35:164, 1975.

58. Raine AEG, Phil D, Erne P, et al: Atrial natriuretic peptide and atrial pressure in patients with congestive heart failure. N Engl J Med 315:533, 1986.

59. Reale A: Acute effects of countershock conversion of atrial fibrillation upon right and left heart hemodynamics. Circulation 32:214, 1965.

60. Richards AM, Ikram H, Yandle TG, et al: Renal, haemodynamic and hormonal effects of human alpha atrial natriuretic peptide in healthy volunteers. Lancet 1:545, 1985.

61. Ross J Jr, Linhart JW, Braunwald E: Effects of changing heart rate in man by electrical stimulation of the right atrium. Circulation 32:549, 1965.

62. Roy D, Paillard F, Cassidy D, et al: Atrial natriuretic factor during atrial fibrillation and supraventricular tachycardia. J Am Coll Cardiol 9:509, 1987.

63. Rozenman Y, Weiss AT, Atlan H, Gosman MS: Left ventricular function during atrial pacing: A radionuclide angiographic study. Clin Cardiol 7:349, 1984.

64. Samet P: Hemodynamic sequelae of cardiac arrhythmias. Circulation 47:399, 1973.

65. Samet P, Castillo C, Bernstein WH, Fernandez P: Hemodynamic results of right atrial pacing in cardiac subjects. Dis Chest 53:133, 1968.

66. Saunders DE Jr, Ord MJW: The hemodynamic effects of paroxysmal supraventricular tachycardia in patients with the Wolff-Parkinson-White syndrome. Am J Cardiol 9:223, 1962.

67. Schlepper M, Weppner HG, Merle H: Haemodynamic effects of supraventricular tachycardias and their alterations by electrically and verapamil induced termination. Cardiovasc Res 12:28, 1978.

68. Scott ME, Patterson GC: Cardiac output after direct current conversion of atrial fibrillation. Br Heart J 31:87, 1969.

69. Sinno MZ, Gunnar RM: Hemodynamic consequences of cardiac dysrhythmias. Med Clin North Am 60:69, 1976.

70. Smith VE, Schulman P, Karimeddini MK, et al: Rapid ventricular filling in left ventricular hypertrophy. II. Pathologic hypertrophy. J Am Coll Cardiol 5:869, 1985.

71. Swiryn S, Pavel D, Byrom E, et al: Assessment of left ventricular function by radionuclide angiography during induced supraventricular tachycardia. Am J Cardiol 47:555, 1981.

72. Swan HJC: Circulatory effects of cardiac arrhythmias. Acta Cardiol [Suppl] 18:107, 1974.

73. Wang Y, Marshall RJ, Shepherd JT: Stroke volume in the dog during graded exercise. Circ Res 8:558, 1960.

74. Waxman MB, Bonet JF, Finley JP, Wald RW: Effects of respiration and posture on paroxysmal supraventricular tachycardia. Circulation 62:1011, 1980.

75. Waxman MB, Sharma AD, Cameron DA, et al: Reflex mechanisms responsible for early spontaneous termination of paroxysmal supraventricular tachycardia. Am J Cardiol 49:259, 1982.

76. Waxman MB, Wald RW, Sharma AD, et al: Vagal techniques for termination of paroxysmal supraventricular tachycardia. Am J Cardiol 46:655, 1980.

77. Waxman MB, Wald RW, Cameron DA: Interactions between the autonomic nervous system and tachycardias in man. In Zipes DP (ed): Cardiology Clinics, Arrhythmias—2. Philadelphia, W. B. Saunders Company, 1983, p 143.

78. Wenkebach KF, Winteberg H: Die Unregelmaessige Herztaetigkeit. Leipzig, Wilhelm V Engelmann, 1927, p 252.

79. Wilson JR, Douglas P, Hickey WF, et al: Experimental congestive heart failure produced by rapid ventricular pacing in the dog: Cardiac effects. Circulation 75:857, 1987.

80. Wood P: Polyuria in paroxysmal tachycardia. Br Heart J 25:273, 1963.

B.   Ventricular Tachycardia

RYSZARD B. KROL *and* SANJEEV SAKSENA

The clinical presentation of patients with cardiac rhythm disturbances varies widely. Whereas ventricular fibrillation is invariably associated with hemodynamic collapse and unconsciousness, the hemodynamic changes that occur during ventricular tachycardia range from minimal impairment to cardiovascular collapse and sudden death.[1, 26, 29, 36, 46, 47, 52, 55, 62, 67] In most patients, ventricular tachycardia is associated with severe symptoms, such as severe hypotension and a loss of consciousness, and usually requires emergent treatment.[1, 26, 29, 36, 47, 52, 62, 67] There have, however, been several reports of patients who experienced mild symptoms associated with ventricular tachycardia and who survived episodes of tachycardia lasting many days.[46, 55] The variable clinical presentation depends mainly on the hemodynamic consequences of the particular arrhythmia.[1, 26, 29, 36, 47, 52, 62, 67] Factors responsible for different hemodynamic responses to ventricular tachycardia in individual patients are not well understood. Investigating the hemodynamics of ventricular tachycardia in humans is difficult owing to the life-threatening character of the arrhythmia. At the present time, there is also no available standard animal model of ventricular tachycardia. In view of these problems, there are relatively few published clinical studies that have evaluated hemodynamic changes during inducible or spontaneous ventricular tachycardia.[29, 30, 33, 41, 59, 61] However, a large body of clinical and experimental information has been obtained by the substitution of rapid ventricular tachycardia with ventricular pacing both in humans and in experimental animals. On the basis of information from both sources, several factors resulting in hemodynamic changes during ventricular tachycardia have been identified: (1) inappropriate increase in heart rate, (2) time relationship between atrial and ventricular systole, (3) asynchrony of ventricular contraction during ventricular tachycardia, (4) reduced end-diastolic volume and systolic ventricular function, (5) myocardial ischemia, and (6) neurohormonal reflex responses to the arrhythmia. This chapter will review individually these factors as well as their complex interactions,

which ultimately decide the hemodynamic consequences of ventricular tachycardia in a particular patient.

ALTERATIONS IN RATE

Rate is probably the most important clinical variable that influences the hemodynamic outcome of ventricular tachycardia.[29, 52] A decline in stroke volume occurs with an increasing heart rate regardless of the type of arrhythmia producing the pathologic tachycardia.[8, 11, 14, 26, 30, 32, 54, 61] There is a good correlation between the decreasing cycle length of ventricular tachycardia and the decline in left ventricular systolic pressure.[61] Ventricular pacing in patients with normal hearts causes progressive decline in stroke volume in a linear fashion as the pacing rate increases.[8, 14, 32, 54] In patients with ventricular tachycardia, ventricular pacing at rates identical with the ventricular tachycardia was shown to produce comparable decrease in cardiac output, left ventricular systolic pressure, and the first derivative of left ventricular pressure (dp/dt)[61] (Fig. 23–3). The cardiac output falls inappropriately despite increases in heart rate. This decline in output is due to abbreviation of the diastolic filling period and the fixed venous return present in a patient at rest.[8, 11, 14, 33, 55, 60, 62]

Despite the widely held belief that extent of resting left ventricular dysfunction is an important determinant of the hemodynamic outcome of ventricular tachycardia, there is little confirmation of this in current literature. Recent studies suggest that the rate of ventricular tachycardia is more important than baseline left ventricular function. There is a lack of direct correlation between baseline right and left ventricular function or individual hemodynamic parameters and the hemodynamic response to ventricular tachycardia.[30, 33, 41, 59] In two studies, only the rate of ventricular tachycardia and a prior history of syncope associated with arrhythmia were predictive of the hemodynamic outcome of inducible ventricular tachycardia.[29, 52] Patients with rates of ventricular tachycardia in excess of 200 beats per

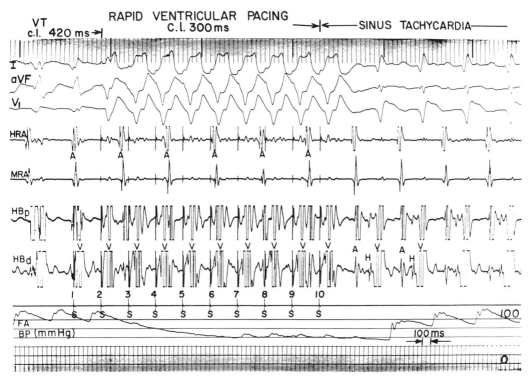

Figure 23–3. Effects of rapid ventricular pacing during ventricular tachycardia (VT) on arterial blood pressure (BP). Note the sudden decrease in arterial blood pressure during rapid overdrive ventricular pacing. I, a V_F, V_1 = electrocardiographic (ECG) leads recorded; HRA = high right atrial electrogram; MRA = mid right atrial electrogram; HBp = proximal His bundle electrogram; HBd = distal His bundle electrogram; FA = femoral artery.

minute had a 65 per cent incidence of syncope or near-syncope, compared with a 15 per cent incidence among patients whose ventricular tachycardia rate was less than 200 beats per minute.[52] Consequently, the rate of ventricular tachycardia is usually faster (over 230 beats per minute) in patients who experience syncope, while most patients with ventricular tachycardia of a rate less than 200 beats per minute are able to maintain blood pressure and remain conscious.[29, 52] However, there is significant overlap in patients with ventricular tachycardia rates of 200 to 230 beats per minute.[52] There is also a marked difference in hemodynamic response to ventricular tachycardia in syncopal and nonsyncopal patients. In both groups of patients, the mean arterial pressure falls within the first 5 seconds.[29] In patients without syncope, arterial pressure shows partial stabilization within 3 to 16 seconds of ventricular tachycardia, while patients with syncope develop profound and progressive hypotension.[29] The importance of rate is also underscored by the effect of antiarrhythmic therapy. Drug-induced slowing of the ventricular tachycardia rate may prevent he-

modynamic deterioration and sudden death in a previously syncopal patient.[1, 29, 36]

TIME RELATIONSHIP BETWEEN ATRIAL AND VENTRICULAR SYSTOLE

Appropriately timed atrial contraction is an important factor in maximizing cardiac output at rest and during exercise in animals and humans. Properly timed atrial systole is mandatory for optimal cardiac output and systemic arterial pressure and results in lower pulmonary or left atrial pressures in patients with normal left ventricular function and in those with decreased left ventricular function.[13, 15, 24, 25, 32, 37–39, 42, 49, 53, 54, 58, 63, 64, 66, 69, 70, 78] Gessel and later Wiggers quantified the effect of atrial systole on systemic arterial blood pressure.[24, 77] In 1911, Gessel demonstrated an increase in arterial blood pressure of 10 to 15 per cent with appropriately timed atrial systole, and later in 1922, Wiggers observed that the atrial contribution to left ventricular filling averaged 20 to 35 per cent. Atrial systole increases left ventricular preload and diastolic fiber length and thus improves left ventricular performance according to the Frank-Starling mechanism.[42, 43, 49] The actual contribution of atrial systole to cardiac output is dependent on a number of factors, including heart rate, time interval between atrial and ventricular systole, functional status of the myocardium, and the presence of valvular disease.[13, 15, 18, 25, 27, 35, 37–39, 42, 43, 49, 53, 58, 63, 64, 66, 69, 70] The hemodynamic effects of atrioventricular (AV) synchrony are significantly modified and considerably different at different ventricular rates.[32, 38, 54] The contribution of atrial contraction decreases with increasing ventricular rate, particularly at fast heart rates in excess of 200 beats per minute. Strikingly deleterious hemodynamic effects have been demonstrated when atria and ventricles contract simultaneously.[32, 53, 54] This effect is most pronounced at short cycle lengths.[32, 53, 54] Augmentation of cardiac output by 30 per cent can be achieved with appropriate AV coordination during ventricular tachycardia, as opposed to asynchronous or simultaneous atrial and ventricular contraction.[13, 38, 63, 64, 70] The importance of the relationship between ventricular rate and AV coordination is also demonstrated by patients in whom supraventricular tachycardias may cause serious hemodynamic deterioration even if they do not have apparent cardiac disease.[26, 32, 47, 62, 67] The altered hemodynamics cannot be ascribed primarily to the rapid rate itself, which is often in the physiologic range of 140 to 160 beats per minute and similar to that seen on physical exertion.[32] Moreover, the observation that there are also patients who suffer serious hemodynamic deterioration as a result of ventricular pacing at heart rates of 70 to 90 beats per minute suggests further that alternative mechanisms may be responsible for some of the adverse hemodynamic effects of various arrhythmias associated with abnormal AV coordination.[18, 35, 53, 69]

During ventricular pacing or ventricular tachycardia, atrial activation may be absent, dissociated from ventricular activity, or improperly coupled to ventricular events by retrograde conduction.[24, 32, 42, 49, 54, 78] Both AV and ventriculoatrial (VA) conduction can be markedly affected by the tachycardia cycle length.[25, 54] A consistent VA activation sequence may be associated with greater hemodynamic compromise than random AV dissociation because of significant decreases in systemic and left ventricular pressures and cardiac output, along with concomitant increases in right atrial, right ventricular, and pulmonary pressures.[32, 53, 54] If the timing of atrial contraction and the resulting cannon waves occur just prior to opening of the AV valve, there is a significant decrease in mitral flow and ventricular end-diastolic volume, as well as a reduction in the magnitude of ventricular contraction.[26, 32, 47, 66] When atrial and ventricular contractions coincide, marked reduction and reversal of superior vena caval flow occur, as well as mitral and tricuspid regurgitation, especially in patients with valvular disease.[18, 25, 64, 69] Patients in whom ventricular pacing produces retrograde atrial activation with elevation of right and left atrial pressures, pulmonary capillary wedge pressure, and cannon "a" waves due to simultaneous atrial contraction during ventricular systole frequently experience hypotension because of vasodepressor reflexes initiated by large atrial pressure waves.[32, 54, 66, 69] In addition, during some tachycardias, there is not only loss of active atrial contribution to ventricular filling but also evidence of a retrograde or negative atrial kick, resulting in cardiodepressant reflexes that further compromise cardiac hemodynamics.[32, 53]

An important physiologic variable influencing the hemodynamic effects of AV synchrony is the intrinsic function of the left ventricle. Left ventricular end-diastolic volume and end-diastolic pressure may affect the augmentation in cardiac output achieved by appropriately timed atrial depolarization.[27] When left ventricular end-diastolic pressure is in the normal range, atrial contribution increases the stroke volume maximally, since the left ventricular pressure-volume function curve is at its steepest point.[60] However, when left ventricular end-diastolic pressure is elevated and the ventricular function curve is in its "flat" portion, further increments in pressure have progressively less effect.[27, 60] Atrial contribution is less important in patients with increased end-diastolic volumes and filling pressures of more than 20 mm Hg.[27] Generally, the amount by which the atrial contribution to left ventricular filling improves left ventricular stroke volume depends on several factors. The increase in the left ventricular end-diastolic volume depends on the pump function of the atrium and the augmentation of stroke volume gained for this increase in end-diastolic volume, as determined by the slope of the pressure-volume function curve.[60] All these factors might be altered in the diseased heart, explaining the observation that atrial systole seems important for one patient but not for another. Thus, the relationship between timing of atrial contraction, rate of tachycardia, intrinsic left ventricular function, and neurohumoral responses to elevated atrial pressures is extremely complex and may help to explain the great variation in hemodynamic responses to ventricular tachycardia among different patients. Providing optimal sequence between atrial and ventricular contraction during ventricular tachycardia can be of significant hemodynamic benefit. Optimally timed atrial pacing during sustained ventricular tachycardia may produce a 10 to 33 per cent increase in the cardiac index and an 18 to 75 per cent increase in the mean arterial pressure and therefore may have important applications in the clinical management of patients with hemodynamically unstable ventricular tachycardia.[30]

ASYNCHRONY OF VENTRICULAR CONTRACTION

In 1925, Wiggers first described the hemodynamic consequences of ectopic cardiac stimulation and believed that a certain "orderliness" in the mode of contraction may be necessary to produce a maximal effect on ventricular pressures.[77] He found that when such asynchrony existed, there was a slower rate of rise of ventricular pressure and less effective cardiac performance. Bourassa and colleagues reported interesting hemodynamic observations in a patient who was in sinus rhythm and who developed intermittent left bundle branch block during the course of cardiac catheterization.[6] The presence of left bundle branch block resulted in the fall of left ventricular systolic pressure, a slower rate of pressure rise in the left ventricle, a decrease in central aortic and peripheral pulse pressure, and a decrease in cardiac output. However, this observation was unusual, and the development of bundle branch block has no major hemodynamic effects in the majority of patients.[7, 11, 79] Lister and associates examined the changes in cardiac hemodynamics that occurred in response to ventricular pacing at various sites in dogs with chronic complete heart block.[45] There was wide variation in cardiac output with pacing from different ventricular sites. Lister concluded that the hemodynamic effectiveness of the site of ventricular pacing was inversely related to the left ventricular muscle mass, which was activated by intraventricular conduction rather than by His-Purkinje conduction.

Corday and coworkers described "benign" and "malignant" ventricular tachycardias based upon the hemodynamic response to apical and basal stimulation of the left ventricle in dogs.[12] Their observations were confirmed by Eber and colleagues, who observed that apically stimulated left ventricular beats were hemodynamically more effective than beats arising from basilar stimulation.[17] Apparent regional expansion of the stimulated portion of the left ventricle has been noted by others.[2, 5, 31, 73–75] The general patterns of contraction observed were unrelated to preload or diastolic filling periods but were determined solely by the point of stimulus application.[31, 75] The severity of the derangement of ventricular contraction is also dependent on the degree of prematurity of the ventricular beat.[11, 76] One echocardiographic study demonstrated that premature ventricular contractions with long coupling intervals of ventricular contraction had normal ejection indices. A distinct regional outward bulging was observed in the region where the extrastimulus had been applied.[74] In contrast, ventricular extrastimuli with short coupling intervals were associated with more significant generalized derangement of systolic ventricular function (Fig. 23–4). All these experimental data can be interpreted to support the viewpoint that the site of the origin of ventricular tachycardia may significantly influence hemodynamics. However, available experimental and clinical evidence questions the primary importance of altered mechanical contraction in the hemodynamic consequences associated with ventricular premature beats and ventricular tachycardia.[7, 11, 13, 65] Canine experiments have demonstrated that AV sequential pacing with an optimal AV interval was able to overcome the adverse hemodynamic effects associated with ectopic activation of the ventricles.[13, 65] Clinical studies do not demonstrate any relationship between the morphology of tachycardia or its site of origin and its hemodynamic consequences. One potential exception is ventricular tachycardia with a right ventricular origin.[56] Radioangiography with phase imaging during ventricular tachycardia may be able to localize the focus of ventricular tachycardia but also failed to demonstrate any relationship between the site of tachycardia and its hemodynamic outcome, which was determined by the rate of tachycardia, the extent of decline in ventricular end-diastolic volume, and the decrease in ventricular ejection fraction.[4, 71] Ventricular pacing at rates comparable with ventricular tachycardia results in an equivalent degree of left

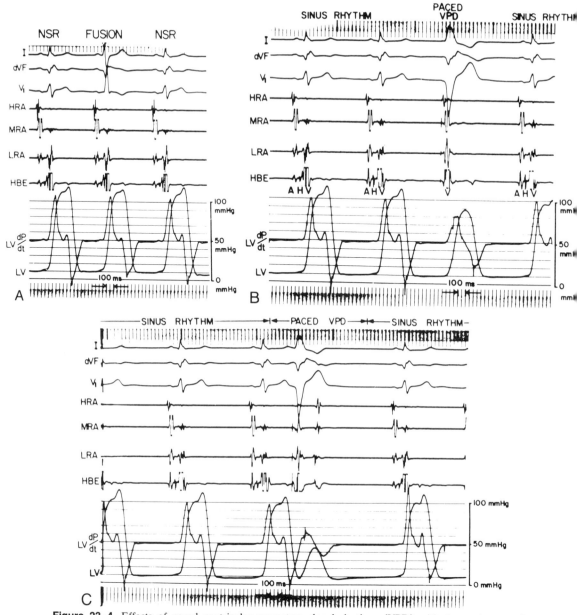

Figure 23–4. Effects of paced ventricular premature depolarizations (VPD) with decreasing coupling interval on left ventricular pressure (LV) and first derivative of left ventricular pressure (dp/dt). *A,* Late VPD resulting in a fusion beat. *B,* Increasing prematurity of the VPD with loss of atrial systole. *C,* Early VPD. Note the progressive decline in LV pressure and dp/dt with shortening of the coupling interval of the VPD. I, aV$_F$, V$_1$ = ECG leads recorded; HRA = high right atrial electrogram; MRA = mid right atrial electrogram; LRA = low right atrial electrogram; HBE = His bundle electrogram; NSR = normal sinus rhythm. (From Saksena S, Ciccone J, Craelius W, et al: Studies on left ventricular function during sustained ventricular tachycardia. J Am Coll Cardiol 4:506, 1984 with permission.)

ventricular dysfunction, decrease in systolic left ventricular pressure, and both positive and negative dp/dt, despite different patterns of ventricular contraction of the two rhythms (Fig. 23–5).[61] Therefore, asynchrony of ventricular contraction seems to be an important factor determining the hemodynamic response to ventricular tachycardia in experimental studies in normal hearts, but clinically, the site of origin of ventricular tachycardia is a factor of much less importance than, for example, tachycardia rate or AV synchrony.

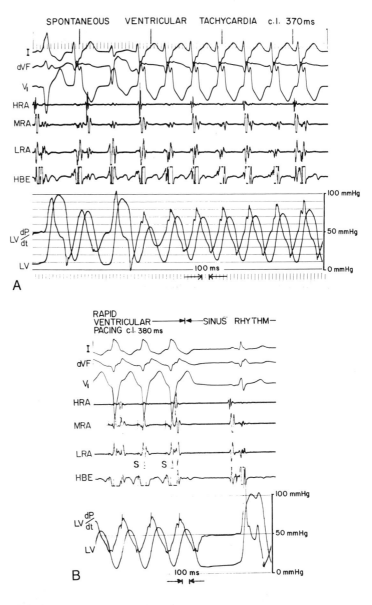

Figure 23–5. Left ventricular hemodynamic variables during sustained VT *(A)* and during ventricular pacing with similar cycle length *(B)* I, aV$_F$, V$_1$ = ECG leads recorded; HRA = high right atrial electrogram; MRA = mid right atrial electrogram; LRA = low right atrial electrogram; HBE = His bundle electrogram; LV = left ventricular pressure; LV dp/dt = first derivative of left ventricular pressure. (From Saksena S, Ciccone J, Craelius W, et al: Studies on left ventricular function during sustained ventricular tachycardia. J Am Coll Cardiol 4:506, 1984 with permission.)

DIASTOLIC AND SYSTOLIC VENTRICULAR FUNCTION DURING VENTRICULAR TACHYCARDIA

The mechanisms that are responsible for the fall in cardiac output during ventricular tachycardia or any other cardiac arrhythmia are related to reduced diastolic filling of the heart or reduced systolic emptying or both. The onset of ventricular tachycardia is characterized by a continuously changing end-diastolic volume, stroke volume, and left and right ventricular systolic and diastolic function, which are all dependent on the effectiveness of ventricular filling.[11, 61] Impairment of left ventricular filling is related to ventricular rate and is caused mainly by shortened diastolic filling time and loss of AV synchrony. There is a close correlation between the end-diastolic volume preceding any given beat and stroke volume. Therefore, beats with a high degree of prematurity irrespective of their origin (atrial or ventricular) are preceded by an incomplete ventricular filling and are initiated by a lower end-diastolic volume, with resultant stroke volume being diminished as well.[11] Other factors are incomplete ventricular relaxation between consecutive tachycardia beats, increased diastolic ventricular stiffness, loss of atrial kick, and neurohumoral reflexes influencing venous return and peripheral vascular resistance.[11, 41, 61] Systolic function of the left

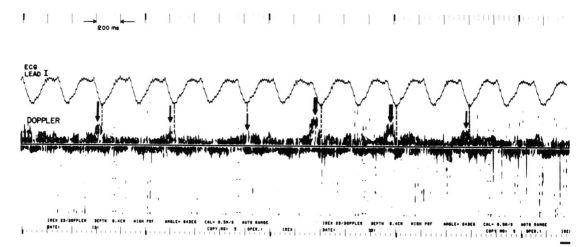

Figure 23–6. Pulse Doppler recording of the velocity of mitral flow during VT. The flow velocity is considerably greater (maximum of 0.9 m/sec, *thick arrows*) when mitral inflow occurs well before the peak of QRS complex, compared with its occurrence very close to or at the peak of the QRS complex (0.5 m/sec, *thin arrows*). (Reproduced from Rosenbloom M, Saksena S, Nanda NC, et al: Two-dimensional echocardiographic studies in sustained ventricular tachycardia. PACE 7:136–142, 1984.)

ventricle during tachycardia is affected by the low initial ventricular volume, discoordinate ventricular contraction, and ischemic myocardial dysfunction in patients with coronary artery disease with secondary development of acute AV valve regurgitation. Reduced mitral flow has been demonstrated in our laboratory by continuous and color flow Doppler studies in patients during sustained ventricular tachycardia (Fig. 23–6).[59, 72] Patients with normal mitral valves developed minimal or no regurgitation during ventricular tachycardia, while patients with preexisting mitral insufficiency demonstrated significant worsening of this condition, which contributed to hemodynamic deterioration. Atrial contraction preceding ventricular contraction improved beat-to-beat mitral blood flow, ventricular ejection fraction, and stroke volume.

End-diastolic volume represents the principal determinant of beat-to-beat stroke volume in a given patient, regardless of whether sinus rhythm or atrial or ventricular arrhythmias are present.[11, 41, 61] The Starling law and, therefore, the end-diastolic myocardial fiber length remain the prime mechanisms governing hemodynamic changes during cardiac arrhythmias. Earlier premature beats of various types are preceded by an incomplete degree of ventricular filling and are thus initiated at a lower than usual end-diastolic volume.[11]

An increase in the heart rate limits the normal process of diastolic filling and relaxation.[8] The diastolic properties of the heart are probably not changed during ventricular tachycardia, but their normal expression is pre-

vented as relaxation is interrupted, which is reflected by the reduction of left ventricular diastolic volume. Lima and colleagues demonstrated the important differences in response to ventricular tachycardia between patients with normal left ventricular function and those with impaired function.[41] In patients with normal left ventricular function, impairment of stroke volume during ventricular tachycardia was caused mainly by interruption of diastolic filling, which was reflected by a reduction of left ventricular cavity size. Other aspects of left ventricular function—in particular, ejection fraction—remain unchanged. In this study patients with impaired left ventricular function also developed profound incoordination of overall pump function. Rosenbloom and associates, who studied only patients with abnormal left ventricular function, demonstrated either a worsening of preexisting wall motion abnormalities or the development of new wall motion abnormalities during ventricular tachycardia in almost all patients.[59] In this study, there was also a significant decrease in ejection fraction during ventricular tachycardia, which was more severe in patients with short cycle lengths of tachycardia.

Asynchronous ventricular relaxation during tachycardia slows the rate of left ventricular pressure decay, which may cause an elevation of diastolic pressures, particularly in the early diastolic period. Discoordinate relaxation may result in an upward shift in the left ventricular diastolic pressure-volume relation during ventricular tachycardia. Therefore, during sustained ventricular tachycardia, left ventricular diastolic pressure is artificially maintained by impaired left ventricular relaxation, leaving an inaccurate impression of adequate left ventricular filling. Radioangiography performed during ventricular tachycardia revealed decreases in end-diastolic volume, stroke volume, and cardiac output, all of which were related to the mean rate of ventricular tachycardia.[4] Hemodynamic deterioration was also related to greater asynchrony in wall motion and lower ejection fraction during ventricular tachycardia.

MYOCARDIAL ISCHEMIA

Myocardial ischemia is one of the precipitating factors for ventricular tachycardia and fibrillation.[22, 51, 57] Myocardial ischemia may occur during programmed ventricular stimulation in patients with coronary artery disease and potentially affects the induction of ventricular tachycardia.[22, 51] However, myocardial ischemia probably has no major effect on the hemodynamic outcome of ventricular tachycardia in most patients. Systolic left ventricular pressure, peak dp/dt, and negative dp/dt decrease markedly with the first beat of tachycardia, and essentially all hemodynamic changes during ventricular tachycardia occur within the first five beats of tachycardia, which is too short a time for the development of significant myocardial ischemia.[29, 61] However, in the later phase of ventricular tachycardia, myocardial ischemia may develop and may potentially be one of the factors that determine whether blood pressure stabilizes and recovers or whether the patient develops progressive hypotension. The development of myocardial ischemia has significant influence on both left ventricular diastolic and left ventricular systolic function.[9, 16, 44, 48] It may cause a decrease in the diastolic compliance of the ventricles and therefore may affect end-diastolic volume, which is probably the most important determinant of stroke volume during ventricular tachycardia, as well as the development of new wall motion abnormalities and a decrease in ejection fraction.[9, 16, 44, 48] Therefore, the development of myocardial ischemia during ventricular tachycardia may either result in further hemodynamic deterioration or prevent hemodynamic recovery. Myocardial hypoperfusion and metabolic abnormalities may lead to degeneration of the ventricular tachycardia to ventricular fibrillation.[23, 28]

NEUROHUMORAL REFLEXES DURING VENTRICULAR TACHYCARDIA

The initiation of ventricular tachycardia typically produces hypotension and elevated filling pressures, which are powerful stimuli to arterial baroreceptors and cardiac mechanoreceptors. The functional response to ventricular tachycardia appears to involve alterations in both left ventricular contractility and peripheral vascular tone. The sudden acceleration of heart rate and decrease in blood pressure can be tolerated by some patients if the vascular bed can adapt to the changes in cardiac output. In experimental animals, a central role of baroreceptor reflexes was implicated in the recovery of systolic blood pressure during tachycardia.[20] Hypotension resulted in increased sympathetic tone, which was manifested by the recovery of blood pressure to control values. There was an increase in vagal tone, which was accompanied by slowing of tachycardia rate and frequently by termination of arrhythmia. In humans, hypotension produced by supraventricular or ventricular arrhythmia causes the activation of adrenergic receptors, partial recovery of systemic blood pressure, and changes in vagal tone that may terminate tachycardia.[26, 76] These observations suggest the importance of the autonomic nervous system in affecting hemodynamic recovery during tachycardia and modifying the rate of tachycardia. Also important are the venomotor tone, blood volume, and other factors that influence venous return to the heart. Experimental studies showed that increased beta-adrenergic tone accelerates left ventricular pressure decay and may have a significant influence on the diastolic pressure-volume relationships during ventricular tachycardia.[9] Ventricular tachycardia frequently occurs in patients with left ventricular dysfunction who have often had myocardial infarction and are receiving adrenergic receptor blocking agents.[10, 40, 68] These patients have decreased responsiveness to adrenergic stimulation, with reduction in beta receptors and elevated levels of circulating catecholamines.[10, 40, 68] In these patients, the upward shift in the diastolic pressure-volume relation during ventricular tachycardia can be partially related to the lack of beta-adrenergic–mediated acceleration of pressure decay. Besides plasma catecholamines, levels of atrial natriuretic factor, vasopressin, and cortisol increase during ventricular tachycardia.[19, 21, 34, 50] The exact effects of these hormonal changes on ventricular tachycardia are unknown at the present time. However, all these substances may potentially influence electrophysiologic properties of the tachycardia substrate or peripheral vascular resistance.

CONCLUSIONS

The hemodynamic consequences of ventricular tachyarrhythmias can now be understood in terms of current principles of cardiovascular physiology. A complex interaction exists between intrinsic cardiac mechanical function resulting from the electrical disorder and extrinsic responses from the autonomic nervous system. Neurohumoral factors and the response of the peripheral vascular circulation can determine the hemodynamic outcome of ventricular tachycardia. This chain of events occurring during ventricular tachycardia can be influenced at many levels for a more favorable hemodynamic result. For example, reduction in the tachycardia rate by antiarrhythmic drug therapy has been associated with improved survival of patients with ventricular arrhythmias, despite persistent recurrences of ventricular tachycardia. AV synchrony achieved by sequential pacing techniques during ventricular tachycardia can improve hemodynamics and permit electrophysiologic procedures, such as cardiac mapping or catheter ablation, during the induced arrhythmia. The role of hormonal influences and autonomic reflexes is just being recognized in humans. Improved understanding of hemodynamic issues can have an important bearing on strategies to reduce the incidence of sudden death due to ventricular tachyarrhythmias. The use of these parameters is being suggested in sensing algorithms for future antitachycardia devices. Implantable sensors for intracavitary pressures have been used acutely and chronically in experimental studies, and their acute clinical application has been reported. The influence of additional noncardiac factors, such as respiration, may be greater for right ventricular hemodynamic function than left ventricular function. Combination sensing algorithms may permit individualized electrical therapy for different patients and for different tachycardias in the same patient.

REFERENCES

1. Armbrust CA, Levine SA: Paroxysmal ventricular tachycardia: A study of one hundred and seven cases. Circulation 1:28, 1950.
2. Bashore TM, Stine RA, Shaffer PB, et al: The non-invasive localization of ventricular pacing sites by radionuclide phase imaging. Circulation 70:681, 1984.
3. Bishop VS, Malliani A, Thoren P: Cardiac mechanoreceptors. *In* Shepherd JT, Abboud FM, Geiger SR (eds): Handbook of Physiology: The Cardiovascular System. Baltimore, The Williams & Wilkins Co, 1983, pp 497–556.
4. Botvinick E, Schechtmann N, Dae M, et al: Scintigraphy provides a thorough evaluation of "electrical" and mechanical events during ventricular tachycardia [abstract]. J Am Coll Cardiol 7:235A, 1986.
5. Botvinick EH, Frais MA, Shosa DW, et al: An accurate means of detecting and characterizing abnormal patterns of ventricular activation by phase image analysis. Am J Cardiol 50:289, 1982.
6. Bourassa MG, Boiteom GM, Allenstein BY: Hemodynamic studies during intermittent left bundle branch block. Am J Cardiol 10:792, 1962.
7. Braunwald E, Morrow AG: Sequence of ventricular contraction in human bundle branch block: A study based on simultaneous catheterization of both ventricles. Am J Med 23:205, 1957.
8. Bristow TD, Ferguson RE, Mintz F, et al: The influence of heart rate on left ventricular volume in dogs. J Clin Invest 42:649, 1963.
9. Brutsaert DL, Rademakers FE, Sys SU: Triple control of relaxation: Implications in cardiac disease. Circulation 69:190, 1984.
10. Cohn JN, Levine TB, Olivari MT, et al: Plasma norepinephrine as a guide to prognosis in patients with congestive heart failure. N Engl J Med 311:819, 1984.
11. Cohn K, Kryda W: The influence of ectopic beats and tachyarrhythmias on stroke volume and cardiac output. J Electrocardiol 14:207, 1981.
12. Corday E, Gold H, DeVera LB, et al: Effect of the cardiac arrhythmias on the coronary circulation. Ann Intern Med 50:535, 1959.
13. Daggett WM, Bianco JA, Powell WJ, et al: Relative contribution of atrial systole–ventricular systole interval and of patterns of ventricular activation to ventricular function during electrical pacing of the dog heart. Circ Res 27:69, 1970.
14. DeMaria AN, Neumann A, Schubert PY, et al: Systematic correlation of cardiac chamber size and ventricular peformance determined with echocardiography during alterations in heart rate in normal persons. Am J Cardiol 43:1, 1979.
15. DiCarlo LA, Morady F, Krol RB, et al: The hemodynamic effects of ventricular pacing with and without atrioventricular synchrony in patients with normal and diminished left ventricular function. Am Heart J 114:746, 1987.
16. Dwyer CM: Left ventricular pressure-volume alterations and regional disorders of contraction during myocardial ischemia induced by atrial pacing. Circulation 42:1111, 1970.
17. Eber LM, Berkovits BV, Matloff JM, et al: Dynamic characterization of premature ventricular beats and ventricular tachycardias. Am J Cardiol 33:378, 1974.
18. Edhag O, Fagrell B, Lagergren H: Deleterious effects of cardiac pacing in a patient with mitral insufficiency. Acta Med Scand 202:331, 1977.
19. Ellenbogen KA, Rogers R, Walsh M, et al: Increased circulating atrial natriuretic factor (ANF) release during induced ventricular tachycardia. Am Heart J 116:1233, 1988.
20. Feldman T, Carroll JD, Munkenbeck F, et al: He-

modynamic recovery during simulated ventricular tachycardia: Role of adrenergic receptor activation. Am Heart J 115:576, 1988.

21. Fromer M, Razi M, Dubue M, et al: Effect of induced ventricular tachycardia on atrial natriuretic peptide in humans. J Am Coll Cardiol 6:1395, 1988.

22. Garan H, Ruskin JN, DiMarco JP, et al: Electrophysiologic studies before and after myocardial revascularization in patients with life-threatening ventricular arrhythmias. Am J Cardiol 51:519, 1983.

23. Gerst PH, Fleming WH, Molin JR: Increased susceptibility of the heart to ventricular fibrillation during metabolic acidosis. Circ Res 19:63, 1966.

24. Gessel RA: Auricular systole and its relation to ventricular output. Am J Physiol 29:32, 1911–1912.

25. Gilmore JP, Sarnoff SJ, Mitchell JH, et al: Synchronicity of ventricular contraction: Observations comparing hemodynamic effects of atrial and ventricular pacing. Br Heart J 28:299, 1963.

26. Goldreyer BN, Kastor JA, Kerschbaum KL: The hemodynamic effects of induced supraventricular tachycardia in man. Circulation 54:783, 1976.

27. Greenberg B, Chatterjee K, Parmley WW, et al: The influence of left ventricular filling pressure on atrial contribution to cardiac output. Am Heart J 98:742, 1979.

28. Guilleminault C, Connolly SJ, Winkle RA: Cardiac arrhythmia and conduction disturbances during sleep in 400 patients with sleep apnea syndrome. Am J Cardiol 52:490, 1983.

29. Hamer AWF, Rubin SA, Peter CT, et al: Factors that predict syncope during ventricular tachycardia in patients. Am Heart J 107:997, 1984.

30. Hamer AWF, Zaher C, Peter CT, et al: Hemodynamic benefits of sequential atrial pacing during ventricular tachycardia in man [abstract]. J Am Coll Cardiol 1(2):636, 1983.

31. Hood WB Jr, Covelli VH, Normal JC, et al: Systolic bulging at sites of left ventricular stimulation. Circulation 38 [Suppl VI]:VI–102, 1968.

32. Hung J, Kelly DT, Hutton BF, et al: Influence of heart rate and atrial transport on left ventricular volume and function: Relationship to hemodynamic changes produced by supraventricular arrhythmia. Am J Cardiol 48:632, 1981.

33. Hunt D, Burdeslaw JA, Baxley WA: Left ventricular volumes during ventricular tachycardia, first post-tachycardia beat, and subsequent beats in normal rhythm. Br Heart J 36:148, 1974.

34. Ikram H, Crozier IG, Nicholls MG: Hemodynamic and hormone changes during ventricular tachycardia in man. Eur Heart J [Suppl] 1:110, 1988.

35. Johnson AD, Laiken SL, Engler RL: Hemodynamic compromise associated with ventriculoatrial conduction following transvenous pacemaker placement. Am J Med 65:75, 1978.

36. Josephson ME, Horowitz LN, Farshiti A, et al: Recurrent sustained ventricular tachycardia. I. Mechanisms. Circulation 57:431, 1978.

37. Kappenberger L, Gloor MO, Babotai I, et al: Hemodynamic effects of atrial synchronization in acute and long-term ventricular pacing. PACE 5:639, 1982.

38. Kosowski BD, Scherlag BJ, Damato AN: Reevaluation of the atrial contribution to ventricular function. Am J Cardiol 21:518, 1968.

39. Kruse I, Arnman K, Conradson TB, et al: A comparison of the acute and long-term hemodynamic effects of ventricular inhibited and atrial synchronous ventricular inhibited pacing. Circulation 65:846, 1982.

40. Levine TB, Francis GS, Goldsmith SR, et al: The neurohumoral and hemodynamic responses to orthostatic tilt in patients with congestive heart failure. Circulation 67:1070, 1983.

41. Lima JAC, Weiss JL, Guzman PA, et al: Incomplete filling and incoordinate contraction as mechanisms of hypotension during ventricular tachycardia in man. Circulation 68:928, 1983.

42. Linden RJ, Mitchell JH: Relation between left ventricular diastolic pressure and myocardial segment length and observations on the contribution of atrial systole. Circ Res 8:1092, 1960.

43. Linderer T, Chatterjee K, Parmley WW, et al: Influence of atrial systole on the Frank-Starling relation and the end-diastolic pressure-diameter relation of the left ventricle. Circulation 67:1045, 1983.

44. Linhart JW, Hildner FJ, Barold SS, et al: Left heart hemodynamics during angina pectoris induced by atrial pacing. Circulation 40:485, 1969.

45. Lister JW, Klotz DH, Jomain SL, et al: Effect of pacemaker site on cardiac output and ventricular activation in dogs with complete heart block. Am J Cardiol 14:494, 1964.

46. Mays AT: Ventricular tachycardia of unusually long duration (77 days). Am Heart J 23:119, 1942.

47. McIntosh HD, Morris JJ Jr: The hemodynamic consequences of arrhythmias. Prog Cardiovasc Dis 8:330, 1966.

48. McLaurin LP, Rolett EL, Grossman W: Impaired left ventricular relaxation during pacing-induced ischemia. Am J Cardiol 32:751, 1973.

49. Mitchell JH, Gilmore JP, Sarnoff SJ: The transport function of the atrium: Factors influencing the relation between mean left atrial pressure and left ventricular end-diastolic pressure. Am J Cardiol 9:237, 1962.

50. Morady F, DiCarlo LA, Halter JB, et al: The plasma catecholamine response to ventricular tachycardia induction and external countershock during electrophysiologic testing. J Am Coll Cardiol 8:584, 1986.

51. Morady F, DiCarlo LA Jr, Krol RB, et al: Role of myocardial ischemia during programmed stimulation in survivors of cardiac arrest with coronary artery disease. J Am Coll Cardiol 9:1004, 1987.

52. Morady F, Shen EN, Bhandari A, et al: Clinical symptoms in patients with sustained ventricular tachycardia. West J Med 142:341, 1985.

53. Naito M, Dreifus LS, David D, et al: Reevaluation of the role of atrial systole to cardiac hemodynamics: Evidence for pulmonary venous regurgitation during abnormal atrioventricular sequencing. Am Heart J 105:295, 1983.

54. Ogawa S, Dreifus LS, Shenoy PN, et al: Hemodynamic consequences of atrioventricular and ventriculoatrial pacing. PACE 1:8, 1978.

55. Papadopoulos C, Blazek CJ: Ventricular tachycardia of 70 days' duration with survival. Am J Cardiol 11:107, 1963.

56. Pietras RJ, Mautner R, Denes P, et al: Chronic recurrent right and left ventricular tachycardia: Comparison of clinical hemodynamic and angiographic findings. Am J Cardiol 40:32, 1977.

57. Ricci A, Risson P: Ischemia related ventricular arrhythmias in patients with variant angina pectoris. Eur Heart J 5:1013, 1985.

58. Romero LR, Haffajee CI, Levin W, et al: Noninvasive evaluation of ventricular function and vol-

umes during atrioventricular sequential and ventricular pacing. PACE 7:10, 1984.

59. Rosenbloom M, Saksena S, Nanda NC, et al: Two-dimensional echocardiographic studies during sustained ventricular tachycardia. PACE 7:136, 1984.

60. Ross J Jr: Afterload mismatch and preload reserve: A conceptional framework for analysis of ventricular function. Prog Cardiovasc Dis 18:255, 1976.

61. Saksena S, Ciccone JM, Craelius W, et al: Studies on left ventricular function during sustained ventricular tachycardia. J Am Coll Cardiol 4:501, 1984.

62. Samet P: Hemodynamic sequelae of cardiac arrhythmias. Circulation 47:399, 1973.

63. Samet P, Castillo C, Bernstein WH: Hemodynamic sequelae of atrial ventricular and sequential atrioventricular pacing in cardiac patients. Am Heart J 72:725, 1967.

64. Samet P, Castillo C, Bernstein WH: Hemodynamic consequences of sequential atrioventricular pacing: Subjects with normal hearts. Am J Cardiol 21:207, 1968.

65. Samet P, Bernstein WH, Levine S, et al: Hemodynamic effects of tachycardias produced by atrial and ventricular pacing. Am J Med 35:905, 1965.

66. Samet P, Bernstein WH, Nathan DA, et al: Atrial contribution to cardiac output in complete heart block. Am J Cardiol 16:1, 1965.

67. Schire V, Vogelpoel L: The clinical and electrocardiographic differentiation of supraventricular and ventricular tachycardias with regular rhythm. Am Heart J 49:162, 1955.

68. Schwartz PJ, Zaza A, Massimo P, et al: Baroflex sensitivity and its evolution during the first year after myocardial infarction. J Am Coll Cardiol 12:629, 1988.

69. Scully HD, Bello AG, Beierholm E, et al: The relationship between the atrial systole–ventricular systole interval and left ventricular function. J Thorac Cardiovasc Surg 65:684, 1973.

70. Sowton E: Hemodynamic studies in patients with artificial pacemakers. Br Heart J 26:737, 1964.

71. Swiryn S, Pavel D, Byrom E, et al: Sequential radionuclide phase mapping of radionuclide-gated ventriculograms in patients with sustained ventricular tachycardias: Close correlation with electrophysiologic characteristics. Am Heart J 103:319, 1982.

72. Switzer D, Saksena S, Nanda N, et al: Color and pulsed Doppler flow mapping of mitral blood flow during sustained ventricular tachycardia. PACE 9:301, 1986.

73. Torres MAR, Corday E, Meerbaum S, et al: Characterization of left ventricular mechanical function during arrhythmias by two-dimensional echocardiography. II. Location of the site of onset of premature ventricular systoles. J Am Coll Cardiol 1:819, 1983.

74. Uchiyama T, Corday E, Meerbaum S, et al: Characterization of left ventricular mechanical function during arrhythmias with two dimensional echocardiography. I. Premature ventricular contractions. Am J Cardiol 48:679, 1981.

75. Ueda H, Harumi K, Ueda K: Cineangiocardiographic observations on the asynchronism of cardiac contraction during ventricular pacing. Jpn Heart J 9:295, 1968.

76. Waxman MB, Wald RW, Finley JP, et al: Valsava termination of ventricular tachycardia. Circulation 62:843, 1980.

77. Wiggers LJ: The muscular reactions of the mammalian ventricles to artificial surface stimuli. Am J Physiol 73:348, 1925.

78. Wiggers CJ, Katz LN: The contours of ventricular volume curves under different conditions. Am J Physiol 58:439, 1922.

79. Wong B, Rinkenberger R, Dunn M, et al: Effect of intermittent left bundle branch block on left ventricular performance in the normal heart. Am J Cardiol 39:45, 1977.

24

IMPLANTATION AND INTRAOPERATIVE ASSESSMENT OF ANTITACHYCARDIA DEVICES

DEBRA S. ECHT, JOHN T. LEE, *and* JOHN W. HAMMON

OVERVIEW

As detailed in Chapter 22, careful selection of the patient and thorough preoperative evaluation of the arrhythmias are crucial to the success of the antitachycardia device implantation and its long-term clinical efficacy. This process involves obtaining hard-copy documentation of (ideally) all clinical arrhythmic events, the assessment of coexistent structural cardiovascular abnormalities, electrophysiologic testing, and consideration of all treatment modalities. Such a procedure provides specific information on the numbers, types, clinical manifestations, and mechanisms of the primary arrhythmias; the coexistence of bradycardia or of conduction system or secondary arrhythmic disorders; the relationships of the arrhythmias to underlying cardiac diseases; the hemodynamic consequences of the arrhythmia (or arrhythmias) and pacing; the relative effectiveness of different pacing modes and other therapies; and the type and likelihood of pacemaker-induced arrhythmias (e.g., ventricular tachycardia/fibrillation or atrial fibrillation). These data are fundamental to both the decision to use and the choice of an antitachycardia device. Moreover, they specifically influence all aspects of the implantation operation, the use of concurrent adjunctive or complementary therapies, subsequent complications, long-

term safety and efficacy, and perhaps the patient's survival.

Whereas antitachycardia pacemakers have been utilized predominantly in patients with supraventricular tachycardias, automatic cardioverters/defibrillators are utilized solely in patients with ventricular tachycardia and ventricular fibrillation. Because antitachycardia pacemakers and automatic cardioverters/defibrillators deliver distinctly different pulses and are used for different purposes, there are individual considerations in determining the safety and efficacy requirements for implantation.

Arrhythmia Detection

In regard to antitachycardia pacemakers employing atrial electrodes for the treatment of supraventricular tachycardia, arrhythmia nondetection is generally not life threatening. On the other hand, overdetection by these antitachycardia pacemakers may actually initiate supraventricular tachycardia. For instance, if sinus tachycardia satisfies the detection criteria, the termination attempt may induce the supraventricular tachycardia. Therefore, overdetection may be more problematic than nondetection for supraventricular tachycardias.

With regard to automatic cardioverters/defibrillators, nondetection of a potentially lethal ventricular arrhythmia is generally not acceptable. Therefore, some overdetection of supraventricular tachycardias is acceptable, and cardioverter/defibrillator devices are purposefully designed and specific parameters are selected that are overly sensitive. Arrhythmia detection requires the satisfaction of one or more criteria. The most sensitive device requires only that the rhythm equal or exceed an activation interval or rate.[104] The addition of an electrogram morphology criterion can reject tachycardias with narrow QRS complexes.[30] Other detection criteria that may be incorporated in the near future, sudden onset and rate stability criteria, are currently utilized in antitachycardia pacemakers and are discussed below. These additional criteria further reduce the sensitivity and increase the specificity of the device. It is important to understand the engineering design of the detection mechanisms when selecting the appropriate device and settings for individual patients.

Arrhythmia Termination

There are two major goals in the assessment of tachyarrhythmia termination using both antitachycardia pacemakers and automatic cardioverters/defibrillators. First and foremost is an extension of the physician's creed to "first do no harm." A device must be tested to evaluate the likelihood of accelerating and worsening rather than terminating the tachyarrhythmia and to assess the ability of the device to terminate effectively the subsequent rhythm that the device initiated.[26, 105] In the worst case, a patient with hemodynamically well-tolerated ventricular tachycardia who has never previously experienced ventricular fibrillation could develop ventricular fibrillation as a consequence of an unsuccessful pacing or cardioversion attempt. This concern has severely limited the usefulness of antitachycardia pacemakers for the treatment of ventricular tachycardia. This consideration has led to the standard practice that all patients with ventricular tachycardia undergo testing of the ability of an automatic cardioverter/defibrillator device to terminate ventricular fibrillation successfully.[30, 96] The other major consideration regarding arrhythmia termination is what constitutes a sufficient safety margin for effective termination. The range of stimulus pacing coupling intervals resulting in successful termination can be identified for antitachycardia pacemakers.[76] However, the exact relationship between energy and successful cardioversion

of ventricular tachycardia has not been fully evaluated. Moreover, recent evidence from canine studies and mathematical analyses suggests that there is not a discrete ventricular defibrillation threshold above which all termination attempts are effective and below which none are effective.[19, 67] The bias is to err on the side of delivering too high an energy rather than too low.

The acute assessment of efficacy is complicated because numerous factors can influence the ability to terminate tachyarrhythmias successfully, including the underlying mechanism; the tachycardia rate, morphology, and duration; and the potential interactions of two devices[58, 66] or the presence of concomitant antiarrhythmic drug therapy.[39, 97]

Equipment

For the implantation of any pacemaker or device, the principal prerequisite is a sterile surgical environment. We utilize a standard operating room exclusively, although others alternatively may use a specially cleaned and prepared catheterization or electrophysiologic laboratory. This room must contain all of the standard resources, including oxygen supplies, suction/vacuum lines, and grounded and shielded electrical supplies. A radiolucent patient operating table and fluoroscopic equipment, either permanently installed or portable, must be available. Even when procedures are performed with the patient under local anesthesia, resuscitative equipment should be available, including an external defibrillator, intubation supplies, a mechanical ventilator, suction pumps, and the entire spectrum of antiarrhythmic and other cardioactive drugs. Ideally, the room would be equipped with a cardiopulmonary perfusion system in the unlikely event of a major complication, such as myocardial rupture. Implantation should be performed only in hospitals with facilities for intracardiac surgery. Whereas standard antibradycardia pacemakers are implanted in outpatient surgical centers during 1-day admissions, for the implantation of antitachycardia devices, the patient should be admitted to the hospital.

In the course of implanting either antitachycardia pacemakers or cardioverter/defibrillator devices, extensive intraoperative testing is required to evaluate their ability to sense and terminate various arrhythmias and to assess and optimize their pacing and defibrillation functions. The basic testing equipment needed is similar to that utilized in the clinical electrophysiology laboratory, including a programmable stimulator, a multichannel recording instrument with hard-copy capability, and a commercial external defibrillator. A multichannel physiologic amplifier/recorder is used to record multiple surface electrocardiographic leads as well as intracardiac electrograms and arterial blood pressure. Tachyarrhythmia induction (and sometimes termination) is usually accomplished through a programmed electrical stimulator, which is connected with the patient's heart via separate temporary external pacing leads or the permanent pacemaker/defibrillator leads themselves. In addition, an electrical means to induce ventricular fibrillation rapidly and reproducibly is needed for devices designed for defibrillation. Few programmable stimulators are capable of delivering high output (greater than 20 mA) and short coupling intervals (less than 100 msec), which result in relatively reliable induction of ventricular fibrillation. Most physicians prefer to utilize a device delivering fibrillating alternating current (AC). The commercial defibrillator should be equipped with both internal and external chest defibrillating electrodes. All items contacting the patient—for example, cables, defibrillating paddles, magnets, and probes—must be sterilized. Ideally, an extra set of all components and equipment is available as a backup.

An instrument that enables the efficacy of the electrode system to be tested must be available prior to interrupting the sterility of the packaging for the device. For antitachycardia pacemakers, temporary external "pacing systems analyzers" are often useful for intraoperative testing, since they share many of the same stimulatory and sensing characteristics (e.g., pulse waveform, sensing amplifiers, and filters). By virtue of their diagnostic capabilities and their greater programming flexibility, more extensive system and lead evaluations can be performed prior to the actual implantation of the permanent device. Acute and chronic programming of the pacemaker is then performed using the companion programmer, either a portable computer or a hybrid microprocessor-programming device, which transmits instructions and receives telemetry via a magnetic or radiofrequency transducer.

Specific instruments required for intraoperative testing of the automatic implantable cardioverter/defibrillator (AICD, Cardiac Pacemakers, Inc, St. Paul, MN) have been discussed in detail.[12, 107] These include an AID-CHECK (Cardiac Pacemakers, Inc) interrogating/telemetry probe and device, which monitors AICD activation and charge times; a magnet for AICD activation; an external cardioverter/defibrillator (ECD, Cardiac Pacemakers, Inc), which delivers discharges of various energies for use in determining defibrillation thresholds, and several electrical cables and connectors. When appropriately interfaced with the above electrophysiologic equipment, direct recordings of electrograms and defibrillator outputs are possible, in addition to manual delivery of pacing via the programmed stimulator and pulse discharges from the ECD.

Personnel

Implantation of all these devices requires a close coordinated effort on the part of the clinical electrophysiology team, the cardiac surgical team, and the anesthesia team.[107] This arrangement allows the surgeon to concentrate on the sterile operative procedure and the handling of the actual hardware (generator and leads) while the cardiologist/electrophysiologist operates, programs, and tests the device, as well as performs the electrical/arrhythmia analyses. The third team member, an anesthesiologist, is responsible for the patient's overall welfare, the hemodynamic and physiologic monitoring, and the administration of anesthetic agents (sedatives and oxygen in the case of antitachycardia pacemakers and general anesthesia for cardioverter/defibrillator devices). The supporting nursing and technical staffs must devise a system to ensure that all the equipment needed for the procedure is available in the operating room and appropriately sterilized.

The intraoperative management of the patient must be made by consensus, with the overriding considerations of the patient's safety and, secondarily, of attaining the desired therapeutic objectives. Since patients' arrhythmic disorders are usually chronic, difficult to treat, and often continually evolving, the implantation of a pacemaker or cardioverter/defibrillator should not be viewed as a solitary definitive treatment but rather as one of many complementary modalities. Accordingly, both surgeons and cardiologists must have thorough training and familiarity with the various arrhythmia management options, the nuances of antitachycardia device technology and capabilities, and standard device implantation techniques, to make the appropriate preoperative and intraoperative decisions. This same team approach also proves to be beneficial in the postoperative management and follow-up of patients, particularly those with complex or refractory arrhythmias.

SURGICAL IMPLANTATION

The basic surgical principles for implantation of antitachycardia pacemakers and the AICD are essentially similar to those of standard pacemakers. The electrodes must be placed in a stable and secure anatomic position in which satisfactory thresholds for pacing and sensing are found, and the electrodes and pulse generator have to be securely implanted, with maximal attention paid to basic surgical techniques.

Antitachycardia Pacemakers

Transvenous implantation of these devices is preferred. An incision is made on either side slightly below the clavicle and parallel to it. An introducer device is used to enter the subclavian vein, and a guide wire is advanced into the right atrium. A sheath is passed over the guide wire, and the pacing electrode is passed through the sheath, which is then peeled away. If two leads are to be used for a dual-chamber device, the guide wire is left in the sheath as the pacing electrode is advanced into the vein. As the sheath is peeled away, the guide wire remains and is used for a second sheath for the second catheter. Once the leads have been positioned in the atrium and ventricle, a generous pocket, about twice the size of the device, is made directly anterior to the fascia of the pectoralis major muscle and is packed temporarily with a sponge soaked in povidone-iodine.

In some centers, the cephalic vein is still dissected to gain entrance into the venous system. In about half the patients, the cephalic vein will be too small or unsuitable, and the direct venipuncture technique will have to be used. Meticulous technique and insertion of the needle with the tip of the needle advanced toward the head of the opposite clavicle through the interosseous membrane between the first and second ribs generally guarantee a safe venipuncture. Elevation of the legs in the Trendelenburg position distends the vein and prevents air embolism. If the carotid or subclavian artery is inadvertently punctured, the needle should be immediately withdrawn and

pressure applied to the area for 5 minutes before additional maneuvers are restarted.

The ventricular lead is positioned first because it is usually the most clinically important of the two leads. We prefer to pass the lead into the pulmonary artery to verify its position within the ventricle. Then the lead is slowly withdrawn and made to lie in the apex of the right ventricle. The atrial lead is usually easily positioned in the atrial appendage, with the tip anterior on a lateral fluoroscopic view. A characteristic motion with atrial systole verifies its position. If the patient has had previous cardiac surgery and has no atrial appendage, a screw-on transvenous lead may be utilized for the atrium. Once the lead is in satisfactory anatomic position, threshold testing is performed, and then the leads are stabilized by placing a nonabsorbable suture through the fascia, tying it firmly on both sides of the fixation sleeve and placing an extra throw around the body of the lead. It is important that the lead be secure in its position and that no movement occur with vigorous activity to prevent lead dislodgment. The leads are then connected with the pulse generator and buried in the subcutaneous pocket. A pouch of polyester mesh may be used to enhance the fixation of the pulse generator to the surrounding tissue and prevent migration. The subcutaneous tissue is closed with running absorbable sutures in the skin with a running subcuticular stitch. Sterile strips may be used to bolster this closure.

If, for some reason, the transvenous route is not available, permanent pacing electrodes may be attached to the ventricle by a transpericardial approach. Access to the pericardium can be obtained through a short upper midline abdominal incision, with excision of the xyphoid process. This subxyphoid approach gives good exposure to the inferior surface of the right ventricle. If this approach is used, screw-on electrodes that are of low profile and have two and one-half turns should be used. A left anterior thoracotomy can similarly be utilized for approach to the lateral surface of the left ventricle. This approach is preferable in children and in patients who have had inferior myocardial infarctions or extensive apical ventricular aneurysms. Three and one-half turn screw-on electrodes are preferred. A number of new electrode configurations for epicardial use have been recently introduced, but few have had the extensive testing necessary to ascertain if the chronic threshold problems encountered with other types of epicardial electrodes will also be a problem with these leads.[10] The leads can be tunneled either subcutaneously into the upper abdomen or, in the case of a left anterior thoracotomy, upward and made to lie in the pectoral region on the left. It is important to place a loop of electrode in the chest just outside the pericardium to avoid tension on the leads.

Automatic Implantable Cardioverter/ Defibrillator

Several approaches to the implantation of the AICD device may be used. Basically, all have the disadvantage of requiring general anesthesia and vary in regard to incisions for placement of the myocardial patch electrodes.[101]

Anterolateral thoracotomy is the technique that is preferred in our institution. The patient is placed supine on the operating table, and the left side of the chest is elevated on a folded sheet. The arm is placed at the side of the patient. A small incision is made just beneath the left clavicle, and a needle–introducer device is used to enter the left subclavian vein. With a sheath, the spring lead electrode is then advanced to the junction of the superior vena cava and right atrium. The electrode is secured in place but not tunneled. A left anterolateral thoracotomy is performed, and the chest is entered through the fifth interspace. The left ventricular apex is dissected extrapericardially. The apical patch electrode is sutured to the

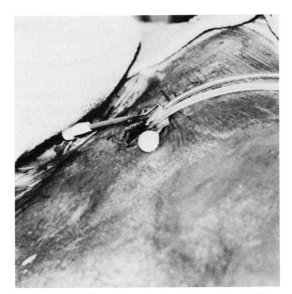

Figure 24–2. When the spring lead is combined with a transvenous right ventricular electrode, a guide wire passed through the first introducer sheath, followed by a second introducer, will prevent the complications of a second venipuncture.

pericardium with nonabsorbable material, and two epicardial screw-on electrodes are used for the ventricular bipolar leads inside the pericardium (Fig. 24–1).

The spring electrode is inserted through a small incision made beneath the left clavicle, and with use of an introducer device, the left subclavian vein is entered and the spring lead advanced to the junction of the superior vena cava and right atrium under the guidance of image-intensification fluoroscopy. If screw-on pacing leads are not preferred, a transvenous electrode can be placed at the same time the spring lead is placed. This practice is advantageous in patients who have a single patch implanted at the time of cardiac surgery and in whom it is not desirable to reopen the chest. In this technique, the guide wire is left in the vein through the peel-off introducer device, and the spring lead is inserted. Another introducer is then passed over the guide wire, and the pacing lead is inserted into the vein (Fig. 24–2).

If desired, because of large cardiac size or the inability to gain satisfactory defibrillation thresholds using a spring-patch configuration, two patch electrodes can be placed outside the pericardium. The first patch is placed as described previously, over the apical posterior portion of the myocardium, and the second patch is placed anteriorly over the right ventricle. The dissection is performed under the

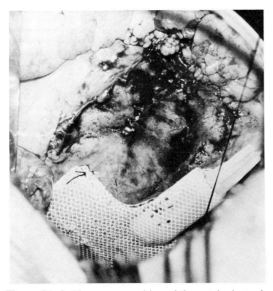

Figure 24–1. The proper position of the patch electrode when an extrapericardial implantation technique is used.

sternum, dividing by electrocautery the attachments between the pericardium and the sternum. This technique can be very hazardous in patients having previous median sternotomy, as the right ventricle is often adherent to the underside of the sternum. This procedure should be done with the utmost care, and provisions should be made for crossing the sternum using a Gigli saw if the right ventricle is inadvertently entered.

Another technique for the placement of the patch electrodes is the subxyphoid technique, which has the two advantages of requiring only a very small incision made in the midline of the abdomen and of not entering the pleural space.[100] With this technique, the patches need to be placed inside the pericardium, which has disadvantages if the system should become infected; moreover, it is very difficult to perform if the patient has had previous cardiac surgery. A third technique for patch implantation that has been recently described involves a single incision in the left upper quadrant of the abdomen parallel to the costal margin.[60] Through this single incision, the subcutaneous pockets for the defibrillator pulse generator and the patch electrodes are made simultaneously. The diaphragm is taken down from its attachments to the rib cage, and through this approach the patch electrodes can be placed either inside or outside the pericardium, although the inside route is easier (Fig. 24–3). Either one or two patches can be placed with relative ease using this technique. Its disadvantages lie in the rather large amount of dissection that is required to take down and reattach the diaphragm and the severe postoperative

pain encountered in many patients that is caused by dividing the rectus abdominus muscle.

In any case, the pulse generator is ordinarily placed in the left upper quadrant of the abdomen, although the right side can be used if there are other incisions or outstanding reasons why the left approach is not feasible. The pulse generator is usually placed over the rectus fascia, and many patients find that the pulse generator is better tolerated if it is placed horizontally rather than vertically in the pocket. The pocket should be made in both men and women so that the patient's beltline is below the pocket. Otherwise, if the patient's belt rubs on the incision or the pulse generator, pain can develop.

Complications of Antitachycardia Devices

Complications related to the placement of pacemakers and AICDs are not common. Three important complications of the direct venipuncture technique of transvenous pacemaker lead implantation are pneumothorax, hemopneumothorax, and massive air embolism. Elevation of the feet during the catheter introduction and adequate sedation to prevent the patient's movement will minimize the chances for these problems. If shortness of breath or hypotension develops, immediate tube thoracostomy on the side operated on is indicated. If air is heard to enter the catheter, the patient should be immediately rolled to the left lateral decubitus position, with the head up to prevent air from entering the heart.

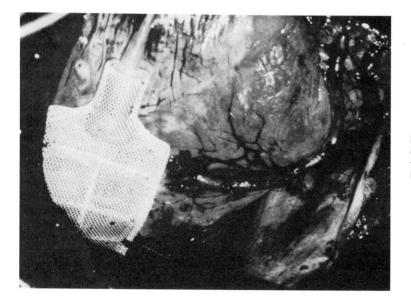

Figure 24–3. Proper intrapericardial patch electrode placement with careful avoidance of a vein bypass graft.

During the intracardiac manipulation of pacemaker leads, inadvertent perforation of the right atrium or ventricle may result. In most cases, these perforations are self-limited and cause no difficulty if the catheter is immediately withdrawn. Pacing of the diaphragm during the manipulation of a right ventricular catheter can alert one to the possibility that the catheter has perforated the ventricular myocardium. Should the patient's blood pressure precipitously drop, in association with distended neck veins and other signs of cardiac tamponade, preparations for immediate thoracotomy must be made. If the pacemaker is being placed in a cardiac catheterization laboratory, it is possible to drain the pericardium using a large-bore needle and to stabilize the patient so that thoracotomy can be performed within the sterile confines of the operating room. In the vast majority of cases, cardiac tamponade due to right ventricular perforation should be approached surgically, not treated expectantly by only tapping the pericardium.

The other serious complication of pacemakers and defibrillators is erosion and infection. If the pulse generator or leads appear to be eroding through the skin, immediate surgical revision is indicated. If formal erosion occurs, surgical revision is indicated if it is performed within the first 12 to 24 hours, with the expectation that chronic infection will result in 25 to 50 per cent of cases. Erosion present for longer periods should be considered infected. If any portion of the lead system or pulse generator becomes infected, it is necessary to remove the entire foreign-body apparatus from the body. This removal becomes difficult in some cases, such as when pacemaker electrodes that have tined tips have been used. In most cases, with use of gentle traction over a period of time, the electrode can be removed from the right ventricular apex and withdrawn from the vein. In some cases, excessive traction will cause collapse of the right ventricle and immediate hypotension. In these cases, the lead can be buried in another subcutaneous pocket and the other incision can be drained. If infection persists, it will be necessary to perform a thoracotomy to remove the lead. If the lead becomes chronically infected with subacute bacterial endocarditis, a formal cardiac procedure for removal of the catheter may be necessary.

If infection complicates AICD insertion, it is necessary to remove the entire lead system, including the patch electrodes. If the electrodes have been placed outside the pericardium, this is usually no problem. Intrapericardial implantation of the leads may require a median sternotomy and full exposure of the heart to remove the electrodes. The incidence of infection requiring removal of hardware ranged from 2.9 to 4.5 per cent in published series.[41, 66, 106] The total perioperative mortality of patients in these same series ranged from 0 to 3.8 per cent.

The remainder of this chapter will discuss electrophysiologic and other considerations for the intraoperative assessment of antitachycardia pacemakers delivering discrete pulses and then will address considerations that apply to automatic cardioverters/defibrillators delivering high energy electrical discharges.

ANTITACHYCARDIA PACEMAKERS

Preimplantation Considerations

The issues affecting the decision to use an antitachycardia pacemaker, the actual choice of device, the appropriate surgical approach for implantation, and the programming of the device are complex and unique to the individual patient. Listed in Table 24–1 and discussed in detail in Chapters 21 and 22 are some of the considerations involved as well as the necessary preoperative data.

A thorough preoperative electrophysiologic evaluation is essential.[43, 79] Objectives that must be met include (1) the characterization of the targeted arrhythmia mechanism; (2) an assessment of the function of the cardiac conduction system and the potential for bradyarrhythmias and conduction disturbances; (3) a search for other, potentially confounding tachyarrhythmias; (4) determination of the effectiveness of pacing to terminate the arrhythmia; (5) identification of the most effective pacing modality, rates, duration, and stimulatory site; (6) evaluation of the likelihood, type, and consequences of pacing-induced complications, including arrhythmia exacerbation and/or induction; and (7) observation of the patient's ability to perceive or sense the arrhythmia and its termination. Other issues include the need for concurrent antiarrhythmic drugs and whether defibrillation capability is required.

Electrophysiologic testing should be exhaustive, with repeated inductions and terminations of the target arrhythmia performed, using a wide variety of pacing algorithms and techniques. Particularly in patients with ventricular tachycardia, some authors advocate at least

TABLE 24–1. FACTORS INFLUENCING THE USE AND TYPE OF ANTITACHYCARDIA DEVICE

I. CLINICAL ARRHYTHMIA CONSIDERATIONS
   A. Target tachyarrhythmia(s)—types, rates, morphologies, lethal versus nonlethal consequences
   B. Hemodynamic and symptomatic manifestations
   C. Response to prior therapies
   D. Other arrhythmias—types, rates, morphologies
   E. Bradyarrhythmias and conduction disturbances—need for pacing, presence of accessory bypass connections
   F. Therapeutic alternatives

II. CARDIAC CONSIDERATIONS
   A. Anatomic problems, including valve prostheses
   B. Structural disease—type, natural history/prognosis
   C. Prior surgical procedures, including devices, pacemakers
   D. Anticipated need for surgical procedures—coronary bypass grafting, valve replacement, aneurysmectomy
   E. Effects of arrhythmias—e.g., ischemia, congestive heart failure

III. ELECTROPHYSIOLOGIC AND PACING CONSIDERATIONS
   A. Arrhythmia induction—ease, type, risks
   B. Arrhythmia termination—ease, best modality, responses, risks
   C. Conducting system function—risk of conduction of rapid pacing
   D. Arrhythmia mechanisms and locations
   E. Effects of antiarrhythmic drugs—arrhythmia frequency, rates, inducibility, termination ease
   F. Automatic versus manual device
   G. Arrhythmia prophylaxis/suppression versus termination
   H. Need for defibrillation

IV. THE PATIENT AND OTHER CONSIDERATIONS
   A. Patient's wishes
   B. Arrhythmia symptoms—type, severity, frequency, duration
   C. Emotional, physical, and intellectual state—recognition of arrhythmia, insight into disease state, manual versus automatic devices
   D. Patient's compliance
   E. Family support
   F. Proximity to medical care
   G. Physician's experience with devices

100 consecutive successful conversions using the intended pacing scheme to ensure consistent results with a low risk of pacer-induced complications.[35] To facilitate this process, use of an external pacing system analyzer, which mimics the intended pacemaker, or an actual device connected with temporary leads is helpful for testing.

Component Selection

The choice of pacemaker generator and lead system is primarily influenced by the arrhythmia type and the results of electrophysiologic testing. Because of the risk of excessive, life-threatening ventricular tachycardia or fibrillation induced or accelerated inadvertently by ventricular pacing, antitachycardia pacemakers are rarely used for ventricular applications and only with extreme caution and serious reservations.[35, 36, 43] For the present time, the AICD is an effective and safer alternative,[30] although several hybrid antitachycardia pacemaker-defibrillator devices will be forthcoming soon. Carefully selected patients with atrial flutter, atrial reentry, AV nodal reentry, or reciprocating bypass tract–mediated arrhythmias can be successfully treated by a variety of antitachycardia pacemakers used in the atrium or, in the last two conditions, by dual-chamber or ventricular devices.[65, 93, 111] When pacing from either chamber is feasible, atrial pacing is preferable owing to the lower risks of atrial arrhythmia induction or aggravation.[31]

The next decision to be made is between patient-activated manual and automatically operating devices.[43, 79] The lack of objective arrhythmia detection capabilities and the longer response times inherent in externally triggered devices mean that the arrhythmias must be hemodynamically well tolerated, not life threatening themselves, not likely to be accelerated or aggravated by pacing, and easily recognized by the patient.[37] Advantages of these devices include the ability to adjust readily the device's functions to deal with varying arrhythmia characteristics, device longevity, and the opportunity to try other termination modalities (e.g., vagal maneuvers) prior to pacemaker use.[78] In contrast, automatic pacemakers are preferable if the patient is physically or mentally incapable of recognizing the arrhythmia, unable to activate the device, or incapacitated by or severely symptomatic from the target tachycardia, or if he or she prefers to avoid the inconvenience of a manual device.[37, 79]

The choice of specific brand, model, and modality of the device is influenced by the many considerations given above. Simplicity of device use, ease of follow-up and programming, prior personal experiences, and the degree of device flexibility and options may contribute to the final decision. The initial choice may be altered in the course of preoperative and intraoperative electrophysiologic testing. The temporary use of the actual pacemakers or their external "pacing systems analyzers," connected with the pacing leads, allows comparisons of several different configurations, modalities, and devices so that the optimal system may be chosen prior to its actual implantation.

The choice of lead types and configurations to be used in a given patient is usually much less difficult. The device chosen and the chamber to be paced largely dictate the options. Most devices currently employ bipolar leads; when a choice is available, bipolar configurations are generally preferred to unipolar systems.[40] As discussed below, and as is the case with conventional pacemakers, bipolar leads have superior signal-to-noise rate characteristics, minimizing many types of oversensing; intracardiac signal detection by both lead types is otherwise comparable.[40] In terms of pacing capabilities, there are probably no differences, except for a greater incidence of extracardiac skeletal muscle (e.g., pectoral, intercostal, and abdominal muscle) pacing with unipolar leads.[40] However, there may be some increased vulnerability to arrhythmia *induction* using anodal pacing (either unipolar or bipolar) compared with cathodal stimulation.[70, 81] The clinical significance of this problem in humans is unclear and is difficult to assess, especially given the greater overall tendency for pacemaker induction of arrhythmias in those patients with known arrhythmic substrates.

The factors influencing the type of lead fixation for antitachycardia pacing are substantially similar to those for conventional pacing. The lead fixation method used—"passive, tined" versus "active, screw-in" endocardial leads or the particular type of epicardial fixation device—depends in part on the particular operative approach used and anatomic constraints such as abnormal cardiac anatomy, altered myocardial trabeculation, previously unsuccessful lead fixation, or the need for atypical pacing sites. The differences in the electrical (sensing and pacing) characteristics of passive- and active-fixation leads are subject to debate and, to an extent, depend upon the brand or model of the leads being compared; any differences present tend to be largely outweighed by personal preferences and the more substantial differences in lead placement stability.

Intraoperative Electrophysiologic Assessment

The intraoperative electrophysiologic assessment should include the standard evaluation of sensing, capture, and lead impedance using the pacing system analyzer. In addition, intra-cardiac electrograms should be examined, and the sensing and capture thresholds should be determined during inherent rhythm and all induced arrhythmias. Most cardiologists program the pacing output for arrhythmia termination to exceed the usual two to three times the safety margin. The efficacy of the selected programmed arrhythmia detection and termination settings should be repeatedly evaluated. If the tachycardia rates induced intraoperatively differ from rates documented clinically owing to altered autonomic tone, retesting and reprogramming of these settings may be necessary prior to hospital discharge. A detailed discussion of considerations in the selection of arrhythmia detection and termination modes follows.

ARRHYTHMIA DETECTION AND SENSING. The simplest forms of antitachycardia pacemakers, those that are manually activated by the patient or by the physician, have no intrinsic detection capabilities, relying instead on the patient's imperfect, subjective recognition of the arrhythmia by characteristic symptoms or by a rapid pulse rate.[78] The arrhythmia can be confirmed by obtaining an electrocardiogram, but this obviously delays therapy substantially. "Automatic" devices, on the other hand, respond more quickly, without active intervention by the patient or physician, following satisfaction of predetermined, objective arrhythmia detection criteria. One or more arrhythmia detection parameters may be utilized, including heart rate, abruptness of heart rate changes, tachycardia rate stability, and tachycardia duration.[11, 80]

Arrhythmia recognition based on cardiac *rate,* either the atrial or the ventricular rate, is the primary criterion used in all automatic devices.[11] When the sensed rate (either absolutely for each cardiac cycle or, more typically, averaged over a number of cardiac cycles) exceeds the rate threshold, the tachycardia is deemed pathologic and a response is generated. Typically, the rate threshold may be programmed over a wide range to accommodate individual variations in the patient's tachycardia and peak sinus rates. In conjunction with cardiac rate, the *tachycardia duration* criterion, sometimes programmable in terms of the number of consecutive cardiac cycles scrutinized, is used to prevent responses to fleeting tachycardias and to allow nonsustained arrhythmias to terminate spontaneously. A number of devices (e.g., Intermedics Cybertach 60, Freeport, TX; Cordis Orthocor II, Miami, FL; Telectronics PASAR 4171, Engle-

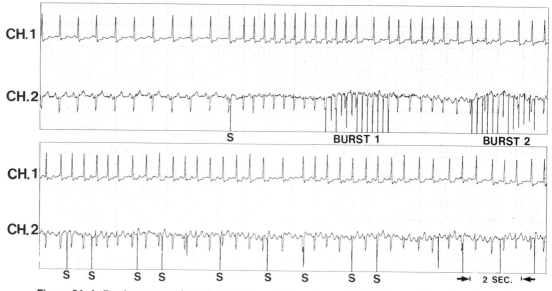

Figure 24–4. Continuous two-channel ambulatory electrocardiographic (ECG) recording of a patient with an automatic atrial burst pacemaker (Intermedics Cybertach-60) for the treatment of supraventricular tachycardia (SVT). In the top panel, an atrial demand paced beat (S), delivered because of sinus P-wave non-sensing, induces SVT. An appropriately delivered atrial burst (BURST 1) converts SVT into atrial fibrillation, followed by an ineffectual atrial burst (BURST 2) and intermittent atrial demand pacing. This figure illustrates undersensing of atrial rhythms, induction and aggravation of arrhythmias, and inability to recognize those atrial tachyarrhythmias not amenable to pace termination. (From Echt DS: Potential hazards of implanted devices. PACE 7:581, 1984; with permission.)

wood, CO; Medtronic Symbios 7008, Minneapolis, MN)[2, 44, 83, 90, 111] determine whether a tachycardia is to be pace-terminated solely by these two parameters. A major limitation of these devices, and of this combined arrhythmia detection modality, is the inability to deal with sinus and other tachycardias that cannot be pace-terminated and that overlap in rate with the targeted tachycardias.[31, 37, 62] An example is the futile attempt of an atrial burst pacemaker to convert atrial fibrillation (Fig. 24–4).

The inclusion of criteria based on cardiac *rate change* and the *stability* of the rate into devices is an attempt to enhance the specificity of arrhythmia discrimination.[37, 80] Activity-related changes in sinus rhythms are typically gradual in onset (and offset), with modest respiration-related fluctuations in the peak heart rate. In contrast, most reentrant (therefore, amenable to pace termination) arrhythmias have more abrupt onsets and little cyclic heart rate variability. Devices with algorithms to assess the abruptness of heart rate changes, in combination with heart rate thresholds (e.g., Intermedics Intertach 262–12; Siemens-Elema Tachylog 651, Solna, Sweden),[89, 99] compare the first tachycardia interval with preceding sinus intervals; the actual cycle length changes necessary to fulfill the criterion may be pro-

grammable as well as the number of preceding sinus intervals. Irregular tachyarrhythmias (e.g., atrial fibrillation) and even marked sinus arrhythmias, both with abrupt onsets, can be further identified and differentiated by rate stability criteria.[80] Those rhythms with considerable beat-to-beat cycle length variability exceeding programmed limits are less likely to be able to be pace-terminated, while those with greater rate consistency are more likely to be reentrant and able to be successfully converted by pacing.

Discrimination of rhythms on the basis of intracardiac electrogram signal characteristics is another approach under consideration.[11, 37, 40, 77] These studies have demonstrated quantitatively small but clear differences in electrogram amplitudes, morphology, duration, and slew rates between normally conducted atrial impulses and those conducted retrograde or aberrantly, using standard pacing leads. More complex multielectrode configurations may provide improved arrhythmia differentiation through differences in their spatial and directional characteristics and their temporal activation sequences.[37, 71] Another proposed scheme utilizes comparisons of atrial and ventricular rates as one level of arrhythmia detection and the ventricular detection of conducted single atrial paced beats as a means of distinguishing between sinus and nonsinus supraventricular mechanisms.[51] Last, incorporation of sensors of other physiologic parameters, such as intracardiac pressure or volume transducers, into the pacemaker lead systems may provide other modalities of arrhythmia detection.[11, 37, 110]

A consideration separate from arrhythmia recognition is the issue of signal detection. Regardless of the diagnostic algorithms used by the devices, underlying them is the pacemaker's ability to detect intracardiac electrograms of the appropriate amplitude and slew rate characteristics. Inappropriate detection of artifact or unintended cardiac activity, "oversensing" in traditional terms, can occur in many ways and with a variety of consequences.[26] The short pacemaker refractory periods necessary to sense rapid rhythms may lead to the overdetection of delayed or fractionated electrograms (e.g., intraventricular conduction delays or slow atrioventricular [AV] conduction) or repolarization activity or both. Lengthening of refractoriness reduces double counting but may preclude recognition of more rapid arrhythmias. Far-field sensing of intrinsic or paced electrograms, noncardiac myopotentials, or electromagnetic noise is particularly likely with unipolar lead configurations; therefore, bipolar lead systems are preferable.

The consequences of oversensing are numerous and diverse. As in antibradycardia systems, oversensing, especially with unipolar leads, of noncardiac signals may inappropriately inhibit the backup bradycardia pacing functions. Other signals, detected as noise, may cause reversion to an asynchronous mode, resulting in unnecessary and competitive pacing during normal rhythms.[62] In these patients, who are prone to pacing induction of tachyarrhythmias, the potential for arrhythmia induction by inappropriate asynchronous pacing is real.[62] Alternatively, noise oversensing may render the device insensitive to the simultaneous presence of a tachyarrhythmia, causing a failure to detect and respond to it. Double counting of nontachycardiac rhythms may trigger unwarranted antitachycardia pacing, resulting in the induction of potentially symptomatic or life-threatening arrhythmias.[62, 89] A final undesirable consequence of antitachycardia pacing due to oversensing is the potential for symptoms and hemodynamic effects directly related to the rapid pacing stimuli.

Undersensing problems in antitachycardia pacemakers are most often due to inadequate electrogram amplitudes and slew rates. Not only must the predominant rhythm (usually sinus) be satisfactorily detected by the pacing system but the target tachyarrhythmia also must be sensed. Because of the different activation sequence and propagation in tachyarrhythmias, the electrograms during tachyarrhythmias may be lower in amplitude and have different frequency or slew rate characteristics.[26, 37, 40, 77] This means that particular attention must be paid intraoperatively to the quality of the electrograms in *all* clinical rhythms and arrhythmias. Undersensing of the tachyarrhythmia can also occur if the arrhythmia rate is lower than the pacemaker's programmed detection rate as a result of physiologic or autonomic changes, alterations in arrhythmia conduction, or concurrently administered cardioactive medications. Inappropriately long pacemaker refractory period settings can also cause undercounting of tachycardia rates.[26] Undersensing of inherent complexes can cause asynchronous bradycardia pacing, which may initiate a tachyarrhythmia[26, 62] (see Fig. 24–4).

ARRHYTHMIA TERMINATION AND EXACERBATION. The overriding problem limiting the use of antitachycardia devices, especially pacemakers, is their lack of uniform antiarrhythmic efficacy combined with their potential for arrhythmia exacerbation. Given the patient's underlying arrhythmic substrate, the same pacing modalities used for tachycardia termination carry an ever-present risk of either inadvertently inducing the same arrhythmia or converting a spontaneously occurring episode into a different form that is less well tolerated.[31] Relatively well tolerated, slower ventricular tachycardias inadvertently may be converted by the pacemaker to faster, hemodynamically unstable, and pacing-resistant arrhythmias, such as ventricular fibrillation, with a disastrous outcome.[36, 43] The prevention of pacemaker-*induced* arrhythmias depends upon improved rhythm detection schemes and the elimination of inappropriate pacing in normal rhythms[37] (see above). Attempts to improve arrhythmia termination rates and reduce the risks of arrhythmia acceleration revolve around the use of a growing number of pacing regimens[73] (Fig. 24–5).

The pacing modalities employed currently all involve the delivery of single or multiple discrete, low-energy pacing impulses in fixed or predetermined sequences. In its simplest form, tachyarrhythmia termination can be

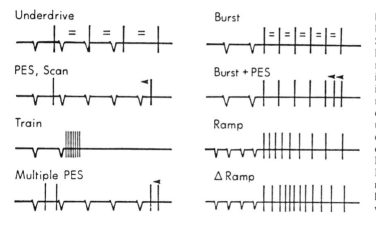

Figure 24–5. Schematic diagrams of basic antitachycardia pacing modes. Spontaneous atrial or ventricular depolarizations during tachyarrhythmias are represented by deflections from the horizontal time line, and pacer stimuli are indicated by vertical lines. The small arrowheads indicate the direction of changes in the timing of successive stimuli. Pacing modes include programmed extrastimuli (PES) and incremental-decremental ramps ($\triangle$ Ramp). (From Fisher JD, Johnston DR, Kim SG, et al: Implantable pacers for tachycardia termination: Stimulation techniques and long-term efficacy. PACE 9:1325, 1986; with permission.)

achieved with *underdrive pacing* by conventional antibradycardia devices. Through either magnet application or programming, temporary asynchronous demand-rate pacing is effective in some patients, particularly those with slower, hemodynamically stable arrhythmias.[102] In slightly more advanced devices, underdrive fixed-rate antitachycardia pacing may occur automatically as a programmed "dual-demand mode."[37, 111] Regardless of these added capabilities, underdrive pacing depends on the delivery of regular, slow-rate stimuli, which fall randomly throughout the arrhythmia cycle until an appropriately timed impulse terminates the tachycardia. By relying on an essentially random terminating event, this modality suffers from relative inefficiency, resulting in time delays in terminating the arrhythmia (especially if manually activated), marginal efficacy rates (particularly in patients with faster tachycardias), and low but possible risk of arrhythmia exacerbation.[102]

Standard pacemakers are also capable of *overdrive suppression* of arrhythmias in certain limited clinical circumstances. Demand-mode pacing can effectively prevent ventricular tachycardias that are specifically related to bradycardia or associated with QT-interval prolongation[37]; and by maintaining proper AV synchrony and timing, dual-chamber pacemakers can suppress bypass tract–mediated reciprocating AV tachycardias.[93]

Overdrive or *burst pacing* termination modalities are more effective than underdrive techniques. The advantages of higher rate pacing include more rapid tachycardia termination and higher levels of success[36, 73] due to burst facilitation of impulse penetration into the arrhythmia circuit and the resetting of tissue refractoriness.[102] As with underdrive pacing, however, the major disadvantage is that of arrhythmia induction by pacing inappropriate

rhythms or arrhythmia exacerbation as a consequence of pacing appropriate tachyarrhythmias.[36, 73] When used for atrial applications, another potential risk involves the unexpectedly rapid conduction of rapid atrial pacing impulses to the ventricle via the AV node or bypass connections, causing an even more rapid heart rate, more hemodynamic compromise, and possibly induction of ventricular arrhythmias.[26, 62]

The simplest burst pacing systems consist of a passive "generator" driven by an external manually activated burst stimulator (e.g., Medtronic RF 5998).[78] Many pacemakers with triggered (VVT, AAT, or DDT) modes will deliver internally powered burst stimuli when triggered transcutaneously by a programmer or an external stimulator (e.g., Cordis Omni-Orthocor) or both.[83] Still others can be acutely programmed to burst pace (e.g., Medtronic Spectrax) or to deliver preprogrammed bursts when manually activated by magnet or programmer or automatically when the arrhythmia rate exceeds the programmed rate threshold (e.g., Medtronic Symbios 7008 and Intermedics Cybertach 60, respectively).[44, 111] The effectiveness of these devices under typical clinical conditions tends to be limited by the inability to modify their function acutely in response to changes in the tachyarrhythmia rate. Burst pacing cycle length generally must be 40 to 50 msec faster than the tachycardia cycle length to ensure myocardial capture.

Devices that deliver *programmed extrastimuli* offer some advantages over the other types described above. A relatively few number of critically timed pacing stimuli can result in satisfactory termination efficacy.[73] If the number of delivered impulses can be limited to one or two, there is potential reduction in the risk of arrhythmia exacerbation.[26, 73] Earlier units (e.g., Telectronics 4151) delivered one or two impulses with systematic "scanning" or preprogrammed stepwise changes in coupling intervals (between a sensed tachycardia beat and the first extrastimulus) over a limited range, until arrhythmia termination was achieved.[91] More recent and complex devices utilize multiple extrastimuli, with either independent or interrelated scanning of each impulse (e.g., Telectronics PASAR 4171, Siemens Tachylog 451, and Cordis Orthocor II).[83, 89, 91] To deal with spontaneously occurring changes in tachyarrhythmia characteristics, capabilities now also exist for "adaptive" changes in the timing and rates of bursts or extrastimuli relative to the tachycardia rate. Further refinements, including adaptive increments in the number of extrastimuli used, ramp pacing, and scanning or shifting burst pacing schemes, are now available in several devices (e.g., Intermedics Intertach).[38, 75]

Objective comparisons between the pacing modalities—their clinical efficacy, applicability, complications, and relative advantages—are difficult because of the limited clinical experiences with most devices.[38, 48, 49] Most reports involve relatively small numbers of highly selected patients, with heterogeneous cardiac and arrhythmic conditions, and nonsystematic comparisons of the pacing techniques. There is, though, general agreement that *overdrive suppression* and *underdrive termination* mode pacemakers have very limited applicability and efficacy in the majority of patients troubled by frequent, recurrent, and symptomatic (presumably reentrant) tachyarrhythmias. *Burst pacing* and *programmed extrastimuli* are substantially more effective.[16, 23, 36, 73] However, no ideal or "universal" antitachycardia pacing mode exists. Extensive testing is needed to individualize therapy. Since arrhythmia characteristics may undergo changes over time, a versatile device is preferable.[22] Other recommendations about optimal pacing modes and specific device preferences await the results of more extensive clinical trials.

Antiarrhythmic Drug Interactions

Although data are not readily available, antiarrhythmic drug use, on an acute and chronic basis, in patients with antitachycardia pacemakers is probably common. As with automatic cardioverter/defibrillators (see below), these agents have the potential for enhancing, complicating, or undermining the operation of the pacemakers.[50]

As a useful adjunct to the pacemaker, antiarrhythmic medications can partially suppress the arrhythmia and reduce the number of tachycardia episodes that require pacemaker responses. With the slowing of the tachycardias that often occurs with most drugs, the arrhythmias are often better tolerated,[50] allowing use of manually activated devices instead of automatic units. Antitachycardia pacing efficacy may be enhanced with slower tachycardia rates and longer vulnerable or "excitable pacing gaps," allowing the use of slower pacing rates or safer, adaptive pacing algorithms or both.[50, 73] This practice, in combination with reduced cardiac tissue excitability, may reduce the likelihood of pacing-induced conversion of rhythms into either flutter or fibrillation.[43]

The same antiarrhythmic drug effects, in other settings, may confound pacer function in several ways. Changes in arrhythmia conduction may result in alterations of electrogram amplitude and morphology, which then fall below programmed or inherent device sensing limitations. More commonly, the slowing of the tachycardia rate (and possibly the changes in the abruptness of the arrhythmia's onset) below the device's primary rate threshold renders the device incapable of responding to an otherwise appropriate tachyarrhythmia. One can speculate that drugs may narrow the excitable gap in some circumstances, diminishing the efficacy of some (e.g., programmed extrastimuli) or all pacing modalities.[50] In extrapolating from limited data on the effects of drugs that increase capture thresholds during demand pacing,[47, 63] a similar effect may be found to exist in antitachycardia settings.

Because of these complex and unpredictable interactions, the testing of anticipated drug-pacemaker combinations is mandatory. Preoperative and intraoperative evaluation of concomitant antiarrhythmic drugs to be used might alter the choice of the device settings or of the drug. Postoperatively, any modification of antiarrhythmic drugs necessitates reevaluation to identify and prevent a potentially undesirable interaction with the pacemaker before discharging the patient to home.

AUTOMATIC CARDIOVERTERS/ DEFIBRILLATORS

Component Selection

Functionally, the device system comprises the electrodes and their arrangement and the type of generator.[21] The electrodes may have a single function (detection or termination) or dual roles. The discharging electrodes are composed of platinum, silver, or titanium conducting material and have surface areas ranging between 2.5 and 28 cm^2. The discharging electrodes of an intracardiac catheter are positioned within the right side of the heart at the atrial or at the ventricular level or both. Extracardiac discharging electrodes are sutured either directly to the epicardial surface or to the internal or external surfaces of the pericardium. The extracardiac electrodes are referred to as patches or plaques and have insulation on the surface facing the lungs and chest wall to focus the current in the direction of the myocardium. The electrode arrangements that have been implanted successfully in patients include a transvenous catheter with a right atrial and a right ventricular intracavitary electrode pair[72]; a right atrial intracavitary spring-coil electrode paired with a left ventricular extracardiac patch electrode; and two extracardiac patch electrodes, with one each over the right and left ventricle.[30, 82] In addition, a promising electrode configuration that has undergone extensive animal testing and is now undergoing clinical investigation is a three-electrode combination of a transvenous catheter with right atrial and right ventricular intracavitary electrodes and either an extracardiac left ventricular or a subcutaneous precordial patch or plaque electrode (Endotak-C, Cardiac Pacemakers, Inc).[13, 52, 53, 85, 86, 103]

The relative efficacy of the various electrode configurations is dependent, in part, upon the distribution of myocardial current density created when energy is applied across the electrode pairs.[42] Results of both animal experimentation and mathematical modeling suggest that successful ventricular defibrillation is associated with electrode configurations that have low but homogeneous current densities over a large myocardial area.[28] Configurations using electrodes with smaller surface areas in intracavitary positions lose current into the intracavitary blood pool and are less energy efficient. Configurations with large total electrode surface area cover greater areas of myocardium and yield higher myocardial current density. Thus, two large extracardiac patches are most efficient for defibrillation.[68, 97] The new three-electrode configuration was developed based on the concept that current pathways in perpendicular directions will result in more homogeneous current density distributions, particularly in localized areas receiving low current flow via a single pathway. This electrode configuration was first developed using sequential delivery of pulses in each of the two current pathways.[52, 86] More recently, the need for sequential pulsing using this electrode configuration has been questioned, with comparable results being obtained in an acute canine study utilizing a single simultaneous pulse discharge in perpendicular directions.[103]

Of the many factors affecting defibrillation energy, including the electrode surface area, electrode material, electrode geometry, pulse waveform, drugs, myocardial disease, and arrhythmia duration, the electrode type and arrangement are the major ones that the physician can choose to optimize individually the performance of the device.[96] In the future, biphasic pulse waveforms will also be an option.[87] At present, the choices of electrodes for the AICD (Cardiac Pacemakers, Inc) are between a spring-coil and patch system or a two-patch system and between standard-sized or large patches. The factors favoring the use of a spring-coil and patch system include the ability to replace the spring-coil electrode using percutaneous technique, should the electrode fail in the future; the avoidance of dissection through chest wall adhesions overlying the right ventricle in patients who have had previous cardiac surgery; and the observation that the transcardiac electrogram utilized for arrhythmia morphology detection may be superior. The factors weighing against the use of the spring-coil and patch electrode configuration include the occurrence of superior vena caval thrombosis due to the large caliber of the electrode, the possibility that corrosive oxidation and fibrotic accumulation on the spring-coil lead may reduce the chronic efficacy of the system, and the incidence of migration of the spring-coil electrode. The major factor in favor of using a two-patch arrangement is that lower energies are required for successful defibrillation. The major consideration against using a two-patch arrangement is the theoretical possibility that myocardial or pericardial constriction may develop; at least one such case has been reported.[1] There is also more difficulty in removing patch leads in the case of late infection requiring explantation of electrodes. The use of two large patches is also associated with the potential hazard that arcing of current could occur if the patches make contact during discharge, essentially short-circuiting the myocardial current pathway.

Ideally, the electrode configuration selected would be one that is associated with the lowest surgical risk and an acceptable safety margin for arrhythmia termination. This strategy might be implemented by first testing an electrode configuration not requiring thoracotomy or a more limited approach. However, should the electrode arrangement selected initially prove to be unsatisfactory during intraoperative testing, repeat testing with electrode repositioning or with another arrangement will be necessary, and it is likely that surgical time will be increased and that one of the original electrodes will have to be discarded. Therefore, many physicians have taken an alternative approach and test two large patches as the initial electrode configuration. The advent of newer electrode configurations will provide alternatives, necessitating a reevaluation of the electrode selection process. One strategy that has been proposed involves first testing a two-electrode transvenous system alone, and, if unsuccessful, then adding a third patch electrode to the system.[96] The patch would initially be positioned subcutaneously in the precordial area but could be repositioned to an extracardiac position if necessary.

At present, the selection of a generator is necessary because of the lack of programmability of available devices. This limitation presents major difficulties, since the device must be preselected and ordered in advance of the intraoperative procedure. The features of the AICD device that must be preselected include the arrhythmia detection rate cut-off, the inclusion of the arrhythmia morphology criterion, and the energy level of the first pulse. Although the availability of noninvasive programmability will soon make preselection obsolete, general guidelines will remain useful to aid in selecting initial settings for future programmable devices.

The preoperative evaluation to aid in the selection of the arrhythmia detection rate cut-off was addressed in Chapter 22. An arrhythmia rate cut-off should be selected that is approximately 10 beats per minute slower than the slowest episode of ventricular tachycardia in the presence of any chronic antiarrhythmic drug therapy. Ideally, the arrhythmia rate cut-off selected would be lower than all sustained ventricular tachycardia episodes and also higher than all supraventricular rhythms, including sinus tachycardia. When the range of supraventricular tachycardia overlaps with the range of ventricular tachycardias, detection of supraventricular rhythms is possible. The added morphology criterion will reject narrow-complex supraventricular tachycardias. However, supraventricular tachyarrhythmias in pa-

tients with an underlying intraventricular conduction delay or with rate-related, aberrantly conducted supraventricular tachyarrhythmias would be detected by the AICD device. Thus, the major advantage of having the morphology criterion is in those patients who have both narrow-complex supraventricular tachycardia and wide-complex ventricular tachycardia at similar rates. In patients with an underlying intraventricular conduction delay or complete bundle branch block, there is no advantage to having the morphology criterion. Since having the morphology criterion frequently extends the arrhythmia detection time and probably shortens the generator battery life, there are several reasons to utilize devices without a morphology criterion in these patients. Similarly, there is little advantage to having a morphology criterion in devices set to arrhythmia detection rate cut-offs greater than 180 beats per minute, since sinus tachycardia and atrial fibrillation rarely exceed this rate. Moreover, supraventricular tachycardias that do exceed 180 beats per minute are usually not hemodynamically tolerated in this particular population of patients, and electrical termination would likely benefit the patient.

The only method to anticipate an individual patient's defibrillation energy needs is to test the defibrillation energy requirement of a transvenous catheter or transvenous catheter plus cutaneous patch electrode system in the clinical electrophysiology laboratory prior to the implantation procedure. Unfortunately, these electrodes are not available to most physicians, and the results of acute testing of one electrode system may not correlate with the results of testing a different electrode system. Thus far, no clinical indicators have been found to identify patients likely to have high or low defibrillation energy needs. Although it seems logical that patients with greatest myocardial mass or chamber size would have the highest energy requirement, a concept that preliminary echocardiographic data support,[14] the clinical experience differs, suggesting that there are other overriding factors.[104] Since it is difficult, if not impossible, to determine individual energy requirements prior to implantation, it is optimal for devices to have a maximal output sufficient to terminate ventricular fibrillation in the vast majority of patients.

Intraoperative Electrophysiologic Assessment

SENSING AND ARRHYTHMIA DETECTION. The intraoperative assessment should include an analysis of intracardiac and transcardiac signals during inherent rhythm and all induced ventricular tachyarrhythmias, the ventricular pacing threshold, the individual lead impedances, cardioversion and defibrillation energy determinations, an assessment of the functional integrity of the generator, and an overall evaluation of the entire system for arrhythmia detection and termination.[12, 27, 96, 107] The transcardiac impedance may also be determined, but this calculation does not appear to have important implications for internal defibrillation,[45] as it may for external defibrillation.[56, 61]

An understanding of the engineering design of the detection algorithms enables the interpretation of the adequacy of the intracardiac signals. In general, the rate detection circuitry for devices designed to detect ventricular tachycardia and fibrillation differs from that of bradycardia pacemakers. The rate detection algorithms employed in bradycardia pacemakers are designed for situations in which slew rate and signal amplitude remain relatively constant. Intracardiac signal amplitude and morphology are markedly and abruptly altered with changes in cardiac rhythm. Rate detection in the AICD device is designed to allow low signal amplitudes and occasional signal dropout.[104] The specific design features include an automatic gain control, which can automatically amplify the signal to detect a signal amplitude as low as 0.1 mV, and rate averaging, which keeps a running total of the signal intervals. The morphology detection criterion in the AICD device utilizes an algorithm referred to as the probability density function (PDF).[59] This signal analysis is complex, and the sensitivity is dependent upon a "window setting." It is not possible for the physician to determine with certainty whether a particular transcardiac electrogram will satisfy the PDF. However, the general principle is that the more time spent away from the isoelectric baseline, the greater the likelihood for detection.

The analysis of the intracardiac and transcardiac signals should involve obtaining unfiltered signals on hard copy at fast paper speed to measure the amplitude and width of the QRS complex, to evaluate qualitatively the signal morphology, and to compare the QRS amplitude with that of a P wave or a T wave (Fig. 24–6). Note in Figure 24–7 that the QRS signal across two patch electrodes during sinus rhythm is generally of narrow width despite the large electrode surface area. The signal during inherent rhythm from a rate-counting electrode pair should be scrutinized for possi-

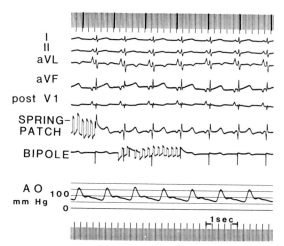

Figure 24–6. Typical intraoperative recordings from a patient receiving a right atrial spring-coil and left ventricular patch AICD electrode configuration. Note that the transcardiac spring-patch electrogram resembles a surface electrogram. I, II, aV$_L$, and posterior V$_1$ are surface electrograms. The recording labeled SPRING-PATCH is the morphology-sensing electrogram. The recording labeled BIPOLE is the rate-sensing electrogram. Calibration markers of 5 mV are shown for the intracardiac electrograms. AO = distal aortic pressure.

ble undersensing of low-amplitude or fragmented signals or double counting of fragmented QRS signals or of the QRS complex and T wave. In patients with large T-wave amplitude, double counting is possible, since the ventricular refractory period of the device must be brief to detect very rapid rates. The signal during inherent rhythm from a morphology-detecting electrode pair should be scrutinized for possible oversensing. A QRS width that exceeds 110 msec may satisfy the morphology criterion regardless of the rate (Fig. 24–8A). However, the device is designed such that satisfaction of the morphology criterion is not sufficient for arrhythmia detection unless the rate criterion is also fulfilled. These signals in the inherent rhythm should then be compared with the same signals during all induced tachyarrhythmias (Fig. 24–8B). The electrogram recorded from the rate-counting pair would optimally retain discrete signals; the amplitude may be adequate, although quite low if the rate-counting circuitry has an automatic gain control. For example, a frequent concern of physicians less familiar with intracardiac electrograms is that ventricular fibrillation might not be detected on the basis of rate because the signals may be of insufficient slew rate and amplitude. However, closely spaced bipolar electrodes produce a local electrogram with discrete signals in the vast ma-

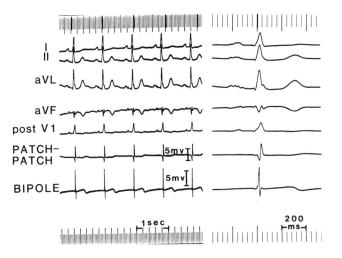

Figure 24–7. Typical intraoperative recordings from a patient receiving a two-patch AICD electrode system. Fast paper speed is shown on the right. Note that the transcardiac patch-patch electrogram resembles the bipolar electrogram with a slightly wider QRS interval. I, II, aV_L, and posterior V_1 are surface electrograms. PATCH-PATCH is the morphology-sensing electrogram. BIPOLE is the rate-sensing electrogram.

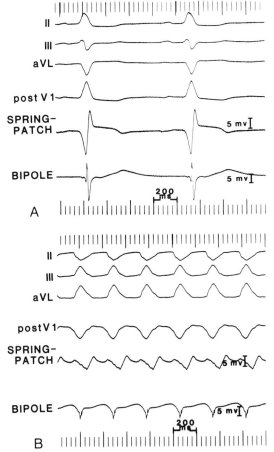

Figure 24–8. Intraoperative recording from a patient with left bundle branch block who received a spring-coil and patch AICD electrode configuration. The electrograms during sinus rhythm are shown in panel *A* and those during ventricular tachycardia in panel *B*. In the morphology-sensing electrogram (labeled SPRING-PATCH), the QRS interval is 120 msec during sinus rhythm and 160 msec during ventricular tachycardia. In the rate-sensing electrogram (labeled BIPOLE), the QRS amplitude is markedly reduced during ventricular tachycardia but retains discrete signals.

jority of instances (Fig. 24–9). Even if occasional signal dropout occurs owing to large variation in signal amplitude, the rate detected exceeds 200 beats per minute except in rare cases.[6] The electrogram across the morphology-sensing electrodes during ventricular tachycardia should have a more prolonged QRS interval than that during a supraventricular rhythm and should have a brief isoelectric component (see Fig. 24–8). A general guideline is that the ratio of the QRS duration to the RR interval should be at least 0.3 (personal communication, Cardiac Pacemakers, Inc., St. Paul, MN).

DEFIBRILLATION ENERGY DETERMINATION. All efforts should be made to perform defibrillation energy testing in all patients, even in those patients who had never previously experienced ventricular fibrillation. This principle is based on results of human testing of cardioversion and defibrillation efficacy.[105] As depicted in Figure 24–10, 1, 5, 10, and 25 J were tested in 33 patients undergoing implantation of the AICD device, and the pooled data were analyzed. A low energy of 1 J was 80 per cent successful for the cardioversion of ventricular tachycardia of stable morphology, and higher energy levels did not result in greater success. Despite the high success rate for cardioversion, there was also a 10 to 25 per cent incidence of acceleration of ventricular tachycardia by cardioversion attempts at all energies between 1 and 25 J (Fig. 24–11). In contrast, successful termination of polymorphic ventricular tachycardia and ventricular fibrillation was correlated with the energy level delivered. In general, the energy needed for successful defibrillation exceeds the energy needed for successful cardioversion, and the determination of successful cardioversion en-

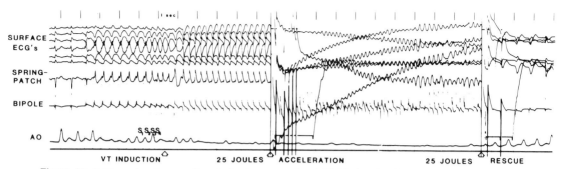

Figure 24–9. Example of a recording during intraoperative defibrillation threshold testing. Recordings are from six surface ECGs (SURFACE ECG's), the transcardiac spring-patch electrode (SPRING-PATCH), the local ventricular bipolar electrode pair (BIPOLE), the aortic pressure (AO), and the programmed stimulus artifacts (S). The local bipolar electrograms have discrete deflections during sinus rhythm, ventricular pacing, ventricular tachycardia, and ventricular fibrillation. (From Echt DS, Winkle RA: Management of patients with the automatic implantable cardioverter/defibrillator. Clin Prog Electrophysiol Pacing 3:11, 1985; with permission.)

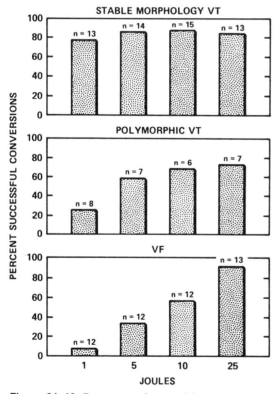

Figure 24–10. Percentage of successful conversions for the 1-, 5-, 10-, and 25-J pulse discharges for termination of ventricular tachycardia of stable morphology (*top*), polymorphic ventricular tachycardia (*middle*), and ventricular fibrillation (*bottom*). Increasing energy from 1 to 25 J did not affect the conversion rate for ventricular tachycardia of stable morphology but did result in an increase in success rate for both polymorphic ventricular tachycardia and ventricular fibrillation. (From Winkle RA, Stinson EB, Echt DS: Measurement of cardioversion/defibrillator thresholds in man by a truncated exponential waveform and an apical patch–superior vena caval spring electrode configuration. Circulation 69:768, 1984; by permission of the American Heart Association, Inc.)

ergy does not predict the energy level necessary for successful defibrillation. However, if ventricular fibrillation cannot be induced with programmed stimulation or AC, testing of a rapid polymorphic ventricular tachycardia may yield similar results.

It is important to realize that intraoperative determination of defibrillation energy needs in patients is a relatively crude approximation. Convincing mathematical and experimental evidence that refutes the concept of an absolute defibrillation threshold is now available.[19, 67] The relationship between defibrillation energy and the incidence of successful defibrillation is better defined by a sigmoid-shaped dose-response curve. The information necessary to construct such a curve is the percentage of effective defibrillation attempts after repeated

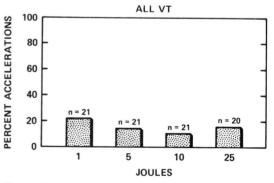

Figure 24–11. Percentage of episodes of stable morphology or polymorphic ventricular tachycardia accelerated by the 1-, 5-, 10-, and 25-J pulse discharges. (From Winkle RA, Stinson EB, Echt DS: Measurement of cardioversion/defibrillator thresholds in man by a truncated exponential waveform and an apical patch–superior vena caval spring electrode configuration. Circulation 69:770, 1984; by permission of the American Heart Association, Inc.)

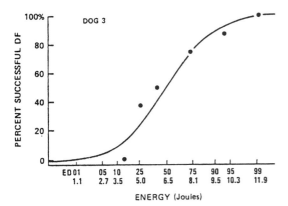

Figure 24–12. Curve of percentage of successful defibrillation versus energy using logistic regression analysis. ED refers to the predicted percentage of success from 1 to 99 per cent. (From Davy J-M, Fain ES, Dorian P, Winkle RA: The relationship between successful defibrillation and delivered energy in open-chest dogs: Reappraisal of the defibrillation threshold concept. Am Heart J 113:79, 1987; with permission.)

attempts are made at a range of energy levels. Figure 24–12 is an example of such a curve derived from logistic regression analysis. In this example, 8 defibrillation attempts were performed at each of the 6 energy levels selected, for a total of 48 determinations. Only the first defibrillation attempt for each episode of induced fibrillation was used for data analysis, to avoid the confounding influence of prolonged arrhythmia duration on defibrillation energy. From this curve, it is possible to determine several pertinent data points, an energy level associated with highly effective defibrillation, and an indication of the slope of the curve. The 80 per cent or 90 per cent effective energy doses (ED80 or ED90) have been used experimentally to indicate a highly successful defibrillation energy value. The difference between the 80 and 90 per cent and the 50 per cent effective energies is an indication of the shallowness or steepness of the slope. These data are extremely helpful in determining a safety margin for defibrillation. Unfortunately, an inordinate number of fibrillation and defibrillation episodes are necessary to define a defibrillation energy curve. In clinical practice, six cardioversion and defibrillation energy determinations, on the average, are obtained to determine the efficacy of the system. With the knowledge that the maximal output of the AICD device is 30 J and the speculation that twice the threshold value is an ideal safety margin, most physicians begin by testing the effectiveness of defibrillating with 15 J. Depending upon the result, the next energy level tested would be of higher or lower

energy. The lowest energy that results in successful defibrillation is generally retested, ideally several times. Alternatively, some physicians will repeatedly test a single energy level 10 to 15 J below the maximal output of the device. With either method, the basic concept is that the likelihood of an energy value's being highly effective increases the more it is tested and is consistently successful.

Another factor in determining an adequate safety margin for successful defibrillation is the stability of the energy requirements over time. Canine studies of the right atrial spring-coil and extracardiac left ventricular patch electrode configuration implanted for 32 days revealed that the defibrillation energy requirements decrease during the first 11 days after implantation and then remain stable.[32] Animal and preliminary human studies suggest that defibrillation energy requirements utilizing spring-coil and patch or two-patch electrodes do not change substantially when results from testing at the time of implantation are compared with those at generator replacement after 15 to 25 months.[15, 21, 45, 69] Animal data suggest that transvenous catheter defibrillating electrodes may dislodge and, if so, are associated with slightly higher defibrillation energy requirements and that the defibrillation energy requirements increase over time until 5 weeks.[55] However, it appears that the defibrillation energy needs with a three-electrode configuration are more stable over time.[54]

Anecdotal human experience and preliminary human data[7] suggest that prolonged durations of ventricular fibrillation due to unsuccessful initial attempts are associated with higher defibrillation energy requirements. Experimental studies have had conflicting results. One canine study[94] found no change in defibrillation current requirements after 10, 20, 30, and 40 seconds of ventricular fibrillation, while a more recent study[9] found significant increases in the defibrillation energy needed after 5, 15, and 30 seconds of ventricular fibrillation. To minimize the potential effects of the arrhythmia duration, it is recommended that consistency be maintained during defibrillation energy testing and that a time that simulates the time period expected during clinical use be selected.

CARDIOVERSION ENERGY DETERMINATION. The basic principles and procedures for determining the energy level associated with reliable cardioversion have been addressed in Chapters 21B and 26B. In summary, the success of low-energy cardioversion is dependent, in part, upon the energy level delivered, the duration of the tachycardia, and the cycle length of the ventricular tachycardia.[85] Ventricular tachycardias with long cycle lengths are most likely to be successfully converted with low energies, and highly selected patients have been successfully treated with a transvenous catheter cardioverter device delivering a maximum of 2 J.[72] The overall incidence of ventricular tachycardia acceleration using a transvenous catheter system is approximately 8 per cent.[17] The incidence of ventricular tachycardia acceleration by the cardioversion pulse is highly dependent upon the tachycardia cycle length, being lowest in patients with ventricular tachycardia of very long cycle lengths. Concomitant antiarrhythmic drug treatment results in improved efficacy, but only because it prolongs the cycle length of the ventricular tachycardia.[17] Most physicians determine the energy requirement for cardioversion by beginning at the lowest energy setting and testing sequentially higher values until termination is successful. However, with this procedure, later attempts are complicated by the possible influence of prolonged tachycardia duration.

GENERATOR ASSESSMENT. The generator should be assessed before surgical implantation to ascertain that it is functional. Ideally, this noninvasive assessment of battery energy, capacitor discharge, and on-off capability is repeated just prior to implantation. After satisfactory testing of the electrode arrangement and generator, the components are attached for final testing of the entire system. The major purpose of this portion of the testing is to evaluate the ability for both successful arrhythmia detection and termination, since the previous testing evaluated termination only and from a testing instrument. Ideally, the successful detection of all clinical ventricular tachyarrhythmias should be observed. On the average, the time necessary to satisfy the rate detection criteria for the AICD device is 2.5 seconds. This time may be substantially lengthened for ventricular tachycardia rates equal to the rate cut-off setting or highly variable intracardiac signal amplitude. This period is followed by a mandatory re-verification time period (nominally 2.5 seconds). The time necessary for satisfaction of the morphology criterion is much less predictable. After all detection criteria are met, the device is committed and charges its capacitors (approximately 5 to 10 seconds); a 1.4-second delay occurs after the capacitors are fully charged, followed by capacitor pulse discharge. Thus,

the arrhythmia duration expected for an AICD device will be at least 11 seconds and is more commonly approximately 15 seconds.

TROUBLESHOOTING. The implanting teams must be prepared for the unexpected. The application of new technology is associated with unique problems that cannot entirely be anticipated despite considerable experience with the particular system. Immediate decisions must be made nonetheless. Some situations can be expected to occur eventually, and general guidelines should be discussed and agreed upon in advance.

One more common situation involves the patient with multiple medical conditions who is a high surgical risk. If the patient's general medical condition mandates limited intraoperative testing, the testing should focus on attaining adequate intracardiac signal quality, consistently successful defibrillation at an energy level below the output of the device, and observation of successful ventricular tachycardia detection by the implanted system.

Another finding in approximately 5 per cent of patients[30] is that the patient's defibrillation energy requirement equals or exceeds the output of the device even after optimizing the electrode arrangement, as discussed above. In this situation, it must be decided whether or not to implant a generator. This is virtually always a difficult decision. One of the major considerations should be the likelihood that the device will actually worsen the patient's clinical arrhythmia. In the case of a patient whose clinical arrhythmia is rapid polymorphic ventricular tachycardia or fibrillation, causing immediate cardiovascular collapse, unsuccessful performance would lead to an ineffective pulse. However, in the case of a patient with a monomorphic ventricular tachycardia causing hypoperfusion but not unconsciousness, there would be the possibility that if the pulse discharge was not only unsuccessful but also resulted in acceleration and worsening of the rhythm, the situation could prove to be worse with the device than without. Therefore, most physicians would favor implantation in the former but not the latter situation. Other factors to be considered include the possible confounding influence of concomitant antiarrhythmic drug therapy (discussed below) or concomitant cardiac surgery (described above). In either case, results of repeat testing performed when the patient is not taking antiarrhythmic agents and at a time remote from the initial procedure are sometimes more satisfactory. It is conceivable that adherence of the patch leads to the underlying tissue contributes to the subsequent improvement in defibrillation efficacy.

The assessment of arrhythmia detection in the AICD device is currently hindered by the lack of an external analyzer that incorporates detection circuitry. Arrhythmia detection cannot be confirmed until the generator is connected with the patient's implanted leads, at which time the resolution of detection is severely limited in nonprogrammable devices. In addition to relying upon devices with lower rate cut-offs and no morphology criterion, electrode repositioning may correct the problem of nondetection. The use of a right atrial spring-coil electrode rather than a right ventricular patch may improve morphology detection.

Finally, a situation occasionally encountered is the inability to initiate either ventricular tachycardia or fibrillation in the operating room, inhibiting the testing of the system. In the case of the inability to induce ventricular tachycardia, the concern is primarily for satisfactory device detection, since cardioversion energy requirements rarely exceed defibrillation energy requirements. Ideally, a device with a lower rate criterion and minimal or no morphology criterion could be implanted, and ventricular tachycardia detection could be verified by electrophysiologic study prior to hospital discharge. The inability to induce ventricular fibrillation is generally due to an inadequate current output or ineffective stimulation technique. Every effort should be made to have available a reliable induction technique or a variety of techniques. Customized current-limiting battery rechargers delivering 120 Hz of unfiltered, full wave rectified AC have been extremely effective. Prolonged rapid pacing with decremental cycle lengths is frequently effective. Single pulses and short pulse trains delivered just beyond the ventricular refractory period usually are effective only when high current (greater than 20 mA) is applied. Antiarrhythmic drugs may prevent the induction of ventricular fibrillation, as discussed below.

Pacemaker Interactions

Until all automatic cardioverters/defibrillators incorporate bradycardia pacing, some patients with both tachycardias and bradycardias will need two devices for treatment. The ability of the available AICD device to distinguish between pacemaker artifacts and two cardiac signals can lead to two major hazardous interactions. To avoid this situation, careful intraoperative assessment is needed and revision of the pacemaker system may be required. The most serious interaction is referred to as detection inhibition.[5, 58] This situation could potentially occur because the rate detection circuitry in each device differs. If the pacemaker fails to sense ventricular tachycardia or fibrillation because the QRS signals have reduced amplitude, the device responds with pacing. The automatic gain control mechanism for rate detection in the cardioverter/defibrillator device would search for the largest signal, which in this case might be the pacemaker stimulus artifact; thus, the underlying tachyarrhythmia could continue undetected (Fig. 24–13). To minimize detection of the pacing artifact by the cardioverter/defibrillator, bipolar pacing is virtually always required. The amplitude of the pacing artifact can be further minimized by placing the rate detection electrodes for the cardioverter/defibrillator close to each other and as far as possible from the ventricular pacemaker lead. Finally, obtaining a low ventricular capture threshold in the pacing lead will enable the programming of a low-amplitude pacing output. After connection of both the pacemaker and the cardioverter/defibrillator systems, provocative testing should then be performed in all patients. Ventricular fibrillation should be induced in all patients to determine whether the pacemaker senses the rhythm appropriately. Even after appropriate performance has been demonstrated, ventricular fibrillation should again be induced while the pacemaker is in an asynchronous pacing mode to observe that appropriate tachyarrhythmia detection can occur despite demand pacing.

The second major potential interaction is double counting of the pacemaker stimulus artifact and the evoked response by the cardioverter/defibrillator device. Double counting could occur if both signals are of sufficient amplitude and reach the rate detection pair of the cardioverter/defibrillator at an interval of at least 150 msec. The rate detection criterion could then be satisfied whenever the paced cardiac rate equaled one-half the actual device cut-off rate. The intracardiac signal across the rate-counting pair of the cardioverter/defibrillator should be scrutinized for possible double counting resulting from a prolonged latency between the pacemaker stimulus artifact and the largest amplitude component of the evoked QRS complex. This latency could occur be-

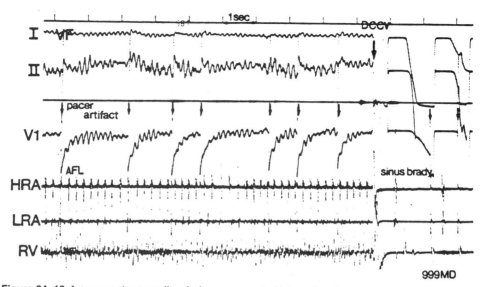

Figure 24–13. Intraoperative recording during assessment of interactions between a permanent pacemaker and automatic defibrillator. A unipolar ventricular pacemaker was not entirely inhibited during ventricular fibrillation (VF), and large pacing artifacts occurred randomly (*arrows* in lead V_1). The automatic implantable cardioverter/defibrillator failed to recognize VF because of these large artifacts. VF was terminated by external direct-current defibrillation (DCCV). HRA = high right atrial electrogram, revealing atrial flutter; LRA = low right atrial electrogram. Surface leads I, II, V_1, and right ventricular electrogram (RV) revealed ventricular fibrillation. (From Kim SG, Furman S, Waspe LE, et al: Unipolar pacer artifacts induced failure of an automatic implantable cardioverter-defibrillator to detect ventricular fibrillation. Am J Cardiol 57:880, 1987; with permission.)

cause of pacemaker stimulus exit block or intraventricular conduction delay. Further confirmation could be obtained with magnet application over the cardioverter/defibrillator generator, which initiates audible beeping of each detected signal. Double counting could also occur if the pacemaker, because of poor sensing, asynchronously paces despite a normal underlying rhythm and the two rates together exceed the rate cut-off of the cardioverter/defibrillator device. This situation might occur immediately following a high-energy pulse discharge if the countershock causes transient loss of pacemaker sensing.

A third potential interaction is the transient loss of pacemaker capture following a defibrillation discharge.[88] This problem is magnified in the presence of antiarrhythmic drugs that increase the pacing capture threshold.[18]

The combination of an antitachycardia pacemaker and an AICD device has been implanted in patients on a chronic basis.[64] The potential hazardous interactions between these two types of devices are partly related to the demand pacing capabilities of the antitachycardia pacemaker, as described above. In addition, if the antitachycardia pacemaker delivered frequent scanning pacing stimuli during ventricular tachycardia, detection by the automatic cardioverter/defibrillator could be in-

hibited despite ongoing tachycardia. Conversely, if the antitachycardia pacemaker delivered long, rapid bursts, the automatic cardioverter/defibrillator could detect the pacing stimulus artifacts as ventricular tachycardia and become committed to discharge despite successful termination by the antitachycardia pacemaker.

Antiarrhythmic Drug Interactions

The majority of patients receiving automatic cardioverter/defibrillator devices also receive antiarrhythmic drug therapy for a variety of indications.[30] Antiarrhythmic drugs that do not suppress arrhythmias may interact with device function by affecting arrhythmia detection, such as slowing the arrhythmia rate, or by affecting arrhythmia termination, such as increasing the energy needed for defibrillation.

The extent to which antiarrhythmic drugs slow the rate of ventricular tachycardia is dependent, in part, upon the specific electrophysiologic effects of the drug and the dose utilized, but marked interindividual variation also exists. Antiarrhythmic agents can also alter the morphology of the ventricular tachycardia. Since most antiarrhythmic agents with sodium channel blocking activity prolong intraventricular conduction time, resulting in wider

QRS complexes during ventricular tachycardia, it would appear that morphology detection should be enhanced by most antiarrhythmic drugs. However, detection is complicated by the fact that the slowing of ventricular tachycardia rate by antiarrhythmic drugs also increases the duration of the isoelectric component. Thus, it is difficult to predict the ultimate effect of antiarrhythmic drugs on morphology detection.

The effects of antiarrhythmic drugs on the defibrillation energy have been evaluated for many drugs in animal studies, but there are only anecdotal reports in humans. Experimental evidence suggests that lidocaine,[4, 8, 25, 57] quinidine,[20, 24, 25, 108] encainide,[34] and propranolol[84] increase the energy required for defibrillation, while procainamide,[29] bretylium,[24, 57, 95] and d-sotalol[20] either lower or do not affect the energy required for defibrillation. Although anecdotal evidence suggests that amiodarone increases the defibrillation energy needs in patients,[39] experimental data are conflicting.[33, 46] At this time, it appears necessary to evaluate the possible interactions of antiarrhythmic agents and automatic cardioverter/defibrillators in each patient.[109] There is no uniform agreement regarding whether this testing should be performed during intraoperative implantation of the device or subsequently. However, several factors favor performing intraoperative testing in the absence of antiarrhythmic agents. For example, cases of amiodarone pulmonary toxicity, manifested as acute respiratory distress syndrome, have occurred postoperatively in patients with no preoperative evidence of pulmonary toxicity.[74] Further, the extraordinarily long elimination half-life of amiodarone precludes the reduction of tissue levels prior to surgery, but plasma levels can be substantially reduced after several days.[92]

Some antiarrhythmic agents, primarily those that markedly prolong action potential duration, impair the ability to initiate or sustain ventricular fibrillation, thus inhibiting the determination of intraoperative defibrillation energy. Although this characteristic is a very desirable one, it can only be speculated that the drug will also reliably prevent the clinical occurrence of ventricular fibrillation. Therefore, an evaluation of defibrillation energy seems prudent in these patients. The presence of an antiarrhythmic agent also complicates the ability to interpret the results of intraoperative defibrillation energy testing. Should the defibrillation energy requirement be unacceptably high, the possible contribution of the antiarrhythmic agent to raising the energy requirement would have to be seriously considered. In this situation, the patient is likely to leave the operating room without a device and undergo a second operative procedure for retesting after drug clearance. Intraoperative testing in the presence of antiarrhythmic drug therapy is indicated in the case of a patient in whom it is absolutely necessary to continue that specific agent and dosage. This circumstance occurs infrequently, since patients receiving a cardioverter/defibrillator device are being treated with antiarrhythmic agents as adjunctive therapy and several drugs can usually provide an adequate effect. Another rationale for performing intraoperative testing in the presence of antiarrhythmic drug therapy is to avoid performing another electrophysiologic study in patients prior to hospital discharge.

A further complicating issue is that anesthetic agents such as pentobarbital, enflurane, and fentanyl may affect the defibrillation energy.[98] However, the experimental results have been conflicting.[3] To avoid this potential confounding factor, we utilize a combination of narcotic benzodiazepine derivatives and muscle relaxants.

In summary, the clinical strategy for patients receiving a nonprogrammable device with concomitant antiarrhythmic drug therapy is to select and evaluate the specific agent prior to implantation. Intraoperative testing would ideally be performed when the patient is not taking any antiarrhythmic drugs, to avoid the confounding influence of drugs on ventricular tachycardia and fibrillation. Postoperative electrophysiologic testing would then be performed, with the patient receiving the antiarrhythmic drug and dosage for long-term use. Alternatively, the patient could undergo intraoperative testing on the long-term drug regimen.

Postoperative Electrophysiologic Testing

The necessity for performing a postoperative electrophysiologic study in all patients is controversial.[12, 27, 41, 66, 82] The rationale for repeat testing of the functioning of the device in all patients is that it allows the patient to experience a high energy pulse in the presence of the attending physician. Advocates feel that this practice alleviates the patient's anxiety, since the unknown is generally worse than the known. Other physicians feel that the anxiety is not a serious problem in patients who have not experienced a high energy pulse. There is general agreement among physicians that electrophysiologic studies performed before discharge from the hospital are needed to evaluate antiarrhythmic drug interactions (unless testing of the long-term regimen was evaluated intraoperatively) and to reassess detection and termination if the intraoperative testing was not totally satisfactory or complete.

ANTITACHYCARDIA DEVICES: FUTURE CONSIDERATIONS

Several advances can be expected in the near future that will modify the intraoperative assessment of antitachycardia devices. The availability of programmable rate and morphology criteria will obviate preimplantation antiarrhythmic drug testing and will increase the extent of intraoperative and postoperative testing to optimize settings. Improved external instruments for arrhythmia detection will remove much of the guesswork from the interpretation of intracardiac signals. With the advent of low-energy cardioversion and antitachycardia pacing modalities, there will be an increased use of concomitant antiarrhythmic drugs to slow the rate of ventricular tachycardia. New lead configurations employing three electrodes may prove to be highly advantageous. As with the advent of sophisticated bradycardia pacemakers, advanced antitachycardia devices will be more complex, requiring more extensive intraoperative evaluation.

ACKNOWLEDGEMENT: The authors wish to thank Mary Ellen Niland for her assistance in preparing this chapter.

REFERENCES

1. Almassi GH, Chapman PD, Troup PJ, et al: Constrictive pericarditis associated with patch electrodes of the automatic implantable cardioverter-defibrillator. Chest 92:369–371, 1987.
2. Arzbaecher R, Bump T, Jenkins J, et al: Automatic tachycardia recognition. PACE 7:541–547, 1984.
3. Babbs CF: Effect of pentobarbital anesthesia on ventricular defibrillation threshold in dogs. Am Heart J 95:331–337, 1978.
4. Babbs CF, Yim GKW, Whistler SJ, et al: Elevation of ventricular defibrillation threshold in dogs by antiarrhythmic drugs. Am Heart J 98:345–350, 1986.
5. Bach SM Jr: Technical communication: AID-B Cardioverter-defibrillator possible interactions with pacemakers. Intec Systems, Pittsburgh, PA, August 29, 1983.
6. Bardy GH, Ivey TD, Stewart R, et al: Failure of the automatic implantable defibrillator to detect ventricular fibrillation. Am J Cardiol 58:1107–1108, 1986.
7. Bardy GH, Stewart RB, Ivey TD, et al: Potential risk of low energy cardioversion attempts by implantable defibrillations [abstract]. J Am Coll Cardiol 9:168A, 1987.
8. Black JN, Barbey JT, Echt DS: Modulation of lidocaine effects on ventricular defibrillation [abstract]. J Am Coll Cardiol 9:166, 1987.
9. Black JN, Barbey JT, Echt DS: Ventricular fibrillation duration affects defibrillation [abstract]. J Am Coll Cardiol 9:142, 1987.
10. Bognolo D, Stokes K, Weibush W, et al: Experimental and clinical study of a new permanent atrial sutureless pacing lead. PACE 6:113–118, 1983.
11. Camm AJ, Davies DW, Ward DE: Tachycardia recognition by implantable electronic devices. PACE 10:1175–1190, 1987.
12. Cannom DS, Winkle RA: Implantation of the automatic implantable cardioverter defibrillator (AICD): Practical aspects. PACE 9:793–809, 1986.
13. Chang MS, Inque H, Kallok MJ, Zipes DP: Double and triple sequential shocks reduce ventricular defibrillation threshold in dogs with and without myocardial infarction. J Am Coll Cardiol 8:1393–1405, 1986.
14. Chapman PD, Sagar KB, Wetherbee JN, Troup PJ: Echocardiographic left ventricular mass and defibrillation threshold for the automatic implantable cardioverter-defibrillator [abstract]. Circulation 72:III–383, 1985.
15. Chapman PD, Troup PJ, Wetherbee JN, et al: The implanted defibrillator: Defibrillation threshold stability over time [abstract]. J Am Coll Cardiol 9:168A, 1987.
16. Charos GS, Haffajee CI, Gold RL, et al: A theoretically and practically more effective method for interruption of ventricular tachycardia: Self-adapting autodecremental overdrive pacing. Circulation 73:309–315, 1986.
17. Ciccone JM, Saksena S, Shah Y, Pantopoulos D: A prospective randomized study of the clinical efficacy and safety of transvenous cardioversion for termination of ventricular tachycardia. Circulation 71:571–578, 1985.
18. Datorre S, Bondke H, Brinker J, et al: Increased pacing threshold after an automatic defibrillator shock: Effects of antiarrhythmic drugs [abstract]. Circulation 76:IV–310, 1987.
19. Davy J-M, Fain ES, Dorian P, Winkle RA: The relationship between successful defibrillation and delivered energy in open-chest dogs: Reappraisal of the "defibrillation threshold" concept. Am Heart J 113:77–83, 1987.
20. Dawson AK, Steinberg MI, Shapland JE: Effect of Class I and Class III drugs on current and energy required for internal defibrillation [abstract]. Circulation 72:III–384, 1985.
21. Deeb GM, Griffith BP, Thompson ME, et al: Lead systems for internal ventricular fibrillation. Circulation 64:242–245, 1981.
22. Den Dulk K, Brugada P, Wellens HJJ: A case report demonstrating spontaneous change in tachycardia terminating window. PACE 7:867–870, 1984.

23. Den Dulk K, Kersschot IE, Brugada P, Wellens HJJ: Is there a universal antitachycardia pacing mode? Am J Cardiol 57:950–955, 1986.

24. Dorian P, Fain ES, Davy J-M, Winkle RA: Effect of quinidine and bretylium on defibrillation energy requirements. Am Heart J 112:19–25, 1985.

25. Dorian P, Fain E, Davy J-M, Winkle RA: Lidocaine causes a reversible, concentration-dependent increase in defibrillation energy. J Am Coll Cardiol 8:327–332, 1986.

26. Echt DS: Potential hazards of implanted devices for the electrical control of tachyarrhythmias. PACE 7:580–587, 1984.

27. Echt DS, Winkle RA: Management of patients with the automatic implantable cardioverter/defibrillator. Clin Prog Electrophysiol Pacing 3:4–16, 1985.

28. Echt DS, Sepulveda NG, Wikswo JP: Development of a mathematical model of defibrillation current distributions [abstract]. Circulation 73:II–341, 1986.

29. Echt DS, Coxe DR, Black JN, Sewell EC: Procainamide does not affect ventricular defibrillation in dogs [abstract]. J Am Coll Cardiol 9:166, 1987.

30. Echt DS, Armstrong K, Schmidt P, et al: Clinical experience, complications and survival in 70 patients with the automatic implantable cardioverter/defibrillator. Circulation 71:291–296, 1985.

31. Fahraeus T, Lassvik C, Sonnhag C: Tachycardias initiated by automatic antitachycardia pacemakers. PACE 7:1049–1054, 1984.

32. Fain ES, Billingham M, Winkle RA: Internal cardiac defibrillation: Histopathology and temporal stability of defibrillation energy requirements. J Am Coll Cardiol 9:631–638, 1987.

33. Fain ES, Lee J, Winkle RA: Effects of acute and chronic amiodarone on defibrillation energy requirements. Am Heart J 114:8–17, 1987.

34. Fain ES, Dorian P, Davy J-M, et al: Effects of encainide and its metabolites on energy requirements for defibrillation. Circulation 73:1334–1341, 1986.

35. Fisher JD, Matos JA, Kim SG: Antitachycardia pacing and stimulation. In Josephson ME, Wellens HJJ (eds): Tachycardias: Mechanisms, Diagnosis, Treatment. Philadelphia, Lea & Febiger, 1984, pp 413–425.

36. Fisher JD, Mehra R, Furman S: Termination of ventricular tachycardia with bursts of rapid ventricular pacing. Am J Cardiol 41:94–102, 1978.

37. Fisher JD, Kim SG, Furman S, Matos JA: Role of implantable pacemakers in control of recurrent ventricular tachycardia. Am J Cardiol 49:194–206, 1982.

38. Fisher JD, Johnston DR, Kim SG, et al: Implantable pacers for tachycardia termination: Stimulation techniques and long-term efficacy. PACE 9:1325–1333, 1986.

39. Fogoros R: Amiodarone-induced refractoriness to cardioversion. Ann Intern Med 100:699–700, 1984.

40. Furman S, Bradman R, Pannizzo F, Fisher JD: Implantation techniques of antitachycardia devices. PACE 7:572–579, 1984.

41. Gabry MD, Brodman R, Johnston D, et al: Automatic implantable cardioverter-defibrillator: Patient survival, battery longevity and shock delivery analysis. J Am Coll Cardiol 9:1349–1356, 1987.

42. Geddes LA, Bourland JD, Ford G: The mechanism underlying sudden death from electric shock. Med Instrum 20:303–315, 1986.

43. German LD, Strauss HC: Electrical termination of tachyarrhythmias by discrete pulses. PACE 7:514–521, 1984.

44. Griffin JC, Mason JW, Calfee RV: Clinical use of an implantable automatic tachycardia-terminating pacemaker. Am Heart J 100:1093–1096, 1980.

45. Guarnieri T, Levine JH, Enrico P, et al: The defibrillation threshold for the automatic internal cardioverter defibrillator increases chronically: Implications for leads and drugs [abstract]. Circulation 74:II–110, 1986.

46. Haberman RJ, Veltri EP, Mower MM: Amiodarone has a time-dependent effect on increasing defibrillation threshold [abstract]. Clin Res 35:283A, 1987.

47. Hellestrand KJ, Burnett PJ, Milne JR, et al: Effect of the antiarrhythmic agent flecainide acetate on acute and chronic pacing thresholds. PACE 6:892–899, 1983.

48. Holley LK, Cooper M, Uther JB, Ross DA: Safety and efficacy of pacing for ventricular tachycardia. PACE 9:1316–1319, 1986.

49. Holt P, Crick JCP, Sowton E: Antitachycardia pacing: A comparison of burst overdrive, self-searching and adaptive table scanning programs. PACE 9:490–497, 1986.

50. Horowitz LN: Drugs and pacemaker therapy. Cardiovasc Clin 14:177–187, 1983.

51. Jenkins J, Noh KH, Bump T, et al: A single atrial extrastimulus can distinguish sinus tachycardia from 1:1 paroxysmal tachycardia. PACE 9:1063–1068, 1986.

52. Jones DL, Klein GJ, Kallok MJ: Improved internal defibrillation with twin pulse sequential energy delivery to different lead orientations in pigs. Am J Cardiol 55:821–825, 1985.

53. Jones DL, Klein GJ, Guiradon GM, et al: Internal cardiac defibrillation in man: Pronounced improvement with sequential pulse delivery to two different lead orientations. Circulation 73:484–491, 1985.

54. Kallok MJ, Olson WH, Marcaccini SJ, Almquist CK: Temporal stability of sequential pulse defibrillation threshold. PACE 9:1361–1366, 1986.

55. Kallok MJ, Wibel FH, Bourland JD, et al: Catheter electrode defibrillation in dogs: Threshold dependence on implant time and catheter stability. Am Heart J 109:821–826, 1985.

56. Kerber RE, Jensen SR, Gascho JA, et al: Determinants of defibrillation: Prospective analysis of 183 patients. Am J Cardiol 52:739–745, 1983.

57. Kerber RE, Pandian NG, Jensen SR, et al: Effect of lidocaine and bretylium on energy requirements for transthoracic defibrillation: Experimental studies. J Am Coll Cardiol 7:397–405, 1986.

58. Kim SG, Furman S, Waspe LE, et al: Unipolar pacer artifacts induced failure of an automatic implantable cardioverter/defibrillator to detect ventricular fibrillation. Am J Cardiol 57:880–881, 1985.

59. Langer A, Heilman MS, Mower MM, Mirowski M: Considerations in the development of the automatic implantable defibrillator. Med Instrum 10:163–167, 1976.

60. Lawrie GM, Morris CG Jr, Howell JF, DeBakey ME: Left subcostal insertion of the sutureless myocardial electrode. Ann Thorac Surg 21:350–353, 1976.

61. Lerman BB, Halperin HR, Tsitlik JE, et al: Relationship between canine transthoracic impedance and defibrillation threshold. J Clin Invest 80:797–803, 1987.

62. Lerman BB, Waxman HL, Buxton AE, et al: Tachy-

arrhythmias associated with programmable automatic atrial antitachycardia pacemakers. Am Heart J 106:1029–1035, 1983.

63. Levick CE, Mizgala HF, Kerr CR: Failure to pace following high dose antiarrhythmic therapy—reversal with isoproterenol. PACE 7:252–256, 1984.

64. Luderitz B, Gerckens U, Manz M: Automatic implantable cardioverter/defibrillator (AICD) and antitachycardia pacemaker (Tachylog): Combined use in ventricular tachyarrhythmias. PACE 9:1356–1360, 1986.

65. Luderitz B, d'Alnoncourt CN, Steinbeck G, Beyer J: Therapeutic pacing in tachyarrhythmias by implanted pacemakers. PACE 5:366–371, 1982.

66. Marchlinski FE, Fores BT, Baxton AE, et al: The automatic implantable cardioverter-defibrillator: Efficacy, complications, and device failures. Ann Intern Med 104:481–488, 1986.

67. McDaniel WC, Schuder JC: The cardiac ventricular defibrillation threshold: Inherent limitations in its application and interpretation. Med Instrum 21:170–176, 1987.

68. Mead RH, Echt DS, Stinson EB, et al: The automatic implantable defibrillator: Improved defibrillation and lowered impedance using two large patch leads [abstract]. J Am Coll Cardiol 5:455, 1985.

69. Mead RH, Ruder M, Schmidt P, et al: Improved defibrillation efficacy with chronically implanted defibrillation leads [abstract]. Circulation 74:II–110, 1986.

70. Mehra R, Furman S, Crump JF: Vulnerability of the mildly ischemic ventricle to cathodal, anodal, and bipolar stimulation. Circ Res 41:159–166, 1977.

71. Mercando AD, Furman S: Measurement of differences in timing and sequence between two ventricular electrodes as a means of tachycardia differentiation. PACE 9:1069–1078, 1986.

72. Miles WM, Prystowsky EN, Heger JJ, Zipes DP: The implantable transvenous cardioverter: Long-term efficacy and reproducible induction of ventricular tachycardia. Circulation 74:518–524, 1986.

73. Naccarelli GV, Zipes DP, Rahilly GT, et al: Influence of tachycardia cycle length and antiarrhythmic drugs on pacing termination and acceleration of ventricular tachycardia. Am Heart J 105:1–5, 1983.

74. Nalos PC, Kass RM, Gang ES, et al: Life-threatening postoperative pulmonary complications in patients with previous amiodarone pulmonary toxicity undergoing cardiothoracic operations. J Thorac Cardiovasc Surg 93:904–912, 1987.

75. Nathan AW, Creamer JE, Davies DW, Camm AJ: Clinical experience with a software based tachycardia reversion pacemaker. PACE 9:1312–1315, 1986.

76. Nathan AW, Camm AJ, Bexton RS, et al: Initial experience with a fully implantable, programmable, scanning, extrastimulus pacemaker for tachycardia termination. Clin Cardiol 5:22–26, 1982.

77. Pannizzo F, Amikam S, Bagwell P, Furman S: Discrimination of antegrade and retrograde atrial depolarization by electrogram analysis. Am Heart J 112:780–786, 1986.

78. Peters RW, Shafton E, Frank S, et al: Radiofrequency-triggered pacemakers: Uses and limitations. Ann Intern Med 88:17–22, 1978.

79. Platia EV, Brinker JA: Tachyarrhythmias and pacemaker therapy. In Platia EV (ed): Management of Cardiac Arrhythmias: The Nonpharmacologic Approach. Philadelphia, JB Lippincott Co, 1987, pp 201–218.

80. Pless BD, Sweeney MB: Discrimination of supraventricular tachycardia from sinus tachycardia of overlapping cycle length. PACE 7:1318–1324, 1984.

81. Preston TA: Anodal stimulation as a cause of pacemaker-induced ventricular fibrillation. Am Heart J 86:366–372, 1973.

82. Reid PR, Mirowski M, Mower MM, et al: Clinical evaluation of the internal automatic cardioverter-defibrillator in survivors of sudden cardiac death. Am J Cardiol 51:1608–1609, 1983.

83. Rothman MT, Keefe JM: Clinical results with Omni-Orthocor, an implantable antitachycardia pacing system. PACE 7:1306–1312, 1984.

84. Ruffy R, Schechtman K, Monje E, Sandza J: Adrenergically mediated variations in the energy required to defibrillate the heart: Observations in closed-chest, nonanesthetized dogs. Circulation 73:374–380, 1986.

85. Saksena S, Parsonnet V, Pantopoulos D, Rothbart ST: Implantation of a cardioverter/defibrillator without thoracotomy using a triple electrode system. JAMA 259:69–72, 1988.

86. Santel DJ, Kallok M, Tacker WA Jr: Implantable defibrillator electrode systems: A brief review. PACE 8:123–131, 1985.

87. Schuder JC, Gold JH, Stoeckle H, et al: Defibrillation in the calf with bidirectional trapezoidal wave shocks applied via chronically implanted epicardial electrodes. Trans Am Soc Artif Intern Organ 37:467–470, 1981.

88. Slepian M, Levine JH, Watkins L Jr, et al: Automatic implantable cardioverter defibrillator/permanent pacemaker interaction: Loss of pacemaker capture following AICD discharge. PACE 10:1194–1197, 1987.

89. Sowton E: Clinical results with the tachylog antitachycardia pacemaker. PACE 7:1313–1317, 1984.

90. Spurrell RAJ, Nathan AW, Camm AJ: Clinical experience with implantable scanning tachycardia reversion pacemakers. PACE 7:1296–1300, 1984.

91. Spurrell RAJ, Nathan AW, Bexton RS, et al: Implantable automatic scanning pacemaker for termination of supraventricular tachycardia. Am J Cardiol 49:753–760, 1982.

92. Staubli M, Bircher J, Galeazzi RL, et al: Serum concentration of amiodarone during long term therapy: Relation to dose, efficacy, and toxicity. Eur J Clin Pharmacol 24:485–495, 1983.

93. Sung RJ, Styperek JL, Castellanos A: Complete abolition of the reentrant supraventricular tachycardia zone using a new modality of cardiac pacing with simultaneous atrioventricular stimulation. Am J Cardiol 45:72–79, 1980.

94. Tacker WA, Babbs CF, Parris RL, Bourland JD: Effect of fibrillation duration on defibrillation threshold in dogs using a pervenous catheter-electrode designed for use with an automatic implantable defibrillator. In Proceedings of the Fourth Purdue Conference on Cardiac Defibrillation and Cardiopulmonary Resuscitation, W. Lafayette, Indiana, 1981, pp 9–10.

95. Tacker WA, Niebauer MJ, Babbs CF, et al: The effect of newer antiarrhythmic drugs on defibrillation threshold. Crit Care Med 8:177–180, 1980.

96. Troup PJ: Lead system selection, implantation, and testing for the automatic implantable cardioverter-

defibrillator. Clin Prog Electrophysiol Pacing 4:260–276, 1986.

97. Troup PJ, Chapman PD, Olinger GN, Kleinman LH: The implanted defibrillator: Relation of defibrillating lead configuration and clinical variables to defibrillation threshold. J Am Coll Cardiol 6:1315–1321, 1985.

98. Wang MJ, Dorian P: Defibrillation energy requirements differ between anesthetic agents [abstract]. PACE 10:446, 1987.

99. Warren J, Martin RO: Clinical evaluation of automatic tachycardia diagnosis by an implanted device. PACE 9:1079–1083, 1986.

100. Watkins L, Mirowski M, Mower MM: Implantation of the automatic defibrillator: The subxyphoid approach. Ann Thorac Surg 34:515–520, 1982.

101. Watkins L, Mower MM, Reid PR, et al: Surgical techniques for implanting the automatic implantable defibrillator. PACE 7:1357–1362, 1984.

102. Wellens HJJ, den Dulk K, Brugada P: Pacemaker management of cardiac arrhythmias. Cardiovasc Clin 14:165–175, 1983.

103. Wetherbee JN, Chapman PD, Klopfenstein JH, Bach SM Jr: Nonthoracotomy internal defibrillation in dogs: Threshold reduction using a subcutaneous chest wall electrode with a transvenous catheter electrode. J Am Coll Cardiol 10:406–411, 1987.

104. Winkle RA, Bach SM Jr, Echt DS, et al: The automatic implantable defibrillator: Local ventricular bipolar sensing to detect ventricular tachycardia and fibrillation. Am J Cardiol 52:265–270, 1983.

105. Winkle RA, Bach SM, Echt DS, et al: Defibrillation/cardioversion energy requirements using the implantable apical patch–superior vena caval spring leads. Circulation 69:766–777, 1984.

106. Winkle RA, Mead RH, Ruder MA, et al: Five year experience with the automatic implantable defibrillator in 157 patients. J Am Coll Cardiol 9:167A, 1987.

107. Winkle RA, Stinson EB, Echt DS, et al: Practical aspects of automatic cardioverter/defibrillator implantation. Am Heart J 108:1335–1346, 1984.

108. Woolfold DI, Chaffee WR, Cohen W, et al: The effect of quinidine on electrical energy required for ventricular defibrillation. Am Heart J 72:659–663, 1966.

109. Zipes DP: Electrical treatment of tachycardia. Circulation 75[Suppl III]:190–193, 1987.

110. Zipes DP, Prystowsky EN, Miles WM, Heger JJ: Future directions: Electrical therapy for cardiac tachyarrhythmias. PACE 7:606–610, 1984.

111. Zipes DP, Prystowsky EN, Miles WM, Heger JJ: Initial experience with Symbios Model 7008 pacemaker. PACE 7:1301–1305, 1984.

25

FOLLOW-UP TECHNIQUES FOR PATIENTS WITH IMPLANTED ANTITACHYCARDIA DEVICES

JERRY C. GRIFFIN

The process of device selection and implantation is only the beginning of pacemaker or defibrillator therapy for recurrent arrhythmias. Careful follow-up of the patient contributes significantly to effective long-term therapy. Success is best ensured by the proper organization of a dedicated follow-up program using appropriate equipment and techniques. Regular assessment will allow the physician to provide the most appropriate prescription for device function and to coordinate the interactions of devices and other arrhythmia therapies.

Goals and Function

The goals of follow-up vary with the type of device implanted[9] (Table 25–1). The principal purpose of follow-up of patients with devices for supraventricular tachycardia is the assessment of efficacy. Since these patients are generally not pacemaker dependent, battery life and the anticipation of battery depletion are of little consequence. In contrast, the assessment of battery status is the most important

TABLE 25–1. FUNCTIONS OF A FOLLOW-UP PROGRAM DEVICES FOR ARRHYTHMIA MANAGEMENT

1. Assessment of efficacy
2. Assessment of system integrity
3. Education and counseling of the patient
4. Information collection and retrieval

reason for serial evaluation of patients with the implanted defibrillator. The safety of these individuals does indeed depend on adequate device function.

For both types of patients, the follow-up clinic can provide a continuing program of education. This need not be formal but should, at a minimum, consist of a survey of patients' concerns at each clinic visit and a thorough explanation of any questions raised by the patient. The benefits of this sort of psychologic and emotional support may be quite significant. Rarely, patients with devices for life-threatening arrhythmias may require more in-depth counseling.[3, 5]

Finally, a follow-up program should serve as a source and repository of data regarding the patient, the reasons for device utilization, implant characteristics, and follow-up performance. If such data are simply entered into the general hospital record, much important information may be lost or not retrieved during some critical assessment of the implanted system. More important, physicians who are following up the patients may miss important trends in device performance.

Organization

Follow-up programs for tachycardia-terminating devices are highly specialized, usually serving a relatively small number of patients.[8] Such care is most easily delivered in a setting in which facilities and personnel are focused on this problem. Separate device follow-up records should be independent of the general medical record, though it should contain summaries of each follow-up encounter. Having a separate device database allows one to focus quickly and easily on needed data. It is worthwhile to retain representative portions of raw data, such as electrocardiographic recordings, telemetry printouts, electrograms, and so forth. Frequently, when a problem is being evaluated, these serial data provide additional helpful clues that might not have been retained in a more concise encounter record.

Evaluation encounters generally take longer than those for patients with bradycardia pace-makers, and a significant amount of time must be allotted for each patient's visit. It is the responsibility of the clinic to pursue patients who fail to appear for an appointment. One must be as certain as possible that patients are not left without follow-up. It is our practice to telephone patients the same day as a missed appointment to reschedule or discuss the patients' provisions for alternative follow-up.

Frequency of follow-up is a function of the clinical circumstances and of the device implanted; however, some general guidelines can be given. Patients with devices for supraventricular tachycardia termination should be seen within 1 month of implantation for the testing of thresholds and assessment of efficacy. Then they may be seen every 3 months for 1 year and every 6 months thereafter. Patients with

SUMMARY OF FOLLOW-UP TEST GUIDELINES

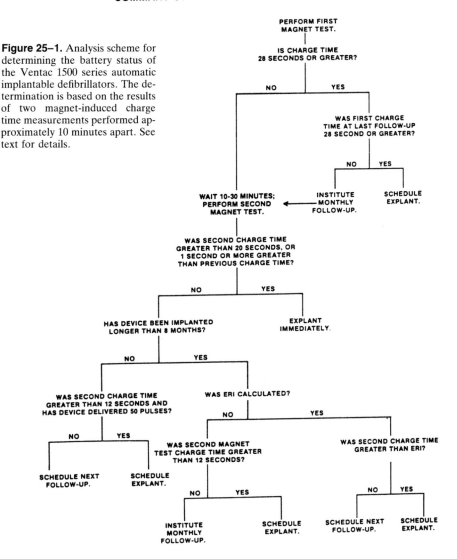

Figure 25–1. Analysis scheme for determining the battery status of the Ventac 1500 series automatic implantable defibrillators. The determination is based on the results of two magnet-induced charge time measurements performed approximately 10 minutes apart. See text for details.

the implanted defibrillator are also seen within 1 month of implantation and every 2 months for the first year of follow-up or until a significant rise in the first charge time is noted (Fig. 25–1). Thereafter, patients are seen monthly until the unit is replaced.[14] Patients are also seen after the first out-of-hospital defibrillator discharge and following any unusual or atypical series of discharges.

In contrast to patients with pacemakers for bradyarrhythmias, transtelephone follow-up plays less of a role in the follow-up of patients with devices for tachycardia control. Reliability, the longevity of devices for supraventricular tachycardia, and the level of pacemaker dependence are such that the risk from undetected battery depletion or other system failure is minimal. Currently, the battery status of the implanted defibrillator cannot be assessed by telephone. It is hoped that future devices will feature this capability, since this might significantly reduce the frequency of clinic follow-up encounters. Transtelephonic electrocardiographic monitoring to evaluate the patient's symptoms can provide important information and significant psychologic support for some individuals.

The area in which follow-up is to be performed should be adequately equipped for cardiac resuscitation, including external defibrillation. A standard electrocardiograph is necessary, preferably one that is multichannel. Some method for recording and displaying the stimulus artifact is helpful in the differential diagnosis of pacing system problems. This recording of the stimulus artifact may be done with a standard industrial oscilloscope or with an electrocardiograph machine appropriately equipped (Fig. 25–2). Magnets should be available but stored in a way that patients cannot inadvertently come in contact with them. Digital counters for the accurate assessment of interpulse intervals should be available. Programmers and other necessary test devices must be on hand for each device to be assessed. The clinic facility should also have access to the full range of noninvasive cardiovascular diagnostic tools, including echocardiography, Holter monitoring, radiography, and cardiac fluoroscopy. Less commonly, computed tomography may be helpful in the assessment of patch or lead placement.[9]

TECHNIQUES FOR DEVICE FOLLOW-UP

General

A careful interval history is very important in the follow-up of patients with devices for tachycardia control. The interval occurrence of tachycardia episodes, near-syncope, syncope, and device usage should all be carefully studied and serve as the basis for the estimation of device efficacy. In addition to a general appreciation of the cardiovascular status, the physical examination allows an assessment of wound healing, the integrity of the skin over and around the implanted device, and any signs of venous thrombosis or phlebitis. As in any medical encounter, general screening evaluations, such as systolic and diastolic blood pressure determinations, should be performed.

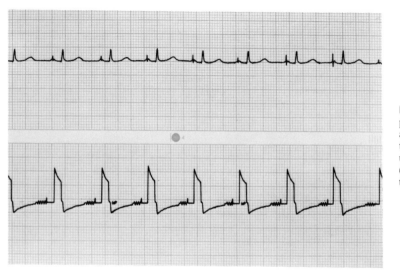

Figure 25–2. Recording of a pacemaker stimulus artifact using a specially equipped digital electrocardiographic (ECG) cart. The upper trace is that of the ECG (lead II), and the bottom trace is the time-expanded stimulus pulse.

Assessment of Devices for Supraventricular Tachycardia Control

The first programming step at any clinic encounter should be interrogation of the device. At a minimum, this will provide a list of the currently programmed values. Three additional types of data may also be available, depending upon the device: measured data, such as battery voltage and lead impedance; calculated data, such as current and energy delivered; and stored monitoring or incidence data regarding tachycardia or device activity. Some devices are able to offer a significant amount of monitoring information, such as tachycardia cycle length (or lengths), the number of arrhythmia episodes, the types of termination methods used, or the algorithm used for detection. Such data help to establish that the device is working properly or to determine the reason for device failure (Fig. 25–3). Measured data provide accurate estimates of battery status and lead/insulation integrity.

The determination of thresholds for pacing and sensing is even more important than with bradycardia devices. Ideally, one should determine the thresholds both in sinus rhythm and in supraventricular tachycardia. The programmed level for accurate sensing frequently changes during supraventricular tachycardia. This may be due to a different activation sequence of the atrium or to the superimposition of the ventricular component of the atrial endocardial electrogram on the atrial component, with cancellation. Threshold testing is begun in sinus rhythm. In easily induced patients, asynchronous pacing may initiate episodes of supraventricular tachycardia. If so, pulse generator sensitivity is increased until the device detects and terminates the tachycardia. Pacing threshold can be determined in tachycardia in the same fashion. Because it is frequently necessary to pace at cycle lengths that encroach on the relative refractory period, a safety margin for output, wider than customary for bradycardia pacing, is commonly used. The energy needed to excite the myocardium rises progressively the earlier one paces in the relative refractory period.[12, 17] Therefore, to

```
262-14-003046              DEC 01 '87 12:10 PM
        DIAGNOSTIC DATA CONTINUED


HIGH RATE CRITERION MET..............    207 TIMES
SUDDEN ONSET CRITERION MET..........    255 TIMES
RATE STABILITY CRITERION MET........    155 TIMES
SUSTAINED HIGH RATE CRITERION MET..      0 TIMES

PRIMARY ANTITACH MODALITY USED......    199 TIMES
SECONDARY ANTITACH MODALITY USED...      0 TIMES
SECONDARY MODALITY USED FIRST......      0 TIMES


MOST RECENT PRIMARY MODALITY:
MEASURED TACHYCARDIA INTERVAL......    492  MSEC
BURST CYCLE LENGTH..................    394  MSEC
DELAY (TS1).........................    420  MSEC

MOST RECENT SECONDARY MODALITY:
MEASURED TACHYCARDIA INTERVAL......    N/A   *
BURST CYCLE LENGTH.................    N/A   *
DELAY (TS1).........................    N/A   *
```

Figure 25–3. Monitoring data from a tachycardia-terminating pacemaker implanted for control of ventricular tachycardia. The device features four separate tachycardia identification algorithms. Monitoring data are acquired for each algorithm, whether or not it is currently activated. These data were collected over a period of 6 weeks and represent 199 episodes of tachycardia. All were terminated by the primary pacing technique; the backup or secondary mode was not required. By comparing the number of times the high-rate criterion was met with the number of times the primary modality was used, one can determine the average number of attempts necessary with this modality to achieve termination. In this case, on only eight occasions were two or more tries necessary.

achieve adequate coupling intervals, higher outputs may be needed.[17] After thresholds have been assessed and appropriate adjustments made, a number of episodes of supraventricular tachycardia should be induced and the current programmed settings observed for their ability to terminate the tachycardia efficiently. Devices vary in their provision for tachycardia induction from simple asynchronous pacing to very sophisticated programmed stimulation. Adjustments should be made in the termination protocol until the device is able to terminate induced episodes consistently with one or two bursts of pacing.

After an optimal pacing scheme is adopted, the memory registers, if present, should be cleared. The final step in any programming session should be an interrogation of the device and a careful review of the programmed values. Devices for supraventricular tachycardia termination are quite complex, and one must be certain that each parameter has been reprogrammed appropriately.

Ventricular Tachycardia

Patients with devices implanted for management of ventricular arrhythmias are at risk for ventricular fibrillation. Care should be taken that all appropriate personnel and provisions for complete cardiac resuscitation be available before such patients are evaluated. It is our practice not to perform noninvasive ventricular tachycardia induction and termination in the clinic setting even if the means are available. If the history and telemetry data suggest that such is needed, the patient is transferred to the electrophysiology laboratory, where such testing can be carried out more safely.

The lack of programmability of the currently available automatic implantable defibrillator limits what can be accomplished during routine follow-up visits. Unlike with devices for supraventricular tachycardia, the most important goal of automatic implantable cardioverter/defibrillator (AICD) follow-up is detection of system failure or battery depletion. The only other testable parameter is the accuracy of sensing. End-of-life testing must be done carefully and according to specific protocols. It is recommended that the manufacturer's literature be consulted regularly to ensure safe practices.[14] Battery status is estimated by measuring the length of time required to charge the capacitors using a device called an AID-CHECK (Cardiac Pacemakers, Inc., St. Paul, MN). This small hand-held unit times the

charging cycle and records the cumulative number of discharges delivered to the patient's terminals.

All manipulation of the device is done with a magnet. To measure a charge time, the device must be turned on. If the device is off, turning it on may be accomplished by placing the magnet over it for approximately 30 seconds. When the magnet is in the appropriate position, the upper right-hand corner near the epoxy header (Fig. 25–4), the device will make a continuous tone. The change in state is registered by a sudden absence of the tone. After a few seconds, the device will begin to sense and produce a tone synchronous to each R wave. At that point, if the magnet is removed, and no charge time is registered after magnet removal, the device is activated. It is important to place the wand of the AID-CHECK in its appropriate position, the upper left-hand corner of the device, any time the magnet is brought into proximity. If a charge time is registered during an on-off sequencing, the device should be turned off and on again until no charge time is registered. To invoke a charge time cycle, the magnet is placed over the device for at least 5 but less than 25 seconds and then is removed. Upon its removal, a continuous tone will sound from the AID-

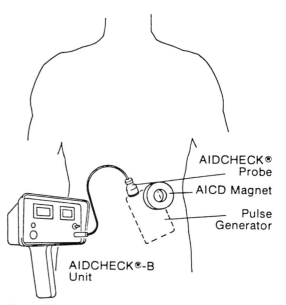

Figure 25–4. Illustration of the proper positioning of the magnet and the pickup coil of the AIDCHECK unit for performing a charge time. The magnet is placed over the upper right corner (the leads insert in the upper end), and the wand is placed over the upper left corner. The orientation of the pulse generator should be noted before hospital discharge and recorded in the chart for future reference.

CHECK, and numbers will begin to accumulate in the left-hand screen. At the end of the charging cycle, the display will freeze, recording the data. The total number of patient pulses emitted will appear in the right-hand register. If the figure "7" flashes in the right-hand screen, an inaccurate transmission has occurred, and the patient's pulse data are not reliable. If another charge time is desired, one should wait 10 minutes before performing it. Following the final charge time, the device should be turned off and then back on, again without registering a charge cycle.[14]

Magnets should be used with great caution around patients with implanted defibrillators. It is sometimes possible to activate the reed switch from a distance of several inches from the skin. Since the device can respond in one of several ways to magnet proximity, accidental activation of the reed switch must be avoided. The magnet should be brought to the device in one smooth motion from a distance of more than 2 feet. Its removal should also be accomplished in a smooth, continuous motion, and the magnet should be placed more than 2 feet away from the device until it is to be used again.

The currently recommended elective replacement indicator (ERI) is based on the second charge time obtained 8 months after implantation. This value in seconds is multiplied by 1.2 to obtain the ERI. If the 8-month charge time is not available, the manufacturer suggests a scheme based on initial and second observed charge times (Fig. 25–1). The validity of the ERI continues to be examined; therefore, one should periodically consult the latest manufacturer's recommendations.[14]

When the magnet is placed over a device in the activated mode, a tone sounds synchronous to each sensed R wave, and the defibrillating output is inhibited. This feature can be used to assess the patient for both undersensing and oversensing. On occasion, it is useful to record this activity, which can be accomplished with a phonocardiogram pickup placed near the device. The synchronous tone can be compared with a simultaneous surface electrocardiogram. This technique may be used to detect a variety of conditions, such as lead fracture, P- or T-wave sensing, sensing of an implanted pacemaker spike and its evoked R wave, or the sensing of two components of a wide endocardial electrogram.[1]

In selected patients, it may be necessary to combine the automatic implanted defibrillator with a pacemaker for ventricular tachycardia termination or for bradycardia pacing. The pacemaker must be assessed carefully to prevent accidental activation of the implanted defibrillator.[10] It is possible, in some cases, for the AICD to sense the pacemaker stimulus as well as the R wave. This may lead to problems in circumstances such as a pacing threshold testing in which subthreshold stimuli occur or during a sensing test in which asynchronous stimuli are provided in the refractory period of the ventricle but not of the AICD. This "double counting" may raise the aggregate sensed event rate of the AICD above its threshold.

In the future, implanted defibrillators will possess much more programmability and will include or exceed the pacing capabilities of today's tachycardia-terminating pacemakers. The value and challenge of effective follow-up evaluations will increase commensurately.

DEVICE PRESCRIPTION FOR TACHYCARDIA CONTROL

Supraventricular Tachycardias

An important issue in programming pacemakers for supraventricular tachycardia termination is selection of the basic mode of pacing. If bradycardia pacing is not necessary, as is the case in most patients, it should be programmed off if possible. We have had improved results, with fewer episodes of pacemaker-induced tachycardias, using the OAO mode (with tachycardia termination features programmed on). Using this approach, a single undersensed P wave will not result in an asynchronous atrial pace event having the potential to induce a run of supraventricular tachycardia.

In general, the output and sensitivity values that are chosen provide a greater safety margin than those used with bradycardia pacing. The duty cycle of pacemakers for tachycardia termination is low, and premature battery depletion due to excessive output is not a concern. This advantage should not be taken to extremes, since the overutilization of voltage and current may increase the risk of acceleration or fibrillation. If backup pacing is provided, an appropriate rate should be chosen based on the patient's bradyarrhythmia and hemodynamic status. In some patients, more rapid pacing may be useful in the suppression of ectopy and tachycardia episodes.[7]

Although newer devices provide a variety of

algorithms for defining a pathologic tachycardia, a minimal tachycardia rate is the fundamental value that must be selected, and the majority of patients can be managed using this criterion alone. More complex algorithms should be avoided if they are not needed; though they provide increased specificity, it is only at the cost of decreased sensitivity. However, if there is overlap between the peak physiologic rates and the minimal tachycardia rates, other criteria may be helpful. These are linked in boolean fashion, that is, criterion A + B, A + B + C, A + (B or C), and so on. Some devices can track succeeding RR intervals and detect a sudden change in rate. This algorithm is designed to recognize sinus tachycardia but has only moderate specificity.[15] It may also produce false-negative results if a tachycardia is initiated in the midst of a subthreshold sinus tachycardia, as in the following example. A patient who has a device for supraventricular tachycardia with a rate criterion of 140 beats per minute is exercising at a heart rate of 130 beats per minute. If a supraventricular tachycardia with a rate of 150 beats per minute occurs, the sudden-onset criterion, if greater than 20 beats per minute, will not be met. This is a significant problem, since exercise and excitement are frequent causes of both sinus and pathologic tachycardias. Electrograms sensed during atrial fibrillation may also meet sudden-onset criteria.

A second algorithm, rate stability, is excellent for rejecting atrial fibrillation as a rhythm appropriate for pacing. On the other hand, it is frequently not successful in detecting spontaneous rate variations during exercise-induced sinus tachycardia. It has few false-negative results, since most paroxysmal arrhythmias that can be terminated by pacing are rate stable.[15]

Finally, it is important to include some "fail-safe" criterion, such as a period of sustained high rate. This allows the pacemaker to activate the tachycardia-terminating sequence if a tachycardia meeting the minimal rate criterion continues for longer than a specified duration. Such a fail-safe criterion permits the pacemaker to recover from a tachycardia generating a false-negative response from either sudden-onset or rate stability algorithms. In general, it is our practice to link this algorithm to the sudden-onset criterion. In the future, even more sophisticated criteria using atrial/ventricular relationships as well as electrogram pattern recognition may aid substantially in making these critical device decisions.

The most useful devices offer a wide variety of pacing patterns for tachycardia termination. To some extent, these can be simplified by recognizing that only four decisions must be made. The most fundamental decision is whether the pacing cycle lengths will be selected at the time of programming or whether they will occur at some fraction of the measured tachycardia cycle length. Changes in autonomic tone and circulating catecholamine levels may significantly alter the tachycardia rate. As the overall tachycardia cycle length changes, the window for tachycardia termination also changes. Therefore, adaptive behavior is desirable and probably provides a more efficient and effective termination scheme.[4] We employ adaptive pacing routinely in patients with supraventricular tachycardia. Effective termination can usually be achieved by pacing at 70 to 85 per cent of the tachycardia cycle length. Individual testing is required to determine the fraction most suitable to a given patient.

The next decision is whether one to three programmed extrastimuli or a burst of rapid pacing will be employed. It has been demonstrated that bursts of rapid pacing are more effective over a wider range of tachycardia cycle lengths.[16]

The third decision is whether each train of pacing will be fixed in cycle length or will shorten from one stimulus to the next within a train, that is, decremental pacing. Recent studies suggest that decremental pacing or variants of it provide more effective termination than simple, fixed burst pacing. This principle seems to hold true for both ventricular and supraventricular tachycardia.[2, 4] We routinely use adaptive decremental pacing, and it appears to be more effective than ordinary adaptive bursts.

Finally, the pacing pattern selected above may be repeated without change if the tachycardia persists or is scanned over a range of cycle lengths.

Some devices also offer the capability of multitiered therapy. That is, one can program a less aggressive pacing pattern as an initial attempt. Even if the likelihood of success is less than 100 per cent, this first approach may also be less likely to produce acceleration of the tachycardia or fibrillation. After some number of unsuccessful attempts, or if certain criteria are met (e.g., tachycardia in excess of a certain rate), the device will automatically progress to a more aggressive approach.

Ventricular Tachycardias

Unfortunately, the present generation of implanted defibrillators lacks programmable features other than an on-off toggle. Therefore, the only opportunity for changing functional characteristics is at the time of implantation or device replacement. It is critical that a particular patient's needs regarding detection rate criteria, the need for rate plus probability density function (PDF) versus rate only, and the need for increased initial pulse output be carefully considered prior to implantation.

With increasing experience, we have tended to select higher rate criteria and to add a tachycardia-terminating pacemaker if slower ventricular tachycardias occur.[11] Sinus tachycardia and paroxysmal atrial fibrillation with ventricular response rates in the range of 150 to 165 beats per minute are sufficiently frequent to make these tachycardia detection rates too often problematic. If it is known in advance that a tachycardia-terminating pacemaker is also to be used, a rate cut-off of 205 beats per minute is generally chosen. The pacemaker is then programmed to provide pacing termination with the primary modality using rates

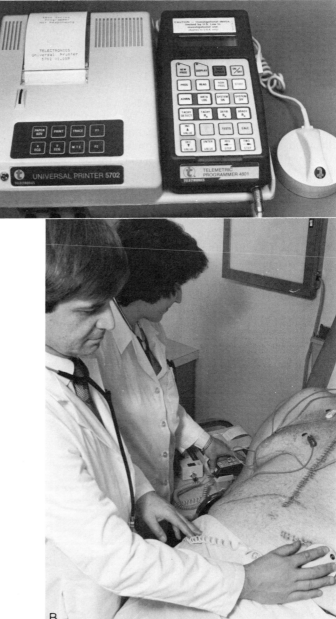

Figure 25–5. *A,* Multifunction programmer and printer for Telectronics Model 4201 pacemaker-cardioverter-defibrillator. Programmable parameters include pacemaker output, sensitivity, cardioverter/defibrillator output and sensing, and tachycardia detection parameters. The programming head is on the right-hand side. *B,* Interrogation and programming is accomplished by placing the programming head over the device pulse generator. This permits noninvasive evaluation and programming of this first-generation hybrid device. (Courtesy of S. Saksena.)

below 205 or short periods of pacing. If tachy-cardias at rates less than 205 result in hemodynamic compromise, the secondary modality is generally used to accelerate the tachycardia to a rate that will guarantee defibrillator activation. The current combination of two devices is cumbersome but can provide considerable benefit if patients are carefully selected and the devices are programmed appropriately (see Fig. 25–3).

In general, the comments regarding the programming of pacemakers for supraventricular tachycardia control are applicable to pacemakers for ventricular tachycardia as well. Mode selection is the parameter that is most often difficult. The VVI mode is more frequently selected than OVO in patients with ventricular tachycardia. There is generally a greater margin of safety in ventricular sensing and less concern about undersensing. These devices are also implanted in conjunction with the automatic defibrillator, and postshock bradycardias may be significant. The OVO mode may be used if sensing of the pacemaker stimulus tends to occur or if there is concern about false inhibition of the defibrillator due to the sensing during ventricular fibrillation of pacing stimuli occurring at the bradycardia rate. Future generations of implantable cardioverter-defibrillators, which are currently in clinical investigation, provide programmable sensing as well as pacing and shock output (see Chapter 26). External programmers with capability for interrogation, display, and reprogramming have been developed for this purpose (Fig. 25–5).

One must also be careful when providing a prescription for therapies other than devices. The administration of antiarrhythmic drugs may significantly affect tachycardia cycle length and the ability to pace-terminate the rhythm.[13] Some drugs may also affect defibrillation threshold.[6] Therefore, it is critical that whenever antiarrhythmic drugs are added, stopped, or changed in dose, the effect on tachycardia termination be investigated. One must also be very careful in the selection and implantation of any pacemaker in a patient already having an automatic defibrillator. Only bipolar pacemakers should be used; unipolar pacemakers are contraindicated.[14] It is preferable that the lead be placed as far as possible from the sensing lead of the defibrillator. When the pacemakers are programmed, the minimal effective output should be used and extra sensing margin provided. This practice will decrease the likelihood of the AICD's oversensing the stimulus artifact or being falsely inhibited by bradycardia pacing stimuli

emitted from the pacemaker owing to a failure to sense ventricular flutter or fibrillation.

REFERENCES

1. Chapman PD, Troup P: The automatic implantable cardioverter-defibrillator: Evaluating suspected inappropriate shocks. J Am Coll Cardiol 7:1075–1078, 1986.
2. Charos GS, Haffajee CI, Gold RL, et al: A theoretically and practically more effective method for interruption of ventricular tachycardia: Self-adapting autodecremental overdrive pacing. Circulation 73:309–315, 1986.
3. Cooper DK, Luceri RM, Thurer RJ, Myerburg RJ: The impact of the automatic implantable cardioverter defibrillator on quality of life. Clin Prog Electrophysiol Pacing 4:306–309, 1986.
4. Den Dulk K, Kersschot IE, Brugada P, Wellens HJJ: Is there a universal antitachycardia pacing mode? Am J Cardiol 57:950–955, 1986.
5. Echt DS, Winkle RA: Management of patients with the automatic implantable cardioverter/defibrillator. Clin Prog Electrophysiol Pacing 3:4–16, 1985.
6. Fain ES, Dorian P, Davy J-M, et al: Effects of encainide and its metabolites on energy requirements for defibrillation. Circulation 73:1334–1341, 1986.
7. Fisher JD, Teichman SL, Ferrick A, et al: Antiarrhythmic effects of VVI pacing at physiologic rates: A crossover controlled evaluation. PACE 10:822–830, 1987.
8. Glasso D, Gallagher R, Parsonnet V, et al: A special outpatient clinic for following patients with implanted tachyarrhythmia devices. PACE 10:1168–1174, 1987.
9. Griffin JC, Schuenemeyer TD: Pacemaker follow-up: An introduction and overview. Clin Prog Electrophysiol Pacing 1:30–39, 1983.
10. Kim SG, Furman S, Matos JA, et al: Automatic implantable cardioverter/defibrillator: Inadvertent discharges during permanent pacemaker magnet tests. PACE 10:579–582, 1987.
11. Manz M, Gerckens U, Funk HD, et al: Combination of antitachycardia pacemaker and automatic implantable cardioverter/defibrillator for ventricular tachycardia. PACE 9:676–684, 1986.
12. Mehra R, Furman S: Comparison of cathodal, anodal, and bipolar strength-interval curves with temporary and permanent pacing electrodes. Br Heart J 41:468–476, 1979.
13. Naccarelli GV, Zipes DP, Rahilly GT, et al: Influence of tachycardia cycle length and antiarrhythmic drugs on pacing termination and acceleration of ventricular tachycardia. Am Heart J 105:1–5, 1983.
14. Physician's Manual for the Automatic Implantable Cardioverter Defibrillator. St Paul, MN, Cardiac Pacemakers, Inc, CPI Document #16J0155, Revision A, August 1986, pp 1–48.
15. Tomaselli G, Scheinman M, Griffin J: The utility of timing algorithms for distinguishing ventricular from supraventricular tachycardias [abstract]. PACE 415, 1987.
16. Ward DE, Camm AJ, Spurrell RAJ: The response of regular reentrant supraventricular tachycardia to right heart stimulation. PACE 2:586–595, 1979.
17. Waxman HL, Cain ME, Greenspan AM, Josephson ME: Termination of ventricular tachycardia with ventricular stimulation: Salutary effect of increased current strength. Circulation 65:800–804, 1982.

26

CLINICAL RESULTS WITH IMPLANTED ANTITACHYCARDIA PACEMAKERS

A. Clinical Results with Antitachycardia Pacemakers

JOHN D. FISHER

Up to the present time, pacing in the acute setting with temporary devices (discussed in Chapter 21) has differed fundamentally from antitachycardia pacing using implanted devices. In acute settings, physicians can and often must be bold. They are faced with an acute problem but are surrounded with immediate backup provisions for cardiopulmonary resuscitation and countershock, if needed. An implanted device assumes that patients will spend the vast majority of their time in places relatively remote from quick rescue. For most patients with supraventricular tachycardias, the penalties for failure of antitachycardia pacing are a sustained tachycardia or perhaps acceleration to atrial fibrillation. In the ventricle, the penalty for failure is potentially much greater, since acceleration to ventricular fibrillation is likely to prove fatal. This last issue is now being addressed by the implantation of an antitachycardia pacer with a backup implantable defibrillator placed separately[51] or in the same unit. Nevertheless, the decision to implant an antitachycardia pacer is not undertaken lightly, and the number of patients receiving this type of therapy has remained relatively limited.

The section of Chapter 21 on pacing in the acute setting includes antitachycardia pacing techniques suitable for such settings, emphasizing simple methods. In this section of the chapter, more sophisticated techniques will be

outlined, together with pacemakers capable of delivering such treatments. Some of the many detection algorithms for automatic antitachycardia pacers will be reviewed. A summary then follows of clinical results with implanted antitachycardia pacemakers for both supraventricular tachycardia (SVT) and ventricular tachycardia (VT).

PACEMAKER TERMINATION AND ACCELERATION OF TACHYCARDIAS

General principles of termination have been covered elsewhere in this volume. Detailed explanations of both termination and acceleration mechanisms have appeared recently in the literature,[16, 19, 23–25] and readers wishing to delve more deeply into this area are referred to those sources.

ANTITACHYCARDIA PACING STIMULATION PATTERNS

Techniques of antitachycardia pacing have evolved from simple competitive underdrive pacing to complex patterns of stimuli. The following is a brief survey of techniques from the original publications referenced and condensed from a more narrowly focused review.[31] Specific implantable devices capable of certain antitachycardia pacing patterns are mentioned.

UNDERDRIVE (Fig. 26–1). Slow, asynchronous (underdrive) pacing during tachycardia can be done with conventional pacemakers.[55] Automatic underdrive pacers include "dual-demand" and "upside-down demand" units.[18, 48] The former paces if the heart rate moves below or above prescribed limits, and the latter becomes active only during tachycardia. The fixed cycle length between successive stimuli competes with faster tachycardia, gradually scanning the tachycardia cycle unless the tachycardia is exactly twice or three times (and so on) the rate of the underdriving stimuli. This approach is simple, with a low risk of acceleration.[22] Successful application requires a slow, well-tolerated tachycardia, susceptible to single-capture termination; these conditions are often absent, especially in patients with VTs.[22]

PROGRAMMED EXTRASTIMULI (PES) OR SCANNING METHODS (Fig. 26–1).[57] Successive stimuli are delivered with predetermined alterations in timing within the tachycardia cycle, a major increase in efficiency compared with the underdrive approach. Some devices "remember" the timing of the extrastimulus, resulting in termination. An example is the Telectronics PASAR 4151 (Telectronics, Englewood, CO). There are many others.

ULTRARAPID TRAIN STIMULATION (Fig. 26–1).[26, 71] The termination zone almost always

begins immediately after the effective refractory period in tachycardias susceptible to single-capture termination.[26] Thus, a train of ultrarapid stimuli (cycle length of 10 to 20 msec, equivalent to 3000 to 6000 beats per minute) beginning during the refractory period, but of a duration causing only a single capture, produces termination on the first attempt. An example is the Intermedics Intertach (Intermedics, Freeport, TX).

MULTIPLE PES (Fig. 26–1).[42, 73] Double, triple, or more extrastimuli can be programmed with such devices. An example is the Teletronics PASAR 4151 and 4171, as well as several others.

BURST PACING (Fig. 26–1).[20] Burst pacing delivers multiple stimuli at a fixed cycle length shorter (faster) than the tachycardia. Risks of acceleration are minimized by keeping both the number and the rate of stimuli as low as possible. Risks are higher than for single-capture methods, even with slow, well-tolerated tachycardias.[22] Examples include Medtronic 5998 radiofrequency (RF) (Medtronic, Minneapolis, MN); Intermedics Cybertach and Intertach; and many more.

BURST PLUS PES (Fig. 26–1).[35, 44] Burst pacing is followed by one or more PES. A slower burst rate may be effective when PES are added. Acceleration may remain a risk.[44]

RAMP PACING (Fig. 26–1).[14, 21] The rapid pacing rate is continuously altered, from faster to slower (rate decremental, or tune down), as shown in Figure 26–1, or in the opposite direction (cycle length decremental). Ramping may be less prone to result in acceleration than burst pacing. Examples are Cordis Orthocor II (Cordis, Miami Lakes, FL), and Intermedics Intertach.

CHANGING RAMPS (Fig. 26–1).[21] The ramp is changed from slower to faster to slower or the opposite. A gradual increase to a rapid rate, followed by a decrease in pacing rate, may be less "jolting" than very rapid bursts.

ADAPTIVE BURSTS (Fig. 26–2).[21] The burst cycle length is a preset percentage of the tachycardia cycle length. This method provides changing burst rates to accommodate for changes in tachycardias. There is a change in the tachycardia cycle length in Figure 26–2, panels a and b; the burst rate increases but remains a fixed percentage of the tachycardia cycle length. Examples include Intermedics Intertach and others.

SHIFTING BURST (Fig. 26–2). The burst rate is fixed, but the first stimulus is introduced progressively earlier in the cycle. Teletronics PASAR 4171 is an example.

SCANNING BURST (Concertina/Accordion)

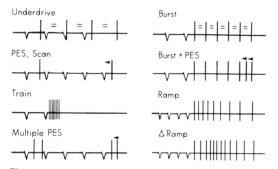

Figure 26–1. Basic stimulation patterns for tachycardia termination. In this and in Figures 26–2 and 26–3, spontaneous atrial or ventricular depolarizations are represented by "V"-like deflections from the baseline, and pacer stimuli are indicated by vertical lines. Small arrowheads at the top of the pacer stimulation line represent the direction of changes in the timing of successive stimuli. Tachycardia depolarizations are omitted after termination has occurred, or when they might obscure the stimulation pattern. See text and reference 31 for an explanation of each technique. PES = programmed extrastimulus. (From Fisher JD, Johnston DR, Kim SG, et al: Implantable pacers for tachycardia termination: Stimulation techniques and long-term efficacy. PACE 9:1325–1333, 1986; with permission.)

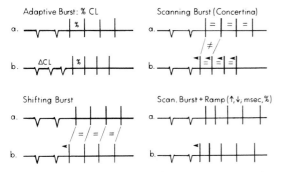

Figure 26–2. Automatic stimulation patterns available in implantable antitachycardia pacers. Conventions are as for Figure 26–1. See text for details. CL = cycle length. (From Fisher JD, Johnston DR, Kim SG, et al: Implantable pacers for tachycardia termination: Stimulation techniques and long-term efficacy. PACE 9:1325–1333, 1986; with permission.)

(Fig. 26–2).[73] The timing of the first stimulus decrements on successive attempts, as with the shifting, but with this technique the cycle length of successive bursts also decreases. Examples are Teletronics PASAR and Intermedics Intertach, as well as others.

SCANNING BURSTS WITH RAMP PACING (Fig. 26–2). The timing of the first beat of the ramp changes during successive termination attempts. In some pacers, the ramp can be incremental or decremental, with changes determined in milliseconds or as a percentage of the tachycardia cycle length (adaptive). Cordis Orthocor II and Intermedics Intertach are examples.

INCREMENTAL-DECREMENTAL (CENTRIFUGAL) SCAN (Fig. 26–3).[42, 70] The first stimulus (S2) timing increments and decrements on successive termination attempts, with the variation programmable in milliseconds or percentage of tachycardia cycle length (adaptive).

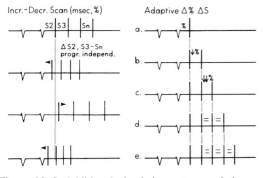

Figure 26–3. Additional stimulation pattern variations as detailed in the text and in reference 31. Conventions are as for Figures 26–1 and 26–2. Decr. = decremental; Incr = incremental; S = stimulus. (From Fisher JD, Johnston DR, Kim SG, et al: Implantable pacers for tachycardia termination: Stimulation techniques and long-term efficacy. PACE 9:1325–1333, 1986; with permission.)

Single or multiple extrastimuli can be used, in turn independently programmable to increment or decrement on successive attempts. Examples include the Siemens Tachylog (Siemens, Solna, Sweden) and Intermedics Intertach.

ADAPTIVE PACING WITH CHANGES IN THE NUMBER OF STIMULI (Fig. 26–3).[7, 10, 11] With one method,[11] the first extrastimulus is delivered at a selected percentage of the tachycardia cycle length. If the arrhythmia persists, a second extrastimulus is delivered at a slightly smaller percentage of the cycle length. If the tachycardia continues, successive stimuli will be introduced without further decrement. An alternative approach is to start with larger numbers of stimuli, for example, five, all at successively shorter cycle lengths, and then to continue adding stimuli and shortening the cycle length until preset limits are reached.[7] An example is the Medtronic SP0500 Interactive Tachy System.

EXOTIC PACING TECHNIQUES.[76] Subthreshold pacing may be effective in some instances of SVT or VT.

CONVENTIONAL PACERS. Pacers marketed for the treatment of bradycardias may have significant antitachycardia capability.[27, 52, 75] Some can be used for programmed stimulation or burst pacing using special programmers[75]; others have specific modes that permit noninvasive programmed stimulation and antitachycardia pacing.[27]

MEDICATIONS. Concurrent administration of antiarrhythmic drugs may be required for successful antitachycardia pacing. When used as adjuvant rather than primary therapy, drug doses may be smaller and less likely to cause side effects.[6, 29, 46, 56]

Detection Algorithms

This subject is specific to individual devices and thus outside the purview of this discussion. For an individual discussion of detection algorithms, see references 3, 4, 8, 9, 13, 21, 28, 29, 32–34, 38, 43, 47, 48, 53, 54, 57, 58, 62, 70, and 73.

THE PATIENT. The patient remains the initial diagnostic entity for manually activated systems. Some patients become overconfident in their abilities and may initiate therapy inappropriately.

A host of algorithms have been considered, and all have limitations. First, *rapid rate*[29, 48, 57, 58, 73] may not distinguish sinus from pathologic tachycardias. Second, *sudden onset*[13, 38, 62, 70] or *constancy of cycle length*[62] may not distinguish SVT from VT, or atrial fibrillation (AF) from other rhythms in patients with Wolff-Parkinson-White (WPW) syndrome and dual atrioventricular (AV) nodal pathways or rarer forms of VT. Third, overlap can occur in *endocardial signal amplitude, slew rate, morphology, frequency content, or sequence.*[3, 4, 8, 21, 28, 32–34, 47, 53] Fourth, the *probability density function*[43] detects fibrillation better than regular tachycardia. Fifth, *responses to extrastimuli*[3, 4] are known for only a few tachycardias. Timing of termination zones can change spontaneously[26, 54] or with changes in activity state or posture,[9] invali-

dating the therapy "remembered" by the pacer. To meet these challenges, multiple programmable *types* of detection algorithms will be required.

Long-Term Antitachycardia Pacing with Implantable Devices

CANDIDATES. Choice of candidates is an area subject to much debate, centered on the risk-benefit ratios and how to predict efficacy.

TABLE 26–1. SVT TERMINATION

INVESTIGATOR	NO. OF PATIENTS	PACER MODEL	PACER TYPE	NO. OF PRE-IMPLANTATION TESTS	NO. OF POST-IMPLANTATION TESTS
Bertholet[5]	13	Telectronics PASAR 4151; Medtronic SPO 500	Automatic; scan, PES; manual, extrastimuli, H bursts	At least 100	q 1 mo × 3, then q 3 mos
Spurrell[73]	21	Telectronics PASAR 4151 and 4171	Automatic; shift, scan, bursts	NS	NS
Den Dulk[13]	1	Cordis Orthocor	Manual, scan, bursts	Extensive evaluation	NS
Sowton[70]	16	Siemens-Elema Tachylog	Automatic, scan, PES, bursts	NS	NS
Zipes[78]	21	Medtronic Symbios 7008	Automatic, scan, PES, bursts	NS	NS
Moss[55]	2	Medtronic 5842, 1317A	Manual, magnet	NS	NS
Goyal[36]	1	Medtronic 5998	Manual, burst	NS	NS
Wyndham[77]	1	Medtronic 5998	Manual, burst	NS	NS
Solti[69]	1	Medtronic 5998	Manual, burst	NS	NS
Peters[61]	10	Medtronic 5998	Manual, burst	At least 50	
O'Keefe[60]	1	Telectronics 150 B (custom device)	Automatic, underdrive	NS	NS
Den Dulk[12]	12	Medtronic SPO 500	Manual, PES	NS	NS
Portillo[63]	8	Medtronic DVI-Mn	Automatic	NS	NS
Spurrell[72]	1	Devices 4271	Automatic, VAT	NS	NS
Abinader[1]	1	—	Manual, magnet	NS	NS
Arbel[2]	1	Cordis Atricor	Automatic, coupled	NS	NS
Fahraeus[15]	8	Telectronics PASAR 4151	Automatic, scan	NS	NS 1 exercise test
Luderitz[49]	9	Intermedics Cybertach	Automatic, manual, underdrive, burst	NS	NS
Nilsson[59]	1	Cardiac Pacemakers, Inc (CPI) Micro Lith	Automatic, synchronized ventricular pacing	NS	NS
Preston[64]	1	Medtronic 5998	Automatic	NS	NS
Mandel[50]	1	Am Opt custom	Manual, ramp	NS	NS
Saksena[68]	2	Cordis Orthocor I	Manual, burst	≥10	Many
Krikler[48]	2	Ela Stanium	Automatic VVT or AAT	NS	NS
Fisher[30]	16	Miscellaneous	Miscellaneous	100	100
Kahn[45] (multicenter)	12	Medtronic 5998	Manual, burst	NS	NS
Griffin[37] (multicenter)	91	InterMedics Cybertach	Automatic, burst	NS	NS
Rothman[66] (multicenter)	16	Cordis Orthocor	Manual, burst	NS	NS

AF = Atrial fibrillation; CHF = congestive heart failure; CVA = cardiovascular accident; NS = not significant; PES = programmed extrastimuli; SVT = supraventricular tachycardia; WPW = Wolff-Parkinson-White syndrome; ( ) = initially.
Modified and expanded from Fisher JD, Johnston DR, Kim SG, et al: Implantable pacers for tachycardia termination: Stimulation techniques and long-term efficacy. PACE 9: 1325–1333, 1986.

Pacers can provide long-term therapy, with low-risk surgery and minimal need for the patient's compliance. Medications and their side effects can often be reduced or eliminated altogether. It may be easier to change a drug than a pacemaker (debatable in view of the highly programmable devices currently available), and pharmacologic *prevention* may be preferable to electrical *intervention*.

Candidates for antitachycardia pacers in our institution are given the same antiarrhythmic drugs, if any, that are planned for long-term therapy. At least 100 episodes of tachycardia are induced, and the results of attempts to terminate these episodes are evaluated.[30, 70] Pacemaker implantation in patients with VT raises serious concerns. Because acceleration can prove fatal in patients with VT,[9] criteria for pacemaker implantation are more stringent. Patients are considered for an implantable device only after exhaustive drug trials.[21] Alternatives such as surgery, ablation, and certainly an implantable defibrillator are considered. A backup implantable defibrillator

BY IMPLANTED PACERS

CONCURRENT DRUG ADMINISTRATION	DURATION OF FOLLOW-UP (MO)	RESULTS			
		Excellent	Good	Poor	Comments
5	5–30	7	3	3	—
8	2–40	16	—	—	2 sudden death, 3 deactivated plus surgical therapy
No	3	1	—	—	—
3	5–19	14	—	—	2 surgical therapy for WPW with rapid AF
NS	NS	21	—	—	—
No	2–7	2	—	—	—
Yes	8	1	—	—	—
Yes	21	—	1	—	Some problems with AF
NS	>11	1	—	—	—
4	24–60	6	1	3	—
Yes	6	1	—	—	—
8	3–26	8	4	—	—
2	4–20	5	—	—	3 pt did not have SVT + implant
Yes	10	1	—	—	—
Yes	>16	—	(1)	—	SVT became unresponsive after 16 mo
NS	Up to 48	1	—	—	CHF and cardiomegaly resolved 4 mo after implant
2	NS	4	—	—	Sinus tachycardia/SVT rate overlap caused inappropriate stimulation
Yes	NS	5	4	—	—
Yes	NS	—	—	—	—
Yes	5.5	1	—	—	Rapid A pacing with 2:1 or 4:1 conduction
NS	7	1	—	—	Ramp pacing to 300 beats per minute
No	20	2	—	—	—
1	18	2	—	—	—
Yes	6–177	12	4	—	Not all patients had 100 pre- and postimplant trials
8	15–36	10	—	—	1 explant, 2 chronic pericarditis, 1 died of CVA
NS	>21	—	82%	—	8 units explanted due to inadequate sensing
NS	1–40	88%	—	—	

would currently be used with an antitachycardia pacer in patients with VT causing syncope or those who have had any episode accelerated. Patients with well-tolerated tachycardias may be considered for manually activated units for use only in the presence of medical backup.

Pacing for Supraventricular Tachycardia: Long-Term Results

A three-decade survey, although nonexhaustive, yielded 27 reports on SVT in 270 patients (Table 26–1) (see also references 1, 2, 5, 12, 13, 15, 30, 36, 37, 45, 48–50, 55, 59–61, 63, 64, 66, 68–70, 72, 73, 77, and 78). Only six studies provided data on the number of preimplant or postimplant trials of the selected antitachycardia pacing mode. Follow-up periods ranged from 1 to 177 months (average of 12 to 15 months). Most investigators reported

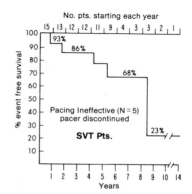

Figure 26–4. Actuarial efficacy of pacing for termination of supraventricular tachycardia (SVT). All 15 patients had episodes of SVT terminated by their implanted device. The endpoint "event" was discontinuation of pacing for any reason other than an unrelated death of the patient. Pts. = patients. (From Fisher JD, Johnston DR, Furman S, et al: Long-term efficacy of antitachycardia pacing for supraventricular and ventricular tachycardias. Am J Cardiol 60:1311–1316, 1987; with permission.)

TABLE 26–2. VENTRICULAR TACHYCARDIA

INVESTIGATOR	NO. OF PATIENTS	PACER MODEL	PACER TYPE	NO. OF PRE-IMPLANTATION TESTS	NO. OF POST-IMPLANTATION TESTS
Reddy[65]	1	Telectronics 4151 PA-SAR	Automatic, scanning PES	Many	Several
Bertholet[5]	3	Medtronic SPO 500	Manual, scanning, burst	At least 100	NS
Spurrell[73]	1	Telectronics PASAR 4151	Automatic, shifting	NS	NS
Sowton[70]	9	Siemens-Elema Tachy-log	Automatic, scanning, PES, burst	NS	NS
den Dulk[12]	6	Medtronic SPO 500	Manual, variable modes	NS	NS
Moss[55]	1	Medtronic 5842	Manual via magnet	NS	NS
Hartzler[39]	2	Medtronic 5998	Manual RF	>30–100	>50–70
Ruskin[67]	3	Medtronic 5998	Manual RF	>100 each	100
Herre[40]	28	Medtronic 5998	Manual RF	NS	125 EP studies
Peters[61]	6	Medtronic 5998	Manual RF	NS	NS
Strasberg[74]	2	Medtronic 5998	Manual RF	NS	NS
Tanabe[75]	1	Medtronic Spectrax	Manual	NS	NS
Higgins[41]	1	Telectronics PASAR 4151	Automatic, scan, burst, PES	NS	NS
Luderitz[49]	3	2 magnet	Manual underdrive	NS	
Saksena[68]	11	Cordis Orthocor I	Manual burst	NS	NS
Fisher[30]	20	Miscellaneous	Miscellaneous	>100	>100
Griffin[37] (multicenter)	52	InterMedics Cybertach	Automatic, burst	NS	NS
Rothman[66] (multicenter)	53	Cordis Orthocor	Manual, burst	NS	NS

EP = electrophysiologic; NS = not significant, miscellaneous; PES = programmed extrastimuli; RF = radiofrequency; VF = ventricular fibrillation; VT = ventricular tachycardia.

Modified and expanded from Fisher JD, Johnston DR, Kim SG, et al: Implantable pacers for tachycardia termination: Stimulation techniques and long-term efficacy. PACE 9: 1325–1333, 1986.

using antiarrhythmic agents in 20 to 50 per cent of their patients (range of 0 to 100 per cent), and most expressed satisfaction with antitachycardia pacing, judging results to be excellent or good. Results were considered poor in 10 patients (3.7 per cent). The percentage of each investigator's patients with SVT who received antitachycardia pacers was rarely stated. In our series,[30] 7 per cent of patients referred for SVT studies received antitachycardia pacers. These had a continuing efficacy rate of 93 per cent at 1 year and 78 per cent at 5 years (Fig. 26–4).

Pacing for Ventricular Tachycardia: Long-Term Results

Table 26–2 lists 18 papers describing 203 patients with VT who have antitachycardia pacers (see also references 15, 30, 37, 39, 40,

45, 50, 55, 60, 65–67, 69, 70, 73–75). Data were scanty on methods of efficacy assessment used prior to discharge and on follow-up details. Follow-up averaged about 12 to 15 months, ranging from unstated to 92 months. Most of these patients with VT also received antiarrhythmic drugs. Results were generally felt to be good to excellent, with poor results in eight patients (3.9 per cent). Compared with patients who have SVT, those with VT had a higher overall mortality, related to both sudden death and other causes, though pacemakers were rarely implicated directly as a cause of death. The need for a backup defibrillator was widely perceived in the more recent publications. In our own series of patients studied for VT, only 3.5 per cent received a pacer for VT termination.[30] Actuarial efficacy was 78 per cent at 1 year and 55 per cent at 5 years (Figs. 26–5 and 26–6).

TERMINATED BY IMPLANTED PACERS

CONCURRENT DRUGS ADMINISTRATION	DURATION OF FOLLOW-UP (MO)	RESULTS			
		Excellent	Good	Poor	Comments
Yes	6	1	—	—	—
Yes	17–30	3	—	—	—
NS	NS	1	—	—	Unit explanted after patient free of VT
3	6–14	5	—	—	—
5	6–20	4	2	—	—
?	6	1	—	—	No VT after pacer rate increased
Yes	1–11	1	—	—	1 patient had VF at 4 wk—died
Yes	Mean, 13.6	3	—	—	1 died of lung cancer
18	1–25	97% success in 9 patients	—	—	No spontaneous VT in 19 patients, 1 patient experienced sudden death
Yes	3–36	1	5	—	2 acceleration, 3 refractory
NS	—	—	—	—	1 patient no recurrence, 1 patient 1 recurrence
NS	—	—	—	—	—
No	16	—	1	—	—
Yes	NS	2	1	—	—
Yes	2–92	16	2	2	1 explant at 1 mo, 4 disarmed at 1 mo, 4 sudden, not pacer-related deaths
NS	12	—	58% alive and use device	—	14 nontachycardia deaths, 4 sudden deaths
NS	1–41	—	84% tachycardia terminated ≥ once	—	3 sudden deaths, 3 documented VT/VF deaths

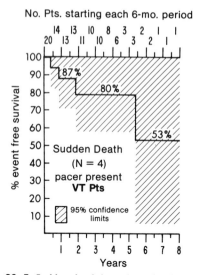

No. Pts. starting each 6-mo. period

Figure 26–5. Sudden death in patients (Pts.) with pacers for ventricular tachycardia (VT) termination. Among the 20 patients in this series, sudden death occurred in 20 per cent by the fifth year. This actuarial efficacy is much less than would be expected with an implantable cardioverter/defibrillator. Most of these deaths occurred in patients for whom no other options were available and prior to the availability of the automatic implantable cardioverter/defibrillator. Actuarial efficacy in patients with well-tolerated VT has been much better. None of these deaths could be attributed to actual use of antitachycardia pacing. (From Fisher JD, Johnston DR, Furman S, et al: Long-term efficacy of antitachycardia pacing for supraventricular and ventricular tachycardias. Am J Cardiol 60:1311–1316, 1987; with permission.)

CONCLUSIONS

Remarkable advances have been achieved in the design of pacemakers able to carry out sophisticated antitachycardia pacing. Nevertheless, pacing has not captured a large portion of the tachycardia "market" for many reasons. Pacing for prevention of tachycardias remains a largely unexplored realm, with unknown potential. Implantation of devices for periodic noninvasive programmed electrical stimulation to assess continuing drug efficacy or tachycardia stability can be useful but is not yet included in standard pacemaker implantation guidelines. Antiarrhythmic medications are often required in conjunction with antitachycardia pacers, so that many physicians would prefer to exhaust the medical options before turning to an implanted device. It is true that drug doses can often be reduced substantially when used with antitachycardia pacers, but this has not yet been widely appreciated as a point in favor of pacing. Many physicians have been frustrated by the detailed workups leading to the implantation of an antitachycardia pacemaker, for both patients with SVT and those with VT. With SVT there is often a continual reprogramming of the unit until it behaves properly as the patient moves from rest to exercise, from supine to upright position, and from being an inpatient to an outpatient. For patients with VT, there is always the specter of tachycardia acceleration or precipitation of ventricular fibrillation. The actuarial efficacy of antitachycardia pacing[30] has been reasonably good but for most patients does not provide a lifelong therapy. Pacing also has an "image" problem. Many patients with tachycardia are young and have an impression of patients with pacemakers as elderly and debilitated. Modern pacemakers are small, but for some patients, cosmetic concerns are important enough that they prefer to exhaust medical options before moving on to any type of surgery. Investigators may also have been unwitting participants in the continuing relatively low use of antitachycardia pacemakers. Scientific reports are often not up to the standards required in other areas. Reports tend to be long on enthusiasm and short on numbers, details, protocols, and data, a situation prompting the recent publication of suggested guidelines for reports on antitachycardia pacing.[17]

The low use of pacemakers for termination of SVT has been an area of surprise. When very sophisticated antitachycardia pacemakers were introduced, it was felt that they might be a major force in controlling SVTs. Except in certain patients such as those with the WPW syndrome, it was expected that anti-SVT pacing had relatively little potential for doing harm and would be a satisfactory substitute for the side effects of pharmacologic treatment. For many of the reasons outlined above, the move to anti-SVT pacers did not take place. In many instances, devices developed primarily for control of SVT, and approved by federal agencies for routine implantation only in patients with SVT, were in fact implanted primarily in patients with VT. It remains to be seen whether still more sophisticated anti-SVT pacemakers, perhaps with an increased emphasis on prevention, will alter this situation or whether the treatment of SVT will remain in the province of pharmacology, surgery, or other ablative techniques.

VT is less susceptible than SVT to the vagaries of neurohumoral tone. Particularly in the case of relatively slow VT, with rates under about 200 beats per minute, termination

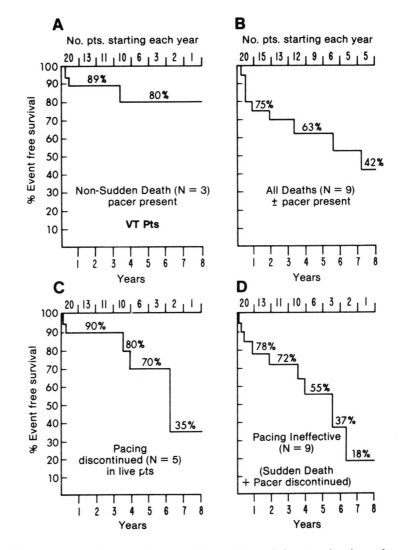

Figure 26–6. Other actuarial endpoints in patients with pacers for termination of VT. *A,* Nonsudden death in patients with pacemakers present. *B,* All deaths in this series, whether or not the pacemaker was present. *C,* Pacing discontinued in this series of 20 patients. Pacing was discontinued in 5 subjects because of inefficacy, an increase in VT frequency, or acceleration of VT. *D,* Overall actuarial efficacy of anti-VT pacing. Endpoint events here were ineffective pacing, resulting in discontinuation of the pacer, together with the occurrence of sudden death. (From Fisher JD, Johnston DR, Furman S, et al: Long-term efficacy of antitachycardia pacing for supraventricular and ventricular tachycardias. Am J Cardiol 60:1311–1316, 1987; with permission.)

should be possible in over 90 per cent of episodes. Nevertheless, when pacing is used in multiple episodes, many patients experience at least occasional acceleration of VT; and this has limited widespread application of this otherwise effective technique. Combinations of automatic implantable cardioverters/defibrillators (AICDs) and antitachycardia pacemakers in the same unit have been recognized for several years as a solution. As usual, widespread acceptance of such a combined device will be greater with the availability of relatively small units that do not require a thoracotomy for implantation.

It is likely that implanted antitachycardia pacemakers will find increasing employment. Techniques for prevention of tachycardias and longitudinal assessment of tachycardias (noninvasive programmed electrical stimulation) will be increasingly emphasized. In contrast to original projections, it now seems likely that

most pacemakers designed for termination of tachycardias will be used in the ventricle, in combination with implantable cardioverters/defibrillators.

REFERENCES

1. Abinader EG: Recurrent supraventricular tachycardia: Success and subsequent failure of termination by implanted endocardial pacemaker. JAMA 236:2203–2205, 1976.
2. Arbel ER, Cohen CH, Langendorf R, Glick G: Successful treatment of drug-resistant atrial tachycardia and intractable congestive heart failure with permanent coupled atrial pacing. Am J Cardiol 41:336–340, 1978.
3. Arzbaecher R, Bump T, Jenkins J, et al: Automatic tachycardia recognition. PACE 7:541–547, 1984.
4. Aubert AE, Denys BG, Ector H, DeGeest H: Detection of ventricular tachycardia and fibrillation using ECG processing and intramyocardial pressure gradients. PACE 9:1084–1088, 1986.

5. Bertholet M, Demoulin JC, Waleffe A, Kulbertus H: Programmable extrastimulus pacing for long-term management of supraventricular and ventricular tachycardias: Clinical experience in 16 patients. Am Heart J 110:582–589, 1985.

6. Camm J, Ward D, Washington HG, Spurrell RAJ: Intravenous disopyramide phosphate and ventricular overdrive pacing in the termination of paroxysmal ventricular tachycardia. PACE 2:395–402, 1979.

7. Charos GS, Haffajee CI, Gold RL, et al: A theoretically and practically more effective method for interruption of ventricular tachycardia: Self-adapting autodecremental overdrive pacing. Circulation 73:309–315, 1986.

8. Davies DW, Wainwright RJ, Tooley MA, et al: Detection of pathological tachycardia by analysis of electrogram morphology. PACE 9:200–208, 1986.

9. Den Dulk K, Brugada P, Wellens HJJ: A case report demonstrating spontaneous change in tachycardia terminating window. PACE 7:867–870, 1984.

10. Den Dulk K, Kersschot IE, Brugada P, Wellens HJJ: Is there a universal antitachycardia pacing mode? Am J Cardiol 57:950–955, 1986.

11. Den Dulk K, Bertholet M, Brugada P, et al: A versatile pacemaker system for termination of tachycardias. Am J Cardiol 52:731–738, 1983.

12. Den Dulk K, Bertholet M, Brugada P, et al: Clinical experience with implantable devices for control of tachyarrhythmias. PACE 7:548–556, 1984.

13. Den Dulk K, Brugada P, Waldecker B, et al: Automatic pacemaker termination of two different types of supraventricular tachycardia. J Am Coll Cardiol 6:201–105, 1985.

14. Escher DJW, Furman S: Emergency treatment of cardiac arrhythmias: Emphasis on use of electrical pacing. JAMA 214:2028–2034, 1970.

15. Fahraeus T, Lassvik C, Sonnhag C: Tachycardias initiated by automatic antitachycardia pacemakers. PACE 7:1049–1054, 1984.

16. Fisher JD: Electrical devices for the treatment of tachyarrhythmias. Cardiol Clin 4:527–542, 1986.

17. Fisher JD: Antitachycardia devices: Minimum report standards. PACE 11:2–4, 1988.

18. Fisher JD, Furman S: Automatic termination of tachycardia by an implanted "upside down" demand pacemaker [abstract]. Clin Res 26:231a, 1978.

19. Fisher JD, Kim SG, Mercando AD: Electrical devices for treatment of arrhythmias. Am J Cardiol 61:45A–57A, 1988.

20. Fisher JD, Mehra R, Furman S: Termination of ventricular tachycardia with bursts of ventricular pacing. Am J Cardiol 41:94–102, 1978.

21. Fisher JD, Kim SG, Furman S, Matos JA: Role of implantable pacemakers in control of recurrent ventricular tachycardia. Am J Cardiol 49:194–206, 1982.

22. Fisher JD, Kim SG, Matos JA, Ostrow E: Comparative effectiveness of pacing techniques for termination of well-tolerated sustained ventricular tachycardia. PACE 6:915–922, 1983.

23. Fisher JD, Kim SG, Matos JA, Waspe LE: Pacing for ventricular tachycardia. PACE 7:1278–1290, 1984.

24. Fisher JD, Kim SG, Matos JA, Waspe LE: Pacing for tachycardias: Clinical translations. In Zipes D, Jalife J (eds): Electrophysiology and Arrhythmias. Orlando, FL, Grune and Stratton, 1985, pp 507–511.

25. Fisher JD, Kim SG, Waspe LE, Matos JA: Mechanisms for the success and failure of pacing for termination of ventricular tachycardia: Clinical and hypothetical considerations. PACE 6:1094–1105, 1983.

26. Fisher JD, Ostrow E, Kim SG, Matos JA: Ultrarapid single-capture train stimulation for termination of ventricular tachycardia. Am J Cardiol 51:1334–1338, 1983.

27. Fisher JD, Furman S, Kim SG, et al: DDD/DDT pacemakers in the treatment of ventricular tachycardia. PACE 7:173–178, 1984.

28. Fisher JD, Goldstein M, Ostrow E, et al: Maximal rate of tachycardia development: Sinus tachycardia with sudden exercise vs. spontaneous ventricular tachycardia. PACE 6:221–228, 1983.

29. Fisher JD, Johnston DR, Furman S, et al: Long-term stability of antitachycardia devices. Clin Res 34:298A, 1986.

30. Fisher JD, Johnston DR, Furman S, et al: Long-term efficacy of antitachycardia pacing for supraventricular and ventricular tachycardias. Am J Cardiol 60:1311–1316, 1987.

31. Fisher JD, Johnston DR, Kim SG, et al: Implantable pacers for tachycardia termination: Stimulation techniques and long-term efficacy. PACE 9:1325–1333, 1986.

32. Furman S, Pannizzo F: The role of implantable pacemakers in the therapy of tachycardias. Arch Mal Coeur 78:29–34, 1985.

33. Furman S, Fisher JD, Pannizzo F: Necessity of signal processing in tachycardia detection. In Barold SS, Mugica J (eds): The Third Decade of Cardiac Pacing. New York, Futura, 1982.

34. Furman S, Brodman R, Pannizzo F, Fisher JD: Implantation techniques of antitachycardia devices. PACE 7:572–579, 1984.

35. Gardner MJ, Waxman HL, Buxton AE, et al: Termination of tachycardia: Evaluation of a new pacing method. Am J Cardiol 50:1338–1345, 1982.

36. Goyal SL, Lichstein E, Gupta PK, Chadda KD: Refractory reentrant atrial tachycardia: Successful treatment with a permanent radio frequency triggered atrial pacemaker. Am J Med 58:586–590, 1975.

37. Griffin JC, Sweeney M: The management of paroxysmal tachycardia using the Cybertach-60. PACE 7:1291–1295, 1984.

38. Griffin JC, Mason JW, Calfee RV: Clinical use of an implantable automatic tachycardia-terminating pacemaker. Am Heart J 100:1093–1096, 1980.

39. Hartzler GO: Treatment of recurrent ventricular tachycardias by patient-activated radiofrequency ventricular stimulation. Mayo Clin Proc 54:75–82, 1979.

40. Herre JM, Griffin JC, Nielsen AP, et al: Permanent triggered antitachycardia pacemakers in the management of recurrent sustained ventricular tachycardia. J Am Coll Cardiol 6:206–212, 1985.

41. Higgins JR, Swartz JD, Dehmer GJ, Beddingfield GW: Automatic scanning extrastimulus pacemaker to treat ventricular tachycardia. PACE 8:101–109, 1985.

42. Holt P, Crick JCP, Sowton E: Antitachycardia pacing: A comparison of burst overdrive, self-searching and adaptive table scanning programs. PACE 9:490–497, 1986.

43. Jenkins J, Bump T, Munkenbeck F, et al: Tachycardia detection in implantable antitachycardia devices. PACE 7:1273–1277, 1984.

44. Jentzer JH, Hoffmann RM: Acceleration of ventricular tachycardia by rapid overdrive pacing combined with extrastimuli. PACE 7:922–924, 1984.

45. Kahn A, Morris JJ, Cintron P: Patient-initiated rapid atrial pacing to manage supraventricular tachycardia. Am J Cardiol 38:200–204, 1976.
46. Keren G, Miura DS, Somberg JC: Pacing termination of ventricular tachycardia: Influence of antiarrhythmia-slowed ectopic rate. Am Heart J 107:638–643, 1984.
47. Klementowitz PT, Furman S: Selective atrial sensing in dual chamber pacemakers eliminates endless loop tachycardia. J Am Coll Cardiol 7:590–594, 1986.
48. Krikler DM, Curry PVL, Buffet J: Dual-demand pacing for reciprocating atrioventricular tachycardia. Br Med J 1:1114–1116, 1979.
49. Luderitz B, d'Alnoncourt CN, Steinbeck G, Beyer J: Therapeutic pacing in tachyarrhythmias by implanted pacemakers. PACE 5:366–371, 1982.
50. Mandel WJ, Laks MM, Yamaguchi I, et al: Recurrent reciprocating tachycardias in the Wolff-Parkinson-White syndrome: Control by the use of a scanning pacemaker. Chest 69:769–774, 1976.
51. Manz M, Gerckens U, Funke HD, et al: Combination of antitachycardia pacemaker and automatic implantable cardioverter/defibrillator for ventricular tachycardia. PACE 9:676–684, 1986.
52. Medina-Ravell V, Castellanos A, Portillo-Acosta B, et al: Management of tachyarrhythmias with dual-chamber pacemakers. PACE 6:333–345, 1983.
53. Mercando AD, Furman S: Measurement of differences in timing and sequence between two ventricular electrodes as a means of tachycardia differentiation. PACE 9:1069–1078, 1986.
54. Mirowski M: The automatic implantable cardioverter-defibrillator: An Overview. J Am Coll Cardiol 6:461–466, 1985.
55. Moss AJ, Rivers RJ: Termination and inhibition of recurrent tachycardias by implanted pervenous pacemakers. Circulation 50:942–947, 1974.
56. Naccarelli GV, Zipes DP, Rahilly GT, et al: Influence of tachycardia cycle length and antiarrhythmic drugs on pacing termination and acceleration of ventricular tachycardia. Am Heart J 105:1–5, 1983.
57. Nathan AW, Camm AJ, Bexton RS, et al: Initial experience with a fully implantable, programmable, scanning, extrastimulus pacemaker for tachycardia termination. Clin Cardiol 5:22–26, 1982.
58. Neumann G, Funke H, Simon H, et al: Successful treatment of supraventricular reentry tachycardia by implantation of demand overdrive pacemakers. Toulouse, France, Societé de la Nouvelle Imprimerie Fournie, 1978, pp 193–196.
59. Nilsson G, Ringqvist I: Long-term control of reciprocating paroxysmal tachycardia by ventricular pacing in a case of Wolff-Parkinson-White syndrome. Br Heart J 47:609–612, 1982.
60. O'Keefe DB, Curry PVL, Sowton E: Treatment of paroxysmal nodal tachycardia by dual demand pacemaker in the coronary sinus. Br Heart J 45:105–108, 1981.
61. Peters RW, Scheinman MM, Morady F, Jacobson L: Long-term management of recurrent paroxysmal tachycardia by cardiac burst pacing. PACE 8:35–44, 1985.
62. Pless BD, Sweeney MB: Discrimination of supraventricular tachycardia from sinus tachycardia of overlapping cycle length. PACE 7:1318–1324, 1984.
63. Portillo B, Medina-Ravell V, Portillo-Leon N, et al: Treatment of drug resistant A-V reciprocating tachycardias with multiprogrammable dual demand A-V sequential (DVI, MN) pacemakers. PACE 5:814–825, 1982.
64. Preston TA, Haynes RE, Gavin WA, Hessel EA: Permanent rapid atrial pacing to control supraventricular tachycardia. PACE 2:331–334, 1979.
65. Reddy CP, Todd EP, Kuo CS, DeMaria AN: Treatment of ventricular tachycardia using an automatic scanning extrastimulus pacemaker. J Am Coll Cardiol 3:225–230, 1984.
66. Rothman MT, Keefe JM: Clinical results with Omni-Orthocor,® an implantable antitachycardia pacing system. PACE 7:1306–1312, 1984.
67. Ruskin JN, Garan H, Poulin F, Harthorne JW: Permanent radiofrequency ventricular pacing for management of drug-resistant ventricular tachycardia. Am J Cardiol 46:317–321, 1980.
68. Saksena S, Pantopoulous D, Parsonnet V, et al: Usefulness of an implantable antitachycardia pacemaker system for supraventricular or ventricular tachycardia. Am J Cardiol 58:70–74, 1986.
69. Solti F, Szabo Z, Czako E, et al: Refractory supraventricular reentry tachycardia treated by radiofrequency atrial pacemaker. PACE 5:275–277, 1982.
70. Sowton E: Clinical results with the tachylog antitachycardia pacemaker. PACE 7:1313–1317, 1984.
71. Spurrell RAJ, Sowton E: Pacing techniques in the management of supraventricular tachycardia. J Electrocardiol 8:287–295, 1975.
72. Spurrell RAJ, Sowton E: An implanted atrial synchronous pacemaker with a short atrioventricular delay for the prevention of paroxysmal supraventricular tachycardias. J Electrocardiol 9:89–96, 1976.
73. Spurrell RAJ, Nathan AW, Camm AJ: Clinical experience with implantable scanning tachycardia reversion pacemakers. PACE 7:1296–1300, 1984.
74. Strasberg B, Fetter J, Palileo E, et al: Postoperative electrophysiologic studies with a modified radiofrequency system. Technical aspects and clinical usefulness. PACE 5:688–693, 1982.
75. Tanabe A, Ikeda H, Fujiyama M, et al: Termination of ventricular tachycardia by an implantable atrial pacemaker and external pacemaker activator. PACE 8:532–538, 1985.
76. Von Leitner R, Linderer T: Subthreshold burst pacing: A new method for termination of ventricular and subventricular tachycardia [abstract]. J Am Coll Cardiol 3:472, 1984.
77. Wyndham CR, WU D, Denes P, et al: Self-initiated conversion of paroxysmal atrial flutter utilizing a radiofrequency pacemaker. Am J Cardiol 41:1119–1122, 1978.
78. Zipes DP, Prystowsky EN, Miles WM, Heger JJ: Initial experience with Symbios model 7008 pacemaker. PACE 7:1301–1305, 1984.

B. Clinical Results with Transvenous Cardioversion

LAWRENCE S. KLEIN, WILLIAM M. MILES,
JAMES J. HEGER, ERIC N. PRYSTOWSKY,
and DOUGLAS P. ZIPES

Although pharmacologic treatment remains the mainstay of therapy for ventricular arrhythmias, many patients experience recurrence of arrhythmias despite therapy with multiple antiarrhythmic agents. Therefore, many investigators have become interested in implantable devices to terminate ventricular tachycardia (VT) and ventricular fibrillation (VF) in patients presumed to be high risk. Mirowski and colleagues showed that a catheter electrode system could effectively terminate VF in humans.[7] These investigators subsequently modified their system to include an electrode of large surface area introduced by thoracotomy and placed over the apex of the heart to defibrillate humans reliably.[6, 8] We and others have demonstrated that VT may be safely and reproducibly terminated in dogs[3] and human patients[17, 19, 20] with synchronized shocks using low energy and delivered through a catheter electrode. Synchronization of these shocks to the QRS complex has been found to be critical, since, as with transthoracic cardioversion, energy delivered during ventricular repolarization can precipitate VF. Therefore, we developed a system for transvenous cardioversion that employed a permanent cardioverter, implanted with the patient under local anesthesia, similar to implantation of a permanent transvenous pacemaker.[18] In addition, we used this prototype device to gather data on the long-term efficacy of transvenous, low-energy cardioversion in 11 patients,[4, 5] anticipating that future models with backup defibrillation capabilities would soon be available for investigation. Last, repeated induction of VT performed noninvasively on multiple occasions over long periods was possible using the device, and therefore, the stability of VT induc-

tion characteristics and other electrophysiologic measurements could be investigated.

THE FIRST-GENERATION IMPLANTABLE CARDIOVERTER
(Fig. 26–7)

The implantable cardioverter (Medtronic model 7210, Medtronic, Minneapolis, MN) is encased in a hermetically sealed titanium case measuring 57 by 73 by 19 mm and it weighs 95 grams. It is powered by two independent lithium battery sources. The device delivers truncated exponential waveforms of 3 to 10 msec duration that can be programmed from 0.6 to 2.0 J, synchronized to the QRS complex over a single No. 10 French tined lead (Medtronic 6882) placed in the right ventricle. The lead contains distal and proximal pairs of electrodes, which are separated by 100 to 150 mm. During cardioversion, the distal electrodes serve as a cathode in the right ventricular apex, and the proximal pair serves as the anode. The spacing of the electrodes may vary, depending upon the patient's heart size, in the positioning of the proximal electrodes near the superior vena caval–right atrial junction. Shocks may be delivered automatically via a rate detection algorithm, or the device may be discharged manually by an external programmer. When set in the automatic mode, the device delivers the first shock at the programmed energy settings. If tachycardia persists, two more shocks are delivered at the programmed energy setting prior to two final shocks, which are delivered at 2 J.

The device has three programmable tachycardia detection indices: (1) A critical cardiac cycle length (205 to 545 msec) must be present for the device to recognize tachycardia; (2) the number of consecutive tachycardia intervals at the triggered cycle length (2 to 32) must be satisfied; and (3) an optional criterion is the change in cycle length from the last normal beat to the tachycardia cycle (0 to 200 msec).

Supported in part by the Herman C. Krannert Fund, Indianapolis; by grants HL-06308 and HL-07182 from the National Heart, Lung, and Blood Institute of the National Institutes of Health, Bethesda, MD; by the Attorney General of Indiana Public Health Trust and by the Roudebush Veterans Administration Medical Center, Indianapolis.

Figure 26–7. Posteroanterior (*left*) and lateral (*right*) chest radiographs showing the implanted transvenous cardioverter. The distal electrodes are in the right ventricular apex, and the proximal electrodes are at the superior vena caval–right atrial junction. The pulse generator is implanted below the left clavicle. (Reprinted by permission of the New England Journal of Medicine [311; 485–490, 1984].)

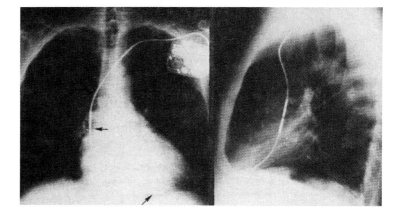

The first and second criteria must always be met for a shock to be delivered automatically. The third criterion may be programmed either on or off and is based on the assumption that the change from sinus rhythm to tachycardia is abrupt. Once these tachycardia recognition parameters are satisfied, the unit charges to the programmed energy setting and delivers the shock synchronized to the next detected QRS complex. The charge time varies both with the energy of the shock and with the amount of time since the last discharge. In our 11 patients with long-term follow-up, the mean charge time was 12.9 seconds (range of 2.5 to 40.3 seconds) for the first shock delivered on any given day and 3.5 seconds (range of 1.1 to 7.8 seconds) for the second shock, with the difference attributable to battery and capacitor characteristics. If tachycardia persists, the unit is programmed to deliver the second shock and so on for a total of five shocks. At that point, no more shocks are delivered automatically unless the device senses a cycle length longer than the trigger interval (i.e., an indication that tachycardia has terminated), and the tachycardia detection criteria are once again satisfied.

The cardioverter also functions as a bradycardia pacemaker and has programmable demand ventricular pacing (VVI mode) at rates between 30 and 100 per minute. The pulse width and QRS sensitivity are programmable. In addition, temporary ventricular pacing in the asynchronous (VOO) mode at rates of 30 to 400 per minute can be performed. After a drive train of VOO pacing at programmable duration and cycle lengths, 1 or more (up to 99) premature ventricular extrastimuli at programmable intervals can be introduced to perform programmed ventricular stimulation for induction of VT. We have used this feature of the cardioverter to test cardioversion efficacy of the device over long periods and to examine the reproducibility of induction of VT (Figs. 26–8 and 26–9). In addition, these premature extrastimuli can also be used to terminate tachycardia, should spontaneous tachycardia occur. These are all under telemetric control via the external programmer. Finally, bidirectional telemetry provides a print-out of the cardioverter settings, marker pulses, electrograms, and battery end-of-life indicators (Fig. 26–10).

SELECTION OF PATIENTS

Patients were considered suitable candidates for the implantable transvenous cardioverter if they had recurrent, sustained, monomorphic VT and no history of spontaneous VF in the absence of acute myocardial infarction. All patients recognized the onset of VT, and in all except one patient who had syncope, VT was tolerated for several hours without hemodynamic embarrassment, allowing adequate time for medical attention. Each patient in the study had required repeated transthoracic cardioversions despite therapy with multiple antiarrhythmic agents, both conventional and investigational. Patients either had refused or were considered unsuitable candidates for surgical treatment of ventricular tachycardia, usually because of poor left ventricular function. Each patient had a successful preoperative response to catheter cardioversion at the time of electrophysiologic study.

With consideration of the above criteria, a very select group of patients was obtained for implantation of the permanent transvenous cardioverter. Thirteen patients had the device implanted at Indiana University; however, two patients refused follow-up VT induction. For that reason, long-term follow-up of the cardio-

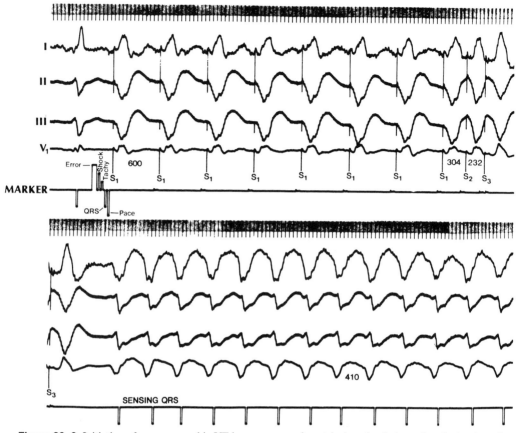

Figure 26–8. Initiation of a monomorphic VT by programmed ventricular stimulation using the implanted device. Surface leads I, II, III, and VI are shown. A marker channel is telemetered from the device and is displayed underneath the surface leads. In the first panel, calibration of the marker channel results in recorded displacements of differing size and shape, representing error, shock, tachycardia detection, normal QRS detection, and ventricular pacing, respectively. In the example shown, a train of eight ventricular pacing stimuli (S_1) is followed by two ventricular extrastimuli (S_2 and S_3). No marker channel deflections occur during programmed stimulation because pacing instructions are being telemetered to the device from the external programmer. Ventricular tachycardia having a left bundle branch block morphology, a rightward axis, and a cycle length of 410 msec is induced, and the marker channel indicates that each QRS complex is being appropriately sensed. The last complex of the first panel is reproduced as the first complex of the second panel. (Reprinted by permission of the New England Journal of Medicine [311; 485–490, 1984].)

verter is available for 11 patients, all but 1 male. The age range was 44 to 67 years (mean of 62 years). All patients had coronary artery disease and had had at least one prior myocardial infarction. Five of the patients had undergone prior cardiac surgery, and five had left ventricular aneurysms. No patient had had a myocardial infarction or cardiac surgery within 6 months prior to implantation of the cardioverter or during the follow-up period. All patients were receiving pharmacologic antiarrhythmic therapy during follow-up. In all but two patients (patients 5 and 8), drug therapy remained unchanged over the duration of follow-up.

PERIOPERATIVE ELECTROPHYSIOLOGIC EVALUATION

Patients underwent electrophysiologic evaluation in the awake and nonsedated state while receiving the antiarrhythmic drug regimen that best controlled their VT and that they would most likely receive during long-term follow-up. A No. 10 French temporary lead (Medtronic 6880) similar to the permanent cardioversion lead and an external cardioverter unit (Medtronic 5350), which delivers shocks that are similar to the implanted unit, were employed. The catheter electrode was inserted

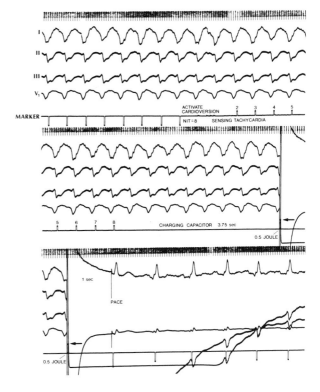

Figure 26–9. Cardioversion of VT. The cardioverter is activated manually via the external programmer. The marker channel then indicates that it interprets the QRS complexes as tachycardia and counts eight complexes. In the second panel, the counting is completed, and the capacitor charge time is 3.75 seconds. A shock of 0.5 J is delivered synchronously to the QRS complex. After a 1-second pause, the unit paces once, but normal sinus rhythm returns, and the marker channel shows sensing of normal QRS complexes. The last complex of each panel is reproduced in the subsequent panel. (Reprinted by permission of the New England Journal of Medicine [311; 485–490, 1984].)

```
*TELEMETRY READ_OUT*
 TEMP MODE = DEMAND
 PERM MODE = DEMAND
 ICT   = OFF       PERM
 TTI   = 505 MS    PERM
 NIT   =  32       PERM
 CPE   = 0.5  JOULE
 RATE  =  45 PPM PERM
 PW    = 0.5  MS PERM
 SENS  = 1.5 MV   PERM
 TELEMETRY = MARKER
 BATTERY   = OK

   ** CONFIRMED **
 NIT  =   8       PERM



   ACTIVATED CARDIOV.
```

Figure 26–10. Print-out of device settings: TEMP MODE = temporary mode (VVI pacing); PERM MODE = permanent mode (automatic cardioversion is turned off); ICT = interval change threshold (cycle length shortening at onset of tachycardia—turned off); TTI = tachycardia trigger interval (cycle length to trigger tachycardia recognition—505 msec); NIT = number of intervals to trigger (consecutive cycles meeting TTI criteria—32); CPE = cardioversion pulse energy (0.5 J); RATE = rate for VVI pacing (45 per minute); PW = pulse width for VVI pacing (0.5 msec); SENS = sensitivity for ventricular sensing (1.5 mV); TELEMETRY = telemetry on marker channel; battery is OK. (From Zipes DP, Heger JJ, Miles WM, et al: Preliminary experiences with the transvenous cardioverter. PACE 7:1325–1330, 1984; with permission.)

through an arm or internal jugular vein after local lidocaine anesthesia and was positioned in the apex of the right ventricle under fluoroscopic guidance. Programmed ventricular stimulation (via the 6880 lead) was utilized to induce the patient's clinically occurring monomorphic VT, after which shocks, similar to those produced by the implantable cardioverter, were delivered via the external unit, which was connected to the lead. The shocks were synchronized to the QRS complex by triggering from the electrogram recorded from the distal pair of electrodes.

Initial shocks were 0.05 J and were gradually increased in intensity until VT termination occurred. The cardioversion threshold was defined as the minimal energy required for consistent termination of VT. If an energy level above 1.7 J was required to terminate VT, or if a synchronized shock accelerated VT by more than 15 beats per minute or resulted in more than three repetitive ventricular complexes after the shock, the patient was considered an unsuitable candidate for permanent cardioverter implantation. At least three episodes of VT were successfully terminated in each patient prior to implantation of the permanent cardioverter. The VT induced at implantation of the device in this group of patients was relatively slow (range of 400 to 510 msec; mean of 453 msec). Five patients (2, 4, 8, 10, and 11) had two distinct monomorphic VT morphologies inducible before implantation of the cardioverter.

At the time of implantation of the cardioverter, the permanent lead was inserted under lidocaine anesthesia through a No. 10 French introducer placed in a cephalic or subclavian vein. Pacing and sensing thresholds were determined to ensure adequate lead tip position. With use of the permanently implanted lead, VT was induced by programmed ventricular stimulation and subsequently terminated by synchronous cardioversion using the temporary external cardioverter unit to be sure that cardioversion threshold and VT response to the shocks were similar to those at the initial electrophysiologic study. If not, the lead position was changed until adequate termination occurred. The permanent lead was then connected with the implanted device, and VT was again induced and then terminated with synchronous shocks given via the device while the patient was still in the operating room. A subcutaneous pocket was created inferior to the clavicle, and the cardioverter was implanted in a manner similar to a standard pacemaker.

The cardioverter was programmed to operate in the automatic mode during the remaining hospitalization only when the patient was being monitored in the coronary care unit. Because the cardioverter cannot terminate VF, automatic tachycardia detection and cardioversion were programmed to be off at the time of hospital discharge, and the device functioned solely as a demand ventricular pacemaker. The referring physicians caring for the patients in the study, who were trained in the use of the programmer, activated the implanted device in an emergency room setting with appropriate defibrillation equipment. Thus, safety and efficacy of the device continued to be tested, a reasonable approach in patients who tolerated VT for several hours without hemodynamic instability. Because of the potential for VT acceleration, the device was only rarely placed in the automatic mode.

LONG-TERM ELECTROPHYSIOLOGIC EVALUATION

Programmed ventricular stimulation was performed noninvasively via the cardioverter

at the time of implantation and 1 week, 1 month, and every 3 months thereafter unless spontaneous VT occurred in the interim and was subsequently successfully terminated with the cardioverter. The VT induction protocol included a structured hierarchy of one to three ventricular extrastimuli introduced after drive trains of eight paced complexes at three pacing cycle lengths.

The mode of VT induction for the 11 patients with long-term follow-up available is illustrated in Figure 26–11. Sustained VT could not be reproducibly induced in patient 1 and was inconsistent in patient 8, although several spontaneous episodes of VT subsequently occurred in patient 8. In the remaining patients,

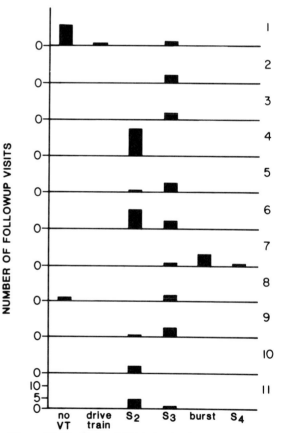

Figure 26–11. Mode of VT induction immediately after implantation and at each of the follow-up visits for each of the 11 patients, numbered at the right of the figure. The height of each bar represents the number of follow-up visits at which VT was induced by the pacing drive train, one ventricular extrastimulus (S_2), two ventricular extrastimuli (S_3), burst ventricular pacing, or three ventricular extrastimuli (S_4). (From Miles WM, Prystowsky EN, Heger JJ, Zipes DP: The implantable transvenous cardioverter: Long-term efficacy and reproducible induction of ventricular tachycardia. Circulation 74:518–524, 1986; by permission of the American Heart Association, Inc.)

the mode of VT induction remained stable over time, with only slight variation. Comparison of the first VT induction after implantation of the cardioverter with subsequent modes of induction disclosed that only patient 7 demonstrated a tendency toward requiring a more aggressive pacing technique to induce the clinical arrhythmia.

Figure 26–12 illustrates VT cycle length data for both spontaneous and induced episodes. Where applicable, tachycardias of different

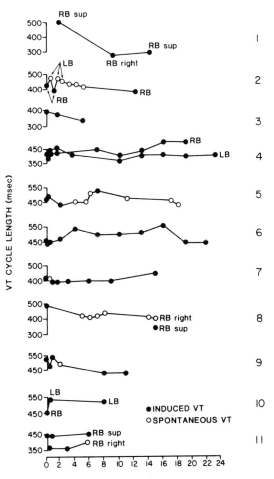

Figure 26–12. VT cycle length in each of the 11 patients over the duration of follow-up. The filled circles represent induced VT, and the unfilled circles, spontaneous VT. Where applicable, VT morphology is noted. LB = left bundle branch block morphology; RB = right bundle branch block morphology; right = right-axis deviation, sup = superior-axis deviation. (From Miles WM, Prystowsky EN, Heger JJ, Zipes DP: The implantable transvenous cardioverter: Long-term efficacy and reproducible induction of ventricular tachycardia. Circulation 74:518–524, 1986; by permission of the American Heart Association, Inc.)

morphologies have been separated. Patients 1 and 8 had inconsistent VT induction during follow-up, with intermittent induction of more rapid tachycardia (thought to be either nonclinical or possibly related to a change in drug therapy in patient 8). The remaining nine patients demonstrated less variation in the cycle length of induced VT. The cycle length of induced VT was comparable to that which had occurred spontaneously. In patients 2, 10, and 11, tachycardia cycle lengths depended on the morphology of tachycardia.

The morphology of VT could be analyzed for most episodes in each of the 11 patients. Five patients (3, 5, 6, 7, and 9) had one monomorphic VT identified, and four patients (2, 4, 10, and 11) had VT with two different morphologies. In the remaining two patients (2 and 8), the more rapid induced VTs were thought to be nonclinical. In all patients with two tachycardia morphologies, intracardiac cardioversion was successful for both morphologies.

Cardioverter sensing was evaluated by measuring the interval in milliseconds between the onset of the QRS complex during tachycardia and the delivery of the shock or the ventricular endocardial sensing marker. Figure 26–13 shows cardioverter sensing over the duration of follow-up for patients in whom monomorphic VTs were available for comparison. The sensing values for each VT morphology tended to show little change during the follow-up.

Patient 4, however, demonstrated transient (≤40 seconds) loss of VT sensing after unsuccessful shocks on two occasions despite stable time to sensing during the follow-up of 24 months. The ventricular pacing threshold remained excellent in this patient (a pulse duration of <0.1 msec). Neither this patient nor any other patient demonstrated loss of ventricular pacing capture when pacing was required immediately after a shock. Reliable sensing and capture over long periods are important, as some authors have suggested that there may be changes in thresholds after transvenous catheter shocks.[16]

Figure 26–14 demonstrates right ventricular effective refractory period determinations that were available in seven patients who had not undergone a change in antiarrhythmic medications during the follow-up period. In patient 1, over a 27-month follow-up period, the right ventricular effective refractory period at pacing cycle lengths 600 and 500 msec was stable after a small initial rise. Shorter follow-up periods

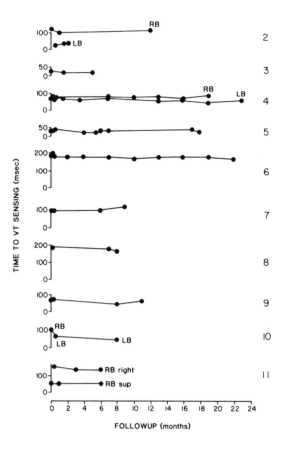

Figure 26–13. Cardioverter sensing over the follow-up period for patients in whom monomorphic VTs were available for comparison. Patient 1 is excluded because two of the three induced tachycardias were thought to be nonclinical arrhythmias. In patients 2, 4, 10, and 11, the sensing for two tachycardia morphologies is shown. The time in milliseconds from the earliest QRS deflection during tachycardia to the ventricular endocardial sensing marker or cardioversion impulse is plotted for each patient. (From Miles WM, Prystowsky EN, Heger JJ, Zipes DP: The implantable transvenous cardioverter: Long-term efficacy and reproducible induction of ventricular tachycardia. Circulation 74:518–524, 1986; by permission of the American Heart Association, Inc.)

Figure 26–14. Right ventricular effective refractory period determinations were available on more than one occasion in seven patients. Drive train pacing cycle lengths of 600 msec (filled circles) and 500 msec (unfilled circles) are illustrated. (From Miles WM, Prystowsky EN, Heger JJ, Zipes DP: The implantable transvenous cardioverter: Long-term efficacy and reproducible induction of ventricular tachycardia. Circulation 74:518–524, 1986; by permission of the American Heart Association, Inc.)

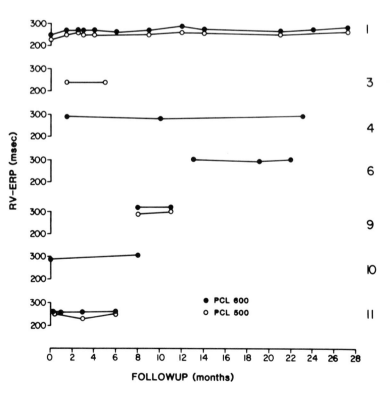

in six other patients also disclosed little variation in the effective refractory period of the right ventricle.

EFFICACY OF LONG-TERM VENTRICULAR TACHYCARDIA CARDIOVERSION (Table 26–3)

At each follow-up visit, the cardioverter delivered a shock at an intensity that had been demonstrated previously to terminate VT effectively. There was no attempt to reestablish cardioversion thresholds over long periods because this would have necessitated multiple shocks at each visit for each patient. All 11 patients had induced VT terminated and 6 of the 11 patients had spontaneous VT terminated by the implanted device. The energy required for successful VT cardioversion was unchanged from initial study in six patients. Four patients required an increase in energy over the duration of follow-up, but successful cardioversion was still reliably achieved. In patients 5, 9, and 11, cardioversion energy was increased by 0.3 to 0.5 J. However, as these were the next highest programmable settings, this apparent increase in energy requirement

may represent only a minimal increase in cardioversion threshold. Patient 8 had one episode of VT that was not terminated with 2 J, but six subsequent episodes were cardioverted successfully with 2 J. There was no evidence that an increase in cardioversion threshold was related to an increased ventricular pacing threshold.

A mean of 1.3 shocks was required to terminate each episode of tachycardia, as VT was not always terminated with the first shock. VT was accelerated on three occasions in patient 3. In addition, this patient also experienced VT acceleration from a synchronized transthoracic shock on a subsequent occasion. VT was also transiently accelerated in both patients 3 and 11, which is a contraindication to leaving the device in the automatic mode. In addition, atrial fibrillation was induced by appropriately timed shocks on at least one occasion each in patients 2 and 5 (Fig. 26–15). Patient 2 had multiple cardioversion discharges during atrial fibrillation (AF) with a rapid ventricular response, while the device was programmed in the automatic mode. One of these discharges was inappropriately synchronized to the QRS complex and precipitated VF (though the patient was successfully resuscitated).

TABLE 26–3. EFFICACY OF CARDIOVERSION

| PATIENT | FOLLOW-UP (MO) | CARDIOVASCULAR ENERGY (J) | | EPISODES OF VT TERMINATED | | COMMENTS |
		At Implantation	At Last Follow-up	Total	Spontaneous VT	
1	27	0.20	0.20	3	0	—
2	13	0.50	0.50	>20	>13	AF once; improperly timed shock during rapid ventricular response to AF precipitated VT on one occasion
3	5	0.20	0.2–0.5	2	0	VT acceleration three times
4	24	1.75	1.75	20	0	—
5	18	0.50	1.00	30	21	AF three times
6	22	0.20	0.20	16	0	—
7	15	0.50	0.50	12	5	—
8	15	0.50	2.00	8	5	Unable to terminate spontaneous VT on one occasion; transient VT acceleration once
9	11	0.50	1.00	8	1	—
10	8	0.50	0.50	5	0	—
11	6	0.20	0.50	13	4	Transient VT acceleration once

AF = atrial fibrillation; VT = ventricular tachycardia.

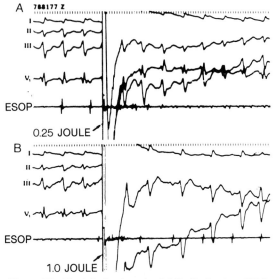

Figure 26–15. *A,* Induction of atrial fibrillation by a QRS-synchronized catheter shock of 0.25 J. Surface leads I, II, III, and V_1 are displayed with an esophageal recording. The low-energy shock is unsuccessful at terminating ventricular tachycardia but occurs during the vulnerable period of the atrium, inducing atrial fibrillation. *B,* The format is identical with that of panel *A.* A second shock of 1.0 J synchronized to the QRS complex successfully terminates both ventricular tachycardia and atrial fibrillation. (From Zipes DP, Heger JJ, Miles WM, et al: Synchronous intracardiac cardioversion. PACE 7:522–533, 1984; with permission.)

CLINICAL IMPLICATIONS

To summarize, long-term cardioversion efficacy was demonstrated by termination of VT on each occasion in nine patients and on eight of nine occasions in one patient. Potential hazards of transvenous cardioversion included acceleration of VT on three of five occasions in one patient and induction of AF in two patients.

Few studies have investigated the stability of electrophysiologic parameters in patients over long periods. Schoenfeld and associates[13] performed two electrophysiologic evaluations in 17 patients in the drug-free state at a mean of 18 months (range of 2 to 42 months) to address long-term reproducibility of ventricular arrhythmias. In their 11 patients with coronary artery disease, VT morphology and induction mode were reproducible, but in patients with heart disease other than coronary artery disease, reproducibility was poor. Without the ability to perform programmed electrical stimulation noninvasively, evaluation of VT reproducibility on multiple occasions over a long period is impractical.

Our data confirm the observations of Schoenfeld. In patients in whom transvenous, low-energy, synchronized cardioversion is effective prior to implantation of a permanent device, the efficacy is likely to continue over the duration of follow-up. Thus, low-energy cardioversion may be a valuable feature in future devices, even though defibrillation backup would be essential. We did not attempt to compare transvenous, synchronized, low-energy cardioversion with pacing techniques for termination of VT.[12, 14] A potential advantage of low-energy cardioversion over pacing is that it does not have to be tailored as carefully to any particular patient or specific arrhythmia and may be employed more quickly than antitachycardia pacing.

The patients in our series represented a select population with slow, monomorphic, sustained VT initially responsive to catheter cardioversion.[2] All patients had stable coronary artery disease, had prior myocardial infarctions, and were receiving antiarrhythmic medications. No patient suffered a myocardial infarction or underwent cardiac surgery during the follow-up period. Thus, the reproducibility of VT characteristics demonstrated in this study population may not necessarily be applicable to all patients with VT.

The presence of more than one monomorphic VT in the same patient is common and adds to the complexity of both the preimplantation evaluation and the subsequent follow-up. Changes in VT activation sequence (VT morphology) may alter the energy required for internal cardioversion, but no distinct VT morphology or sensing time (interval from the beginning of the QRS complex to the onset of the shock) predicted low cardioversion thresholds.[10] Among our six patients with two VT morphologies, both tachycardias could be terminated with low-energy, synchronized cardioversion.

ADVANTAGES AND DISADVANTAGES OF THE CURRENT DEVICE

The transvenous route of insertion and its small size give this early device a clear advantage over other devices that require thoracotomy and placement of an epicardial electrode(s), especially in patients who may be more ill. The low energies delivered by the transvenous cardioverter are usually well tolerated by most patients; shocks below 0.5 J are described as "large hiccups." Cardioversion energies between 1.0 and 2.0 J are associated with more discomfort but are usually well tolerated by most patients. The bradyarrhythmia pacing ability of the device may be important, especially for bradycardias that may occur immediately following termination of VT.

Programmability of tachycardia detection parameters and cardioversion energy increases the flexibility of the device once it has been implanted. The ability to perform noninvasive electrophysiologic studies enables one to test repeatedly the unit for efficacy of cardioversion and for lack of acceleration of VT. Serial electrophysiologic evaluations may also be easily performed in patients if changes in drug therapy become necessary.

A major disadvantage of the device currently in use is the potential complication of VT acceleration, even by a shock synchronized to the QRS complex. Acceleration of VT did occasionally occur in our patients, though they had been carefully screened. Backup defibrillation capabilities are necessary because (1) antitachycardia pacing or low-energy, synchronized cardioversion may accelerate VT to an arrhythmia that cannot be terminated with low energy; (2) a patient who has slow, stable VT on one occasion may have rapid VT or spontaneous VF on another occasion; and (3) if the unit does not properly sense a cardiac impulse, a cardioversion impulse might be delivered at a time other than during the QRS complex, precipitating VF. Attempts at achieving defibrillation capabilities with a transvenous unit are ongoing; sequential shocks over multiple pathways may defibrillate with use of a transvenous lead and a patch, possibly subcutaneous in location.[1] Recently, a biphasic, truncated exponential waveform was found to lower defibrillation energies in humans.[15] In fact, another study showed that transvenous cardioversion of rapid VT (mean cycle length of <300 msec) was effective in 92 per cent of VT episodes using 20 J of energy and dual current pathways—a common right ventricular apical cathode and two anodes (superior vena cava and a skin patch electrode).[11]

AF is a known complication of any implantable antitachycardia device that delivers a shock to the heart. Ventriculoatrial dissociation often occurs during VT. Thus, even though a cardioversion impulse may be synchronized to the ventricular complex, it may occur during the atrial vulnerable period and induce AF (see Fig. 26–15). The algorithm for tachycardia detection of the implanted cardioverter may be unable to differentiate the rapid ventricular response during AF or other supraventricular arrhythmias from VT.

The transient loss of sensing capabilities is a possibility when the same electrode is used for both cardioversion and QRS sensing but does not appear to be a common problem with this device.[16]

FUTURE DIRECTIONS

Smaller and more effective devices will be available as advances in battery, capacitor, and lead technology occur. Future devices will provide several modes for tachycardia termination, including pacing (ventricular extrasystoles or bursts), low-energy, synchronous cardioversion, and defibrillation. The mode and parameters within each mode will be programmable. Escalation to another mode if the first is ineffective will be essential. Tachycardia detection will need to be improved over the present device so that nonsustained VT and supraventricular tachycardias can be reliably recognized. The device will ideally be small and not require a thoracotomy for implantation. It will have the ability to record what it sees and does (telemetry) so that appropriate function can be confirmed. Drug administration may be possible (i.e., lidocaine for an episode of VF). Pacing methods to prevent VT before it occurs may also be developed.[9]

CONCLUSIONS

In patients with inducible, monomorphic, and hemodynamically stable VT, the tachycardia usually remains inducible with similar pacing techniques. VT induction mode, cycle length, morphology, QRS sensing, and ventricular effective refractory period remain stable. Low-energy, synchronized cardioversion, if effective at the time of implantation, can be expected to remain stable, although acceleration of VT may occasionally occur. Reproducibility of VT induction over time by means of noninvasive programmed electrical stimulation will continue to be useful for assessing long-term efficacy of implanted antitachycardia devices.

REFERENCES

1. Chang MS, Inoue H, Kallok MJ, Zipes DP: Double and triple sequential shocks reduce defibrillation

threshold in dogs with and without myocardial infarction. J Am Coll Cardiol 8:1393–1405, 1986.

2. Ciccone JM, Saksena S, Shah Y, Pantopoulos D: A prospective randomized study of the clinical efficacy and safety of transvenous cardioversion for termination of ventricular tachycardia. Circulation 71:571–578, 1985.

3. Jackman WM, Zipes DP: Low-energy synchronous cardioversion of ventricular tachycardia using a catheter electrode in a canine model of subacute myocardial infarction. Circulation 66:187–195, 1982.

4. Miles WM, Heger JJ, Prystowsky EN, Zipes DP: Long-term results of internal low energy cardioversions. *In* Iwa T and Fontaine G: Cardiac Arrhythmias—Recent Progress in Investigation and Management. The Netherlands, Elsevier Science Publishing Co, pp 367–378, 1988.

5. Miles WM, Prystowsky EN, Heger JJ, Zipes DP: The implantable transvenous cardioverter: Long-term efficacy and reproducible induction of ventricular tachycardia. Circulation 74:518–524, 1986.

6. Mirowski JF, Reid PR, Mower MM, et al: Termination of malignant ventricular arrhythmias with an implanted automatic defibrillator in human beings. N Engl J Med 303:322–324, 1980.

7. Mirowski M, Mower MM, Gott VL, Brawley RK: Feasibility and effectiveness of low-energy catheter defibrillation in man. Circulation 47:79–85, 1973.

8. Mirowski M, Mower MM, Langer A, et al: A chronically implanted system for automatic defibrillation in active conscious dogs: Experimental model for treatment of sudden death from ventricular fibrillation. Circulation 58:90–94, 1978.

9. Prystowsky EN, Zipes DP: Inhibition in the human heart. Circulation 68:707–713, 1983.

10. Prystowsky EN, Miles WM, Heger JJ, Zipes DP: Intracavitary cardioversion of ventricular tachycardia in man: Importance of ventricular tachycardia activation sequence on energy requirements for termination [abstract]. J Am Coll Cardiol 5:458, 1985.

11. Saksena S, Calvo RA, Pantopoulos D, et al: A prospective evaluation of single and dual current pathways for transvenous cardioversion in rapid ventricular tachycardia. PACE 10:1130–1141, 1987.

12. Saksena S, Chandran P, Shah Y, et al: Comparative efficacy of transvenous cardioversion and pacing in patients with sustained ventricular tachycardia: A prospective, randomized, crossover study. Circulation 72:153–160, 1985.

13. Schoenfeld MH, McGovern B, Garan H, Ruskin JN: Long-term reproducibility of responses to programmed cardiac stimulation in spontaneous ventricular tachyarrhythmias. Am J Cardiol 54:564–568, 1984.

14. Waspe LE, Kim SG, Matos JA, Fisher JD: Role of a catheter lead system for transvenous countershock and pacing during electrophysiologic tests: An assessment of the usefulness of catheter shocks for terminating ventricular tachyarrhythmias. Am J Cardiol 52:477–484, 1983.

15. Winkle RA, Mead RH, Ruder MA, et al: Improved low energy defibrillation efficacy in man using a biphasic truncated exponential waveform [abstract]. J Am Coll Cardiol 9:142, 1982.

16. Yee R, Jones DL, Klein GJ: Pacing threshold changes after transvenous catheter countershock. Am J Cardiol 53:503–507, 1984.

17. Yee R, Zipes DP, Gulamhusein S, et al: Low energy countershock using an intravascular catheter in an acute care setting. Am J Cardiol 50:1124–1129, 1982.

18. Zipes DP, Heger JJ, Miles WM, et al: Early experience with an implantable cardioverter. N Engl J Med 311:485–490, 1984.

19. Zipes DP, Jackman WM, Heger JJ, et al: Clinical transvenous cardioversion of recurrent life-threatening ventricular tachyarrhythmias: Low energy synchronized cardioversion of ventricular tachycardia and termination of ventricular fibrillation in patients using a catheter electrode. Am Heart J 103:798–794, 1982.

20. Zipes DP, Prystowsky EN, Browne KF, et al: Additional observations on transvenous cardioversion of recurrent ventricular tachycardia. Am Heart J 104:163–164, 1982.

C. Clinical Results with an Implantable Defibrillator

MORTON M. MOWER, IGOR SINGER, E. P. VELTRI, *and* M. MIROWSKI

Over the past two decades, malignant ventricular arrhythmias have gone from being usually fatal to being effectively treatable entities, and this despite generally disappointing experiences with most of the available therapeutic modalities. Many patients are refractory to antiarrhythmic medications, and even those

who are treated with as effective a drug as amiodarone have 1-year mortality rates of 10 to 20 per cent.[13, 25, 28] In addition, the side effects of most of the drugs can be serious, with noncompliance an ever-present possibility. Even more worrisome is the increasing evidence that some of the pharmacologic agents in use may actually be arrhythmogenic and thus aggravate rather than prevent the arrhythmia.[35, 40] With regard to antiarrhythmic surgery, the mortality associated with the procedure alone is approximately 10 per cent, and recurrences are noted in some 20 per cent of surviving patients.[18]

In large part, the major improvement in outlook for the high-risk patient has been due to the introduction into clinical practice of the automatic implantable cardioverter/defibrillator (AICD), which has markedly increased our therapeutic capabilities.[19, 22] This device was approved for widespread use by the United States Food and Drug Administration (FDA) in October 1985. The AICD is an electronic unit intended to prevent sudden cardiac death in high-risk patients. It is designed to sense when ventricular tachycardia (VT) or ventricular fibrillation (VF) occurs and automatically terminate them with high-energy, synchronized electrical shocks.

The concept of a fully implantable automatic system for recognition and treatment of VF was first suggested in 1970.[22, 36] At that time, figures had become available indicating that each year some 450,000 people were dying suddenly of coronary problems in the United States alone.[15] Growing awareness that survival depended on prompt defibrillation led to proliferation of mobile rescue systems and coronary care units.[2, 6, 27] The resulting experiences indicated that VF was the arrhythmia responsible for sudden cardiac death. Then when substantial numbers of resuscitated patients were available to be followed, it was soon realized that VT was frequently the heart rhythm precipitating the arrests and that it would then often quickly degenerate to fibrillation. The accepted effectiveness of external defibrillation and the belief that someday, in some way, the high-risk patient would be able to be identified provided the rationale for the development of an automatic implantable device. Indeed, the prospect of identifying patients seems now at hand. Recent information in this regard in a prospective study of 102 patients after myocardial infarction revealed good progress with combinations of tests,[11] although electrophysiologic testing alone in patients with aborted sudden death may prove to be disappointing.[9]

The early work aimed at developing this device took place at Sinai Hospital of Baltimore, where, in 1969, the first experimental prototype of the system was built and successfully tested in dogs.[21] The first implantation of the device in a human being was performed in February 1980 at The Johns Hopkins Hospital in Baltimore.[24] For the following year, implantations were performed only at that institution, but this was expanded to Stanford University Medical Center in March of 1981. In subsequent years, the number of centers was increased markedly to the present number of 130 throughout the world. To date, almost all AICD implantations in the United States have been performed at centers with a major interest in electrophysiology. Thus, virtually all patients receiving these devices have undergone electrophysiologic and usually angiographic study, and those with inducible arrhythmias have failed serial antiarrhythmic drug testing. These patients are therefore highly refractory to conventional treatment.[45]

DESCRIPTION OF DEVICES

The initial clinical model of the automatic implantable defibrillator (AID) was designed to detect and treat VF only. When it became evident, however, that many patients at high risk of arrhythmia-caused death suffered from VT that occasionally degenerated into VF, the sensing algorithm of the device was modified (AID-B and AID-BR Cardiac Pacemakers, Inc, St Paul, MN) in 1982, by adding cardioverting capabilities.[31, 46] Another technologic milestone was recorded in December 1986, when the first fully integrated circuit version of the device, the Ventak (Cardiac Pacemakers, Inc, St Paul, MN), was first implanted in patients.[29] This latest model, currently in clinical use, weighs 250 grams, occupies a volume of 148 cc, and is hermetically sealed in a titanium case. The system consists of a pulse generator and three electrode leads (Fig. 26–16). Two electrodes sense the morphology of the ventricular electrical activity and are also used for cardioversion and defibrillation. Several electrode systems are available for clinical use, but the most frequent one consists of a pair of epicardial patches. A superior vena cava electrode paired to a single patch on the left ventricle is not used as frequently now. An additional bipolar catheter electrode with two closely spaced rings on its tip wedged into the right ventricular apex or, alternatively, a pair of myocardial screw-in electrodes serves for heart rate determination and R-wave synchronization.

The sensing of a life-threatening arrhythmia is usually based on heart rate analysis and

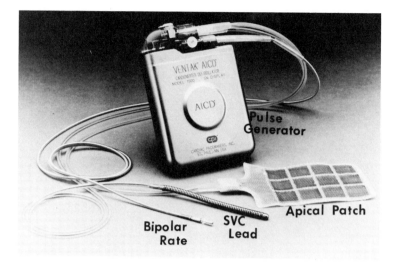

Figure 26–16. The Ventak model of the automatic implantable cardioverter/defibrillator (AICD). From left to right are displayed bipolar right ventricular, superior vena caval (SVC), and apical patch electrodes.

waveform configuration[16]; however, devices having their detection algorithm derived from rate determination alone are also available and, because of their greater sensitivity, are preferred by some investigators. When a "treatment-requiring" arrhythmia is detected, the capacitors are charged by specially designed lithium batteries to approximately 720 V, with the device delivering a truncated exponential pulse of 25-J intensity. If the initial discharge is ineffective, the device recycles, delivering as many as three additional shocks of 30-J intensity during a single arrhythmic episode.

Noninvasive communication with the device before and after implantation is accomplished through magnetically triggered coded audio signals and by use of an external analyzer, the AIDCHECK (Cardiac Pacemakers, Inc, St Paul, MN) (Fig. 26–17). Placement of a ring magnet over the device initiates the charging cycle, the duration of which is measured with an electromagnetic transducer. Progressive increases in charging time indicate battery depletion, while failure to initiate the cycle suggests abnormal operation of the device. The AIDCHECK's digital display shows the cumulative number of pulses delivered by the unit to the patient. During these tests, the pulse generator's energy is diverted into a built-in resistor rather than being allowed to go through the leads to the patient's heart. Using the magnet, one can also deactivate and activate the device at will.

THE POPULATION OF PATIENTS

Until recently, potential implantees had to have a history of at least one episode of VF

or hemodynamically unstable VT not associated with acute myocardial infarction, as well as evidence of incomplete protection by antiarrhythmic medications, as determined by arrhythmia inducibility during electrophysiologic or stress testing or by the inability to suppress complex ventricular arrhythmias on Holter recordings. Recent information, how-

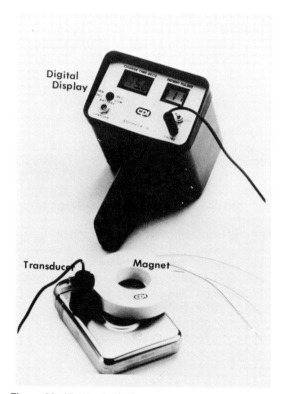

Figure 26–17. The defibrillator analyzer with magnet and electromagnetic transducer placed over the pulse generator. The digital display on the left indicates the capacitor charge time, and that on the right shows the number of discharges delivered by the device to the patient.

ever, strongly suggests that survivors of arrhythmia-produced cardiac arrest who are noninducible also have a very poor prognosis and can benefit from AICD implantation.[42]

As of February 1987, more than 1500 patients with life-threatening ventricular arrhythmias unresponsive to conventional therapy had been treated with the AICD at 79 centers throughout the world, and over 12,700 months of use had been accumulated (personal communication, Cardiac Pacemakers, Inc, St Paul, MN, 1987). These figures change rapidly with each passing month, and because the clinical base is so large, our experience with the device is expanding almost exponentially. As of August 1987, with some 7 years of clinical use internationally and, so far, over 2000 patients treated, in excess of 26,000 device-months have now been logged (personal communication, Cardiac Pacemakers, Inc, St Paul, MN, 1987). It is striking that the mortality from arrhythmias in these implantees has been virtually eradicated.

The clinical profile of the group of patients has been fairly stereotyped. Virtually all implantees have been survivors of multiple cardiac arrests. The great majority suffer from coronary artery disease, but in approximately 20 per cent of the implantees, the underlying disease process was nonischemic cardiomyopathy of a variety of types; a few patients had prolonged QT interval syndrome or primary electrical disease. Congestive heart failure was present in 32 per cent. Most patients have had markedly compromised left ventricular function, with a mean ejection fraction of 32 per cent. Similar patients described in the literature have had 1-year arrhythmia-associated mortality rates ranging from 30 to 60 per cent.[4, 7, 12, 26, 32, 33, 34, 39]

IMPLANTATION OF THE DEVICE

At least four surgical approaches are available. Because of the need to place the electrodes over the heart, insertion of the AICD patches requires some form of thoracotomy. Whenever indicated, coronary artery bypass grafting or antiarrhythmic surgery or both are done at the same time the device is implanted. In general, median sternotomy is preferred when these concomitant cardiac procedures are to be performed, while left thoracotomy is done in patients who have had previous cardiac surgery.[43] Subxiphoidal or subcostal approaches are employed when implantation of the AICD is the only procedure to be performed.[17, 44]

Intraoperative testing for adequacy of sensing and energy requirements is an important part of implantation. In many centers, determining the energy requirement for conversion of VT as well as VF is an integral part of the procedure. It has been shown, for example, that pacemaker interaction and drug effects may lead to interference with sensing or to a raising of the reversion thresholds. Unipolar pacemakers, in particular, are incompatible with the AICD because they inhibit the device's sensing ability. As a result, only bipolar pacemakers should be used in conjunction with the AICD.[1]

Routine determination of the defibrillation threshold during implantation is also most helpful in finding the optimal electrode configuration and placement. Excessive energy levels can be caused by metabolic disorders such as hyperkalemia and by the patient's pharmacologic regimen. For example, amiodarone has been shown to raise the defibrillation threshold.[10, 14] In the rare instances when all efforts fail to reduce a high threshold for defibrillation, the system should not be implanted unless the patient's clinical arrhythmia is VT and uniformly successful cardioversion has been demonstrated.

CLINICAL RESULTS

Under the controlled conditions of the electrophysiology laboratory, the diagnostic ability to identify VT and VF was virtually 100 per cent; the relatively rare instances of misdiagnosis were usually due to lead malposition, 60-cycle interference, or interaction with implanted unipolar pacemakers, all of which were easily identified and corrected. Arrhythmia conversion was usually achieved with a single 25-J shock; the AICD occasionally recycled to achieve reversion. The time interval between onset of the arrhythmia until termination ranged between 11 and 36 seconds (mean of 17 seconds).[31] An example of malignant arrhythmia conversion is depicted in Figure 26–18.

In general, internal discharges are well tolerated, even when delivered to conscious patients, most of whom describe them as moderate blows to the chest resulting in momentary discomfort. No serious emotional problems occur unless the patient receives a large num-

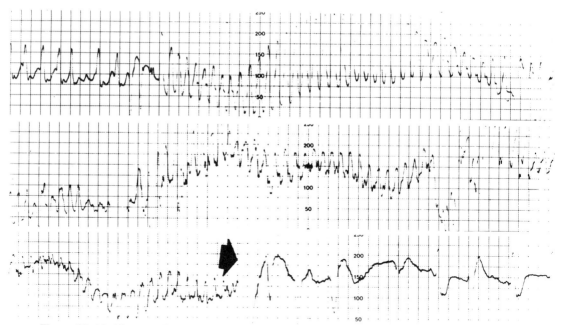

Figure 26–18. Electrocardiogram (ECG) of an implantee who developed atrial flutter of 28 minutes' duration. The device remained silent during this time. The last few beats of this supraventricular rhythm, seen in the left portion of the upper strip, are followed by two spontaneous premature ventricular contractions, which induce ventricular flutter or fibrillation. Twenty-three seconds later (*arrow*), both the atrial flutter and the ventricular fibrillation were automatically terminated with a single 25-J discharge. The strips are continuous.

ber of discharges in a very short period. In this event, it is advisable to deactivate the unit temporarily and stabilize the cardiac rhythm in a hospital setting by pharmacologic or other means. Most patients adapt well to the device and accept it. A degree of emotional lability, depression, and fear are common problems that decrease with time and can be helped by education, counseling, and relaxation techniques.[3, 30]

RISKS AND COMPLICATIONS

The potential risks and complications associated with AICD therapy may be classified broadly into those that are related to surgery or anesthesia and those that are associated with the device or result from drug-pacemaker interactions. The incidence of both kinds of complications differs from center to center and at the present time often reflects the learning curve of the implanting team. The first category includes pocket and systemic infections, low-output state, and blood loss requiring transfusion. Transient pericardial friction rub is ubiquitous during the first days after implantation, but large pericardial effusion is rare.

Complications associated with the device

itself have also often reflected a learning curve, but one of new technology. Pulse generator or lead extrusion and migration may occur. Lead fracture and migration, frequent a few years ago, were remedied by improved construction and fixation techniques. Nine per cent premature battery depletion rates in the early experience were reduced with the application of Teflon to the glass insulator area in the feedthrough connectors. Thromboembolic phenomena are infrequent and have been satisfactorily treated with anticoagulant or antiplatelet drugs. Occasional device malfunctions, such as misdirects, loss of hermeticity, and random component failures, happen. False-positive discharges also occur sometimes but do not result in permanent harm. Rarely, the tachyarrhythmia may be aggravated into an incessant type. Perioperative mortality is low (2 to 5 per cent) (personal communication, Cardiac Pacemakers, Inc, St Paul, MN, 1987).

Arrhythmia acceleration or degeneration may occur whenever VT is treated with electrical discharges, as, for example, during external or transvenous cardioversion and with antitachycardia pacing. Under these circumstances, the tachycardia, rather than being terminated, may become faster and less organized and may even degenerate into VF. This life-threatening complication is independent of the energy levels used. The AICD is the only implantable system capable of controlling acceleration or degeneration through recycling, recognizing the new rhythm de novo and correcting it automatically with one or more subsequent internal discharges.

COST OF THERAPY

The cost of the AICD device alone is approximately $14,000. An analysis of overall hospital charges and costs information has shown an average hospital charge of more than $51,000 for an initial implantation and $18,000 for a replacement unit. Although both types of cases involve implantation of the same device, most patients receiving an initial implant have this procedure done at the end of a long hospitalization, frequently filled with an extensive workup, including multiple electrophysiologic studies, and have been refractory to multiple drug trials. In addition, some patients who receive an AICD implant have other cardiac surgery performed at the same time or during the same hospitalization. For example, patients with VT or VF may have a discrete site on the heart that can be identified as the source of the arrhythmia. At the time they undergo excision or ablation of the site, they may also have an AICD lead implanted. If the cardiac surgery is found not to eliminate the arrhythmia, the complete system may then be implanted. Another type of cardiac surgery that patients receiving AICDs frequently undergo is coronary artery bypass grafting. Such patients will also have higher charges than patients having an AICD implant alone. It should be realized, however, that overall costs for treating patients with arrhythmias may decline as the AICD decreases subsequent hospitalizations for arrhythmic breakthrough and the patients become fairly easy to manage as outpatients.

The Health Care Financing Administration (HCFA) began studying the AICD for the Medicare program in 1985 in regard to issues of insurance coverage and reimbursement. The HCFA announced in March of 1986 a decision for Medicare to pay for cases involving implantation of a "complete defibrillator system" as if they fell into diagnosis-related group (DRG) 104 (cardiac surgical procedure) and to pay for "less comprehensive procedures such as lead or pulse generator replacements" as if grouped to DRG 117 (pacemaker replace-

ment). It was recommended, however, that the AICD should ultimately be assigned to its own unique DRG (personal communication, Cardiac Pacemakers, Inc, St Paul, MN, 1987).

IMPACT ON MORTALITY

In a 6-year cumulative experience with the AICD, approximately 50 per cent of patients had at least one out-of-hospital AICD discharge that was classified as an "appropriate" discharge based on hypotensive symptoms or AICD discharge during sleep.[41] In addition, approximately 20 per cent of patients have experienced an AICD discharge in the absence of any prodromal symptoms, and some 20 per cent of these have been documented by continuous electrocardiographic monitoring to be due to ventricular tachyarrhythmias.[38]

The impact of the AICD on the mortality rates of the implantees has been examined by a number of investigators and is remarkably consistent. Although the expected mortality rate of the type of patients operated upon ranges in historical controls between 27 and 66 per cent,[4, 5, 12, 37] actuarial analysis has shown the 1-year sudden death mortality in the AICD implantees to be about 2 per cent or less. For example, in a study of 70 such patients treated with the AICD at Stanford University Hospital, 1-year mortality due to arrhythmia was 1.8 per cent.[8] In 151 Baltimore patients treated with the AICD, the 1-year sudden death mortality was 2.1 per cent; it was 1.4 per cent when patients whose devices were inactive at the time of death were excluded.[23] Data submitted by the manufacturer of the device prior to approval by the FDA were derived from the analysis of 618 patients[8] and showed virtually identical results, 1.9 per cent. Most recently, analysis of 1100 patients worldwide[20] continues to show the same results (Fig. 26–19). In this analysis, sudden deaths, cardiac deaths (which include arrhythmias as well as entities such as heart failure), and total mortality (including all of the above) are plotted separately. The 1-year death rates due to sudden death, cardiac death, and all deaths are seen to be 1.8 per cent, 8 per cent, and 12 per cent, respectively.

NEED FOR PULSE GENERATOR REPLACEMENT

The available data on long-term follow-up of patients with AICDs who were treated at

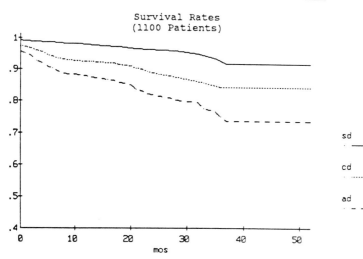

Figure 26–19. Kaplan-Meier curves for sudden death (*solid line*), arrhythmia-related death (*dotted line*), and total mortality (*dashed line*) in 1100 patients worldwide. Note rates of 1.8 per cent, 8.0 per cent, and 12.0 per cent, respectively, at 1 year following implantation. Sd = Sudden death; cd = cardiac death; ad = all deaths.

the Johns Hopkins and Sinai Hospitals in Baltimore would support the need for AICD pulse generator replacement at battery end of life, even in the absence of appropriate AICD discharge during the first or second year post implantation. Of the first 148 patients with AICDs recently analyzed, 46 per cent experienced the first appropriate AICD discharge during the first year and 21 per cent during the second year post implantation. Aside from these patients with appropriate AICD discharge, who are at very high risk of recurrent AICD discharge—namely, 43 per cent at subsequent 18-month follow-up—it is extremely important to note, however, that in 8 to 10 per cent of instances, the first AICD discharge occurred in the third, fourth, and fifth years post implantation. Thus, in light of this very high incidence of first arrhythmic events late after initiation of AICD therapy, we recommend that all patients have pulse generator replacements (E. P. Veltri, unpublished data).

APPLICATION TO GROUPS AT LESSER RISK

It seems evident that the AICD can successfully detect and correct VT and VF. The use of this therapeutic modality has resulted in an impressive decrease in sudden death mortality. The potential risks and dangers associated with the AICD in these high-risk patients are moderate and often unavoidable.

Although we have no evidence indicating that the clinical benefit of the device would be greater or longer lasting for patients with less advanced left ventricular dysfunction than in those treated so far, studies of AICD effectiveness in such lower-risk groups may well be warranted now. Certainly, it would be worthwhile to risk-stratify patients even before a first arrhythmic event and consider the very highest-risk groups as prospective candidates for implantation.

The total number of patients needing AICD implantation will probably rise remarkably in the future. Thus, it is probably fair to say that as of this time the full potential of this exciting new treatment to save lives has yet to be realized.

REFERENCES

1. Bach SM: Cardioverter-Defibrillator: Possible Interaction with Pacemakers. Pittsburgh, Intec Systems Technical Bulletin, 1983.
2. Brown KWG, MacMillan RL, Forbath N, et al: Coronary unit: An intensive-care centre for acute myocardial infarction. Lancet 2:349–352, 1963.
3. Bryant JM, Pardoe P: Care of the patient with an automatic implantable cardioverter-defibrillator. *In* Reigel B, Purcell JA, Brest AN, Dreifus FA (eds): Dreifus' Pacemaker Therapy: An Interprofessional Approach. Philadelphia, FA Davis, 1986, pp 189–200.
4. Cobb LA, Werner JA, Trobaugh GB: Sudden cardiac death. Mod Concepts Cardiovasc Dis 49:31–36, 1980.
5. Cobb LA, Baum RS, Alvarez H, III, Schaffer WA: Resuscitation from out-of-hospital ventricular fibrillation: 4 years follow-up. Circulation 52 (Suppl III):223–228, 1975.
6. Day HW: An intensive coronary care area. Dis Chest 44:423–427, 1963.
7. Denniss AR, Baijens H, Cody DV, et al: Value of programmed stimulation and exercise testing in predicting one-year mortality after acute myocardial infarction. Am J Cardiol 56:213–220, 1985.

8. Echt DS, Armstrong K, Schmidt P, et al: Clinical experience: Complications and survival in 70 patients with the automatic implantable cardioverter-defibrillator. Circulation 71:289–296, 1985.
9. Eldar M, Sauve MJ, Scheinman MM: Electrophysiologic testing and follow-up of patients with aborted sudden death. J Am Coll Cardiol 10:291–298, 1987.
10. Forgoros RN: Amiodarone-induced refractoriness to cardioversion. Ann Intern Med 100:699–700, 1984.
11. Gomes JA, Winters SL, Stewart D, et al: A new noninvasive index to predict sustained ventricular tachycardia and sudden death in the first year after myocardial infarction: Based on signal-averaged electrocardiogram, Radionuclide ejection fraction and Holter monitoring. J Am Coll Cardiol 10:349–357, 1987.
12. Graboys TB, Lown B, Podrid PJ, Desilva R: Long-term survival of patients with malignant ventricular arrhythmias treated with antiarrhythmic drugs. Am J Cardiol 50:437–443, 1982.
13. Green HL, Graham EL, Werner JA, et al: Toxic and therapeutic effects of amiodarone in the treatment of cardiac arrhythmia. J Am Coll Cardiol 2:1114–1128, 1983.
14. Haberman RJ, Veltri EP, Mower MM: The effect of amiodarone on defibrillation threshold. PACE 10:406, 1987.
15. Kuller L: Sudden death in atherosclerotic heart disease: The case for preventive medicine. Am J Cardiol 24:617, 1969.
16. Langer A, Heilman MS, Mower MM, Mirowski M: Considerations in the development of the automatic defibrillator. Med Instrum 10:163–167, 1976.
17. Lawrie GM, Griffin JC, Wyndham CRC: Epicardial implantation of the automatic implantable defibrillator by left subcostal thoracotomy. PACE 7:1370–1374, 1984.
18. Miller JM, Kienzle MG, Harken AH, Josephson ME: Subendocardial resection for ventricular tachycardia: Predictors of surgical success. Circulation 70:624–631, 1983.
19. Mirowski M: Prevention of sudden arrhythmic death with implanted automatic defibrillators. Ann Intern Med 97:606–608, 1982.
20. Mirowski M: Worldwide experience with low and high energy cardioversion/defibrillation devices in recurrent ventricular tachycardia. In Abstracts of the NASPE Policy Conference on The Clinical Investigation of New Implantable Antitachycardia Devices, Dallas, 1986.
21. Mirowski M, Mower MM, Langer A, et al: A chronically implanted system for automatic defibrillation in active conscious dogs: Experimental model for treatment of sudden death from ventricular fibrillation. Circulation 58:90–94, 1978.
22. Mirowski M, Mower MM, Staewen WS, et al: Standby automatic defibrillator: An approach to prevention of sudden coronary death. Arch Intern Med 126:158–161, 1970.
23. Mirowski M, Mower MM, Veltri EP, et al: Clinical experience with the automatic implantable cardioverter-defibrillator. In Cardiac Arrhythmias—Recent Progress in Investigation and Management. The Netherlands, Elsevier Science Publishing Co, [in press].
24. Mirowski M, Reid PR, Mower MM, et al: Termination of malignant ventricular arrhythmias with an implanted automatic defibrillator in human beings. N Engl J Med 303:322–324, 1980.
25. Morady F, Sauve MJ, Malone P, et al: Long-term
26. Multicenter Postinfarction Research Group: Risk stratification and survival after myocardial infarction. N Engl J Med 309:331, 1983.
27. Pantridge JF, Geddes JS: A mobile intensive-care unit in the management of myocardial infarction. Lancet 2:271–273, 1967.
28. Peter T, Hamer A, Weiss D, et al: Prognosis after sudden cardiac death without associated myocardial infarction: One year follow-up of empiric therapy with amiodarone. Am Heart J 107:209–213, 1984.
29. Physicians Manual for the CPI AICD. St Paul, MN, Cardiac Pacemakers Inc, 1986.
30. Pycha C, Gulledge AD, Hutzler J, et al: Psychological responses to the implantable defibrillator: Preliminary observations. Psychosomatics 27:841–845, 1986.
31. Reid PR, Mirowski M, Mower MM, et al: Clinical evaluation of the internal automatic cardioverter-defibrillator in survivors of sudden cardiac death. Am J Cardiol 51:1608–1613, 1983.
32. Richards DA, Cody DV, Denniss AR, et al: Ventricular electrical instability: A predictor of death after myocardial infarction. Am J Cardiol 50:23–29, 1982.
33. Roy D, Marchand E, Theroux P, et al: Programmed ventricular stimulation in survivors of an acute myocardial infarction. Circulation 72:487–494, 1985.
34. Ruskin JN, DiMarco JP, Garan H: Out-of-hospital cardiac arrest: Electrophysiologic observations and selection of long-term antiarrhythmic therapy. N Engl J Med 303:607–613, 1980.
35. Ruskin JN, McGovern B, Garan H, et al: Antiarrhythmic drugs: A possible cause of out-of-hospital cardiac arrest. N Engl J Med 309:1302–1306, 1983.
36. Schuder JC, Stoeckle H, Gold JH, et al: Experimental ventricular defibrillation with an automatic and completely implanted system. Trans Am Soc Artif Organs 16:207–212, 1970.
37. Schulze RA, Jr, Strauss HW, Pitt B: Sudden death in the year following myocardial infarction: Relation to ventricular premature contractions in the late hospital phase and left ventricular ejection fraction. Am J Med 62:192–199, 1977.
38. Guarnieri T, Strickberger A, Magiros E, et al: Is an asymptomatic automatic implantable cardioverter-defibrillator (AICD) discharge a false positive? PACE 10:II–983, 1987.
39. Swerdlow CD, Winkle RA, Mason JW: Determinants of survival in patients with ventricular tachyarrhythmias. N Engl J Med 308:1436–1442, 1983.
40. Velebit V, Podrid P, Lown B, et al: Aggravation and provocation of ventricular arrhythmias by anti-arrhythmic drugs. Circulation 65:886–894, 1982.
41. Veltri EP, Mower MM, Guarnieri T, et al: Clinical efficacy of the automatic implantable defibrillator: 6 year cumulative experience. Circulation 74 [Suppl II]:109, 1986.
42. Veltri EP, Mower MM, Mirowski M, et al: Clinical outcome of patients with noninducible ventricular tachyarrhythmias and the automatic implantable defibrillator. Circulation 74 [Suppl II]:109, 1986.
43. Watkins L Jr, Mirowski M, Mower MM, et al: Automatic defibrillation in man: The initial surgical experience. J Thorac Cardiovasc Surg 82:492–500, 1981.
44. Watkins L Jr, Mirowski M, Mower MM, et al: Im-

efficacy and toxicity of high-dose amiodarone therapy for ventricular tachycardia or ventricular fibrillation. Am J Cardiol 52:975–979, 1983.

plantation of the automatic defibrillator: The subxi-phoidal approach. Ann Thorac Surg 34:515–520, 1982.

45. Winkle RA, Thomas A: The automatic implantable cardioverter defibrillator: The U.S. experience. Brugada P, Wellens HJJ (eds): *In* Cardiac Arrhyth-mias: Where to Go from Here. Mount Kisco, Futura Publishing Co, 1987, pp 663–680.

46. Winkle RA, Bach SM, Echt DS, et al: The automatic implantable defibrillator: Local ventricular bipolar sensing to detect ventricular tachycardia and fibril-lation. Am J Cardiol 52:265–270, 1983.

D. Implantable Antitachycardia Devices—The Next Generation

SANJEEV SAKSENA

Implantable devices designed to terminate tachyarrhythmias have been under development for nearly two decades. Implantable cardioverter/defibrillators are being increasingly employed as chronic therapy for patients with sustained ventricular tachycardia (VT) and ventricular fibrillation (VF).[37, 39] In contrast, implantable devices for termination of supraventricular tachycardia (SVT), such as antitachycardia pacemakers, have not achieved comparable popularity.[51] The approval of the first implantable cardioverter/defibrillator (Automatic Implantable Cardioverter-Defibrillator or AICD, Cardiac Pacemakers Inc, St Paul, MN) in 1985 for general clinical application was a major step in the treatment of VT and VF. Continuing widespread application confirms its clinical efficacy in reducing from arrhythmic mortality in short-term and long-term studies.[40] However, increasing clinical experience has uncovered a myriad of issues that remain to be addressed. The need for epicardial electrode systems, frequent exposure of the patient to uncomfortable high-energy shocks, inappropriate device activation, nonprogrammability, absence of pacing and monitoring capabilities, limited battery life with an oversized pulse generator, and considerations of surgical risk during device implantation continue to plague the current-generation device. Careful analysis of individual center experiences[22, 32] confirms these limitations and are detailed in Chapter 27. The next-generation device is designed to address many of these issues. This section will examine the basis of future development in these areas as well as currently available information on second-generation implantable cardioverter/defibrillators.

THE SECOND-GENERATION IMPLANTABLE CARDIOVERTER/ DEFIBRILLATOR

Tachycardia Termination

The combination of an implantable pacemaker with a cardioverter/defibrillator has long been suggested.[67] The rationale for such devices is based on the frequent clinical association of bradyarrhythmias requiring demand pacing with recurrent ventricular tachyarrhythmias. Furthermore, some patients with recurrent VT and VF will manifest transient but symptomatic bradyarrhythmias after cardioversion and defibrillation. Finally, selected VT episodes can be cardioverted by painless rapid pacing modes, which thus can eliminate the discomfort associated with direct-current (DC) shock cardioversion.[52] The efficacy of asynchronous rate-adaptive burst pacing is comparable to that of low-energy intracavitary shocks for VT termination and has superior tolerance by the patient.[52] Early prototype devices used for the treatment of patients with recurrent SVT and VT employed pacing for bradycardia rate support and tachycardia termination.[19, 41, 56] These devices were applicable only to highly selected patients, and tachycardia acceleration with the potential for fibrillation remained an ever-present hazard. Induction of VF in patients with recurrent VT, or atrial fibrillation (AF) in patients with Wolff-Parkinson-White syndrome and rapid, antegradely conducting bypass tracts, has culminated in sudden death.[59, 60] Two combination prototype devices have also been evaluated, and their clinical experiences are detailed in the second and third sections of this chapter. The first implantable cardioverter/defibrillator had combined cardioversion and defibrillation capabilities using a high-energy direct-current shock for both purposes but lacked pacing therapy. Another first-generation device (Medtronic model 7210, Medtronic, Minneapolis, MN) had a capability for transvenous pacing and low-energy direct-current shock delivery and was used in patients with recurrent VT. Clinical evaluation demonstrated similar concerns and limitations as previously described for antitachycardia pacemakers.[36, 68] Safety concerns, particularly with respect to VT acceleration, precluded use of this device in an automatic mode or in an unsupervised clinical setting. This device was also not applicable to patients with rapid VT or VF. Second-generation implantable cardioverters/defibrillators seek to correct these device limitations. Important objectives include (1) applicability to a more diverse population of patients with ventricular tachyarrhythmias; (2) rational combination of therapeutic electrical modes; and (3) improving ease and safety of device implantation.

Nonepicardial Electrode Systems

Current investigative efforts have attempted to examine combination electrical therapy in the electrophysiology laboratory. Acute studies combining pacing and shock therapy in our laboratory have utilized wholly transvenous or combined transvenous and cutaneous electrode systems. Pacing is usually performed via bipolar right ventricular endocardial electrodes. Shocks have been delivered through dual or triple electrode systems, permitting single (unidirectional) or dual (bidirectional) current pathways, respectively. Triple electrode systems permit simultaneous or sequential energy delivery into each current pathway.

Typically, two catheter electrodes and one cutaneous electrode are employed for shock delivery (Fig. 26–20). Prototype tripolar electrode catheters used in these studies included the Medtronic 6880 (Medtronic, Minneapolis, MN) and the Endotak C (Cardiac Pacemakers Inc, St Paul, MN) systems (Figs. 26–21 and 26–22). Both catheters are inserted transvenously and have two defibrillation electrodes at varying interelectrode distances. The distal electrode at the catheter tip can be positioned in the right ventricular apex. Another electrode 100 to 150 mm proximal to the distal electrode is positioned in the right atrium or superior vena cava. The two electrode catheters differ significantly with respect to surface area of the defibrillation electrode. The Medtronic 6880 defibrillating electrodes have a surface area of 125 mm^2, while the Endotak C has surface areas of 400 mm^2 and 800 mm^2 for its distal and proximal electrodes, respectively. Subsequent generations of this device have somewhat smaller surface areas. The distal right ventricular defibrillation electrode in the Medtronic 6880 actually consists of two electrodes, which become common for shock delivery but can be used separately for bipolar pacing. The third electrode in the Endotak C catheter is a porous-tip electrode that can be used for pacing and sensing. Bipolar stimulation and recording are achieved using the distal defibrillation electrode as the second electrode. A modified version of the Medtronic 6880 (Medtronic model 6882) with active-fixation properties was used in conjunction with the prototype pacemaker/cardioverter (Medtronic model 7210).[36] The Endotak C catheter has been implanted in conjunction with the AICD.[47]

Non-Epicardial Electrode System for ICD's

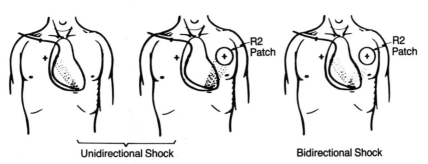

Unidirectional Shock   Bidirectional Shock

Figure 26–20. Different shock delivery patterns are feasible with nonepicardial electrode systems consisting of two catheter electrodes and one chest wall electrode. Unidirectional shocks employ any two electrodes, while bidirectional shocks employ a triple electrode system. Additional configurations for bidirectional shocks (e.g., using both catheter electrodes or patch electrodes as one anode or cathode) and alternative patch locations (apical, posterior, and left lateral) are also possible.

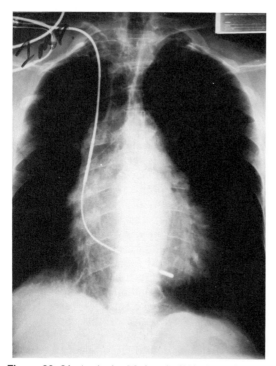

Figure 26–21. A tripolar Medtronic 6880 electrode catheter is introduced in the right subclavian vein, and its distal tip is positioned in the right ventricular apex. The distal two electrodes (total surface area, 125 mm²) are used for pacing and become common during shock delivery. The proximal electrode is common with an identical surface area and is separated by a distance of 12.5 cm from the distal electrodes. It is positioned at the high right atrial–superior vena caval junction.

Early, controlled prospective studies using the Medtronic 6880 catheter and unidirectional shocks demonstrated that effective VT cardioversion was related to tachycardia cycle length

and absolute shock energy[9] (Fig. 26–23). Low-energy shocks (up to 2.7 J) terminated 56 per cent of all VT episodes, while intermediate-energy shocks (up to 10 J) terminated 72 per cent of all VT episodes.[9] However, tachycardia acceleration occurred in 31 per cent of these episodes, and results were especially poor for episodes with cycle lengths below 300 msec. More than 25 per cent of these rapid VT episodes failed to terminate at energies of 20 J.[46, 49] Later studies employing the Endotak C and unidirectional shocks of 15 J using two catheter electrodes demonstrated a failure to cardiovert 25 per cent of rapid VT episodes.[1] Thus, the use of low-energy transvenous shocks in future programmable devices is likely to be limited. Randomized, controlled studies have shown comparable efficacy of right ventricular burst pacing, with inferior tolerance by the patient.[52] The incidence of VT acceleration is slightly lower with burst pacing.[48] Considerable concordance in efficacy of the two modes is also present.[52] Availability (i.e., selected based on tachycardia cycle length) of burst pacing modes in future devices should relegate low-energy transvenous shocks to a secondary therapeutic mode, which will be useful in selected patients.

Subsequent investigations at our center indicated that the addition of a cutaneous patch electrode to the two Medtronic 6880 catheter electrodes permitted dual current pathways during single and sequential bidirectional shock delivery.[30, 50, 57] In several studies, a right ventricular common cathode with dual anodes (superior vena caval and cutaneous electrodes) was employed. VT cardioversion thresholds

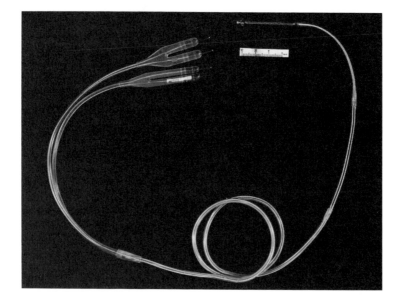

Figure 26–22. A tripolar Endotak C electrode catheter is introduced into the left subclavian vein. The distal electrode is a porous-tip pacing electrode narrowly separated from a distal cardioversion/defibrillation spring electrode (surface area, 400 mm²). The distal tip electrode is used in conjunction with the distal spring for bipolar pacing. A proximal spring electrode, separated by 10 to 13 cm from the distal electrode, has a surface area of 800 mm² and is also positioned at the superior vena caval–right atrial junction. (From Saksena S, Lindsay BD, Parsonnet V: Development of future implantable cardioverters and defibrillators. Pacing Clin Electrophysiol 10:1350, 1987; with permission.)

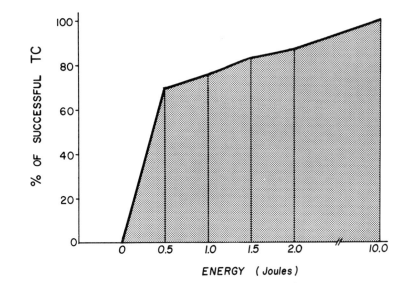

Figure 26–23. Frequency of successful termination of VT at different shock energy levels with transvenous cardioversion. Successful termination was achieved in 62 per cent of all VT episodes with unidirectional shocks up to 10 J in this study. (Ciccone JM, Saksena S, Shah Y, et al: A prospective, randomized study of the clinical efficacy and safety of transvenous cardioversion for ventricular tachycardia termination. Circulation 71:577, 1985; by permission of the American Heart Association, Inc.)

declined, and efficacy of cardioversion increased at each energy level with this approach[50, 57] (Figs. 26–24 and 26–25). With this electrode system, VT can be cardioverted by 25-J bidirectional shocks, regardless of rate and drug therapy.[30, 48, 57] However, reliable defibrillation was possible in fewer than 40 per cent of all VF episodes with the Medtronic 6880 catheter, using 25-J bidirectional shocks.[30, 57] This energy level approaches the maximal potential output for implantable devices. Catheter electrodes of larger surface area improve efficacy of ventricular defibrillation with this triple electrode configuration.[57] A pilot study with the Endotak C catheter demonstrated reliable defibrillation with 25-J bidirectional shocks[57] (Fig. 26–26). The effectiveness of unidirectional shocks using one catheter and one cutaneous apical patch electrode has also been studied. This configuration

is inferior to bidirectional shocks with both catheter systems.[1, 49] Cardioversion of rapid VT with this electrode system was achieved in 57 per cent of episodes at the 15-J level with the Endotak C catheter and in fewer than 35 per cent of episodes with the Medtronic 6880 catheter.[1, 46, 49] In some studies, this configuration has been inferior to the two catheter electrodes alone for each system.[1] As optimal lead arrays are defined for nonepicardial lead systems, it may be possible to reduce energies required for reliable cardioversion and defibrillation. The use of bidirectional shocks is of value in this regard. Studies using epicardial electrodes also suggest reduction in defibrillation threshold with single and sequential bidirectional shocks.[3, 6, 27, 53] Sequential shocks offer the advantage of controlled energy delivery into each current pathway. Future devices may need to be programmed for differential energy

Figure 26–24. Efficacy of unidirectional shocks (6880 catheter electrodes only) compared with bidirectional shocks (right ventricular [RV] apical cathode to superior vena cava and cutaneous patch anodes) for rapid VT (cycle length < 300 msec) cardioversion at different energy levels. Bidirectional shocks have higher efficacy at 10 J and 20 J. Note the need for high-energy delivery for improved efficacy rates. However, the VT mean cardioversion energy in the 2.7- to 10.0-J range is significantly lower ($P < .05$) for bidirectional shocks than for unidirectional shocks. (From Saksena S, Lindsay BD, Parsonnet V: Development of future implantable cardioverters and defibrillators. Pacing Clin Electrophysiol 10:1347, 1987; with permission.)

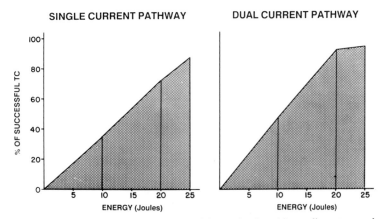

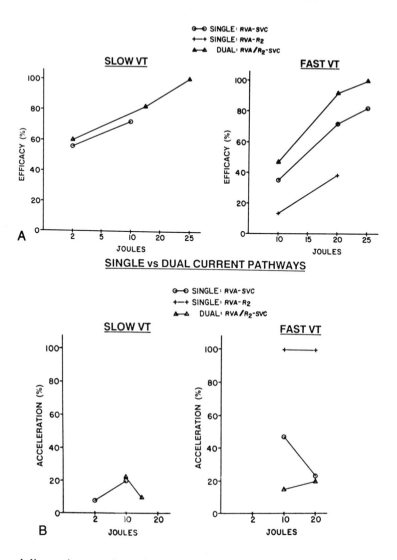

Figure 26–25. Efficacy (*A*) and safety (*B*) of unidirectional (single current pathway) and bidirectional (dual current pathway) shocks for slow and rapid VT cardioversion. Note that the RV apex (cathode) to apical R$_2$ patch (anode) unidirectional current pathway had the lowest efficacy rate and frequently resulted in VT acceleration that could only be infrequently terminated at 20 J. RVA = right ventricular apex; SVC = superior vena cava. (From Saksena S, Lindsay BD, Parsonnet V: Development of future implantable cardioverters and defibrillators. Pacing Clin Electrophysiol 10:1349, 1987; with permission.)

delivery into each pathway to maximize efficiency of defibrillation with conservation of pulse generator energy stores. Experimental support for the use of more than two current pathways for energy delivery is at present unavailable.[6]

Combined Pacemaker–Cardioverter/Defibrillator

It is clearly recognized that implantable cardioverter/defibrillators constitute palliative therapy and permit recurrences of symptomatic VT and VF. Therefore, combined therapy with antiarrhythmic drugs is often advocated to reduce the frequency and symptoms of recurrent arrhythmias. Combined pacing and shock algorithms for VT cardioversion have been examined in the presence and ab-

sence of antiarrhythmic drug therapy. These algorithms have been based largely on tachycardia rate. The rationale for this approach is based on the observations that clinical symptomatology, hemodynamic tolerance for the arrhythmia, and effectiveness of pacing and shock interventions are all related to this parameter.[9, 18, 53] A properly designed electrical algorithm should seek to minimize serious symptomatology associated with the arrhythmia recurrence while permitting maximal tolerance by the patient and effectiveness of the therapy. It has been previously demonstrated that single extrastimuli have lower efficacy than multiple extrastimuli, which in turn are less effective than burst pacing for VT cardioversion.[18, 42] Recently, rate-adaptive burst pacing alone or in conjunction with adaptive stimulus train length has been proposed.[8, 14]

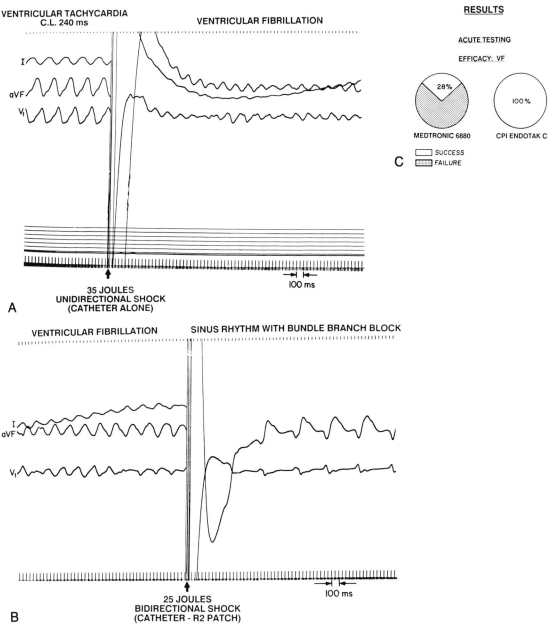

Figure 26–26. Acute testing of unidirectional and bidirectional shocks with Endotak C catheter and cutaneous R_2 patch in a patient who subsequently underwent implantation of a permanent nonepicardial lead system for defibrillation in conjunction with the AICD. *A,* Rapid VT episode is accelerated to ventricular fibrillation (VF) by a 35-J unidirectional shock employing Endotak C catheter electrodes only. *B,* VF episode is terminated by a simultaneous bidirectional shock using the distal RV apical electrode as cathode and proximal catheter electrode at the superior vena caval–right atrial junction and cutaneous R_2 patch (location: midaxillary line at fourth intercostal space) as two separate anodes. *C,* Frequency of successful VF termination with 25-J bidirectional shocks using the Medtronic 6880 and Endotak C catheter electrode catheters in conjunction with a cutaneous patch electrode. (*B* from Saksena S, Lindsay BD, Parsonnet V: Development of future implantable cardioverters and defibrillators. Pacing Clin Electrophysiol 10:1351, 1987; with permission.)

Comparative data on these modes are currently unavailable. To date, three different electrical algorithms have been reported from our laboratory using nonepicardial electrode systems.[4, 5, 30, 48] The VT rate cut-off has varied from 200 to 215 beats per minute in these reports. Slower episodes have been treated with sequential pacing and shock therapy, while faster episodes have been directly exposed to incremental unidirectional or bidirec-

TABLE 26–4. ELECTRICAL ALGORITHMS USING A COMBINATION OF THERAPEUTIC MODES*

PACING THERAPY: ASYNCHRONOUS BURSTS AT ADAPTIVE RATES (90%, 80%, AND 70% OF VT CYCLE LENGTH)

Method A	Method B	Method C
10 and 15 stimuli, applied twice	15 stimuli, applied once	5 stimuli at 90%, 8 stimuli at 80%, 10 stimuli at 70%, applied twice

SHOCK THERAPY:

Method A	Method B	Method C
Unidirectional, 2.7, 5.4, and 10 J	Bidirectional, 5, 15, and 25 J	Bidirectional, 25 J

*Individual steps in three sequential transvenous pacing and shock algorithms investigated during clinical electrophysiologic studies. Slow ventricular tachycardia (VT) was defined as tachycardia cycle lengths of more than 280 msec for method A and more than 300 msec for methods B and C. Rapid VT cycle lengths were less than 270 msec in method A and less than 290 msec in methods B and C. Sequential pacing and shock therapy were used for slow VT and shocks alone for rapid VT.

tional shocks. Table 26–4 illustrates the individual steps in these three different algorithms. Rate-adaptive, asynchronous burst pacing was used in each method. In method A, only unidirectional shocks were employed, while bidirectional shocks were used in the remaining two methods. The clinical results are illustrated in Figure 26–27. Method A had substantial efficacy in slow VT episodes but was inadequate for fast episodes. Method B increased efficacy at both tachycardia rates, but

acceleration to VF was frequently observed with intermediate-energy shocks (5 and 15 J).[30, 48] Elimination of these intermediate energies in method C resulted in complete resolution of this safety hazard.[48] The use of rate- and train-adaptive versus rate-adaptive pacing bursts alone does not increase efficacy and shows a trend toward greater risk of acceleration. Adjunctive therapy with antiarrhythmic medications prolongs the cycle length of the tachycardia, rendering it more amenable to termination with pacing techniques and thus reducing exposure to high-energy shocks.[57] The incidence of successful pacing termination of VT nearly doubles after antiarrhythmic drug therapy in individual patients.[57] Prior experience with antitachycardia pacemakers in these patients has also shown that concomitant antiarrhythmic drug therapy is nearly always required for this purpose.[17, 19, 26, 56] It has also been suggested, but remains to be established, that antiarrhythmic drug therapy reduces the frequency of VT or VF.[62] Should this be proved, the use of concomitant drug therapy with programmable devices could improve the patient's acceptance of combination therapy and prolong the life of the device. Table 26–5 outlines general considerations and suggests suitable electrical algorithms for VT cardioversion with nonepicardial electrode configurations for programmable devices. Similar approaches would be appropriate for devices with one or more epicardial electrodes. One potential concern with the use of antiarrhythmic drugs has been an increase in cardioversion or defibrillation thresholds.[15, 28] Although single

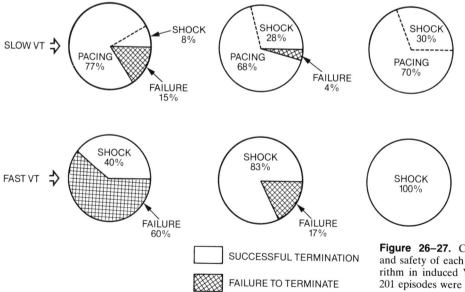

Figure 26–27. Clinical efficacy and safety of each electrical algorithm in induced VT. A total of 201 episodes were evaluated.

case reports and experimental studies suggest
that this may indeed occur, clinical studies do
not indicate major differences in these parameters in a larger population of patients with or
without drug therapy. We have not observed
significant changes in cardioversion thresholds
in drug-free and drug-treated patients when
tachycardia episodes are matched for rate and
morphology.[9] The risk of tachycardia acceleration with or without drugs does not appear
to be significantly altered at identical tachycardia rates. However, carefully controlled clinical studies are lacking, and limited alterations
in these parameters may indeed be elicited.
These do not appear at the present time to
have a major clinical impact.

Tachycardia Detection

Prototype implantable antitachycardia devices had limited tachycardia detection parameters. These were based primarily on the atrial
or ventricular rate during the SVT or VT,
respectively. Although tachycardia detection
rates and duration were programmable in recent antitachycardia pacemakers and in the
prototype pacemaker/cardioverter,[44, 55, 68] this
feature was not available in the AICD. Inability to differentiate SVT from VT at comparable tachycardia rates often resulted in inappropriate device activation.[22, 32] The AICD had an
additional parameter in some models, referred
to as the probability density function. This
parameter continuously analyzes the period of
isoelectric activity in the RR interval as sensed
by the defibrillating electrodes. Significant re-

duction and even elimination of this period is
observed during wide QRS tachycardias and
VF. Unfortunately, aberrantly conducted SVT
may fulfill this criterion, and should it meet
rate and duration criteria, device activation
results. The specificity of this parameter has
recently been questioned.[13] Rarely, narrow
QRS complexes during VT will not meet this
parameter, resulting in failure of device activation. The duration for which these criteria
need to be met is also fixed in these prototype
devices. Whereas the antitachycardia pacemaker or the Medtronic pacemaker/cardiover-
ter delivers tachycardia termination therapy
instantaneously or within seconds of complet-
ing detection, the AICD requires a significant
charge time for its high-energy pulse. Spontaneous tachycardia termination during the
charging cycle fails to interrupt shock delivery,
resulting in unnecessary therapy. In the absence of adequate interrogation or monitoring
capabilities in the current device, the frequency of these unnecessary device discharges
cannot be assessed. However, it is clear that
they can reduce pulse generator longevity and
the patient's tolerance for electrical therapy
and in some instances can induce serious ventricular tachyarrhythmias.[33] Improved tachycardia detection methods are clearly necessary.

A number of subsidiary parameters have
been examined to enhance the effectiveness of
rate detection criteria. The "sudden-onset"
criterion, defined as a minimal percentage decrease in RR interval over a specified number
of cycles in conjunction with rate criteria, may
help differentiate physiologic from paroxysmal
tachycardias.[20] Separating automatic from
reentrant rhythms may or may not be feasible
in individual instances. Detailed analysis of
single or multiple intracardiac electrograms,
which are usually monitored by implantable
devices, has also been suggested. A number
of parameters derived from single intracardiac
electrograms have been studied. In a previous
publication, we noted that the frequency spectra of bipolar ventricular electrograms shift to
lower frequencies during sustained VT[10, 54]
(Fig. 26–28). Furthermore, antegrade and retrograde atrial activation can be differentiated.[11] More recently, changes in intracardiac
ventricular electrogram morphology during VT
have been reported.[29] Camm and coworkers
have simplified this approach by examining
only the number of electrical potential reversals across the isoelectric line during SVT and
VT.[12] They have reported that this parameter
reliably differentiates VT from SVT. The ability to sense and analyze the timing of two

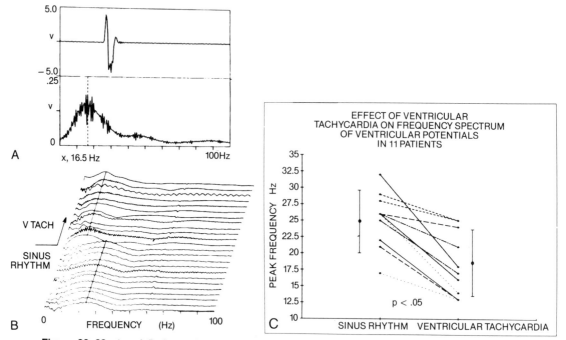

Figure 26–28. *A* and *B,* Spectral analysis of ventricular potentials during VT. Panel *A* (*upper portion*) shows ventricular potential recorded during VT. Lower portion of Panel *A* shows averaged spectrum of eight potentials as shown above. Panel *B* shows spectra obtained on filtered potentials in sinus rhythm from another patient (*lower portion*). Spectra obtained during VT begin at the arrow. Note the regularity of peaks at 22.5 Hz obtained during sinus rhythm and the shift to 13 Hz during VT. (From Saksena S, Craelius W, Hussain SM, et al: Intraoperative spectral analysis of ventricular electrograms during sinus rhythm and ventricular tachycardia. *In* Steinkopff D [ed]: Cardiac Pacing. Darmstadt, Federal Republic of Germany, GmbH & C. Verlag, 1983, p 680.)

intracardiac electrograms has been present in dual-chamber pacemakers for some time. Similar approaches have been suggested for antitachycardia devices. Availability of two intracardiac signals from the same chamber or from right atrium and right ventricle has been examined.[34, 58] In the former category is the use of orthogonal lead systems to differentiate antegrade or retrograde atrial activation.[24, 25] Alternatively, two spatially different electrodes may show alteration in activation sequences during antegrade and retrograde atrial activation or in the ventricle during VT.[35, 61] Furthermore, if atrial and ventricular signals are present, the presence of ventriculoatrial dissociation or abrupt change in activation sequence during VT and VF activation could be used in individual patients for arrhythmia detection.[58, 61]

The hemodynamic and metabolic consequences of VT can also be considered as potential tachycardia detection parameters, analogous to the use of these systems during rate-responsive pacing. However, it must be noted that hemodynamic changes are instanta-

neous,[53] while metabolic changes may be considerably slower. Early studies on sensors for the AICD examined the use of right ventricular systolic pressure as a possible parameter.[38] Inconsistent changes in this parameter and nonavailability of a reliable implantable pressure transducer precluded this approach. In 1983, we observed that there was an immediate decline in left ventricular dp/dt and negative dp/dt at the onset of VT[53] (Fig. 26–29). This phenomenon was due to alterations in left ventricular filling and the ventricular electrical activation sequence. We subsequently noted similar changes in the right ventricular dp/dt and negative dp/dt during VT[63] (Fig. 26–30). Preliminary studies suggest that a 25 per cent or greater decline in this value occurs during VT and VF. Another alternative includes analysis of changes in cardiac impedance, detected by a transvenous right ventricular catheter, to calculate stroke volume, which can decline in VT and VF.[2] Metabolic parameters could be evaluated, including alteration in blood pH, partial pressure of oxygen, or temperature. Developments in tachycardia detection algo-

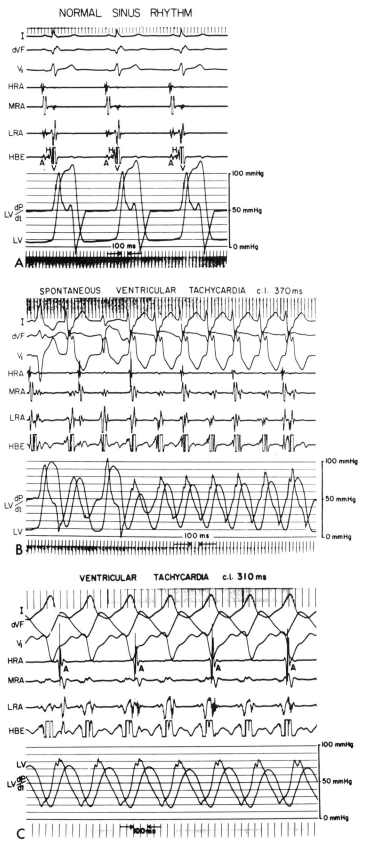

Figure 26–29. Left ventricular hemodynamic variables during sinus rhythm (*A*), during spontaneous VT (*B*), and during sustained VT (*C*). Note that the decline in left ventricular (LV) systolic pressure during spontaneous and induced VT is accompanied by little change in LV end-diastolic pressure but a major decrease in LV dp/dt and LV negative dp/dt. Fortuitous atrial contractions preceding the QRS (panel *B*, complex 3) improves pressures and dp/dt. c.l. = cycle length; dP/dt = first derivative of LV pressure; HBE = His bundle electrogram; HRA = high right atrium; LRA = low right atrium; MRA = mid right atrium. (From Saksena S, Ciccone J, Craelius W, et al: Studies on left ventricular function during sustained ventricular tachycardia. J Am Coll Cardiol 4:506, 1984; with permission.)

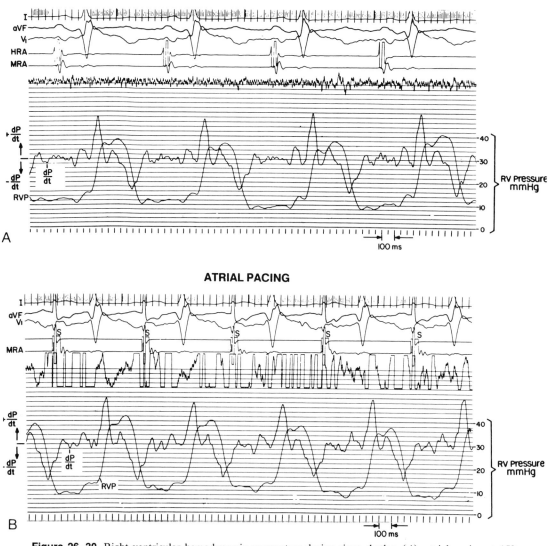

Figure 26–30. Right ventricular hemodynamic parameters during sinus rhythm (*A*), atrial pacing at 150 beats per minute (*B*), ventricular pacing (*C*), and sustained VT (*D*). Note that RV pressure, RV dp/dt, and RV negative dp/dt are preserved in panels *A, B* and *C* but decline rapidly at the onset of VT and remain depressed during the arrhythmia. HRA = high right atrium; MRA = mid right atrium; RVP = right ventricular pressure tracing; S = pacing stimuli.

rithms can be expected in two stages. Initially, further sophisticated analysis of rate, as well as single or multiple intracardiac electrograms for tachycardia detection, will be included in second- and third-generation devices. The use of novel and distinct subsidiary detection parameters will probably await the development of future generations of implantable antitachycardia devices.

Tachycardia Monitoring

The effectiveness and safety of implantable antitachycardia devices have hitherto been judged by clinical parameters alone. These parameters (survival of patients, symptomatology, and need for additional therapy) have been used in the absence of resources for accurate detection of all tachycardia recurrences and their outcome. This lack of resources is largely due to the inability to develop external long-term tachycardia monitoring capabilities. Transtelephonic or 24-hour ambulatory electrocardiographic monitoring fails to detect paroxysmal arrhythmias and can provide information only for a limited duration. Thus, internal tachycardia monitoring capabil-

VENTRICULAR PACING

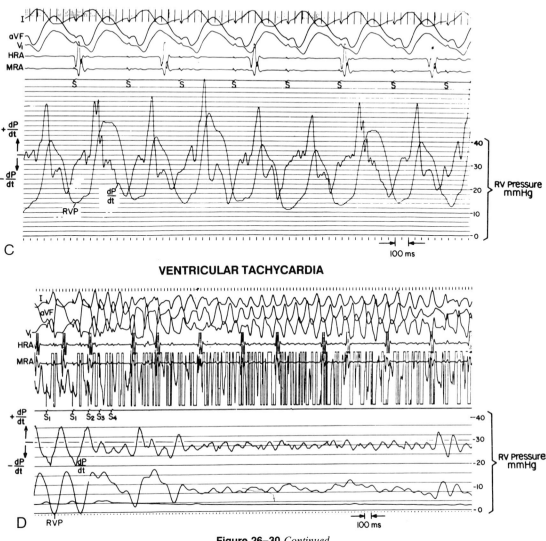

Figure 26–30 *Continued*

ities in the implanted device have been proposed. These have been used in second-generation implantable antitachycardia pacemakers and the prototype pacemaker/cardioverter.[49, 55, 68] Capabilities for monitoring and displaying ventricular rate, tachycardia events, and duration are based on preprogrammed detection criteria and delivered therapy and have been included in these devices. Figure 26–31 is an example of monitoring information obtained from an implanted Cordis model 284A (Cordis, Miami Lakes, FL) antitachycardia pacemaker in a patient with recurrent VT. Information on heart rate and tachycardia events, as well as programmed values, can be obtained. The prototype implantable pacemaker/cardioverter provides information on delivered therapies in its telemetry (see the second section of this chapter). This information can be derived from internally sensed or output data from the implanted device. It is invaluable for analyzing the clinical tachycardia recurrences and following this form of therapy longitudinally. Differentiation of unnecessary from therapeutic shocks has been a major follow-up problem for the AICD. Cumbersome clinical techniques with variable sensitivity have been proposed for this purpose.[7] The need for reprogramming of antitachycardia devices during outpatient follow-up has been emphasized in individual reports.[23, 55, 64] This monitoring information is essential for programming purposes. A recent report on the efficacy of combined antitachycardia pace-

<u>PACING MONITORS</u>
(DATA COLLECTED FROM PACER TELEMETRY)

TIME PERIOD

	AVG. RATE (BPM)	PERCENT SENSED	NUMBER OF EPISODES	MAX. DURATION (SECONDS)	MAX. RATE (BPM)
LAST 256 DAY(S)	64	59.9	40	24	226
LAST 154 MIN.	61	35.2	0	0	130
PREVIOUS 4 HOURS	60	17.6	0	0	95
4 - 8 HOURS	60	23.4	0	0	116
8 - 12 HOURS	60	12.5	0	0	82
12 - 16 HOURS	60	28.7	0	0	120
16 - 20 HOURS	61	26.4	0	0	110
20 - 24 HOURS	64	90.3	0	0	140
24 - 28 HOURS	67	69.5	0	0	197
28 - 32 HOURS	60	19.8	0	0	132
32 - 36 HOURS	60	20.9	0	0	97
36 - 40 HOURS	60	17.0	0	0	101
40 - 44 HOURS	61	35.4	0	0	116
44 - 48 HOURS	61	23.8	0	0	187

Figure 26–31. Pacing monitor data obtained from a Cordis model 284A antitachycardia pacemaker in a patient with recurrent, sustained VT. The number of VT episodes, duration, and heart rate can be obtained and are valuable in assessing efficacy of therapy. (From Saksena S, Lindsay BD, Parsonnet V: Development of future implantable cardioverters and defibrillators. Pacing Clin Electrophysiol 10:1356, 1987; with permission.)

maker and AICD implantation noted that pacemaker monitoring data revealed that multiple VT episodes were terminated by pacing without need for high-energy shocks.[31] Figure 26–32 shows such an example in our institution of a patient who has an implanted Orthocor II (Cordis, Miami Lakes, FL) antitachycardia pacemaker and automatic implantable cardioverter/defibrillator. Frequent slower but symptomatic VT below the defibrillator sensing rate could be terminated by the pacemaker. This feature will be essential to the future development of electrical therapy.

Demand and Triggered Pacing

The need for rate support in patients with recurrent tachycardias has been recognized. Coexistence of intrinsic or drug-induced bradycardias in patients with SVT or VT is frequent. Bradycardias after tachycardia termination have been noted. Ten to 20 per cent of patients undergoing AICD implantation need permanent pacing. In a multicenter report, permanent pacemakers were required in 5 per cent of patients with implanted devices.[16] Transvenous shocks also induce transient but significant bradycardias in 23 per cent of VT

VT Termination by Antitachycardia Pacemaker in

Patient With Implanted Defibrillator

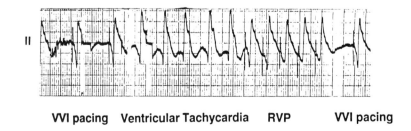

VVI pacing   Ventricular Tachycardia   RVP   VVI pacing

Figure 26–32. Combined implantation of an automatic antitachycardia pacemaker (Cordis model 284A, Orthocor II) and AICD in a patient with frequent recurrent VT. The tachycardia rate was usually below rate selection criteria of the defibrillator but could be terminated by burst pacing, as shown. Occasionally, tachycardia acceleration was observed and terminated by the defibrillator shock.

episodes terminated by this method.[9] These are accompanied by transient increases in local pacing thresholds.[66] Prolonged bradyarrhythmias are less frequent (3 per cent). The frequent presence of significant left ventricular dysfunction in patients with ventricular tachyarrhythmias magnifies the hemodynamic and clinical consequences of these bradyarrhythmias. Rate support is particularly desirable in these patients. In addition, pacemaker stimuli and evoked ventricular electrograms can be individually sensed, resulting in oversensing of beat rate and inappropriate device activation. Double and triple sensing for dual-chamber pacemakers can occur.[7] Engineering concerns regarding the potential for double sensing of the pacing stimulus and evoked ventricular electrograms, as well as increases in local pacing threshold at the shock electrode site, require use of separate pacing electrodes and shielded sensing circuits.[49]

An additional valuable pacing mode for patients with recurrent tachycardias is the triggered mode. This mode has been used in the past to overdrive the pacemakers externally for tachycardia termination. This mode can also be used for tachycardia induction when coupled to a programmed stimulator, which can deliver critically timed chest wall stimulation.[55, 56, 62] Figure 26–33 is an example of noninvasive tachycardia induction and termination in a patient with an implanted Cordis model 284A antitachycardia pacemaker. The ability to induce tachycardia in a noninvasive manner permits serial evaluation of the persistence of inducible tachycardia as well as the efficacy of electrical termination modes. This feature will be invaluable for assessing effectiveness of future implantable antitachycardia devices and will permit serial evaluation of the

clinical history of tachyarrhythmias. This ability, in time, will further the development of antiarrhythmic therapy.

Second-Generation Implantable Cardioverter/Defibrillators: Future Directions

The next generation of implantable cardioverter/defibrillators has been under development. Table 26–6 outlines some major features of three of these devices, which are currently under clinical investigation. Sensing remains dependent on bipolar ventricular electrograms. Rate sensing is universally used; morphology sensing is available in the Ventak-P (Cardiac Pacemakers, Inc, St Paul, MN), and patterns of rate change are used in the other two devices as secondary criteria. Pacing for bradycardia and tachycardia control is being added. Figures 26–34A and B show examples of cardioversion of VT and defibrillation of VF by the Telectronics Guardian Model 4201 programmable pacemaker-cardioverter-defibrillator (Telectronics, Englewood, CO). Differences in defibrillation shock energy patterns and energy output are also present in these devices. These reflect the present uncertainty regarding the most efficient defibrillation pulse and electrode configuration. Nonepicardial electrode systems are currently available for one device and expected for the other two devices. An example of a chronically implanted nonepicardial electrode system, reproduced from a recent report,[47] is shown in Figures 26–35 to 26–37. The Endotak C electrode catheter was implanted in conjunction with a submuscular patch electrode in the left lateral chest wall. A Y connector was used to connect the proximal catheter electrode in the right atrium and the

Figure 26–33. Noninvasive induction using chest wall stimulation and termination of sustained ventricular tachycardia by a Cordis Orthocor II antitachycardia pacemaker programmed to the triggered mode (see text for details). Ventricular tachycardia is induced noninvasively by rapid ventricular burst pacing. Once the arrhythmia is induced, the magnet is removed. The pacemaker senses the tachycardia after 10 beats and automatically delivers a rapid pacing burst to terminate the tachycardia. NSR = normal sinus rhythm; VVT = ventricular pacing, ventricular sensing, triggered mode; MGT. = magnet; NIEPS = noninvasive electrophysiologic study; RV = right ventricle; c.l. = cycle length (in milliseconds); VT = ventricular tachycardia; S = pacing stimulus artifact. (From Pract Cardiol 14:58, 1988; with permission.)

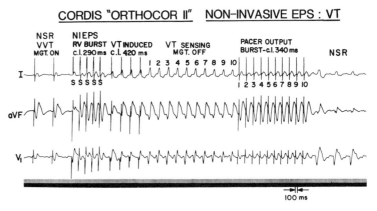

CORDIS "ORTHOCOR II"   NON–INVASIVE EPS : VT

TABLE 26–6. MAJOR FEATURES OF SECOND-GENERATION IMPLANTABLE CARDIOVERTERS/DEFIBRILLATORS*

FEATURE	CPI VENTAK-P	MEDTRONIC MODEL 7216	TELECTRONICS MODEL 4201
Electrode system	Dual or triple	Triple	Dual or triple
Shock pattern	Single, truncated exponential pulse	Sequential, truncated exponential pulse	Single, truncated exponential pulse
	Monophasic	Monophasic	Monophasic
Programmable sensing rate	Present	Present	Present
VT/VF reconfirmation	Absent	Present	Present
Antitachycardia pacing	Absent	Present	Present
Demand pacing	Absent	Present	Present
Low-energy cardioversion	Present	Present	Present
Maximal energy	30–35 J	30 J	30 J
Nonepicardial electrode system	Available	Expected	Expected

*Under clinical investigation, 1988–1989.

IMPLANTABLE PACEMAKER-CARDIOVERTER-DEFIBRILLATOR

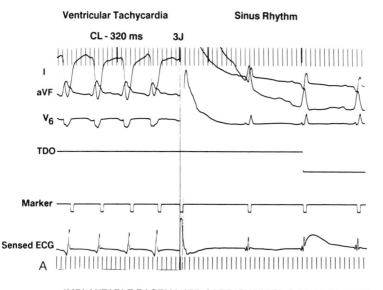

IMPLANTABLE PACEMAKER-CARDIOVERTER-DEFIBRILLATOR

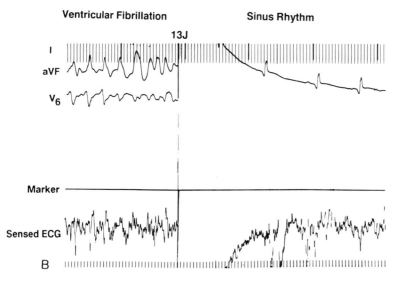

Figure 26–34. *A,* Cardioversion of VT by implanted pacemaker-cardioverter-defibrillator (Telectronics Model 4201). A 3-J shock terminates sustained VT in this patient. *B,* Termination of VF with a 13-J shock from the same implanted pacemaker-cardioverter-defibrillator as in *A.* CL = cycle length; TDO = tachycardia detection output.

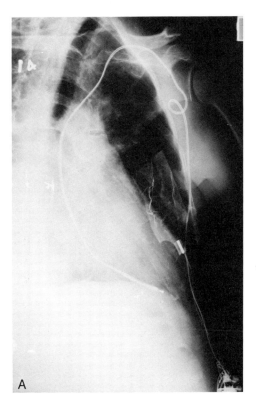

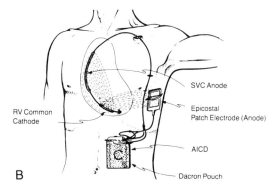

B

Figure 26–35. *A,* Chest roentgenogram (posteroanterior view) showing tripolar electrode catheter positioned in right ventricular apex and subcutaneous patch electrode in left midaxillary line at fourth intercostal space. Cables from transvenous catheter and patch electrodes have been tunneled into abdominal pocket of AICD. *B,* Diagrammatic representation of nonepicardial electrode system used in conjunction with AICD and spatial vectors of bidirectional shock. Note dual anodes and single, right ventricular (RV) common cathode. Bipolar sensing electrogram is derived from tip and distal spring electrodes, and the shock is delivered simultaneously using right ventricular, superior vena caval (SVC), and patch electrodes. (From Saksena S, Parsonnet V: Implantation of a cardioverter/defibrillator without thoracotomy using a triple electrode system. JAMA 259:70, 1988; with permission. Copyright 1988, American Medical Association.)

Figure 26–36. Postoperative induction of VF at electrophysiologic study 3 days after AICD implantation. Note that duration of sensing and charging time is 14 seconds and the first discharge induces supraventricular rhythm with bundle branch block pattern. Aberrant conduction subsided within a few seconds, and normal sinus rhythm was restored. RVA = right ventricular apex; ICDC = internal cardioversion/defibrillation catheter. (From Saksena S, Parsonnet V: Implantation of a cardioverter/defibrillator without thoracotomy using a triple electrode system. JAMA 259:70, 1988; with permission. Copyright 1988, American Medical Association.)

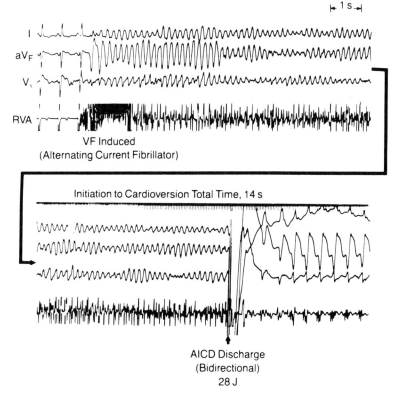

AICD WITH TRIPLE ELECTRODE NON-EPICARDIAL LEAD SYSTEM

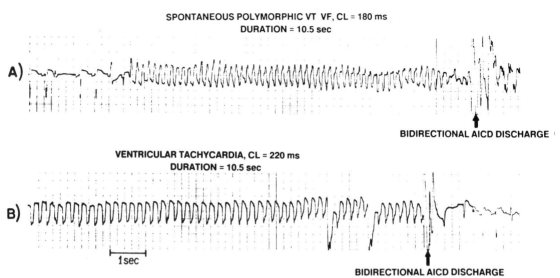

Figure 26–37. Telemetric ECG recording obtained during a spontaneous episode of sustained polymorphic ventricular tachycardia in the same patient as in Figures 26–35 and 26–36 6 months after implantation of the nonepicardial electrodes. The patient was minimally symptomatic, and the tachycardia was terminated by the second AICD discharge. VT = ventricular tachycardia; VF = ventricular fibrillation; AICD = automatic implantable cardioverter/defibrillator; CL = cycle length. (From Saksena S, et al: Initial clinical experience with endocardial defibrillation using an implantable cardioverter defibrillator with a triple electrode system. Arch Intern Med. In press.)

submuscular patch electrode as dual anodes into the anodal input of a standard AICD. The distal catheter electrode positioned in the

TABLE 26–7. IMPLANTABLE CARDIOVERTER/DEFIBRILLATOR: NONEPICARDIAL LEAD SYSTEM

Patient Population
1. 7 patients with recurrent VT/VF
2. All were men
3. Age: range 60 to 72 (mean 67) years
4. All had CAD
5. LV ejection fraction: 20 to 45 (mean 32) %
6. NYHA Class
     Class II, 4 patients
     Class III, 2 patients
     Class IV, 1 patient
7. Arrhythmia
     Symptomatic refractory sustained VT, 4 patients
     Cardiac arrest with documented VF, 3 patients
8. Prior antiarrhythmic drug trials: 2 to 8 (mean 5)
9. Prior EPS: 1 to 14 (mean 5)
10. Additional medical conditions
     Severe lung disease, 2 patients
     Prior cardiac surgery, 4 patients
        CABG, 3 patients
        CABG and MVR, 1 patient
     Advanced renal failure, 1 patient

VT = ventricular tachycardia; VF = ventricular fibrillation; CAD = coronary artery disease; LV = left ventricular; NYHA = New York Heart Association; EPS = electrophysiologic study; CABG = coronary artery bypass graft; MVR = mitral valve replacement.

right ventricular apex functioned as a common cathode. A single bidirectional shock was thus delivered in two spatially distinct planes. Figure 26–35 shows a chest radiograph of such an implanted lead system in this patient.[47] The defibrillation threshold with bidirectional studies in this patient was 10 J, compared with more than 25 J for unidirectional shocks. Figure 26–36 shows induction of VF with alter-

DEFIBRILLATION THRESHOLDS
Monophasic vs. Biphasic Shocks

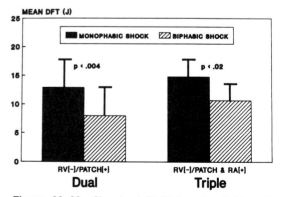

Figure 26–38. Chronic defibrillation thresholds with monophasic and biphasic shocks with dual and triple nonepicardial electrode systems. Note the marked reduction in threshold values.

TABLE 26–8. IMPLANTABLE CARDIOVERTER/ DEFIBRILLATOR: TRANSVENOUS CATHETER/ PATCH LEAD SYSTEM

Preimplantation
1. General anesthesia (continuous/intermittent)
2. Percutaneous cannulation of right subclavian vein
3. Catheter: distal tip = RV apex; proximal electrode = HRA/SVC
4. R_2 patch mapping
   Infraclavicular
   Left lateral
   Apical
   Left scapular region
5. VT/VF induction
6. 20-J external cardioverter/defibrillator shock
   Bidirectional
   Unidirectional
7. Defibrillation threshold determination

Intraoperative Procedure
1. General anesthesia (continuous/?intermittent)
2. Percutaneous cannulation of left subclavial vein
   Catheter tip = RV apex
   Proximal electrode = HRA/SVC
3. SQ patch insertion
   Subcostal location based on R_2 map
4. Evaluate signals
5. VT/VF induction
6. Sensing and defibrillation threshold determination
7. For defibrillation threshold ≤ 20 J (?25 J)
   VT/VF reinduction and ICD response (sensing and arrhythmia termination)

Postimplantation
1. Cardiac monitoring (24 to 48 hr)
2. Stress test (48 to 72 hr)
3. Predischarge EPS (48 to 72 hr)
4. Follow-up EPS (3 to 6 mo; ?noninvasive)

RV = right ventricular; HRA = high right atrium; SVC = superior vena cava; VT = ventricular tachycardia; VF = ventricular fibrillation; ICD = implantable cardioverter/defibrillator; EPS = electrophysiologic study.

nating current (AC) at a postimplantation electrophysiologic study. The VF is sensed by the implanted cardioverter/defibrillator, which terminates it after 14 seconds. Spontaneous VT termination in this patient was documented, as shown in Figure 26–37, several months later.[45] Table 26–7 summarizes the initial clinical experience with this lead system.[69–71] The technique of implantation has been described in detail elsewhere but is summarized in Table 26–8.[47] In nearly all instances, a triple electrode configuration with dual anodes (RA and patch) and common cathode (RV) provided optimal and low defibrillation thresholds. Three of the initial seven patients have experienced spontaneous discharges. Device longevity is expected to improve with these products. However, device size is not anticipated to be significantly different from that at present. Several innovations are expected that may impact on this parameter. The use of biphasic instead of monophasic defibrillating

waveforms is one such possibility.[65] Figure 26–38 shows the effect of biphasic shock energy delivery in defibrillation threshold with different nonepicardial lead configurations.[72] There is a significant reduction in canine defibrillation threshold in this controlled study. The use of nonepicardial electrode systems is expected to improve the patient's and physician's acceptance of this therapy. These systems will be preferred as the lead systems of choice, as is seen in current pacemaker implantation. These advances will enhance the use of electrical therapy in the management of ventricular tachyarrhythmias.

REFERENCES

1. An HL, Saksena S, Pantopoulos D: Prospective comparison of combined transvenous catheter and cutaneous electrodes with catheter electrodes alone for ventricular tachycardia cardioversion. Pacing Clin Electrophysiol 11:492, 1988.
2. Bardy GH, Olson WH, Fishbein DP, et al: Transvenous right ventricular impedance during spontaneous ventricular arrhythmias in man. Circulation 72[Suppl III]:III–474, 1985.
3. Bourland JD, Tacker WA, Wessale JL, et al: Energy reduction for implantable defibrillation using a sequential pulse method to decrease generator size and increase safety. Circulation 70[Suppl II]:II–100, 1984.
4. Calvo R, Saksena S, Pantopoulos D: Sequential transvenous pacing and shock therapy for termination of sustained ventricular tachycardia. Am Heart J 115:569, 1988.
5. Calvo R, Saksena S, Rothbart ST, et al: Efficacy and safety of a combined pacing and transvenous cardioversion algorithm in ventricular tachycardia: A prospective randomized study [abstract]. Circulation 72[Suppl III]:III–383, 1985.
6. Chang M, Inoue H, Kallok MJ, et al: Double and triple sequential shocks reduce ventricular defibrillation threshold in dogs with and without myocardial infarction. J Am Coll Cardiol 8:1393, 1986.
7. Chapman PD, Troup P: The automatic implantable cardioverter-defibrillator: Evaluating suspected inappropriate shocks. J Am Coll Cardiol 7:1075, 1986.
8. Charos GS, Haffajee CI, Gold RL, et al: A theoretically and practically more effective method for interruption of ventricular tachycardia: Self-adapting autodecremental overdrive pacing. Circulation 73:309, 1986.
9. Ciccone JM, Saksena S, Shah Y, et al: A prospective, randomized study of the clinical efficacy and safety of transvenous cardioversion for ventricular tachycardia termination. Circulation 71:571, 1985.
10. Craelius W, Saksena S, Pantopoulos D, et al: Frequency analysis of cardiac potentials: A new technique for ventricular tachycardia detection [abstract]. J Am Coll Cardiol 3:581, 1984.
11. Craelius W, Saksena S, Pantopoulos D, et al: Frequency characteristics of antegrade and retrograde

human atrial potentials [abstract]. J Am Coll Cardiol 3:582, 1984.

12. Davies WD, Wainwright RJ, Tooley MA, et al: Detection of pathological tachycardia by analysis of electrogram morphology. Pacing Clin Electrophysiol 9:200, 1986.

13. DeBorde R, Levine JH, Griffith LSC, et al: Exercise stress testing to prevent asymptomatic automatic implantable cardioverter discharges. Pacing Clin Electrophysiol 10:983, 1987.

14. Den Dulk K, Kersschot IE, Brugada P, et al: Is there a universal antitachycardia pacemaker? Am J Cardiol 57:950, 1986.

15. Dorian P, Fain ES, Davy JM, et al: Lidocaine causes a reversible concentration-dependent increase in defibrillation energy requirements. J Am Coll Cardiol 8:327, 1986.

16. Echt DS, Armstrong K, Schmidt P, et al: Clinical experience, complications and survival in 70 patients with the automatic implantable cardioverter/defibrillator. Circulation 71:289, 1985.

17. Fisher JD, Furman S, Kim SG: Implanted automatic burst pacemakers for termination of ventricular tachycardia. Am J Cardiol 45:458, 1980.

18. Fisher JD, Mehra R, Furman S: Termination of ventricular tachycardia with bursts of rapid ventricular pacing. Am J Cardiol 41:94, 1978.

19. Fisher JD, Kim SG, Furman S, et al: Role of implantable pacemakers in control of recurrent ventricular tachycardia. Am J Cardiol 49:194, 1982.

20. Fisher JD, Kim SG, Furman S, et al: Maximal rate of tachycardia development of sinus tachycardia with sudden exercise in spontaneous ventricular tachycardia. Pacing Clin Electrophysiol 6:221, 1983.

21. Fogoros RN: Amiodarone-induced refractoriness to cardioversion. Ann Intern Med 100:699, 1984.

22. Gabry MD, Brodman R, Johnston D, et al: Automatic implantable cardioverter-defibrillator: Patient survival, battery longevity and shock delivery analysis. J Am Coll Cardiol 9:1349, 1987.

23. Galasso D, Gallagher R, Parsonnet V, et al: A special out-patient clinic for following patients with implanted tachyarrhythmia devices. Pacing Clin Electrophysiol 10:1168, 1987.

24. Goldreyer BN, Shapland E, Cannon DS, et al: A new lead for improved atrial sensing in DDD pacing. Circulation 68[Suppl III]:III–379, 1983.

25. Goldreyer BN, Shapland E, Wyman MG, et al: Atrial activation sequencing in the recognition of ventriculoatrial conduction. Circulation 68[Suppl III]:III–379, 1983.

26. Herre JM, Griffin JC, Nielsen AP, et al: Permanent triggered antitachycardia pacemakers in the management of recurrent sustained ventricular tachycardia. J Am Coll Cardiol 7:206, 1985.

27. Jones DL, Klein GJ, Kallok MJ: Improved internal defibrillation with twin pulse sequential energy delivery to different lead orientations in pigs. Am J Cardiol 55:821, 1985.

28. Kerber RE, Pandian NG, Jensen SR, et al: Effect of lidocaine and bretylium on energy requirements for transthoracic defibrillation: Experimental studies. J Am Coll Cardiol 7:397, 1986.

29. Langberg JJ, Griffin JC: Arrhythmia identification using the morphology of the endocardial electrogram. Circulation 72[Suppl III]:III–474, 1985.

30. Lindsay BD, Saksena S, Rothbart ST, et al: Prospective evaluation of a sequential pacing and high-energy bidirectional shock algorithm for transvenous cardioversion in patients with ventricular tachycardia. Circulation 76:601, 1987.

31. Manz M, Greckens U, Funke HD, et al: Combination of antitachycardia pacemaker and automatic implantable cardioverter/defibrillator for ventricular tachycardia. Pacing Clin Electrophysiol 9:876, 1986.

32. Marchlinski FE, Flores BT, Buxton AE, et al: The automatic implantable cardioverter-defibrillator: Efficacy, complications and device failures. Ann Intern Med 104:481, 1986.

33. Marinchak RA, Friehling TD, Kline RA, et al: Effect of antiarrhythmic drugs on defibrillation threshold: Case report of an adverse effect on mexiletine and review of literature. Pacing Clin Electrophysiol 11:7, 1988.

34. Mercando AD, Furman S, Fisher JD, et al: Stability of activation sequence measured by two ventricular electrodes during supraventricular tachycardia. J Am Coll Cardiol 5:393, 1985.

35. Mercando A, Gabrey M, Klementowicz P, et al: Detection of ectopy by measurement of ventricular activation sequence using two electrodes. J Am Coll Cardiol 7:184, 1986.

36. Miles WM, Prystowsky EN, Heger JJ, et al: The implantable transvenous cardioverter: Long-term efficacy and reproducible induction of ventricular tachycardia. Circulation 74:518, 1986.

37. Mirowski M: Prevention of sudden arrhythmic death with implanted automatic defibrillators. Ann Intern Med 97:606, 1982.

38. Mirowski M, Mower MM, Staewen WS, et al: The development of the transvenous automatic defibrillator. Arch Intern Med 129:773, 1972.

39. Mirowski M, Reid PR, Mower MM, et al: Termination of malignant ventricular arrhythmias with an implanted automatic defibrillator in human beings. N Engl J Med 303:322, 1980.

40. Mirowski M, Reid PR, Watkins L, et al: Clinical treatment of life-threatening ventricular tachyarrhythmias with the automatic implantable defibrillator. Am Heart J 102:265, 1981.

41. Moss AJ, Rivers RJ: Termination and inhibition of recurrent tachycardias by implanted pervenous pacemakers. Circulation 50:942, 1974.

42. Naccarelli GV, Zipes DP, Rahilly GT, et al: Influence of tachycardia cycle lengths and antiarrhythmic drugs on pacing termination and acceleration of ventricular tachycardia. Am Heart J 105:1, 1983.

43. Pannizzo F, Furman S: Automatic discrimination of retrograde P waves for dual chamber pacemakers. J Am Coll Cardiol 5:393, 1985.

44. Rowland E, Rickards AF, Greco C, et al: Clinical experience with the Intermedics 262-12 antitachycardia pacemaker. Clin Prog Electrophysiol Pacing [Suppl]4:100, 1986.

45. Saksena S: The use of non-epicardial electrode systems for implantable cardioverter-defibrillators. New Trends Arrhythmias 4:501, 1988.

46. Saksena S, Calvo R: Transvenous cardioversion and defibrillation of ventricular tachyarrhythmias: Current status and future directions. Pacing Clin Electrophysiol 8:715, 1985.

47. Saksena S, Parsonnet V: Implantation of a cardioverter/defibrillator without thoracotomy using a triple electrode system. JAMA 259:69, 1988.

48. Saksena S, An HL, Pantopoulos D: Rapid transvenous cardioversion of sustained ventricular tachycardia by programmable implantable cardioverter-defibrillators. J Am Coll Cardiol 11:209A, 1988.

49. Saksena S, Lindsay BD, Parsonnet V: Development of future implantable cardioverters and defibrillators. Pacing Clin Electrophysiol 10:1342, 1987.

50. Saksena S, Calvo RA, Pantopoulos D, et al: A prospective evaluation of single and dual current pathways for transvenous cardioversion in rapid ventricular tachycardia. Pacing Clin Electrophysiol 10:1130, 1987.

51. Saksena S, Camm AJ, Bilitch M, et al: Clinical investigation of implantable antitachycardia devices: Report of the Policy Conference of the North American Society of Pacing and Electrophysiology. J Am Coll Cardiol 10:225, 1987.

52. Saksena S, Chandran P, Shah Y, et al: Comparative efficacy of transvenous cardioversion and pacing in patients with sustained ventricular tachycardia: A prospective randomized crossover study. Circulation 72:153, 1985.

53. Saksena S, Ciccone J, Craelius W, et al: Studies on left ventricular function during sustained ventricular tachycardia. J Am Coll Cardiol 4:501, 1984.

54. Saksena S, Craelius W, Hussain SM, et al: Intraoperative spectral analysis of ventricular electrograms during sinus rhythm and ventricular tachycardia. *In* Steinkopff D (ed): Cardiac Pacing. Verlag, 1983, p 677.

55. Saksena S, Heselmeyer T, Batsford W, et al: Long-term clinical experience with a versatile antitachycardia pacemaker for tachycardia termination, induction and monitoring: A multicenter study. Pacing Clin Electrophysiol 11:493, 1988.

56. Saksena S, Pantopoulos D, Parsonnet V, et al: Usefulness of an implantable antitachycardia pacemaker system for supraventricular and ventricular tachycardia. Am J Cardiol 58:70, 1986.

57. Saksena S, Parsonnet V, Pantopoulos D, et al: Transvenous cardioversion and defibrillation of ventricular tachyarrhythmias using bidirectional shocks: Acute feasibility studies and chronic device implantation [abstr]. Circulation 76[Suppl II]:IV–311, 1987.

58. Schuger CD, Jackson K, Steinman RT, et al: Atrial sensing to enhance ventricular tachycardia detection by the automatic implantable cardioverter defibrillator: A utility study. J Am Coll Cardiol 11:209A, 1988.

59. Sowton E: Clinical results with the Tachylog antitachycardia pacemaker. Pacing Clin Electrophysiol 7:1313, 1984.

60. Spurrell RAJ, Nathan AW, Camm AJ: Clinical experience with implantable scanning tachycardia reversion pacemakers. Pacing Clin Electrophysiol 7:1296, 1984.

61. Timmis GC, Westvee DC, Bakalyar DM, et al: Discrimination of anterograde from retrograde atrial electrograms for physiologic pacing. Pacing Clin Electrophysiol 11:130, 1988.

62. Veltri EP, Mower MM, Mirowski M, et al: Clinical outcome of patients with ventricular tachyarrhythmias treated with automatic implantable defibrillator without concomitant drug therapy [abstract]. J Am Coll Cardiol 9:168A, 1987.

63. Wasty N, Pantopoulos D, Rothbart ST, et al: Detection of sustained ventricular tachyarrhythmias using right ventricular hemodynamic parameters: A prospective study [abstr]. J Am Coll Cardiol 9:141A, 1987.

64. Wasty N, Saksena S, Parsonnet V, et al: Long-term efficacy and complications of antitachycardia pacemakers compared with implantable defibrillators [abstract]. J Am Coll Cardiol 9:143A, 1987.

65. Winkle RA, Mead RH, Ruder MA, et al: Improved low energy defibrillation efficacy in man using a biphasic truncated exponential waveform. J Am Coll Cardiol 9:142A, 1987.

66. Yee R, Jones DL, Klein GJ: Pacing threshold changes after transvenous catheter countershock. Am J Cardiol 53:503, 1984.

67. Zipes DP: Electrical therapy of cardiac arrhythmias. N Engl J Med 309:1179, 1983.

68. Zipes DP, Jackman WM, Heger JJ, et al: Clinical transvenous cardioversion of recurrent life-threatening tachyarrhythmias: Low energy synchronized cardioversion of ventricular tachycardia and termination of ventricular fibrillation in patients using a catheter electrode. Am Heart J 103:789, 1982.

69. Saksena S: New developments in implantable antitachycardia devices. *In* Alliegro A (eds): Progress in Clinical Pacing. Amsterdam, Excerpta Medica, 1988, pp 315–325.

70. Saksena S, Tullo NG, Krol RB, et al: Clinical evaluation of an implantable cardioverter/defibrillator with nonepicardial leads in patients with refractory ventricular tachyarrhythmias. J Am Coll Cardiol [in press].

71. Saksena S, Tullo N, Parsonnet V, et al: Initial clinical experience with an implantable cardioverter-defibrillator using a nonepicardial electrode system. Circulation 78[Suppl II]:II–20, 1988.

72. Saksena S, Scott S, Accorti P, et al: Improved pacing and internal difibrillation using a porous electrode catheter with biphase unidirectional and bidirectional shocks. PACE 12:663, 1989.

27

COMPLICATIONS OF IMPLANTABLE ANTITACHYCARDIA DEVICES: Diagnosis and Management

MARK E. ROSENTHAL, FRANCIS E. MARCHLINSKI, *and* MARK E. JOSEPHSON

Technologic advances during the past decade have produced a number of nonpharmacologic therapeutic options for patients with refractory tachyarrhythmias. Among these is a group of implantable antitachycardia devices that function to terminate tachyarrhythmias when they arise, rather than to prevent their occurrence. Included in this group are antitachycardia pacemakers, the automatic implantable cardioverter/defibrillator (AICD), and the automatic transvenous cardioverter. As with any form of therapy, experience in the clinical setting with each of these devices has uncovered a list of potential complications, which are, in some cases, generic to any implanted device (e.g., infection) and are, in other instances, unique to the particular device being considered. This chapter will review the problems that have been recognized with each of the previously described antitachycardia devices and will provide strategies for the physician in managing or overcoming these problems.

Supported in part by grants HL00361 and HL24278 from the National Heart, Lung, and Blood Institute, Bethesda, MD, and grants from The American Heart Association, Southeastern Pennsylvania Chapter, Philadelphia, PA.

ANTITACHYCARDIA PACEMAKERS

Invasive electrophysiologic studies have demonstrated that properly timed programmed extrastimuli delivered during a sustained tachyarrhythmia can terminate the abnormal rhythm in some cases.[15, 16, 19, 24, 39, 45, 46] Such rhythms are generally thought to be due to a reentrant mechanism. In such a tachycardia, the wave front of activation of a premature stimulus may enter the reentrant circuit and collide in a retrograde direction with the wave front already propagating around the circuit, at the same time it is encountering refractory tissue within the circuit in an antegrade direction.[24, 39, 45, 46, 48, 49] Rhythms for which this technique for tachycardia termination has been shown to be successful include both supraventricular tachyarrhythmias (e.g., atrial flutter, atrioventricular [AV] nodal reentry, and circus movement tachycardia utilizing an accessory AV pathway)[39, 45, 49] and uniform, sustained ventricular tachycardia (VT).[15, 16, 19, 24, 39, 49]

As the feasibility of pacing techniques for tachycardia termination became increasingly appreciated, advances in pacemaker technology spurred an interest in incorporating this modality into fully implanted devices. The first type of device developed was a patient-activated unit that utilized an externally placed radiofrequency transmitter to trigger the delivery of bursts of pacing from the implanted unit. To overcome the need for the patient's recognition of arrhythmias as well as the patient's interaction with the device, fully automatic antitachycardia devices were developed with tachycardia recognition algorithms that could signal the pacemaker to deliver programmed extrastimuli to terminate the tachycardia. In each type of device, extensive electrophysiologic testing was mandatory to document the efficacy of a particular pacing modality as well as any propensity of pacing to accelerate a previously well-tolerated arrhythmia or cause it to degenerate into a more malignant form. This section will deal with the clinical experience of using these antitachycardia pacemakers with respect to complications encountered and means to avoid or correct them.

Generic Complications

Permanent transvenous pacemakers possessing the ability to treat tachyarrhythmias would be expected to possess problems similar to those that are encountered in routine permanent pacemaker implantation and follow-up. Phibbs and Marriott recently reviewed the complications of permanent transvenous pacing[36] and noted vascular complications and infection to be the most common problems encountered. The incidence of serious thrombotic or embolic complications (including superior vena cava syndrome, intracavitary thrombi, pulmonary embolism, and upper extremity thrombosis) was 2 per cent, and the incidence of infection of the pacing system ranged from 1 to 7 per cent. Anecdotal reports of ventricular perforation, tricuspid valve insufficiency, and pacemaker pocket fibrosis were also described. In experienced hands, these problems can be minimized and, in and of themselves, should not preclude consideration of pacing therapy. A more detailed dis-

cussion of the complications associated with permanent transvenous pacemakers and their management is presented elsewhere in this text (see Chapter 26).

Problems with Tachycardia Detection

PATIENT-ACTIVATED DEVICES. Recognition of abnormal rhythms can be a major problem with this type of device. For radiofrequency-triggered pacemakers to be clinically effective, patients not only must be able to tolerate their arrhythmias hemodynamically but also must be able to distinguish with reliability sinus tachycardia or the presence of spontaneous, isolated premature beats from sustained tachyarrhythmias. In addition, recognition of rhythms not amenable to pacing termination (e.g., atrial fibrillation) must be distinguished from the tachycardia for which the device was intended to be used.

The appropriate strategy in preventing this problem is in the proper selection of patients. Obviously, patients who have problems in identifying whether their tachyarrhythmia is present or absent should not be considered candidates for this type of device.

AUTOMATIC ANTITACHYCARDIA PACEMAKERS. A major challenge in the development of fully automatic devices for pacing termination of tachycardias has been tachycardia detection. The most commonly used criteria of high rate cut-off cannot distinguish sinus tachycardia or atrial fibrillation from rhythms that can be terminated by pacing therapy when there is an overlap of rates (Fig. 27–1). As a result of inappropriate initiation of pacing in response to these other rhythms, actual pacemaker-induced initiation of the patient's tachycardia may occur[10, 13, 20, 27] (Figs. 27–2 and 27–3).

Careful electrophysiologic evaluation prior to implantation is necessary to avoid this problem in fully automatic units. Characteristics of the tachycardia such as rate, mode of onset,

Figure 27–1. Holter recording demonstrating exercise-induced sinus tachycardia (143 beats per minute), which triggers bursts of rapid atrial pacing in a permanently implanted antitachycardia pacemaker. In this figure, three bursts of rapid atrial pacing (rate, 240 beats per minute; duration, 2.7 seconds) are delivered, since the sinus rate exceeds the device's high rate cut-off for supraventricular tachycardia (SVT) detection (137 beats per minute). (From Lerman BB, Waxman HL, Buxton AE, et al: Tachyarrhythmias associated with programmable automatic atrial antitachycardia pacemakers. Am Heart J 106:1029, 1983; with permission.)

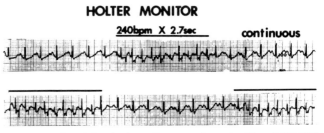

HOLTER MONITOR

240bpm X 2.7sec   continuous

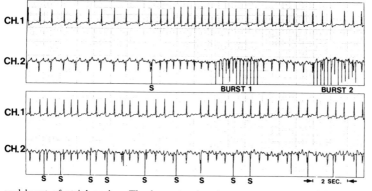

Figure 27–2. Two-channel Holter recording demonstrating atrial undersensing with subsequent pacemaker-mediated induction of SVT. In this figure, channels 1 and 2 are simultaneous, and the upper and lower tracings are continuous. In the upper panel, atrial undersensing leads to an asynchronous atrial paced beat (or beats), which initiates SVT. Atrial burst pacing is automatically initiated by the pacemaker (BURST 1), which converts the SVT to atrial fibrillation. The atrial high rate cut-off is satisfied by the atrial fibrillation, with the subsequent delivery of an ineffectual second burst of atrial pacing. The lower tracing demonstrates poor atrial sensing of atrial fibrillation, with the occasional delivery of ineffectual atrial stimuli (S). (From Echt DS: Potential hazards of implanted devices for the electrical control of tachyarrhythmias. PACE 7:580, 1984; with permission.)

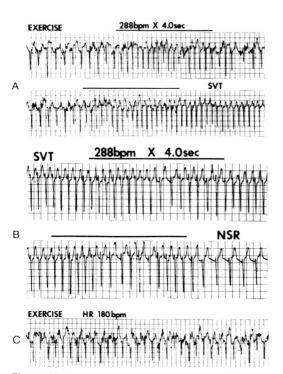

Figure 27–3. Pacemaker-initiated induction of SVT following inappropriate triggering of atrial burst pacing during exercise. In *A,* sinus tachycardia during exercise reaches 180 beats per minute and exceeds the high rate cut-off of the atrial antitachycardia pacemaker. A burst of rapid atrial pacing (rate, 288 beats per minute; duration, 4 seconds) initiates SVT. In *B,* two further bursts of atrial pacing are delivered, with subsequent termination of SVT and resumption of normal sinus rhythm. In *C,* exercise-induced sinus tachycardia (rate, 180 beats per minute) fails to initiate SVT with the antitachycardia pacing modality turned off. (From Lerman BB, Waxman HL, Buxton AE, et al: Tachyarrhythmias associated with programmable automatic atrial antitachycardia pacemakers. Am Heart J 106:1029, 1983; with permission.)

and regularity both in the baseline state and with changes in adrenergic tone and body position must be documented. In addition, the maximal sinus rate with exercise or after isoproterenol or atropine administration should be known to determine if overlap with the tachycardia rate exists. In patients with substantial rate overlap between arrhythmias conducive to pacing termination and episodes of sinus tachycardia or atrial fibrillation, automatic devices with only high rate criteria for tachycardia detection should not be used. However, new devices have been developed with improved recognition algorithms incorporating a number of programmable features in addition to a high rate cut-off (Table 27–1).[37] Although pacemaker programming becomes more complex with these devices, this newly introduced flexibility allows the cardiologist to conform the detection algorithm more effectively to known features of the patient's arrhythmia.

TABLE 27–1. PROGRAMMABLE ALGORITHMS FOR DISCRIMINATION OF SUPRAVENTRICULAR TACHYCARDIA FROM SINUS TACHYCARDIA OR ATRIAL FIBRILLATION*

High rate only
High rate and sudden onset
High rate and rate stability
High rate and (sudden onset or rate stability)
High rate and (rate stability or sustained high rate)
High rate and (sudden onset and rate stability)
High rate and (sudden onset and rate stability or sustained high rate)
High rate and (sudden onset or rate stability or sustained high rate)

*The Intertach device, Intermedics, Freeport, TX.

Figure 27–4. Atrial undersensing leading to SVT initiation in an atrial antitachycardia pacing system. Asynchronous atrial pacing *(upight arrows)* due to atrial undersensing occurs with atrial capture (atrial premature depolarization [APD]), leading to initiation of SVT. Subsequently, three bursts of rapid atrial pacing are delivered (rate, 240 beats per minute; duration, 2.7 seconds), with the first two being ineffectual and the third terminating the SVT. (From Lerman BB, Waxman HL, Buxton AE, et al: Tachyarrhythmias associated with programmable automatic atrial antitachycardia pacemakers. Am Heart J 106:1029, 1983; with permission.)

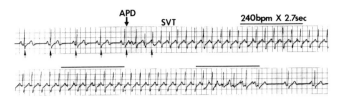

Another difficulty in tachycardia detection with fully automatic devices arises from problems with sensing of intracardiac electrograms. Although great care may be taken intraoperatively to ensure adequate amplitude and slew rate of intracardiac signals during sinus rhythm, the features of these electrograms may change during tachycardia. As a result, undersensing may develop, preventing tachycardia detection. Undersensing has been described with both atrial and ventricular electrograms during tachycardia, with the former being more common.[10, 18, 20, 27, 41] In addition, undersensing during sinus rhythm, resulting from either poor signal quality or inappropriate programming, may lead to asynchronous pacing in devices with backup demand modes. This asynchronous pacing may lead to pacemaker induction of tachycardia[10, 27] (Fig. 27–4).

Problems with undersensing must be promptly dealt with in all automatic antitachycardia pacemakers. Documentation of the amplitude and slew rate of sensed electrograms during *both* sinus rhythm and tachycardia should be done intraoperatively to determine appropriate sensitivity settings for the implanted device. This practice would require tachycardia induction at the time of pacemaker implantation by an electrophysiologist so that signal characteristics could be evaluated with the pacing system analyzer of the appropriate pacemaker manufacturer. Future devices with the ability to print out intracardiac recordings may allow for determination of signal characteristics during postimplantation tachycardia

induction if suspected sensing problems should develop.

Oversensing by the automatic antitachycardia pacemaker may result in false tachycardia recognition and inappropriate initiation of pacing. In devices relying on a high rate criterion for tachycardia detection, myopotential sensing may occur and may initiate pacing during sinus rhythm, with subsequent tachycardia induction[10, 27] (Fig. 27–5). In addition, far-field sensing of signals from another cardiac chamber may result in "double counting" by the pacemaker, with resultant satisfaction of the high rate criterion and triggering of the pacing response.[10] In both cases, the oversensing problem is almost exclusively confined to unipolar pacing systems and can be avoided with bipolar lead systems.

An important problem with tachycardia detection may occur in patients who begin concomitant therapy with antiarrhythmic agents after pacemaker implantation and initial programming. In addition to known alterations in pacing thresholds with certain antiarrhythmic agents (e.g., flecainide), physicians should be aware of changes in tachycardia characteristics following the initiation of drug therapy. The tachycardia rate during recurrences on antiarrhythmic medication may be slowed; in some instances, the rate may not exceed the pacemaker's high rate cut-off, and tachycardia recurrences may go unrecognized. Therefore, programmed stimulation to induce the tachycardia should be performed after any alteration in pharmacologic antiarrhythmic therapy to

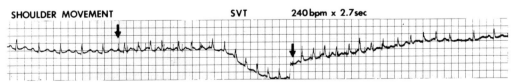

Figure 27–5. Oversensing of skeletal myopotentials with shoulder movement results in the delivery of a burst of rapid atrial pacing by an automatic atrial antitachycardia pacemaker. SVT is initiated and subsequently results in the delivery of a burst of rapid atrial pacing, which terminates the SVT. (From Lerman BB, Waxman HL, Buxton AE, et al: Tachyarrhythmias associated with programmable automatic atrial antitachycardia pacemakers. Am Heart J 106:1029, 1983; with permission.)

document changes in tachycardia cycle length. It is desirable to have flexibility in programming the high rate cut-off in the detection algorithms of all automatic antitachycardia pacemakers.

Proarrhythmic Effects of Antitachycardia Pacing

In the context of this discussion, proarrhythmic effects of antitachycardia pacemakers refer to either tachycardia induction by the pacemaker or acceleration or degeneration of the tachycardia to a hemodynamically less well tolerated form during attempted pacing termination (Table 27–2). The former was discussed in the last section; the latter remains a feared complication of antitachycardia pacing, particularly in ventricular pacing systems in which VT can be converted to ventricular fibrillation (VF).

SUPRAVENTRICULAR TACHYCARDIA (SVT). Other than patients with reentrant SVT utilizing accessory AV pathways, atrial pacing systems are most commonly used to effect termination of SVT. Therefore, atrial arrhythmias are the most common arrhythmias precipitated during attempted pacing termination of SVT, with atrial fibrillation being the most common[25, 33, 34, 43] (see Fig. 27–2). In a study of 111 patients with SVT, Waldecker and colleagues noted an overall incidence of atrial fibrillation or flutter induction of 8 per cent during trials of attempted pacing termination involving 30 per cent of the group of patients.[44] In 75 per cent of instances, the atrial fibrillation

or flutter was sustained. In patients with retrogradely functioning accessory AV pathways, ventricular pacing to terminate SVT may also initiate atrial fibrillation.[9, 18, 44]

In selected patients, the precipitation of atrial fibrillation or flutter may have dire hemodynamic consequences. In addition to patients with hypertrophic or dilated cardiomyopathy, mitral stenosis, and coronary artery disease, patients with SVT and ventricular preexcitation due to the Wolff-Parkinson-White (WPW) syndrome are at the greatest risk. AV accessory pathways with short antegrade effective refractory periods can conduct impulses to the ventricle during atrial fibrillation, leading to a very rapid ventricular response and subsequent VF. Spurrell and associates described two patients with WPW syndrome who experienced sudden cardiac death following implantation of a ventricular antitachycardia pacing system.[42] As a result of these considerations, antitachycardia pacing is not recommended in patients with WPW syndrome and a history of spontaneous or induced atrial fibrillation or a history of cardiac arrest. In selected patients with the WPW syndrome, patient-activated devices may be considered with the provision that they are to be activated only in the presence of a physician with backup defibrillation capability available. Obviously, patients with frequent SVT recurrences or with episodes of insufficient duration to allow the patient to get to a hospital are not candidates for this form of therapy.

VENTRICULAR TACHYCARDIA. Both acceleration of the rate of a previously tolerated

TABLE 27–2. INCIDENCE OF PROARRHYTHMIC EFFECTS OF ANTITACHYCARDIA PACEMAKERS IMPLANTED FOR SUPRAVENTRICULAR AND VENTRICULAR ARRHYTHMIAS

STUDY	YEAR	NO. OF PATIENTS	DEVICE	PROARRHYTHMIC EFFECT	MISCELLANEOUS
Supraventricular Tachycardia					
Kahn et al.[25]	1976	12	PA	Atrial fibrillation, 2 Atrial flutter, 2	—
Peters et al.[35]	1978	10	PA	Atrial fibrillation, 3	—
Hartzler et al.[22]	1981	8	PA	None	—
Nathan et al.[33]	1983	15	Auto	Atrial fibrillation, 3	—
Spurrell et al.[42]	1984	22	Auto	Not known	Sudden death in 2 WPW patients
Ventricular Tachycardia					
Peters et al.[35]	1978	6	PA	VT accel, 2	—
Ruskin et al.[40]	1980	3	PA	None	—
Hartzler et al.[22]	1981	9	PA	None	—
Freedman et al.[18]	1982	18	Auto	Not known	Sudden death in 2 with prior VT accel
Falkoff et al.[14]	1986	2	Auto	VT accel, 1	—

Abbreviations: Accel = accelerated; Auto = automatic; PA = patient activated; VT = ventricular tachycardia; WPW = Wolff-Parkinson-White syndrome.

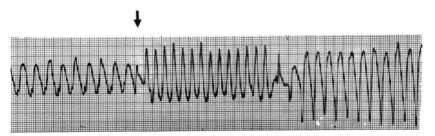

Figure 27–6. Delivery of a burst of right ventricular pacing *(arrow)* with a cycle length of 200 msec during sustained, uniform ventricular tachycardia (VT) with a cycle length of 300 msec. Following the discontinuation of pacing, the tachycardia cycle length decreases to 250 msec and the QRS morphology changes. (From Josephson ME, Seides SF: Evaluation of therapeutic modalities: Antiarrhythmic agents and pacing. *In* Clinical Cardiac Electrophysiology. Philadelphia, Lea & Febiger, 1979, p 308.)

uniform VT and degeneration of VF are well-described complications of pacing therapy for VT[7, 10, 14–16, 18, 23, 34, 39] (Fig. 27–6). Although Fisher and coworkers found rapid bursts of ventricular pacing to be an effective mode of VT termination (89 per cent efficacy), 4 per cent of pacing trials resulted in tachycardia acceleration or degeneration to VF.[10] More important, the latter complication occurred at least once in 43 per cent of the patients. Roy and colleagues found that incorporation of multiple extrastimuli in pacing algorithms for VT termination correlated with increased efficacy for termination as well as increased incidence of VT acceleration or degeneration; only 1.2 per cent of pacing trials incorporating a single ventricular extrastimulus resulted in VT acceleration compared with 3.2 per cent of trials using two extrastimuli, 13 per cent of trials using three extrastimuli, and 35 per cent of trials using rapid pacing.[39] Although some investigators have not reported this problem,[22, 40] it is apparent that one cannot be totally assured that this will not occur in an individual patient at some time during follow-up.

With the prior considerations in mind, we do not recommend antitachycardia pacing alone in patients with sustained VT. A backup defibrillator capability is required to protect the patient from the infrequent, but potentially lethal, proarrhythmic effects of attempted pacing termination of sustained VT. In selected patients with infrequent, prolonged episodes of hemodynamically tolerated VT in which pacing therapy has been shown to be effective without adverse consequences, consideration may be given to a patient-triggered device. As described previously, these patients should activate the device only under the supervision of a physician with ready access to external defibrillators, should a rapid VT or VF be precipitated.

Alterations in Effectiveness of Antitachycardia Pacing

Long-term experience with implantable antitachycardia pacemakers has suggested that in individual patients the efficacy of a particular pacing algorithm for tachycardia termination may change with time.[9, 14, 16, 33–35, 43] This phenomenon is predicted from experience in the electrophysiology laboratory showing that the reproducibility of tachycardia termination may vary from day to day with spontaneous changes in the "window" with which extrastimuli may terminate tachycardias. In addition, changes in body position from supine to upright as well as exercise may alter the effectiveness of a particular pacing modality previously deemed efficacious during testing.[9, 33, 43, 44]

Management of this situation may be difficult. In many instances, the problem of changes in efficacy of the pacing algorithm is related to alterations in tachycardia cycle length in response to physiologic stimuli. Newer antitachycardia pacemakers are "adaptive" in that they adjust the coupling intervals of extrastimuli to the tachycardia rate by delivering them as percentage values of the tachycardia cycle length rather than as preset intervals.[9, 13, 18, 25, 33, 34, 37, 41, 43, 44] Further experience is required to determine if this modality overcomes this problem. Nevertheless, careful preimplantation evaluation, including assessment of the effect of changes in body position or of exercise (or isoproterenol infusion) on tachycardia termination, is essential.

AUTOMATIC IMPLANTABLE CARDIOVERTER/DEFIBRILLATOR (AICD)

Since its introduction for clinical trials in 1980, the automatic implantable defibrillator

TABLE 27–3. COMPLICATIONS OF THE AUTOMATIC IMPLANTABLE CARDIOVERTER/DEFIBRILLATOR

COMPLICATION	NO. OF PATIENTS
Early Postoperative Problems	
Atelectasis/pneumonia	4
Large pleural effusion	3
Pneumothorax	2
Coronary artery erosion	1
Seromas of generator pocket	3
Subcutaneous hematoma	1
Subclavian vein thrombosis	1
Superficial wound infection	1
Embolic cerebrovascular accident following cardioversion	1
Late Problems	
Asymptomatic discharge	11
Documented rhythm	
Sinus tachycardia	1
Atrial fibrillation	1
Nonsustained VT	1
Unknown	6
Sensed myopotentials	2
Spring lead migration	3
Pocket infection	1
Early generator failure	4
Inability to defibrillate VF postoperatively	3
Postoperative VT less than rate cut-off	3
Detection inhibition by pacemaker	1

Of the 33 patients at the Hospital of the University of Pennsylvania, Philadelphia, 26 patients had a full system implanted (spring lead–patch, 14; patch-patch, 12) and 7 patients had the patch only.

VF = ventricular fibrillation; VT = ventricular tachycardia.

Data from Marchlinski FE, Flores BT, Buxton AE, et al: The automatic implantable cardioverter-defibrillator: Efficacy, complications, and device failures. Ann Intern Med 104:481, 1986.

has been shown to be an effective means for prolonging life in survivors of cardiac arrest due to VT or VF.[12, 31] As the experience with this device has accumulated, its limitations and associated complications have become known to the clinical investigators studying it. However, with the Food and Drug Administration (FDA) approval of the current model of the device, it is increasingly important for physicians who will be caring for patients with the AICD to be aware of these problems as well. This section will focus on reported complications of the AICD during the periimplantation period and during clinical follow-up (Table 27–3), with suggested management strategies.

Perioperative Complications

Implantation of the AICD requires entering the thoracic cavity to expose the cardiac surface for placement of one or two defibrillating patches. Commonly, lateral thoracotomy or subcostal or medial sternotomy incisions are used. The last is used in patients undergoing concomitant coronary artery bypass grafting or

arrhythmia surgery. Most commonly, two defibrillating patches (either 10 cm^2 or 20 cm^2 in area) are used for energy delivery. Previously, one patch was ordinarily used in combination with a spring lead tunneled subcutaneously and inserted in the subclavian vein, with final positioning of the tip at the junction of the superior vena cava and right atrium. Rate detection is accomplished via a separately positioned rate-sensing lead system, which can be endocardially or epicardially located and is bipolar in configuration. The current AICD generator (Ventak 1530, Cardiac Pacemakers, Inc., St. Paul, MN), weighing approximately 250 grams and measuring 10.8 by 7.6 by 2.0 cm, is positioned in an abdominal subcutaneous pouch and is connected with the previously mentioned lead systems via an epoxy header.

The operative procedure of AICD implantation should not be underestimated with respect to its potential for producing complications. In the initial report of our experience at the Hospital of the University of Pennsylvania with patch lead implantation by both lateral thoracotomy and median sternotomy, 33 patients were included (26 with a full system implanted and 7 with only a patch implanted). Of these, 4 patients developed atelectasis with probable pneumonia, 2 patients had a pneumothorax during the first 24 postoperative hours, and 3 patients manifested large pleural effusions.[29] In addition, in 1 patient a 10-cm^2 patch eroded a small marginal branch of the circumflex artery, resulting in severe postoperative bleeding and the requirement for repeat sternotomy and surgical repair 6 hours postoperatively. This patient died 36 hours later, and at autopsy, no evidence of myocardial infarction was seen. The overall operative mortality of AICD implantation has been estimated to be 2 to 3 per cent.[5]

Local problems related to the abdominally located subcutaneous generator pocket have also been described. Large seromatous accumulations over the generator were observed in 4 patients in our experience within 4 days after surgery, with 1 patient requiring needle drainage.[29] Subcutaneous hematomas were noted in 2 of 112 patients reported by Mirowski and colleagues[30] and in 1 patient in our series.[29] Pocket infection is a serious complication that may require explantation of the entire system. This infection occurred in 1 patient in our series, who required explantation[29]; 1 patient in the Stanford University series of 70 patients, who required subsequent explantation[12]; and

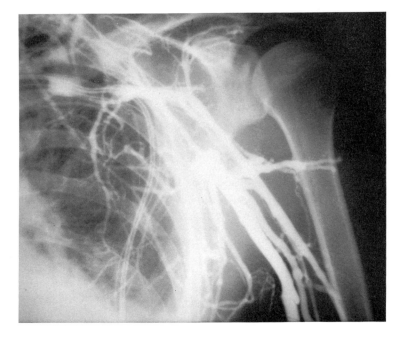

Figure 27-7. Venogram demonstrating subclavian vein thrombosis and occlusion in a patient in whom a superior vena caval spring lead and an endocardial bipolar sensing lead were present in the subclavian vein.

in 4 of 112 patients reported by Mirowski, with 2 of the patients requiring explantation of the AICD to eradicate the infection.[30]

With the increasing use of two-patch AICD defibrillating systems in lieu of a combination patch–spring lead system, vascular complications are less frequent. However, with earlier use of the large-caliber spring lead and bipolar sensing leads positioned transvenously, symptomatic subclavian vein thrombosis at the site of lead insertion occurred with an incidence of 7 per cent in the series of Marchlinski and associates[29] and Reid and coworkers[38] (Fig. 27-7). In both series, intravenous heparinization was utilized, with subsequent resolution of the problem.

An unusual but important embolic event occurred following intraoperative testing of the AICD in one patient in our series who had longstanding atrial fibrillation in addition to serious ventricular arrhythmias.[29] After conversion of VF, the patient also converted from atrial fibrillation to normal sinus rhythm. The patient had not received anticoagulation treatment during the perioperative period; 48 hours following AICD implantation, he suffered a presumed embolic cerebrovascular accident.

In a number of studies, migration of the superior vena caval spring electrode occurred (Fig. 27-8). This was noted in 3 of 14 patients in our study[29] and in 2 of 57 in the Stanford University study.[12] The overall incidence of this complication has been estimated at 2 to 3

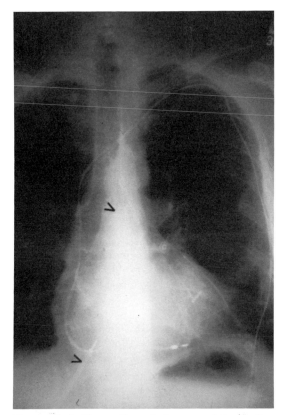

Figure 27-8. Chest radiograph demonstrating migration of a superior vena caval spring electrode to a subdiaphragmatic location in the inferior vena cava in a patient with an automatic implantable cardioverter/defibrillator (AICD). The lead is delineated by arrowheads.

per cent.[5] Improved techniques of lead fixation at the subclavian incision site have essentially eliminated this problem.

Complications Related to Arrhythmia Detection

The AICD detects VT or VF using a high rate cut-off criterion either alone or in combination with a probability density function (PDF), which indexes time during a rhythm away from the electrocardiographic baseline. In both cases, rhythms other than VT or VF may satisfy this detection criteria and inappropriately cause the AICD to discharge. Both sinus tachycardia and atrial fibrillation may trigger the AICD if the rate cut-off is exceeded (devices with high rate criterion only) or if aberrant conduction is present in combination with a sufficiently rapid ventricular response (devices with both high rate criterion and PDF).

Once a rhythm has satisfied the AICD's criterion for tachycardia detection and has begun to charge its capacitors, the impending discharge is irreversible. As a result, nonsustained VT with a rate sufficiently high to meet existing detection algorithms may trigger the AICD and cause it to discharge at a time when the rhythm has stopped[29] (Fig. 27–9). The concern with such a circumstance is not only for the patient's discomfort but also for AICD-induced VT or VF, which may lead to hemodynamic collapse (Fig. 27–10).

In addition to inappropriate sensing of supraventricular tachyarrhythmias, sensing of noncardiac signals has been reported to trigger AICD discharge. In our series, two patients had discharges secondary to sensed myopotentials; in one patient the AICD discharged during shivering and in a second patient during arm motion.[29] Others have reported similar occurrences.[5] In addition, electromagnetic interference produced by surgical electrocautery may also satisfy detection criteria, leading to inappropriate AICD discharge.[5]

Rarely, the AICD may fail to detect VT or VF. Spontaneous fluctuations in VT cycle length may occur. If the high rate cut-off is too close to the tachycardia rate, it is possible for minor decreases in the VT rate to result in failure of arrhythmia sensing. Antiarrhythmic agents begun following AICD implantation may slow VT rate during recurrences and may similarly increase the VT cycle length, so that the high rate criterion is not met.[5, 29, 50] Bardy and colleagues reported a case in which excessive variability in the electrogram size (2 to 39 mV) during VF prevented the automatic gain of the AICD to adjust rapidly enough to sense the low-amplitude signals following the large, high slew rate electrograms.[2] VF detection was prevented in much the same manner as that which can occur during asynchronous unipolar pacing during VF (see below).

The following recommendations may prevent or solve the preceding problems:

1. Prior to implantation, all patients should undergo exercise tolerance testing to document the maximal achievable heart rate. With this information one can determine the degree of overlap between VT rate and maximal sinus tachycardia rate so that the feasibility of AICD implantation can be ascertained. If sufficient separation is present, an AICD device with an appropriate rate cut-off could be chosen. If the maximal sinus rate with exercise approaches the rate cut-off of the device, adjunctive therapy with beta blockers to lower the maximal sinus rate can be used. Current AICD models come with a preset rate cut-off, and this feature is not programmable.

2. Extensive ambulatory and telemetric monitoring of cardiac rhythm should be performed preoperatively to detect concomitant supraventricular tachyarrhythmias as well as nonsustained episodes of VT, which could potentially trigger the AICD to deliver a coun-

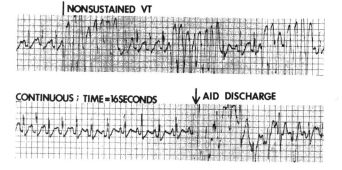

Figure 27–9. Continuous electrocardiographic (ECG) recording demonstrating triggering of an AICD discharge by bursts of spontaneous, nonsustained VT.

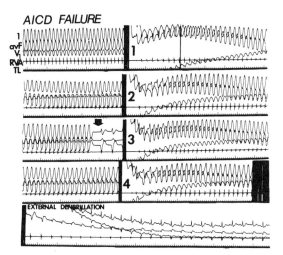

Figure 27–10. AICD failure during postoperative electrophysiologic testing. Surface ECG leads I, aV_F, V_1 and the electrogram recorded from the right ventricular apex (RVA) are displayed. AICD discharges 1 and 2 are ineffectual in terminating induced uniform VT in a patient in whom intraoperative testing had demonstrated an adequate defibrillation threshold. In the third panel, VT terminates spontaneously; however, the AICD discharges following termination of VT and reinitiates it. Discharge 4 is ineffectual, and in the final panel external cardioversion is required.

tershock inappropriately. Antiarrhythmic medications should be administered preoperatively to suppress these arrhythmias.

3. It is recommended that if antiarrhythmic medication is to be given, all electrophysiologic studies should be performed while the patient is receiving that agent. In this way, the electrophysiologic characteristics of the induced ventricular arrhythmia, particularly cycle length, can be determined prior to AICD selection. In addition, theoretical alterations in defibrillation threshold by antiarrhythmic agents could be assessed intraoperatively. If an antiarrhythmic agent is to be added at a later time or the regimen is to be changed, it is recommended that repeat electrophysiologic testing with tachycardia induction be performed to ensure that the tachycardia has not been slowed below the device's rate cut-off and to ensure that the defibrillation threshold is not increased so as to render the device ineffective.

4. If inappropriate sensing leading to AICD discharge is suspected, it can be verified by deactivating the device with a magnet and then leaving the magnet in place over the AICD generator. In this mode, a tone will be emitted with each sensed event. This pattern can be correlated with the patient's electrocardiographic tracing to determine if extracardiac

signals are being sensed by the device. If specific maneuvers are thought to be correlated with myopotentials, these actions can be performed with the magnet in place. Chapman and Troup have recommended simultaneous phonocardiographic recordings of the tones emitted by the AICD and electrocardiographic tracings of cardiac rhythm to document the correlation on a hard-copy tracing.[6] In addition, prolonged ambulatory monitoring is indicated in this situation, since patients may have appropriate discharges of the device at a time when they are asymptomatic.

5. The AICD should be deactivated before any procedures in which the potential for electromagnetic interference is high, such as surgical procedures in which electrocautery is used.

Interactions Between the AICD and Permanent Pacemakers

Signals produced by permanent transvenous pacemakers may adversely affect the ability of the AICD to operate effectively. In an alert distributed in 1983 by the manufacturer of the device, three situations were outlined[1]:

1. *Detection inhibition:* In this instance, the pacemaker would function in an asynchronous mode during VF or VT owing to failure to sense the low-amplitude ventricular electrograms in these rhythms (Fig. 27–11 and 27–12). The higher-amplitude pacemaker stimulus artifacts would be sensed by the AICD, with the automatic gain control of the device being unable to adjust rapidly enough to the rapid, low-amplitude VF electrograms. As a result, the AICD would be "fooled" into sensing the cardiac rate as being identical to the asynchronous paced rate and would fail to sense VF. This problem is confined almost exclusively to unipolar pacing systems, with their attendant high-amplitude stimulus artifacts, although experience with bipolar devices is more limited.

2. *Double counting:* In patients with dual-chamber pacemakers with AV sequential pacing, both the atrial and the ventricular pacemaker stimulus artifacts may also be inappropriately sensed as ventricular electrograms, leading to an apparent doubling of the true rate by the AICD sensing circuitry. A similar situation may occur during atrial pacing with intact AV conduction; the AICD may sense the atrial stimulus artifact and the ventricular electrogram as separate signals and thus double the true rate.[6] In both instances, unipolar

UNIPOLAR PACING DURING VENTRICULAR FIBRILLATION

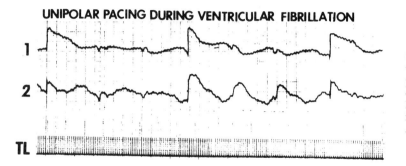

Figure 27-11. Undersensing of ventricular fibrillation (VF) in a patient with a unipolar ventricular demand pacemaker, leading to large unipolar pacing artifacts during intraoperative evaluation for AICD implantation.

pacing systems are generally to blame, although the latter circumstance has been noted in bipolar units.

Double counting may also occur when excessive latency exists between the pacemaker stimulus artifact and the provoked ventricular electrogram. Since the refractory period of the AICD sensing circuitry is short, 150 msec, a stimulus to electrogram interval exceeding this could potentially lead to sensing of both the stimulus artifact and the ventricular electrogram in a ventricular demand pacemaker. Only unipolar pacemaker stimulus artifacts are generally large enough to cause this phenomenon.

3. *Countershock-induced pacemaker sensing error:* Transient undersensing in ventricular pacemakers following AICD discharge has been reported.[8] With failure to sense, the units may function asynchronously. In this instance, large unipolar pacemaker spikes may be sensed in addition to ventricular electrograms, leading to overestimation of the true rate by the AICD and the potential for subsequent inappropriate discharge.

Specific recommendations have been developed to deal with these problems:

1. Because of the large size of the stimulus artifact in unipolar pacing systems, only bipolar leads and pacemakers should be utilized in patients with the AICD. If a unipolar unit was implanted prior to AICD implantation, it should be programmed to the lowest stimulus

amplitude that will ensure adequate pacing. During intraoperative testing, VT or VF should be induced with the pacemaker in an asynchronous mode to see if detection inhibition occurs at these settings. If it does, revision of the pacing system with implantation of a bipolar lead system is recommended. Similarly, during intraoperative testing with either a unipolar or a bipolar system in place, VT or VF should be induced with the pacemaker in the demand mode to see if asynchronous pacing occurs during these rhythms.

2. The AICD rate detection leads should be placed as far as possible from the leads used for pacing. If right ventricular endocardial pacing is to be done, the AICD epicardial sensing leads should be placed on the posterolateral left ventricle using a narrow (1 cm) interelectrode spacing. Placement of pacing and AICD sensing leads endocardially in the right ventricle should be avoided.

3. AICD sensing positions in which the latency between the pacing stimulus artifact and the evoked electrogram exceeds 150 msec should be avoided, especially in unipolar systems.

4. After AICD discharge or intraoperative testing, the pacemaker's pacing and sensing thresholds should be rechecked, and if necessary, reprogramming should be done to ensure adequate safety margins.

Routine pacemaker programming during

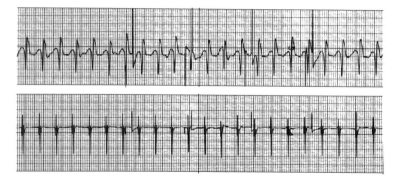

Figure 27-12. Undersensing of VT in a patient with a dual-chamber unipolar pacemaker. The upper tracing is recorded from the two patch leads during AICD implantation, and the lower tracing is recorded from the bipolar endocardial sensing lead. Note asynchronous atrioventricular (AV) pacing artifacts during VT.

follow-up may also lead to adverse interactions with the AICD. A number of pacemaker programmers have a magnet in the programming head. Inadvertent positioning of the head near the AICD generator could lead to internal discharge of the device and the potential risk of VT or VF induction if the countershock is delivered to the patient. If the head is left near the AICD for more than 30 seconds, the AICD could inadvertently be deactivated by the magnet. It is therefore advisable to deactivate the AICD prior to pacemaker programming, with subsequent reactivation after this is accomplished.

Early AICD Failure

The original automatic implantable defibrillator was manufactured with an expected life of 18 months. However, early device failure occurred. In our experience, this failure was noted in 4 of 26 patients, with the mean time to premature failure being 12.5 months.[29] An electrochemical glass corrosion in the AICD battery was identified as the primary cause of this premature depletion in 1983. A protective feedthrough coating of ethylenetetrafluoro-ethylene was incorporated in all AICD batteries shipped after January 1, 1984, with the elimination of this problem. Other generator component failures have been rare.

Failure to Terminate Ventricular Tachycardia or Ventricular Fibrillation

In occasional patients, an adequate defibrillation threshold is difficult to obtain in the operating room. In our experience, this is more commonly seen in patients with large, dilated hearts. Utilization of the two-patch system as opposed to the spring lead–patch system may overcome this problem. So, too, may use of large (27 cm^2) patches instead of the smaller ones (10 cm^2). In some patients, minor variations in patch position also can aid in lowering the defibrillation threshold (DFT), as can alteration of the patch polarity. Generally, a DFT less than 20 J should be sought to provide some safety margin between the maximal energy delivered by the AICD and the defibrillation threshold. When a threshold less than 20 J cannot be achieved, one runs the risk of having only intermittent success of the AICD during postoperative testing or during actual recurrent arrests. Marchlinski and colleagues recently reported a 100 per cent success rate during postoperative AICD testing in patients with intraoperative DFTs less than or equal to 15 J, compared with only a 70 per cent success rate during postoperative AICD testing in patients with DFTs greater than or equal to 20 J.[28] Problems with high DFTs are being addressed by the release of higher-energy devices capable of delivering greater than 30 J.

Another consideration in patients with an AICD that can no longer cardiovert VT or VF is adjunctive antiarrhythmic therapy. Although the data are not unequivocal, it appears that different pharmacologic agents may alter the defibrillation threshold. In canine experiments, lidocaine[4] and amiodarone[17] increase the defibrillation threshold, while procainamide has little effect.[11] The clinical relevance of these findings is as yet uncertain.

Problems During AICD Follow-up

A major concern of cardiologists involved in the follow-up of patients with AICDs is the selection of appropriate time for elective device replacement to avoid leaving the patient unprotected. The current device utilizes an elective replacement indicator (ERI), which uses the charge time of the device following brief magnet application. The charge time is digitally displayed on a commercially available AIDCHECK device (Cardiac Pacemakers, Inc., St. Paul, MN). The AICD will then deliver the stored charge to an internal load. In rare instances, the stored energy may be inadvertently delivered to the patient with the potential for arrhythmia induction. As a result, external defibrillators should be on hand during all magnet tests.

During follow-up studies, it became clear that the first charge time often exceeded the ERI. However, a second charge time, obtained 10 minutes after the first, would give a shorter charge time. This phenomenon was due to the need for reformation of the AICD's capacitors by the first magnet test. It was still clear that the ERI determined by the second charge time early in the life of the device was too conservative. As a result, the manufacturers of the AICD have revised the ERI determination and have suggested the following formula:

$$\text{ERI} = \text{second charge time at 8-month} \\ \text{follow-up visit} \times 1.2$$

If data at 8 months are not available, elective replacement should be scheduled if the second magnet test exceeds 12 seconds. The time to end of life is 3 ± 1 months when the former criterion is met and 3 ± 3 months for the latter. As a result, with the latter criterion, some patients will have little battery reserve when this ERI is met. Further refinements in ERI for future generations of the AICD are expected.

Psychologic Considerations with the AICD

As might be expected, patients with both life-threatening arrhythmias and an implanted device, whose adequate function stands between survival and possible sudden death, are prone to severe anxiety and depression. Such findings have been documented in patients with permanent transvenous pacemakers[36] and is magnified in the AICD population. A number of patients in our care have required concomitant psychiatric consultation in an attempt to lead a normal existence after AICD implantation. In addition, an informal support group composed of the patients with AICDs, their families, and medical professionals has been organized at our institution to help these patients cope with their unique situation. This example of the team approach to caring for these patients has been successful in our experience and should be considered at any institution implanting the AICD.

TRANSVENOUS CARDIOVERTER

In 1984, Zipes and colleagues reported their initial experience with a fully implantable transvenous device capable of terminating VT with a low-energy endocardial countershock.[51] Use of this device followed a number of studies in the electrophysiology laboratory that documented this technique to be successful in terminating up to 85 per cent of episodes of sustained, uniform VT, with at least one attempt being effective in up to 75 per cent of patients.[21, 26, 47] The device had mixed degrees of success in terminating various forms of SVT[3, 21, 32] and was generally not reliably effective for terminating VF.

Although the transvenous cardioverter has not been approved for clinical use, a consideration of the problems associated with its use is important, since this modality may be incorporated into future antitachycardia devices. Acceleration of VT following attempted catheter cardioversion has been reported in up to 16 per cent of termination trials,[47] with ventricular flutter or VF induced in 5 per cent.[26]

In the clinical study of Zipes and colleagues in which the implanted device was used, documentation of VT acceleration or degeneration to VF during preimplantation trials was employed as an exclusion criterion.[51] Nevertheless, one of the seven patients reported had four episodes of significant VT acceleration, while a second patient had multiple discharges of the device during atrial fibrillation as well as a countershock delivered on the ST segment during VT, which resulted in ventricular flutter and ultimately VF.

A second feature of the transvenous cardioverter that should be considered is the reported discomfort associated with the low-energy shocks. This device had been considered only for patients with hemodynamically tolerated, sustained VT. As a result, patients are conscious at the time of attempted cardioversion. Tolerance of the patient to device discharge is variable but is generally inversely proportional to the amount of energy delivered. Discharges greater than 0.5 to 1.0 J were poorly tolerated.[21, 32, 47, 52]

In summary, this device suffers from the same potential proarrhythmic problems as antitachycardia pacemakers and is no more effective. As currently designed, it is not capable of terminating VF effectively, and therefore it cannot stand alone as a device for terminating VT. Incorporation of a backup defibrillatory capability will be needed before further clinical trials can be attempted.

CONCLUSIONS

Physicians dealing with patients who have cardiac arrhythmias are turning increasingly toward nonpharmacologic modes of therapy. Implantable devices such as antitachycardia pacemakers and the AICD have selected indications but stand as forerunners of future universal antiarrhythmic devices. Until the necessary advances are made, physicians must deal with the realities of the present and the limitations and complications associated with the devices now available. The recognition of these problems and the management strategies that have been devised can serve as useful guidelines for the present as well as aids in the design of future devices.

REFERENCES

1. Bach SM: AID-B Cardioverter-Defibrillator: Possible Interaction with Pacemakers. Pittsburgh, Intec Systems, 1983.

2. Bardy GH, Ivey TD, Stewart R, et al: Failure of the automatic implantable defibrillator to detect ventricular fibrillation Am J Cardiol 58:1107, 1986.
3. Benditt DG, Kriett JM, Tobler HG, et al: Cardioversion of atrial tachyarrhythmias by low energy transvenous technique [abstract]. PACE 6:A–133, 1983.
4. Black JN, Barbey JT, Echt DS: Modulation of lidocaine effects on ventricular defibrillation [abstract]. J Am Coll Cardiol 9:166A, 1987.
5. Cannom DS, Winkle RA: Implantation of the automatic implantable cardioverter defibrillator (AICD): Practical aspects. PACE 9:793–809, 1986.
6. Chapman PD, Troup P: The automatic implantable cardioverter-defibrillator: Evaluating suspected inappropriate shocks. J Am Coll Cardiol 7:1075, 1986.
7. Charos GS, Haffajee CI, Gold RL, et al: A theoretical and practically more effective method for interruption of ventricular tachycardia: Self-adapting autodecremental overdrive pacing. Circulation 73:309, 1986.
8. Cohen A, Wish M, Miller F, et al: Interactions between the automatic implantable defibrillator and implanted pacemakers. Circulation 74:111, 1986.
9. Den Dulk K, Kersschot IE, Brugada P, Wellens HJJ: Is there a universal antitachycardia pacing mode? Am J Cardiol 57:950, 1986.
10. Echt DS: Potential hazards of implanted devices for the electrical control of tachyarrhythmias. PACE 7:580, 1984.
11. Echt DS, Robertson-Coxe D, Black JN, Sewell E: Procainamide does not affect ventricular defibrillation in dogs [abstract]. J Am Coll Cardiol 9:166A, 1987.
12. Echt DS, Armstrong K, Schmidt P, et al: Clinical experience, complications and survival in 70 patients with the automatic implantable cardioverter/defibrillator. Circulation 71:289, 1985.
13. Fahraeus T, Lassuik C, Sonnhag C: Tachycardias initiated by automatic antitachycardia pacemakers. PACE 7:1049, 1984.
14. Falkoff MD, Barold SS, Goodfriend MA, et al: Long-term management of ventricular tachycardia by implantable automatic burst tachycardia-terminating pacemakers. PACE 9:885, 1986.
15. Fisher JD, Mehra R, Furman S: Termination of ventricular tachycardia with bursts of rapid ventricular pacing. Am J Cardiol 41:94, 1978.
16. Fisher JD, Kim SG, Matos JA, Ostrow E: Comparative effectiveness of pacing techniques for termination of well-tolerated sustained ventricular tachycardia. PACE 7:915, 1983.
17. Frame LH, Hoffman N, Kolenik SA, Sheldon JH: Oral loading with amiodarone increases ventricular defibrillation threshold in dogs [abstract]. J Am Coll Cardiol 7:82A, 1986.
18. Freedman RA, Griffen JC, Rothman MT, Mason JW: Safety and efficacy of an automatic tachycardia terminating device [abstract]. Circulation 66:217, 1982.
19. Gardner MJ, Waxman HL, Buxton AE, et al: Termination of ventricular tachycardia—evaluation of a new pacing method. Am J Cardiol 50:1338, 1982.
20. Griffin JC, Sweeney M: The management of paroxysmal tachycardias using the Cybertach-60. PACE 7:1291, 1984.
21. Hartzler GO, Kallok MJ: Low energy transvenous intracavitary cardioversion of tachycardias [abstract]. PACE 6:A–144, 1983.
22. Hartzler GO, Holmes DR, Osborn MJ: Patient activated transvenous cardiac stimulation for the treatment of supraventricular and ventricular tachycardia. Am J Cardiol 47:903, 1981.
23. Jentzer JH, Hoffman RM: Acceleration of ventricular tachycardia by rapid overdrive pacing combined with extrastimuli. PACE 7:922, 1984.
24. Josephson ME, Horowitz LN, Farshidi A, Kastor JA: Recurrent sustained ventricular tachycardia. I. Mechanisms. Circulation 57:431, 1978.
25. Kahn A, Morris JJ, Citron P: Patient-initiated rapid atrial pacing to manage supraventricular tachycardia. Am J Cardiol 38:200, 1976.
26. Kallok MJ, Fisher JD, Fletcher RD, et al: Intracavitary cardioversion and defibrillation: A multicenter study [abstract]. Circulation 68:89, 1983.
27. Lerman BB, Waxman HL, Buxton AE, et al: Tachyarrhythmias associated with programmable automatic atrial antitachycardia pacemakers. Am Heart J 106:1029, 1983.
28. Marchlinski FE, Flores B, Miller JM, Hargrove WC: Is postoperative testing of the automatic implantable defibrillator necessary [abstract]? PACE 10:438, 1987.
29. Marchlinski FE, Flores BT, Buxton AE, et al: The automatic implantable cardioverter-defibrillator: Efficacy, complications, and device failures. Ann Intern Med 104:481, 1986.
30. Mirowski M, Mower MM, Veltri EP, et al: Recent clinical experience with the automatic implantable cardioverter-defibrillator. Cardiol Clin 3:623, 1985.
31. Mirowski M, Reid PR, Winkle RA, et al: Mortality in patients with implanted defibrillators. Ann Intern Med 98:585, 1983.
32. Nathan A, Bexton R, Hellestrand K, et al: Internal "microshock" for arrhythmia termination [abstract]. PACE 6:A–129, 1983.
33. Nathan A, Hellestrand K, Bexton R, et al: Problems with patient activated pacemakers for tachycardia termination [abstract]. PACE 6:A–137, 1983.
34. Peters RW, Scheinman MM, Morady F, Jacobson L: Long-term management of paroxysmal tachycardia by burst overdrive pacing [abstract]. J Am Coll Cardiol 3:473, 1984.
35. Peters RW, Shafton E, Frank S, et al: Radiofrequency-triggered pacemakers: Uses and limitations. Ann Intern Med 88:17, 1978.
36. Phibbs B, Marriott HJL: Complications of permanent transvenous pacing. N Engl J Med 312:1428, 1985.
37. Pless BD, Sweeney MB: Discrimination of supraventricular tachycardia from sinus tachycardia of overlapping cycle length. PACE 7:1318, 1984.
38. Reid PR, Mirowski M, Mower MM, et al: Clinical evaluation of the internal automatic cardioverter-defibrillator in survivors of sudden cardiac death. Am J Cardiol 51:1608, 1983.
39. Roy D, Waxman HL, Buxton AE, et al: Termination of ventricular tachycardia: Role of tachycardia cycle length. Am J Cardiol 50:1346, 1982.
40. Ruskin JN, Garan H, Poulin F, Harthorne JW: Permanent radiofrequency ventricular pacing for management of drug resistant ventricular tachycardia. Am J Cardiol 46:317, 1980.
41. Sowton E: Clinical results with the Tachylog antitachycardia pacemaker. PACE 7:1313, 1984.
42. Spurrell RAJ, Nathan AW, Camm AJ: Clinical experience with implantable scanning tachycardia reversion pacemakers. PACE 7:1296, 1984.
43. Spurrell RAJ, Nathan AW, Bexton RS, Hellestrand KJ: Implantable automatic scanning pacemaker for termination of supraventricular tachycardia. Am J Cardiol 49:753, 1982.

44. Waldecker B, Brugada P, den Dulk K, et al: Arrhythmias induced during termination of supraventricular tachycardia. Am J Cardiol 55:412, 1985.
45. Waldo AL, McLean WAH, Karp RB, et al: Entrainment and interruption of atrial flutter with atrial pacing: Studies in man following open heart surgery. Circulation 56:737, 1977.
46. Waldo AL, Plumb VJ, Arciniegas JG, et al: Transient entrainment and interruption of the atrioventricular bypass type of paroxysmal atrial tachycardia. Circulation 67:73, 1983.
47. Waspe LE, Fisher JD, Kim SG, Matos JA: Reliability of transvenous shocks for termination of ventricular tachycardia and ventricular fibrillation [abstract]. J Am Coll Cardiol 1:595, 1983.
48. Wellens HJJ, Durrer DR, Lie KI: Observations on mechanisms of ventricular tachycardia in man. Circulation 54:237, 1976.
49. Wellens HJJ, den Dulk K, Brugada P: Pacemaker management of cardiac arrhythmias. *In* Dreifus LD (ed): Pacemaker Therapy. Philadelphia, FA Davis, 1983, p 165.
50. Winkle RA, Stinson EB, Echt DS, et al: Practical aspects of automatic cardioverter/defibrillator implantation. Am Heart J 108:1335, 1984.
51. Zipes DP, Heger JJ, Miles WM, et al: Early experience with an implantable cardioverter. N Engl J Med 311:485, 1984.
52. Zipes DP, Jackman WM, Heger JJ, et al: Clinical transvenous cardioversion of recurrent life-threatening ventricular tachyarrhythmias: Low energy synchronized cardioversion of ventricular tachycardia and termination of ventricular fibrillation in patients using a catheter electrode. Am Heart J 103:789, 1982.

28

RECOGNITION OF TACHYARRHYTHMIAS BY IMPLANTABLE DEVICES

A. JOHN CAMM, VINCE PAUL, *and* D. E. WARD

There is no doubt that electrical methods of tachycardia termination are effective.[22] The development of the implantable defibrillator, with its potential combination with pacemaker techniques, provides a therapeutic modality that is not otherwise available for the treatment of malignant and life-threatening ventricular arrhythmias. It may well be that the number of devices implanted for the reversion or control of tachycardia will eventually exceed those implanted for the prevention of bradycardia. However, although the methods of tachycardia termination are now well developed, the automatic recognition of pathologic tachyarrhythmias is still difficult and unreliable. The utility of implantable devices for the management of serious tachyarrhythmias hinges on the prompt and certain automatic recognition of the origin and hemodynamic consequences of spontaneous tachycardia.

Until recently, implanted or semi-implanted devices were designed to be used for tachycardia termination when activated by the patient in response to an abnormal tachycardia (Table 28–1). This design is inadequate when tachycardia induces syncope or hemodynamic and functional collapse. To some extent this problem was addressed by advocating device activation by physician, relative, or friend, but this requires that a patient must rely on another person to achieve tachycardia termination. Patient-activated devices are also not ideal when the tachycardia is asymptomatic. Occasionally, patients may perversely initiate their tachycardias by activating the pacemaker during sinus rhythm. For this reason, devices were developed that needed both activation by

the patient and automatic recognition and confirmation of tachycardia. This development, as well as the appreciation that effective and useful tachycardia termination should be as immediate as possible and not reliant on the development of symptoms that the treatment was intended to avoid, stimulated the search for methods to detect the onset of tachycardia automatically and to distinguish physiologic and benign forms from pathologic and malignant varieties.

TACHYCARDIA RECOGNITION

There are several settings in which automatic analysis of the cardiac rhythm, hemodynamic situation, and electrophysiologic circumstance is required (Table 28–2). Tachycardia may develop in a specific setting that might be capable of detection and correction. For example, tachycardia could be dependent on

TABLE 28–1. MANUAL ACTIVATION OF TACHYCARDIA TREATMENT DEVICE

ADVANTAGES	DISADVANTAGES
Operation is simple.	Symptoms are essential for operation.
Activation can be restricted to a physician.	Severe symptoms disable the patient.
	Activation is delayed.
Activation can be restricted to a safe setting (hospital or clinic).	Deliberate *initiation* of tachycardias is possible.
Several forms of tachycardia may be recognized as abnormal.	Patient cooperation is essential.
	An external device (magnet pacer or programmer) is needed.

589

TABLE 28–2. AUTOMATIC RECOGNITION OF RHYTHM

1. Events preceding tachycardia (sinus tachycardia, premature beats, loss of preexcitation)
2. Onset of tachycardia
3. Hemodynamic consequences of tachycardia (e.g., stroke output or arterial pressure)
4. Physiologic circumstances of tachycardia (e.g., during exertion), as assessed by piezoelectric crystal signals
5. Moment of tachycardia termination (e.g., during burst pacing)
6. Continuation of tachycardia (after electrical intervention or immediately before delayed treatment)
7. Restoration of normal rhythm (sinus rhythm or atrial fibrillation)

adrenergic activation and would consequently occur in the setting of relative sinus tachycardia associated with little or no physical activity. Such a circumstance might easily be detected by the combination of rate and activity sensors. Alternatively, tachycardia might arise from a background of bradycardia, which could easily be avoided by bradycardia prevention pacing techniques. An increase in the frequency or complexity of premature beats might signal imminent tachycardia initiation. Such a circumstance is detectable and potentially treatable. Thus far, this aspect of tachycardia control has not been much applied.

The onset of tachycardia can be detected relatively easily by simple rate criteria (Table 28–3). Confounding this, however, is the possibility of confusing myocardial electrograms with other myopotentials or extraneous electromagnetic interference. Developments in

TABLE 28–3. CRITERIA FOR AUTOMATIC DIAGNOSIS OF TACHYARRHYTHMIAS

Rate	Rate; rate of change of rate; rate stability; duration of high rate; percentage of beats at high rate
Electrogram	Amplitude; slew rate; frequency content; electrogram timing; multiple electrogram differential timing Gradient pattern detection (GPD); intrinsic timing (IT); autocorrelation; probability density function (PDF); area of difference (AOD); temporal electrogram analysis (TEA)
Hemodynamics	Impedance; arterial pressure; intramyocardial pressure; ventricular dp/dt; preejection period
Activity sensing	Piezoelectric detection of body activity respiration

bradycardia pacing technology have improved the security of detecting and analyzing myocardial electrograms by the incorporation of filters and noise elimination circuits and by the use of specific electrode types and arrangements. In this regard, bipolar electrode configurations are particularly important for reducing the likelihood of detecting myopotentials and external interference. Almost all automatic antitachycardia devices have utilized bipolar sensing techniques.

The mere presence of tachycardia should not be a sufficient trigger for initiation of a tachycardia reversion therapy. Tachyarrhythmias should be assessed in terms of origin (sinus, supraventricular, ventricular, and so on), type (e.g., tachycardia, flutter, or fibrillation), hemodynamic consequence (normal, depressed, and so forth), and stability (unchanging or deteriorating). A combination of rate, electrogram, activity, and hemodynamic and metabolic sensors may eventually be required to characterize arrhythmias sufficiently accurately to allow specific therapy to be administered.

During the delivery of pacing therapy, it may be possible to detect the exact moment at which tachycardia terminates. All present-generation devices fail to explore this possibility. In response to atrial burst pacing in a patient with Wolff-Parkinson-White (WPW) syndrome, orthodromic reentrant atrioventricular (AV) tachycardia termination might be signaled by the occurrence of preexcited beats in response to atrial pacing. Appropriate electrogram analysis could reveal this and result in timely termination of the atrial burst. Similarly, during a slowly accelerating burst of pacing it should be possible to recognize entrainment and "broken entrainment," that is, termination, of other tachycardias, provided that critical electrode placement is employed. During an attempted pacing intervention, the evoked response could be analyzed (see Table 28–5). Such an analysis could be used to detect the relative refractory period[8] (increased stimulus latency) and to optimize pacing energy, perhaps to a value marginally above the diastolic threshold.[6] The timing of beats following a pacing intervention should also be measured to detect the provocation of ectopic beats, possibly warning of the degeneration of tachycardias, or to assess tachycardia reset or nonreset, which might then be used to influence the direction of a pacemaker scan.[42]

After a therapeutic intervention, it is necessary to confirm the continuation of the pathologic tachycardia or to recognize the resumption of the normal rhythm. It is also essential to reanalyze the rhythm immediately before a therapy, which, although appropriately triggered by an arrhythmia, will be delayed before being administered. For example, the charging of a defibrillator occurs when tachycardia is first recognized, but prior to its discharge, some seconds later, it should be necessary to confirm that the arrhythmia is still present. Reconfirmation of tachycardia is difficult because it must be achieved rapidly, cannot rely on tachycardia onset criteria, and might involve the recognition of an arrhythmia somewhat different from that originally diagnosed. Immediately after a termination event, a pathologic tachycardia may be unstable (e.g., varying cycle lengths), sinus tachycardia may occur, or low-amplitude electrograms may be undetected (e.g., after a defibrillator discharge). These changes may make difficult the confirmation of persistent tachycardia or diagnosis of the resumption of sinus rhythm.

HEART RATE CRITERIA

Because the rates of physiologic and pathologic tachycardias may be similar, the use of heart rate alone to differentiate them will often be inadequate. Furthermore, the rates of both pathologic and physiologic tachycardia may vary with posture, autonomic influences, drugs, and disease progression; therefore, previously established differences between these tachycardias may not be maintained. To overcome these difficulties, other features, presumed specific to the pathologic tachycardia, are incorporated into the diagnostic algorithm.

One such feature is the rate of onset or acceleration of tachycardia. Fisher and colleagues[21] found that the rate of onset of sinus tachycardia in volunteers was generally slower than that of spontaneously occurring ventricular tachycardia (VT) in patients, although some overlap was seen. More recently, the same group has compared the onset of sinus tachycardia with the onset of VT or supraventricular tachycardia (SVT) in the same subjects and found no overlap.[31] This differentiation is used by the "delta heart rate" algorithm, which is incorporated in several commercially available pacemakers and which determines the decrease in cycle length occurring immediately or over several cycles at the onset of tachycardia. The alteration in cycle length required to satisfy the criteria of arrhythmia onset may be programmed as an absolute figure or as a proportion of the preceding cycle lengths. This algorithm appears to improve the specificity of diagnosing pathologic tachycardias,[14] although it may be invalidated when the arrhythmia commences against the background of sinus tachycardia, rapid atrial fibrillation, or frequent ventricular extrasystoles.

Another rate parameter in current use is that of rate stability. Instability of the ventricular rate suggests the diagnosis of atrial fibrillation or ventricular fibrillation (VF), polymorphic ventricular tachycardia (possibly including *torsades de pointes*), sinus tachycardia with frequent ventricular extrasystoles, or any form of SVT with a variable AV conduction response. None of these circumstances would warrant a ventricular pacing attempt to terminate tachycardia. Atrial rate instability suggests atrial fibrillation, which would not respond to an atrial pacing intervention. An inherent problem with a rate stability criterion is the need to analyze successive cycles, which will result in a delayed diagnosis and response. The likelihood of successful termination may also be reduced because of the delay introduced by assessing this criterion. It should also be noted that paroxysmal tachycardias may show marked cycle length variations shortly after their initiation.[23]

RATE CRITERIA FOR THE DIAGNOSIS OF VENTRICULAR FIBRILLATION

The amplitude and cycle length of VF are so variable that on occasions long cycle lengths or low-amplitude electrograms might give the impression that fibrillation has terminated. For this reason, rate algorithms that are designed to diagnose fibrillation are usually "probabilistic," that is, only a proportion of cycle lengths (e.g., 10 of 12 or 18 of 20) must be shorter than the cycle length that distinguishes VF (fibrillation detection interval) from VT (Fig. 28–1).[36] In forthcoming versions of the implantable defibrillator, this probabilistic approach will be utilized, and the sampling period and required proportion will probably be programmable.

The sensitivity of the recording is vital[35] in this system because oversensing may lead to incorrect diagnosis of fibrillation, while undersensing will result in failure to recognize the arrhythmia.

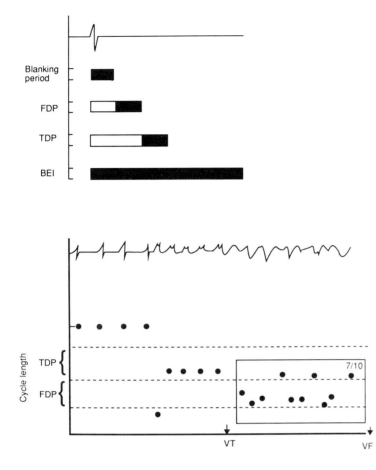

Figure 28–1. The RR intervals of successive beats are measured. Those beats with an RR interval falling in the tachycardia detection period (TDP) are counted, and when a consecutive programmed number of beats are detected, ventricular tachycardia (VT) is diagnosed. Conversely, only a proportion of successive beats need to have an RR interval falling within the fibrillation detection period (FDP) for ventricular fibrillation (VF) to be diagnosed. When no beat falls before the end of the bradycardia escape interval (BEI), bradycardia support pacing occurs.

MORPHOLOGY OF THE ELECTROCARDIOGRAM

These methods involve analysis of the suspect electrogram either by comparison of individual complexes with a previous recorded template or by comparison of a period of the electrogram after a discrete time shift with the original recording before the shift. The means of comparison varies between methods—those of greater complexity requiring considerable computational power—but all suffer the same limitations.

The *intrinsic deflection* time represents the interval between earliest recorded ventricular depolarization and the depolarization at the tip of the electrode (evidenced by dv/dt_{max}) and is dependent on the position of the electrode, the intraventricular conduction, and the degree of far-field sensing (Fig. 28–2). Davies[16] showed that the difference in intrinsic deflection time between sinus rhythm and VT allowed adequate discrimination in 10 of 11 cases.

With reference to *amplitude* and *slew rate,* the electrogram has been evaluated mainly in the differentiation of anterograde from retrograde P waves. Amikam and Furman[2] found slew rates always to be faster in anterograde conduction in 6 cases studied and the ampli-

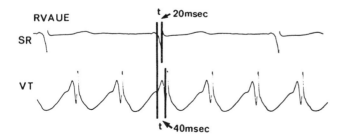

Figure 28–2. The time, t, from the onset of the far-field deflection to the intrinsic deflection is 20 msec during sinus rhythm (SR) and 40 msec during ventricular tachycardia (VT). Tachycardia diagnosis by this method relies on automatic detection of this difference. RVAUE = right ventricular apical unipolar electrogram.

tude to be greater in anterograde than retrograde conduction in 14 of 16 cases. However, the value of these parameters is known to vary considerably with exercise and heart rate,[11] which may account for the greater overlap observed in other studies.[47] These parameters also appear to be of less discriminatory value when applied to ventricular electrograms.[47]

Temporal electrocardiogram analysis (TEA), which, like intrinsic deflection time, has the advantage of requiring low computing power, characterizes the electrocardiogram according to the sequence and time spent by the signal outside threshold rails set above and below the isoelectric line (Fig. 28–3). This method, which largely transposes the electrogram to its time components and minimizes the effect of amplitude variation, has not yet been fully evaluated.

Gradient pattern detection (GPD) is also concerned with the timing and amplitude of events within the electrocardiogram but analyzes a computerized equivalent of the first derivative (with respect to time) after analog to digital conversion. The sequence of turning points is specific for each morphology (Fig. 28–4), and the pattern of the suspect electro-

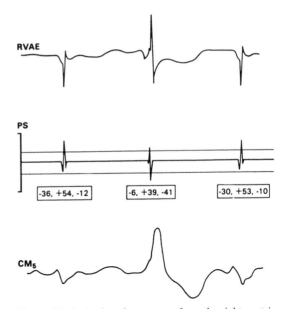

Figure 28–4. Analog electrograms from the right ventricular apex *(upper trace)*, the first-time derivative of the original electrograms *(middle trace)*, with the boxed digital values representing the major turning points of each signal and the surface electrocardiographic (ECG) lead CM₅ *(lower trace)*. A ventricular ectopic beat is different from the sinus beats, which are similar to each other. This difference is retained in the processed signal (in which the baseline is stable), allowing automatic distinction of the two rhythms. The digits illustrate how this can be done. A sequence with a signal of +30 followed by −39 (shown by the thin horizontal lines in the middle panel) differentiates the ectopic beat from sinus rhythm. PS = processed signal; RVAE = right ventricular apical electrogram.

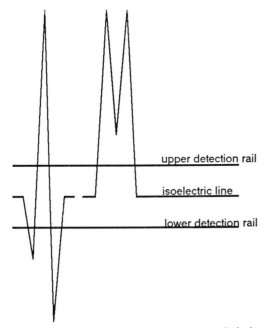

Figure 28–3. The timing of the electrogram as it deviates from the isoelectric line (above and below) is recorded for each complex. The sequence of events is different for varying morphologies. The approximation of the sampling lines to the isoelectric line minimizes any difference that occurs because of changing slew rates. Thus, with this temporal method of analysis, the electrogram is reduced to a series of turning points that are largely independent of amplitude.

cardiogram is compared with a recorded pattern obtained during sinus rhythm. This method, like intrinsic deflection time, has been shown to be highly sensitive[17] in differentiating between sinus rhythm and VT. Furthermore, unlike with many other parameters under investigation, the effect on the recordings of physiologic variables such as exercise and posture has been assessed.

More complex methods of morphologic comparison involve the use of *template matching*. The electrocardiogram is digitized and sampled for a set period of time (40 to 80 msec), centering on the point of maximal dv/dt. A template of the ventricular electrocardiograms during sinus rhythm is next constructed by signal averaging. This template is then compared with the suspect electrocardiogram either by correlation waveform analysis or by measuring area of difference (Fig. 28–5).[24, 44]

In *autocorrelation* the electrogram is compared with itself after a number of discrete time shifts, and a correlation value is obtained after each shift. Regular rhythms will retain a

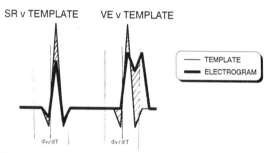

SR v TEMPLATE   VE v TEMPLATE

——— TEMPLATE
━━ ELECTROGRAM

dv/dT   dv/dT

Figure 28–5. The electrogram under consideration is compared with a previously recorded template. The sampling window is set at 40 msec on either side of the fiducial point, and the area of difference *(shaded area)* is then calculated. A sinus (SR) beat shows little variation from the template compared with a ventricular extrasystole (VE).

periodicity, with gradual decrease in amplitude, while an irregular rhythm will give a fragmented and variable trace (Fig. 28–6). A modification of this technique was suggested by Ohm,[45] who proposed that the suspect electrogram should be compared with itself after a shift of 100 msec. The amplitude of the original recording is plotted against the amplitude of the shifted electrogram, and a "phase angle" is calculated. The electrogram of a normally conducted sinus beat will have an amplitude close to zero at 100 msec after the dv/dt_{max}, and plotting this against the shifted electrogram will give a low "phase angle." The electrogram of a broad-complex rhythm (such as VT) will have an amplitude appreciably different from zero at 100 msec after dv/dt_{max}; thus, the phase angle produced by plotting this value against that of the shifted electrogram would be greater (Fig. 28–7). This method,

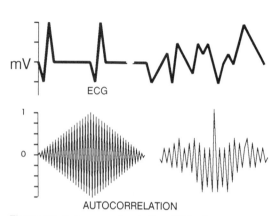

SR   VF

mV

ECG

1

0

AUTOCORRELATION

Figure 28–6. In a regular rhythm (SR), the comparison of the electrogram with itself at all phases of the cycle will show a simple harmonic pattern. In an irregular rhythm (such as VF), this pattern is lost.

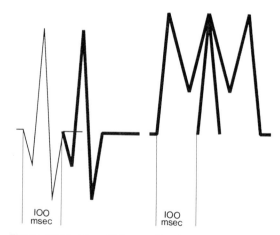

100 msec   100 msec

Figure 28–7. At multiple sampling intervals, the amplitude of the electrogram is plotted against the amplitude of the electrogram after a single time shift of 100 msec, and the angle from the origin is calculated. Narrow-complex beats tend to have smaller, less variable angles than do broad-complex beats.

like other forms of morphologic comparison, has been claimed to be 100 per cent sensitive in discriminating VT from sinus rhythm. However, in only a few studies[29] has the influence of aberrant conduction in sinus rhythm been considered, and in no study has the algorithm been shown to distinguish between different pathologic tachycardias.

Recently, Langberg and colleagues[28] described a method of comparing electrograms using the *area of difference* between all or part of the electrograms associated with sinus rhythm and pathologic tachycardia. They showed that adequate sensitivity could be retained with digitization of the signal at 250 Hz with high pass filtering at no more than 5Hz. Comparing a sample window of 80 msec allowed consistent and reliable distinction between VT and sinus rhythm. However, the signals were collected only under ideal circumstances: when the subject was at rest, supine, and breathing quietly.

As morphologic comparison requires the electrograms to be aligned, a clear reference point is essential to analysis. Thus, markedly irregular or chaotic rhythms may not be clearly identified, making comparison impossible. The ability of these methods to differentiate between two abnormal rhythms or to recognize aberrant conduction de novo seems limited at present.

DERIVED SIGNALS

The use of rate analysis is supplemented in implantable defibrillators by the addition of an

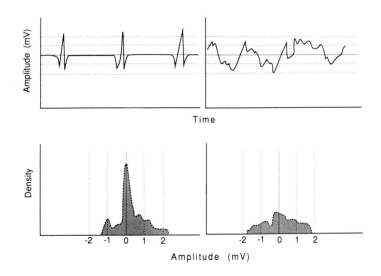

Figure 28–8. The time that the electrogram spends at any given amplitude is plotted as "the density" against that amplitude. Between regular complexes the electrogram spends most of its time at or near the isoelectric line, and as such there is a peak density at amplitude zero. Fast and chaotic rhythms will spend less time at the isoelectric line, and as such the peak density at zero amplitude is lost.

algorithm based upon *probability density analysis*.[32] This function considers the proportion of time that the electrocardiogram signal spends outside amplitude limits set close to the isoelectric line. During sinus rhythm, the signal spends relatively short periods away from the isoelectric line, while in VF the electrogram continually oscillates, spending a greater amount of time away from the isoelectric line (Fig. 28–8). However, at more rapid rates, regardless of the etiology, the proportion of time spent on the isoelectric line between complexes is reduced, and the signal may incorrectly be interpreted as VF. This has proved to be a problem clinically,[20] particularly during atrial fibrillation with a fast ventricular response. In addition to lack of specificity, several studies have reported a low sensitivity in the detection of ventricular arrhythmias other than VF.[4]

Another technique that has recently been applied for distinguishing fibrillatory (atrial or ventricular) from nonfibrillatory tachycardias (sinus, supraventricular, and ventricular) is the *coherence spectrum*.[40] Essentially, this technique can successfully distinguish organized from disorganized rhythm but as yet is not feasible for incorporation into implantable devices.

The application of *fast Fourier analysis* enables the electrocardiogram to be transformed into its frequency spectra (Fig. 28–9). Attempts to discriminate objectively between the different spectra obtained from varying rhythms, on the basis of peak frequency, magnitude, band width, and cut-off frequency, have met with variable success. Pannizzo[38] was able to differentiate between VT and sinus rhythm on the basis of frequency analysis in 85 per cent of cases. Aubert[5] accurately discriminated VF from other rhythms and showed that the power spectra peak was at higher frequencies (4 to 6 Hz) in VF than in sinus rhythm (1 to 4 Hz). Lin[29] obtained a maximal sensitivity in such circumstances of only 60 per cent. However, the spectral content obtained does depend on the recording electrode used,[5] and this may account for some of the discrepancies. As with morphologic analysis, it is likely that problems will arise in differentiating abnormal rhythms.

MONOPHASIC ACTION POTENTIALS

Brachmann and colleagues[10] analyzed the dominant frequency in monophasic action potential (MAP) recordings obtained from dogs, revealing a lower frequency during VT of 4 to 6 Hz compared with 10 to 12 Hz during VF. In the same study, it was noted that the actual duration of the signals was 18 per cent shorter during VT than sinus rhythm and 41 per cent shorter during VF than sinus rhythm; VF was further characterized by the onset of the MAP before completion of the preceding signal. Ward[49] also noted a reduction in duration of the signal during VT in patients but recorded regular MAPs of 170 to 200 msec during VF. MAPs, because of the current of injury, are essentially acute phenomena and are unlikely to be useful with chronically implanted lead systems.

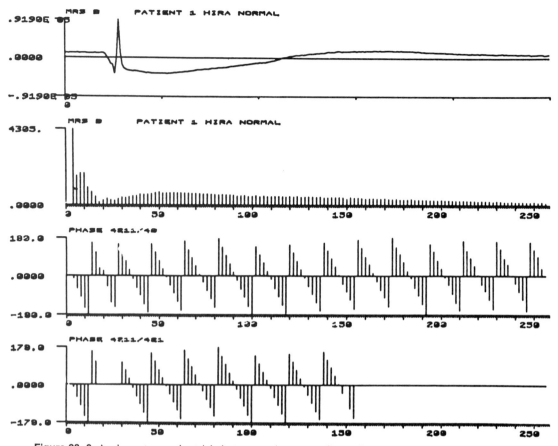

Figure 28–9. Analog anterograde atrial electrogram *(upper panel)*, amplitude fast Fourier transform (FFT) of the anterograde electrogram *(middle panel)*, and phase FFT of the anterograde atrial electrogram *(bottom panel)*. HIRA = high right atrium.

SEQUENTIAL ANALYSIS

The analysis of sequential depolarization from dual-chamber or transcardiac systems[18, 25] has been proposed as a method of differentiating rhythms with partial or complete AV dissociation (Fig. 28–10). Such a method will not reliably distinguish between sinus tachycardia and a pathologic tachycardia with 1:1 AV activation. Paroxysmal supraventricular (or AV) tachycardia usually manifests with a PR interval that is different from the PR interval associated with sinus tachycardia at a similar rate in the same patient. Thus, the AV interval could theoretically be used to distinguish appropriate sinus tachycardia from an inappropriate tachycardia mechanism. For example, the PR interval associated with atrial tachycardia is usually longer than that associated with sinus tachycardia, while during AV nodal tachycardia the P and R waves usually occur simultaneously. In the orthodromic tachycardia associated with the WPW syndrome, the PR interval is usually longer than that found with sinus tachycardia. However, the exact difference will depend on the electrode location. For example, with an orthodromic AV reentrant tachycardia (AVRT) that utilizes a left lateral accessory pathway, location of the sensing electrode in the atrial appendage remote from the tachycardia circuit often results in PR interval measurements that do not distinguish AVRT from sinus tachycardia (Fig. 28–11).[43] Obviously, atrial fibrillation, flutter, or tachycardia with associated AV conduction block will be easily diagnosed using combined atrial and ventricular electrode sensing.[48] Munkenbeck and associates[33] described a system of distinguishing between these by analyzing the timing of ventricular depolarization following an atrial extrastimulus delivered 80 to 100 msec prematurely. In sinus tachycardia the ventricular complex was premature by 30 to 50 msec, while in the pathologic tachycardias the next ventricular complex was not premature by more than 10 msec (Fig.

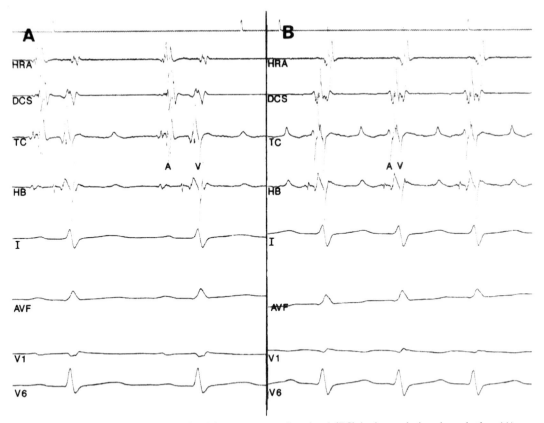

Figure 28–10. The recording obtained from a transcardiac signal (TC) is shown during sinus rhythm *(A)* and during atrioventricular nodal reentrant tachycardia (AVNRT) *(B)*. The transcardiac signal gives a high-frequency signal for both the atrial and the ventricular components, facilitating the measurement of the atrioventricular (AV) delay, which in this case is markedly reduced during tachycardia. HRA = high right atrium; DCS = distal coronary sinus; HB = His bundle electrocardiogram.

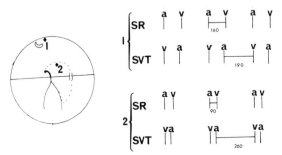

Figure 28–11. In sinus rhythm (SR), atrial (a) activation occurs first and the AV delay depends upon the antero-grade conduction time. In an orthodromic AV reentrant tachycardia (AVRT), the atrial activation follows ventric-ular (v) activation and the AV delay is longer than during sinus tachycardia because the rate is inappropriately fast for physiologic needs. However, the atrial recording po-sition is crucial for detecting the difference in the AV interval. For example, in AVRT due to a left lateral bypass tract, the high right atrial electrogram *(position 1)* will tend to be late in recording the atrial signal during tachycardia. Thus, the AV interval during this form of AVRT will be artifactually shortened and possibly indis-tinguishable from that of sinus tachycardia. Recording within the tachycardia cycle *(position 2)* will tend to accentuate the differences between sinus rhythm and AVRT. SVT = supraventricular tachycardia.

28–12). However, the sinus tachycardia was produced by pharmacologic means, and the efficacy of this algorithm in physiologic condi-tions has yet to be established.

SVT may be distinguished from 1:1 VT on the basis of the differences in sequence and timing of depolarization recorded from two different ventricular electrodes.[30] The use of multiple epicardial ventricular electrodes has also been described by Davies[15] as a sensitive method of distinguishing VT from sinus rhythm and of detecting the onset of VF in patients undergoing bypass surgery. The reli-ability of such a system will depend on the positioning of the electrodes and may require an epicardial approach to increase the area available for comparison.

HEMODYNAMIC CRITERIA

Although not providing a precise morpho-logic diagnosis, the assessment of hemody-

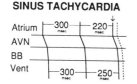

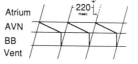

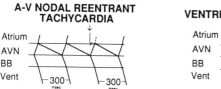

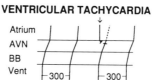

Figure 28–12. Tachycardia may be diagnosed by its response to an atrial premature beat. During sinus tachycardia, a late coupled premature beat is conducted to the ventricles with little additional AV delay. However, during other forms of SVT or VT it is unusual for AV conduction to occur. AVN = atrioventricular node; BB = bundle branch.

namic status permits an appreciation of the functional effect of tachyarrhythmias.

Olson[37] studied the changes in right ventricular pressure in dogs following the induction of VF. The pressures were recorded from chronically implanted pacing leads with additional pressure transducers. Within the first 10 seconds after the onset of VF, the pressure had decreased by an average of 82 per cent, from 23.9 ± 13.0 mm Hg to 3.7 ± 2.1 mm Hg. After defibrillation, baseline right ventricular pressures were equaled or exceeded within 5 seconds. Although the effect of VT was not specifically studied, monomorphic ventricular flutter was induced in one subject with only a comparatively small reduction (52 per cent) in right ventricular pressure. Aubert[5] recently reported the combination of electrocardiogram analysis and aortic pressure recording in 22 patients undergoing implantation of an automatic implantable cardioverter/defibrillator (AICD). In these patients, electrogram analysis differentiated between sinus rhythm and VF on all occasions but failed to recognize ventricular flutter in 7 of 22 cases and VT in 6 of 29 cases. Including aortic pressure in the detection algorithm allowed 100 per cent recognition of VT and ventricular flutter.

The measurement of intracardiac impedance, which is being assessed for use in rate-responsive pacing, may be of value in detecting hemodynamic deterioration associated with arrhythmias. In 1985, Olson and associates[34] studied the effect of induction of VT and VF on intracardiac impedance in 15 patients undergoing electrophysiologic studies. In each of the five patients in whom VF was induced, the intracardiac impedance decreased substantially (average of 27 per cent), but in VT, reductions were smaller and inconsistent.

Whether the decrease in impedance during VT reflected changes in the patient's clinical state is not noted, and postural effects were not considered. However, Bardy[7] found in six patients with a history of failed sudden death that the reduction in ventricular impedance during induced VT or VF correlated with the reduction in mean arterial pressure recorded simultaneously. The greater reduction (44 per cent) in impedance observed by Bardy may have been a reflection of the tendency of these patients to experience hemodynamic deterioration during tachycardia.

Shapland and colleagues[41] have recently reported the hemodynamic consequences of VT induced at electrophysiologic study in nine patients. The arterial pressure, right ventricular systolic pressure, and right ventricular stroke volume (impedance change) all fell during tachycardia, whereas they did not during sinus rhythm in the same patients. These changes were most marked when the tachycardia cycle length was less than 250 msec (>240 beats per minute).

Measurements of pressure or impedance are more easily applicable to the right ventricle, although in practical terms this may be a disadvantage, as the potential exists for a delay in diagnosis if ventricular dissociation occurs, during which time the right ventricle may function normally, or nearly normally, despite left VF. How right ventricular distention due to congestive failure or acute engorgement would affect the recording is not clear.

The measurement of intramyocardial pressure (possibly in the septum) might prevent these complications and is a technique that has been available for many years (Fig. 28–13). In 1984, Denys[19] suggested its use for the detection of VF, and recently, Aubert and Denys[3]

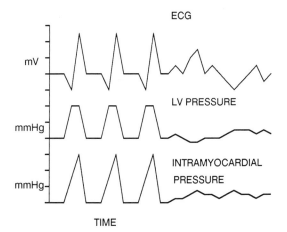

Figure 28–13. At the onset of VF, there is a rapid fall in both the left ventricular (LV) pressure and the intramyocardial pressure. These marked changes in pressure may be used as indicators of a hemodynamically significant arrhythmia.

reported using a combination of electrocardiographic analysis and intramyocardial pressure recording to differentiate among sinus rhythm, VT, and VF in 11 acute open-chest dog experiments. They concluded that the combination of electrocardiographic and hemodynamic parameters improved sensitivity. Van den Bossche[46] has also used a combination of electrocardiographic analysis and hemodynamic parameters (intramyocardial pressure and left ventricular impedance) to differentiate VT and VF from sinus rhythm in seven animal experiments. Again, a high sensitivity was achieved, but the relative importance of the different parameters within the algorithm was not described.

Recently, Kresh[27] has reported the measurement of intramyocardial pressure in patients undergoing bypass grafting surgery. During sinus rhythm, systolic intramyocardial pressure was 90.0 ± 12.5 mm Hg, and diastolic intramyocardial pressure was less than 10 mm Hg, while during VF the intramyocardial pressure exhibited random oscillations, with excursions between 43.0 ± 20.5 and 86.7 ± 39.2 mm Hg. Such variations seem initially to entail the same problems of differentiation as are inherent in electrogram analysis.

BIOSENSORS

In recent years, a number of sensors have been used to control the discharge rate of so-called rate-responsive bradycardia support pacemakers. Of these activity sensors (usually piezoelectric crystals), temperature sensors (thermistors), respiratory sensors (transthoracic impedance-based systems), and evoked potential sensors (stimulus to T wave or ventricular electrogram "gradient") are the most popular and well developed.

Table 28–4 reviews these sensors from the perspective of their possible inverse application to the diagnosis of inappropriate tachycardia. Central venous temperature reacts too slowly to exercise for the absence of such changes to signal a pathologic tachycardia. Chirife and colleagues[13] have suggested that the preejection period should be used to distinguish sinus tachycardia from pathologic tachycardia. The preejection period or some derivation of this was assessed using a combination of electrographic, impedance (volume), and possibly pressure measurements.[9] Chirife found that the preejection period shortened physiologically with sinus tachycardia but did not shorten when abnormal SVT or VT was induced.

Both activity and respiration sensors could theoretically distinguish those tachycardias that occur outside the setting of exercise. However, not all physiologic tachycardias are exercise induced. Nevertheless, these sensors would provide important contributory information for a complex algorithm based on multiple inputs.

The possible analysis of potentials evoked during tachycardia is particularly attractive. Table 28–5 details several uses of such potentials. The safety, efficacy, and diagnostic capacity of implantable devices could be improved by analysis of these signals.

TABLE 28–4. BIOSENSOR USE FOR TACHYCARDIA DIAGNOSIS

RESPONSE	ACTIVITY	RESPIRATION	TEMPERATURE	EVOKED POTENTIALS
Response to exertion	Immediate	Intermediate	Delayed	Intermediate
Response to other situations associated with sinus tachycardia	Nil	Moderate	Little	Moderate
Response to pathologic tachycardia	Nil	Moderate	Nil	Moderate

TABLE 28–5. POSSIBLE USE OF EVOKED POTENTIALS FOR TACHYCARDIA DETECTION

1. Diagnosis of tachycardias
2. Determination of tachycardia termination
3. Avoidance of "vulnerable period" pacing
4. Reset versus nonreset for determination of extrastimulus timing (self-searching pacemaker)

LIMITATIONS OF STUDIES TO DATE

Most studies have been involved in assessing potential algorithms in restricted and unphysiologic conditions, which though useful in initial evaluation, do not address the clinical problems that must be overcome for any system to succeed.

The differentiation of sinus tachycardia from a pathologic tachycardia has often been neglected, as many investigations have compared the pathologic rhythm only with basic sinus rhythm. When sinus tachycardia has been compared with the pathologic tachycardia, it has been produced pharmacologically rather than by exercise.[33] The effects of other physiologic variables such as posture, respiration, and emotion on the recorded parameter have also been neglected, although it is known that posture and exercise may affect amplitude of the intracardiac signal and intracardiac conduction.[11]

Often, the problem presented to the sensing algorithm under review has been that of retrospective distinction between a normally conducted sinus rhythm and a clearly abnormal rhythm. Not surprisingly, many investigators have claimed high sensitivity for their algorithms. Usually, the specificity of an algorithm in differentiating abnormalities of rhythm not requiring intervention from pathologic tachycardias has not been tested. Such criticism is particularly relevant to those algorithms that are based on differences in the electrocardiogram morphology, for which difficulties would be expected in distinguishing aberrantly conducted tachycardias or multiple ventricular extrasystoles from VT.

Other possible complications of the use of intracardiac electrogram morphology are the effects of acute ischemia, myocardial distention, drugs, and electrolyte disturbance. All these features are likely to be a problem in a proportion of those patients considered suitable candidates for antitachycardia pacing, yet their influence on the intracardiac signal is unknown.

Most studies have been conducted in the acute situation (during an operation, during electrophysiologic testing, or as an open-chest animal experiment) with acute placement of temporary electrodes. Although the long-term reliability of electrodes is established and chronic recordings do not appear to differ greatly from those taken acutely,[39] the requirements for reprogramming post implantation must be assessed.

IMPLANTABLE HOLTER MONITORING

In recent years, some implantable pacemakers have contained primitive "Holter" functions. Devices may count the number of paced beats, the number of sensed beats, and other variables related to these fundamental events—for example, the interval between consecutive sensed or paced beats. Advanced tachycardia termination devices have also been capable of logging simple information about tachycardia events, the intervention of the pacemaker, and its results. Recent experience with the implantable defibrillator has emphasized that it is essential to record and analyze the antecedent and postdischarge electrocardiographic events so that the appropriateness of the discharge can be evaluated. Because current technology does not allow an implantable device to retain substantial periods of electrographic data, reconstructed information (electrograms plus the duration of intervening isoelectric periods) or merely the time intervals between recognized events are remembered for subsequent telemetry. Short periods of electrocardiographic data can be stored for later analysis.

It is increasingly acknowledged that external Holter and electrophysiologic stimulation techniques are essential for the optimal therapy of cardiac arrhythmias, particularly VT. During the course of their illness, patients may require hundreds of Holter recordings and occasional electrophysiologic studies. An implantable device could theoretically perform both studies in addition to providing possible therapy for spontaneous arrhythmias. It is therefore necessary to develop further the Holter capacity of implantable devices. Short segments of the complete cardiac rhythm can be reviewed, but for long periods of data collection (days, weeks, or even months) events must be stored, together with their time of occurrence. For this purpose, the device must accurately sense heart rate and electrogram characteristics.

IMPLANTABLE ANTIARRHYTHMIC DRUG INFUSION PUMPS

Implantable drug infusers have been developed, particularly for the controlled administration of insulin. Recently, it has become possible to deliver antiarrhythmic drugs using an implanted mechanical pump. One such pump has a capacity of 12 ml and can deliver bolus doses of 0.05 ml to 0.25 ml.[1] Specific reports have noted the use of disopyramide for medical conversion of atrial fibrillation.[12, 26] Release of the drug could be achieved by "manual" activation[1] or, more conveniently, by automatic diagnosis of the arrhythmia by the implantable device. In the future, automatic drug infusion and electrotherapy may be combined in a single implantable device.

CONCLUSIONS

For the most part, the presence of a pathologic tachycardia may be diagnosed when a fast heart rate is present. However, apparently fast heart rates may result from myopotential or electromagnetic interference, from sinus tachycardia, or from tachycardias other than those intended or suitable for treatment with an implantable device. To refine and improve the diagnostic capability of automatic tachycardia-terminating devices, it has been necessary to introduce more sophisticated diagnostic criteria based upon an analysis of heart rate or electrogram morphology and content. In theory, at least, specific tachycardias can now be accurately diagnosed and distinguished from each other.

It is apparent that not only the tachycardia but also its autonomic, metabolic, and hemodynamic circumstances and effects must be sensed, and this information must be used to design and prescribe specific therapeutic interventions.

An important goal of antitachycardia electrotherapy is to prevent the occurrence of tachycardias. It is increasingly obvious that many tachycardias emerge from a specific electrophysiologic background, which could theoretically be detected and corrected by electrical or pharmacologic techniques.

In terms of number of patients affected, tachycardia is a far greater problem than bradycardia. Simple drug therapy for tachycardia is often inadequate for the control of symptoms and for the improvement of prognosis. Electrotherapy delivered by implantable devices is both efficacious and safe. Provided that tachycardias and their prodromes and consequences can be accurately sensed, implantable devices will be used increasingly for the successful management of a wide range of tachyarrhythmias.

REFERENCES

1. Abdul-Noir F, Cannon R, Jaafrin MY: A new mechanical bolus implantable pump. PACE 11:975, 1988.
2. Amikam S, Furman S: A comparison of anterograde and retrograde atrial depolarization in the electrogram. PACE 6:A–111, 1983.
3. Aubert AE, Denys BG, Ector H, et al: Detection of ventricular tachycardia and fibrillation using ECG processing and intramyocardial pressure gradients. PACE 9:1084, 1986.
4. Aubert AE, Goldreyer BN, Wyman MG, et al: Detection of ventricular fibrillation during AICD implantation using electrogram analysis. PACE 11:524, 1988.
5. Aubert A, Goldreyer BN, Wyman MG, et al: Frequency analysis during AICD implantation. PACE 11:486, 1988.
6. Baig W, Boute W, Wilson J, et al: Use of the evoked response in the determination of pacing threshold. PACE 11:822, 1988.
7. Bardy GH, Olson WH, Fishbein, et al: Transvenous right ventricular impedance during spontaneous ventricular arrhythmias in man. Circulation 72:III–474, 1985.
8. Begemann MJS, Boute W: Automatic refractory period. PACE 6:820, 1988.
9. Bennett T, Beck R, Erickson M: Right ventricular dynamic pressure parameters for differentiation of supraventricular and ventricular rhythms. PACE 10:415, 1987.
10. Brachmann J, Stroobandt R, Aidonidis I, et al: Analysis of monophasic action potentials facilitates differentiation of ventricular tachyarrhythmias. PACE 9:308, 1986.
11. Bricker JT, Ward KA, Zinner A, et al: Decreases in canine endocardial and epicardial voltages with exercise: Implications for pacemaker sensing. PACE 9:282, 1986.
12. Bump T, Arzbaecher R: Automatic implantable drug delivery for conversion of experimental atrial fibrillation. PACE 11:973, 1988.
13. Chirife R: The pre ejection period: A physiologic signal for rate responsive pacing and tachycardia diagnosis in automatic pacemakers. PACE 11:821, 1988.
14. Creamer JE, Davies DW, Nathan AW: Clinical experience with the Intertach pacemaker. PACE 10:996, 1987.
15. Davies DW, Nathan AW, Wainwright RJ, et al: Recognition of ventricular tachycardia and fibrillation from epicardial electrogram timings. Circulation 72:III–475, 1985.
16. Davies DW, Wainwright RJ, Tooley MA, et al: Electrogram analysis for the automatic recognition of ventricular tachycardia. Circulation 72:III–474, 1985.
17. Davies DW, Wainwright RJ, Tooley MA, et al: De-

tection of pathological tachycardia by analysis of electrogram morphology. PACE 9:200, 1986.

18. Della Bella P, Brugada P, Lemery R, et al: A transcardiac lead system for identification and termination of supraventricular and ventricular tachycardia. Am J Cardiol 60:1043, 1987.

19. Denys BG, Aubert AE, Ector H, et al: Intramyocardial pressure as a trigger for automatic implantable defibrillators. Eur Heart J 5:256, 1984.

20. Echt DS, Armstrong K, Schmidt P, et al: Clinical experience, complications, and survival in 70 patients with the automatic implantable cardioverter/defibrillator. Circulation 71:289, 1985.

21. Fisher JD, Goldstein M, Ostrow E, et al: Maximum rate of tachycardia development: Sinus tachycardia with sudden exercise vs spontaneous ventricular tachycardia. PACE 6:221, 1986.

22. Fisher JD, Johnston DR, Furman S, et al: Long term efficacy of antitachycardia pacing for supraventricular and ventricular tachycardia. Am J Cardiol 60:1311, 1987.

23. Geibel A, Zehender M, Brugada P: Changes in cycle length at onset of sustained tachycardias—importance for anti-tachy pacing. Am Heart J 115:589, 1988.

24. Griffin JC, Nielsen AP, Finke WL, et al: A new method of rhythm identification: Endocardial electrogram morphology. Circulation [Suppl II]:201, 1984.

25. Jenkins J, Wu D, Arzbaecher R: Computer diagnosis of supraventricular and ventricular arrhythmias. Circulation 60:977, 1979.

26. Jenkins J, Poiger G, Bump T, et al: Computerized drug delivery system for termination of atrial tachycardia during electrophysiologic studies. PACE 11:973, 1988.

27. Kresh JY, Brockman SK: Intramyocardial pressure during arrhythmias and fibrillation in man. PACE 10:701, 1987.

28. Langberg JL, Gibb WJ, Auslander DM, et al: Identification of ventricular tachycardia with use of the morphology of the endocardial electrogram. Circulation 77:1363, 1988.

29. Lin D, DiCarlo L, Jenkins J: Identification of ventricular tachycardia using intracavity electrograms: Analysis of time and frequency domain patterns. PACE 11:1592, 1988.

30. Mercando AD, Furman S: Measurement of differences in timing and sequence between two ventricular electrodes as a means of tachycardia differentiation. PACE 9:1069, 1986.

31. Mercando AD, Gableman G, Fisher JD: Comparison of the rate of tachycardia development in patients: Pathologic vs sinus tachycardia. PACE 11:516, 1988.

32. Mirowski M, Mower WM, Staewen WS, et al: The development of the transvenous automatic defibrillator. Ann Intern Med 129:773, 1973.

33. Munkenbeck FC, Bump TE, Arzbaecher R: Differentiation of sinus tachycardia from paroxysmal 1:1 tachycardias using single late diastolic atrial extrastimuli. PACE 9:53, 1986.

34. Olson WH, Miles WM, Zipes DP: Intracardiac electrical impedance during ventricular tachycardia and fibrillation in man. Circulation 72:III, 1985.

35. Olson WH, Bardy GH, Lund J, et al: Sensing and detection of ventricular fibrillation from human epicardial electrograms for an implantable pacer-cardioverter-defibrillator. PACE 11:485, 1988.

36. Olson WH, Bardy GH, Mehra R, et al: Tachycardia detection algorithm for an implantable cardioverter and defibrillator. Circulation 74:II-110, 1986.

37. Olson WH, Bennett TD, Huberty KP, et al: Automatic detection of ventricular fibrillation with chronically implanted pressure sensors. J Am Coll Cardiol 7:182A, 1986.

38. Pannizzo MS, Furman S: Optimal tachycardia sensing for cardiac pacemakers. PACE 8:298, 1985.

39. Pannizzo F, Wanliss, Furman S: The consistency of NSR/VT electrograms from acute and chronic permanent leads. PACE 9:304, 1986.

40. Ropella KM, Sahakian AV, Baerman JM, et al: Discrimination of fibrillatory from nonfibrillatory rhythms: Coherence spectra. PACE 11:485, 1988.

41. Shapland JE, Bach SM, Baumann L, et al: New approaches for tachycardia discrimination. PACE 11:821, 1988.

42. Sowton E: Clinical results with the tachylog antitachycardia pacemaker. PACE 7:1313, 1984.

43. Sponzilli C, Davies DW, Cornu EB, et al: Is recognition of junctional reentry tachycardia possible by analysis of atrioventricular relationships? PACE 11:519, 1988.

44. Tomaselli GF, Neilsen AP, Finke WL, et al: Morphological differences of the endocardial electrogram in beats of sinus and ventricular origin. PACE 12:254, 1988.

45. Tronstad A, Hoff PI, Ohm OJ: A new method for the detection of ventricular tachyarrhythmias. PACE 10:754, 1987.

46. Van den Bossche J, Van de Voorde P, Verryt A, et al: Electrogram and hemodynamic parameter analysis for the automatic detection of ventricular tachycardia and fibrillation. Circulation 74:II-109, 1986.

47. Wainwright R, Davies W, Tooley M: Ideal atrial lead positioning to detect retrograde atrial depolarization by digital slope analysis of the atrial electrogram. PACE 7:1152, 1984.

48. Walsh CA, Singer LP, Mercando AD, et al: Differentiation of supraventricular and ventricular rhythms in the dog by ventricular activation sequence and timing. PACE 11:821, 1988.

49. Ward DE: Usefulness of monophasic action potential recordings during ventricular tachycardia. *In* Proceedings of the VIIIth Asian-Pacific Congress of Cardiology, 1983, p 65.

29

ELECTRICAL STIMULATION TECHNIQUES FOR PREVENTION OF VENTRICULAR TACHYARRHYTHMIAS

RAHUL MEHRA

Techniques that can prevent the onset of tachyarrhythmias can significantly improve the prognosis of patients with high-grade symptomatic and malignant arrhythmias. The initiation of a tachyarrhythmia usually requires the presence of a "trigger" with or without an "electrophysiologic substrate" in which the tachyarrhythmia can be sustained. To prevent tachyarrhythmias, one or both of these factors must be altered. The most common methods for prevention of tachyarrhythmias include use of pharmaceutical agents, surgical resection of the substrate responsible for the tachyarrhythmia, and ablation techniques. Surgical removal of diseased myocardial tissue or its ablation can alter the substrate as well as eliminate the trigger. Drugs can also prevent arrhythmias by altering both these factors. Each of these techniques, however, has its associated advantages and disadvantages. For example, the proarrhythmic effect of certain drugs and their undesirable side effects are well appreciated, and the surgical methods can have significant risk and are not always efficacious. Therefore, the use of electrical stimulation provides an attractive alternative. Electrical stimulation techniques can alter the trigger mechanism or change the electrophysiologic properties of the substrate, or both, and hence prevent the arrhythmia. Prevention can also be accomplished by aborting the tachyarrhythmia before it progresses to a sustained rhythm. However,

very few methods have been shown to be efficacious in preventing spontaneous clinical arrhythmias. Overdrive ventricular pacing for suppression of ventricular tachyarrhythmias has been practiced in coronary care units since the 1950s, although few well-controlled scientific studies have investigated the relative merit of this technique and the mechanism responsible for its success. Electrical methods for the prevention of ventricular tachyarrhythmias would be useful not only in coronary care units but also in implantable devices that control tachyarrhythmias. These prevention techniques could reduce the number of tachyarrhythmias that need to be terminated by high-energy shocks and therefore could increase the longevity and reduce the size of such devices.

The techniques for preventing ventricular tachyarrhythmias have been developed based on several approaches. The first approach is based on the electrocardiographic observations of the initiation of tachyarrhythmias. Clinical and animal studies have demonstrated that there is frequently an association between heart rate and initiation of tachyarrhythmias, and therefore optimizing heart rate could suppress arrhythmias. In patients with repolarization abnormalities, electrocardiographic recordings have also shown that abrupt changes in RR interval (short-long cycle lengths) are associated with the onset of malignant arrhythmias. Even though the cause-effect relationship is difficult to isolate in such cases, these observations have led to the development of techniques for prevention of tachyarrhythmias. In animals, direct modulation of the autonomic nervous system by electrical stimulation of the central or peripheral nerves has demonstrated antiarrhythmic effects. Another approach has been based on theoretical considerations and experimental observations of the effects of electrical stimulation on cardiac tissue. Techniques such as "preexcitation of ischemic tissue" were based on simple conceptual models of reentrant activity and have subsequently been tested in animals and patients. Prevention of tachyarrhythmias has also been demonstrated when a high-voltage stimulus is delivered to cardiac tissue within a narrow "protective zone" of the QRS complex. Each one of these techniques will now be discussed in greater detail.

PREVENTION OF HEART RATE–DEPENDENT VENTRICULAR TACHYARRHYTHMIAS

The association between heart rate and premature ventricular beats (PVBs) or ventricular tachycardia has been well documented with 24-hour ambulatory electrocardiographic recordings.[3, 16, 29, 51, 56] Complex relationships between heart rate and PVBs have been observed in patients with coronary artery disease as well as in apparently healthy patients. In some patients the PVBs increase with increasing heart rate, and in others they increase at lower heart rates. Some patients also exhibit a window of heart rate above and/or below which the extrasystoles are reduced (Fig. 29–1). In patients with monomorphic idiopathic ventricular extrasystoles, it was shown that the upper and lower limits of this window change with the mean sinus rate and indicate a dynamic phenomenon under the influence of the autonomic system.[16] This relationship between heart rate and PVB frequency has also been shown to predict the response of certain antiarrhythmic drugs, such as diltiazem. The drug reduced the mean heart rate and was successful in suppressing arrhythmias in patients in whom a positive correlation between heart rate and arrhythmias existed prior to antiarrhythmic drug therapy.[22] This phenomenon may also explain "spontaneous" variability in premature beat frequency, sleep suppression of arrhythmias, and the antiarrhythmic effect of beta blockers. Another clinical observation of interest is that prior to spontaneous episodes of malignant tachyarrhythmias there is frequently an increase in spontaneous heart rate.[26, 39, 43] In one study of 20 patients who died of sudden cardiac death related to tachyarrhythmias, there was an increase in heart rate from a mean of 78.6 ± 11.6 beats per minute during the first hour of monitoring to 96.4 ± 8.2 beats per minute in the last hour preceding ventric-

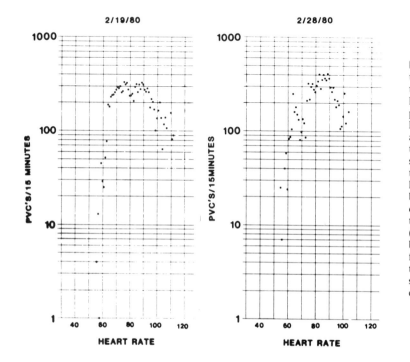

Figure 29–1. The relationship between frequency of premature ventricular complexes (PVCs) and heart rate in a 68-year-old man. This patient demonstrated a complex relationship between PVC frequency and heart rate. At heart rates of 55 to 80 beats per minute, there was a striking increase in ventricular ectopic beat frequency, whereas at heart rates above approximately 90 beats per minute, there was a reduction in PVC frequency. The pattern was reproducible over 9 days. (From Winkle RA: The relationship between ventricular ectopic beat frequency and heart rate. Circulation 66:439–445, 1982; by permission of the American Heart Association, Inc.)

ular tachycardia or ventricular fibrillation because of the increased sympathetic drive.[26] In all these situations, whether the change in heart rate was responsible for the arrhythmia or both were by-products of a fundamental electrophysiologic change as a result of autonomic modulation is not known.

The relationship between arrhythmogenicity and heart rate has been investigated in a few animal studies during acute ischemia caused by sudden ligation of the left anterior descending coronary artery.[1, 19, 44] The studies clearly indicate that a relationship does exist. One study showed that at stable rates between 110 and 150 beats per minute the frequency of ventricular arrhythmias was much less than at slower rates of 60 to 90 beats per minute.[1] At rates above 180 beats per minute, the incidence of ectopic beats again increased dramatically and provoked ventricular tachycardia or fibrillation. There appeared to be an optimal intermediate rate for maximal antiarrhythmic effect. Han and associates showed a similar relationship during acute ischemia and sudden elevation of aortic pressure.[19] The mechanisms for these complex relationships is not clear, and both reentry and ectopic firing may play a role. It has been shown that an increase in heart rate can reduce conduction velocity, especially in ischemic tissue. The formation of an arc of block, in conjunction with slower conduction, would favor reentrant excitation. On the other hand, triggered activity may also be responsible for inducing arrhythmias when the rate is increased.[37] In the 1-day-old model of myocardial infarction in the dog, the amplitude of the delayed afterdepolarization increases at shorter cycle lengths, and at a critical cycle length, triggered activity can be initiated.[12] The bradycardia-related premature beats are not compatible with the reentry as the underlying mechanism and are more likely to be related to early afterdepolarization. Purkinje fibers exposed to acidosis or cesium have demonstrated bradycardia-dependent triggered firing.[2, 6] These hypotheses do not exclude the possibility that the tachyarrhythmia may be perpetuated by a reentrant mechanism after being initiated by a triggered beat.

If there is a causal relationship between arrhythmias and heart rate, then it is reasonable to expect that they can be suppressed clinically by altering the heart rate. The heart rate can be raised by pacing, and there are many clinical studies that suggest that tachyarrhythmias can be suppressed by increasing the heart rate to rates greater than the spontaneous sinus rate. In one study by Fisher and colleagues, a crossover controlled evaluation of VVI pacing was done at rates 10 to 15 beats per minute above the mean daily heart rate.[14] Pacing significantly reduced the number of premature beats, couplets, and runs of ventricular tachycardia in 13 patients, and the greatest reduction was in couplets and ventricular tachycardias. In another study of seven patients with recurrent ventricular tachycardia and fibrillation, speeding the heart rate to 110 beats per minute or more contributed to a temporary suppression of the arrhythmia.[15] Eventual failure of this technique in some patients indicates that other mechanisms (including hemodynamic compromise at high rates) frequently limit its chronic efficacy. In 1966, McAllister and coworkers were the first to report on a patient who had a permanent pacemaker implanted for control of ventricular tachyarrhythmias.[31] The patient was a 59-year-old man with evidence of ischemic heart disease who had recurrent ventricular tachycardia and fibrillation and was refractory to drug therapy. A permanent epicardial pacemaker with a rate of 90 beats per minute was implanted in this patient to control his arrhythmias. Chronic high-rate atrial pacing in patients with normal atrioventricular (AV) conduction and overdrive pacing in the immediate postoperative period after open heart surgery[18, 20] has been successful in controlling ventricular arrhythmias. Employment of an activity-based rate-responsive pacemaker whose rate increases during exercise has also demonstrated suppression of exercise-induced PVBs in patients with AV block.[24]

The concept of increasing the heart rate to suppress tachyarrhythmias has already been incorporated into some implantable or external devices. The concept of "dynamic overdrive" attempts to increase the pacing rate whenever PVBs are observed and is available in an implantable device. This mode is designed to prevent tachyarrhythmias by continually overdriving the patient's spontaneous rhythm. Whenever a spontaneous beat is sensed, the pacing interval is reduced by a programmable amount. The pacing interval is then gradually increased by lengthening each subsequent pacing interval by a preprogrammed value. This process continues until either the basic rate has been reached or another spontaneous beat is sensed. One clinical study with dynamic overdrive showed that in 5 of 10 patients, a reduction in PVBs of more than 80 per cent was achieved.[52] Some concerns about myocardial insufficiency due to chronic high-rate pacing still remain, especially in patients with reduced left ventricular performance.

Another concept very similar to dynamic overdrive is called "automatic frequency adjustment." In such an external device, every premature beat increases the pacing rate, and the time spent at the new rate is dependent on the frequency of premature beats. If the PVBs are suppressed at the high rate, the pacing rate automatically begins to decrease in a stepwise manner until the chosen standby rate or spontaneous rhythm is reached. When PVBs do not decrease after the maximal rate is reached, the system automatically ceases to increase the rate. A few case reports illustrating suppression of ventricular tachycardia with this concept do exist.[55]

PREVENTION OF PAUSE-DEPENDENT TACHYARRHYTHMIAS

Malignant clinical arrhythmias are frequently preceded by a beat with a long cycle length.[23, 27] This phenomenon has been termed "short-long" and is observed in patients with a long QT syndrome as a result of antiarrhythmic drugs or hypokalemia (Fig. 29–2). The long cycle causes a significant QT prolongation that leads to *torsades de pointes* rhythm. Holter monitor recordings in such patients frequently show an associated bradycardia rhythm. Even patients without the long QT syndrome who die suddenly following a sustained monomorphic or polymorphic ventricular tachycardia that degenerates into fibrillation display the "short-long" phenomenon. In one study of 45 cases of ventricular fibrillation recorded on the Holter monitor, the arrhythmia occurred after a long cycle length in 20 of them, usually owing to a postatrial or PVB compensatory pause.[4] After the long cycle length, PVBs with a small prematurity index have been shown to be more likely to induce the arrhythmia than are those with a long prematurity index. Even in the electrophysiology laboratory, abrupt changes in pacing cycle length from short to long facilitate initiation of sustained ventricular tachycardia. In one report, 13 of 21 patients in whom ventricular tachycardia could not be induced at constant cycle lengths were found to be inducible with the short-long sequence.[8] In that study, the investigators hypothesized that an increase in the dispersion of refractory periods between ventricular muscle and His-Purkinje system for the beat following the long pause was responsible for the arrhythmia. The induction of arrhythmias by the short-long pacing sequence has been mapped in the canine subacute infarction model.[11] The isochronal maps show that the short-long pairing sequence increases the conduction delay around a functionally blocked region, facilitating reentry. Both these models fail to explain the origin of the spontaneous premature beat, since in each study the paced premature stimulus was the artificial "trigger." Recently, on the basis of transmembrane recordings in isolated tissue, it has been hypothesized that the pause-dependent premature beats may be caused by early afterde-

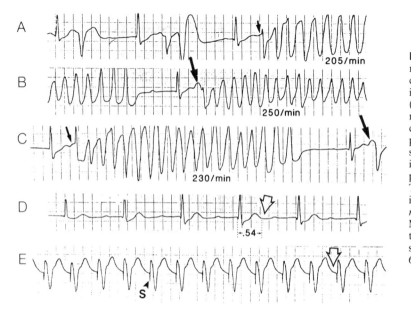

Figure 29–2. Imipramine-induced runs of *torsades de pointes* tachycardia occur following long pauses in the RR interval in this patient (panels *A, B,* and *C*). Solid arrows mark postpause U waves. Electrocardiographic (ECG) tracing in panel *E* shows complete suppression of the tachyarrhythmias during temporary right ventricular pacing at 100 beats per minute. There is also a marked decrease in U-wave amplitude (*open arrow*). (From Jackman WM, Clark M, Friday KJ, et al: Ventricular tachyarrhythmias in the long QT syndrome. Med Clin North AM 68:1079–1109, 1984.)

polarizations.[5, 23] This triggered arrhythmia could sustain itself or, in the presence of an abnormal electrophysiologic substrate, induce reentrant beats. Even in acutely ischemic animals, atrial pacing with intermittent, abrupt pauses results in induction of ventricular arrhythmias, beginning after the second conducted beat following each pause.[21] This electrocardiographic pattern is different from what is frequently observed clinically in the long QT syndrome, since it requires the presence of two supraventricular beats after the pause. Onset of arrhythmias, in this model, was associated with an increased delay in activation of ischemic epicardium and fractionation of the electrogram of the second conducted impulse, indicating reentry. It is quite likely that the second supraventricular beat acted as a premature beat, since the refractory period of the first beat would be very long because of the pause.

One of the simplest ways to prevent these abrupt changes in cycle length is by constant pacing. Kay and colleagues showed that in 32 patients in whom the beginning of the *torsades de pointes* arrhythmia was pause related, temporary overdrive pacing was the only consistently effective therapy.[25] In such studies, although it was difficult to prove that the effect is due to elimination of the pauses and is not the result of other electrophysiologic or hemodynamic effects of ventricular pacing, the former is the more likely mechanism. Jackman and associates reported that temporary pacing at rates of 50 to 110 beats per minute reduced the amplitude of the U waves in patients with pause-dependent or acquired long QT syndrome and prevented the recurrence of the tachyarrhythmias.[23] Permanent cardiac pacing is also beneficial in some patients with idiopathic long QT syndrome. In these patients, profound bradycardia frequently precedes the initiation of *torsades de pointes* tachyarrhythmia.[10] It is important to note that with permanent pacing at rates between 70 and 80 beats per minute, the duration of the pause following premature beats may sometimes be too long to prevent the induction of all *torsades*

de pointes rhythms. In such cases, constant high-rate pacing would be hemodynamically compromising, and alternative algorithms for pacing may be required.

PREVENTION OF VENTRICULAR ARRHYTHMIAS BY MODULATION OF THE AUTONOMICS

It is well appreciated now that the autonomic nervous system can play a significant role in the genesis of malignant arrhythmias, a role that has been dealt with in recent reviews.[45] The effects of sympathetic stimulation can be dependent on the induced changes in heart rate or can be independent of it and caused by the direct action of norepinephrine on the electrophysiologic properties of the substrate,[48] as illustrated in Figure 29–3. Electrical stimulation of the various areas of the brain has also resulted in a diversity of cardiac arrhythmias mostly mediated by the activation of the sympathetic nervous system.[36] The role of vagal activity in ventricular arrhythmogenesis is still controversial. Reduction in heart rate may play a large role in vagal stimulation–induced antiarrhythmic effects. A clinical study showed that phenylephrine-induced suppression of ventricular arrhythmias was primarily dependent on heart rate.[49] Similar results were obtained in a conscious animal model of exercise-induced spontaneous fibrillation.[7] Verrier and Lown have provided evidence that the protective result of increased vagal activity may also occur by opposing the arrhythmogenic influence of adrenergic activity.[46]

If vagal stimulation does provide an antiarrhythmic effect, then electrical stimulation of the vagus could be used for prevention of tachyarrhythmias. Vagal stimulation would be initiated when precursors to the onset of tachyarrhythmias are sensed. To elicit the same response, it may also be possible to stimulate certain "fat pads" on the epicardium that are innervated with postganglionic cell populations.[41] Although the functional anatomy of these fat pads has been investigated in animals, their existence in humans is not yet verified.

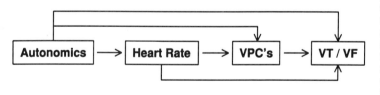

Figure 29–3. This block diagram illustrates that the autonomic nervous system can affect the inducibility of ventricular tachycardia or fibrillation (VT/VF) by affecting the heart rate; the ventricular premature contractions (VPCs) that can initiate VT/VF; or by directly affecting the substrate responsible for the tachyarrhythmias.

"PREEXCITATION" OF ISCHEMIC TISSUE FOR PREVENTION OF VENTRICULAR ARRHYTHMIAS

In the past few years, isochronal mapping studies have elucidated the mechanism of tachyarrhythmias produced by premature beats. In the canine subacute infarction model, as well as in clinical studies, epicardial and intramural activation mapping has shown that unsustained and sustained runs of tachyarrhythmias can occur owing to reentrant activation.[9, 35, 53] Wave fronts produced by premature beats block in the region of the prolonged refractory period and circumvent this block from either side of an arc or surface of block. This arc of block forces the conduction path to be prolonged. At the same time, the conduction velocity of the premature beat is decreased in the ischemic area. The increase in the conduction path and the decrease in conduction velocity both increase the time taken by the wave front to reach the tissue distal to the arc of block. If by this time the tissue proximal to the block has expended its refractoriness, it can be reexcited, giving rise to an extra beat. On the basis of this simple model, it can be argued that pacing or "preexciting" the ischemic site with a prolonged refractory period may be able to prevent the occurrence of reentrant tachyarrhythmias. If the dispersion of recovery of repolarization is responsible for unidirectional block,[17] then preexciting the tissue with a prolonged refractory period should decrease this dispersion, reduce the length of the arc of block, and/or improve conduction in the ischemic zone, since the wave front would be infringing on less refractory tissue. This situation would, in turn, decrease the conduction time around the arc of block and thereby reduce the likelihood of a reentrant beat, as illustrated in Figure 29–4.

The best test for this hypothesis would be in a model of spontaneous arrhythmias. Pacing would be done from a normal ventricular site, and the incidence of arrhythmias would be compared with the incidence in a situation when pacing is done from the ischemic site at the same rate. However, since adequate models for spontaneous arrhythmias do not exist, all the studies to test this hypothesis have been conducted in a model of artificially induced arrhythmias.[30, 33, 34, 42] In these studies, the site of delivery of the premature beat was in normal tissue and held constant, and its ability to induce arrhythmias was compared when pacing was done from the normal tissue or when dual-site pacing was done from the ischemic and the normal tissue (Fig. 29–5). The degree of preexcitation was varied in some of the experiments. In one study, the efficacy of dual ventricular stimulation for the prevention of ventricular tachyarrhythmias was investigated 3 to 5 days after left anterior descending coronary artery occlusion, and computerized epicardial mapping was conducted to delineate the mechanism.[34] Arrhythmias could be induced when premature beats during pacing were delivered from the base of the right ventricle. To prevent the arrhythmias, simultaneous dual ventricular pacing (S1–S1) was performed from the base of the right ventricle and at a site from within the ischemic zone. Specific sites from the ischemic zone were able to prevent the arrhythmias, whereas dual pacing from two normal sites was unsuccessful. The results of one such experiment are illustrated in Figure 29–6. The left-hand panel shows the control, with the induction of a reentrant beat by two premature stimuli at a coupling of 190 and 165 msec. For the S1 beat, the epicardium is activated within 60 msec. During S2, a functional arc of block is observed, and the epicardial activation occurs in 100 msec. With S3, the arc of block gets longer, and the wave front travels clockwise and counterclockwise around the ends of the block. The common wave front arrives on the distal side

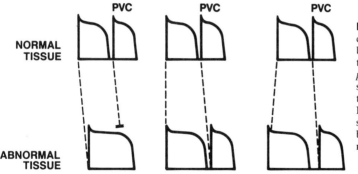

PVC   **PVC**   **PVC**

NORMAL TISSUE

ABNORMAL TISSUE

Figure 29–4. A spontaneous PVC occurring in the normal zone would be blocked in the abnormal tissue where the refractory period is prolonged (*left panel*). If the abnormal tissue is excited simultaneously (*middle panel*) or prior to the normal zone (*right panel*), and if the PVC occurs in the normal tissue at the same coupling as before, then it would be less likely to be blocked in the abnormal tissue.

STIMULATION PROTOCOL

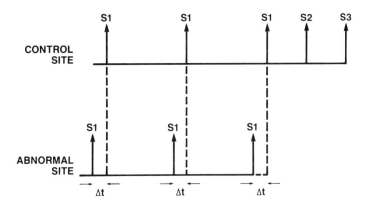

Figure 29–5. Stimulation protocol for prevention of ventricular tachyarrhythmias. For induction of arrhythmias, S1-S1 pacing was performed from a normal control site, and one (S2) or two (S2 and S3) premature beats were delivered. To prevent these arrhythmias, the control site was paced, and the abnormal or ischemic site was paced earlier than the control site by Δt; Δt is the "preexcitation" interval. S2 and S2 and S3 were again delivered from the control site only, and their ability to initiate tachyarrhythmias was assessed.

of the arc of block at 160 msec, and a reentrant beat is initiated because the tissue proximal to the block has recovered by then and is excitable. To prevent this beat, simultaneous dual-site pacing is conducted from the control site A and a site B within the ischemic zone. The surface electrocardiogram shows that when S2 and S3 are given at the same coupling, a

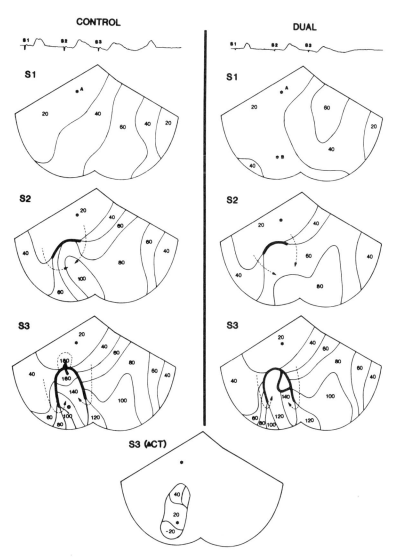

Figure 29–6. Isochronal maps of epicardial activation. The dark, thick line denotes the arc of functional conduction block. The epicardial surface is depicted as if the ventricles were folded out after a cut was made from the crux to the apex. The left-hand panel shows the isochronal maps for the S1, S2, and S3 beats during the control when pacing and premature stimuli are delivered from site A. A single reentrant beat is initiated following the S3 stimulus. During dual-site pacing from sites A and B (*right panel*), the premature S2 and S3 stimuli from site A fail to induce a reentrant beat. The lowest epicardial surface representation displays the difference in conduction time for the S3 beat—S3 (ΔCT)—between the "control" and "dual" pacing modes. See text for discussion.

reentrant beat is not initiated. As one would expect, the epicardial activation of the S1 beat and its QRS morphology are altered. During S2, conduction in the ischemic zone is enhanced, and epicardial activation occurs in 80 msec, as opposed to 100 msec, in the control situation. For the S3 beat, the shape of the arc of block is similar to that occurring before, but conduction in the ischemic zone between the arc of block is significantly increased. Most of this area is activated at 120 msec. By this time, the area proximal to the block has not recovered, and hence reentry is prevented. The lowest panel shows the change in conduction time for the S3 beat in the two situations. (Only differences greater than 10 msec are identified. For example, 20 indicates that conduction time is enhanced by > 10 msec and < 20 msec.) It is clear that conduction is enhanced in the ischemic area around site B, where dual stimulation is performed. Figure 29–7 illustrates a case in which dual stimulation is performed from two normal sites and reentry is not prevented. During dual stimulation, the epicardial map of the S1 beat is significantly altered, but the map of the S2 beat is virtually identical. It is important to note that site B in this case is located early in the reentrant circuit, whereas in the previous case it was much later. Quantitative analyses of the effect of refractory periods and conduction time during dual stimulation in this canine model have been conducted and reported.[42] In that study, it was concluded that prevention of reentry can result from a reduction in the length of the arc of block, early activation of regions distal to the arc, a shift in the arc of block toward the ischemic zone, or any combination of the above.

The previous discussion illustrates the mechanism of preventing ventricular reentry by dual-site pacing. The effect of electrical "preexcitation" of the ischemic zone during dual-site pacing on the coupling time window during which premature stimuli induce arrhythmias was investigated in another study.[33] In the same canine model, the ischemic site was paced earlier than the control site; the preexcitation was varied from 0 to 50 msec, and the premature stimuli were delivered from the control site. It was shown that as the degree of preexcitation was increased from 0 to 50 msec, the coupling window for induction of tachyarrhythmias decreased from 30 ± 12 msec to 9 ± 5 msec (Fig. 29–8). Each was significantly less than the control window of 66 ± 11 msec, and in about 60 per cent of the dogs, a maximal preexcitation of 50 msec protected the animals against tachyarrhythmias, even with the most premature stimuli. This finding illustrates the beneficial effect of the preexcitation of ischemic tissue. In this protocol, it is imperative that the maximal preexcitation be limited by the conduction time of the wave front from the ischemic to the control site. However, in situations in which spontaneous arrhythmias occur, this concept indicates that pacing the ischemic site would have the most antiarrhythmic effect.

This technique for prevention of ventricular

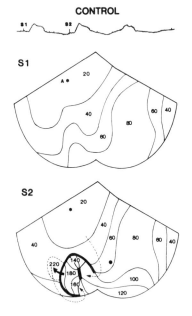
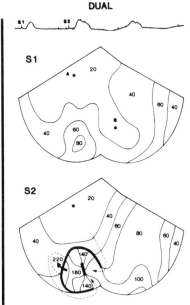

Figure 29–7. Epicardial activation during S1 and S2 stimuli delivered from site A in the base of the right ventricle (*left panel*). A single reentrant beat occurs at 220 msec after the S2 stimulus. During dual-site pacing from control site A and another normal site B, the reentrant beat still occurs when the premature S2 stimulus is delivered (*right panel*). See text for details.

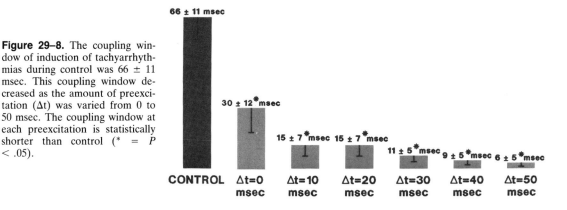

Figure 29–8. The coupling window of induction of tachyarrhythmias during control was 66 ± 11 msec. This coupling window decreased as the amount of preexcitation (Δt) was varied from 0 to 50 msec. The coupling window at each preexcitation is statistically shorter than control (* = P < .05).

arrhythmias has also been tested clinically.[30] The abnormal area of slow conduction for preexcitation was delineated by determining the "site of origin" of the ventricular tachycardia. In 11 cases, this was a site that demonstrated the earliest recorded electrical activity, as determined by left ventricular endocardial mapping. Simultaneous pacing was done from the site of origin and the normal site, and premature stimuli were delivered through the normal control site. This is equivalent to a preexcitation of 0 msec. In 5 of the 11 cases, this technique completely prevented the induction of tachyarrhythmias at any premature coupling interval. In three cases, a tachycardia of a different morphology was initiated, and no effect was observed in another two cases. It is encouraging that with a preexcitation of 0 msec prevention occurred in 45 per cent of the cases. At the same time, this study highlights a potential limitation of the technique. Preexcitation at one site may block one exit route for the wave front, but alternative reentrant pathways may exist in some patients, as indicated by initiation of a tachycardia with a different morphology.

For this technique to find practical utility, the safety and efficacy of ischemic site pacing for preventing spontaneous ventricular arrhythmias need to be assessed. At the same time, some of the practical limitations need to be addressed. The technique requires that the substrate responsible for sustaining the arrhythmia be anatomically defined. If it is in the left ventricle, then pacing would have to be done from the epicardial surface. If it is in the left side of the septum, which is usually the case, then pacing at high current outputs from the right side of the septum may be able to preexcite this tissue. The stimulus could be synchronized to the atrial complex and delivered at a shorter AV interval than the conduction time through the normal conduction path-

way. Second, as pointed out by the clinical study, several potential reentrant circuits could exist in the same patient. One may require multisite pacing or pacing at very high current outputs to preexcite all of them. This requirement may not always be practically feasible, and hence the efficacy of this technique could vary significantly from patient to patient. Future studies need to be conducted to answer these questions.

PREVENTION OF VENTRICULAR TACHYARRHYTHMIAS BY STIMULATION IN THE "PROTECTIVE ZONE"

It is known that a high-output stimulus delivered in the vulnerable period initiates ventricular fibrillation in dogs. In 1972, Wolf and colleagues and subsequently other investigators showed that a second large stimulus delivered within a "protective zone" can prevent this arrhythmia.[13, 47, 54] In their studies, the protective zone typically began 10 to 40 msec after the end of the vulnerable period and had a duration of 25 to 90 msec. This method of inducing arrhythmias by a high-energy stimulus does not have a clinical correlate, and therefore its application to the clinical setting was ambiguous. In recent studies, this concept was expanded to a more physiologic model of ventricular tachyarrhythmias.[32] It was shown that a high-voltage subthreshold stimulus delivered immediately after premature electrical stimuli could prevent ventricular arrhythmias. In the chronic canine ischemic model, arrhythmias were induced by premature stimuli delivered to the epicardial surface of the right ventricle during ventricular pacing. The stimulus for preventing these arrhythmias was delivered across an endocardial right ventricular lead and an epicardial patch electrode sutured on

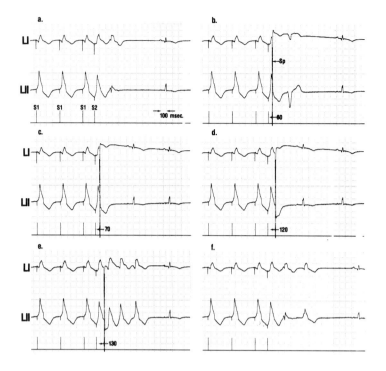

Figure 29–9. In each panel, surface ECG leads I and II are shown with stimulus markers at the bottom. Panels *a* and *f* show induction of multiple responses by S1 and S2 of 200 msec in which the first unstimulated response is reproducible. The arrhythmia could not be prevented by a 0.05-J Sp (protective) stimulus when it occurred at an interval less than or equal to 60 msec following S2 (*panel b*). At delays between 70 and 120 msec, the Sp stimulus prevented the arrhythmia (*panels c* and *d*), and at 130 msec it became suprathreshold, giving rise to multiple beats (*panel e*).

the anteroseptal infarct. We found that in all dogs the ventricular arrhythmia could be prevented if the protective stimulus (Sp) was delivered in a critical coupling window after the last premature stimulus (Fig. 29–9). The Sp stimulus in the "protective zone" did not give rise to a propagated response, as seen on the surface electrocardiogram, and was therefore subthreshold. Figure 29–9 illustrates that when the Sp coupling interval was longer than the outer boundary of the protective zone, it became suprathreshold. With the amplitude of the protective stimulus between 20 and 70 V, the duration of the protective zone had a mean value between 40 and 57 msec. It was also demonstrated that the duration of the protective zone was dependent on the prematurity of the S2 stimulus used to induce the ventricular tachyarrhythmia. Greater prematurity of the S2 beat reduced the duration of the protective zone, but its onset with respect to the pacing (S1) stimulus was not altered (Fig. 29–10). This observation indicates that the onset of the protective zone may represent the Sp stimulus falling just outside the repolarization phase of the S1 beat and hence outside the vulnerable period. Similarly, since the protective zone became shorter with increased prematurity of S2, the outer limit of the protective zone may represent the beginning of the vulnerable period of the S2 premature beat. Sp stimuli falling outside the protective zone were

frequently arrhythmogenic. This feature is one of the major drawbacks of this concept and could limit its practical application.

One possible hypothesis to explain the existence of the protective zone is illustrated in Figure 29–11. Computerized isochronal mapping of activation in this animal model has shown that the mechanism of arrhythmias is reentrant. As discussed previously, the wave front of the premature beat encounters conduction block at the border of the ischemic zone because of its prolonged refractoriness. The wave fronts travel around this arc of block, and for reentry to occur, the conduction time around the arc of block $(T_1 - T_2)$ must exceed

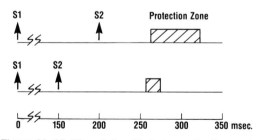

Figure 29–10. The relationship between the "protective zone" and the S1-S2 coupling when it is 200 msec (*top*) and when it is 150 msec (*bottom*). At an S1-S2 of 150 msec, the duration of the protective zone is much shorter. The onset of the protective zone, as measured from S2, occurs much later at an S1-S2 of 150 msec (110 versus 70 msec). When measured from S1, the onset of the protective zone is not significantly different in the two cases.

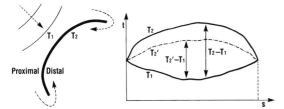

Figure 29–11. The left-hand panel shows an advancing wave front encountering an arc of functional conduction block. The wave front first excites tissue on the proximal side of the arc of block (at T_1). The activation times T_1 and T_2 vary along the length of the arc of block, as shown in the right-hand panel. The ordinate, s, denotes distance along the arc of block and the abscissa, t, the time of activation on the proximal (T_1) and the distal (T_2) side of the arc of block. In this idealized diagram, T_1 is shortest in the central segment of the proximal side of the arc of block because it is activated earliest, whereas the same region is activated latest on the distal side, giving rise to the longest T_2. For reentry to occur, $(T_2 - T_1)$, for example, the conduction time around the arc of block must be greater than the RP1, which is the refractory period of tissue on the proximal side of the arc of block. Hence, reentry occurs through the segment that satisfies this condition. It is hypothesized that the protective stimulus shortens the excitation time at the distal side of the arc of block to T_2' and thereby decreases $(T_2' - T_1)$. Reentry is blocked because nowhere along the arc of block is $(T_2' - T_1)$ greater than the RP1.

the refractory period of the tissue proximal to the block (RP1). In our experiments, the Sp stimulus potentially gave rise to two wave fronts, one from underneath the epicardial patch electrode and the other from the endocardial lead. When the Sp stimulus is given in the protective zone, the normal tissue underneath the endocardial lead could already be excited from the premature S2 beat, and hence the Sp stimulus would fall on refractory tissue. Since conduction of the premature beat to the ischemic tissue underneath the patch electrode occurs more slowly, it is likely that the Sp stimulus excites this tissue before the wave front of the premature beat can reach there. This wave front created by the Sp stimulus would excite the tissue distal to the area of block prematurely at T_2' as opposed to T_2. If $(T_2' - T_1)$ is less than the refractory period of the tissue proximal to the arc of block (RP1), reentry would be blocked. This fact also explains why Sp would appear as subthreshold on the surface electrocardiogram.

The technique of stimulation in the protective zone has not yet been attempted clinically. One major reason for this has been the concern that the Sp stimulus may become arrhythmogenic if it is not delivered at the correct time interval. At the same time, delivering a high-

energy stimulus after every PVB may not be possible in an implantable device owing to the limited available energy. One solution would be to reduce the intensity of the Sp stimulus. This practice could also conserve energy and make the ventricle less susceptible to arrhythmias if the stimulus is incorrectly timed. However, this requires delivering the stimulus at the critical area of slow conduction of the reentrant pathway and makes the technique much more site specific. Another issue that needs to be investigated is the efficacy of the technique if the stimulus is delivered after the second or third premature beat rather than the first. This delivery after the second or third premature beat could significantly reduce the number of "protective stimuli" that need to be delivered, as the frequency of couplets and triplets is typically much less than the number of single PVBs. Even in the most susceptible patient, every PVB does not degenerate into a sustained arrhythmia. Unless techniques can be developed to isolate the PVBs that will degenerate, delivering the stimulus in the protective zone of the second or third premature beat would be desirable.

OTHER TECHNIQUES

Apart from the four techniques mentioned above, there have been case reports and speculation about other methods for prevention of tachyarrhythmias. Subthreshold electrical stimulation, delivered within the refractory period, has been shown to inhibit the response to extrastimuli that normally give rise to a propagated response.[40] Its mechanism is related to increased local refractoriness, and it has been hypothesized that subthreshold stimulation may be useful in preventing ventricular tachyarrhythmias.[50] The effects of subthreshold stimulation are very localized, and it is possible that if the stimulation is performed at a critical site, alteration of the refractory periods at that site could prevent arrhythmias.

In a case report,[38] it was shown that delivery of a suprathreshold stimulus following a premature beat could prevent induction of ventricular tachycardia in a 60-year-old man with an inferior myocardial infarction. In that patient, the S2 stimulus initiated unsustained ventricular tachycardia, but the delivery of an S3 stimulus at a critical time aborted the arrhythmia. Similar results have been obtained in the coronary care unit, where delivery of a suprathreshold stimulus following a spontaneous premature beat has prevented sustained tachyarrhythmias. It is important to note that this technique is significantly different from protective zone stimulation, in which the S3 stimulus is subthreshold.

CONCLUSIONS

This chapter indicates that an understanding of electrical stimulation techniques for preventing ventricular tachyarrhythmias is still in its infancy. Several potentially useful techniques have been described. Some of these techniques, if they are found to be safe and efficacious, would be easy to implement technically in implantable devices or could be useful in the coronary care unit setting. Since the substrate responsible for tachyarrhythmias is frequently dynamic, it is unlikely that any of these techniques would be effective all the time. They will not, therefore, completely eliminate the use of termination techniques in implantable devices but, rather, will complement them. Use of these stimulation techniques could significantly reduce the size of such devices as well as increase their longevity. A reduction in the number of high-energy defibrillation shocks for terminating tachyarrhythmias would greatly improve the quality of life experienced by patients with these devices. Clinical testing and refinement of these techniques should continue to meet these objectives.

REFERENCES

1. Chadda KD, Banka VS, Helfant RS: Rate dependent ventricular ectopia following acute coronary occlusion: The concept of an optimal antiarrhythmic heart rate. Circulation 49:654–658, 1974.
2. Corabouef E, Deroubaix E, Coulombe A: Acidosis induced abnormal repolarization and repetitive activity in isolated dog Purkinje fibers. J Physiol (Paris) 76:97–106, 1980.
3. Coumel P, Leclercq JF, Slama R: Repetitive monomorphic idiopathic ventricular tachycardia. In Zipes DP, Jalife J (eds): Cardiac Electrophysiology and Arrhythmias. Orlando, FL, Grune and Stratton, 1985, p 457.
4. Coumel P, Leclercq JF, Zimmerman M, Funck-Brentano JL: Antiarrhythmic therapy: Noninvasive guided strategy versus empirical or invasive stratagies. In Brugada P, Wellens HJJ (eds): Cardiac Arrhythmias: Where to go from here? Mount Kisco, NY, Futura Publishing Co, 1987.
5. Cranefield PF, Aronson RS: Torsade-de-pointes and other pause induced ventricular tachycardias: The short-long-short sequence and early afterdepolarizations. PACE 11:670–678, 1988.
6. Damiano BP, Rosen MR: Effects of pacing on triggered activity induced by early after depolarizations. Circulation 69:1013–1025, 1984.
7. De Farrari GM, Vanoli E, Stramba-Badiale M, et al: Vagal stimulation and sudden death in conscious dogs with healed myocardial infarction. Circulation 76[Suppl IV]:107, 1987.
8. Denker S, Lehmann M, Mahmud R, et al: Facilitation of ventricular tachycardia induction with abrupt changes in ventricular cycle length. Am J Cardiol 53:508–515, 1984.
9. Downar E, Harris L, Mickleborough LL, et al: Endocardial mapping of ventricular tachycardia in the intact human ventricle. J Am Coll Cardiol 11:783–791, 1988.
10. Eldar M, Griffin JC, Abbott JA, et al: Permanent cardiac pacing in patients with long QT syndrome. J Am Coll Cardiol 10:600–607, 1987.
11. El-Sherif N, Gough WB, Restivo M, Kowtha VJ: The mechanism by which abrupt changes in cycle length facilitate the induction of reentrant rhythms. Circulation 72[Suppl II]:279, 1985.
12. El-Sherif N, Gough WB, Zeiler RH, Mehra R: Triggered ventricular rhythms in 1 day old myocardial infarction in the dog. Circ Res 52:566–579, 1983.
13. Euler DE, Moore EN: Continuous fractionated electrical activity after stimulation of the ventricles during the vulnerable period: Evidence for local reentry. Am J Cardiol 46:783, 1980.
14. Fisher JD, Tichman SL, Ferrick A, et al: Antiarrhythmic effects of VVI pacing at physiologic rates: A crossover controlled evaluation. PACE 10:822–830, 1987.
15. Friedberg CK, Lyon LJ, Donoso E: Suppression of refractory recurrent ventricular tachycardia by transvenous rapid atrial pacing and antiarrhythmic drugs: Report of seven cases. Am Heart J 79:44–50, 1970.
16. Funck-Brentano C, Coumel P, Lorente P, et al: Rate dependence of ventricular extrasystoles: Computer identification and quantitative analysis. Cardiovasc Res 22:101–107, 1988.
17. Gough WB, Mehra R, Restivo M, et al: Reentrant ventricular arrhythmias in the late myocardial infarction period in the dog. 13. Correlation of activation and refractory maps. Circ Res 57:432–442, 1985.
18. Haft JJ: Treatment of arrhythmias by intracardiac electrical stimulation. Prog Cardiovasc Dis 16:539–567, 1974.
19. Han J, DeTraglia J, Millet D, Moe GK: Incidence of ectopic beats as a function of basic drive in the ventricle. Am Heart J 72:632–639, 1966.
20. Harris PD, Malm JR, Bowman FO, et al: Epicardial pacing to control arrhythmias following cardiac surgery. Circulation 37, 38 [Suppl II]:178–183, 1968.
21. Hope RR, Scherlag BJ, Lazzara R: The induction of ventricular arrhythmias in acute myocardial ischemia by atrial pacing with long-short cycle sequences. Chest 71:5, 651, 1977.
22. Ito M, Tsumabuki S, Maeda Y, et al: Suppression of ventricular premature contractions possibly related to triggered activity by oral diltiazem and atenolol. Jpn Circ J 51:217–229, 1987.
23. Jackman WM, Friday KJ, Anderson JL, et al: The long Q.T. syndromes: A critical review, new clinical observations and unifying hypothesis. Prog Cardiovasc Dis 31:115–172, 1988.

24. Jordaens E, Vandekerckhove Y, Van Wassenhove E, et al: Does rate responsive pacing suppress exercise-related ventricular arrhythmias? Stimucoeur 14:93–98, 1986.

25. Kay GN, Plumb VC, Arciuicgas JG, et al: Torsade de pointe: The long-short initiating sequence and other clinical features. Observations in 32 patients. J Am Coll Cardiol 2:806, 1983.

26. Kempf FC, Josephson ME: Cardiac arrest recorded on ambulatory electrocardiograms. Am J Cardiol 53:1577–1582, 1984.

27. Leclercq JF, Zimmerman M, Coumel P: Is it possible to prevent ventricular tachyarrhythmias by pacing? In Breithardt G, Borggrefe M, Zipes DP (eds): Nonpharmacological Therapy of Tachyarrhythmias. Mount Kisco, NY, Futura Publishing Co, 1987, pp 395–408.

28. Leclercq JF, Coumel P, Maisonblanche P, et al: Mise en evidence des mécanismes déterminants de la morte subite. Arch Mal Coeur 7:1028–1033, 1986.

29. Leclercq JF, Rosengarten MD, Attuel P, et al: L'extrasystolie ventriculaire idiopathique: Une parasystolie ventriculaire droite non protegée du rhythme sinusail? Arch Mal Coeur 74:1249, 1981.

30. Marchlinski FE, Buxton AF, Miller JM, Josephson ME: Prevention of ventricular tachycardia induction during right ventricular programmed stimulation by high current strength pacing at the site of origin. Circulation 76:332–342, 1987.

31. McAllister BD, McGron DC, Connolly DC: Paroxysmal ventricular tachycardia and fibrillation without complete heart block. Am J Cardiol 18:898, 1966.

32. Mehra R, Santel D: Can a high voltage shock delivered immediately after premature beats prevent subsequent ventricular arrhythmias? In Belhassen B, Feldman S, Cooperman Y (eds): Cardiac Pacing and Electrophysiology. Israel, R & L Creative Communications, Tel Aviv, 1987, pp 425–432.

33. Mehra R, Santel D: Electrical preexcitation of ischemic tissue for prevention of ventricular tachyarrhythmias. PACE 9:282, 1986.

34. Mehra R, Gough WB, Zeiler R, El-Sherif N: Dual ventricular stimulation for prevention of reentrant ventricular arrhythmias. J Am Coll Cardiol 2:272, 1984.

35. Mehra R, Zeiler RH, Gough WB, El-Sherif N: Reentrant ventricular arrhythmias in the late myocardial infarction period. 9. Anatomic electrophysiologic correlation of reentrant circuits. Circulation 67:11–24, 1983.

36. Melville KI, Bunn B, Suister HE, Silver MD: Cardiac ischemic changes and arrhythmias induced by hypothalamic stimulation. Am J Cardiol 12:781, 1963.

37. Mendez C, Delmar M: Triggered activity: Its possible role in cardiac arrhythmias. In Zipes DP, Jalife J (eds): Cardiac Electrophysiology and Arrhythmias. Orlando, FL, Grune and Stratton, 1985, p 311.

38. Miller SM, Deal BJ, Seagliotti D, et al: Prevention of ventricular tachycardia induction by introduction of a second extrastimulus. Am J Cardiol 57:881–882, 1986.

39. Pratt CM, Francis MJ, Luck JC, et al: Analysis of ambulatory electrocardiograms in 15 patients during spontaneous ventricular fibrillation with special reference to preceding arrhythmic events. J Am Coll Cardiol 2:789, 1983.

40. Prystowsky EN, Zipes DP: Inhibition in the human heart. Circulation 68:707–713, 1983.

41. Randall WC, Ardell JL: Functional anatomy of the cardiac efferent innervation. In Kulbertus HE, Franck G (eds): Neurocardiology. Mount Kisco, NY, Futura Publishing Co, 1988, pp 3–24.

42. Restivo M, Gough WB, El-Sherif N: Reentrant ventricular rhythms in the late myocardial infarction period: Prevention of reentry by dual stimulation during basic rhythm. Circulation 77:429–444, 1988.

43. Roelandt J, Klootwijk P, Lubsen J, et al: Sudden death during long term ambulatory monitoring. Eur Heart J 5:7, 1984.

44. Scherlag BJ, Hope RR, Williams DO, et al: Mechanism of ectopic rhythm formation due to myocardial ischemia: Effects of heart rate and ventricular premature beats. In Wellens HJJ, Lie KI, Janse MJ: The Conduction System of the Heart. Leiden, Stenpert Kroese BV, 1976, pp 633–649.

45. Verrier RL: Neural factors and ventricular electrical instability in sudden death. In Kulbertis HE, Wellens HJJ (eds): Sudden Death. The Hague, Martinus Nijhoff, 1980, p 137.

46. Verrier RL, Lown B: Autonomic nervous system and malignant cardiac arrhythmias. In Wiener H, Hofer MA, Stunkard AJ (eds): Brain, Behavior and Bodily Disease. New York, Raven Press, 1981, p 239.

47. Verrier RL, Lown B: Prevention of ventricular fibrillation by use of low-intensity electrical stimuli. Ann NY Acad Sci 382:355–369, 1982.

48. Verrier RL, Thompson P, Lown B: Ventricular vulnerability during sympathetic stimulation: Role of heart rate and blood pressure. Cardiovasc Res 8:602–610, 1974.

49. Weiss TG: The role of heart rate in the phenylephrine induced suppression of premature ventricular beats [abstract]. Eur J Clin Invest 9:39, 1979.

50. Windle JR, Miles WM, Zipes DP, Prystowsky EN: Subthreshold conditioning stimuli prolong human ventricular refractoriness. Am J Cardiol 57:381, 1986.

51. Winkle RA: The relationship between ventricular ectopic beat frequency and heart rate. Circulation 66:439–446, 1982.

52. Winter UJ, Behrenbeck DW, Brill TH, et al: Hemodynamic and antiectopic effects of long term dynamic overdrive pacing in implanted VVI pacemakers. In Behrenbeck DW, Sowton E, Fontaine G, Winters UJ (eds): Cardiac Pacemakers. New York, Springer-Verlag, 1985, pp 291–297.

53. Wit AL, Allessie MA, Bonke FIM, et al: Electrophysiologic mapping to determine the mechanism of experimental ventricular tachycardia initiated by premature impulses: Experimental approach and initial results demonstrating reentrant excitation. Am J Cardiol 49:166–185, 1982.

54. Wolf M, Scroppian E, Lown B, et al: Protective zone for ventricular fibrillation. Am J Cardiol 29:298, 1972.

55. Zacouto F, Juillard A, Gerbaux A: Prevention of ventricular tachycardias by automatic rate pacing. Rean Art Org 8:3–11, 1982.

56. Zimmerman M, Maisonblanche P, Cauchemez B, et al: Determinants of spontaneous ectopic activity in repetitive idiopathic ventricular tachycardia. J Am Coll Cardiol 7:1219, 1986.

IV

ELECTRICAL THERAPY FOR TACHYCARDIAS: ABLATION

30

PHYSICAL AND EXPERIMENTAL ASPECTS OF ABLATION WITH DIRECT-CURRENT SHOCKS

P. M. HOLT *and* E. G. C. A. BOYD

The electrical ablation technique was discovered, like many important advances, by accident. In 1979, Vedel and colleagues[57] reported the production of atrioventricular (AV) block by electric shock. It occurred during a routine electrophysiologic study in which a patient required cardioversion for a refractory tachycardia. The current from the defibrillator was thought to have flowed through the His bundle investigation catheter. Subsequently, this effect was confirmed in animals[22, 23] and humans.[19, 51] Eight years later the procedure is routinely used for the management of patients with paroxysmal supraventricular or ventricular tachycardias who find drug therapy ineffective or productive of unacceptable side effects.

Unfortunately, electrical ablation is not without its own complications. These include arrhythmias,[46] cardiac tamponade,[11] coronary sinus rupture and thrombosis,[18] circumflex artery lesions,[11] impaired ventricular function,[1, 52] and sudden death.[14a] Efforts have been made to improve the efficiency of the energy delivery and reduce these side effects. These include the use of active-fixation electrodes,[31] suction electrodes,[48] anodal instead of cathodal energy impulses,[7, 55] bipolar energy delivery,[45] or a second intracardiac electrode as the indifferent pole.[16]

The objective of any ablation procedure is to interrupt electrical conduction or activity permanently in a region of cardiac tissue within approximately 1 cm of the electrode tip. For this reason, the basic research has concentrated on the physical processes occurring around the electrode during energy delivery. There are obvious difficulties with in vivo research; therefore, most of this basic research has been conducted using in vitro models. These investigations are imperfect patient analogs, but they do allow comparative assessments to be made and can indicate potentially fruitful avenues for further research.

This chapter is divided into four parts: (1) the results of the in vitro tank experiments, (2) the cardiovascular effects of high-energy delivery, (3) potential changes in ablation electrodes and energy delivery systems, and (4) a discussion of the possible therapeutic mechanism of the endocardial ablation technique.

IN VITRO TANK INVESTIGATIONS

In vitro studies may be performed using either clear physiologic solutions or opaque whole blood. The former—for example, saline, Ringer's solution, or Tyrode's solution—allow direct observation of the electrode tip. If whole blood is used, it is more difficult to observe the optical effects, but not impossible. The information gained from the use of clear media, whole blood, and viable tissue is reviewed below.

Investigations Using Clear Media

Recently, the unipolar ablation technique has been investigated using a simple laboratory apparatus.[6] A standard defibrillator back paddle and a catheter were immersed in a tank filled with Ringer's solution. The electrodes were connected, respectively, with the anodal and cathodal outputs of a standard cardioversion unit. Through an observation port, the catheter electrodes were visible. Delivery of impulses into this system between the electrodes produced an intense flash of light, a loud report, and the generation of gas bubbles around the electrode. After several discharges, marked local roughening of the electrode was found.

The visual effects produced during energy delivery were initially recorded using 35-mm time exposures and video tape. Subsequently, high-speed cine film at 4000 fps was used. During these experiments, the voltage between the catheter electrode and back paddle, plus the current through the system, was measured and recorded on magnetic tape. The pressure wave produced was measured by a piezoelectric crystal mounted on a back plate for mechanical support.

The sequence of events occurring when a 400-J impulse was delivered to the system using a No. 6 French USCI bipolar catheter electrode (CR Bard Inc, Billerica, MA) is illustrated in Figure 30–1. During the delivery of the shock, an incandescent globe was produced around the electrode tip. The globe expanded to reach its maximal diameter in 5 msec. This time corresponded approximately to the peak current flow time; thereafter, the globe collapsed.

The incandescence continued during the contraction phase for the period of the flow of current. With the extinction of the glow, there remained a diffuse, cloudlike structure around the electrode, which coalesced into minute bubbles. These bubbles became larger and fewer in number moving away from the catheter tip.

Simultaneous measurements of pressure 3 cm from the electrode tip showed that the initial emission of energy from the catheter tip resembles an explosion, with the generation of a large, positive-pressure wave. This is followed by a negative-pressure wave and a rapid collapse of the fireball into discrete gas bubbles. These positive and negative pressure excursions have peak-to-peak values of over 1 atm with 400-J deliveries. Subsequent reports[3] showed that with higher-frequency response pressure transducers even higher short-duration pressure pulses were present, over 500 psi.

Voltage and current recordings taken during the electrical impulse delivery showed a generally smooth current waveform with a discon-

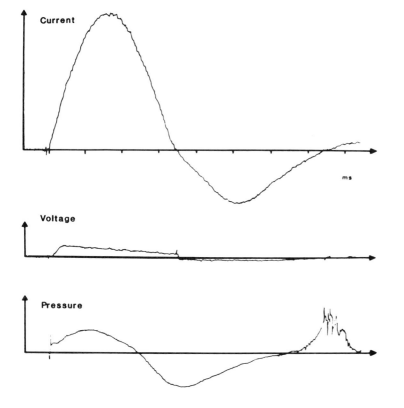

Figure 30–1. The voltage, current, and pressure effects produced by a 400-J cathodal impulse delivered from the distal electrode of a bipolar No. 6 French catheter electrode.

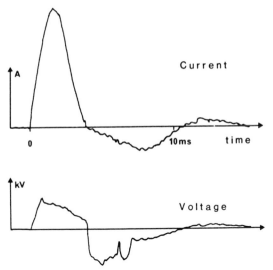

Figure 30–2. The simultaneous voltage and current recordings for a 50-J impulse in a clear medium. It can be seen that the current profile is relatively smooth, whereas the voltage trace is highly discontinuous, indicating voltage breakdown or arcing effects.

tinuous and irregular voltage waveform. Figure 30–2 shows the voltage and current recordings taken for a 50-J impulse in a clear medium.

Reliable and accurate measurements of the temperature at the electrode tip during the brief electrical impulse are difficult to obtain, primarily because of the high voltages and currents present. However, experiments in which the electrode tips have fused indicate that temperatures in excess of 1700°C occur. It is likely that even greater temperatures are present.

These simple experiments show that the environmental conditions around the catheter tip electrode during an ablation pulse are extremely harsh. As the therapy occurs within this local environment, it is important to gain an understanding of the various physical processes involved. A sequence of events occurring during the energy delivery can be proposed. At the onset of the current flow, there is a maximal dissipation of energy in the medium around the electrode tip, which causes the temperature of the medium to rise rapidly. When its temperature reaches boiling point, vapor forms on the electrode surface, probably as discrete bubbles. As the last of the liquid in contact with the electrode vaporizes, it will be heated very rapidly due to the concentration of the current in the remaining liquid medium. The high field strength in the last of the vapor film to be formed may be sufficient to initiate ionization, producing plasma tracks in the vapor volume surrounding the electrode.

The formation of plasma arcs should generate localized high temperatures next to the electrode, optical emission, and intraelectrode impedance discontinuities. The temperatures are probably higher than 1700°C, since plasma arc temperatures are seldom less than 5000°C. The second phenomenon of optical emission is certainly observed, and since the light is generated by electrical discharges, it will be over a broad spectral band extending into the infrared and ultraviolet regions. The intraelectrode voltage-current relationships show pronounced discontinuities.

With a further increase in the current, more energy is dissipated in the liquid medium, producing further vaporization. This would account for the expanding incandescent globe. The initial rapid expansion of the bubble would generate a positive mechanical pressure wave. Once the current has passed its peak value, energy loss is no longer balanced by electrical energy input. The bubble expansion rate falls, and the vapor starts to condense. This activity accounts for the reported negative pressure wave.[3, 6] Similar pressure characteristics are also found during the cavity formation in tissue simulants by speed missile penetration. The generation of high-pressure impulses by capacitor discharges underwater is not unexpected. This method has been used for underwater survey techniques for many years as an alternative to chemical explosives. These light, pressure, voltage, and current effects are all reduced by delivering impulses at lower energy.

Investigations Using Whole Fresh Blood

The generation of gas in clear solutions suggested that bubbles might also be released in blood and that the presence of high temperatures and large pressure pulses could produce red cell damage. A pilot study in which impulses were delivered to a small volume of fresh human blood showed that hemolysis and gas production occurred.[5] This finding was later confirmed in vivo.[49] Hemolytic damage and gas production in fresh heparinized pig's blood have been measured in the test tank.[28] Both cathodal and anodal shocks were delivered through the distal electrodes of No. 6 French USCI catheters immersed in the blood using energies from 10 to 400 J.

In this study, a total of 4000 J was delivered at each energy, first in an ascending energy order and then in a descending sequence to

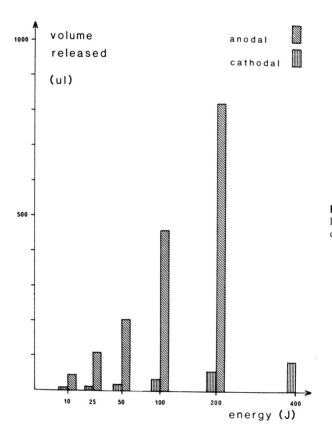

Figure 30–3. The calculated volumes of gas released per impulse for anodal and cathodal deliveries in 7 L of fresh pig's blood.

remove any systematic error in electrode or blood deterioration. The volume of gas liberated per single impulse at each energy was calculated for anodal and cathodal deliveries and is illustrated in Figure 30–3. For cathodal impulses, mean gas production over the energy range of 10 to 50 J was 0.50 μl/J, falling to 0.29 μl/J in the higher range of 100 to 400 J. Anodal impulses liberated greater gas volumes at a rate of 4.34 μl/J from 10 to 200 J. Unfortunately, the gas-collecting apparatus could not withstand the pressure shock wave produced when 400 J was delivered anodally, and the energy was limited to 200 J for this polarity.

Analysis of the gas samples was performed using gas chromatography and is shown in Figure 30–4. The volumes collected were composed predominantly of hydrogen and nitrogen. Values of hydrogen for cathodal and anodal energy delivery, respectively, were 50 to 69 per cent and 66 to 69 per cent. The corresponding figures for nitrogen were 21 to 39 per cent and 12 to 17 per cent. Oxygen and carbon dioxide were present in much smaller amounts. As the impulse energy increased, the percentage of nitrogen and oxygen rose and that of hydrogen and carbon dioxide fell. For anodal delivery, in addition to the above gases,

small quantities of carbon monoxide were present.

With use of either electrode polarity, hemolysis was found to be directly proportional to the impulse energy. The hemolysis produced per single impulse is illustrated in Figure 30–5. Expressed as blood hemolyzed per joule delivered, the rates were 1.37 μl/J for cathodal electrodes and 4.48 μl/J for anodal electrodes. Analysis of blood films after delivery of high-energy impulses showed evidence of cellular clumping or aggregation. However, there was no significant change in hematocrit or hemoglobin.

The results of delivering energy anodally differ markedly from those produced by cathodal energy delivery. Gas production is 8.7 to 15.0 times greater using anodal energy delivery, and hemolysis is three times greater using anodal compared with cathodal polarity.

Faraday's law of electrolysis predicts the formation of hydrogen around a negative electrode. Calculations based on the charge transported per impulse suggest that the volume of hydrogen evolved would be 2.1 to 13.2 μl for 10- to 400-J impulses. The amount detected was considerably greater. Theoretically, no hydrogen should be evolved with a positive

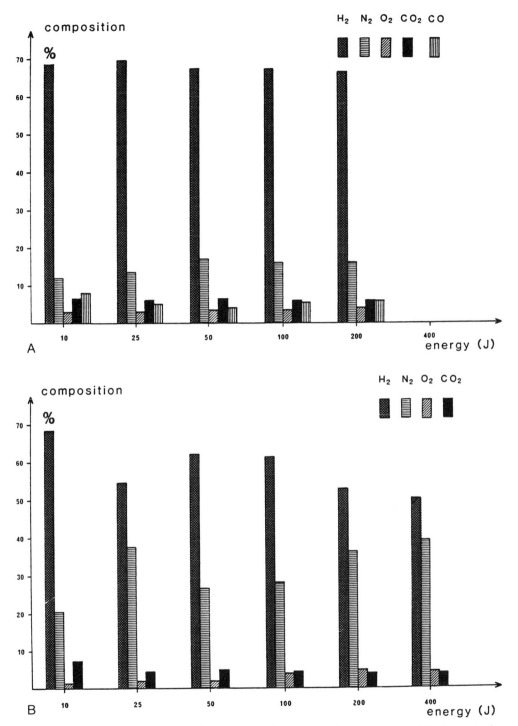

Figure 30–4. *A,* The gas composition for anodal impulses delivered to fresh pig's blood in vitro over the range 10 to 200 J. *B,* The gas composition for cathodal impulses delivered to fresh pig's blood in vitro over the range 10 to 400 J.

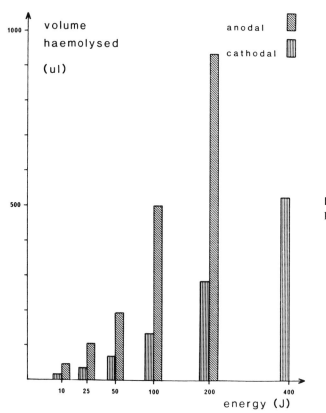

Figure 30–5. The calculated hemolysis produced per impulse for anodal and cathodal deliveries.

electrode, whereas it forms more than 60 per cent of the total volume. Both these findings provide additional evidence of plasma within the fireball around the electrode. Plasma temperatures may be high enough to promote direct thermal dissociation of water, releasing hydrogen, oxygen, and various species of free radicals.

With a cathodal electrode polarity, oxygen would be released only after establishment of the electrical plasma, that is, after fireball production, whereas with anodal electrode polarity, oxygen could be produced initially by electrolysis before the fireball had formed. It would then be available for oxidation reactions during the later phases of the fireball development. The heat of reaction of this anodal process could increase the local environmental temperature around the electrode and could enhance the initial energy dissipation. This effect may account for the more violent pressure effects observed when using anodal electrodes.

Although carbon monoxide is produced during anodal discharges, the maximal volume produced was 0.16 ml for 400 J delivered in 10-J impulses. The volume created for single shocks of 10 to 200 J is therefore below that causing clinical toxicity.[40] However, the vol-

ume of gas produced experimentally during anodal delivery of high-energy impulses may prove to be a potential source of emboli. This finding could be important in procedures involving the left ventricle.

Investigations Using Isolated Tissue

Recently, excised viable tissue has been subjected to ablation impulses over a wide range of energies in the test tank. Experiments in which shocks of 100 J were delivered to isolated, perfused guinea pig hearts and in which shocks of 400 J were administered to dog hearts perfused using the Langendorff technique[26] failed to show any macroscopic endocardial lesion produced acutely.[27] This is the case despite high arc temperatures of thousands of degrees centigrade. Direct measurements of the temperature in vitro at the endocardium and at different depths within the myocardium have been made.[5] This study showed that as long as the endocardium remained in contact with liquid, such as saline or blood, then tissue temperatures remained low. Earlier, Anderson and associates[2] had measured temperature changes under defibrillator electrodes and did not find any substantial temperature increase at the site of injury. This observation may be due to two factors. If 400 J is stored in the defibrillator, the delivered energy is not sufficient to raise 1 gram of water by 100°C. The second factor is the thermal insulating properties of the protective gas film adjacent to the endocardial wall.

Pressure recordings, taken at various depths in the myocardium, show that significant pressure pulses are generated in the cardiac wall.[5] The use of hearts from freshly killed sheep suspended in the tank of oxygenated Ringer's solution provided an even more graphic demonstration of the physical effects occurring during the ablation technique. Figure 30–6

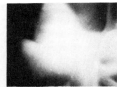
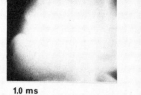
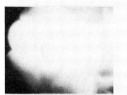
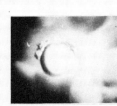
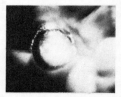
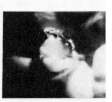
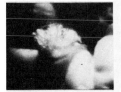
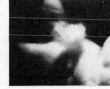
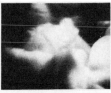
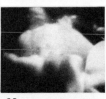
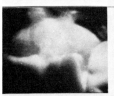
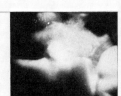
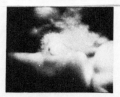
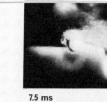
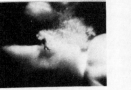
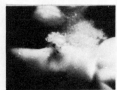
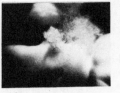
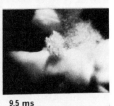

0.0 ms	0.5 ms	1.0 ms	1.5 ms
2.0 ms	2.5 ms	3.0 ms	3.5 ms
4.0 ms	4.5 ms	5.0 ms	5.5 ms
6.0 ms	6.5 ms	7.0 ms	7.5 ms
8.0 ms	8.5 ms	9.0 ms	9.5 ms

Figure 30–6. Prints of individual frames of a high-speed cine film, taken at 4000 fps, of a 200-J delivery to the coronary sinus of a viable sheep heart in oxygenated Ringer's solution.

shows single frames from a high-speed cine film recorded when 200 J was delivered via the distal pole of a No. 6 French USCI electrode positioned in the coronary sinus of a freshly killed sheep's heart. The time interval from impulse delivery is indicated under each frame. Following delivery of the 200-J shock, a fireball is produced around the electrode tip. This fireball can be seen extending laterally down the lumen of the coronary sinus. The initiation of this fireball resembles an explosion. The effects of this positive-pressure wave can be clearly seen on the free wall of the coronary sinus, which expands and then ruptures 2.5 msec after energy delivery. Following the initial "explosive" energy delivery, the flash of light condenses into a definite ball, which further contracts into vapor and gas bubbles, which can be seen escaping from the ruptured coronary sinus into the surrounding fluid medium.

Coltorti and colleagues[10] showed in a study using 20 dogs that 200-J impulses delivered in either unipolar or bipolar mode invariably produced microscopic rupture in the coronary sinus internal elastic membrane. Gross coronary sinus rupture induced cardiac tamponade and resulted in the immediate death of three dogs.

CARDIOVASCULAR EFFECTS

The cardiovascular effects of the high-energy ablation technique will be considered in two sections: first, the gross effects on cardiac tissue and, second, the in vivo effects on impedance in human subjects.

The Cardiac Effects of Endocardial Ablation

Experiments in which energies of different values (10 to 200 J) have been delivered via various catheter electrodes to the ventricles of dogs have been performed.[29] Delivery of such impulses produced both acute and chronic complications. The acute complications consist of ventricular arrhythmias and sudden death due to global myocardial failure.

Evidence suggests that the mechanism of the arrhythmias may be enhanced automaticity rather than reentry.[24] The etiology of these acute arrhythmias may be high field strength or current density. Previous work by Jones and coworkers[33, 36] on cultured chick embryo cells showed that a field strength of 60 to 80 V/cm

induced action potentials that were followed by incomplete repolarization and a number of rapid action potentials of reduced amplitude. Ventricular arrhythmias have been seen in other animal studies[8] as well as in humans. The latter have been shown to be unrelated to synchrony or nonsynchrony of the discharge with the R wave.[56] If high field strength or current density is responsible for the arrhythmias, then using lower energies should prove less arrhythmogenic.

The second and most important acute complication encountered in our animal experiments was that of death due to inexorable deterioration of ventricular function despite all resuscitation attempts. Myocardial rupture had not occurred, and there were no signs of myocardial injury distant from the site of energy delivery. No coronary artery abnormalities were detected. This phenomenon of electromechanical dissociation immediately after energy delivery has also been reported in humans.[50]

It is possible that pressure waves generated during energy delivery[6] may have been responsible for myocardial failure by halting endocardial flow or, by baroreflex, reducing coronary artery flow.[21] The shock waves are almost certainly responsible for the acute myocardial rupture reported during ablation procedures in humans.[52]

An alternative explanation for the acute impairment of ventricular function seen in this experiment and also reported in humans is, again, the presence of high current densities. During animal studies on defibrillator safety, Geddes and associates[20] reported myocardial depression related to high current densities. This was termed "current overdose." Cells receiving such high-intensity shocks exhibit pronounced changes in their ultrastructure.[38] One hypothesis to explain these findings is that transient microlesions are produced in the sarcolemma owing to compression of the membrane by the electric field.[34] Therefore, the occurrence of ventricular failure following a single shock of 400 J could be due to high field strength.

The results from the dogs surviving 5 months showed only one major complication. This was the formation of a small, thin-walled aneurysm following the delivery of 50 J via a USCI electrode to a right ventricle approximately 4 mm thick. The development of such lesions after clinical ablation procedures may explain the late sudden deaths reported, which were apparently unrelated to arrhythmias.[50, 52]

Although significant ventricular arrhythmias occurred immediately after the acute study, they did not prove to be a chronic problem. The sites of ablation in those dogs surviving 5 months did not produce an arrhythmogenic focus. No significant abnormality could be detected in the electrograms, nor was ventricular tachycardia (VT) inducible.

Reducing the energy delivered produces smaller pressure waves and lower current densities and should increase the safety of the technique. Although the results in dogs pertain to normal myocardium, the effects seen have their parallel in clinical ablation procedures.

Our experiment suggests that ablation techniques should be applied to the ventricles with great caution. Large energies or multiple pulses via the USCI electrode may cause sudden death from apparent acute myocardial failure. Long-term myocardial effects may be important, the most notable example being the formation of an aneurysm in the thin-walled right ventricle. Diffuse impairment of ventricular function was not observed by us in dogs surviving 5 months, nor were the chronic lesions arrhythmogenic.

The choice of electrode is important. Active-fixation electrodes are probably safer, since they produce myocardial lesions at low energies similar to those produced at higher energies using standard electrodes.

Effects on Impedance During Clinical Ablation Procedures

In principle, all the in vitro measurements may be carried out on canine models. In practice, the technical problems are formidable. The easiest physical measurements that can be made in animals, as well as in human subjects, are voltage and current recordings. From these data, it is possible to calculate impedance, power, and energy delivered. By comparison with the in vitro measurements, some estimate of the intracardiac physical effects may be made.

The calculated impedance for patients is generally higher than that recorded in the tank using whole blood or clear solutions. Figure 30–7 shows calculated impedance curves for the initial, or primary, pulse for a patient and the tank filled with whole fresh blood and a clear solution. These records show that the simple tank is not a perfect patient analog. It does not include a serial impedance element to simulate the myocardial tissue and the extracardiac thoracic structures. However, im-

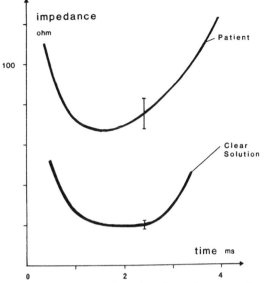

Figure 30–7. The calculated impedance-time curves for 50-J impulses delivered to a patient and to a clear medium in the test tank. In both cases, the electrode was a No. 6 French bipolar USCI energized through the distal electrode.

pedances in both the tank and the patient show marked nonlinearities during the current pulses. Measurements of the impedance of the fireball show that it has a low value, less than approximately 10 ohms for 50- to 400-J impulses. It is almost certainly the major factor controlling the observed nonlinearity of the impedance.

The fireball has the effect of increasing the electrode size. At higher energies, the fireball has a greater diameter. The extent of the endocardium covered by the fireball becomes larger as the energy is increased. It might be expected that the almost perfectly spherical shape of the fireball freely expanding in a large volume of liquid would be hemispheric when in contact with a solid surface. Figure 30–8 shows a 200-J delivery through an electrode partially embedded in a clear acrylic cylinder. The shape of the fireball is not a perfect hemisphere. There is a lateral portion that appears to spread along the solid-liquid interface. The low impedance and the shape of the fireball have implications concerning the development of the ablation electrodes and the energies involved if the therapy is controlled by current density. It has been calculated from the high-speed cine film records that the current density at the liquid-gas interface falls dramatically during the current pulse, and despite high absolute current magnitudes, the current density is only moderate at peak power delivery.[30]

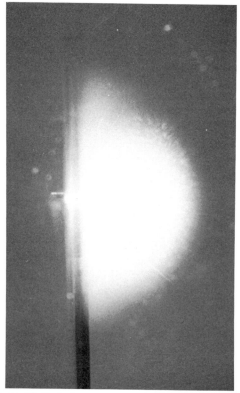

Figure 30–8. A time exposure taken of a 200-J delivery to a half-embedded USCI catheter in the test tank. It can be seen that the fireball is not exactly hemispheric.

MODIFICATIONS OF THE ELECTRODES AND ENERGY DELIVERY SYSTEM

Electrodes

Most clinical ablation procedures employ USCI catheter electrodes, which were designed and manufactured for low-current and low-voltage pacing applications. They have been shown to withstand safely the repeated delivery of high-energy, direct-current (DC)

impulses from standard defibrillators. Nevertheless, it is essential that any electrode intended for use in clinical ablation procedures should undergo extensive in vitro investigation, possibly using the technique described above.[6] This is necessary, since testing different leads has revealed considerable variations in high-voltage and high-current capabilities among manufacturers and for different models from the same manufacturer.[17] Failures can occur near the electrodes or in the lead. Figure 30–9A shows the effect of internal electrical breakdown. The distal electrode was energized, but energy is seen to emerge from the proximal electrode and through the intervening insulation. Typical damage to a lead is shown in Figure 30–9B. This aperture was probably formed by a localized high-energy dissipation within the body of the lead, possibly caused by overheating at a localized high-resistance portion of the conductor. The high-temperature gases that were generated softened and ruptured the outer covering of the catheter. The damage to the catheter cover was not as a result of dielectric breakdown through the outer covering, as the lead was in free air at the time of impulse delivery.

The highest electrical field stress in a dielectric is produced by the smallest radius of curvature of a conductor in contact with the dielectric. In the case of standard, non–active-fixation leads, this is usually at the base of the distal electrode. Flash or arc initiation will occur at the sharpest part or parts of this ring. As these arcs provide low-impedance paths for the current flow, they will concentrate the current in these regions. If, by modification of the electrode shape, the sharpest radius of curvature is not at its base, then the sites of flash initiation can be altered, producing a flash-directable catheter.

Different catheter electrodes currently mar-

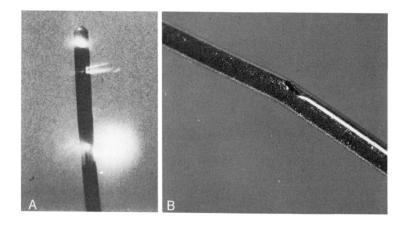

Figure 30–9. Catheters intended for low-voltage pacing applications may fail electrically during the application of the high-voltage ablation pulses. *A,* A failure local to the electrodes. *B,* A lead failure.

keted for temporary or permanent pacing have been evaluated in terms of their ability to withstand high-energy impulses and to investigate whether the geometry of the electrode influences the position and direction of the flash produced. Nine electrodes were studied.[36] The results showed that independent of the electrode geometry the shape of the fireball was always nearly spherical when high energy was delivered. However, at lower energies of 50 J or less the flash was different, depending on the shape of the electrode being tested. It was concluded that some of the active-fixation, or screw-type, electrodes could present low energies more efficiently to the tissue than could the plain, rounded electrode. Unfortunately, the catheter electrodes with active-fixation properties have been designed for use in permanent pacing systems, and their torque characteristics make them difficult to position. Temporary pacing wires, such as the USCI, are much easier to position.

Recently, a method of fixing the smooth, rounded electrode type has been devised using suction. This method appears to be more efficient, allowing ablation of His bundle conduction with lower energy requirements.[48] Further experimental data on the low-energy suction catheter have been published by Saksena et al.[49b] Other workers[44a] have attempted to improve safety by delivering small energy shocks via conventional catheter electrodes. This tends to modify conduction rather than abolish it.

With the use of currently available leads and energies higher than 100 J, there is a considerable risk of coronary sinus rupture, and most workers do not advocate attempting ablation procedures from the mid or distal coronary sinus, especially when this is a small structure. An attempt has been made to produce a catheter electrode capable of directing energy laterally, as a focused beam. The in vitro performance is shown in Figure 30–10. This catheter electrode is a 16-pole device and is intended to deliver low energies. It has been repeatedly tested with 400-J impulses and has not failed. However, this device is not yet capable of ablating conduction in accessory AV pathways using energies less than 100 J. Various catheter electrode designs continue to be investigated. No definitive solution has yet been achieved.

The Energy Delivery System

THE ENERGY SOURCE. Most groups use the standard DC defibrillator to store and deliver the high-energy electrical charge during trans-

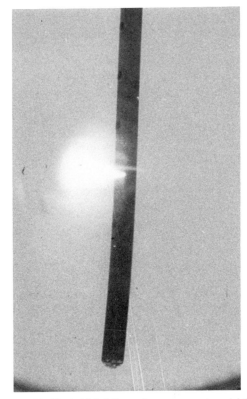

Figure 30–10. A 25-J delivery from an experimental 16-pole energy-directable coronary sinus electrode.

catheter ablation procedures. The development of the modern defibrillator is given in several references.[25, 47, 54] Lown and coworkers developed the form of the modern DC defibrillator by using a capacitor discharging through an inductor. This produced a damped sinusoidal current flow through the subject.[44] Alterations in the degree of damping in the Lown waveform produce the Edmark and Pantridge current profiles. In addition to the damped sine wave, there are two other waveshapes, the exponential and the truncated exponential, which have been investigated and incorporated into commercial defibrillator instruments. There are no reports comparing clinical evaluations of the relative efficiency of the various defibrillator designs available for abalation therapy. It has been recognized that the energy source is an important element in the technique, and its design is currently under review at several centers. The first instrument specifically constructed for ablation purposes was produced by ODAM. The output waveform was similar to a conventional defibrillator but with a finer control over the energy selected. It also had other refinements to make it suitable for use in the electrophysiology laboratory.

The second type of unit marketed for ablation therapy was the National Heart Hospital Ablater. This instrument utilized the same capacitor discharge principle but without the series inductor to control the current delivery. The theory underlying its design is an attempt to maximize the thermal effect by maximizing the peak power output. However, with short duration pulses of approximately one millisecond, the temperature rises in tissue are governed primarily by the total energy delivered; the peak power controls the speed by which these temperatures are reached, not the final temperature achieved. Initial in vivo trials in patients have shown that this design can reduce energy requirements. It is important to keep the energy from this device below the plasma arcing threshold, otherwise greater pressure pulses may be produced. It is understood that refinements in the instrument and the delivery electrode are currently being studied in further animal trials.

A third novel energy delivery system has been under active investigation. The design of this instrument is based on an electrical field theory tissue damage mechanism.[6] This theory suggests that the tissue damage is induced by electrical current flow. A low mean energy delivery rate may be used to minimize the possibility of generating a pressure pulse by plasma arcing. The electrical design is considerably more sophisticated than a standard defibrillator, as pulses as short as 10 microseconds can be delivered at currents and voltages up to 30 amperes and 3000 volts, respectively. Initial in vivo animal investigations have shown that this energy delivery system produces complete heart block as predicted by the theory. Permanent complete heart block has been produced with impulse energies of 0.65J. There have been no recorded postoperative complications. It is expected that the energy requirements may be further reduced by developments in the electrode tip geometry. The complete absence of a pressure effect should allow the treatment of anomalous pathways accessible via the coronary sinus without the frequent complications of rupture and tamponade.

UNIPOLAR VERSUS BIPOLAR IMPULSES. In unipolar ablation, all the current passes through the heart muscle and the thoracic structures. The energy density is highest near the electrode surface of the intracardiac catheter. In a bipolar ablation procedure, both electrodes are within the heart, and the current is restricted to the tissue adjacent to the path between the electrode surfaces. There are two methods of applying bipolar ablation impulses. Some investigators use two electrodes on the same catheter,[45] while others use an electrode on two separate catheters.[16] The former method is usually employed for coronary sinus procedures, while the latter is used in transseptal AV ablation. Intercatheter energy delivery produces higher peak currents and greater tissue damage than catheter to back plate energy delivery.[10, 39] Therefore, smaller energies should be used clinically when impulse delivery occurs between two catheter electrodes.

Bipolar catheters have been shown to withstand energies up to 400 J when the distal electrode is used in unipolar mode ablation. Unfortunately, the internal conductor to the proximal electrode is usually less electrically robust, and using these electrodes in single-catheter bipolar ablation mode energies above approximately 100 J can cause conductor or insulation failures. Tank failures have occurred with energies as low as 25 J with some bipolar electrodes.

ANODAL OR CATHODAL IMPULSES. Although energy delivery with the catheter electrode connected with the cathodal output of a defibrillator is widely used, some groups are employing anodal energy delivery.[7, 55] The hematologic effects measured in vitro show that hemolysis and gas production are much greater for anodal than cathodal impulses. More important, anodal energy delivery produces much larger shock waves than do cathodal impulses.[3, 28]

The surface appearance of electrodes subjected to repeated anodal and cathodal impulses suggests that the arc discharges are different for the two electrode polarities. The anodal electrode surface appears to have a relatively small number of discrete foci, suggesting a small number of stable arc initiation points. The cathodally eroded electrode shows a more uniform surface appearance, which suggests a "sheet"-type discharge mechanism. The importance of these observations warrants further attention. Electrode erosion rates are also different for the two polarities. However, the amount of platinum released during clinical ablation procedures is not significant for either electrode polarity.

THE THERAPEUTIC MECHANISM

During a high-energy ablation impulse delivery, there are four physical phenomena that may be readily observed or measured. They are light, heat, mechanical pressure waves, and electrical current intensity. It is important to know which is most likely to be responsible for the therapeutic effects on the cardiac conduction system.

The delivery of high-energy impulses via standard pacing catheter electrodes does produce energy in the visible spectrum even in blood, as shown in Figure 30–11. Light energy in the form of neodymium yttrium-aluminum-garnet (Nd-YAG) lasers[9] has been investigated in coronary artery disease[41] and cardiac arrhythmias.[53] The therapeutic effects produced acutely by these lasers have the appearance of craters with photocoagulation, indicating the conversion of light energy into an intensely heated focus. Argon laser energy[49a] or excimer laser energy[32a] produces tissue vaporization. Lesions of this type are not seen following electrical ablation. Such thermal effects are unlikely to be implicated in the acute therapeutic response, since the rise in tissue temperature beneath the endocardium is very small and would not account for the endocardial and epicardial effects observed. A recent study has compared the thermal effects of laser and electrical ablation and found much smaller endocardial temperature changes with the latter technique.[42]

There has been speculation on the role of barotrauma in the ablation of conduction.[58] Shock waves have been shown to initiate depolarization in conducting tissue.[59] Experiments with shock or blast injuries have shown that the pressure changes generated by the shock waves can produce myocardial lesions.[12] Such lesions are due to shearing stresses. These stresses produce myocardial contusions that not only occur immediately on the point of impact but also are apparently distant from the impact, most commonly adjacent to major coronary vessels, along the interventricular groove.[13] The pathologic findings in animal experiments involving the high-energy ablation technique are localized to the site of energy delivery. These acute lesions showed no signs of rupture of the myocardial cells. These histologic appearances, although not conclusive, suggest that barotrauma is not the primary mechanism responsible for the acute lesion or the modification of conduction in the high-energy ablation technique.

Electric countershock studies on chick embryo myocardial cells have related cellular effects to field intensity.[33] It was found that the field modified the action potentials and the cellular mechanical contractions. After the application of electrical field stresses below 20 V/cm, action potentials of normal amplitude were followed by complete repolarization. A shock of 200 V/cm produced an extrasystole, followed by temporary arrest. A contracture of approximately 75 per cent of the normal contraction amplitude developed, accompanied by nonsustained cellular fibrillation.[35, 37] In addition to these electrical and mechanical disturbances, there were associated changes in the cellular ultrastructure.[38] High-intensity shocks of 200 V/cm produced pronounced aggregation of mitochondria, with alteration of mitochondrial structure. Other changes include contracture with occasional disorganization of myofibrils, separation of the nuclear membranes, and swelling of the endoplasmic reticulum. These changes are consistent with those reported following application of shocks of similar voltage gradients to dog[15] and guinea pig

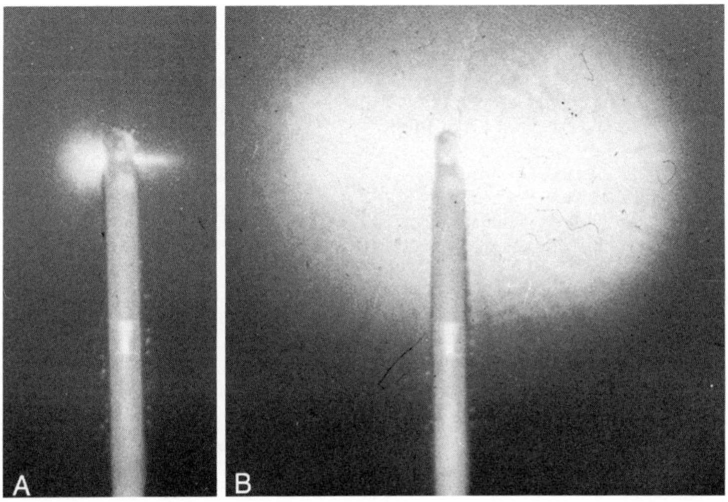

Figure 30–11. With use of modified tank apparatus, it is possible to photograph the flash produced in opaque blood. A, The equivalent of a 25-J delivery. B, The equivalent of a 100-J delivery.

myocardium[32] and exhibit dose dependence similar to that reported by other workers.[14, 27]

One hypothesis to explain these findings is that transient microlesions are produced in the sarcolemma by the generation of a critical transmembrane electrical field stress.[33, 24] Such a dielectric breakdown would lead to membrane depolarization and postshock arrest over a volume related to the shock intensity. This theory is supported by investigations with pharmacologic agents[37] and labeled dextrans.[33] Additional evidence for cellular membrane involvement is provided by in vivo studies using ablation electrodes.[43]

The current density is probably responsible for the acute effect on cardiac conducting tissue seen during delivery of high-energy electrical impulses. This may explain why successful ablation of AV nodal conduction can occur with the use of much lower energies, when shielded USCI electrodes[22] or active-fixation electrodes[31] are used. Although depression of myocardial function[1, 55] may be related to barotrauma, it could be due to "overdose" of the current density.[20] Measures designed to decrease the amount of energy required for successful ablation will reduce the former effect, and efficient targeting of the therapeutic current could reduce the latter effect. The energy delivery system, the catheter electrodes, and the optimal location will be involved.

REFERENCES

1. Abbott JA, Eldar M, Segar JJ, et al: Noninvasive assessment of myocardial function following attempted catheter ablation of ventricular tachycardia foci [abstract]. Circulation 72:III–388, 1985.
2. Anderson HN, Reichenbach D, Steinmetz GP Jr, et al: An evaluation and comparison of alternating and direct current discharges on canine hearts. Ann Surg 160:251–262, 1966.
3. Bardy GH, Coltorti F, Ivey TD, et al: Some factors affecting bubble formation with catheter-mediated defibrillator pulses. Circulation 73:525–538, 1986.
4. Bennett DH: In Symposium on Endocardial Ablation. British Pacing Group, Royal College of Physicians, London, June 1985.
5. Boyd E, Holt P: Haematological and tissue affects of high energy ablation. [abstract]. Br Heart J 53:99, 1985.
6. Boyd EGCA, Holt P: An investigation into the electrical ablation technique and a method of electrode assessment. PACE 8:815–824, 1985.
7. Breithardt G, Borggrefe M, Karbenn U, et al: Catheter ablation of ventricular tachycardia. Eur Heart J 6 [Suppl 1]:19, 1985.
8. Chapman PD, Klopfenstein S, Troup PJ, Brooks HL: Evaluation of a percutaneous catheter technique for ablation of ventricular tachycardia in a canine model. Am Heart J 110:1–8, 1985.
9. Colles MJ: Lasers in medicine. Physics Bull 35:430–432, 1984.
10. Coltorti F, Bardy GH, Reichenbach D, et al: Effects of varying electrode configuration with catheter-mediated defibrillator pulses at the coronary sinus orifice in dogs. Circulation 73:1321–1333, 1986.
11. Conde AX, Perez Gomez F, Harguindey LS: Endocardial ablation. In Perez Gomez F (ed): Cardiac Pacing, Electrophysiology, and Tachyarrhythmias. Madrid, Editorial Group, 1985, pp 1545–1558.
12. Cooper GJ, Maynard RC, Pearse BP, et al: Cardiovascular distortion in experimental nonpenetrating chest impacts. J Trauma 24:188–200, 1984.
13. Cooper GJ, Pearse BP, Strainer MC, et al: The biomechanical response of the chest wall to impact with particular reference to cardiac injuries. J Trauma 22:994–1008, 1982.
14. Dahl CF, Gwy GA, Warner ED, Thomas ED: Myocardial necrosis from direct current countershock: Effect of paddle electrode size and time interval between discharges. Circulation 50:956–961, 1974.
14a. Davies DW, Nathan AW, Camm AJ: Three sudden deaths after attempted high-energy catheter ablation of ventricular tachycardia. Br Heart J 55:506–507, 1986.
15. Davis JS, Lie JT, Bentinck DC, et al: Cardiac damage due to electric current and energy: Light microscopic and ultrastructural observations of acute and delayed myocardial cellular injuries. In Proceedings of the Cardiac Defibrillation Conference, Purdue University, West Lafayette, IN (Engineering Station Document No. 00147), 1975, pp 27–32.
16. De la Asuncion MA, Guillen L, Almeria C, et al: Low energy endocardial His Bundle ablation method using two intracardiac electrodes: Preliminary results. In Perez-Gomez F (ed): Cardiac Pacing, Electrophysiology, and Tachyarrhythmias. Madrid, Editorial Group, 1985, pp 1605–1610.
17. Fisher JD, Brodman R, Johnston DR, et al: Non-surgical electrical ablation of tachycardias: Importance of prior in vitro testing of catheter leads. PACE 7:74–81, 1984.
18. Fisher JD, Brodman R, Kim SG, et al: Attempted non-surgical electrical ablation of accessory pathways via the coronary sinus in the Wolff-Parkinson-White syndrome. J Am Coll Cardiol 4:685–694, 1984.
19. Gallagher JJ, Svenson RH, Kassell JH, et al: Catheter technique for closed chest ablation of the atrioventricular conduction system. N Engl J Med 306:194–200, 1982.
20. Geddes LA, Niebauer MJ, Babbs CF, Bourland JD: Fundamental criteria underlying the efficiency and safety of defibrillating current waveforms. Med Biol Eng Comput 23:122–130, 1985.
21. Gerova M: Autonomic innervation of the coronary vasculature. In Kalsner S (ed): The Coronary Artery. 1982, pp 189–215.
22. Gonzales R, Scheinman M, Bharati S, Lev M: Closed chest permanent atrioventricular block in dogs. Am Heart J 105:461–470, 1983.
23. Gonzales R, Scheinman M, Margaretten W, Rubinstein M: Closed-chest electrode-catheter technique for His bundle ablation in dogs. Am J Physiol (Heart Circ Physiol 10) 241:H283–H287, 1981.
24. Hauer AN, Pobles de Medina E, Borst C: Mechanism and origin of ventricular arrhythmias following electrical catheter ablation. J Am Coll Cardiol 7:130A, 1986.
25. Higgins S: Defibrillation: What You Should Know. Redmond, WA, Physio-Control Corp, 1978.

26. Hoerter JH, Opie LH: Perinatal changes in glycolytic function in response to hypoxia in the incubated or perfused rat heart. Biol Neonate 33:144–161, 1978.

27. Holt PM, Boyd EGCA: Endocardial ablation: The background to its use in ventricular tachycardia [abstract]. Br Heart J 51:687, 1984.

28. Holt P, Boyd EGCA: Haematological effects of the high energy endocardial ablation technique. Circulation 73:1029–1036, 1986.

29. Holt PM, Boyd EGCA: The role of electrode geometry in successful low energy ablation [abstract]. Br Heart J 57:64–65, 1987.

30. Holt PM, Boyd EGCA: The biophysical effects of the high energy, direct current endocardial ablation technique. In Scheinman M (ed): Catheter Ablation of Cardiac Arrhythmias. Boston, Martinus Nijhoff Publishing, pp 1–36, 1987.

31. Holt P, Boyd EGCA, Crick JCP, Sowton E: Low energies and Helifix electrodes in the successful ablation of atrioventricular conduction. PACE 8:639–645, 1985.

32. Homburger H, Rossner JA, Antoni H: Ultrastructural findings after injury of isolated heart muscle tissue of the guinea pig by direct currents [in German]. Bietr Ersten Hife Bahandl Unfallen Elektr Strom 7:140–181, 1976.

32a. Isner JM, Donaldson RF, Deckelbaum LI, et al: The excimer laser. J Am Coll Cardiol 6:1102–1109, 1985.

33. Jones JL, Jones RE: Determination of safety factor for defibrillator waveform in cultured heart cells. Am J Physiol (Heart Circ Physiol 11) 242:H662–H670, 1982.

34. Jones JL, Jones RE: Decreased defibrillator induced dysfunction with biphasic rectangular waveforms. J Physiol (Heart Circ Physiol 16) 247:H792–H796, 1984.

35. Jones JL, Lepeschkin E, Jones R, Rush S: Cellular fibrillation appearing in cultured myocardial cells after application of strong capacitor discharges [abstract]. Am J Cardiol 39:273, 1977.

36. Jones JL, Lepeschkin E, Jones RE, Rush S: Response of cultured myocardial cells to countershock-type electric field stimulation. Am J Physiol 235:H214–H222, 1978.

37. Jones JL, Lepeschkin E, Rush S, Jones R: Depolarisation induced arrhythmias following high intensity electric field stimulation of cultured myocardial cells. Med Instrum 12:54, 1978.

38. Jones JL, Proskauer CC, Paull WK, et al: Ultrastructural injury to chick myocardial cells in vitro following "electric countershock." Circ Res 46:387–394, 1980.

39. Kadish AH, Spear JF, Prood C, et al: Intercatheter energy delivery for ablation of ventricular myocardium. J Am Coll Cardiol 7:237A, 1986.

40. Koch-Weser J: Common poisons. In Wintrobe, MM, et al (eds): Harrison's Principles of Internal Medicine. 7th ed. New York, McGraw-Hill, 1974.

41. Lee G, Ikeda RM, Theis JH, et al: Acute and chronic complications of laser angioplasty: Vascular wall damage and formation of aneurysms in the atherosclerotic rabbit. Am J Cardiol 53:290–293, 1984.

42. Lee NI, Notargiacoma A, Fletcher RD, et al: The thermal response of ventricular endocardium to laser and electrical ablation and the disparate effects of different superfusion media. J Am Coll Cardiol 7:37A, 1986.

43. Levine JH, Spear JF, Weisman HF, et al: The cellular electrophysiologic changes induced by high-energy electrical ablation in canine myocardium. Circulation 73:818–829, 1986.

44. Lown B, Neuman J, Amarasingham R, Berkovits BV: Comparison of alternating current with direct current electroshock across the chest. Am J Cardiol 10:223, 1962.

44a. McComb JM, McGovern B, Garmon H, Ruskin JN: Management of refractory supraventricular tachyarrhythmias using low-energy transcatheter shocks. Am J Cardiol 58:959–963, 1976.

45. Morady F, Scheinman M, Winston S, et al: Efficacy and safety of transcatheter ablation of posteroseptal accessory pathways [abstract]. Circulation 72 [Suppl III]:III–389, 1985.

46. Nathan AW, Ward DE, Bennett DH, et al: Catheter ablation of atrioventricular conduction. Lancet 1:1280–1284, 1984.

47. O'Dowd WJ: Defibrillator design and development—a review. J Med Eng Technol 7:5–15, 1983.

48. Polgar P, Bolnar P, Worum F, et al: Closed chest ablation of the His Bundle: A new technique using suction electrode catheter and DC shock. In Steinbach K (ed): Cardiac Pacing. Darmstadt, Federal Republic of Germany, Steinkopff Verlag, 1983, pp 883–890.

49. Rowland E, Foale R, Nihoyannopoulos P, et al: Intracardiac contrast echoes during transvenous His bundle ablation. Br Heart J 53:240–242, 1985.

49a. Saksena S, Ciccone JM, Chandran P, et al: Laser ablation of normal and diseased human ventricle. Am Heart J 112:52–60, 1986.

49b. Saksena S, Tarjan PP, Bharati S, et al: Low-energy transvenous ablation of the canine atrioventricular conduction system with a suction electrode catheter. Circulation 76:394, 1987.

50. Scheinman MM, Davies JC: Catheter ablation for treatment of tachyarrhythmias: Present role and potential promise. Circulation 73:10–13, 1986.

51. Scheinman MM, Morady F, Hess DS, Gonzales R: Catheter-induced ablation of the atrioventricular junction to control refractory supraventricular arrhythmias. JAMA 248:851–855, 1982.

52. Shofield PM, Bowes RJ, Laurence G, et al: Impaired right ventricular function following transvenous fulguration of atrioventricular conduction [abstract]. Br Heart J 55:506, 1986.

53. Svenson RH, Gallagher JJ, Selle JG, et al: Successful intraoperative Nd:YAG laser ablation of ventricular tachycardia. J Am Coll Cardiol 7:237A, 1986.

54. Tacker WA Jr, Geddes LA: Electrical Defibrillation. Boca Raton, FL, CRC Press, 1980.

55. Tonet JL, Fontaine G, Frank R, Grosgogeat Y: Treatment of refractory ventricular tachycardias by endocardial fulguration [abstract]. Circulation 72:III–388, 1985.

56. Tonet JL, Barata M, Fontaine G, et al: Ventricular arrhythmias during endocardial catheter fulguration of ventricular tachycardias. J Am Coll Cardiol 7:236A, 1986.

57. Vedel J, Frank R, Fontaine G, et al: Bloc auriculoventriculaire intra-Hisien definitif induit au cours d'une exploration endoventriculaire droite. Arch Mal Coeur 72:107, 1979.

58. Ward DE, Davis M: Transvenous high energy shock for ablating atrioventricular conduction in man: Observations on the histological effects. Br Heart J 51:175–178, 1984.

59. Wehner HD, Sellier K: Compound action potentials in the peripheral nerve induced by shock waves. Acta Chir Scand [Suppl] 508:179–184, 1982.

31

PATHOLOGIC ASPECTS OF ELECTRICAL ABLATION

SAROJA BHARATI *and* MAURICE LEV

Ablation of the atrioventricular (AV) junction involving the AV node or the His bundle is, at present, an accepted procedure in the management of intractable supraventricular arrhythmias.[3, 4] The closed-chest transvenous catheter approach delivery of direct-current (DC) energy at the AV junction for the creation of complete heart block in the human has practically replaced the open-chest surgical methods that were in vogue.

In this chapter, we will deal mostly with the pathologic findings of the ablated area of the AV junction that was done experimentally in dogs. We will also discuss our pathologic findings in one case of a human who died suddenly 6 weeks after ablation of AV junction by means of electric shock for intractable supraventricular arrhythmias. Our experience includes all our work with the innovative electrophysiologists in our country who pioneered the AV junctional ablation by various means. The AV junction was ablated by the following closed-chest catheter techniques to create varying degrees of AV block:
1. Electric shock
   a. Pulsed, synchronized electric shocks—to produce complete heart block.
   b. DC shocks through tissue-fixation catheters—to impair AV conduction.
   c. Suction electrode catheter—deliver low-energy DC shocks to record the His bundle electrogram, pace, and ablate the His bundle to produce complete AV block.

2. Argon laser energy—to produce complete heart block.
3. Radiofrequency energy
   a. Creation of complete AV block.
   b. Creation of prolonged PR interval

ELECTRIC SHOCK

Creation of Complete Atrioventricular Block by Means of Closed-Chest Catheter Techniques[5]

Pulsed, synchronized electric shocks (35 J) were delivered at the His bundle region, and complete AV block was created in 9 of 10 dogs. The dogs were sacrificed 3 months after the procedure.

At a gross level, fibroelastosis of the myocardium in the AV junction was seen extending between the coronary sinus and the septal leaflet of the tricuspid valve. There were no perforations or thrombus formation. The fibroelastosis was focal and smaller in size when a single shock was used (Fig. 31–1). On the other hand, with multiple shocks, the area of fibroelastosis was quite diffuse (Fig. 31–2).

There was marked fibrosis with chronic inflammatory cells in the approaches to the AV node, in the AV node, and in the bundle. In some cases, the node was separated by fat from the surrounding atrial muscle. Occasionally, there was calcification in the approaches to the AV node. The aortic and tricuspid valves showed an increase in and vacuolization of the spongiosa. Despite the extensive changes seen pathologically, the dogs were not

Aided by grant HL 30558-05 from the National Institutes of Health, National Heart, Lung, and Blood Institute, Bethesda, MD.

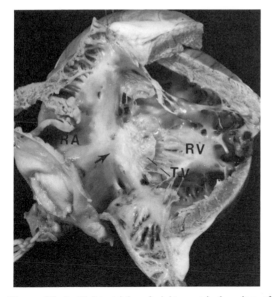

Figure 31–1. Right atrial and right ventricular view of dog's heart after delivery of one shock. RA = right atrium; RV = right ventricle; TV = tricuspid valve. Arrow points to whitened area produced by the shock. (From Gonzalez R, Scheinman M, Bharati S, Lev M: Closed chest permanent atrioventricular block in dogs. Am Heart J 105:464, 1983; with permission.)

in congestive heart failure, nor did they require a pacemaker.

The dogs that received single shocks showed less damage to the bundle, bundle branches, and the summit of the ventricular septum (Fig. 31–3) than did those that received multiple shocks (Fig. 31–4).

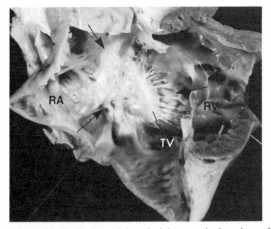

Figure 31–2. Right atrial and right ventricular view of dog's heart after delivery of multiple shocks. RA = right atrium; RV = right ventricle; TV = tricuspid valve. Arrows point to the whitened area produced by the multiple shocks. (From Gonzalez R, Scheinman M, Bharati S, Lev M: Closed chest permanent atrioventricular block in dogs. Am Heart J 105:465, 1983; with permission.)

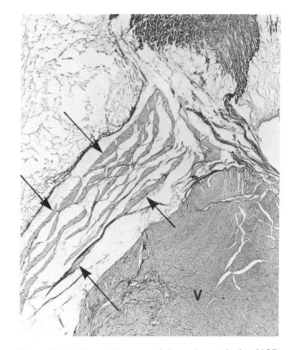

Figure 31–3. Branching part of the atrioventricular (AV) bundle, intact after delivery of one shock. Weigert–van Gieson stain × 45. V = ventricular septum. Arrows point to the AV bundle. (From Gonzalez R, Scheinman M, Bharati S, Lev M: Closed chest permanent atrioventricular block in dogs. Am Heart J 105:470, 1983; with permission.)

Electric Shock with Impairment of Atrioventricular Conduction[12]

DC shocks were delivered through barbed, tipped tissue-fixation catheters at the His bundle area to impair AV conduction and thereby avoid pacemaker dependence in the management of supraventricular arrhythmias.

Six mongrel dogs received 20- to 240-J DC shocks that resulted in acute AV block, with return of 1:1 AV conduction in all animals. The dogs were sacrificed 2 to 3 weeks later. Grossly, only focal fibrosis was present in the AV nodal area, and there were no perforations. The septal leaflet of the tricuspid valve was swollen.

Microscopically, in general, the approaches to the AV node, the AV node, and the bundle showed marked fibrosis with chronic inflammatory cells with low-energy shocks (20 to 180 J) (Fig. 31–5). Greater damage to the His bundle and the involvement of the bundle branches were observed with larger shocks (Fig. 31–6).

This study clearly shows that considerable damage to the conduction system may be seen pathologically but that AV conduction is main-

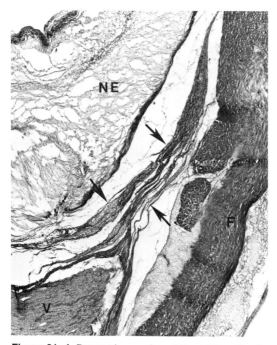

Figure 31–4. Penetrating portion of the AV bundle after multiple shocks. Weigert–van Gieson stain × 45. Arrows point to the bundle. Note almost complete replacement of bundle by fibroelastic tissue. NE = necrosis of subendocardium beneath the aorta on the left side; F = fibrous prong of central fibrous body going to the tricuspid valve; V = ventricular septum. (From Gonzalez R, Scheinman M, Bharati S, Lev M: Closed chest permanent atrioventricular block in dogs. Am Heart J 105:469, 1983; with permission.)

tained functionally with minimal changes. Thus, a large safety margin exists between the amount of tissue damage and the functions of conduction.

Low-energy Transvenous Ablation of the Atrioventricular Conduction System Using a Suction Electrode Catheter[11]

In this method, a single electrode catheter was used to record and pace the His bundle, and low energy (20 to 30 J) was used to ablate the bundle. The electrode was actively fixed to the atrial endocardium at the His bundle level. Electrophysiologic studies were performed both acutely and chronically (more than 40 days) after the procedure. Persistent complete heart block in five and paroxysmal second-degree and third-degree AV block in two dogs were observed.

Grossly, a white plaque was present immediately adjacent to the septal leaflet of the tricuspid valve. There were no perfora-

tions. Microscopically, the conduction system showed fibrosis of the penetrating (Fig. 31–7) and branching bundle in all with minimal AV node and atrial involvement. The dogs who received one or two additional shocks showed, in addition, significant proximal right bundle branch fibrosis. There was marked fatty infiltration or degeneration of the central fibrous body. The base of the tricuspid and aortic valves showed an increase in amount of spongiosa, as well as vacuolization of it, but the integrity of the valve rings and leaflets was preserved. Calcification or cartilage formation and fibrosis of the summit of the ventricular septum were present in all.

In summary, this method suggests that a single suction electrode catheter may be used for His bundle recording, pacing, and ablation. Varying degrees of AV block may be produced with low energy, which creates focal injury to the target area of the conduction system. Recently this catheter has been used in conjunction with radiofrequency energy for ablation of the AV junction in experimental and clinical studies.

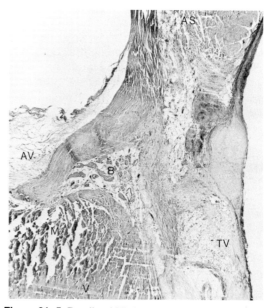

Figure 31–5. Bundle of His in dog with low-energy shock (20 J), showing dissolution of tissue with space formation. Also visible are the degeneration of the spongiosa of annulus of aortic valve and tricuspid valve and coagulative necrosis of some myocardial fibers in summit of ventricular septum. Weigert–van Gieson stain × 30. B = bundle of His; AV = aortic valve; TV = tricuspid valve; M = myocardial fibers; V = ventricular septum; AS = atrial septum. (From Scheinman MM, Bharati S, Wang YS, et al: Electrophysiologic and anatomic changes in the atrioventricular junction of dogs after direct-current shocks via tissue fixation catheters. Am J Cardiol 55:196, 1985; with permission.)

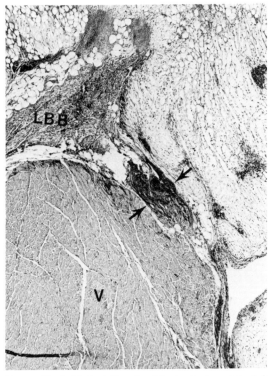

Figure 31–6. Marked fibrosis of the beginning of the left bundle branch and the right bundle branch in a dog that received high-energy shocks (200 J). Arrows point to the beginning of the right bundle branch. LBB = beginning of the left bundle branch; V = ventricular septum. Weigert–van Gieson stain × 63. (From Scheinman MM, Bharati S, Wang YS, et al: Electrophysiologic and anatomic changes in the atrioventricular junction of dogs after direct-current shocks via tissue fixation catheters. Am J Cardiol 55:197, 1985; with permission.)

ARGON-ION LASER RADIATION OF THE HIS BUNDLE[1, 10]

With this technique, short bursts (10 to 60 seconds) of argon laser were delivered (2.5 W) at the His bundle area, which resulted in "split" His bundle potentials with an unchanged AH (50 msec) and H'V interval of 20 msec. At the gross level, a small zone of hemorrhage was present in the His bundle area.

Histologically, the His bundle showed a microscopic vaporized area at the junction of the penetrating and branching portions of the His bundle. The vaporized zone was surrounded by coagulation necrosis and hemorrhage, as well as a thin rim of black, carbon-lined edges. The vaporized zone thus divided the His bundle into superior and inferior portions (Fig. 31–8), which retained continuity with proximal

and distal portions of the His bundle. The AV node, the proximal penetrating and distal branching bundle, and the bundle branches were intact except for superficial loss of left bundle branch fibers.

In the use of argon-ion laser, it must be recalled that acutely this can create fistulous tracts between chambers of the heart or between a large vessel, such as the aorta, and the right ventricle. Chronically, it may result in the formation of granulation tissue, fibrosis, extensive hemorrhage, and giant cell reaction. It appears that if granulation tissue proliferates to a considerable extent, this may occlude or narrow the vaporized zones at a later date.

RADIOFREQUENCY ENERGY

Induction of Complete Atrioventricular Block[6, 7]

Complete AV block was induced both acutely and chronically by using this method. Pathologically, distinct areas of necrosis in the

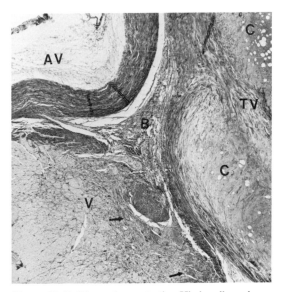

Figure 31–7. Fibrosed, penetrating His bundle and cartilage in the annulus of the tricuspid valve; a small, fibrotic scar on the summit of the ventricular septum; and swelling of the spongiosa of the tricuspid and aortic valves. Weigert–van Gieson stain × 46.5. Arrows point to the fibrotic lesion in the ventricular septum. B = bundle of His; V = ventricular septum; AV = aortic valve; TV = tricuspid valve; C = cartilage. (From Saksena S, Tarjan PP, Bharati S, et al: Low energy transvenous ablation of the atrioventricular conduction system using a suction electrode catheter. Circulation 76:401, 1987; by permission of the American Heart Association, Inc.)

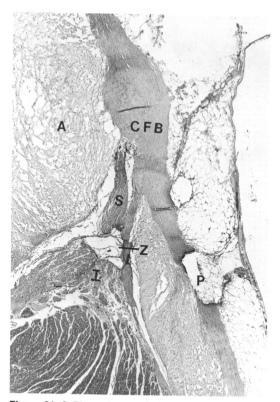

Figure 31–8. Photomicrograph showing laser cut dividing bundle of His into superior and inferior portions. The ventricular septum is intact. Hematoxylin-eosin stain × 45. A = swollen spongiosa of aortic annulus and endocardium; CFB = central fibrous body; I = inferior part of bundle of His; P = zone of penetration of second laser cut into tricuspid prong of central fibrous body; S = superior part of bundle of His; Z = zone of His bundle tissue dissolution and its division into superior and inferior segments. (From Narula OS, Bharati S, Chan MC, et al: Microtransection of the His bundle with laser radiation through a pervenous catheter—correlation of histologic and electrophysiologic data. Am J Cardiol 54:190, 1984; with permission.)

AV node, His bundle, and the summit of the ventricular septum (very close to the His bundle) were seen acutely. The chronic lesions were characterized by discrete areas of fibrosis, chronic inflammatory cell infiltration and cartilage formation, and an increase in amount as well as vacuolization of the spongiosa of the aortic and tricuspid valves (Fig. 31–9). There were no ventricular arrhythmias from the nearby scar areas at the end of 3 months.

Induction of PR Prolongation[9]

Radiofrequency energy may also induce first-degree AV block with well-localized lesions in the approaches to the AV node and the AV node, with minimal or moderate involvement of the surrounding structures.

SUDDEN DEATH AFTER CATHETER-INDUCED ATRIOVENTRICULAR JUNCTIONAL ABLATION IN THE HUMAN[2, 8]

A 56-year-old woman with recurrent atrial fibrillation, refractory to medical management, had AV junctional ablation with two shocks (500 J), which produced complete AV block. Six weeks later, her electrocardiogram and exercise tolerance test showed infrequent premature ventricular contractions, third-degree AV block, and paced ventricular rhythm with 100 per cent capture. At this time, she suddenly collapsed and was found to be in ventricular fibrillation; she died. The conduction system showed marked fatty infiltration of the approaches to the AV node with almost complete separation of atrial musculature from the node (Fig. 31–10). A partially fibrotic atrio-Hisian connection was present. Fibroelastosis with chronic inflammatory cells was seen in the AV node, His bundle,

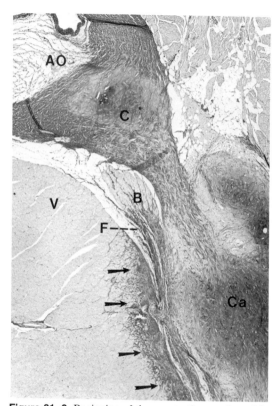

Figure 31–9. Beginning of the penetrating portion of the partially fibrosed His bundle by radiofrequency energy. The bundle is being pressed by the cartilaginous replacement of the AV nodal region. Arrows point to the localized area of fibrosis on the summit of the ventricular septum on the right side, immediately adjacent to the penetrating portion of the His bundle. Weigert–van Gieson stain × 45. AO = aorta; B = penetrating portion of the His bundle; C = central fibrous body; Ca = cartilaginous replacement of the AV nodal region; F = fibrosis; V = summit of the ventricular septum. (From Huang SK, Bharati S, Lev M, Marcus FI: Electrophysiologic and histologic observations of chronic atrioventricular block induced by closed-chest catheter desiccation with radiofrequency energy. PACE 10:813, 1987; with permission.)

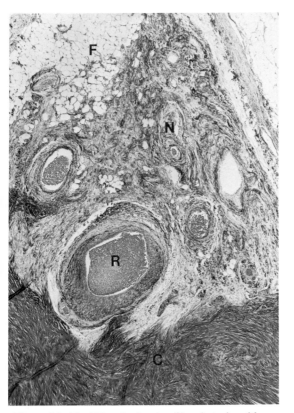

Figure 31-10. AV node showing fibroelastosis, with replacement of the approaches by fat. Weigert–van Gieson stain × 45. C = central fibrous body; R = ramus septi fibrosi; N = AV node; F = fat. (From Bharati S, Scheinman MM, Morady F, et al: Sudden death after catheter-induced atrioventricular junctional ablation in the human. Chest 88:886, 1985; with permission.)

and the bundle branches. In addition, examination of the summit of the ventricular septum and the atrial septum revealed many inflammatory cells with fibrosis (Fig. 31–11), and there were degenerative changes in the aortic and tricuspid valves. The atrio-Hisian connection or the inflammatory changes with fibrosis in the conduction system and the summit of the ventricular septum, or both, could have formed a base for arrhythmogenicity and caused the sudden death in this patient.

This case was one of the first few in the world literature in which the AV junction was ablated in a human and in which pathologic studies were performed. This case occurred early in the experience with ablation, and since then, the techniques have been modified. Today, complete AV block can be produced in a human by ablating the AV junction with less than 400 J. It is very likely that injury to the conduction system and the surrounding structures will be less severe in nature with lesser amounts of energy.

CONCLUSIONS

On the basis of our experience with the pathologic findings of the AV junction after various types of ablation procedures to induce complete AV block or modify AV conduction, we conclude the following:

1. The closed-chest transvenous electrode technique of creating AV block by electric shock, laser, or radiofrequency is a relatively safe procedure.

2. Multiple electric shocks produce extensive damage to the conduction system.

3. A single electric shock causes less severe damage to the conduction system.

4. Low-energy electric shock may produce transient AV block with a return to 1:1 normal AV conduction. Pathologically, low energy produces predominant lesions in the approaches to the AV node, the AV node, and common bundle.

5. Larger shocks create diffuse damage involving the bundle branches as well.

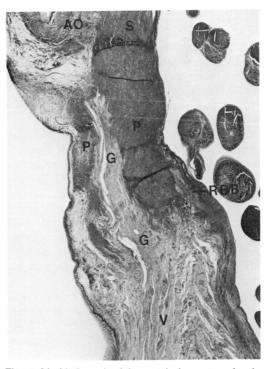

Figure 31-11. Summit of the ventricular septum showing marked fibrosis, with thickened pars membranacea. Weigert–van Gieson stain × 15. V = ventricular septum; P = thickened pars membranacea; S = scar behind aorta meeting pars membranacea; AO = base of aorta at sinus of Valsalva; G = granulation tissue; RBB = right bundle branch. (From Bharati S, Scheinman MM, Morady F, et al: Sudden death after catheter-induced atrioventricular junctional ablation in the human. Chest 88:886, 1985; with permission.)

6. Despite the histologic evidence of damage to the AV junction, only minimal changes in AV conduction are present clinically. Thus, there is a large safety margin for AV conduction.

7. A single suction electrode catheter may be used to record and pace the His bundle as well as to ablate the His bundle with low energy (20 to 30 J), with the production of maximal pathologic changes in the His bundle and fewer changes in the AV node.

8. The argon laser produces acutely precise, local microtransection of the His bundle. However, it may also create macro (large) channels between the aorta and the right ventricle.

9. The chronic effects of laser ablation may be in the form of marked granulation tissue formation.

10. Radiofrequency energy (low power) can produce complete AV block of a permanent nature with well-delineated, clear-cut focal areas. The healing is by granulation tissue and cartilage formation in the dogs.

11. Radiofrequency energy can produce first-degree AV block.

The common denominators seen pathologically with the use of all methods are as follows:

1. Healing occurs by granulation tissue, with fat deposition and chronic inflammatory cells.

2. Areas near the targeted areas can be involved, such as the central fibrous body, the membranous septum, the summit of the ventricular septum, and the aortic and tricuspid valves. The long-term effects of this involvement are unknown at present. Involvement of these structures is probably unavoidable but should be kept to a minimum.

3. Cartilage formation in dogs is frequently noted with low energy rather than with high energy. This may be a normal tissue reaction to a certain type of injury in this animal. Human tissue may react differently in the long run.

4. Finally, laser energy can produce precise, localized microvaporized zones. However, without the development of a fiberoptic laser instrument, the use of laser energy is questionable. On the other hand, radiofrequency energy creates well-delineated zones of lesions, and the energy level can be quite low. Thus, radiofrequency probably will be the tool for future management of intractable supraventricular arrhythmias.

REFERENCES

1. Bharati S, Lev M: Laser irradiation of the normal AV conduction pathway in canines: Preliminary experimental findings. *In* Scheinman MM, Fontaine G (eds): International Symposium on Ablation in Cardiac Arrhythmias. Mount Kisco, NY, Futura Publishing Co, 1987, pp 449–460.
2. Bharati S, Scheinman MM, Morady F, et al: Sudden death after catheter-induced atrioventricular junctional ablation in the human. Chest 88:883, 1985.
3. Davis J, Scheinman M, Ruder MA, et al: Ablation of cardiac tissues by an electrode catheter technique for treatment of ectopic supraventricular tachycardia in adults. Circulation 74:1044, 1986.
4. Evans GT Jr, Scheinman MM, Zipes DP, et al: The percutaneous cardiac mapping and ablation registry: Summary of results. PACE 9:923, 1986.
5. Gonzalez R, Scheinman M, Bharati S, Lev M: Closed chest permanent atrioventricular block in dogs. Am Heart J 105:461, 1983.
6. Huang SK, Bharati S, Lev M, Marcus FI: Electrophysiologic and histologic observations of chronic atrioventricular block induced by closed-chest catheter desiccation with radiofrequency energy. PACE 10:805, 1987.
7. Huang SK, Bharati S, Graham AR, et al: Closed chest catheter desiccation of the atrioventricular junction using radiofrequency energy—a new method of catheter ablation. J Am Coll Cardiol 9:349, 1987.
8. Lev M, Bharati S: Transcutaneous AV junctional ablation in dogs and humans: Histologic observations. *In* Scheinman MM, Fontaine G (eds): International Symposium on Ablation in Cardiac Arrhythmias. Mount Kisco, NY, Futura Publishing Co, 1987, pp 183–190.
9. Marcus FI, Bouin LT, Wharton K, Bharati S: Electrophysiological and pathological assessment of chronic first degree atrioventricular block caused by closed-chest catheter ablation with radiofrequency energy in dogs [abstract]. J Am Coll Cardiol 9:95A, 1987.
10. Narula OS, Bharati S, Chan MC, et al: Microtransection of the His bundle with laser radiation through a pervenous catheter—correlation of histologic and electrophysiologic data. Am J Cardiol 54:186, 1984.
11. Saksena S, Tarjan PP, Bharati S, et al: Low energy transvenous ablation of the atrioventricular conduction system using a suction electrode catheter. Circulation 76:403, 1987.
12. Scheinman MM, Bharati S, Wang YS, et al: Electrophysiologic and anatomic changes in the atrioventricular junction of dogs after direct-current shocks via tissue fixation catheters. Am J Cardiol 55:194, 1985.

32

CATHETER ABLATION FOR PATIENTS WITH SUPRAVENTRICULAR TACHYCARDIA

MELVIN M. SCHEINMAN, FRED MORADY,
and G. THOMAS EVANS

The use of electrode catheters for intracardiac pacing and recording has long been established as an important diagnostic tool. Use of these catheters for therapeutic intervention has opened a new chapter in the management of patients with supraventricular tachycardia refractory to conventional therapy. The purpose of this chapter is to review the present role of catheter ablative techniques in the management of these patients.

MECHANISMS OF CARDIAC DAMAGE

Although catheter ablation techniques utilizing direct-current (DC) shocks, radiofrequency, and laser energy have been studied in the experimental laboratory,[16, 17, 23] to date only high-energy DC shocks have been used in patients. Delivery of a shock of 100 J or more may produce damage to cardiac tissue

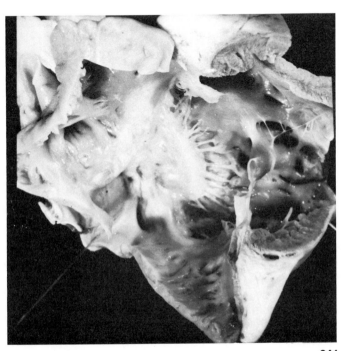

Figure 32–1. Gross examination of a canine heart after multiple direct-current (DC) shocks delivered to the junctional area. Note the wide band of scarring involving the atrial muscle as well as the summit of the ventricular septum in the region of the tricuspid valve.

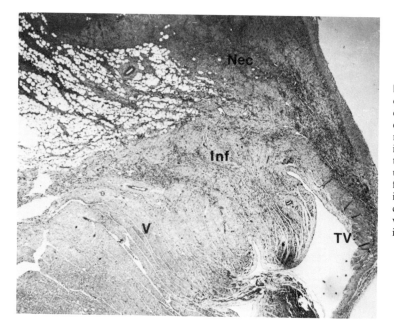

Figure 32–2. Photomicrograph of a cross-section through the lesion caused by a 100-J shock. There is a central area of necrosis with hemorrhage (Nec) closely surrounded by inflammation (Inf). The base of the tricuspid valve (TV) and the ventricular summit (V) are somewhat inflamed. The fat in the coronary sulcus is necrosed, but, on higher magnification, the coronary artery is not involved. (Hematoxylin and eosin, original magnification × 12.5.)

through a variety of mechanisms, including thermal injury,[15] barotrauma,[2] or induction of a dense electrical field.[18] The exact role of each of these mechanisms is currently uncertain, but it is clear that such shocks may produce irreversible injury to the cardiac conduction system or myocardium or both (Figs. 32–1 to 32–3).

RATIONALE FOR CATHETER ABLATIVE PROCEDURES

The rationale for use of ablative shocks includes arrhythmia control through a variety of mechanisms. The most popular approach is catheter ablation of the atrioventricular (AV) junction. In this approach, the clinician attempts to abort the passage of supraventricular impulses, which are funneled into the ventricle. This technique may be applied, for example, in patients with atrial fibrillation, atrial flutter, atrial tachycardia, or AV nodal reentry in whom medical therapy has failed. Although arrhythmia control is achieved, it is accomplished at the expense of sacrificing the AV conduction system and induction of a pacemaker-dependent state.

An alternative approach for some patients with right atrial tachycardia foci is use of catheter ablative shocks to destroy these foci. The advantage of this approach is that it leaves AV conduction intact, but this technique is associated with risk of perforation of the relatively thin right atrial wall by the electrical

discharges. Another approach is to destroy elements of a tachycardia circuit that appear to be critical for maintenance of the tachycardia. For example, the most common tachycar-

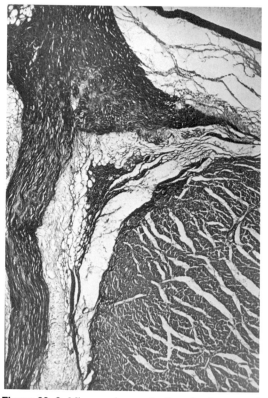

Figure 32–3. Microscopic examination showing necrosis of the bundle branches at their division at the summit of the ventricular septum after shocks delivered to the atrioventricular junction of a dog.

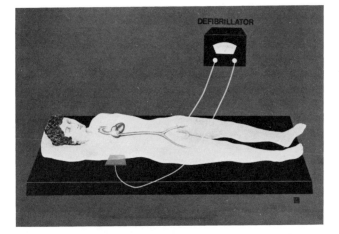

Figure 32–4. Schema showing catheter electrical ablation of the AV junction. The electrode catheter is positioned across the tricuspid valve for optimal His bundle recording. An indifferent plate is placed over the left scapula. Electrical energy is delivered via a defibrillator.

dia mechanism for patients with extranodal accessory pathways involves antegrade conduction over the AV node and retrograde conduction over an accessory bypass tract. Ablative shocks may be delivered either to the AV junction[27] or, in some instances, directly to the bypass tract.[20] Destruction of either of these structures would be expected to control the arrhythmia, since both are necessary components of the tachycardia circuit. Direct ablation of the accessory pathway is far preferable, since it leaves the normal AV conduction system intact.

TECHNIQUE OF CATHETER ABLATION OF THE ATRIOVENTRICULAR JUNCTION

Catheter electrical ablation of the AV junction was first introduced in 1981.[28] This technique involves insertion of a multipolar electrode catheter into the right ventricular apex for purposes of pacing. In addition, a catheter is inserted into a peripheral artery for continuous recording of the arterial pressure. A multipolar electrode catheter is then inserted

across the tricuspid valve for recording the His bundle potential (Fig. 32–4). The catheter is manipulated to record the largest unipolar His bundle potential associated with the largest atrial deflection[13] (Fig. 32–5). One or more shocks of 200 to 300 J are delivered from the electrode showing the largest His bundle deflection to a patch placed over the left scapula via a standard DC defibrillator (Fig. 32–6). A short-acting barbiturate is administered prior to delivery of the shock by an experienced anesthesiologist. The patient is monitored in the catheter laboratory for at least 45 minutes after delivery of the shock to ensure stability of right ventricular pacing, absence of ventricular arrhythmias, and adequate cardiovascular function. After the procedure, the patient is monitored in an intensive care unit for 24 hours to make sure that stable complete AV block has been achieved. A permanent cardiac pacemaker is inserted after this monitoring period.

PRECAUTIONS

Catheter ablation should be performed by personnel experienced in invasive electrophys-

Atrial Fibrillation with Rapid Ventricular Response

Figure 32–5. Simultaneous recordings of leads V_1, I, and III, together with the His bundle electrogram (HBE), in a patient with atrial fibrillation and a rapid ventricular response. CL = cycle length.

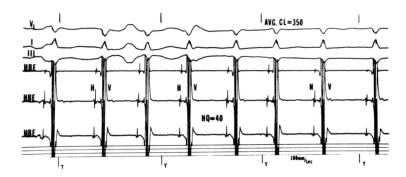

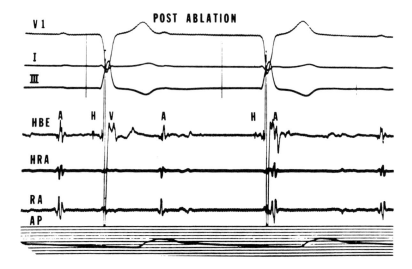

Figure 32–6. Recordings after AV junction ablation in the same patient as in Figure 32–5. Atrial fibrillation has been replaced by sinus rhythm, and complete AV block is present. A His potential precedes each of the QRS complexes. HBE = His bundle electrogram; HRA = high right atrium; RA = right atrium; AP = arterial pressure.

iologic procedures. The patient must undergo complete study prior to the procedure so that the mechanisms of the tachycardia may be discerned and the appropriateness of the approach confirmed. In addition, it is clear that not all electrode catheters are suitable for ablation.[9] We are encouraged that catheters specifically designed to withstand the enormous voltages applied (i.e., between 3 and 4 kV) are currently being made available. Care should be taken not to mistake late atrial potentials for His deflections, to avoid delivery of shocks to the atrial wall. In addition, excessive impingement of the temporary pacing catheter on the right ventricular apex should be avoided, because the force of muscular contraction may cause perforation of the apical myocardium.[27] The procedure should be performed by personnel fully adept at resuscitative procedures, and the team should include an experienced anesthesiologist and a surgeon to handle any acute cardiac catastrophe.

ATRIOVENTRICULAR ABLATION FOR PATIENTS WITH THE WOLFF-PARKINSON-WHITE SYNDROME

Ablation of the AV junction for patients with accessory pathways capable of antegrade bypass conduction deserves special consideration. In those with intractable orthodromic tachycardia, ablation of the AV junction would be expected to result in tachycardia control, but several important factors must be applied before considering this approach. First, this technique should not be used in those with accessory pathways with short refractory periods, since the patient will not be protected

should atrial flutter or atrial fibrillation supervene. In addition, a permanent ventricular pacemaker should be inserted, since the long-term natural history of accessory pathway conduction is not known. We feel that the surgical approach[11] (or direct ablative approach) is preferable for most patients with the Wolff-Parkinson-White syndrome. Use of catheter ablation should be restricted to those who refuse surgical intervention or who are considered high risk for these cardiac electrosurgical procedures.

CLINICAL CHARACTERIZATION OF PATIENTS UNDERGOING ATRIOVENTRICULAR JUNCTIONAL ABLATION

A number of centers have reported results of catheter electrical ablation of the AV junction.[7, 24, 29, 32] The most extensive experience to date has been collected from the Percutaneous Cardiac Mapping and Ablation Registry,[27] which was organized in 1982 to collect data for patients undergoing this procedure. To date, data from 480 patients have been submitted, and the data for the first 367 patients have been recently analyzed.[8] The clinical data for these patients are summarized in Table 32–1. All patients had symptomatic paroxysmal or chronic supraventricular arrhythmias. Episodes of frank syncope or presyncope were recorded in 61 per cent, and 61 patients required one or more external DC shocks for arrhythmia control. The patients proved intolerant of, or the arrhythmia was refractory to, an average of 3.5 drugs. The types of drugs

TABLE 32–1. CLINICAL FINDINGS IN PATIENTS WITH DRUG- AND/OR PACEMAKER-RESISTANT SUPRAVENTRICULAR TACHYCARDIA

HEART DISEASE (type/% of patients)	ARRHYTHMIA (type/% of patients)	SYMPTOMS (type/% of patients)	PRIOR TREATMENT (type/% of patients)
No organic disease/48	Atrial fibrillation/flutter/60	Palpitations/70	Digitalis/82
Coronary artery disease/16	Atrioventricular node	Dizziness/36	Type I/77
Cardiomyopathy/14	reentry/22	Dyspnea/40	Beta blockers/72
Valvular heart disease/12	Atrial tachycardia/13	Syncope/25	Calcium-channel
Hypertensive cardiovascular	Accessory pathway/11	Chest pain/17	blocker/71
disease/8	Permanent JRT/2	Fatigue/17	Amiodarone/56
Cor pulmonale/2	Other/4	Angina/11	Other experimental
Other/6		Other/6	drugs/24
			Antitachycardia
			pacemaker/7

The percentages total more than 100 because more than one parameter may have been present in a given patient. JRT = junctional reciprocating tachycardia; type I = type I antiarrhythmic agents.

used are listed in Table 32–1. Over 50 per cent of patients had associated cardiac disease, with coronary artery disease or cardiomyopathy being among the most frequent diagnoses. The most common arrhythmia requiring AV junctional ablation included chronic or paroxysmal atrial fibrillation or flutter (60 per cent). The procedure was also used in those with AV nodal reentrant tachycardia, AV tachycardia, and atrial and junctional tachycardia.

CLINICAL RESPONSE

The 367 patients were followed for an average of 11 ± 10 months. The results of the catheter ablative procedure are summarized in Figure 32–7. Stable third-degree AV block (including maximal preexcitation for those with accessory pathways) was achieved in 63 per cent of patients. The condition in these patients is at present controlled without antiarrhythmic drugs. In 27 per cent of patients, AV conduction resumed after a mean of 6 ± 18

days following the procedure. In 10 per cent of patients, the ablative shock resulted in sufficient modification of AV conduction so that arrhythmia control was achieved without need for antiarrhythmic drug therapy. An additional 12 per cent had resumption of AV conduction, but previously failed therapy was effective for arrhythmia control. The procedure proved unsuccessful in 15 per cent of patients.

COMPLICATIONS OF ATRIOVENTRICULAR JUNCTIONAL ABLATION

Immediate Complications

The most frequent acute complications occurring after delivery of the electrical shocks were arrhythmic in nature. Six patients developed ventricular tachycardia or fibrillation after application of the shock and required external DC cardioversion. Two additional patients developed ventricular tachycardia within

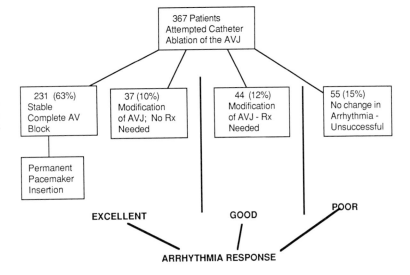

Figure 32–7. Response of patients to attempted catheter ablation of the AV junction (AVJ) is detailed.

24 hours of the procedure. Ventricular arrhythmias may be a result of acute injury to the myocardium. Transient sinus arrest, atrial tachycardia, atrial flutter, and nonsustained ventricular tachycardia (17 patients) were reported, but no specific therapy was required. Hypotension post shock was reported in six patients, three of whom required pressor support. The hypotensive episode was transient in five and persisted for 72 hours in one. No deaths have been reported in the immediate postshock period. Thromboembolic complications included a pulmonary embolus in one, thrombosis of the left subclavian vein in one, and thrombophlebitis in four patients. One patient developed a large right atrial thrombus despite prior anticoagulant therapy. In addition, infectious complications, all related to pacemaker insertion, were recorded in four patients. One patient with presumed immunodeficient state died of overwhelming sepsis. One patient had diaphragmatic pacing and ventricular tachycardia, which resolved on repositioning of the temporary pacing electrode.

Late Complications

Late complications included a cerebrovascular accident 17 months after ablation in a patient with atrial fibrillation; another patient had a probable arterial embolus after the procedure. Long-term pacemaker complications included a pacemaker-mediated tachycardia in three patients, pacemaker tracking of supraventricular tachycardia in two, pacemaker inhibition due to myopotential sensing in one, and symptoms of acute pacemaker failure in two. A slow underlying pacemaker emerged in these last two patients.

FOLLOW-UP MORTALITY STATISTICS AFTER ATRIOVENTRICULAR JUNCTIONAL ABLATION

A total of 19 patients died in the follow-up period. The death was sudden and of natural causes in eight and occurred from 3 days to 13 months after ablation. Seven of these patients had underlying organic cardiac disease, and one was free of known heart disease. Four patients died of severe congestive heart failure, which was present prior to the ablative procedure; one died 2 years after the procedure of infective endocarditis, and one died after surgery in which accessory pathway division was

attempted. Noncardiac deaths resulted from sepsis (after pacemaker revision in one patient), severe chronic lung disease in one, and cerebral hemorrhage in one. The cause of death was unknown in one patient.

CATHETER ABLATION OF ECTOPIC ATRIAL OR JUNCTIONAL FOCI

Catheter electrical ablation of ectopic atrial or junctional tachycardia foci was first reported by Gillette and colleagues in children.[14] This technique involves careful mapping of the right atrium and selected portions of the left atrium during tachycardia. The earliest atrial endocardial potential relative to multiple surface P waves is taken as the exit site of the tachycardia focus. Shocks are delivered to these areas in an effort to ablate these foci. The advantage of this technique is that if successful it allows for preservation of AV conduction and obviates chronic pacemaker therapy.

Our own experience[6] involves use of this technique in six patients with ectopic atrial or junctional tachycardia. Two patients with tachycardia foci localized to the right posterior septum are at present free of arrhythmias without drugs. Two patients with junctional ectopic tachycardia have experienced arrhythmia control but require chronic pacing. The procedure proved ineffective for one patient with right atrial appendage tachycardia and for one with inappropriate sinus tachycardia. The reported experience to date with this procedure is too limited to allow for definitive recommendations.

CATHETER ABLATION OF POSTEROSEPTAL ACCESSORY PATHWAYS

The suitability of currently available catheter ablation techniques for the treatment of patients who have accessory pathways depends in large part on the location of the accessory pathway. The largest experience and highest success rate have been reported for accessory pathways that are posteroseptal in location.

Experimental Background

Because the atrial insertion of posteroseptal accessory pathways is often very near the os of the coronary sinus, catheter ablation of this type of accessory pathway has involved delivery of shocks at the os. The histologic effects in dogs of shocks delivered near the os of the coronary sinus were reported by Coltorti and associates.[4] The proximal pair of electrodes of a quadripolar electrode catheter was positioned at the os of the coronary sinus and connected with the anodal sink of a defibrillator, and a disc electrode on the anterior portion of the chest was connected with the cathodal output. A 200-J shock was delivered in six dogs and a 360-J shock in another six. Histologic examination 4 weeks later demonstrated transmural atrial injury at the level of the coronary sinus over a 10 ± 5 mm length with the 200-J shock and 21 ± 6 mm length with the 360-J shock. These findings suggested that shocks delivered at the os of the coronary sinus produced atrial injury potentially capable of blocking atrial conduction through an accessory pathway.

Technique

Various techniques have been used to ablate posteroseptal accessory pathways. The technique that the authors have employed will be described here.[20] Before ablation is attempted, a careful electrophysiologic study must be performed to ascertain that the patient has a posteroseptal accessory pathway that is either participating in a reciprocating tachycardia circuit or responsible for a rapid rate during atrial fibrillation or flutter. Because approximately 30 per cent of patients who have a posteroseptal accessory pathway may also have a right-sided accessory pathway,[21] the electrophysiologic study should include detailed mapping of the tricuspid annulus to rule out a second accessory pathway.

Surgical backup should be available at the time of the catheter ablation procedure, in the event of coronary sinus perforation and cardiac tamponade. A central lumen catheter is inserted through a subclavian or internal jugular vein and positioned within the coronary sinus. Contrast is injected to visualize the precise location of the os of the coronary sinus. This catheter is then removed and replaced with a No. 6 or 7 French quadripolar catheter (1-cm interelectrode distance), positioned so that the proximal pair of electrodes straddles the os. The two electrodes are made electrically common and connected with the cathodal output of the defibrillator, and a patch electrode positioned on the anterior or posterior portion of chest is connected with the anodal sink of the defibrillator.

Before shocks are delivered, an electrode catheter is positioned within the right ventricle for backup pacing, should transient sinus arrest or AV block occur. The patient then undergoes general anesthesia, and a 200- to 300-J shock is delivered. If accessory pathway conduction is abolished, it has been the practice of the authors to deliver a second shock of similar strength to minimize the chance that accessory pathway conduction will return.

After the catheter ablation procedure, the patient is observed in the hospital with continuous electrocardiographic monitoring for approximately 5 days.

Results

In the authors' initial experience, the technique described above was successful over the long term in eliminating conduction through a posteroseptal accessory pathway in five of seven patients, and in an additional patient, accessory pathway conduction was modified so that the patient no longer had symptomatic tachycardias.[22] The authors' series has now expanded to 20 patients, and the long-term success rate in eliminating or modifying posteroseptal accessory pathway conduction so that symptomatic tachycardias no longer occur has been 75 per cent.

Complications

In 1 of 20 patients who underwent an attempt at catheter ablation of a posteroseptal accessory pathway, a single 300-J shock resulted in cardiac tamponade. This was managed successfully by needle pericardiocentesis. Examination of the electrode catheter revealed several breaks in the insulation, and it was presumed that energy inadvertently was delivered through the distal electrodes within the coronary sinus, resulting in rupture of the coronary sinus. When this patient underwent elective surgical ablation of the posteroseptal accessory pathway 1 month later, a small, healed perforation of the coronary sinus was found 2 to 3 cm from the os. This case demonstrates that serious complications are possible if electrode catheters that cannot withstand high-energy shocks are used. Only electrode catheters that have been demonstrated by in vitro testing to be capable of withstanding 200- to 300-J shocks should be used.[9] No injury or thrombosis of the coronary sinus was noted in 12 of the remaining 19 patients who underwent either angiographic visualization or direct intraoperative inspection of the coronary sinus.

Shocks delivered at the os of the coronary sinus commonly are followed by several minutes of AV block; however no instance of permanent impairment of AV conduction has occurred in the authors' series of 20 patients.

The mean peak creatine phosphokinase MB fraction was 35 IU/L (upper limits of normal, 9 IU/L), indicating a small degree of myocardial necrosis. A pyrophosphate scan was mildly positive in only one patient, and in no patient was there evidence of transmural infarction. No new ventricular arrhythmias have been noted during continuous electrocardiographic monitoring for 5 to 7 days after the procedure. In seven patients who underwent coronary angiography 4 months after the ablation procedure, no abnormalities of the coronary arteries were found.

CATHETER ABLATION OF LEFT AND RIGHT FREE WALL ACCESSORY PATHWAYS

Experimental Background

Brodman and Fisher studied the histologic effects of shocks delivered within the coronary sinus in dogs.[3] In 16 dogs, one to four 35- to 45-J shocks were delivered in the coronary sinus, and morphologic examination 2 to 11 weeks later revealed dense scarring of the left atrial wall adjacent to the shock site in 15 of the 16 dogs. This finding suggested that 35- to 45-J shocks in the coronary sinus may induce enough fibrosis of the adjacent left atrial wall potentially to interrupt conduction through a left-sided accessory pathway. However, the coronary sinus was completely occluded at the shock site in 8 of the 16 dogs and was stenotic in 5. In addition, intimal hyperplasia of the circumflex coronary artery was observed in three dogs. In regard to the risk of coronary sinus perforation, one of five other dogs that received a single 35- to 45-J shock and two of three dogs that received 240-J shocks developed coronary sinus rupture. Therefore, shocks delivered within the coronary sinus are associated with a significant incidence of perforation, occlusion, or stenosis of the coronary sinus.

Ruder and associates studied the effects on the right atrium of shocks delivered near the tricuspid annulus in dogs.[25] Shocks ranging from 50 to 400 J were delivered to various sites near the tricuspid annulus. There were no instances of right atrial perforation or tamponade. Morphologic examination 10 days later

demonstrated that the extent of atrial injury was dependent on the energy of the shocks. The size of the endocardial lesion was 62 mm² with 50-J shocks and 221 mm² with 400-J shocks, and the injury was transmural with shocks greater than 200 J. Therefore, intracardiac shocks may be capable of inducing enough injury to the right atrial wall possibly to interrupt conduction through a right-sided accessory pathway.

Results and Complications

The published experience with catheter ablation of left- and right-sided accessory pathways is extremely limited. Fisher and colleagues reported on their experience with eight patients who had a left-sided accessory pathway and received 2 to 26 shocks of 40 to 150 J within the coronary sinus.[10] Conduction through the accessory pathway was eliminated acutely in each patient but in all cases returned within 10 days, and only one patient remained asymptomatic without antiarrhythmic medications during follow-up; seven of the eight patients required either antiarrhythmic drug therapy or surgical ablation of the accessory pathway. Of note is that one patient in this series developed cardiac tamponade after two shocks of 150 and 100 J were delivered within the coronary sinus. Therefore, the experience of Fisher and colleagues indicates that DC countershock delivered within the coronary sinus has a low efficacy in abolishing conduction over left-sided accessory pathways and is associated with a risk of cardiac tamponade.

In regard to catheter ablation of a right-sided accessory pathway, the procedure was successful in two of seven patients who received two to four shocks of 80 to 300 J against the right atrial wall.[19, 30, 31] No patient developed cardiac tamponade, but one patient who had a right septal accessory pathway developed complete AV block, requiring a permanent pacemaker.[19] The experience with catheter ablation of right-sided accessory pathways is clearly too preliminary to allow any conclusions regarding efficacy or safety.

CONCLUSIONS

Catheter ablation techniques currently play a limited role in the management of patients with supraventricular tachycardia. In patients who are appropriate candidates for ablation of the AV junction, the catheter approach is appropriate, with surgical ablation of the AV junction being reserved for patients who do not respond to attempts at catheter ablation. However, catheter ablation of the AV junction should be viewed as a last resort and not as an alternative to other effective therapeutic modalities.

Among patients who have tachycardias involving an accessory pathway, the initial experience with catheter ablation of posteroseptal accessory pathways suggests that the long-term efficacy is in the range of 75 per cent and that the risk of serious complications is acceptably low. If this initial experience is confirmed in a larger number of patients, catheter ablation may become an appropriate alternative to surgical ablation of posteroseptal accessory pathways.

At present, surgical ablation of left-sided accessory pathways is preferable to the catheter approach. Surgical ablation of left-sided accessory pathways has a success rate of greater than 95 per cent and a low morbidity,[12] whereas the catheter technique utilizing shocks within the coronary sinus has had a very low efficacy and a risk of coronary sinus perforation. Whether new catheter techniques that are as effective as surgical ablation of left-sided accessory pathways can be developed remains to be determined.

No conclusions about the role of catheter techniques for ablation of right-sided accessory pathways or ectopic atrial foci are possible at present. Further experience with these techniques will be required to define their safety and efficacy.

New developments that may broaden the application of catheter ablation techniques for patients with supraventricular tachycardia include modification of the energy waveform to avoid unwarranted barotrauma;[1, 5] the use of alternate energy sources, such as radiofrequency energy and laser;[17, 23] and the creation of new catheters for energy delivery, such as a suction-tip electrode catheter.[26]

REFERENCES

1. Bardy GH, Coltorti F, Stewart RB, et al: Catheter-mediated electrical ablation: The relation between current and pulse width on voltage breakdown and shock-wave generation. PACE 9:1381–1383, 1986.
2. Boyd EGCA, Holt PM: An investigation into the electrical ablation technique and a method of electrode assessment. PACE 8:815, 1985.
3. Brodman R, Fisher JD: Evaluation of a catheter technique for ablation of accessory pathways near

the coronary sinus using a canine model. Circulation 67:923–929, 1983.
4. Coltorti F, Bardy GH, Reichenbach D, et al: Catheter-mediated electrical ablation of the posterior septum via the coronary sinus: Electrophysiologic and histologic observations in dogs. Circulation 72:612–622, 1985.
5. Cunningham D, Rowland E, Rickards AF: A new low energy power source for catheter ablation. PACE 9:1384–1390, 1986.
6. Davis J, Scheinman MM, Ruder MA, et al: Ablation of cardiac tissues by an electrode catheter technique for treatment of ectopic supraventricular tachycardia in adults. Circulation 74:1044–1053, 1986.
7. Davis MJ, Mews GC, Cope GD: Transvenous ablation of atrioventricular conduction for refractory or malignant supraventricular arrhythmias. Aust N Z J Med 14:479–486, 1984.
8. Evans GT Jr, Scheinman MM, the Executive Committee of the Registry: Catheter ablation for control of cardiac arrhythmias: A report of the Percutaneous Cardiac Mapping and Ablation Registry. Personal communication.
9. Fisher JD, Brodman R, Johnston DR, et al: Nonsurgical electrical ablation of tachycardias: Importance of prior in vitro testing of catheter leads. PACE 7:74, 1984.
10. Fisher JD, Brodman R, Kim SG, et al: Attempted nonsurgical electrical ablation of accessory pathways via the coronary sinus in the Wolff-Parkinson-White syndrome. J Am Coll Cardiol 4:685–694, 1984.
11. Gallagher JJ, Gilbert M, Swenson RH: Wolff-Parkinson-White syndrome: The problem, evaluation and surgical correction. Circulation 57:767, 1975.
12. Gallagher JJ, Sealy WC, Cox JL, Kasell JH: Results of surgery for preexcitation in 200 consecutive cases. In Levy S, Scheinman MM (eds): Cardiac Arrhythmias from Diagnosis to Treatment. New York, Futura, 1984, pp 540–569.
13. Gallagher JJ, Svenson RH, Kasell JH, et al: Catheter technique for closed-chest ablation of the atrioventricular conduction system. N Engl J Med 306:194–200, 1982.
14. Gillette PC: Catheter ablation in dysrhythmias. Cardiology 5:67–69, 1984.
15. Gonzalez R, Scheinman M, Bharati S, et al: Closed chest permanent atrioventricular block in dogs. Am Heart J 105:461, 1983.
16. Gonzalez R, Scheinman M, Margaretten W, et al: Closed-chest electrode-catheter technique for His bundle ablation in dogs. Am J Physiol 241:283, 1981.
17. Huang SK, Jordon N, Graham A, et al: Closed-chest catheter desiccation of atrioventricular junction using radiofrequency energy: A new method of catheter ablation [abstract]. Circulation 72:III–389, 1985.
18. Jones JL, Proskauer CC, Paull WK, et al: Ultrastructural injury to chick myocardial cells in vitro following "electric countershock." Circ Res 46:387, 1980.
19. Kunze KP, Kuck KH: Transvenous ablation of accessory pathways in patients with incessant atrioventricular tachycardia [abstract]. Circulation 70 [Suppl II]:164, 1984.
20. Morady F, Scheinman MM: Transvenous catheter ablation of a posteroseptal accessory pathway in a patient with the Wolff-Parkinson-White syndrome. N Engl J Med 310:705, 1984.
21. Morady F, Scheinman MM, DiCarlo LA, Jr, et al: Coexistent posteroseptal and right-sided atrioven-

tricular bypass tracts. J Am Coll Cardiol 5:640–646, 1985.

22. Morady F, Scheinman MM, Winston SA, et al: Efficacy and safety of transcatheter ablation of posteroseptal accessory pathways. Circulation 72:170–177, 1985.

23. Narula OS, Bharati S, Chan MC, et al: Laser microtransection of the His bundle: A pervenous catheter technique [abstract]. J Am Coll Cardiol 3:537, 1984.

24. Nathan AW, Bennett DH, Ward DE, et al: Catheter ablation of atrioventricular conduction. Lancet 1:1280–1284, 1985.

25. Ruder MA, Davis JC, Eldar M, Scheinman MM: Effects of electrode catheter shocks delivered near the tricuspid annulus in dogs [abstract]. J Am Coll Cardiol 7:7A, 1986.

26. Saksena S, Tarjan PP, Bharati S, et al: Low-energy transvenous ablation of the atrioventricular conduction system using a suction electrode catheter. Circulation 76:403–410, 1987.

27. Scheinman MM, Evans-Bell T, The Executive Committee of the Percutaneous Mapping and Ablation Registry: Catheter ablation of the atrioventricular junction: A report of the Percutaneous Mapping and Ablation Registry. Circulation 70:1024–1029, 1984.

28. Scheinman MM, Morady F, Hess DS, Gonzalez R: Catheter-induced ablation of the atrioventricular junction to control refractory supraventricular arrhythmias. JAMA 248:851, 1982.

29. Trantham JL, Gallagher JJ, German LD, et al: Effects of energy delivery via a His bundle catheter during closed chest ablation of the atrioventricular conduction system. J Clin Invest 72:1563–1574, 1983.

30. Weber H, Schmitz L: Catheter technique for closed-chest ablation of an accessory atrioventricular pathway. N Engl J Med 308:653–654, 1983.

31. Weber H, Schmitz L, Hellberg K: Pacemaker-mediated tachycardias: A new modality of treatment. PACE 7:1010–1016, 1984.

32. Wood D, Hammill S, Holmes DR, et al: Catheter ablation of the atrioventricular system in patients with supraventricular tachycardia. Mayo Clin Proc 58:793, 1983.

33

CATHETER ABLATION FOR VENTRICULAR TACHYCARDIA

A. Technology, Physiology, and Early Clinical Application

THOMAS BUDDE, GUNTER BREITHARDT, *and* MARTIN BORGGREFE

Within the last few years, catheter ablation has become an alternative approach to pharmacologic or surgical therapy for life-threatening ventricular tachyarrhythmias. The main goal of this method is to destroy or to modify those structures of the heart that are involved in the generation or propagation of tachycardias. The principle of catheter ablation was discovered incidentally when, in 1979, Fontaine and coworkers[69] observed an accidental induction of atrioventricular (AV) block after external defibrillation of a patient during an electrophysiologic study. Outside the patient's body, the defibrillator electrode had come into contact with a catheter positioned at the AV junction. This effect was correctly interpreted as damage to the AV conductive tissue produced by fortuitous application of direct current (DC). Later, Gallagher[34] and Scheinman,[35, 61] in a series of experimental studies, developed the therapeutic method of catheter ablation. In the beginning, catheter ablation was used mainly to interrupt conduction from the AV node to the His bundle for the treatment of patients with supraventricular tachycardia, especially atrial flutter or fibrillation.[4, 21, 34, 40, 49, 52, 57, 59–61] Subsequently, the indication for catheter ablation was extended to tachycardias involving accessory pathways[5, 7, 8, 20, 25, 26, 39, 51, 53,57,62,70,72] and to ventricular tachycardia (VT).[6, 13–15, 24, 28, 30–32, 36, 43, 45, 50, 57–59, 64, 66]

INDICATIONS AND PREREQUISITES FOR TREATMENT OF VENTRICULAR TACHYCARDIAS

Since catheter ablation of VTs is a relatively new and still experimental approach, the indications are changing in the light of continuously increasing experience. Therefore, any list of indications, such as those in Table 33–1, may change fast. With any new technique, the first experiences generally involve those patients with the severest cases, in whom all other approaches failed or, at least, did not seem feasible. With increasing confidence and predictability, an extension of indications for the procedure will change this situation.

At present, a patient should be considered for catheter ablation only if pharmacologic antiarrhythmic therapy has failed (i.e., spontaneous recurrences in patients taking medication or a failure to respond to antiarrhythmic

Supported by a grant from the Sonderforschungsbereich 242 (Koronare Herzkrankheit—Therapie und Prophylaxe akuter Komplikationen) of the Deutsche Forschungsgemeinschaft, Bonn/Bad Godesberg, Federal Republic of Germany.

TABLE 33–1. INDICATIONS FOR CATHETER ABLATION OF VENTRICULAR TACHYCARDIAS

Sustained Ventricular Tachycardia (VT)
and
1. Ineffective therapy with antiarrhythmic drugs
2. Appearance of intolerable side effects with drug treatment
3. Failure of antitachycardia surgery
4. Previous cardiac surgery of any kind (increased risk of repetitive interventions because of pericardial adhesions and so on)
5. Severe concomitant diseases (e.g., renal or pulmonary dysfunction)
6. Right ventricular dysplasia
7. (Incessant VT?)

drugs during serial electrophysiologic testing). Today, the "ideal" candidate would be the patient in whom antitachycardia surgery for VT has failed and in whom the risk for reoperation would be increased. In addition, if a patient with drug-refractory VT had undergone previous cardiac surgery (i.e., aneurysmectomy, coronary artery bypass grafting, or valve replacement), an attempt at catheter ablation would seem advisable. Concomitant severe disease, such as pulmonary or renal dysfunction, that may increase the risk of surgery would also constitute an appropriate indication. Furthermore, patients presenting with incessant VT in the presence of heart failure may be considered for catheter ablation, as antitachycardia surgery in those patients has been shown to be associated with a high surgical mortality rate (especially in patients without coronary artery disease). Patients with right ventricular dysplasia represent another group in whom catheter ablation might even be preferable to surgery because early recurrences attributable to the diffusely diseased myocardium might occur as well as late recurrences (despite early success) caused by progression of the underlying right ventricular disease. In contrast, the patient with, for example, a large left ventricular aneurysm and left ventricular failure, despite good function in the rest of the ventricle (with or without an additional indication for coronary artery bypass grafting), is *not* the candidate for catheter ablation; however, left ventricular aneurysm and poor function in the rest of the ventricle, without need for bypass surgery, indicate catheter ablation.

Uncertainty exists over whether catheter ablation is advisable when these are multiple sites of origin of VT, as this might mean an extremely long procedure with a potentially increased risk of thromboembolism, damage to the artery used for catheter introduction, radiation exposure to the patient and the staff, and so on. This situation should be considered an argument for antitachycardia surgery (after careful preoperative catheter mapping). However, should surgery fail, in the case of multiple sites of origin with at least one type of VT, an attempt may be made postoperatively to ablate the remaining "focus" if it is not responsive to drugs.

A summary of criteria on which the decision to perform either antitachycardia surgery or catheter ablation may be based is given in Table 33–2.

MAPPING TECHNIQUES

As a prerequisite for catheter ablation, VT has to be hemodynamically tolerated in the catheterization laboratory—at least for a short time—to allow an exact localization of its site of origin (Table 33–3). The origin of VT is best defined by a combined approach using activation mapping, pacemapping (see below), and pacing interventions at the site of interest. Mapping of ventricular endocardial activation during induced or spontaneous VT (activation mapping) aims at identifying the site that shows earliest endocardial activity preceding the onset of the QRS complex (presystolic activity). Pacemapping tries to reproduce the morphology of VT by pacing the ventricles

TABLE 33–2. COMPARISON OF CATHETER ABLATION VERSUS ANTITACHYCARDIA SURGERY

Advantages of Catheter Ablation
1. Heart-lung machine not necessary
2. Intervention generally less extensive than surgery
3. Repetition without increased risk in case of failure of either antitachycardia surgery or primary catheter ablation
4. Risks not markedly increased with concomitant pulmonary or renal dysfunction
5. Reduced staff requirements
6. (Anesthesia not necessary with radiofrequency ablation)

Advantages of Antitachycardia Surgery
1. Removal of tissue under direct visual guidance
2. No exposure to radiation
3. Minor risk of thromboembolic events
4. Minor risk of vascular damage
5. No risk of catheter perforation and acute pericardial tamponade
6. Higher efficacy with multiple origins of VT
7. Preferable in case of a given indication for cardiac surgery for other reasons as, for example, aneurysmectomy or coronary artery bypass grafting

TABLE 33–3. PREREQUISITES FOR CATHETER ABLATION OF VENTRICULAR TACHYCARDIA

1. Circumscribed, localized arrhythmogenic structure
2. Hemodynamically tolerable, sustained VT

from a presumed site of origin either during sinus rhythm or during induced VT.

The first step during endocardial catheter mapping is to record endocardial signals during VT from up to 10 different sites in the ventricles using biplane fluoroscopy. At the site that roughly shows early activation, a more detailed mapping procedure is performed. In some instances, very early activations may not be separable from very late activity, being part of the preceding QRS complex of VT (and representing either potentials from a "deadend pathway" within scarred tissue or signals from the proximal part of slower conduction within the reentrant pathway). Administration of a single stimulus or a train of premature stimuli at this site may help to differentiate between the activations. Besides activation mapping, pacemapping may be used and can be applied either during sinus rhythm or during VT by pacing the ventricle at a rate slightly faster than VT. It is assumed that if an optimal correspondence between spontaneous QRS morphology of VT and the induced QRS complexes is achieved, this is the site of origin of VT. Care should be taken to record as many electrocardiographic leads as possible to prove that the morphology of induced QRS complexes is identical with that of spontaneous (i.e., clinical) VT. Occasionally, an extremely long latency between the stimuli and induced QRS complexes may be present and probably is due to the location of the stimulating electrode proximal to the area of slow conduction. In addition, the application of premature stimuli that interrupt VT by only local capture (not resulting in premature QRS complexes—"noncapture of the ventricles")[33] (A. Podczeck, M. Borggrefe, and G. Breithardt, unpublished observations, 1987) may help to define a site that is proximal to the area of slow conduction. However, whether a site proximal to the area of slow conduction represents the optimal site for application of catheter shocks has not yet been sufficiently evaluated. The advantage of pacemapping is that it can be used even in patients who do not tolerate spontaneous VT sufficiently long to perform activation mapping. In case of rapid VT, "switching" the

tachycardia on and off by programmed ventricular stimulation is often necessary but may cause degeneration into ventricular fibrillation. In these cases, the initial steps of orientation may be based on pacemapping from various sites. However, pacemapping may be less accurate than activation mapping. Therefore, it is mostly used only as an adjunct to activation mapping.

CATHETER ABLATION TECHNIQUES

To devitalize or to modify the tissue involved in the genesis of VT, high-energy DC shocks from conventional defibrillators are passed through electrode catheters. Recently, radiofrequency current has also been used in a limited number of patients (see Chapter 34). After identification of the "site of origin" of VT by catheter mapping, one or more unipolar shocks in the range of 50 to 400 J are delivered between the distal electrode of the catheter used for mapping and an indifferent plate electrode, which is usually positioned at the back. The use of cathodal shocks (the different electrode as cathode and the indifferent electrode as anode) rather than anodal shocks has been recommended[3, 10, 12] because of smaller amounts of gas bubble formation during pulse delivery.

Application of high-energy DC shocks results in localized damage to the myocardium around the catheter electrode.[2, 4, 22, 23, 35, 37, 42, 47, 67, 68] Most experimental studies[3, 4, 10, 22, 29, 52] suggest that this effect on the tissue is mainly mediated by thermal and/or barotraumatic mechanisms. Boyd and Holt[12] additionally emphasized the importance of local electrical effects and especially of current density for the acute effects of ablation on conductive tissue. They described the complex sequence of events during ablation in the following manner. At the onset of current flow, there is a maximal dissipation of energy in the medium around the electrode tip, rapidly increasing the medium temperature. At the boiling point, vapor is formed at the electrode surface. As the last of the liquid in contact with the electrode vaporizes, the current concentration in the remaining medium results in very rapid heating. This high field strength may lead to ionization and may produce plasma tracks in the vapor volume around the electrode. Localized high temperatures of more than 1700°C next to the electrode are generated by plasma arcs. Electrical discharges induce light emission. Afterward, further vaporization, with increasing current density and expansion of the gas bubble, will result in a positive mechanical pressure wave. After passing peak current values, the bubble expansion falls and results in a negative pressure wave. The authors[12] conclude that current density is probably responsible for the acute effect on cardiac tissue seen during delivery of high-energy electrical fields. These mechanisms will be subject to further discussion, because they have direct implications for the clinical situation. One of these aspects is that the application of DC ablation pulses is painful and therefore has to be performed with the patient under general anesthesia. In contrast, radiofrequency currents have been used without general anesthesia and without the need for administration of analgesics.[9, 18]

IMMEDIATE RESULTS OF THE ABLATION PROCEDURE

After each shock applied to the presumed site of origin of VT, an attempt is made to reinduce the "target" VT by programmed ventricular stimulation. If VT is still inducible, the effect of the shock is probably not sufficient to devitalize the arrhythmogenic tissue. However, owing to the use of general anesthesia during the procedure, induction of VT may become less reproducible, mimicking a "true" effect of the shock. In addition, nonclinical forms of VT (those not documented before and those considered to have less clinical significance) may supervene, thus complicating the assessment of the immediate results of the ablation procedure.

If VT is still inducible after the first shock or shocks, another attempt will be considered either at the same site or at a closely neighboring site after another catheter mapping procedure. In this case, however, the risk of perforation has to be kept in mind.

The endpoint of the ablation procedure is reached as soon as the clinical form of VT can no longer be induced. This endpoint is frequently achieved only after more than one shock. In our own experience with 24 patients (see Table 33–4) having chronic, recurrent VT, the VT was inducible before application of shocks in 20 patients; of these 20, clinical VT was no longer inducible at the end of the catheter ablation session in 8; in 6 patients, a nonclinical form of tachycardia was induced.

In the remaining 6 patients, clinical VT was still inducible after ablation (Table 33–4). In 70 per cent of cases, the ablation procedure was thus successful on an acute basis. Data on results of electrophysiologic studies immediately after ablation can hardly be found in the literature because in most publications any result of programmed stimulation during the postablation hospital stay has been reported as an "acute" result. According to the Percutaneous Cardiac Mapping and Ablation Registry (PCMAR) data,[59] inducible VT immediately after ablation was found in 74 of 117 patients (63 per cent). The morphology of the inducible VT in the immediate postablation period was identical with that of the spontaneous VT in 49 patients (42 per cent)[59] (see Table 33–4).

In our own experience, the first week after ablation is a period of increased instability. There were spontaneous recurrences of VT in 10 of 14 patients during the first week, whereas 4 patients had a relapse after more than 1 week. At the end of the first week, clinical VT was again inducible in 18 of 20 patients. In only 2 patients, no VT was inducible. Thus, 12 of 14 patients in whom no clinical tachycardia could be induced at the end of the ablation procedure had inducible VT after 1 week. These changes in the inducibility of VT between the end of the procedure and the end of the first week show the partially transient nature of the effects of DC catheter ablation. Experimental studies have described the histologic and electrophysiologic effects of catheter ablation.[2, 4, 22, 23, 35, 37, 41, 42, 47, 48, 67, 68, 71] The results of these studies support the idea that the alterations produced by catheter ablation might be partially reversible. A resorption of edema was discussed as a cause of "reparative" effects and tissue recovery[4] that may lead to a resumption of arrhythmogeneity. Therefore, another attempt at catheter ablation that includes the same methodologic approach as described above may be considered. Fontaine and colleagues,[32] we,[15] and others[59] have repeated the procedure in some patients. Ten of our 24 patients underwent subsequent ablation procedures because of spontaneous recurrences in 7 cases and reinducibility of VT after 1 week in the remaining 3 patients.

Table 33–4 compares the results in our group of patients with the results of the PCMAR conducted by Evans and Scheinman at San Francisco.[59] Currently, the PCMAR represents the largest data collection on the results of catheter ablation gained by a collaborative study of many centers. In more than

TABLE 33–4. CATHETER ABLATION OF VENTRICULAR TACHYCARDIA—IMMEDIATE RESULTS

	TOTAL NO. OF PATIENTS	NO VT INDUCIBLE	CLINICAL VT INDUCIBLE	NONCLINICAL VT INDUCIBLE
Hospital of the University of Düsseldorf End of ablation procedure (acute results)	20	8	6	6
End of the first week post ablation (subacute results) (Clinical VT inducible before ablation in 20/24 patients)	20	2	18	0

	TOTAL NO. OF PATIENTS	INDUCIBLE VT MORPHOLOGY IN IMMEDIATE POSTABLATION PERIOD SAME AS BEFORE	INDUCIBLE VT MORPHOLOGY IN IMMEDIATE POSTABLATION PERIOD DIFFERENT	NO VT INDUCIBLE IN IMMEDIATE POSTABLATION PERIOD
Percutaneous Cardiac Mapping and Ablation Registry (PCMAR)[59]	117	49 (42%)	25 (21%)	43 (37%)

half of these patients, VT could still be induced after catheter ablation. Only 37 per cent of the patients no longer showed inducible VT in electrophysiologic studies post ablation. However, the morphology of VT was altered in 21 per cent of the patients.

LONG-TERM RESULTS OF CATHETER ABLATION

Table 33–5 gives the long-term results of several centers. These data are listed in the context of the PCMAR data.[59] Because this registry represents a collection of the data of many centers collaborating with PCMAR, there is some overlap between the data reported by these centers and the PCMAR data.

Overall, the long-term results of catheter ablation can be roughly placed into the three categories given in Table 33–6.

The duration of follow-up has ranged between 5 and 43 months. During these relatively short periods, between 35 and 100 per cent of

patients have been free of VT, with 17 to 100 per cent of patients being maintained on a regimen of antiarrhythmic agents (see Table 33–5). In the PCMAR, 24 per cent of patients belonged to category I, 42 per cent to category II, and the remaining 34 per cent to category III.[59] Obviously, any comparison between individual centers has to be made with caution because of the marked differences in the duration of follow-up and in the underlying disease, as well as in the mapping techniques, stimulation protocols, modes of energy delivery, and number of shocks per patient. In addition, some centers have repeated the procedure in case of early failures, whereas others have not.

In our own group of 24 patients with chronic, recurrent VT (mean duration of follow-up, 58 ± 38 weeks), there was one death occurring in the acute period that was related to the procedure. In 9 patients discharged without antiarrhythmic drugs (mean follow-up, 79 ± 31 weeks) and in another 8 patients discharged on a regimen of antiarrhythmic drugs (66 ± 30

TABLE 33-5. CATHETER ABLATION OF VENTRICULAR TACHYCARDIA—LONG-TERM RESULTS

AUTHOR	NO. OF PATIENTS	NO. OF PATIENTS, UNDERLYING DISEASE	EJECTION FRACTION	MAPPING/PACE-MAPPING	NO. OF MORPHOLOGIES	NO. OF SHOCKS	NO. OF SESSIONS	ENERGY (JOULES) PER SHOCK	SUCCESS (PATIENTS WITHOUT/WITH ANTIARRHYTHMIC DRUGS)	FAILURE (PATIENTS)	FOLLOW-UP (MO)
Touboul[66]	16	11, CAD	?	+/+	?	1-6/patient	?	150-300	8/3	5	10 (mean)
Fontaine[32]	38	13, CAD; 12, right ventricular dysplasia; 7, dilated CM; 1, operated on congenital disease; 4, "idiopathic VT"	12 patients, < 30%	+/+	82	167(total)	65	160-280	18*/16*	0*	12-43
Steinhaus[64]	6	6, structural heart disease with LV dysfunction	28% (mean)	+/+	?	2/patient	?	300	2/1	3	5 (mean)
Morady[50]	33	22, CAD; 6, other types of heart disease; 5, no structural heart disease	34% (mean)	+/+	3 patients, > 1	1-4 patient	?	100-300	9/6	18	12 ± 10
Leclerq[45]	10	10, right ventricular dysplasia	?	+/+	5 patients, 1; 5 patients, 2-4	61 (total)	19	?	2/6	2	16 ± 5
Downar[24]	4	4, CAD, severely impaired LVF	?	+/+	6 (?) (total)	?	4	80-350	0/4	0	Up to 18
Belhassen[6]	8	7, CAD; 1, normal heart	?	+/+	?	1-6/patient	?	250-300	5/1	2	7-17
Klein[43]	17	15, CAD; 1, localized left ventricular dysplasia; 1, congestive CM	32% (mean)	+/?	14 patients, 1; 3 patients, 2	87 (total)	17 (?)	400	3/3	11	9.5 (mean)
PCMAR[59]	141	63%, CAD; 2%, hypertensive heart disease; 6%, valvular heart disease; 16%, CM; 6%, no heart disease; 6%, others	?	+/(?)	70%, 1 morphology; 22%, multiple morphologies; 8, VFl/VF	65 patients: 1-29 shocks; 76 patients: "multiple shocks"	78%, 1; 22%, 2-4	160-5200 (total energy)	34/59	48	12 ± 10
Hospital of the University of Düsseldorf	24	12, CAD/3 dilated CM; 7, arrhythmogenic RV or LV disease; 1, Aortic valve disease; 1, operated on Fallot's tetralogy	31 (CAD) and 67% (remaining patients)	+/+	30	139 (total)	35	100-400	9/8	4†	58 ± 38 (wks)

*Two early deaths after first session; two deaths during second session; total of five early deaths; up to three sessions per patient.
†One death from perforation and two sudden deaths (at 8 and 84 wk).
CAD = coronary artery disease; CM = cardiomyopathy; LV = left ventricular; LVF = left ventricular function; RV = right ventricular; ? = not (definitely) mentioned in reference; VF = ventricular fibrillation.

TABLE 33–6. CATHETER ABLATION OF VENTRICULAR TACHYCARDIA—CATEGORIES OF LONG-TERM RESULTS

I. No recurrence of VT during long-term follow-up without the need for antiarrhythmic drugs
II. No recurrence of VT during long-term follow-up with the patient receiving previously ineffective antiarrhythmic drugs
III. Recurrence of VT

weeks), there was no symptomatic relapse of VT. Within a mean follow-up of 19 ± 26 weeks, 4 patients experienced a clinical relapse. Two patients died suddenly after 8 and 84 weeks, respectively. Successful clinical suppression of VT after the last ablation procedure, including the use of antiarrhythmic drugs previously ineffective, was achieved in 7 of 7 patients with a right ventricular origin of the tachycardia and in 9 of 17 patients with a left ventricular origin. All 3 patients who experienced either acute or late sudden death had had VT of left ventricular origin.

REASONS FOR LONG-TERM FAILURE TO ABOLISH VENTRICULAR TACHYCARDIA

The main reasons for failure to abolish VT are listed in Table 33–7. One of the essential points is the transient character of induced lesions, as according to experimental[2, 4, 22, 23, 35, 37, 47, 68] and clinical[71] studies, the histologic and clinical effects of DC ablation are reversible to a certain degree. In animal experiments, 1 month after DC application, the myocardial lesions showed a smaller size than 1 week after ablation.[37] In some of our patients, as well as in other studies,[32, 59] clinical VT could be reinduced at an electrophysiologic follow-up study in patients in whom VT was suppressed at the immediate postablation study. Thus, a "recovery" of the arrhythmogenic tissue has to be assumed. The histologic alterations of DC ablation are characterized by necrosis with crater formation, granulomatous reactions, and fibrosis. The myocytes show either typical

TABLE 33–7. REASONS FOR FAILURE TO ABOLISH VENTRICULAR TACHYCARDIA

1. Inadequate mapping
2. Transient character of induced lesions
3. Multiple sites of origin of VT
4. Occurrence of "new" clinical VT
5. Antiarrhythmic drugs administered during ablation
6. Spontaneous variability of VT inducibility

contraction bands or disruption of fibers and hemorrhage. These alterations suggest that there might be abnormal but still viable cells at the border zone of the ablated tissue that might be able to recover their arrhythmogenic or pathologic conduction properties. As a basic recovery mechanism, the resorption of a postablative edema has been discussed.[4] Although these mechanisms are not yet completely clarified, they are of great practical importance. They obviously limit the value of an immediate postablation electrophysiologic study as a means to predict the long-term efficacy of the procedure. Another limitation is the fact that despite persistent or recurrent inducibility of VT, patients may still show a benign clinical course without recurrences of VT. Thus, in these cases, some modification, but no abolition, of the tissue involved has been achieved but is not apparent from these studies.

PROBLEMS AND COMPLICATIONS OF CATHETER ABLATION

The most frequent complications are listed in Table 33–8. A discussion of the basic mechanisms of action of catheter ablation may lead to a better understanding and therefore may help to prevent these complications as far as possible.

DOSE EFFECT RELATION. Data on the relation between the amount of energy applied and the resultant tissue effect are controversial. Some studies demonstrated that the depth and diameter of lesions increased with higher energies,[22, 37, 41] whereas others did not find a significant correlation.[47] The anatomic properties (myocardial thickness and degree of scarring) of different sites of the ventricles also seem to be important. For instance, a lesion created by a pulse of 30 J in the right ventricle may well be transmural,[37] but much higher energies delivered to left ventricular endocardium may result in only endocardial and subendocardial lesions.[37] Thus, in clinical practice, the area of myocardial injury cannot be precisely predicted on the basis of the amount of energy discharged.

REVERSIBILITY OF TISSUE EFFECTS. The effects of catheter ablation on the tissue may be partly reversible. This has been documented in histologic and electrophysiologic studies[2, 4, 22, 23, 37, 41, 42, 47, 48, 68, 71] that have shown a central zone of necrosis and an encompassing zone of partly reversible effects. Clinical studies have revealed a certain percentage of re-

TABLE 33–8. CATHETER ABLATION OF VENTRICULAR TACHYCARDIA—COMPLICATIONS

AUTHOR	NO. OF PATIENTS	NO. OF REPORTED ACUTE COMPLICATIONS	NO. OF REPORTED LONG-TERM COMPLICATIONS
Touboul[66]	16	1 collapse 3 transient AV block 1 permanent AV block	—
Fontaine[32]	38	25 VF/VT acceleration 28 transient AV block 2 reversible pulmonary edema 1 MI 5 early deaths 1 pacemaker defect	8 late deaths (up to 14 mo later) without recurrence of VT
Steinhaus[64]	6	No major complications	—
Morady[50]	33	2 transient ischemic episodes 1 VF 1 AV block requiring pacemaker implantation 1 brachial artery thrombosis	—
Leclerq[45]	10	4 VF 1 small MI	—
Downar[24]	4	Without important complications No complications	—
Belhassen[6]	8	1 reversible cardiogenic shock 2 nonclinical VT with need of cardioversion 3 intraventricular conduction disturbance 1 permanent LBBB	1 left-sided heart failure 2 marked decrease of LV ejection fraction
Klein[43]	17	2 reversible hemodynamic impairment No major complications during or after ablation	—
PCMAR[59]	88	7 procedure-related deaths 12 symptomatic hypotension 4 pericarditis 3 systemic embolization 2 MI 1 ventricular perforation 2 sepsis	14 sudden deaths, 9 with documented VT (2 wk–23 mo) 7 congestive heart failure 3 noncardiac deaths
Düsseldorf	17	1 pulmonary edema 1 cardiac tamponade + surgery 1 death from cardiac tamponade 7 perforation without tamponade 1 femoral artery occlusion 1 LV thrombus 2 transient AV block 4 transient RBBB/LBBB 7 ST-segment elev. > 0.5 mV 1 atrial tachycardia	2 sudden deaths

AV = atrioventricular; MI = myocardial infarction; LBBB = left bundle branch block; LV = left ventricular; RBBB = right bundle branch block.

lapses after initially successful catheter ablation.[15, 27, 32] These may occur many days and even weeks after the procedure. One possible explanation is a resorption of edema surrounding the ablation site.

CATHETER DURABILITY. Conventional electrode catheters have not been constructed for this application. They have a limited durability after application of high-energy DC pulses. The insulation may show defects that may appear after single or multiple shocks. In catheters with more than one conductor coil, leakage currents between the conductor coils may develop. This effect makes changes of the mapping and ablation catheter necessary even after a small number of shocks. The catheter should frequently be inspected for injuries after shock application and should be tested for insulation failures. It is hoped that more resistant models for catheter ablation will soon be marketed.

FORMATION OF GAS BUBBLES. The formation of gas bubbles around the catheter electrode during the delivery of ablation shocks has been documented.[3, 10, 12, 52] Bubble formation is more extensive with high energies and anodal pulse delivery via the different electrode. Thus, the use of cathodal pulses has been mostly suggested, although the clinical importance of gas bubble formation has not yet been clarified.

BAROTRAUMA. Histologic observations after catheter ablation suggest that a barotrauma is involved in the ablation process.[3, 4, 10, 22, 52] Under certain circumstances, this mechanical effect may cause myocardial perforation, damage to blood components, or thrombus formation. Pressures generated may be higher than 1 atm of pressure[11, 12] and may sometimes even exceed 500 psi.[3]

ARRHYTHMOGENEITY. In animal studies and in clinical studies, an arrhythmogenic effect of DC catheter ablation has been well documented.[8, 22, 37, 39, 46, 47, 59, 63, 73] VT as well as ventricular fibrillation has been observed immediately after or within the first days after catheter ablation. This effect seems to be mediated by the necrotic process at the site of ablation and the subsequent scar formation. Though arrhythmogenic effects induced by the shock itself seem to be less frequent in humans than in animal experiments, continuous electrocardiographic monitoring within the first days after ablation has to be performed to detect these arrhythmias as well as a possible recurrence of the clinical VT.

UNWANTED INDUCTION OF TRANSIENT OR PERMANENT AV BLOCK. Application of high-energy DC pulses for catheter ablation of VT may induce AV block immediately after shock delivery.[32, 59] In the majority of these patients, this AV block has been transient, but the induction of permanent AV block has been reported.[66] It may be due to a closeness of the site of origin of VT to the proximal bundle system or may be due to misdirection of electrical energy after insulation failure. Therefore, immediate ventricular pacing must be available.

PERFORATION. Myocardial perforation and cardiac tamponade may occur at the site of ablation owing to formation of a transmural lesion and the development of pressure waves by the shock.[15, 27, 37] The risk of this complication seems to be related to the use of somewhat "stiff" catheters and to catheter positions that produce a relatively high pressure of the tip against the wall.[27] A site of increased risk for catheter perforation seems to be the apical region of the right ventricle, as pathologic studies[16] have demonstrated a very low wall thickness. In addition, the right ventricular outflow tract seems to be a site at risk if an electrode catheter is introduced via the femoral vein. Because of the straight course of the catheter, it may exert a relatively high pressure at the catheter tip against the wall. Perforation of the ventricular wall at sites distant from that of ablation may occur as well if electrode

catheters used for recording and stimulation take the straight course described above. A major contributing factor in this situation seems to be the vigorous contraction of the heart during shock delivery. In our group of patients, we had two cases of catheter perforation with cardiac tamponade, causing the death of one patient in the acute period and necessitating emergency surgery in another patient (see Table 33–8).

THROMBUS FORMATION. The formation of thrombi at the site of catheter ablation has been documented in experimental[37] and clinical reports.[27, 44] Furthermore, in an experimental study with fresh blood, hemolysis has been observed,[12] whereas clinical studies give no data on this particular problem. The risk of thrombus formation argues for an acute and—at least for a certain period—chronic anticoagulant therapy. However, systematic clinical studies on the efficacy of different anticoagulant regimens after this type of "trauma" are not available. We currently use intravenous heparin for a few days, starting at the time of catheter placement for ablation, followed by an oral anticoagulant treatment with coumarins for at least 3 weeks.

HEMODYNAMIC IMPAIRMENT. The delivery of high-energy DC pulses in the left ventricle may cause hemodynamic impairment as a result of the more or less limited myocardial necrosis. Long-term observations on the clinical relevance of this functional impairment are conflicting.[1, 37, 59] Besides the long-term consequences of a loss in contractile force due to myocardial necrosis, immediate hemodynamic problems during the ablation procedure may arise from the use of general anesthesia (inhibition of circulatory reflexes) and an imbalance of fluids during a long-lasting session. Therefore, the hemodynamic parameters should be carefully monitored during and after the procedure. For long-lasting ablation procedures, a careful balancing of the patient's fluid uptakes and discharges is mandatory. Continuous monitoring of right atrial or pulmonary artery pressures and systemic blood pressure, or both, is recommended during the ablation procedure to detect backward or forward failure as early as possible. The monitoring of arterial pressure also proves valuable if, immediately after shock delivery, electrocardiographic recording is disturbed. Although no study has been done that compares the complication rate of catheter ablation of VT with, for example, antitachycardia surgery, the incidence of the complications mentioned above is sufficiently low to justify the clinical use of catheter ablation in drug-resistant cases. A thorough knowledge of these potential risk factors and of the underlying mechanisms is mandatory. To decrease the potential risk, the clinical use of catheter ablation should be limited to centers with extended experience in clinical cardiac electrophysiology and with facilities for emergency heart surgery, which could become necessary once a complication occurs.

CLINICAL IMPLICATIONS AND FUTURE DEVELOPMENTS

Catheter ablation of VT has still to be regarded as an experimental approach. Many aspects of the procedure need additional experience and carefully designed studies. The dose-effect relationship of the method needs further evaluation. Those factors indicating the probability of relapses and of potential risks, such as thrombus formation, perforation, hemodynamic impairment and so forth, are not yet completely identified. Experimental studies are necessary to define more precisely the amount of tissue that needs to be ablated. A more exact prediction of the success (or failure) of the procedure immediately afterward is mandatory as well as a more precise localization of the origin of tachycardia.

Most recently, as an alternative to DC ablation, other techniques of energy delivery have been suggested to solve existing problems. Radiofrequency ablation[9, 17–19, 38] (see Chapter 34) seems to provide some advantages because of its easy applicability and because it does not require general anesthesia. In vitro studies have shown that the amount of tissue damage appears to be more closely correlated with the energy applied. Post-ablation arrhythmias seem to be rarer than with DC ablation. The absence of major gas bubble formation and the lack of barotraumatic effects are additional advantages of this method. These aspects, however, have to undergo extensive experimental and clinical investigation. Laser ablation, the latest methodologic approach in ablative techniques, has not yet reached the status of applicability with transvenous catheter systems. The first clinical experiences of laser ablation of VT are limited to using the laser beam during open heart surgery,[54–56, 65] in which, under specific conditions, photocoagulation of the tissue can be achieved. Special systems that allow a transcatheter application of the laser fiber and, at the same time, allow recordings of endocardial signals at the site of ablation will be necessary before catheter ablation of VT by laser energy can be applied to clinical practice.

Catheter ablation has become a valuable alternative to other forms of antiarrhythmia therapy, particularly in patients who, up to now, had no alternative to the treatment of their mostly life-threatening tachyarrhythmias and had to accept the major risks of other therapeutic methods. The technique, however, has to be further developed and improved.

REFERENCES

1. Abbot JA, Schiller NB, Ilvento J, et al: Catheter ablation of the atrioventricular junction may improve left ventricular function and cause minimal aortic valve damage [abstract]. PACE 10:411, 1987.
2. Anderson HN, Reichenbach D, Steinmetz GP, Merendino KA: An evaluation and comparison of effects of alternating and direct current electrical discharges on canine hearts. Ann Surg 160:251, 1964.
3. Bardy GH, Coltorti F, Ivey TD, et al: Some factors affecting bubble formation with catheter-mediated defibrillator pulses. Circulation 73:525–538, 1986.
4. Bardy GH, Ideker RE, Kasell J, et al: Transvenous ablation of the atrioventricular conduction system in dogs: Electrophysiologic and histologic observations. Am J Cardiol 51:1775–1782, 1983.
5. Bardy GH, Poole J, Coltorti F, et al: Catheter ablation of a concealed accessory pathway. Am J Cardiol 54:1366–1368, 1984.
6. Belhassen B, Miller IH, Geller E, Laniado S: Transcatheter electrical shock ablation of ventricular tachycardia. J Am Coll Cardiol 7:1347–1355, 1986.
7. Borggrefe M, Breithardt G: Transvenöse Ablation einer akzessorischen Leitungsbahn bei therapierefraktären supraventrikulären Reentry-Tachykardien. Z Kardiol 74:475–479, 1985.
8. Borggrefe M, Breithardt G: Ectopic atrial tachycardia after transvenous catheter ablation of a posteroseptal accessory pathway. J Am Coll Cardiol 8:441–445, 1986.
9. Borggrefe M, Budde T, Podczeck A, Breithardt G: High frequency current ablation of an accessory pathway in humans. J Am Coll Cardiol 10:576–582, 1987.
10. Boyd EG, Holt PM: Advantages of using cathodal impulses for electrical ablation in the left ventricle [abstract]. Circulation 72 [Suppl III]:390, 1985.
11. Boyd EGCA, Holt PM: An investigation into the electrical ablation technique and a method of electrode assessment. PACE 8:815, 1985.
12. Boyd EGCA, Holt PM: The biophysics of catheter ablation techniques. J Electrophysiol 1:62–77, 1987.
13. Breithardt G, Borggrefe M, Karbenn U, Schwarzmaier J: Catheter ablation of ventricular tachycardia. New Trends Arrhythm 2:253–256, 1986.
14. Breithardt G, Borggrefe M, Karbenn U, et al: Therapie refraktärer ventrikulärer Tachykardien durch transvenöse, elektrische Ablation. Z Kardiol 75:80–90, 1986.

15. Breithardt G, Borggrefe M, Podczeck A, et al: Clinical experience with catheter ablation of ventricular tachycardia using defibrillator pulses. *In* Breithardt G, Borggrefe M, Zipes DP (eds): Non-pharmacological Therapy of Tachyarrhythmias. Mount Kisco, NY, Futura Publishing Co, 1987, pp 1299–1374.

16. Brunner P, Weber R, Götz M: Myokardperforationen bei Implantation von Schrittmachersonden. Lebensversicherungsmedizin 3:86–89, 1987.

17. Budde T, Borggrefe M, Podczeck A, et al: Radiofrequency ablation: An improvement of ablation techniques in comparison to direct-current delivery? *In* Breithardt G, Borggrefe M, Zipes DP (eds): Non-pharmacological Therapy of Tachyarrhythmias. Mount Kisco, NY, Futura Publishing Co, 1987, pp 1221–1241.

18. Budde T, Breithardt G, Borggrefe M, et al: First experiences with radiofrequency alternating current ablation of the AV-conduction system in man. Z Kardiol 76:204–210, 1987.

19. Budde T, Jacob B, Langwasser J, et al: Hochfrequenz-Katheterablation: Eine Methode zur Erzeugung dosisabhängiger Koagulationszonen [abstract]. Z Kardiol 75 (Suppl IV):54, 1986.

20. Critelli G, Gallagher JJ, Perticone F, et al: Transvenous catheter ablation of the accessory atrioventricular pathway in the permanent form of junctional reciprocating tachycardia. Am J Cardiol 55:1639–1641, 1985.

21. Critelli G, Perticone F, Coltorti F, et al: Antegrade slow bypass conduction after closed-chest ablation of the His-bundle in permanent junctional reciprocating tachycardia. Circulation 67:687–692, 1983.

22. Davis JC, Finkebeiner W, Ruder MA, et al: Histologic changes and arrhythmogenicity after discharge through transseptal catheter electrode. Circulation 74:637–644, 1986.

23. Doherty PW, McLaughlin PR, Billingham M, et al: Cardiac damage produced by direct current countershock applied to the heart. Am J Cardiol 43:225–232, 1979.

24. Downar E, Parson I, Cameron D, et al: Unipolar and bipolar catheter "ablation" techniques for management of ventricular tachycardia—initial experience [abstract]. J Am Coll Cardiol [suppl] 5:472, 1985.

25. Ellenbogen KA, O'Callaghan WG, Colavita PG, et al: Catheter atrioventricular junction ablation for recurrent supraventricular tachycardia with nodoventricular fibers. Am J Cardiol 55:1227–1229, 1985.

26. Fisher JD, Brodman R, Kim SG, Mercando AD: Nonsurgical ablation of accessory pathways: Physical, anatomical, and clinical considerations. J Electrophysiol 1:47–57, 1987.

27. Fisher JD, Kim SG, Matos JA, et al: Complications of catheter ablation of tachyarrhythmias: Occurrence, protection, prevention. Clin Prog Electrophysiol Pacing 4:292–298, 1985.

28. Fontaine G, Frank R, Tonet JL, et al: Endocardial fulguration in the treatment of resistant chronic ventricular tachycardia. Rev Portugese Cardiol 4:369–374, 1985.

29. Fontaine G, Frank R, Tonet JL, et al: Treatment of resistant ventricular tachycardia by endocavitary fulguration and antiarrhythmic therapy in 111 consecutive patients followed for 18 months. *In* Breithardt G, Borggrefe M, Zipes DP (eds): Non-pharmacological Therapy of Tachyarrhythmias. Mount Kisco, NY, Futura Publishing Co, 1987, pp 1263–1283.

30. Fontaine G, Tonet JL, Frank R, et al: Traitement d'urgence de la tachycardie ventriculaire chronique après infarctus du myocarde par la fulguration endocavitaire. Arch Mal Coeur 7:1037–1043, 1985.

31. Fontaine G, Tonet JL, Frank R, et al: Traitement des tachycardies ventriculaires rebelles par fulguration endocavitaire associée aux anti-arrhythmiques. Arch Mal Coeur 8:1152–1162, 1986.

32. Fontaine G, Tonet JL, Frank R, et al: Electrode catheter ablation of resistant ventricular tachycardia by endocavitary fulguration associated with antiarrhythmic therapy: Experience in 38 patients with a mean follow-up of 23 months. *In* Brugada P, Wellens HJJ (eds): Cardiac Arrhythmias: Where to Go from Here? Mount Kisco, NY, Futura Publishing Co, 1987, pp 1539–1569.

33. Frank R, Tonet JL, Kounde S, et al: Localization of the area of slow conduction during ventricular tachycardia. *In* Brugada P, Wellens HJJ (eds): Cardiac Arrhythmias: Where to Go from Here? Mount Kisco, NY, Futura Publishing Co, 1987, pp 191–208.

34. Gallagher JJ, Svenson RH, Kasell JH, et al: Catheter technique for closed-chest ablation of the atrioventricular conduction system. N Engl J Med 306:194–200, 1982.

35. Gonzalez R, Scheinman M, Margaretten W, Rubinstein M: Closed-chest electrode-catheter technique for His bundle ablation in dogs. Am J Physiol 241:H283–H287, 1981.

36. Hartzler GO: Electrode catheter ablation of refractory focal ventricular tachycardia. J Am Coll Cardiol 2:1107–1113, 1983.

37. Hauer RNW, Straks W, Borst C, et al: Electrical catheter ablation in the left and right ventricular wall in dogs: Relation between delivered energy and histopathologic changes. J Am Coll Cardiol 8:637–643, 1986.

38. Huang SKS: Use of radiofrequency energy for catheter ablation of the endomyocardium: A prospective energy source. J Electrophysiol 1:78–91, 1987.

39. Jackman WM, Friday KJ, Scherlag BJ, et al: Direct endocardial recordings from an accessory atrioventricular pathway: Localization of the site of block, effect of antiarrhythmic drugs, and attempts of nonsurgical ablation. Circulation 68:906–916, 1983.

40. Josephson M: Catheter ablation of arrhythmias. Ann Intern Med 101:234–237, 1984.

41. Kempf F, Falcone R, Waxman H, et al: Anatomic and hemodynamic effects of electrical discharges in the ventricle [abstract]. Circulation 68 [Suppl III]:174, 1983.

42. Kempf FC Jr, Falcone RA, Marchlinski FE, Josephson ME: The electrophysiologic effects of high energy electrical discharges in the ventricle [abstract]. J Am Coll Cardiol 3:554, 1984.

43. Klein H, Trappe HJ, Hartwig CA, et al: Problems and pitfalls with catheter ablation of ventricular tachycardia. New Trends Arrhythm 21:257–263, 1986.

44. Kunze KP, Schlüter M, Costard A, et al: Right atrial thrombus formation after transvenous catheter ablation of the atrioventricular node. J Am Coll Cardiol 6:1428–1430, 1985.

45. Leclerq JF, Chouty F, Coumel Ph, Slama R: Fulguration in ventricular tachycardia due to right ventricular dysplasia: Mean-term results [abstract]. J Am Coll Cardiol 9:250A, 1987.

46. Lee BI, Gottdiener JS, Fletcher RD, et al: Transcatheter ablation: Comparison of laser photoablation and electrode shock ablation in the dog. Circulation 71:579–586, 1985.

47. Lerman BB, Weiss JL, Bulkley BH, et al: Myocardial

injury and induction of arrhythmia by direct current shock delivered via endocardial catheters in dogs. Circulation 69:1006–1012, 1984.

48. Levine JH, Spear JF, Weisman HF, et al: The cellular electrophysiologic changes induced by high-energy electrical ablation in canine myocardium. Circulation 73:818–829, 1986.

49. Lévy S, Bru P: Interruption électrique par voie percutanée de la conduction auriculo-ventriculaire normale. Arch Mal Coeur 8:1145–1150, 1986.

50. Morady F, Scheinman MM, DiCarlo LA Jr, et al: Results of transcatheter ablation of ventricular tachycardia in 33 patients [abstract]. J Am Coll Cardiol 9:250A, 1987.

51. Morady F, Scheinman MM, Winston SA, et al: Efficacy and safety of transcatheter ablation of posteroseptal accessory pathways. Circulation 72:170–177, 1985.

52. Nathan AW, Bennet DH, Ward DE, et al: Catheter ablation of atrioventricular conduction. Lancet 1:1280–1287, 1984.

53. Ruder MA, Mead H, Gaudiani V, Winkle RA: Experience with catheter ablation of accessory pathways [abstract]. J Am Coll Cardiol 9:251A, 1987.

54. Saksena S, Hussain MS, Gielchinsky I, et al: Intraoperative mapping—guided argon laser ablation of malignant supraventricular and ventricular tachycardia [abstract]. J Am Coll Cardiol [Suppl] 9:249A, 1987.

55. Saksena S, Hussain MS, Gielchinsky I, et al: Laser ablation of human atrium and accessory pathways: Experimental observations and early clinical experience [abstract]. PACE 10:427, 1987.

56. Saksena S, Rothbart ST, Gadhoke A, et al: Anatomic, hemodynamic and electrophysiologic effects of argon laser endocardial ablation for refractory ventricular tachycardia in man [abstract]. PACE 10:411, 1987.

57. Scheinman MM: Catheter ablation for patients with cardiac arrhythmias. PACE 9:551–564, 1986.

58. Scheinman MM, Davies JC: Catheter ablation for the treatment of tachyarrhythmias: Present role and potential promise. Circulation 73:10–13, 1986.

59. Scheinman MM, Evans GT Jr: Catheter ablation of cardiac arrhythmias: A summary report of the percutaneous cardiac mapping and ablation registry. In Brugada P, Wellens HJJ (eds): Cardiac Arrhythmias: Where to Go from Here? Mount Kisco, NY, Futura Publishing Co, 1987, pp 529–538.

60. Scheinman MM, Evans-Bell T, the Executive Committee of the Percutaneous Cardiac Mapping and Ablation Registry: Catheter ablation of the atrioventricular junction: A report of the Percutaneous Cardiac Mapping and Ablation Registry. Circulation 70:1024–1029, 1984.

61. Scheinman MM, Morady F, Hess DS, Gonzalez R:

Catheter-induced ablation of the atrioventricular junction to control refractory supraventricular arrhythmias. JAMA 248:851–855, 1982.

62. Smith RT, Gillette PC, Massumi G, McVey P, et al: Transcatheter ablative techniques for treatment of the permanent form of junctional reciprocating tachycardia in young patients. J Am Coll Cardiol 8:385–390, 1986.

63. Steinbeck G, Bach P, Haberl R, Markewitz A: Ventricular preexcitation following catheter ablation of the His bundle in concealed WPW syndrome. Eur Heart J 7:444–448, 1986.

64. Steinhaus D, Whitford E, Stavens C, et al: Percutaneous transcatheter electrical ablation for recurrent sustained ventricular tachycardia [abstract]. Circulation 70 [Suppl II]:100, 1984.

65. Svenson RH, Gallagher JJ, Selle JG, et al: Neodymium-Yag Laser photo coagulation of ventricular tachycardia: Rationale, method of application, and results in 17 patients. In Breithardt G, Borggrefe M, Zipes DP (eds): Non-pharmacological Therapy of Tachyarrhythmias. Mount Kisco, NY, Futura Publishing Co, 1987, pp 181–200.

66. Touboul P, Atallah G, Kirkorian G, et al: Fulguration for refractory ventricular tachycardia: Prediction of results [abstract]. Abstract Book X. World Congress of Cardiology, American Heart Association, 1986, p 118.

67. Van Vleet JF, Tacker WA Jr, Geddes LA, Ferrans VJ: Sequential cardiac morphologic alterations induced in dogs by single transthoracic damped sinusoidal waveform defibrillator shocks. Am J Vet Res 39:271–278, 1978.

68. Van Vleet JF, Tacker WA Jr, Geddes LA, Ferrans VJ: Sequential ultrastructural alterations in ventricular myocardium of dogs given large single transthoracic damped sinusoidal waveform defibrillator shocks. Am J Vet Res 41:493–501, 1978.

69. Vedel J, Frank R, Fontaine G, Grosgogeat Y: Bloc auriculo-ventriculaire intra-Hisien definitif induit au cours d'une exploration endoventriculaire droite. Arch Mal Coeur 72:107–112, 1979.

70. Ward DE, Camm AJ: Treatment of tachycardias associated with the Wolff-Parkinson-White syndrome by transvenous electrical ablation of accessory pathways. Br Heart J 53:64–68, 1985.

71. Ward DE, Davies M: Transvenous high energy shock for ablating atrioventricular conduction in man—observations on the histological effects. Br Heart J 51:175–178, 1984.

72. Weber H, Schmitz L: Catheter techniques for closed chest ablation of an accessory pathway. N Engl J Med 308:653–654, 1983.

73. Westeveer DC, Nelson T, Stewart JR, et al: Sequelae of left ventricular electrical ablation. J Am Coll Cardiol 5:956–960, 1985.

B. Clinical Application

G. FONTAINE, J. TONET, R. FRANK, Y. GALLAIS,
I. ROUGIER, G. FARENQ, M. LILAMAND,
and Y. GROSGOGEAT

EFFICACY AND SAFETY OF FULGURATION FOR THE TREATMENT OF VENTRICULAR TACHYCARDIA

Fulguration (electrode catheter ablation) is a new method used for the radical treatment of ventricular tachycardia (VT). This approach may permanently alter the arrhythmogenic substrate, preventing arrhythmia relapses. This form of therapy is considered when drugs are ineffective, have side effects, or are used for a young and active patient who does not want to take drugs for the remainder of his or her life and when there is a compliance problem.

Fulguration, which uses the effects of a strong electric shock delivered at the tip of an endocardial catheter positioned in the area to be modified, is an ablative technique whose usefulness for interruption of normal atrioventricular (AV) conduction has been extensively explored for the indirect treatment of supraventricular tachycardia.[36, 63] The same electrical energy applied directly on the site of origin of abnormal ventricular activation, as determined by endocardial mapping, in the treatment of chronic VT is a more recent and promising development.[28, 39, 61]

We have been involved in the evaluation of this new form of therapy with a series of 52 consecutive cases.

Clinical Series

We report the analysis of our experience concerning the first 43 cases of fulguration with a follow-up period extending from 2 to 60 months, starting in May 1983. To present our results in perspective, we describe our clinical series in the following way. This group is taken from a larger cohort of 137 consecutive cases representing the totality of major ventricular

arrhythmias observed at Jean Rostand Hospital, Ivry/Seine (near Paris, France) during the same period. This series consists of 6 cases of ventricular fibrillation (VF) and 131 of chronic, recurrent, sustained VT. Almost all these patients were referred from other institutions, where their conditions were considered resistant to treatment. All of them were restudied according to the drug protocols developed at Jean Rostand Hospital, including amiodarone alone or in combination with class I antiarrhythmic drugs and/or beta-blocking agents. Only those patients whose conditions were resistant to the drug regimens given after reevaluation were considered candidates for the fulguration procedure. The cases are consecutive, and there was no exclusion on the basis of age, cardiac or clinical condition, or other factors. The series of patients who underwent fulguration consists of 35 men and 8 women, with an age range of 14 to 74 years (mean age: 43.19 ± 18.81 SD).

The etiologies of VT include 14 patients with VT after an old myocardial infarction (range: minimum of 3 months, maximum of 10 years), 13 patients with arrhythmogenic right ventricular disease, 7 patients with VT complicating an idiopathic dilated cardiomyopathy, 4 patients with right bundle branch block–left axis deviation VT, 2 patients with infundibular idiopathic VT, one patient with VT occurring 7 years after infundibular resection in a congenital anomaly, and 1 patient with myocarditis sequelae. The main clinical features of these cases are summarized in Table 33–9.

In this series of fulguration cases (except in one case submitted to surgery), we did not have to use forms of therapy other than fulguration alone or in association with drug treatment.

Materials

The techniques developed in our department were primarily based on clinical research that profited from a background provided by previous studies of surgery for arrhythmia man-

Supported in part by grants from Centre de Recherche sur les Maladies Cardiovasculaires de l'Association Claude Bernard, La Fondation de Cardiologie, and L'Institut National de la Santé et de la Recherche Médicale (INSERM contrat No. 865005).

TABLE 33–9. CLINICAL FEATURES OF CAUSES OF VENTRICULAR TACHYCARDIA

(FUTV43/TAB-FUTV) 11.06.88   Updated 01 JUNE 88

N°	Age	SX	LOC	FC	EF	TI	NM	NE	LI	SI	INC	Nb	ENERG	RIP	AR	MT	1OD	FOL
ARRHYTHMOGENIC RIGHT VENTRICULAR DYSPLASIA																		
1	35	M	DIAPH	1	-	>20	1	<2	M	-	-	II	240*1	-	-	-	NP	DCOD
2	62	F	DIAPH	2	-	36	2	>20	M	W	-	I	160*5	RM	0	0	RM	54M
3	74	M	INFUN	2	52%	12	1	3	M	M	-	I	160*1	NI	AMIO	PRO	NI	53M
4	37	M	DIAPH	1	58%	6	1	3	M	<D	-	II	240*6	M	0	0	NI	51M
5	27	M	DIAPH	4	25%	120	4	6	Y	I	+	I	160*17	RM	0	0	NP	DC8D
6	56	M	LV	1	45%	84	5	>20	Y	M	-	III	240*4	R	A+Pr	TH	IN	48M
7	41	F	INFUN	1	59%	48	2	16	M	M	-	II	240*1	TL	0	0	RM	48M
8	32	M	INFUN	1	-	4	1	2	W	<D	-	I	210*4	NI	AMIO	PRO	NI	47M
9	30	M	F.W.	1	56%	12	2	2	M	M	-	II	240*2	TL	AMIO	TH	IN	48M
10	38	M	INFUN	-	-	-	2	>20	<Y	D	+	II	240*3	NP	-	-	-	DCOD
11	37	M	INFUN	2	-	408	3	>20	-	-	+	II	240*9	TL	A+Fl	TH	NC	DC7M
12	27	M	RV Fw	2	50%	120	3	>20	-	-	-	II	240*4	M	Bb+QD	TH	NC	35M
13	26	M	SEPTRV	2	59%	96	1	12	Y	M	-	II	280*3	-	0	0	NI	21M
MYOCARDIAL INFARCTION																		
14	60	M	ANTSEP	2	12%	1	2	>20	W	D	+	II	260*1	NI	AMIO	PRO	NP	60M
15	29	M	INF	1	42%	24	3	4	M	M	-	II	260*7	RM	A+Pr	TH	NP	55M
16	73	M	ANTSEP	2	22%	1	2	>20	M	I	+	II	160*1	NP	AMIO	PRO	NP	53M
17	65	M	ANTSEP	2	<30%	1	3	2	W	<D	-	I	160*5	NI	0	0	NI	51M
18	55	M	INF	1	-	12	1	10	M	M	-	IV	240*2	NI	AMIO	PRO	NI	52M
19	60	M	ANTSEP	3	<25%	24	3	10	M	M	-	I	240*2	NP	-	-	-	DC4D
20	67	M	ANTSEP	3	<25%	1	1	2	D	D	-	I	240*2	NP	AMIO	PRO	NP	DC1M
21	74	M	ANTSEP		<30%	-	2	10	M	D	-	I	240*2	NI	AMIO	TH	NI	45M
22	64	M	ANTSEP	2	46%	-	2	14	M	D	+	I	240*2	NC	AMIO	TH	IN	DC22M
23	62	F	ANTSEP	3	26%	4	6	>20	M	I	+	IV	240*3	R	A+Bb	TH	NP	DC9M
24	53	M	ANTPOST	1	<30%	3	2	7	W	M	-	I	240*2	NC	AMIO	TH	IN	DC4M
25	64	M	INF	3	25%	16	2	>20	Y	D	-	I	240*2	NC	A+PM	TH	NP	DC18M
26	55	M	INF	1	<30%	2	3	7	W	D	-	I	280*3	NI	AMIO	PRO	NI	40M
27	52	M	ANTPOST	2	40%	12	2	>20	Y	M	-	I	240*3	NI	AMIO	PRO	NI	23M
28	65	M	LV	3	25%	36	2	>20	M	I	-	II	240*8	NI	A+Bb	TH	NI	17M
IDIOPATHIC CARDIOMYOPATHY																		
29	18	M	ANTSEP	2	<30%	12	1	>20	M	I	+	I	260*5	0	AMIO	TH	NI	DC14M
30	14	F	SEPTLV	3	<20%	168	1	>20	I	I	+	I	160*3	0	0	0	NP	DC2M
31	56	M	LV	2	20%	36	1	6	Y	M	-	I	240*3	NI	AMIO	PRO	NI	DC16M
32	28	M	RV	1	48%	-	3	>20	<Y	D	+	III	240*1	NI	FLEC	TH	IN	46M
33	58	M	RV+LV	1	48%	120	2	>20	M	D	-	III	280*3	NC	QD+Bb	TH	NI	40M
34	21	M	RV APX	1	-	3	1	4	M	D	-	I	240*1	NC	A+Bb	TH	IN	35M
35	16	M	SEPTRV	3	<30%	24	1	>20	-	D	+	I	240*1	0	-	-	NP	DC1D
IDIOPATHIC VENTRICULAR TACHYCARDIA																		
36	53	F	INFUN	1	59%	96	1	>20	M	D	+	II	240*2	NI	0	0	NI	48M
37	26	F	SEPTRV	1	50%	48	1	>20	Y	D	-	I	240*6	TL	QD	TH	NP	29M
VERAPAMIL SENSITIVE VENTRICULAR TACHYCARDIA																		
38	22	M	POSTSEP	1	-	60	1	>20	M	W	-	II	240*2	NI	0	0	NP	48M
39	17	M	SEPTLV	1	70%	40	1	6	Y	D	-	II	240*4	NI	0	0	NI	34M
40	38	M	SEPTLV	1	47%	252	1	>20	W	D	-	I	240*1	NI	0	0	NI	30M
41	22	F	SEPTLV	1	60%	120	1	>20	M	D	-	II	240*2	NI	0	0	NI	19M
CORRECTED CONGENITAL DISEASE																		
42	21	M	INFUN	1	61%	120	4	10	M	D	-	I	240*4	NI	AMIO	PRO	NP	53M
SEQUELAE OF MYOCARDITIS																		
43	23	F	SEPTRV	1	51%	24	1	>20	I	I	+	II	240*3	NI	Dis	TH	NI	20M

LOC: Location of abnormality. DIAPH = diaphragmatic; INFUN = infundibulum; LV = left ventricle; F.W. = free wall; SEPTRV = right ventricular septum; ANTSEP = anteroseptal; ANTPOST = anterior and posterior; INF = inferior; SEPTLV = left ventricular septum; RV = right ventricle; and POSTSEP = posteroseptal.

FC: Functional class (New York Heart Association)

EF: Ejection fraction (echography, angiography, scintigraphy)

TI: Time interval since the first attack of VT (mo).

NM: Number of clinical morphologies of VT.

NE: Total number of VT episodes prior to fulguration.

LI,SI: Longest and shortest interval between two episodes of VT. I = incessant; D = day; W-week; M-month; Y-year.

INC: Incessant VT in the electrophysiologic laboratory.

Nb: Number of fulguration sessions.

ENERG: Joules delivered—160*5 = 5 discharges of 160 J (value concerning the last procedure).

RIP: Reasons for interrupting the procedure. R = changes in rate; M = changes in morphology; NP = programmed pacing not performed; TL = time limit; NC = nonclinical VT; NI = VT not inducible.

AR: Antiarrhythmic prescription upon hospital discharge. AMIO = amiodarone; A+Pr = amiodarone + propafenone; A+Fl = amiodarone + flecainide; FLEC = flecainide; A+Bb = amiodarone + beta blockers; A+PM = amiodarone + pacemaker; QD = quinidine; Dis = Disopyramide

MT: Mode of treatment. PRO = prophylactic treatment; TH = therapeutic treatment.

1OD: Provocative test performed 10 days after fulguration. NP = provocative test not performed; NI = VT not inducible; IN = inducible by programmed stimulation; RM = change in rate and morphology of VT morphology; NC = Nonclinical VT.

FOL: Follow-up. DC = death.

agement in a center dedicated to the treatment of cardiac arrhythmias and to cardiac pacing. The equipment available is therefore important, and only some specific aspects will be presented in this chapter. A more complete description is published elsewhere.[20, 24]

Catheter Technology and Selection

The first step in an endocardial catheter fulguration procedure is the localization by endocardial mapping of the area to be fulgurated. The catheter should be appropriately positioned inside the cavities. This task is frequently more difficult to achieve when the heart is normal in size. An important prerequisite of endocardial catheters is their torque control. In our experience, the USCI catheters (Bard Electrophysiology Division, C. R. Bard Inc., Billerica, MA) are the most suitable, probably because of their unique woven Dacron structure. The problems concerning their steering properties, however, have not been completely solved. Their standard length is not sufficient in cases of a large aneurysm or in older patients with a dilated aortic arch.

Owing to different designs, the steering properties of the different models are not the same. In addition, these design features strongly affect the catheter insulation strength. It has been demonstrated in our own laboratory since 1983[18] and confirmed by others that the regular catheters that have been developed for endocardial recording or pacing are, for the most part, unable to withstand the high peak voltage and current used in the fulguration procedure.[1, 14] The differences in the internal structures of the catheter also explain why the insulation properties of multipolar catheters are generally better than those of bipolar catheters.[20, 24] These insulation properties have also changed as modifications have been made in manufacturing. They affect the weakest link in the insulation strength along the catheter. In a certain series, breakdown of the catheters occurred in the electrode region,[21] which could lead to release of gas and smoke in the blood stream,[22] a situation that could be dangerous if the catheter is located within the left ventricle. It is also probable that the abrupt surge of decomposition products would damage normal myocardium.

Therefore, we developed a method to select catheters prior to their sterilization.[23] Since fulguration shocks are always delivered through the distal electrode to ensure close contact with the endocardium, the number of electrodes is not crucial. Theoretically, a bipolar catheter is sufficient. In practice, we use either tripolar or quadripolar catheters because of better electrical properties. The catheters that were used for mapping are also subsequently used for shock delivery.

In the case of a right-sided VT, catheters are introduced through the femoral vein. Two catheters positioned in the infundibulum and apex are introduced for endocavitary recording and pacing, in addition to a catheter placed in the coronary sinus or against the atrial wall.

For left-sided VT, the catheter used for fulguration and mapping is introduced by a femoral or axillary artery puncture. The use of a guiding tube (Bioptome Sheath 502, 300, Cordis, Miami, FL) pushed beyond the aortic cusps facilitates catheter positioning within the left ventricle and prevents inadvert entry into the ostium of the coronary arteries.

Fulgurator

The preselected discharge energy varied from 160 to 320 J, with the actual value set at an amount equal to 3 J/kg of body weight. This equation was determined from animal experiments that suggested it was appropriate with our equipment.[16] The shock is provided by a piece of equipment developed specifically for this application (Fulgucor ODAM, Wissembourg, France). In its more recent design, this equipment incorporates a capacitor of 45 μF and an inductor of 45 mH, with the internal resistance of this latter component being around 10 ohms. These features are different from those of most "defibrillators." As a result, the waveform is different, and a different biologic effect could be expected. Most defibrillators are not properly recalibrated before the procedure, and variations in their energy output (a parameter not critical for standard defibrillation) could play a significant role when the same equipment is used to modify conduction in a limited zone of myocardium. In our equipment, special attention has been paid to ensure precise and stable energy delivery.

Our equipment also includes an electric circuit that measures both the current and the voltage applied to the fulgurating catheter.[30] When both curves are displayed on a Model 7854 Tektronix oscilloscope with waveform calculator,[24] precise measurements can be made in terms of voltage, current, power, energy, and impedance all along the curves (Fig. 33–1). Polaroid pictures of the screen are taken after each shock. This protocol assumes that the catheter has been able to withstand

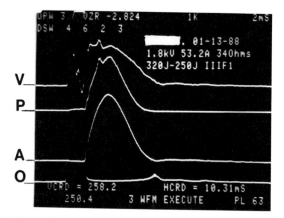

Figure 33–1. Recording of the electrical parameters during the shock delivery. V = voltage curve that is preceded by an electrical artifact indicating the stored voltage.[24] P = power in watts. The area under the curves indicates the energy in Joules applied to the proximal part of the catheter. A = evolution of the current during the impulse (pulse width, 6 msec). O = ohms shows the variation of the impedance. Note that there is a progressive increase of the impedance when the current curve is going back to the zero line.

the energy used for each fulguration. Moreover, a high-voltage electromechanical relay system, developed for our first His bundle ablation procedure, automatically switches the catheter from the recording of the endocardial signals to the capacitor containing the fulgurating energy.[28] Therefore, from a review of the recordings, it may be assumed that when the endocardial electrogram remains the same, the fulgurating electrode tip does not change its position until the shock is delivered.

An electrically completely independent defibrillator is located in the same piece of equipment. It is left in a waiting position charged at 40 J and connected with an anterior patch defibrillating electrode (R_2 Corporation, Morton Grove, IL) made with an adhesive ring positioned on the precordial region. Its other electrode is the indifferent electrode used for the fulguration shock, provided that the indifferent electrode is located on the left side of the patient's back. When the first defibrillation shock is not effective, the energy is switched to 80 or 160 J. The latter value is generally appropriate for the treatment of VF.

Special care is taken to keep all the preceding electric circuits "floating" to avoid leakage of current toward inappropriate electrodes. Such leakage could lead to burns or could deprive the active electrode of part of the current and decrease the shock's effectiveness.

A backup independent defibrillator with reg-

ular paddles is left in the waiting position, ready to be charged at 400 J.

Fluoroscopy and Videotape Recordings

A custom-made video system records either the signal from a camera focused on the areas of catheter entry in the femoral vessels or the video signal generated by the fluoroscopic equipment. Alpha-numeric data concerning the patient's name, the date, and the characteristics of the shocks are superimposed on the video images.

A videotape recorder is connected with the fluoroscopic equipment to store the data from the video system. During the time when the fluoroscope is off, a separate solid-state memory is used to store and display the last image obtained. An electronic arrow provides a manually controlled indication for each point to be mapped. Video recording is done on a videocassette recorder during the entire procedure except for two important periods: the final position of the catheters prior to the shock and the end of the fulguration countdown. This information is stored on a permanent, independent tape kept in the file. The other tape is erased during the next procedure but played back when special investigation is required. Fulguration video recording is frequently played back during the postfulguration resting period to study the behavior of the catheter during the shock. In addition, Polaroid pictures are taken in both the anteroposterior and the left anterior oblique views to keep track of catheter position before each shock.

A specially developed on-line computer program, "Chronos," stores the timing of relevant events throughout the procedure and updates independent clocks, which could be activated and stopped at any time.

Hemodynamic Monitoring

Radial arterial pressure and pulmonary capillary wedge pressure are continuously monitored using a Swan-Ganz catheter. The cardiac output is also studied by thermodilution. These measurements are taken by the anesthesia team. In addition, in cases of patients with poor cardiac contractility, permanent monitoring of the radial artery blood pressure is done by a dedicated team member located in the technical room. The blood pressure signal is displayed on a 5115 storage Tektronix oscilloscope with a 5A14N vertical amplifier and a 5B12N time base plug-in unit, the sweep being adjusted at a slow speed (5 sec/div).

Equipment for Activation Time Measurements

Electrocardiographic leads I, V_F, V_1, and V_6—or I, II, III, and V_1—or any selection of leads that are informative for pacemapping are recorded with an Electronics for Medicine machine (VR 12). Activation times are measured on the 12-channel ink jet paper recorder, Siemens Mingograph (Solna, Sweden). Comparison is made with a digital measurement system from a 5116 Tektronix oscilloscope with a 5A26 vertical amplifier and 5D10 signal sampling and storage unit. We store two channels on the screen. The first is the endocardial mapping signal, and the second is derived from the analogic summation of the absolute value of one to four surface leads. Interval measurements are easily determined on the oscilloscope screen by moving two cursors positioned on the signals' relevant points. Each mapped area is indicated on a schematic representation of the inside of the heart.

Electrocardiographic and endocardial signals are also amplified by a custom-made piece of equipment incorporating analogic low-pass and high-pass filters adapted for both surface electrocardiographic and endocardial signals (ODAM, Wissembourg, France). In the same equipment, two markers indicate QRS detection and positioning of the shock in the cardiac cycle. An automatic calibrating signal for both amplitude and filtering is delivered every 5 to 30 seconds and is interrupted just before the shock. Triggering of the shock can be linked with either the electrocardiogram or an endocardial signal when the surface recording of the QRS complexes during VT shows a rise time that is too smooth to activate the detecting circuit. Surface and endocardial signals are recorded with an EMI SE 7000, 14-channel magnetic tape recorder. A special track is used to record coded time marks, which are also traced on the ink jet recorder.

Five of the 10 people involved in the procedure, 3 in the technical room and 2 in the sterile room, wear microphones and headsets; multiplexing allows recording of all the comments on the same EMI SE 7000 voice recording channel. These comments have proved to be of the utmost importance in the event of major complications.

Precise comparison between documented arrhythmias and pacemapping is made with a 12-lead electrocardiogram by an independent, battery-operated, three-channel microprocessor-based recorder.

Method

Prior to the procedure, class I antiarrhythmic drug therapy is interrupted for a period equivalent to 5 half-lives. When present, amiodarone therapy is not discontinued (about 60 per cent of the cases). Protracted general anesthesia is used because of the duration of the procedure and the frequent need to deliver more than one shock in a single procedure.

Endocardial Mapping

In cases in which VT is not incessant, programmed stimulation (Savita, Paris) is used to induce the arrhythmia. The protocol includes the introduction of progressively more premature stimuli ranging from 1 to 3 extra stimuli and delivered as a paced basic stimulation at a progressively increasing rate. In some cases, isoproterenol is injected to facilitate VT induction. VT induction was not possible during the procedure in only two cases (in one of them, case No. 38, fulguration was based only on pacemapping data). When unstable VT or VF is induced during the pacing protocol, the session is interrupted or postponed and drugs are prescribed to make the arrhythmia easier to manage.

Endocavitary mapping is used to localize the presumed area of the origin of the VT (Figs. 33–2 to 33–4).[33] Confirmation is sought by trying to reproduce the morphology of the

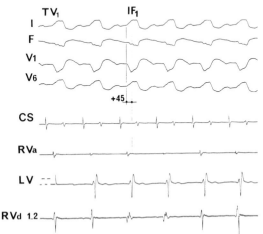

Figure 33–2. Patient with two morphologies of ventricular tachycardia (VT) after myocardial infarction. The first shock (240 J) is delivered in the left ventricle, on a potential that occurs 45 msec after the onset of the VT type 1 QRS complex. In that place, pacemapping was not perfect. This shock (IF_1) did not prevent VT type 1 reinduction. CS = coronary sinus; TV_1 = first VT morphology; RV_a = anterior right ventricle; LV = left ventricle; RVd = distal right ventricle.

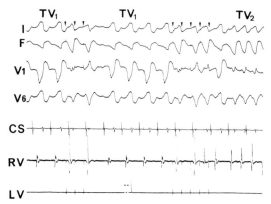

Figure 33–3. Same patient as in Figure 33–1. Pacing is performed in the left ventricle. VT type I (TV₁) is transformed in VT type 2 (TV₂) after the second attempt by a burst of rapid ventricular pacing *(arrows)*.

VT[60] with ventricular pacing during sinus rhythm or VT.[46] Three methods of ventricular pacemapping are used: continuous pacing in sinus rhythm at a rate identical with the tachycardia rate, slight overdrive of VT, and introduction of a premature stimulus during VT. Comparison of QRS morphologies is made using the independent, portable 12-lead recorder. In the most recent studies, special attention was paid to identification of the area of slow conduction and investigation of its role as a necessary link for VT. An interesting marker could be the recording of perfect reproduction of VT morphology after pacing in sinus rhythm at a rate close to the VT rate, provided that ventricular activation is obtained after a delay that is similar to the interval between a distinct presystolic endocardial potential and onset of ventricular QRS complexes during VT (Fig. 33–5).[15] Pacing an area of slow conduction connected with the critical slow conduction pathway of VT could be deduced from more recent electrophysiologic parameters.[19]

Fulguration

Fulguration is delivered at the conclusion of a checklist protocol, which is followed by a countdown, during which every piece of relevant equipment is put into action. The shock is synchronized to the surface QRS complexes or endocardial electrogram during either VT or sinus rhythm. This latter method is now preferred for hemodynamic reasons.[37] As a last resort, a nonsynchronized shock is automatically delivered after 2 seconds. The shock is applied between the distal electrode of the fulgurating catheter, which is used as an anode, and an indifferent electrode, which functions as a cathode and is positioned in the patient's back. One to eight shocks are generally delivered during each session.

In case of AV block, ventricular pacing is performed. In case of acceleration of VT or its degeneration to VF, a defibrillating external shock is immediately delivered.[71] Within a few minutes after fulguration, provided that the catheter has not moved, the pacing threshold studied by the fulgurating catheter returns to a level compatible with stimulation. After completion of the fulguration shock, provided sta-

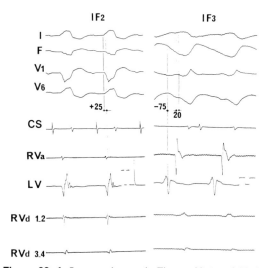

Figure 33–4. Same patient as in Figures 33–1 and 33–2. The second shock (240 J) of the first session (IF₂) shows a coupling of 25 msec with respect to the VT type 1 QRS complex. This shock, however, proved to be unsuccessful. The third shock (IF₃) (240 J) is delivered in a place where it was possible to change from VT-1 to VT-2 after a pacing burst (Fig. 33–2). In this place, which also exhibited prematurity in the VT cycle (−75 msec), a single shock of 240 J (IF₃) ablated both VT-1 and VT-2 (20 msec indicates the zone where the VT onset was not clearly defined).

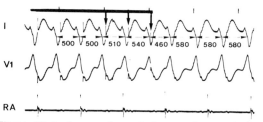

Figure 33–5. A case of ventricular entrainment during pacing the area of slow conduction. Pacing is achieved in the zone proximal to the slow conducting pathway. The last spikes *(last vertical arrow on the right)* fall inside VT QRS complexes but are able to achieve entrainment with unstable intraventricular conduction, leading to beat-to-beat tachycardia variation between 540 and 460 msec. The last QRS complexes are separated by the stable VT basic cycle length of 580 msec. RA = right atrium.

bility of the fulgurating electrode is maintained, it is possible to record flattening of the endocardial potential.[30]

After a 10-minute rest period to permit electrical and hemodynamic stabilization, programmed stimulation is resumed.

The main endpoints of the session are as follows:

1. Failure to induce a stable, monomorphic VT by a programmed pacing protocol equivalent to or more aggressive than that employed for initiating the VT required for mapping.

2. Spontaneous interruption in less than 1 minute of a previously sustained VT.

3. Induction of repeated episodes of acceleration of VT or VF after fulguration.

4. Repeated induction of VT, leading to hemodynamic deterioration.

5. Time limitation due to technical considerations (procedure lasting more than 8 hours).

6. Elective number of preprogrammed shocks in case of reinducibility.

Postoperative Surveillance

The patient's radial artery and venous blood pressures are monitored for 24 hours. A left subclavicular catheter is left at the apex of the right ventricle to permit reassessment of bedside VT reinduction, which is done at or within 10 days after fulguration, provided that no recurrence has happened spontaneously.

Regular electrocardiographic monitoring is done by computer during the 10-day interval, either by cable or by telemetrics (Hewlett-Packard HP 78225 system with the NADIA software, Andover, MA). All alarm signals are recorded. Graphs indicating trends in cardiac rhythm, extrasystole frequency, tachycardia, and so on can be printed out, and the data can be corrected, when necessary, by using the "recall" function.

When VT comparable to previous attacks either occurs spontaneously or is inducible, antiarrhythmic drug therapy is attempted again. This therapy includes amiodarone therapy, at a dosage of 400 mg/day or less, used alone or in combination with class I antiarrhythmic and/or beta-blocking agents. When the latter approach proves ineffective, fulguration therapy is reconsidered. Amiodarone is generally continued in cases in which the previous attacks of VT were life-threatening. In this situation a regimen of 400 mg/day or less is used. This is called "prophylactic" antiarrhythmic treatment (see Table 33–9). This category also includes patients who are taking

amiodarone for treatment of symptomatic extrasystoles. When drugs are necessary to prevent spontaneous or programmed pacing-induced VT, the treatment is called a "therapeutic" antiarrhythmic treatment. Table 33–9 lists the antiarrhythmic drugs administered at hospital discharge, whether therapeutically or prophylactically.

The effectiveness of fulguration is reassessed before the patient's discharge by use of 24-hour Holter recording, stress testing on a stationary bicycle, and programmed stimulation. This reassessment is done using a programmed pacing protocol, incorporating up to three extrastimuli on basic pacing cycles of 400 to 600 msec.

Follow-up

Total coverage of the outcome of this series of patients is based on the general computer (Digital Equipment DEC PDP 11/23+, Andover, MA) data bank of our department. A specialized application program has been developed to facilitate the follow-up. The same computer program is also used to process data obtained from the parallel study group of drug-treated patients who did not undergo fulguration.

Information on the patient given by the patient's physician, cardiologist, or family member is permanently updated in the computer system. In case of an absence of information, direct phone calls to the patient's home or a family member have proved to be the most practical form of follow-up. Despite the fact that one third of our patients were referred from other countries, no patient has been lost to follow-up. Follow-up time was computed from the difference between the first fulguration procedure and the current date. Each death was investigated to determine if it met the definition of "sudden death," which, according to our standard, is an unexpected death occurring within 1 hour after the first symptom.

Results

The 29-survivor follow-up is calculated from the first fulguration date to the current date. It extends from 17 to 60 months (mean value: 41.48 ± 12.55). The follow-up of nonsurvivors is calculated from the first fulguration date to the date of death, excluding early death. It extends from 1 to 22 months (mean value: 9.78 ± 7.48).

Success Rate with Ventricular Tachycardia and Management of Short-term Relapses

In view of the fact that five (case Nos. 5, 14, 16, 23, and 25) of the candidates for fulguration therapy were moribund and two (case Nos. 5 and 16) were already unconscious, the results were surprisingly favorable. Five (case Nos. 1, 5, 10, 19, and 35) early deaths occurred, however, during the learning phase, but none of the deaths seemed to be related to malignant arrhythmia or tamponade or to have occurred as a direct result of the fulguration itself. For reasons explained later, we chose to assess the success rate at 3 months after hospital discharge (Fig. 33–6).

Of the 43 patients on whom a first fulguration procedure was performed, 2 (case Nos. 19 and 35) died within a few days following the procedure. The follow-up study group is therefore limited to 41 cases. During reevaluation of the rhythm disorder after the first fulguration procedure, including the hospital stay and the follow-up period of up to 3 months, no VT relapse was observed in 13 patients. Therefore, a single session without

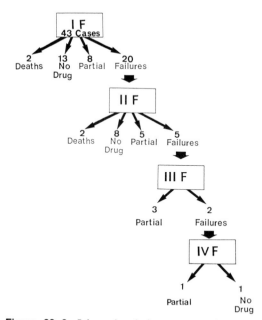

Figure 33–6. Schematic of the representation of the evolution of 43 consecutive cases of fulguration. The fulguration session is indicated in a square. "No drug" indicates that the patient is not receiving a therapeutic treatment to prevent relapses of VT. "Partial" means that VT recurrence has been controlled by drug treatment (the same treatment was not effective before fulguration). "Failures" identify patients who had relapses after a preceding fulguration session and whose condition was not controlled by antiarrhythmic treatment.

the need for drug therapy was able to prevent arrhythmia in 12 of 41 survivors (32 per cent; in this percentage we have included as a success of VT fulguration patient No. 5, who died after 8 days of a noncardiac cause; this case was nevertheless considered a success because this patient was referred while having incessant VT and no arrhythmia recurred before death). Spontaneous or induced VT occurred in 28 patients. Drug therapy, which was not effective before the fulguration procedure, became effective in 8 patients. As a result, the success rate increased to 21 cases (51 per cent) when, in these 8 cases (case Nos. 9, 21, 22, 24, 25, 29, 34, and 38), effective drug therapy after the first fulguration procedure was added.

The remaining 20 resistant patients were submitted to a new attempt. Two patients (Nos. 1 and 10) died during the second fulguration procedure. The study group in which the second fulguration procedure was used was therefore reduced to 18 cases, and the study population was decreased to 39 cases. After the second fulguration procedure, 8 more patients of the 18 survivors were brought under control without therapeutic drugs. At that point, the success rate became 74 per cent. Five more patients were controlled by drug therapy. Therefore, the combination of two fulguration procedures alone and in association with drug therapy led to the control of VT in 34 patients, for a success rate of 87 per cent. Spontaneous or induced VT recurred in 5 patients.

A third fulguration procedure was attempted, but in no case was this third fulguration procedure effective alone. However, drug therapy was effective in three patients. At this point in this analysis, 37 of the study population of 39 cases are considered successfully treated, which gives a success rate of 95 per cent. In only two patients was the VT not controlled. A fourth fulguration attempt was performed in these two last cases. Antiarrhythmic treatment was, however, necessary in both to achieve complete in-hospital prevention of VT. We then reach a success rate for fulguration for VT of 100 per cent. However, early (<3 months) recurrences of VT after discharge, although better tolerated, were observed on several occasions in two patients (Nos. 6 and 18). These cases were originally considered fulguration failures. However, after 3 months, these patients experienced no further episodes of VT despite progressive reduction of their antiarrhythmic treatment, with one now being classified as receiving only prophylactic therapy. He (No. 18) is taking amiodarone alone at 100 mg/day.

In summary, of 39 patients surviving the perioperative period, single or multiple VT was brought under control in all of them by means of one or more fulguration sessions, with 18 (46 per cent) requiring the help of a therapeutic regimen of antiarrhythmics following the fulguration therapy.

Mortality

During the overall period of this study, which extended up to 60 months, 13 deaths were observed, none of which were attributable to fulguration itself.

EARLY DEATH. Five deaths were early (less than 1 month after the procedure).

Cardiac Deaths. Two technically related deaths, leading to low cardiac output, occurred during the procedure. The first of these (case No. 1) involved a case of arrhythmogenic right ventricular dysplasia, successfully operated on 7 years previously but with recent recurrent episodes of life-threatening VT. Death was probably the consequence of a lack of hemodynamic monitoring (at the beginning of our experience) during the procedure. The second patient (No. 10) succumbed from an irreversible low cardiac output associated with a progressive decline of myocardial contractility. A few minutes before the patient died, external heart massage was administered following a single external defibrillation shock for VT acceleration.

Noncardiac Deaths. The first patient (No. 5), referred after multiple episodes of VT following angiography, was unconscious and in a state of incessant VT upon arrival. A series of 17 low-energy (160 J) shocks led to a reduction in the rate of VT, which stopped spontaneously a few hours later without the need for antiarrhythmic therapy. The patient nevertheless succumbed 8 days later from refractory hypoxemia due to preexisting extensive pulmonary infection. No recurrence of VT was observed until death.

Death also occurred in a patient (No. 19) with a low ejection fraction following an old myocardial infarction. He had been rejected as a candidate for surgical treatment. Delay in the resuscitation procedures resulted in irreversible brain damage and death 4 days after fulguration.

The third patient (No. 35) who died had very poor cardiac function due to idiopathic dilated cardiomyopathy; he also had pulmonary hypertension and was in permanent monomorphic VT for 2 years. He went into hemodynamic distress at the induction of anesthesia. This situation was, however, controlled after dopamine administration. Fulguration was therefore performed according to a previously indicated protocol (a single shock of 240 J was delivered). During the following night while the hemodynamic situation was under control, the patient developed hyperacute septic shock of unknown origin, resulting in cardiovascular collapse and anuria. In hyperkalemia, he finally succumbed 1 day after the procedure. VTs of different morphology were also observed before death. Autopsy was not possible.

Anatomic and histologic examinations were performed for patients Nos. 1, 5, and 10. They revealed myocardial modifications, which, when superimposed on the particular histologic structure of the underlying pathology, were similar to histologic lesions found in experimental animals following the application of endocavitary shock therapy.[16, 50]

LATE MORTALITY. Eight late deaths were observed.

CARDIAC DEATH

Sudden Death. Three cases (Nos. 22, 24, and 29) met the criteria for sudden death 4, 14, and 22 months after the fulguration procedure. These deaths were considered the consequence of VT relapses and will be discussed in detail later.

Congestive Heart Failure. Patient No. 20 died 1 month after discharge from acute pulmonary edema without recurrence of VT. The patient, suffering from severe triple-vessel coronary artery disease with poor distal vessels, a low ejection fraction, cardiomegaly, and left-sided ventricular failure, was not a surgical candidate. Patient No. 30 was diagnosed as having idiopathic dilated cardiomyopathy; death resulted from pulmonary edema 3 months following fulguration, with no recurrence of major rhythm disturbance. Patient No. 23 died of cardiac failure 10 months after the fulguration procedure while on an effective therapeutic regimen of antiarrhythmic drugs.

NONCARDIAC DEATH

Two patients (Nos. 11 and 31) died of noncardiac conditions. All the preceding late deaths occurred outside the hospital, and therefore, autopsy was not possible.

Complications

Acute pulmonary edema was observed in 3 patients (Nos. 14, 16, and 28) during the first 10 minutes after fulguration. The problem was, however, manageable with standard therapy.

In one case (No. 6) during the second fulguration session, the patient experienced chest pain associated with modification of the ST segment and transient right bundle branch block. The rise in the Creatine Kinase (CK) and particularly the CK, MB fraction, was 140 IU, greater than that observed in the other patients treated (37 ± 15 SD).

Transient complete AV block was frequently observed in the course of the procedure and occurred immediately after the shocks (17 per cent of 167 shocks). In two cases (Nos. 14 and 16) only, it persisted after the session and resolved in a maximum of 2 hours (case No. 16). Intraventricular conduction anomalies of short duration were also noted (167 shocks, 8 per cent left bundle branch block and 5 per cent right bundle branch block).

VT acceleration and VF were observed equally in 15 per cent of the shocks immediately following the initial electrical discharge. The patients were easily defibrillated,[71] except for two (Nos. 19 and 35), one of whom was in acute hemodynamic cardiac failure (No. 19) and the other of whom was in hypoxia. However, no malignant arrhythmia resistant to defibrillation was observed following fulguration.

One pacemaker patient (No. 20) in whom the fulguration shocks were delivered close to the ventricular pacing electrode needed generator replacement.

Long-term Relapse of Ventricular Tachycardia

According to the previous definition of success rate, long-term relapses mean relapses occurring more than 3 months after discharge. Relapses could be classified in the following categories:

RELAPSES BETTER TOLERATED AND DISREGARDED

This situation was observed in three patients (Nos. 22, 24, and 29), of whom one (No. 22) was asymptomatic (this term means that the patient was not able to detect a relapse of VT by the feeling of rapid heart rate or palpitation despite possible indirect signs like dyspnea, fatigue, and gastrointestinal disorders). Patient No. 29 died suddenly 14 months after fulguration, when he was in a major phase of heart failure, owing to the terminal stage of an idiopathic dilated cardiomyopathy. Patient No. 24 had two forms of sustained VT elicited during programmed pacing. A fulguration procedure was performed and seemed to be effective for one form. The nonfulgurated VT was still inducible at the time of discharge, but the attacks were slower and better tolerated. Nondocumented sudden death occurred 4 months after the procedure, and it is unknown if this was due to recurrence of the fulgurated VT, degeneration of the nonfulgurated VT, or a different complication. Patient No. 22 was in incessant VT when the fulguration procedure was performed. Relapse was observed a few hours later, and at that time VT could be terminated by pacing. It was reproducibly demonstrated that a class Ic antiarrhythmic drug was then able to prevent VT. This drug had not been effective prior to the procedure. One year later, the patient was reevaluated by programmed pacing 1 week after discontinuation of the class Ic drug and was found to be noninducible. The patient took amiodarone only. Holter monitoring revealed nonsymptomatic VT at 110 beats per minute. Class Ic drug therapy was resumed without reinvestigation at Jean Rostand Hospital. The patient died suddenly 4 months later.

RELAPSES CONTROLLED BY DRUGS

Relapses controlled by drugs were observed in three cases. In case No. 34, a modification in drug therapy led to the control of the arrhythmia. This patient had a first relapse 12 months after fulguration during an attempt at reducing dosages of the two drugs given as treatment. Two more episodes were later observed after resumption of the original therapy. Finally, replacement of class Ic antiarrhythmic drugs by a beta-blocking agent continues to appear to prevent relapses.

In the second case (No. 27), amiodarone therapy used alone at a dosage of 200 mg/day controlled the arrhythmia. After 9 months, this drug was interrupted. The patient experienced relapse 1 month later. After a short hospital stay by the patient, amiodarone therapy was resumed and controlled the arrhythmia.

In case No. 6, several episodes of VT, some necessitating direct-current (DC) shocks, recurred after 34 months, when the patient was not receiving antiarrhythmic treatment. A dosage of 200 mg of amiodarone a day proved effective with a 9-month follow-up.

RELAPSES CONTROLLED BY REFULGURATION

This approach was used in six cases, with the second procedure proving successful, although in patient No. 12 some additional episodes were observed and finally disappeared. This pattern suggests the previously mentioned evolution of some of our early relapses. Patient No. 39 had relapses identical with previous episodes after 4 months and underwent successful refulguration. Patient No. 13 experienced frequent relapses of the same VT morphology 5 months after the first session. A new fulguration procedure performed in the same area proved successful with a follow-up of 15 months. Patient No. 38 experienced a syncopal relapse of VT 24 months after the fulguration. He denied this event for 10 months for professional reasons. Later, relapses became more frequent, and this patient has undergone a second fulguration procedure. Twenty-four month follow-up indicates that the patient benefited from the second attempt.

A relapse after 31 months was observed with patient No. 9. A new fulguration procedure controlled the arrhythmia with a follow-up of 16 months; however, five short episodes of nonsustained VT were observed transiently after 2 months. Amiodarone therapy was prescribed and proved to be successful.

Patient No. 41 had a first relapse after 6 months; the attacks became more and more frequent, and after a few months a situation identical with the initial situation was observed. A third procedure using three shocks at 240 J (higher energy than the previous attempts) was tried, and for 3 months the patient, who is not receiving drug therapy, has not experienced any new relapse.

Discussion of Results

In a larger population and with a longer follow-up, the overall results of our previous series confirm the favorable results reported by both Hartzler, in patients with idiopathic VT and to a lesser extent those with coronary artery disease,[39, 40] and Puech,[61] in a patient with arrhythmogenic right ventricular dysplasia. These authors reported the first cases of fulguration for the treatment of VT, adapting to this form of cardiac arrhythmia a technique derived from His bundle fulguration for indirectly treating supraventricular tachycardia.[36, 38, 64-66]

Other investigators have reported irregular

results in the management of VT with this technique.[4, 10, 12, 42, 48, 59, 62, 68, 75] In view of the very poor cardiac condition of most of our patients, we do not think that differences in the population of patients explain why we observed better results. We think, rather, that these differences could be explained by a difference in the selection of the equipment and methods. At the beginning of our experience (No. 14, second patient in the VT series) we observed that the vast majority of the regular USCI catheters were not able to withstand the high peak current and voltage necessary to create a sufficient effect on the endocardium. Discovery of the catheter problem was the result of a research protocol previously developed in the experimental laboratory in which endocardial signal amplitude and pacing threshold were evaluated before and after each shock. Failure to pace and to record in the bipolar mode when pacing and recording were possible at the same values in the unipolar mode indicated that the bipolar catheter was in short circuit. With the catheter being used in the unipolar mode for ablation, something difficult to understand did happen.[22] Because no alternative equipment was available, despite a screening of commercial catheters, we developed a technique for selection of USCI tripolar or quadripolar catheters by a nondestructive high-voltage test.[22, 23] As a result, we were able to demonstrate in some cases that a successful outcome could be obtained using a relatively low fulgurating energy delivered in a single shock.[29]

A second difference is that we originally decided to use the active electrode as an anode instead of a cathode because in vitro studies of the effect of shocks demonstrated that anodal shocks provided a stronger mechanical effect. We also observed, with electron microscopy, and recently with light microscopy, acute rupture of myofibrils at a distance of 1 cm from the fulguration site. Since it is well known that the stretch of myocardial fibers modifies cardiac conduction,[43] we choose to incorporate this parameter in our protocol. Recently, we have observed that the variation in waveforms generated by different types of defibrillators should also be taken into account. Limited in vitro experiments have shown that anodal shocks with fast rise times lead to stronger mechanical effects and tissue damage.

These three technical points (catheter selection, anodal shocks, and shock impulse waveform) therefore make difficult any comparison

between our group and others concerning the results obtained in animal experiments or in clinical situations. Results comparable to ours have been reported only recently by Warin and colleagues.[74] It is interesting that this group is using the same equipment in terms of defibrillator basic circuit and also is careful in regard to catheter selection. Therefore, we could not recommend the fulguration procedure as a simple technique that could be used in any place with any equipment. Further studies are necessary to elucidate the differences on a more scientific basis between our technique and the technique of the other groups.[13]

THE FULGURATION PROCESS

Physics

The technique of VT fulguration is still in a discovery phase, and many of its most basic aspects are at the present time only partially understood.[3, 32, 44, 45, 51, 52] The energy used for the fulguration procedure (several hundred Joules) is similar to the energy used for external defibrillation. However, in the fulguration procedure, the catheter tip is relatively small compared with a defibrillator paddle. Therefore, a large amount of energy is concentrated on a small area.

A high-temperature spark, estimated to be in the range of 5000 to 10,000°C, is produced. This temperature raises the surrounding water to the boiling point. Subsequently, a short-lived (10 msec) ionized vapor globe several centimeters in diameter is produced abruptly, giving rise to a first shock wave of small amplitude. When the bubble is built, a phenomenon known as a "cavitation bubble" is observed. After a phase of maximal expansion involving a second less rapid but stronger mechanical event, the cavitation bubble, which is in a definite lack of thermic balance compared with the surrounding medium and which is no longer receiving energy, begins to condense, loses ionization, shrinks in on itself, and finally collapses (Fig. 33–7). At that very moment, a second shock wave of larger amplitude (third mechanical event) is produced. During this phenomenon, nitrogen is extracted from the surrounding blood.[2] This collapse phenomenon is so strong that one or several cavitation bubbles could be observed (at least in saline) as a mechanical rebound.

The behavior of the cavitation bubble is

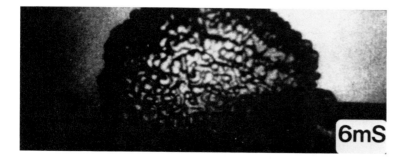

Figure 33–7. Immediately before the implosion (at the terminal phase of the cavitation bubble). The look of the vapor globe is extremely irregular. The surface irregularity could probably be related to an electrolysis phenomenon, which occurred at the periphery of the bubble.

different when it is produced against a wall as opposed to an unbounded fluid. In case of collapse of a bubble close to a solid wall, a reentrant jet with strong mechanical effects is produced.[8, 69] When the same experiment is made against a soft wall like a piece of myocardium, the bubble expansion produces a first phase of compression followed by a phase of suction and finally a phase of relaxation. All these phenomena are over within 10 msec. Therefore, a shearing effect, which could dissociate myocardial fibers, is produced. The resulting damage should largely exceed the size of the catheter tip.

Recently we have incorporated into our experiments a fiberoptic superimposing the timing of one or two electrical events on the photographic pictures recorded with high-speed cinematography. It is therefore possible to correlate the onset of the current flow with the beginning of bubble formation. This information, which was not available previously, demonstrated that for energies used clinically, development of the bubble is observed to be in the range of 400 to 1400 μsec or microseconds after the initial flow of current.

Therefore, before the growth of the cavitation bubble, an increasing amount of current flows from the catheter tip to the myocardium with a high current density. In contrast, as soon as the bubble is built, the current density around the sphere decreases rapidly, although in the absolute a larger amount of current is delivered.

During bubble growth, high-speed shadow cinematography has demonstrated a nonuniform lightening within the vapor globe, suggesting that at the end of the discharge the production of plasma inside the bubble is an unstable event. To investigate this phenomenon more thoroughly, we developed a technique in which the shocks were delivered against a wall of methylpolymethacrylate constituting the transparent bottom of a tank against which the electrode was applied. The bubble generated against the wall was hemi-

spheric, and its inside could be observed without optical distortion. A mirror inclined at 45 degrees reflected this image toward the high-speed camera. It was therefore observed that after a first phase of plasma formation unstable strands of plasma of different morphologies connected the electrode tip with the periphery of the bubble. This finding suggests that the flow of electricity at the periphery of the bubble is not homogeneous.

Therefore, the two main parameters of the fulguration procedure seem to be, on one hand, the flow of electricity with high density around the electrode tip at the beginning of the discharge and then the building of a cavitation bubble, which irradiates the current with a lower and irregular density around the bubble. This flow of electric current is grossly oriented between the active and the indifferent electrodes (only a part of it is, in fact, crossing the myocardium). On the other hand, the second parameter consists of at least two shock waves and a less abrupt but potentially more important phenomenon of gas expansion. Although the effect of electric current on the myocardium has been extensively discussed with respect to external defibrillation,[9, 11, 53, 67, 73] the same is not true for its endocavitary application.[50] The respective parts played by electrical and mechanical agents in the process of fulguration remain to be clarified.

Gross Pathologic Effects

The effect of the fulguration procedure on myocardium is better assessed after 1 or 2 weeks, when the size of the lesion created by the procedure can be evaluated and above all the development of or replacement by connective tissue can be observed. After an initial period during which shocks were delivered to dogs, we chose to perform the procedure on 80-kg pigs. We mainly studied the effects of 240-J shocks, this energy being the most frequently used in the clinical situation. Shocks were delivered by either tripolar or quadripolar USCI catheters selected to withstand voltages and currents used for fulguration or Cordis experimental unipolar catheters.

Shocks delivered in the right ventricle produced a transmural scar, and the epicardial aspect showed an ellipse of fibrous tissue softly bulging out with a length of 1.5 to 2.0 cm on the long axis and 1.0 to 1.5 cm along the short axis. In the left ventricle, the scar tissue was rarely transmural and generally involved three quarters of the lateral wall. In a particular experiment, shocks of high energies were delivered to the lateral wall, with the indifferent electrode located on the right posterior aspect of the thorax; gross examination indicated that the fibrotic tissue surrounded the place where the electrode was located but also extended within the middle of the free wall toward the position of the indifferent electrode.

Histologic Studies

In an acute study, the animal being sacrificed at the end of the experiment, electron microscopic studies performed 1.5 cm away from the catheter electrode tip showed, among other things, signs of rupture of myofibrils, a pattern strongly suggestive of a mechanical effect. We have more recently observed the possible equivalent with light microscopy. If these findings are confirmed, they could in part explain the problems with cardiac conduction produced by the shocks.

In a chronic study on the effect of the shocks, giant cells and particles were demonstrated in the area where the electrode tip was located, which could be the result of platinum vaporization produced by the shocks. In any case, the distinction between modified and the nonmodified tissues was clear cut, suggesting that the shocks were not supposed to be able to create a new arrhythmogenic substrate. However, in the pig, in which high-energy shocks were delivered, a patchy zone of normal and abnormal myocardium was observed. This finding could probably explain why this animal exhibited major ventricular arrhythmias during programmed pacing performed before sacrifice.

ELECTROPHYSIOLOGY

Ventricular Tachycardia Morphologies

The induction of VT by programmed pacing may lead to varied results. It is now well accepted that some forms of nonsustained or polymorphic VT induced by programmed pacing may not have clinical significance.[7] Therefore, only sustained, monomorphic VTs have been considered. However, programmed pacing can also induce episodes of VT not previously documented, the so-called "nonclinical" VTs. Because all the class I antiarrhythmic treatments are interrupted several days before the fulguration procedure, it is unlikely that they would alter the morphology of VT induced during the fulguration procedure.[47] We think that in most cases clinical as well as nonclinical VT should be considered for fulguration treatment.[57, 72] This recommendation was the result of strict analysis of some of our initial cases. One patient (No. 2) suffering from recurrent VT related to arrhythmogenic right ventricular dysplasia had two VT morphologies: One was clinically documented to originate in the diaphragmatic zone of the right ventricle, and the other, of different morphology, was induced only during programmed pacing and originated in the infundibular area. Fulguration was performed on the patient with clinical diaphragmatic VT. Programmed pacing both after 10 days and 1 month exhibited the nonclinical (nonfulgurated) VT. No spontaneous episode of this VT was observed during the follow-up (54 months). We therefore concluded after this initial case that only those patients with clinical episodes should be considered for the fulguration procedure.

A second patient (No. 7) was referred with similar clinical and electrophysiologic patterns. However, in this case the so-called nonclinical (nonfulgurated) VT recurred spontaneously a few weeks later, leading to a second fulguration procedure, which proved successful. It was therefore concluded that nonclinical VT could become clinical in the long run and should be considered for treatment. The next patient (No. 15) had several morphologies of VT; a thorough analysis of the data demonstrated that several fulguration procedures were necessary to ablate each VT morphology. It was thus confirmed that each sustained, monomorphic VT morphology, clinical as well as nonclinical, required fulguration.

The second change in our protocols, suggested by this finding and confirmed by case No. 15, was to concentrate on VT morphology in the evaluation of the results. Therefore, we judged the efficacy of the procedure in terms of the effect of ablation on each VT morphology instead of on the occurrence of any relapse of VT.[72] On this basis, it is possible to understand that generally speaking, patients with multiple VT morphologies will require more shocks and more sessions than patients with single, monomorphic VTs.

On the other hand, we have also observed patients in whom a single shock was able to ablate more than one VT morphology (case No. 26, reported in Figures 33–2 and 33–4).

Endocardial Catheter Mapping

Evaluation of the endocavitary potential as a marker for determining the fulguration site yielded bleak findings. However, we came to the conclusion that the absence of presystolic activity led invariably to failures. On the other hand, our results indicate that success was generally greater in cases in which high-amplitude presystolic VT potential had a definite prematurity.[30]

Manipulation of the catheter all over the large area of the endocardium, although theoretically possible, requires expertise and appropriate training. Thorough investigation of the endocardium in preparation for fulguration seems to be more critical than the endocardial mapping needed prior to an open heart surgical procedure. In this latter situation, the direct view of the lesions provides an additional marker. In addition, surgical action of any type is, in fact, never restricted to the limited area of endocardium determined by mapping.[55] The area of resection is extended by the resection of an amount of scar tissue based on anatomic criteria. Therefore, the area of endocardial resection is larger than the area determined by either the preoperative or the perioperative mapping. This observation probably partly explains the questionable long-term results reported recently.[56]

RESULTS OF FULGURATION

Success Rate

Fulguration appears to be a new milestone in the treatment of chronic, stable VTs. We have seen that a success rate for VT of 100 per cent was finally achieved. This confirmed, with a *significant* series of patients, our former views concerning the effectiveness of limited physical action for the long-term prevention of VT. However, this result was achieved with great pains by a group that invested a lot of time and expertise in the management of difficult cases.

There is now no doubt that at least in some cases the procedure is effective. In seven cases (Nos. 3, 7, 14, 16, 32, 34, and 40), a single fulguration shock of an amplitude varying between 160 and 240 J was sufficient to prevent recurrence of VT without the need for therapeutic administration of antiarrhythmic agents. This finding suggests that the injury produced by a single shock is able to modify the pathologic substrate that was the basis of a life-threatening arrhythmia. This finding also confirms a previously reported similar observation that a minor surgical action (simple ventriculotomy) was able to prevent recurrence of resistant VT.[25, 27] However, because of the limited endocardial surface modified by the shock, we have to stress that precise endocardial mapping is probably a crucial prerequisite for the success of the procedure. On a theoretical basis, it should be more appropriate to deliver the fulgurating shock to the area of slow conduction, provided that this area is indeed a necessary link for the perpetuation of the arrhythmia rather than the "site of origin" of VT, which is, in any case, located near normal myocardium. Recent data from our laboratory suggest that this goal could be achieved successfully in at least some cases.[17, 34, 58]

On the other hand, the need for several shocks per session, the need for several sessions in some cases, and a relatively high rate of early relapses requiring antiarrhythmic therapy or refulguration suggest that fulguration is not, for the time being, an "ideal" form of therapy.

Early Relapses

In some cases, recurrences are easily ascribed to technical difficulties involving the catheter,[22] leading to insufficient energy output (case No. 14), on the one hand, and fulguration performed too far from the zone of origin of the VT, on the other (cases Nos. 16 and 18). Other recurrences are less easily accounted for and allow only the formulation of hypotheses: inadequate mapping; arrhythmogenic area extending beyond the zone benefiting from fulguration, thus partially inhibiting abnormal activation; and increasing sensitivity to antiarrhythmic agents. The chances of a favorable, spontaneous evolution of the disease need to be yet determined. However, the fact that some patients were cured after a transient period of relapses led us to postulate that fulguration has delayed effects. Several investigators have seen the late development of AV conduction impairment several weeks or months after a seemingly inadequate fulguration procedure aimed at His bundle ablation.

Late Relapses

Late relapses are frequently difficult to analyze, as are postsurgical results. It is quite possible that in some patients the recurrences could be due to healing of the tissue transiently modified by the shocks; again, a similar behavior has been observed after initially successful His bundle ablation. It could also be that in the long run a new zone of slow conduction, which was not previously fulfilling the conditions for reentry, could become operative. This is probably another phenomenon related to the small myocardial damage produced by the fulguration procedure. When a new VT is created, it could be hemodynamically acceptable and manageable by regular drug therapy. However, it could be also life threatening.

Experience gained during follow-up prompted us to realize the need for an implantable device for both arrhythmia detection and possible temporary treatment.

Three patients died suddenly during the follow-up, 17 patients (45 per cent) required two or more sessions, and 15 patients (44 per cent) needed antiarrhythmic therapy. Two points should be mentioned. (1) The current precision of mapping is probably not sufficient; this is suggested by the need for several shock sessions and for antiarrhythmic therapy in most of the cases. (2) The amount of modified tissue is probably too restricted. The condition of myocardial contractility after the shock and the small amount of CK MB fraction suggest that a more aggressive physical agent could be employed.

From a practical standpoint, the present techniques require general anesthesia and a large number of personnel and are long and difficult; therefore, this technique is limited to dedicated centers. Despite the fact that fulguration itself could be perfected, other ablative techniques should be considered.

This new update of our series incorporates five more patients. The surprisingly good results obtained at the beginning of our experience, despite the extremely poor condition of some patients, have probably contributed to the referral of less critical cases. Therefore, it is now possible to present data concerning a special form of VT difficult to treat by regular antiarrhythmic agents. This is a verapamil-sensitive VT observed in young patients with an otherwise normal heart.[70] Despite the need for more than one session in three of the four cases, fulguration seems to be an appropriate form of therapy in this particular subgroup.

Mortality

Owing to the experimental character of this study, patients referred at the beginning of our investigations were mainly in a high-risk group for whom the fulguration procedure was a last resort. Therefore, their cardiac function was generally poor. In the overall series, an ejection fraction below 30 per cent was documented in 15 cases. This finding mainly explains the high mortality observed at the beginning of this study. On the other hand, unexpected good results obtained in desperate cases prompted us to concentrate all our efforts on the study of this new and surprising technique.

Three patients (Nos. 5, 14, and 16) were moribund when effective fulguration was performed. At least 11 cases (Nos. 5, 10, 14, 16, 19, 20, 23, 25, 29, 30, and 35) involved prohibitive surgical risks. None died of the immediate effect of the endocardial electric shocks.

It is possible that two deaths early in the study could have been avoided: the first (No. 1) by hemodynamic monitoring and the second (No. 19) by avoiding a real-time modification of an anesthetic protocol that was not properly reviewed. However, these cases were thoroughly reviewed, the mechanism of the catastrophe was understood, the protocols were subsequently modified, and the same situation was no longer observed. The six deaths (Nos. 5, 10, 20, 23, 30, and 35) have been interpreted as consequences of the evolution of preexistent pathologic processes. In the first case (No. 5) and in the second (No. 10), death was foreseen as inevitable in view of a precarious hemodynamic situation. It should be recalled that the cases included in the series were consecutive. No patient was excluded. In four cases (Nos. 20, 23, 30, and 35), clinical evidence of deterioration of myocardial function apart from the rhythm disorder had been observed during the period preceding fulguration.

The three last patients (Nos. 22, 24, and 29) died suddenly. The death of patient No. 24 was critical. In this patient, the nonfulgurated, less rapid VT was still inducible at the time of discharge; recurrences did happen but were better tolerated. In retrospect, this patient, who was not in definite cardiac failure, would have been a candidate for other investigational forms of therapy (implantable defibrillator or another fulguration procedure). The sudden death of patient No. 22 is also critical; this patient had an ejection fraction of 46 per cent, and the cardiac failure observed at the time of nonsymptomatic VT was probably related more to the arrhythmia than to intrinsic cardiac contractility. The question of out-of-hospital patient surveillance must be raised; some form of continuous Holter monitoring with an implantable device is mandatory. In any case, this patient should have had this arrhythmia completely reevaluated when the nonsymptomatic VT was discovered. Here again, an implantable defibrillator or a new fulguration procedure could have been considered. In case No. 29, sudden death occurred 14 months after the procedure. Despite documented episodes of VT, preterminal deterioration of cardiac function did not prompt us to attempt a repeat fulguration; a new fulguration procedure or an implantable defibrillator could have been considered.

This experience of sudden death in three patients with symptoms or documented episodes of VT relapses led us to change our policy and to consider refulguration in case of late relapses.

Secondary Effects

Cardiac Output

In some cases, cardiac function was assessed 7 days after the procedure by two-dimensional echocardiography and yielded normal values. However, the results of hemodynamic studies demonstrate that there is a temporary drop in cardiac output after the procedure but that output reverts to its control values within 10 to 15 minutes after the shocks.[37] In addition, the small amount of CK MB fraction, obtained after the shocks made this concern less important. This finding was also in agreement with some experimental data from our laboratory that indicate that following endocavitary fulguration delivered to a healthy endocardium (pig weighing 80 kg), the left ventricular cardiac output decreases by 10 to 15 per cent for approximately 10 minutes. One of the cases of acute pulmonary edema (No. 14) in our series was, however, probably related to the fulguration of nearly normal myocardium distant from the area of infarction.

Arrhythmias

Episodes of VT acceleration or VF brought on by fulguration or occurring during pro-

grammed VT activation were occasionally observed; all of these arrhythmias represented minor electrophysiologic events and were immediately brought under control by instant defibrillation.[71] Such episodes further demonstrate the necessity of situating the defibrillating electrode in an anterior position to avoid emergency removal of sterile surgical fields and fluoroscopic equipment.

No malignant ventricular arrhythmia was observed after the procedure. However, extrasystoles were frequent, and new forms of sustained VT were even observed in some patients, especially in those without coronary artery disease; but these arrhythmias disappeared after a few days and did not seem to represent the creation of a new arrhythmogenic substrate.

Myocardial Infarction

The case of myocardial infarction (No. 6) observed during the fulguration procedure was the consequence of difficulty encountered during manipulation of the catheter in the root of the aorta in an attempt to reenter the ventricle after inadvertent withdrawal. Subsequent review of the magnetic tapes revealed that during the left-sided catheter insertion the patient, who was not yet asleep, complained of chest pain, which was rapidly followed by progressive ST-segment modification and right bundle branch block. At the same time, voice channel data from the magnetic tape recorder indicated that the catheter tip appeared to be blocked in the root of the aorta. Myocardial ischemia, resulting in a definite increase in the CK isoenzyme, MB fraction, was therefore produced. Modification of the technique employed subsequently eliminated this risk, which could be critical. Our experimental studies have shown that a discharge of 240 J in the coronary artery of an 80-kg pig resulted in instantaneous irreversible hemodynamic failure caused by rupture of this vessel and subsequent tamponade.

Effect on a Permanent Pacemaker and Implantable Defibrillator

A defect in the functioning of one patient's pacemaker (No. 20) at the time of fulguration required replacement of the generator. This risk is higher in case of a unipolar device, and malfunctioning might not be obvious after the shock. Thorough evaluation of pacemaker pacing safety margin and sensing and programming functions is mandatory before as well as after the fulguration procedure.[6, 31]

Despite the fact that no systematic study has

been made, it is probable that an implantable defibrillator could be rendered completely ineffective. Since any patient who has an implantable defibrillator could present with incessant episodes needing a more radical approach because of repeated episodes of VT or VF, it may be necessary to disconnect the implantable defibrillator temporarily before delivering the fulgurating shocks.

Alternative Therapy and Patient Selection

Selection of patients for the fulguration procedure was one of the most difficult parts of our approach. In most cases, this therapeutic approach was in competition with the alternative drug treatment, for which we had ongoing studies evaluating investigational antiarrhythmic agents. Major decisions were taken after a staff meeting including the three most experienced members of the group (G. Fontaine, R. Frank, and J. Tonet).

We have learned from some cases that so-called resistant and almost incessant VT is not the result of ineffectiveness of drug therapy but rather the proarrhythmic effect of the drugs. Two examples illustrate this point. A case of ischemic cardiomyopathy involving three-vessel disease studied with the arrhythmia monitoring computer system demonstrated a direct relationship between the amount of a class Ic antiarrhythmic agent given in combination with amiodarone and the number of nonsustained episodes of VT or extrasystoles or both. Reduction in the dosage of the class Ic antiarrhythmic agent led to a decrease in the number of shorter runs of nonsustained VT, followed by obvious clinical improvement. Heart transplant was nevertheless indicated and performed, but the patient was referred to the surgical department in a definitely better clinical condition without need of the fulguration procedure originally planned by the referring center.

In another patient treated with multiple antiarrhythmic drugs for VT after a myocardial infarction and finally referred as a good candidate for fulguration, study of documented episodes of VT showed that *torsades de pointes*–like VT was preceded by QT prolongation. This pattern was mixed with other VT monomorphic in nature preceded by a normal QT interval. Interruption of treatment with antiarrhythmic agents led to suppression of most of the VTs and to clinical improvement in a few days. After that time only mono-morphic VTs were observed and were easily treated with a loading dose followed by a maintenance dose of amiodarone. No fulguration was necessary.

These examples stress the importance of correctly evaluating the arrhythmia before the procedure; should these patients have undergone fulguration, the interruption of drug therapy would have led to an absence of relapses wrongly interpreted as successful fulguration.

To put our results in perspective, we compared them with the overall results in terms of global mortality and relapse from the original cohort of 117 consecutive patients with chronic, stable VTs. Almost all of these so-called resistant cases were reevaluated in terms of antiarrhythmic treatment. It appeared that only one third needed the fulguration procedure. This finding suggests that two thirds of cases were controlled by drug therapy (only one patient was referred for surgery). This study has already been presented in part[26] and was done from a review of the outcome of patients not undergoing fulguration, available in April 1986. Therefore, this comparison is valid vis-á-vis the results of 31 fulguration cases in the same period.

The global mortality in the group of patients not undergoing fulguration was 15 cases (21 per cent), with 6 cases of sudden death (8 per cent). Relapses were observed in five patients who survived and six patients who died, yielding a relapse rate of 15 per cent.

In the population undergoing fulguration, a suitable comparison should omit the patients who died because of inappropriate protocols (three cases: Nos. 1, 19, and 35). The global mortality was 7, calculated from 35 survivors (20 per cent), and sudden death occurred in 3 patients (8 per cent). Long-term relapses were observed in 4 patients out of 35 survivors (11 per cent).

Finally, despite the small number of patients in each series and the relatively short follow-up, it was possible to conclude in April 1986 that the fulguration procedure associated with drug therapy yields results comparable to those with drug treatment alone. However, because fulguration was performed only in patients resistant to drug therapy and in particularly poor condition, it is suggested that this form of treatment provides a definite adjunct in the management of ventricular arrhythmias. It is also concluded that refulguration should clearly be considered when a patient who has previously undergone fulguration presents with relapses.

Limitations of the Study

On the basis of our studies, we conclude that fulguration is a safe and effective form of therapy for VT. Nevertheless, many points could be criticized. A limited number will now be mentioned:

1. There is a bias in the population of patients. For instance, since our population was a second or third generation of so-called resistant cases, it does not provide a valid sampling of the population at large and represents only a high-risk group.

Because of the unpredictable outcome of the fulguration procedure, as suggested by some clinical reports[5, 35, 39, 41, 49, 54] and laboratory experiments, preselection of patients was particularly restricted at the beginning of our experience. The technique was used as a last resort, and its use was restricted to the most resistant and difficult cases that were beyond operability; some patients were even moribund when the fulguration procedure was performed.[29]

Observing how well the procedure was tolerated, we extended its use to the most difficult cases of dilated idiopathic cardiomyopathy to learn about the possible limits of this method (case Nos. 30 and 35).

2. Patients referred to us tended to be a particular type with a primary electrical disease and in whom other indications of cardiac surgery were not present (rather, we had to treat some patients who had VT after surgery for cardiac revascularization or even after antiarrhythmia surgery).

3. The experience accumulated over years with surgical procedures tends to bring to our centers patients with VT related to noncoronary diseases like arrhythmogenic right ventricular disease and right bundle branch block with left-axis VT in young adults.[70] In other countries, and especially in the United States, patients with post–myocardial infarction VT are primarily considered. This observation could also reflect the prevalence of the basic disease, which is different in different countries. In addition, it is obvious that the arrhythmogenic substrate is different if we compare the borderline zone of an old myocardial infarction with the right ventricular wall in a case of arrhythmogenic right ventricular dysplasia. Therefore, it may be appropriate to adapt the endocardial shock procedure to the underlying disease.

4. Some bias could also be introduced in each step of our study that does not follow the same antiarrhythmic protocol. It could be that a combination of drugs that was effective after fulguration could have been effective before the procedure if the same combination had been used.

5. The learning phase has introduced some variations concerning both the protocols and the equipment.

6. A limitation in the evaluation of arrhythmia control also results from the fact that after treatment a previously symptomatic patient could become asymptomatic owing to a slower rate of tachycardia, negative inotropic effect of antiarrhythmic treatment, or spontaneous degeneration of cardiac function. Later reevaluation by invasive methods was performed in one case (No. 22), and rehospitalization and monitoring were necessary in another case (No. 33) 1 year after the procedure. In one case (No. 2), attempts to reinduce VT were done with burst pacing through a radiofrequency pacemaker connected with a catheter located at the right ventricular apex during the few months following the procedure.

7. When a patient with incessant VT enters the electrophysiologic laboratory, complete disappearance of the arrhythmia is a clear-cut effect of the treatment (the possible proarrhythmic effects of antiarrhythmic drugs have been already discussed). This situation was observed in 90 per cent of the cases in this series. An algorithm to determine when a VT should be considered ablated is not available at the present time. To figure out the clinical impression of the VTs observed in this series, we have included in Table 33–9 the number of VT episodes, the shortest as well as the longest time elapsed between two VT episodes, and the paroxysmal or incessant nature of the arrhythmia.

A particular problem concerns the long-term evaluation of the effectiveness of the procedure. Case No. 9 is an example. This patient had only two episodes of badly tolerated VT, with a time interval between attacks of 6 months. One documented relapse of VT with the same morphology occurred 3 months after discharge and then disappeared. Recently, a new relapse was observed 25 months after the last episode. In the same episode, two morphologies were observed. One was similar to the previous documented episode, and the other happened to exhibit a new morphology. Was this a new VT due to the evolution of an unstable myocardium (arrhythmogenic right ventricular disease) or was it the relapse of the fulgurated VT?

8. The fact that treatment with antiarrhythmic agents is frequently needed is not in our view a sign of failure but, rather, a sign of incomplete effectiveness of the procedure, in the same way that several shocks are frequently needed in the same session or that several sessions are needed for a particular patient.

Many questions concerning the treatment of VT by fulguration remain to be answered. Little is known about the cellular modification of the arrhythmogenic substrate resulting from the electrical discharge. The various mechanical factors involved need clarification. How important is the positioning of the indifferent electrode? Which electrical parameters are the most reliable? What should be the size and shape of fulguration electrodes? What are the best criteria for choosing the fulguration target?[49]

Despite the fact that the pacemapping technique needs to be fully perfected, it nevertheless has proved to be highly valuable in some cases when VT could not be induced during the session. With the guidance of this method, it was possible to deliver discharges that proved to be effective in some patients.

The predictive value of VT reinduction during sessions is relatively unreliable. In general, it seemed at first view that 50 per cent of recurrences took place in patients in whom it was not possible to reinduce VT at the end of the session. However, a more thorough analysis of VT morphology demonstrated that the recurrences were mainly observed in the non-fulgurated VTs,[72] and in all of the patients who remained inducible, a spontaneous recurrence was observed. Better results were obtained, however, 10 days after fulguration, although fulguration completely failed in one case (No. 18). Nor can the protocol of reevaluation on the tenth day account for modifications apt to develop over a longer period. It might be too early for long-term evaluation, since stabilization of the lesion on myocardium generally needs a longer time. In addition, the possible modifications induced inside the fibrous tissue created by the procedure may need an even longer time, which could be extended to several months before the stage of stable, retractile fibrosis is reached. As usual, it is difficult to extrapolate to humans results obtained in animal experiments. In this latter situation, shocks have generally been delivered to normal myocardium.

Measurement of the myocardial isoenzyme CK MB fraction revealed low values (38 ± 15 IU) comparable to the values obtained after invasive explorations like angiography and electrophysiologic study, confirming what we noted in experimental studies: The myocardial area altered by the endocavitary shock is limited to a small zone of myocardium.[50] Consequently, fulguration may be performed without danger one or more times when the result has not been adequate on the first attempt, before the procedure is determined to be ineffective. In our experience, another attempt at fulguration was always preferred by the patients to its cardiovascular surgical counterpart!

CONCLUSIONS

In conclusion, the experience with VT fulguration collected over a 6-year period suggests that fulguration is effective in preventing VT relapses and is a promising alternative to drug treatment and other forms of palliative as well as curative therapy. However, although the results are dramatic, the technique is generally difficult. Data suggest that by a modification of the technique a simpler procedure could be developed in which a greater area of tissue could be modified. We think that in the management of VT, surgery is effective but is limited to a selected group of patients and is probably too damaging a procedure; in contrast, fulguration seems to produce too little damage to be easily effective.

REFERENCES

1. Bardy GH, Coltorti F, Ivey TD, et al: Effect of damped sine-wave shocks on catheter dielectric strength. Am J Cardiol 56:769–772, 1985.
2. Bardy GH, Coltorti F, Ivey TD, et al: Some factors affecting bubble formation with catheter-mediated defibrillator pulses. Circulation 73:525–538, 1986.
3. Bardy GH, Coltorti F, Ivey TD, et al: Effects of high-energy electrical shocks delivered to the ostium of the coronary sinus. In Scheinman MM (ed): Catheter Ablation of Cardiac Arrhythmias. Boston, Martinus Nijhoff, 1988, pp 67–96.
4. Belhassen B, Miller HI, Geller E, Laniado S: Transcatheter electrical shock ablation of ventricular tachycardia. J Am Coll Cardiol 7:1347–1355, 1986.
5. Bharati S, Scheinman MM, Morady F, et al: Sudden death after catheter-induced atrioventricular junctional ablation. Chest 88:883–889, 1985.
6. Bowes RJ, Bennett DH: Effect of transvenous atrioventricular nodal ablation on the function of implanted pacemakers. PACE 8:811–814, 1985.
7. Brugada P, Green M, Abdollah H, Wellens HJJ: Significance of ventricular arrhythmias initiated by programmed ventricular stimulation: The importance of the type of ventricular arrhythmia induced

and the number of premature stimuli required. Circulation 69:87–92, 1984.

8. Chahine GL: Etude locale du phénomène de cavitation: Analyse des facteurs régissant la dynamique des interfaces. Thèse de Doctorat ès Sciences, Paris, 1979.

9. Dahl CF, Ewy GA, Warner ED, Thomas ED: Myocardial necrosis from direct current countershock: Effect of paddle electrode size and time interval between discharges. Circulation 50:956–961, 1974.

10. Downar E, Parson I, Cameron DA, et al: Unipolar and bipolar catheter ablation techniques for management of ventricular tachycardia: Initial experience. J Am Coll Cardiol 5:472, 1985.

11. Ehsani A, Ewy GA, Sobel BE: Effects of electrical countershock on serum creatine phosphokinase (CPK) isoenzyme activity. Am J Cardiol 37:12–18, 1976.

12. Evans GT, Scheinman MM: Catheter ablation of ventricular tachycardia foci: a report of the Percutaneous Cardiac Mapping and Ablation Registry [abstract]. Circulation 74[Suppl II]:460, 1986.

13. Fisher JD, Brodman R, Waspe LE, Kim SG: Nonsurgical electrical ablation (fulguration) of tachycardias. Circulation 75[Suppl III]:194–199, 1987.

14. Fisher JD, Brodman R, Johnson D, et al: Nonsurgical electrical ablation of tachycardia: Importance of in vitro testing of catheter leads. PACE 7:74–81, 1984.

15. Fontaine G: Prevention of sudden arrhythmic death: Catheter ablation. In Proceedings of the 1985 Sydney Opera House Symposium. Sydney, Telectronics Vectors, October 1986, pp 18–21.

16. Fontaine G: The effects of high-energy DC shocks delivered to ventricular myocardium. In Scheinman MM (ed): Catheter Ablation of Cardiac Arrhythmias. Boston, Martinus Nijhoff, 1988, pp 97–114.

17. Fontaine G: Du lieu d'origine á la zone á conduction lente: Application au traitement de la tachycardie ventriculaire. Arch Mal Coeur 81:145, 1988.

18. Fontaine G, Cansell A: Potential risk of using multipolar catheters for the treatment of tachycardias. Stimarec Bull 5–6:1, 1983.

19. Fontaine G, Frank R, Tonet J, Grosgogeat Y: Ablating the slow conduction zone during ventricular tachycardia: Criteria for the critical circuit [abstract]. PACE [in press].

20. Fontaine G, Cansell A, Frank R, et al: Catheter ablation techniques for ventricular tachycardia. In Samet P, El-Sherif N (eds): Cardiac Pacing and Electrophysiology. New York, Grune and Stratton, [in press].

21. Fontaine G, Cansell A, Lampe L, et al: Endocavity fulguration (electrode catheter ablation): Equipment—related problems. In Fontaine G, Scheinman MM (eds): Ablation in Cardiac Arrhythmias. Mount Kisco, NY, Futura Publishing Co, 1987, pp 85–100.

22. Fontaine G, Cansell A, Lechat P, et al: Les chocs electriques endocavitaires: Problèmes lies au materiel. Arch Mal Coeur 77:1307–1314, 1984.

23. Fontaine G, Cansell A, Lechat P., et al: Method of selecting catheters for endocavitary fulguration. Stimucoeur 12:285–289, 1984.

24. Fontaine G, Cansell A, Tonet JL, et al: Techniques and methods for catheter endocardial fulguration. PACE 11:592–602, 1988.

25. Fontaine G, Frank R, Bonnet M, et al: Methode d'étude expérimentale et clinique des syndromes de Wolff-Parkinson-White et d'ischemie myocardique par cartographie de la depolarisation ventriculaire epicardique. Coeur Med Interne 12:105, 1973.

26. Fontaine, G, Frank R, Tonet JL, et al: Treatment of resistant ventricular tachycardia by endocavitary fulguration and antiarrhythmic therapy in 111 consecutive patients followed for 18 months. In Breithardt G, Borggrefe M, Zipes DP (eds): Nonpharmacological Therapy of Tachyarrhythmias. Mount Kisco, NY, Futura Publishing Co, 1987, pp 263–284.

27. Fontaine G, Guiraudon G, Frank R, et al: La cartographie épicardique et le traitement chirurgical par simple ventriculotomie de certaines tachycardies ventriculaires rebelles par réentree. Arch Mal Coeur 68:113–124, 1975.

28. Fontaine G, Tonet JL, Frank R, et al: La fulguration endocavitaire: Une nouvelle méthode de traitement des troubles du rhythme? Ann Cardiol Angeiol 33:543–561, 1984.

29. Fontaine G, Tonet JL, Frank R, et al: Traitement d'urgence de la tachycardie ventriculaire chronique après infarctus du myocarde par la fulguration endocavitaire. Arch Mal Coeur 78:1037–1043, 1985.

30. Fontaine G, Tonet JL, Frank R, et al: Traitement des tachycardies ventriculaires rebelles par fulguration endocavitaire associée aux anti-arythmiques. Arch Mal Coeur 79:1152–1162, 1986.

31. Fontaine G, Touil F, Frank R, et al: Defibrillation, fulguration et cardioversion: Effets sur les pacemakers. Stimucoeur 12:91, 1984.

32. Fontaine G, Volmer W, Nienaltowska E, et al: Approach to the physics of fulguration. In Fontaine G, Scheinman MM (eds): Ablation in Cardiac Arrhythmias. Mount Kisco, NY, Futura Publishing Co, 1987, pp 101–116.

33. Frank R, Fontaine G, Baraka M, et al: Catheter endocardial mapping in fulguration. In Aliot E, Lazzara R (eds): Ventricular Tachycardias: From Mechanism to Therapy. Dordrecht, the Netherlands, Martinus Nijhoff, 1987, pp 390–402.

34. Frank R, Tonet JL, Kounde S, et al: Localization of the area of slow conduction during ventricular tachycardia. In Brugada P, Wellens HJJ (eds): Cardiac Arrhythmias: Where to Go from Here? Mount Kisco, NY, Futura Publishing Co, 1987, pp 191–208.

35. Gallagher JJ: Ablation by transcatheter shock: Current status. Chest 88:804–806, 1985.

36. Gallagher JJ, Svenson RH, Kasell JH, et al: Catheter technique for closed-chest ablation of the atrioventricular conduction system. N Engl J Med 306:194–200, 1982.

37. Gallais Y, Touzet M, Gateau O, et al: Anesthésie et surveillance dans la fulguration endocavitaire pour le traitement radical des tachycardies ventriculaires. Ann Cardiol Angeiol 35:539–549, 1986.

38. Gonzalez R, Scheinman MM, Margaretten W, Rubinstein M: Closed chest electrode—catheter technique for His bundle ablation in dogs. Am J Physiol 241:H283–H287, 1981.

39. Hartzler GO: Electrode catheter ablation of refractory focal ventricular tachycardia. J Am Coll Cardiol 2:1107–1113, 1983.

40. Hartzler GO, Giorgi LV: Electrode catheter ablation of refractory ventricular tachycardia: Continued experience. J Am Coll Cardiol 3:512, 1984.

41. Hartzler GO, Giorgi LV, Diehl AM, Hamaker WR: Right coronary spasm complicating electrode catheter ablation of a right lateral accessory pathway. J Am Coll Cardiol 6:250–253, 1985.

42. Henthorn RW, Cohen M, Anderson PG, et al: Pathological and clinical observations after catheter fulguration in man [abstract]. J Am Coll Cardiol 7:236, 1986.
43. Hoffman BF, Cranefield PF: Electrophysiology of the Heart. Mount Kisco NY, Futura Publishing Co, 1976.
44. Holt PM, Boyd EGCA: Hematologic effects of the high-energy endocardial ablation technique. Circulation 73:1029–1036, 1986.
45. Holt PM, Boyd EGCA: Bioelectric effects of high-energy, electrical discharges. *In* Scheinman MM (ed): Catheter Ablation of Cardiac Arrhythmias. Boston, Martinus Nijhoff, 1988, pp 1–36.
46. Holt PM, Smallpeice C, Deverall PB, et al: Ventricular arrhythmias: A guide to their localisation. Br Heart J 53:417–430, 1985.
47. Horowitz LN, Vetter VL, Harken AH, Josephson ME: Electrophysiologic characteristics of sustained ventricular tachycardia occurring after repair of tetralogy of Fallot. Am J Cardiol 46:446–452, 1980.
48. Huang SK, Marcus FI, Ewy GA: Clinical experience with endocardial catheter ablation for refractory ventricular tachycardia. J Am Coll Cardiol 5:473, 1985.
49. Josephson ME: Catheter ablation of arrhythmias. Ann Intern Med 101:234–237, 1984.
50. Lechat P, Fontaine G, Cansell A, Grosgogeat Y: Epicardial and endocardial myocardial damage related to catheter ablation techniques [abstract]. Eur Heart J 5 [Suppl 1]:258, 1984.
51. Lee BI, Rodriguez ER, Notargiacomo A, et al: Thermal effects of laser and electrical discharge on cardiovascular tissue: Implications for coronary artery recanalization and endocardial ablation. J Am Coll Cardiol 8:193–200, 1986.
52. Levine JH, Spear JF, Weisman HF, et al: The cellular electrophysiologic changes induced by high-energy electrical ablation in canine myocardium. Circulation 73:818–829, 1986.
53. Mandecki T, Giec L, Kargal W: Serum enzyme activities after cardioversion. Br Heart J 32:600–602, 1970.
54. Marchlinski FE, Flores BT, Buxton AE, et al: The automatic implantable cardioverter-defibrillator: Efficacy, complications and device failures. Ann Intern Med 104:481–488, 1986.
55. Mason JW, Stinson EB, Winkle RA, et al: Relative efficacy of blind left ventricular aneurysm resection for the treatment of recurrent ventricular tachycardia. Am J Cardiol 49:241–248, 1982.
56. McGiffin DC, Kirklin JK, Plumb VJ, et al: Survival and relief of life-threatening ventricular tachycardia after direct operations [abstract]. Circulation 74 [Suppl II]:460, 1986.
57. Miller JM, Kienzle MG, Harken AH, Josephson ME: Morphologically distinct sustained ventricular tachycardias in coronary artery disease: Significance and surgical results. J Am Coll Cardiol 4:1073–1079, 1984.
58. Morady F, Frank R, Kou WH, et al: Identification and catheter ablation of a zone of slow conduction in the reentry circuit of ventricular tachycardias in humans. J Am Coll Cardiol [in press].
59. Morady F, Scheinman MM, DiCarlo LA Jr, et al: Catheter ablation of ventricular tachycardia with intracardiac shocks: Results in 33 patients. Circulation 75:1037–1049, 1987.
60. O'Keefe DB, Curry PVL, Prior AL, et al: Surgery for ventricular tachycardia using operative pace mapping. Br Heart J 43:116, 1980.
61. Puech P, Gallay P, Grolleau R, Koliopoulos N: Traitement par électrofulguration endocavitaire d'une tachycardie ventriculaire récidivante par dysplasie ventriculaire droite. Arch Mal Coeur 77:826–835, 1984.
62. Scheinman MM: Electrical ventricular endocardial ablation: A tomato ripe or rotted? J Am Coll Cardiol 5:961–962, 1985.
63. Scheinman MM, Evans-Bell GT: Catheter ablation of the atrioventricular junction: A report of the Percutaneous Mapping and Ablation Registry. Circulation 70:1024–1029, 1984.
64. Scheinman MM, Morady F, Shen EN: Interventional electrophysiology: Catheter ablation technique. Clin Prog Pacing Electrophysiol 1:375–381, 1983.
65. Scheinman MM, Morady F, Hess DS, Gonzalez R: Catheter-induced ablation of the atrioventricular junction to control refractory supraventricular arrhythmias. JAMA 248:851–855, 1982.
66. Scheinman MM, Morady F, Hess DS, Gonzalez R: Transvenous catheter technique for induction of damage to the atrioventricular junction in man [abstract]. Am J Cardiol 49:1013, 1982.
67. Slodki SJ, Falicov RE, Katz MJ, et al: Serum enzyme changes following external direct current shock therapy for cardiac arrhythmias. Am J Cardiol 17:792–797, 1966.
68. Steinhaus D, Whitford E, Stavens C, et al: Percutaneous transcatheter electrical ablation for recurrent sustained ventricular tachycardia. Circulation 70 [Suppl II]:100, 1984.
69. Tidd MJ, Webster J, Cameron Wroght H, Harrison IR: Mode of action of a surgical electronic lithoclast high speed pressure, cinematographic and Schlieren recordings following an ultrashort underwater electronic discharge. Biomed Eng 1:5–11, 1976.
70. Tonet JL, Frank R, Fontaine G, Grosgogeat Y: Ventricular tachycardia responsive to verapamil: Treatment by catheter fulguration [abstract]. Circulation 74 [Suppl II]:461, 1986.
71. Tonet JL, Baraka M, Fontaine G, et al: Ventricular arrhythmias during endocardial catheter fulguration of ventricular tachycardias [abstract]. J Am Coll Cardiol 7:236A, 1986.
72. Tonet JL, Baraka M, Frank R, et al: Endocardial catheter fulguration of ventricular tachycardias: Pitfalls of the clinical and nonclinical approach [abstract]. Circulation 72 [Suppl III]:388, 1985.
73. Van Vleet JF, Tacker WA, Geddes LA, Ferrans VF: Acute cardiac damage in dogs given multiple transthoracic shocks with a trapezoidal wave-form defibrillator. Am J Vet Res 38:617–626, 1977.
74. Warin JF, Haissaguerre M, Le Metayer P, et al: Catheter ablation of ventricular tachycardia: Report of 20 patients [abstract]. Circulation 74 [Suppl II]:461, 1986.
75. Winston SA, Morady F, Davis JC, et al: Catheter ablation of ventricular tachycardia. Circulation 70 [Suppl II]:412, 1984.

34

ABLATION USING RADIOFREQUENCY CURRENT AND LOW-ENERGY DIRECT-CURRENT SHOCKS

NICHOLAS G. TULLO, HUANLIN AN, *and* SANJEEV SAKSENA

The treatment of cardiac tachyarrhythmias has become progressively challenging because of the myriad of therapeutic options now available to the cardiologist. Ablation of cardiac tissues responsible for arrhythmogenesis may offer the patient the greatest potential for long-term "cure." Surgical ablation of cardiac tissues, such as the atrioventricular (AV) junction, accessory AV bypass tracts, atrial myocardium, or ventricular myocardium, is a major surgical procedure with significant morbidity and mortality. An alternative to this approach is percutaneous catheter ablation.[29, 68, 78–80] Until recently, catheter ablation was solely performed using high-energy direct-current (DC) shocks delivered from a standard defibrillator through an electrode catheter. Tissue destruction with high-energy DC shock ablation involves three physical mechanisms, namely, thermal injury, barotrauma, and electrical field effects.[43] Reported complications of DC shock ablation include ventricular and supraventricular arrhythmias, permanent complete AV block, hypotension, congestive heart failure, cardiac rupture, coronary sinus rupture, pericardial tamponade, thrombus formation, cerebral emboli, and septicemia.[11, 21, 23, 32, 43, 52, 61, 62, 68, 78, 79, 83] In addition, this procedure is painful and must be done with the patient under general anesthesia, which may further increase risk. Reported efficacy has been low for pa-

tients with ventricular tachycardia and higher in patients with supraventricular tachyarrhythmias.[5, 21, 33, 53, 69, 79] The procedure may need to be repeated several times, since local edema produced by the shock has transient electrophysiologic effects, which resolve after several hours or days. Modifications of the current DC shock technique with respect to the energy source, waveform, or catheter delivery system have been under investigation. Radiofrequency (RF) current, laser energy, and low-energy–modified DC shocks have been proposed as alternative energy sources. It is the purpose of this chapter to discuss new techniques for electrode catheter ablation.

RADIOFREQUENCY ENERGY— A HISTORICAL PERSPECTIVE

Radiofrequency (RF) electrical energy is an alternating electric current with frequencies ranging from 100,000 cycles per second to 5 million cycles per second. The use of high-frequency alternating electric current in medicine is a well-established practice, particularly in surgery. Electrosurgery offers certain advantages over the surgical scalpel. Tissue division can be performed with simultaneous hemostasis of the incised tissues at the surgical site.

The initial human application of high-frequency electrical energy was in 1893 by d'Arsonval. He passed RF current through a circuit including a light bulb and two human subjects.[19] The light bulb glowed brightly, and the subjects noted a sensation of warmth. In 1911, Clark reported using high-frequency alternating current (AC) to cut and coagulate human tissue.[16] Subsequently, WT Bovie popularized the use of RF energy in collaboration with the neurosurgeon Harvey Cushing.[18] RF energy was first applied to cardiac tissues accidentally through an intracardiac catheter, and this induced ventricular fibrillation.[30] Early in vivo experiments were abandoned owing to a high incidence of atrial and ventricular perforation.[24] In 1971, RF energy was successfully used intraoperatively to ablate a localized area of the right ventricle in a patient with incessant ventricular tachycardia.[72]

The original "Bovie knife" RF generators were bulky devices that produced a sinusoidal electrical waveform.[65] Varying the output voltage resulted in either a cutting (high-output) or a coagulating (low-output) effect on tissues. Subsequently, RF electrosurgical devices based on solid-state technology were developed. This advance resulted in a decrease in generator size and weight, with greater versatility of biologic effects. Available effects include cutting, coagulation, desiccation, fulguration, or combinations of the above. The precise effect on the tissue depends on the magnitude, frequency, and waveform characteristics of the RF current applied.

PHYSICAL AND BIOLOGIC ASPECTS OF RADIOFREQUENCY ENERGY[31, 37, 42, 51, 71]

The basic RF electrosurgical waveform is a sinusoidal waveform with a frequency between 100 kHz and 5 MHz (Fig. 34–1). Most modern devices are limited to the narrower frequency range of 400 to 700 kHz. The sinusoidal waveform may be modulated in amplitude by solid-state circuits. This modulation in amplitude results in an interrupted waveform consisting of bursts of exponentially decaying sinusoidal RF waveforms. The burst repetition rate is at a lower frequency of 30 to 80 kHz (Fig. 34–2). The proportion of the "active" or oscillating portion of a modulated waveform to the total waveform (including active and quiescent portions) is referred to as the "duty cycle." The ratio of the maximal (peak-to-peak) amplitude of the waveform to the root mean square (RMS) amplitude is known as the "crest factor." The crest factor for a pure sine wave is 1.4 and for a highly modulated waveform may approach 10.0 or greater. In addition, sinusoidal and modulated sinusoidal waveforms can be combined by certain solid-state devices. This combining results in hybrid waveforms made up of components of each basic waveform. Devices often have a "blend" setting that produces such a hybrid waveform.

When an electrosurgical probe is placed in contact with biologic tissue, electrical contact is established and RF current flows through the tissue. A large voltage drop occurs across the tissue, since the impedance of biologic tissue is much greater than that of the electrode and connecting cables. This impedance to current flow results in the production of heat within the tissue. This process differs from electrocautery, in which electricity is used to heat the electrode itself, and the heat is conducted from the electrode to the tissue. The magnitude of the heat produced in the tissue is related to the current density, the duration of current application, and the impedance of the tissue. The current density is a function of

Figure 34–1. A diagrammatic representation of a sinusoidal waveform produced by an electrosurgical radiofrequency (RF) generator used in the cutting mode.

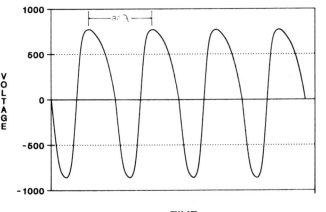
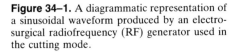

TIME

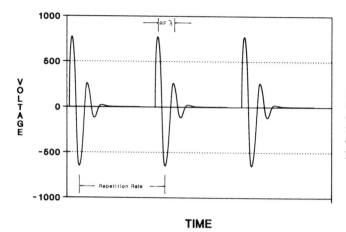

Figure 34–2. A diagrammatic representation of a highly modulated sinusoidal waveform produced by an electrosurgical RF generator used in the coagulation mode. The repetitive bursts of RF energy have relatively long quiescent periods between them.

the surface area of the electrode-tissue interface. Additional heat production may occur owing to the rapid oscillation of tissue ions in synchrony with the alternating electrical field. Initially, tissue heating results in protein denaturation and a fall in impedance. Extravascular blood begins to coagulate, and the tissue begins to blanch. With further heating, the intracellular and extracellular fluids are driven from the tissues, resulting in desiccation. The desiccation phase produces tissue and blood vessel contraction and results in hemostasis. It is accompanied by a rise in impedance and generally leaves a soft brown eschar. If higher current density is used, tissue heating occurs rapidly and intracellular fluids are turned into steam. This activity causes the cells to burst and results in destruction of tissue architecture and a cutting effect. If sufficient steam is produced by the RF current, a bubble of steam forms an insulating barrier or dielectric between the tissue and the electrode, resulting in a marked increase in impedance. If the RF voltage is high enough to ionize the molecules in the steam barrier, the current will pass across the ionized steam, producing a spark (arcing) at the thinnest point of the steam barrier. This activity results in marked tissue destruction and a deep, penetrating, cutting effect. Sinusoidal waveforms give the smoothest cutting action with little desiccation or hemostasis because of the almost continuous arcing across a thin steam barrier. The electrode can appear to float on a cushion of steam.

With modulated sinusoidal waveforms (particularly with "blend" settings on RF generators), RF current is interrupted at regular intervals. This periodic stalling of the current results in a collapse of the steam barrier, and thus electrical contact of the electrode and the tissue is resumed. With the next waveform

burst, the tissue repeats the initial desiccation phase and steam production before arcing can occur again. This results in simultaneous cutting and coagulation. Highly modulated waveforms have a low duty cycle and a high crest factor, and their peak-to-peak voltage can be very high (nearly 1000 V). This situation enables very long sparks to form. In addition, there is a tremendous current density during arcing because of the small area of ionization (typically less than 1 mm²). This high current density may cause tissue charring (fulguration), which generally forms a hard black eschar. Occasionally, fulguration causes adhesion of the electrode to the tissue, resulting in marked deep tissue destruction. Fulgurating waveforms may also cause carbonization and charred tissue products to be deposited on the electrode, which can lead to a marked decrease in current flow. Though AC has the ability to excite depolarizable cells, such as muscular, neural, and cardiac cells, the maximal excitation effect is seen at frequencies of 50 to 1000 Hz. This "faradic effect" is abolished at frequencies above 300,000 Hz. Thus, RF AC does not cause significant contraction of muscle tissue or stimulation of nervous tissue.

Some RF current generators (e.g., the HAT 100 [Fig. 34–3], Oscor Medical Corporation, Palm Beach, FL) have detection circuits that monitor current and voltage. Sudden increases in impedance and decreases in current suggest formation of either a steam barrier or an insulating layer of blood degradation products.[84] These detection circuits can interrupt the RF output and thus prevent significant arcing. These circuits are useful in the ablation of cardiac tissues to avoid fulguration and crater formation (Fig. 34–4). RF energy may be applied to tissues via a unipolar or a bipolar electrode system. In a unipolar system, an

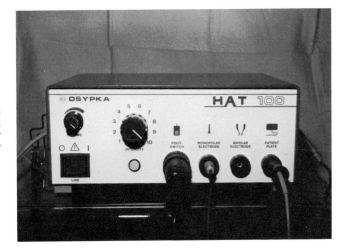

Figure 34–3. The HAT 100 RF generator used in conjunction with a catheter delivery system for tachycardia ablation. A graduated power output and unipolar or bipolar energy delivery is possible.

"active" electrode in the shape of a needle, a blade, or a catheter electrode is brought into contact with the tissue. The RF current passes through this active electrode into the tissues and returns to the RF generator through a much larger "passive," "dispersive," or "indifferent" patch electrode located on the patient's skin at a distance from the operative site. The surface area of the passive electrode is much larger than that of the active electrode, so the density of the RF current at the passive electrode is too low to produce a significant effect. In a bipolar electrode system, the RF current is passed between two adjacent electrodes that are both in contact with the tissue. Bipolar electrodes may be fashioned from surgical instruments such as forceps or from multipolar catheters. In unipolar systems, proper electrical contact between the passive electrode and the patient's skin must be ensured by using sufficient conducting gel or paste. Otherwise, the surface area may be decreased, the current density may thus be increased, and surface burns may result.[13] In addition, RF current generators must have an output that is properly isolated from ground, to prevent electrocution from current leakages flowing through the patient or from the patient to the operating room staff through an alternative pathway to ground.[82]

EXPERIMENTAL OBSERVATIONS

Histologic findings of myocardial lesions produced by RF energy application in vitro include shrinkage of endocardium and subendocardial muscle layers (desiccation) without damage to cell architecture at low and medium energy levels. At higher energy levels, extensive destruction of endocardium and subendocardium occurs, with formation of multiple vesicles[12, 75] (Fig. 34–5A and B). In vivo studies confirm coagulation necrosis at the AV junction without surrounding hemorrhage or mural thrombus.[47, 67] A thin layer of endocardial thrombus has been observed following the in vivo application of RF energy to right and left ventricular myocardium, but large thrombi have not been observed.[70]

The minimal threshold for inducing myocardial damage with a bipolar RF discharge may be as low as a power of 5 W with a pulse duration of 5 seconds.[46] The major determinants of the extent of myocardial damage are pulse duration and power[12, 34, 46, 76] (Fig. 34–6). The total dimensions and volume of the RF

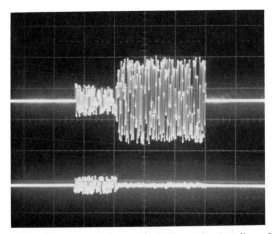

Figure 34–4. A simultaneous oscilloscopic recording of voltage (*top tracing*) and current (*bottom tracing*) during an RF discharge into normal myocardium in vitro. The tracings indicate a large increase in voltage accompanied by a decrease in current flow resulting from a sudden increase in impedance across the electrode-tissue interface. This commonly occurs because of arcing.

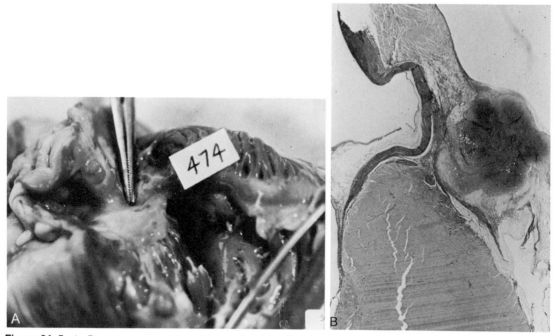

Figure 34–5. *A*, Gross appearance of a lesion produced by the application of RF energy to the atrioventricular (AV) node of a dog through a custom-designed suction catheter. There is an area of thickening and whitening of the median leaflet of the tricuspid valve (at tip of clamp). The lesion extends to the area of the AV node and His bundle. (From Circulation 76:400, 1987; by permission of the American Heart Association, Inc.) *B*, Histologic appearance of a lesion produced by RF energy. The micrograph shows fibrosis and vacuole formation in the penetrating His bundle and the cartilage in the annulus of the tricuspid valve. Weigert-van Gieson stain; original magnification, × 14.25. (From Saksena S, Tarjan PP, Bharati S et al: Low-energy transvenous ablation of the canine atrioventricular conduction system with a suction electrode catheter. Circulation 76:401, 1987; by permission of the American Heart Association, Inc.)

lesion are related to total delivered energy. At medium and high power levels, the depth of the lesion can be controlled by using the pulse duration.[34, 84] Lesion depth is also directly related to catheter contact pressure.[39, 46] The in vivo, unipolar application of RF energy appears to produce larger lesions than does bipolar application of RF energy.[27] In vitro, interrupted (pulsed) application of RF energy appears to be comparable to continuous application in terms of lesion size.[1] However, in vivo observations suggest that pulsed RF energy application requires less energy than does continuous application to produce the same lesion.[25] Higher-frequency RF energy may be more suited to myocardial ablation owing to the decreased impedance of muscle tissue at higher frequencies.[81] Experimentally, the waveform crest factor appears to have no effect on lesion size.[46] Lesions produced in the left ventricle in vivo may be greater in volume than lesions produced in the right ventricle when equivalent energy output is used.[25] Monitoring catheter tip temperature with a thermistor incorporated into the catheter tip may also be

useful in gauging lesion size. Impedance changes cannot be used to guide the size of the RF lesion.[1, 40] The in vitro effects of RF energy on diseased myocardium (scar) appear to be significantly less than those on normal myocardium.[75] This finding has been disputed by one in vivo study.[26] The size of RF lesions is often limited by acute increases in electrode-tissue impedance, which may be due to the deposition of a thin, insulating layer of blood degradation products[73, 84] or to arcing.[1] Larger lesions in vitro may be obtained by the use of a saline-cooled porous catheter, which prevents sudden increases in impedance,[85] but myocardial cooling may decrease lesion size.[15]

Transcatheter ablation of cardiac tissues with RF energy has been extensively studied in closed-chest animal models, and the results have been generally favorable (Table 34–1). The immediate success rate for induction of complete AV block has been reported to be 85 per cent to 100 per cent, with long-term persistence of complete heart block seen in 75 per cent to 100 per cent of animals treated with this technique.[3, 47, 50, 55] The remainder

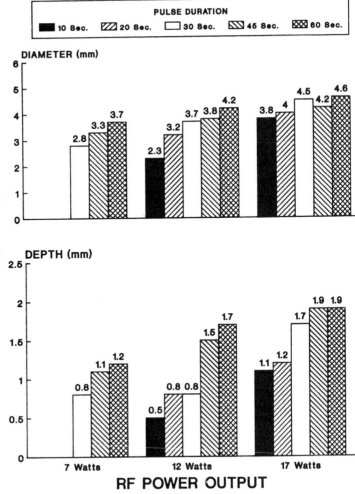

Figure 34–6. The relationship between RF lesion size and pulse duration and power. Lesion diameter and depth, particularly depth, are increased with longer pulse duration and higher power settings. Pulse duration appears to have a more marked effect on lesion depth than on lesion diameter.[1]

usually show a measurable modification of AV conduction with first- or second-degree AV block.[47] In addition, delayed complete heart block, occurring several hours to days after the procedure, can be observed.[47] In animals who recover 1:1 AV conduction, there is usu-ally a persistent first- or second-degree AV block with increased AH intervals and decreased Wenckebach rates.[3, 47] Complete AV block may be more easily induced with lower total energy requirements if higher-power settings (greater than 20 W) are used initially.[55]

TABLE 34–1. EXPERIMENTAL RESULTS OF RADIOFREQUENCY ABLATION OF THE AV JUNCTION

AUTHOR	IMMEDIATE RESULTS			LONG-TERM RESULTS	
	Number of Animals	Complete AV Block (%)	First-Degree or Second-Degree AV Block (%)	Complete AV Block (%)	First-Degree or Second-Degree AV Block (%)
Aubert et al[3]	12	12 (100)	0 (0)	9 (75)	3 (25)
Huang et al[47]	13	11 (85)	2 (15)	10 (77)	2 (15)
Langberg et al[55]	14	14 (100)	0 (0)	14 (100)	0 (0)
Iwa[50]	15	13 (87)	2 (13)	13 (87)	2 (13)
TOTAL	54	50 (93)	4 (7)	46 (85)	7 (13)

AV = atrioventricular.
Numbers in parentheses are percentages of the total number of animals reported in each series.

RF lesions have also been produced in right and left ventricular myocardium in closed-chest dogs by the application of RF energy through a transvenous catheter.[70] The size of the lesions may not correlate well with total energy delivered as observed in vitro, possibly because of variable contact pressure.

Discrete lesions on the tricuspid annulus of dogs can be produced with RF energy,[60] which makes this well suited for the ablation of right-sided AV bypass tracts. RF lesions have also been produced in the coronary sinus of dogs without the complications associated with DC ablation, such as coronary sinus rupture, pericardial tamponade, and damage to the circumflex coronary artery.[35, 48, 56] Rarely, coronary sinus occlusion[56] or stenosis[35] has been observed as a late complication. The feasibility of atrial ablation has also been examined. Discrete lesions, which are frequently extensive or transmural or both, can be produced, but atrial perforation has not been seen.[14, 15, 59, 60] Endocardial thrombi within the right atrium have been observed after RF ablation.[14, 15]

The development of late arrhythmias is a complication of DC catheter ablation. Many studies suggest that RF ablation is less likely to induce late arrhythmias.[58] This observation may be related to the homogeneity of the histologic and electrophysiologic effects of RF ablation.[28] Presumably, a heterogeneous lesion, such as that seen with DC ablation, might have a potential for reentry and thus can be more arrhythmogenic.

CLINICAL EXPERIENCE

RF energy has been used to ablate cardiac tissues in patients with refractory supraventricular and ventricular tachycardia (Table 34–2). The reported success rate for AV junctional ablations varies from 33 to 100 per cent (Fig. 34–7A and B), with subsequent recovery of 1:1 AV conduction ranging from 0 to 50 per cent (unpublished observations, Saksena and colleagues; references 9, 10, 12, 20, 33, 49, 57, and 77). Often, modification of AV conduction without the production of permanent complete heart block obviates permanent pacemaker implantation (unpublished observations, Saksena and colleagues; reference 54). Figure 34–8 illustrates RF catheter ablation of the AV junction in one of our patients with dual AV nodal pathways and AV nodal reentry tachycardia. AV nodal conduction can be altered, thus eliminating the tachycardia, despite the persistence of 1:1 AV conduction. Complete AV block may develop after a delay of up to 5 days in patients in whom RF ablation initially appeared to be inadequate.[76] Occasionally, right bundle branch block is inadvertently produced.[33, 57]

Ventricular ablation in patients with refractory ventricular tachycardia has been associated with variable success rates (range of 0 to 100 per cent[7, 10, 12, 20, 33]) (Table 34–2). In general, the results are markedly inferior to those achieved with AV junctional ablation. This finding may be a result of a smaller lesion size due to the limited effects of RF current in diseased (scarred) myocardium and the need for more extensive tissue damage for successful ventricular tachycardia ablation. Selective ablation of the right bundle branch or the left bundle branch in patients with bundle branch reentrant tachycardia is possible.[10]

Right-sided accessory AV pathways have been successfully modified or ablated with RF energy.[8, 9, 12, 33] Occasionally, the effects may be only temporary, with bypass tract conduction resuming several hours after ablation.[9, 12] Success appears to be dependent on accurate localization of the bypass tract and adequate catheter fixation (unpublished observations, Saksena and colleagues). Right-sided and posteroseptal Kent bundles are more easily localized by catheter, but RF energy has also been delivered within the coronary sinus without major complications.[49, 56] Information on RF ablation for refractory atrial tachycardia is scant.[9]

SAFETY OF RADIOFREQUENCY CATHETER ABLATION

The major advantage of RF energy lies in the relative safety of its cardiac application. Active-fixation and passive-contact catheters placed in contact with atrial and ventricular myocardium during continuous RF energy applications at a power of 50 W for durations of up to 180 seconds do not produce myocardial perforation.[1] At contact pressures of 30 grams, however, crater formation and left ventricular perforation have been observed in dogs.[39] Crater formation and coring out of myocardium have also been described with suction catheters,[1] probably because of their small surface area and the resultant high current density. At 25 W of power, the formation of gas bubbles at the electrode-tissue interface has been ob-

TABLE 34–2. CLINICAL STUDIES IN RADIOFREQUENCY ABLATION

CARDIAC TISSUE	AUTHOR	IMMEDIATE RESULTS			LONG-TERM RESULTS	
		Number of Patients	Complete Success (%)	Partial Success (%)	Complete Success (%)	Partial Success (%)
AV junction	Goy[33]	3	1 (33)	0 (0)	1 (33)	0 (0)
	Lavergne et al[57]	2	1 (50)	0 (0)	1 (50)	1 (50)
	Huang et al[49]	1	1 (100)	0 (0)	1 (100)	0 (0)
	Davis et al[20]	3	2 (67)	0 (0)	1 (33)	0 (0)
	Scanu et al[77]	3	3 (100)	0 (0)	3 (100)	0 (0)
	Borggrefe et al[9]	10	6 (60)	2 (20)	5 (50)	1 (10)
	Bowman et al[10]	3	3 (100)	0 (0)	3 (100)	0 (0)
	Saksena et al (unpublished observations)	4	3 (75)	0 (0)	1 (25)	2 (50)
	TOTAL	29	20 (69)	2 (7)	16 (55)	4 (14)
Bypass tract	Goy[33]	3	1 (33)	0 (0)	1 (33)	1 (33)
	Huang et al[49]	1	0 (0)	0 (0)	0 (0)	0 (0)
	Borggrefe et al[9]	7	2 (29)	0 (0)	1 (14)	0 (0)
	Saksena et al (unpublished observations)	1	0 (0)	0 (0)	0 (0)	0 (0)
	TOTAL	12	3 (25)	0 (0)	2 (17)	1 (8)
Ventricular myocardium	Goy[33]	1	0 (0)	0 (0)	0 (0)	0 (0)
	Davis et al[20]	1	1 (100)	0 (0)	1 (100)	0 (0)
	Bowman et al[10]	2	2 (100)	0 (0)	2 (100)	0 (0)
	Borggrefe et al[7]	5	3 (60)	0 (0)	3 (60)	0 (0)
	TOTAL	9	6 (67)	0 (0)	6 (67)	0 (0)
Atrial myocardium	Borggrefe et al[9]	2	0 (0)	0 (0)	0 (0)	0 (0)

Numbers in parentheses are percentages of the total number of patients in each series.

CATHETER ABLATION WITH RADIOFREQUENCY ENERGY

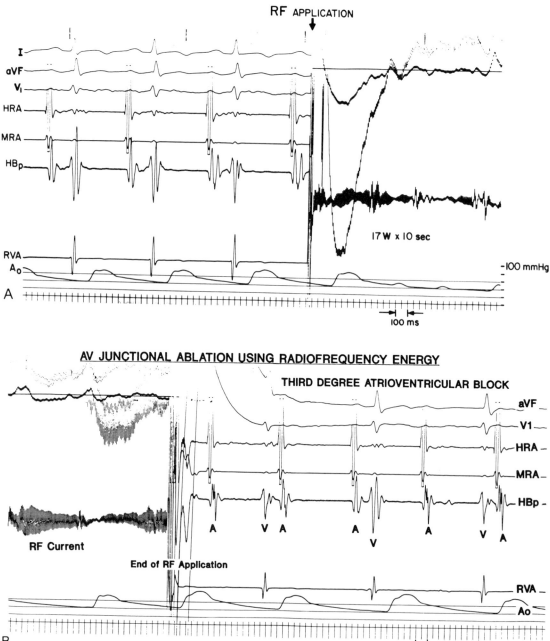

Figure 34–7. *A*, Electrophysiologic recordings from a patient with drug-refractory AV nodal reentry tachycardia undergoing RF ablation of the AV junction. The left side of the figure is recorded during normal sinus rhythm, and the right side shows the onset of RF application through the distal pair of electrodes, which were used to record the His bundle electrogram. The top three traces are of surface electrocardiographic (ECG) leads I, aV$_F$, and V$_1$. HRA = high right atrium; MRA = mid right atrium; HBp = His bundle catheter, proximal pair of electrodes; RVA = right ventricular apex; A$_o$ = aortic pressure; RF = radiofrequency energy; W = watts; sec = seconds; ms = milliseconds. *B*, Electrophysiologic recordings from the patient in *A* immediately after the application of RF energy. The electrograms demonstrate third-degree AV block produced by RF ablation. HRA = high right atrium; MRA = mid right atrium; HBp = His bundle catheter, proximal pair of electrodes; RVA = right ventricular apex; Ao = aortic pressure; RF = radiofrequency energy; ms = milliseconds; A = atrial depolarization; V = ventricular depolarization.

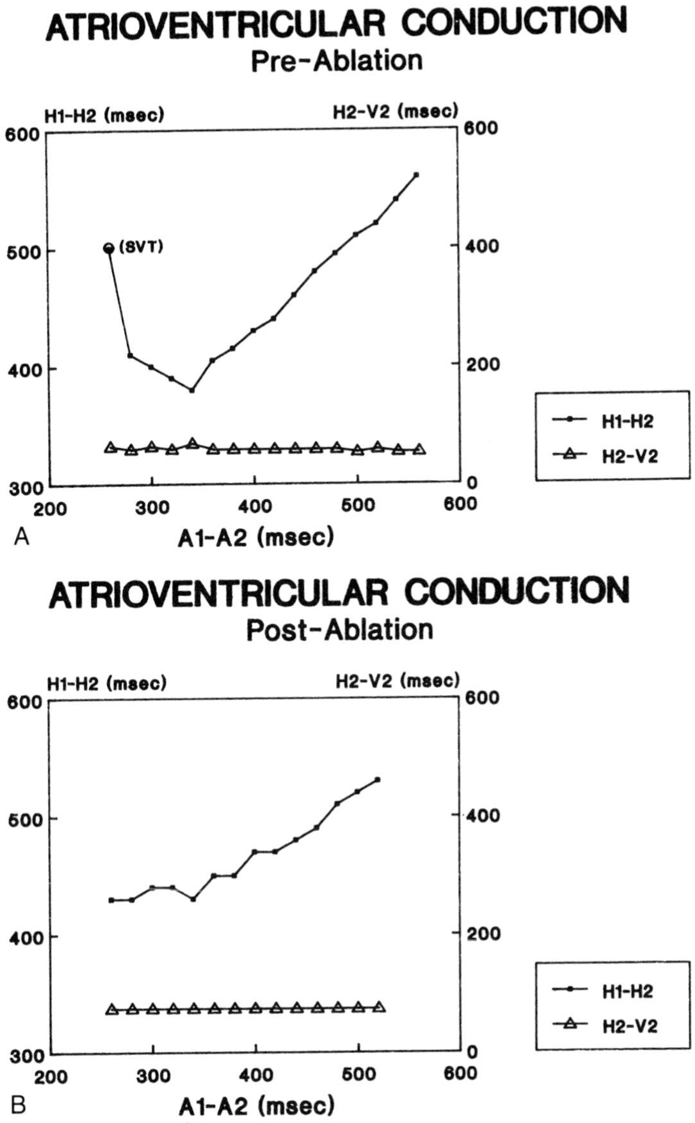

ATRIOVENTRICULAR CONDUCTION
Pre-Ablation

ATRIOVENTRICULAR CONDUCTION
Post-Ablation

Figure 34–8. *A*, AV-conduction curves derived prior to AV junction ablation in a patient with inducible AV nodal reentrant tachycardia. There is decremental conduction through the AV node with programmed, single atrial extrastimuli, beginning at the functional refractory period (A1-A2 of 340 msec). At an A1-A2 coupling interval of 260 msec (circled point), there is a discontinuity in AV conduction and a sudden prolongation in the atrial to His (AH) interval, consistent with dual AV nodal pathways. At that point, AV nodal reentry tachycardia is induced. *B*, AV conduction curves from the patient referred to in *A*, derived after AV junctional ablation. One-to-one AV conduction persists, but evidence for dual AV nodal pathways is no longer present. This situation indicates favorable modification of AV conduction without the induction of complete heart block, which may eliminate the need for a permanent pacemaker.

served in vitro.[12] In vitro studies also suggest that clot formation is uncommon.[12]

Ventricular fibrillation during the application of RF energy has been observed in animals by a number of investigators.[3, 4, 27, 66, 70] It appears that modulated waveforms that are asymmetric (those that do not have geometrically identical parts above and below the baseline), such as those produced by the newer solid-state RF generators, may be more likely to cause ventricular fibrillation than the older arc-type devices.[3] In addition, bipolar RF application may be more likely to induce ventricular tachycardia or ventricular fibrillation than would unipolar application.[27] Ventricular fibrillation has been induced in humans during RF electrode catheter ablation of the AV junction, mainly with high-energy pulses (un-

published observations, Saksena and colleagues) (Fig. 34–9).

RF energy delivery is well tolerated by patients.[9, 12, 54, 57] Our patients have been awake and have generally felt no discomfort from the procedure. There has been no mortality reported from RF ablation in humans.[12] Insignificant increases in serum creatine phosphokinase-MB fraction have been observed after RF ablation (unpublished observations, Saksena and colleagues; reference 77). Long-term follow-up is not yet available in most studies.

Catheters used in DC ablation are frequently damaged by the current pulse,[22] but RF pulses up to a cumulative energy of 1500 J generally do not affect catheter integrity.[47] Permanent pacemakers subjected in vitro to RF energy have been shown to be inhibited or accelerated

RF CATHETER ABLATION

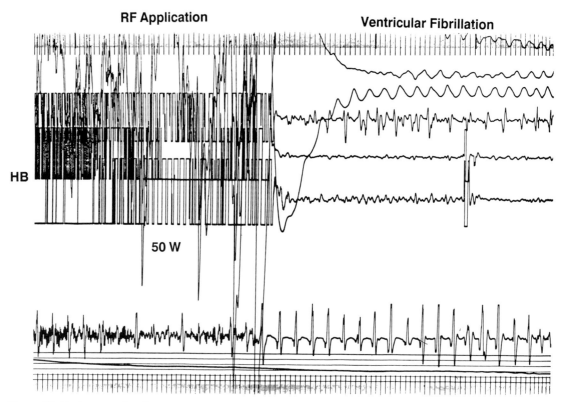

Figure 34–9. An example of an acute complication of RF ablation of the AV junction. Ventricular fibrillation was induced in this patient during the delivery of a 50-W pulse of RF energy.

or to have temporary loss of sensing, or they may revert to magnet mode.[2] Thus, consideration should be given to the use of a temporary backup pacemaker during RF ablation in patients with permanent pacemakers. However, RF catheter AV junctional ablation has been performed in patients with implantable defibrillators without adverse effects.

CATHETER DELIVERY SYSTEMS

A number of delivery systems have been used for RF catheter ablation, including standard multipolar electrode catheters in both unipolar and bipolar configurations, screw-in electrode catheters, custom-designed catheters, and suction electrode catheters. Generally, a linear relationship exists between the size of the coagulation zones produced by unipolar RF pulses and the amount of energy applied[1, 12, 46, 76] (Fig. 34–10). However, when screw-in catheters are used with the screw extended, this linear relationship can be lost, probably because of excessive arcing due to

inconsistent surface areas.[12] Near-transmural lacerations and crater formation have been observed with screw-in electrodes.[1, 12] Suction catheters have been used successfully for AV junctional ablation in humans[57] (Fig. 34–11), but these catheters also suffer from the disadvantage of a nonlinear relationship between lesion size and delivered energy.

An optimal catheter delivery system for use in RF catheter ablation has yet to be devised. There is evidence to suggest that the most efficient catheter design will have a large enough electrode surface area to produce lesions at low power and will also be thermally and electrically insulated from the blood stream.[6] Standard ring electrode catheters are very difficult to maintain in position in vivo, and adequate contact between the electrode and the tissue, a prerequisite for effective catheter ablation, is impossible to assess during the procedure. A method of active fixation, with either suction or a screw-in helix, may help to ensure that adequate electrical contact be maintained throughout the duration of the RF pulse. However, exact fixation in the target

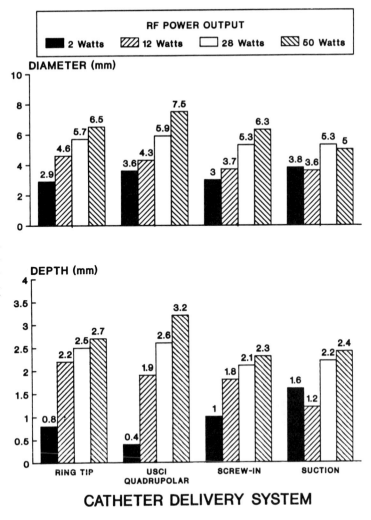

Figure 34–10. The relationship of different catheter delivery systems to RF lesion diameter and depth at different power settings. Lesion size remains relatively linear for different catheter delivery systems, with the exception of the suction catheter, which has the propensity for arcing because of a small surface area.[1]

ablation zone must be obtained. The development of effective, low-impedance, durable, dependable leads, preferably with some means of active fixation, will be a very important milestone in RF current delivery to cardiac tissues.

INNOVATIONS IN DIRECT-CURRENT SHOCK CATHETER ABLATION

DC catheter ablation is generally carried out using a standard defibrillator and energy levels of 200 to 500 J. Investigators using low-energy (under 50 J) DC shocks delivered through standard USCI multipolar catheters (USCI Division, Billerica, MA) as well as through active-fixation electrode catheters have been successful in producing complete AV block.[45, 64] More important, low-energy shocks appear to

be useful in modifying antegrade or retrograde AV conduction without producing complete AV block.[64] This situation may result in either suppression of supraventricular tachycardia or modification of AV conduction, so that the tachycardia will be associated with a much slower ventricular response. In patients with supraventricular tachycardia who underwent high-energy DC electrode catheter ablation, modification of AV conduction, indicated by increases in PR and atrium-His (AH) intervals without the production of complete heart block, was associated with clinical success.[74] Thus, modification of AV conduction can obviate potentially toxic antiarrhythmic medications. Using lower energies may also reduce the complication rate of DC shocks.

The standard defibrillator used for DC catheter ablation delivers a damped sinusoidal waveform.[63] This waveform results from the high-voltage discharge of a capacitor through

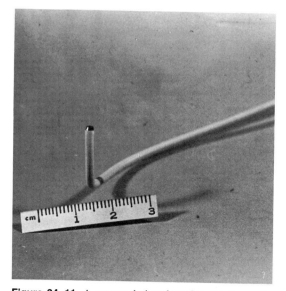

Figure 34–11. A custom-designed suction ablation catheter. The catheter has a central lumen with a suction port and two electrodes. There are two perpendicular curves at its distal end. The initial curve places the catheter across the septal leaflet of the tricuspid valve, and the second curve allows perpendicular attachment to the endocardium after application of suction. The two electrodes are separated by a distance of 15 mm. (From Saksena S, Tarjan PP, Bharati S et al: Low-energy transvenous ablation of the canine atrioventricular conduction system with a suction electrode catheter. Circulation 76:395, 1987; by permission of the American Heart Association, Inc.)

the patient in series with an inductance load. This inductance limits the peak current. To maximize local myocardial damage with a minimal total energy delivery, modifications in the current waveform have been investigated. New energy sources that deliver large peak currents with short pulse widths have been used successfully for low-energy catheter ablation of the AV node.[17] Complete heart block was attained with as little as 0.5 J using single pulses from this new energy source. Altering the current waveform also seems to decrease the tendency for arcing and can minimize barotrauma and gas formation associated with DC catheter ablation. The use of a series of high-current impulses of 10 μsec each has resulted in the production of complete heart block in experimental animals with the use of 0.65 J.[44] The impulses are too brief to allow arcing to occur. Thus, modification of the catheter delivery system, the energy source, or both, may increase the usefulness and decrease the complication rate of DC catheter ablation.

REFERENCES

1. An HL, Saksena S, Janssen M, Osypka P: Radiofrequency ablation of ventricular myocardium using active fixation and passive contact catheter delivery systems. Am Heart J 118:69–77, 1989.
2. Aouate JM, Lavergne T, Guize L, et al: In vitro effects of transcatheter radiofrequency energy on pacemaker functions [abstract]. PACE 11:916, 1988.
3. Aubert AW, Gewillig M, Joossens J, et al: A new method of catheter ablation of the atrioventricular junction using high frequency energy. *In* Belhassen B, Feldman S, Cooperman Y (eds): Cardiac Pacing and Electrophysiology: Proceedings of the VIIIth World Symposium on Cardiac Pacing and Electrophysiology, Tel Aviv, 1987.
4. Beazell JW, Adomian GE, Furmanski M, et al: Experimental production of complete heart block by electrocoagulation in the closed chest dog. Am Heart J 104:1328, 1983.
5. Belhassen B, Miller HI, Geller E, et al: Transcatheter electrical shock ablation of ventricular tachycardia. J Am Coll Cardiol 7:1347, 1986.
6. Blouin LT, Marcus FI: Effect of electrode design on efficiency of delivery of radiofrequency energy to cardiac tissue in vitro [abstract]. PACE 11:906, 1988.
7. Borggrefe M, Budde T, Podczeck A, Breithardt G: Application of transvenous radiofrequency alternating current ablation in humans [abstract]. Circulation 76[Suppl IV]:IV–406, 1987.
8. Borggrefe M, Budde T, Podczeck A, Breithardt G: High frequency alternating current ablation of an accessory pathway in humans. J Am Coll Cardiol 10:576, 1987.
9. Borggrefe M, Podczeck A, Budde T, et al: Catheter ablation of supraventricular tachycardia [abstract]. PACE 11:910, 1988.
10. Bowman A, Fitzgerald D, Friday K, et al: Catheter ablation of selected segments of the AV conduction system using radiofrequency current [abstract]. PACE 11:908, 1988.
11. Brodman R, Fisher JD: Evaluation of a catheter technique for ablation of accessory pathways near the coronary sinus using a canine model. Circulation 67:923, 1983.
12. Budde T, Borggrefe M, Podczeck A, et al: Radiofrequency ablation: An improvement of ablation techniques in comparison to direct current delivery? *In* Breithardt G, Borggrefe M, Zipes D (eds): Non-pharmacological Therapy of Tachyarrhythmias. Mount Kisco, NY, Futura Publishing Co, 1987.
13. Burton CV: RF lesion generation: International Symposium on Radiofrequency Lesion Making Procedures. Appl Neurophysiol 39:77, 1976/77.
14. Chauvin M, Dumont P, Di Francesco G, Brechenmacher C: Trans-catheter radiofrequency ablation of atrial myocardium: An anatomical examination in dogs [abstract]. PACE 11:523, 1988.
15. Chauvin M, Wihlm JM, Dumont P, et al: The ablation of canine atrial tissue by high-frequency currents: Anatomical and histological findings. J Electrophysiol 2:407, 1988.
16. Clark W: Oscillatory desiccation in the treatment of accessible malignant growths and minor surgical conditions. J Adv Therap 29:169, 1911.
17. Cunningham D, Rowland E, Rickards AF: A new

low energy power source for catheter ablation. PACE 9:1384, 1986.

18. Cushing H, Bovie WT: Electro-surgery as an aid to the removal of intracranial tumors. Surg Gynecol Obstet 47:751, 1928.

19. D'Arsonval A: Action physiologique des courants alternatifs à grand frequence. Arch Physiol Norm Pathol 5:401, 1893.

20. Davis MJE, Murdock CJ, Cope GD, et al: Radiofrequency catheter ablation for refractory arrhythmias [abstract]. PACE 11:918, 1988.

21. Evans GT Jr, Scheinman MM, Executive Committee of the Registry: Catheter ablation of ventricular tachycardia foci: A report of the Percutaneous Cardiac Mapping and Ablation Registry. Circulation 74[Suppl II]:II–1835, 1986.

22. Fisher JD, Brodman R, Johnston DR, et al: Nonsurgical electrical ablation of tachycardias: Importance of prior in vitro testing of catheter leads. PACE 7:74, 1984.

23. Fisher JD, Brodman R, Kim SG, et al: Attempted nonsurgical electrical ablation of accessory pathways via the coronary sinus in the Wolff-Parkinson-White syndrome. J Am Coll Cardiol 4:685, 1984.

24. Fontaine G, Lechat P, Cansell A, et al: Advance in the treatment of cardiac arrhythmias in the last decade: Definition and role of ablative techniques. In Fontaine G, Scheinmann MM (eds): Ablation in Cardiac Arrhythmias. Mount Kisco, NY, Futura Publishing Co, 1987.

25. Franklin JO, Langberg JJ, Herre JM, et al: Pulsed and continuous radiofrequency catheter ablation in the canine ventricle [abstract]. PACE 11:523, 1988.

26. Franklin JO, Langberg JJ, Landzberg JS, et al: Radiofrequency catheter ablation in the canine ventricle [abstract]. Circulation 76[Suppl IV]:IV–407, 1987.

27. Franklin JO, Oeff M, Langberg JJ, et al: Arrhythmias during unipolar and bipolar radiofrequency catheter ablation in the canine ventricle [abstract]. PACE 11:489, 1988.

28. Gagey S, Lavergne T, Le Heuzey J-Y, et al: Cellular electrophysiological effects of radiofrequency ablation in rabbit sino-atrial preparation [abstract]. PACE 11:915, 1988.

29. Gallagher JJ, Svenson RH, Kasell JH, et al: Catheter technique for closed-chest ablation of the atrioventricular conduction system: A therapeutic alternative for the treatment of refractory supraventricular tachycardia. N Engl J Med 306:194, 1982.

30. Geddes LA, Tacker WA, Cabler PO: A new electrical hazard associated with the electrocautery. Med Instrum 9:112, 1975.

31. Gerhard G, Elliott W, Selikowitz S: A programmable variable waveshape generator for electrosurgical research. Med Instrum 20:150, 1986.

32. Gonzalez R, Scheinman RR, Margaretten W, Rubinstein M: Closed-chest electrode catheter technique for His bundle ablation in dogs. Am J Physiol 241:H283, 1981.

33. Goy J-J, Kappenberger L: Different techniques of catheter ablation [abstract]. PACE 11:910, 1988.

34. Grogan EW, Nellis SH: Catheter ablation using radiofrequency energy: Control of lesion volume and shape by varying power and duration of ablation [abstract]. J Am Coll Cardiol 9:128A, 1987.

35. Grogan IW Jr, Subramanian R, Whitesell L, Nellis S: Catheter ablation in the coronary sinus using radiofrequency energy [abstract]. PACE 11:523, 1988.

36. Haines DE, Watson DD, Halperin C: Monitoring electrode tip temperature during radiofrequency fulguration of ventricular myocardium is strongly predictive of lesion size [abstract]. Circulation 76[Suppl IV]:IV–406, 1987.

37. Harris F: Desiccation As a Key to Understanding Electrosurgery. Boulder, CO, Valleylab, Inc, 1977.

38. Haverkamp W, Hindricks G, Rissel U, et al: Monitoring catheter tip temperature during radiofrequency coagulation of ventricular tissue to estimate lesion size in vivo [abstract]. PACE 11:916, 1988.

39. Haverkamp W, Hindricks G, Rissel U, et al: Radiofrequency-coagulation of ventricular myocardium: Significance of catheter contact pressure [abstract]. PACE 11:916, 1988.

40. Hindricks G, Haverkamp W, Rissel U, et al: Significance of tissue impedance for lesion size during coagulation of ventricular myocardium using radiofrequency energy [abstract]. PACE 11:906, 1988.

41. Hindricks G, Haverkamp W, Schostok M, et al: Fluid-supported radiofrequency coagulation of ventricular myocardium [abstract]. PACE 11:905, 1988.

42. Hoenig WM: The mechanism of cutting in electrosurgery. IEEE Trans Biomed Eng BME p.58, 1975.

43. Holt P, Boyd E: Endocardial ablation as an antiarrhythmic technique: The background to its application to ventricular tachycardia [abstract]. Br Heart J 53:687, 1985.

44. Holt PM, Boyd EGCA: His bundle ablation using impulses below one joule [abstract]. J Am Coll Cardiol 11:16A, 1988.

45. Holt PM, Boyd EGCA, Crick J, Sowton E: Low energies and Helifix electrodes in the successful ablation of atrioventricular conduction. PACE 8:639, 1985.

46. Hoyt RH, Huang SK, Jordan N, Marcus F: Factors influencing trans-catheter radiofrequency ablation of the myocardium [abstract]. Circulation 72 [Suppl III]:III–473, 1985.

47. Huang SK, Bharati S, Graham AR, et al: Closed chest catheter desiccation of the atrioventricular junction using radiofrequency energy—a new method of catheter ablation. J Am Coll Cardiol 9:349, 1987.

48. Huang SK, Graham AR, Bharati S, et al: Chronic effect of radiofrequency catheter ablation of the coronary sinus [abstract]. Circulation 76 [Suppl IV]:IV–406, 1987.

49. Huang SKS, Lee MA, Bazgan ID, Gorman G: Initial experience with radiofrequency catheter ablation for intractable cardiac arrhythmias in man [abstract]. PACE 11:919, 1988.

50. Iwa T: Radiofrequency catheter ablation of the atrioventricular conduction system in a canine model [abstract]. PACE 11:914, 1988.

51. Janssen M: Annotated bibliography on Radiofrequency Energy for Endocardial Ablation. West Palm Beach, FL, Oscor Medical Corporation, 1986.

52. Kempf FC, Falcone RA, Iozzo RV, Josephson ME: Anatomic and hemodynamic effects of catheter-delivered ablation energies in the ventricle. Am J Cardiol 56:373, 1985.

53. Klein H, Trappe HJ, Frank G, et al: Is fulguration of ventricular tachycardia really a new promising therapeutic approach? PACE 9:95, 1986.

54. Kuck K-H, Kunze K-P, Geiger M, Schluter M: Modulation of AV nodal conduction in man by radiofrequency current [abstract]. PACE 11:909, 1988.

55. Langberg JJ, Chin MC, Franklin JO, et al: Complete

AV block using radiofrequency catheter ablation: Energy requirements [abstract]. PACE 11:490, 1988.

56. Langberg J, Griffin JC, Bharati S, et al: Radiofrequency catheter ablation in the coronary sinus [abstract]. J Am Coll Cardiol 9:99A, 1987.

57. Lavergne T, Guize L, Le Heuzey J-Y, et al: Transvenous ablation of the atrio-ventricular junction in human with high-frequency energy [abstract]. J Am Coll Cardiol 9:99A, 1987.

58. Lavergne T, Le Heuzey J-Y, Bruneval P, et al: Comparative effects of electrical catheter ablation and radiofrequency dessication in the canine right ventricle [abstract]. Circulation 74 [Suppl II]:II–186, 1986.

59. Lavergne T, Prunier L, Guize L, et al: Transcatheter radiofrequency ablation of atrial tissue using a suction catheter [abstract]. PACE 11:906, 1988.

60. Lee MA, Huang SK, Graham AR, et al: Radiofrequency catheter ablation of the canine atrium and tricuspid annulus [abstract]. Circulation 76 [Suppl IV]:IV–406, 1987.

61. Lerman BB, Weiss JL, Bulkley BM, et al: Myocardial injury and induction of arrhythmia by direct current shock delivered via endocardial catheters in dogs. Circulation 69:1006, 1984.

62. Levy S, Bru P, Aliot E, et al: Long-term follow-up of transcatheter ablation of the atrioventricular junction [abstract]. PACE 11:909, 1988.

63. Lown B, Crampton RS, DeSilva R: New method for terminating cardiac arrhythmias. JAMA 182:548, 1962.

64. McComb JM, McGovern MB, Garan H, Ruskin JN: Management of refractory supraventricular tachyarrhythmias using low-energy transcatheter shocks. Am J Cardiol 58:959, 1986.

65. McLean A: The Bovie electrosurgical current generator. Arch Surg 18:1863, 1929.

66. Mitsui T, Ijima H, Okamura K, et al: Transvenous electrocautery of the atrioventricular connection guided by the His electrogram. Jpn Circ J 42:313, 1977.

67. Moquet B, De Muret A, Fauchier JP, et al: Radiofrequency catheter ablation: Preliminary study in swine [abstract]. PACE 11:913, 1988.

68. Morady F: A perspective on the role of catheter ablation in the management of tachyarrhythmias. PACE 11:98, 1988.

69. Morady F, Scheinman MM, DiCarlo LA Jr, et al: Catheter ablation of ventricular tachycardia with intracardiac shocks: Results in thirty-three patients. Circulation 75:1037, 1987.

70. Naccarelli GV, Kuck K-H, Pitha J, et al: Selective catheter ablation of canine ventricular myocardium with radiofrequency current [abstract]. J Am Coll Cardiol 9:99A, 1987.

71. Organ L: Electrophysiologic principles of radiofrequency lesion making: International Symposium on Radiofrequency Lesion Making Procedures. Appl Neurophysiol 39:69, 1976/77.

72. Petitier H, Polu J-M, Dodinot B, et al: Tachycardie ventriculaire irréductible traitement par électrocoagulation après localisation du foyer. Arch Mal Coeur 64:331, 1971.

73. Ring ME, Huang SK, Gorman G, Graham AR: Determinants of impedance rise during catheter ablation with radiofrequency energy [abstract]. Circulation 76 [Suppl IV]:IV–406, 1987.

74. Saksena S, An HL, Herman S, Marcantuono D: Clinical outcome of patients with intact atrioventricular conduction after atrioventricular junction ablation for refractory supraventricular tachyarrhythmias [abstract]. J Am Coll Cardiol 11:177A, 1988.

75. Saksena S, Gadhoke A, Pantopoulos D, Osypka P: Radiofrequency ablation of arrhythmogenic diseased human ventricle [abstract]. Circulation 74 [Suppl II]:II–461, 1986.

76. Saksena S, An HL, Marcantuono D, et al: Pulsed radiofrequency ablation with a conventional electrode catheter: Experimental studies and early clinical observations [abstract]. PACE 11:489, 1988.

77. Scanu P, Guilleman D, Belin A, et al: Radiofrequency catheter ablation of the atrioventricular junction in humans [abstract]. PACE 11:913, 1988.

78. Scheinman MM: Catheter ablation for patients with ventricular tachycardia [abstract]. Clin Prog Electrophysiol Pacing 4:34, 1986.

79. Scheinman MM, Evans-Bell T: Catheter ablation of the atrioventricular junction: A report of the percutaneous mapping and ablation registry. Circulation 70:1024, 1984.

80. Scheinman MM, Morady F, Hess DS, Gonzalez R: Catheter induced ablation of the atrioventricular junction to control refractory supraventricular arrhythmias. JAMA 248:851, 1982.

81. Schlter M, Antz M, Kuck K-H, et al: Radiofrequency current: Frequency dependence of the impedance of different cardiac tissues [abstract]. J Am Coll Cardiol 11:59A, 1988.

82. Watson A, Loughman J: The surgical diathermy: Principles of operation and safe use. Anaesth Intensive Care 4:310, 1978.

83. Westveer DC, Nelson T, Stewart JR, et al: Sequelae of left ventricular electrical endocardial ablation. J Am Coll Cardiol 5:956, 1985.

84. Wittkampf FH, Hauer RN, Robles de Medina EO: Controlled growth of radiofrequency lesions by power regulation [abstract]. J Am Coll Cardiol 11:16A, 1988.

85. Wittkampf FH, Hauer RN, Robles de Medina EO: Radiofrequency ablation with a cooled porous electrode catheter [abstract]. J Am Coll Cardiol 11:17A, 1988.

INDEX

Note: Page numbers in *italic* refer to illustrations; page numbers followed by a *t* refer to tables.